MW00559690

Orthopaedic Knowledge Update

OKU 13

Wolters Kluwer
Philadelphia • Baltimore • New York • London
Buenos Aires • Hong Kong • Sydney • Tokyo

AAOS
American Academy of Orthopaedic Surgeons

Orthopaedic Knowledge Update

OKU 13

EDITED BY

Javad Parvizi, MD, FRCS

James Edwards Professor of Orthopaedic Surgery
Department of Orthopaedic Surgery
Rothman Institute
Philadelphia, Pennsylvania

Wolters Kluwer
Philadelphia • Baltimore • New York • London
Buenos Aires • Hong Kong • Sydney • Tokyo

AAOS
American Academy of Orthopaedic Surgeons

Staff

American Academy of Orthopaedic Surgeons

Anna Salt Troise, MBA, *Chief Education Strategist*

Hans Koelsch, PhD, *Director, Publishing Partner Relationships*

Lisa Claxton Moore, *Senior Manager, Editorial*

Steven Kellert, *Senior Editor*

Wolters Kluwer Health

Brian Brown, *Director, Medical Practice*

Stacey Sebring, *Senior Development Editor*

Emily Buccieri, *Senior Editorial Coordinator*

Erin Cantino, *Portfolio Marketing Manager*

David Saltzberg, *Senior Production Project Manager*

Stephen Druding, *Design Coordinator*

Beth Welsh, *Senior Manufacturing Coordinator*

TNQ Technologies, *Prepress Vendor*

ISBN 978-1-9751-2952-1

Library of Congress Control Number: Cataloging in Publication data available on request from publisher.

Printed in China

Published 2021 by the

American Academy of Orthopaedic Surgeons

9400 West Higgins Road

Rosemont, Illinois 60018

CCS0120

ACKNOWLEDGMENTS

DEDICATION

To all our patients who in their endurance of pain and disabilities have shaped our profession.

To our families who sacrifice so much to allow us to pursue our dreams.

CONTRIBUTORS

Mark R. Adams, MD
Associate Professor
Department of Orthopaedic Surgery
Rutgers-New Jersey Medical School
Newark, New Jersey

Samuel B. Adams, MD
Co-Chief, Division of Foot and Ankle Surgery
Director of Foot and Ankle Research
Associate Professor
Department of Orthopaedic Surgery
Duke University Medical Center
Durham, North Carolina

Christopher S. Ahmad, MD
Professor of Orthopaedic Surgery
Vice Chair of Clinical Research
Sports Medicine Service Chief
Columbia Irving University Medical Center, NYP
Head Team Physician, New York Yankees
New York, New York

Benjamin A. Alman, MD
James Urbaniak Professor and Chair
Department of Orthopaedic Surgery
Duke University
Durham, North Carolina

Kimberly K. Amrami, MD
Professor
Vice Chair, Department of Radiology
Mayo Clinic
Rochester, Minnesota

Lindsay M. Andras, MD
Assistant Professor
Children's Orthopedic Center
Children's Hospital Los Angeles
Keck School of Medicine of USC
Los Angeles, California

Andrew K. Battenberg, MD
Department of Orthopaedic Surgery
Kaiser Permanente Vacaville Medical Center
Vacaville, California

Hany Bedair, MD
Assistant Professor, Orthopaedic Surgery
Harvard Medical School
Massachusetts General Hospital/Newton Wellesley Hospital
Boston, Massachusetts

Marschall B. Berkes, MD
Assistant Professor
Department of Orthopaedic Surgery
Washington University School of Medicine
St. Louis, Missouri

Nitin Bhatia, MD
Chairman
Department of Orthopaedic Surgery
University of California, Irvine
Irvine, California

Craig M. Birch, MD
Clinical Instructor
Department of Orthopedic Surgery
Boston Children's Hospital
Harvard Medical School
Boston, Massachusetts

Allen T. Bishop, MD
Professor of Orthopedic and Neurosurgery
Mayo Clinic
Rochester, Minnesota

Philip Blazar, MD
Chief of Hand Surgery
Department of Orthopaedic Surgery
Brigham Health
Associate Professor
Harvard Medical School
Boston, Massachusetts

David M. Brogan, MD, MSc
Assistant Professor
Department of Orthopaedic Surgery
Washington University in St. Louis
St. Louis, Missouri

Wesley H. Bronson, MD, MSB
Assistant Professor
Mount Sinai Hospital and Health System
New York, New York

Scot A. Brown, MD
Assistant Professor
Adult Joint Reconstruction
Orthopaedic Oncology
Thomas Jefferson University
Rothman Institute
Philadelphia, Pennsylvania

Sean V. Cahill, BA
Associate Research Assistant
Department of Orthopaedics and Rehabilitation
Yale University School of Medicine
New Haven, Connecticut

Ryan P. Calfee, MD, MSc
Associate Professor
Department of Orthopedic Surgery
Washington University in St. Louis
Saint Louis, Missouri

Caitlin C. Chambers, MD
Assistant Professor
Department of Orthopedic Surgery
University of Minnesota
Minneapolis, Minnesota

Chung Ming Chan, MD, MBBS
Assistant Professor
Department of Orthopaedics and Rehabilitation
University of Florida
Gainesville, Florida

Marcus P. Coe, MD, MS, FAOA
Assistant Professor
Department of Orthopaedic Surgery
Geisel School of Medicine, Dartmouth
Lebanon, New Hampshire

H. John Cooper, MD
Associate Professor
Department of Orthopedic Surgery
Columbia University Irving Medical Center
New York, New York

P. Maxwell Courtney, MD
Assistant Professor of Orthopaedic Surgery
Rothman Institute at Thomas Jefferson University
Philadelphia, Pennsylvania

Allison E. Crepeau, MD
Assistant Professor of Orthopedic Surgery
UConn School of Medicine
Elite Sports Medicine at Connecticut Children's Medical Center
Farmington, Connecticut

Michael B. Cross, MD
Assistant Attending Orthopaedic Surgeon
Department of Orthopaedic Surgery
Hospital for Special Surgery
New York, New York

Chris Culvern, MS
Research Director for the Joint Replacement Division
Midwest Orthopaedics at Rush University Medical Center
Chicago, Illinois

Scott D. Daffner, MD
Professor
Department of Orthopaedics
West Virginia University
Morgantown, West Virginia

Mark Dales, MD
Clinical Associate Professor
Seattle Children's Hospital Department of Orthopedics and Sports Medicine
University of Washington
Seattle, Washington

Craig J. Della Valle, MD
Professor of Orthopaedic Surgery
Chief, Section of Adult Reconstruction
Rush University Medical Center
Chicago, Illinois

Meng Deng, PhD
Assistant Professor
Department of Agricultural and Biological Engineering
School of Materials Engineering
Weldon School of Biomedical Engineering
Bindley Bioscience Center
Purdue University
West Lafayette, Indiana

Vishal Desai, MD
Assistant Professor
Department of Radiology
Thomas Jefferson University
Philadelphia, Pennsylvania

Christopher Doro, MD
Clinical Assistant Professor
Department of Orthopedics and Rehabilitation
University of Wisconsin School of Medicine and Public Health
Madison, Wisconsin

Maureen K. Dwyer, PhD, ATC
Director, Office of Clinical Research
Newton-Wellesley Hospital
Newton, Massachusetts

Ryan D. Endress, MD
Assistant Professor
Department of Plastic Surgery
University of Kansas School of Medicine
Kansas City, Missouri

Vahid Entezari, MD, MMSc
Associate Staff
Department of Orthopaedic Surgery
Cleveland Clinic
Cleveland, Ohio

Saif Aldeen Farhan, MD
Assistant Professor
Department of Orthopedic Surgery
University of California
Irvine, California

Wolfgang Fitz, MD
Assistant Professor
Department of Orthopedic Surgery
Harvard University
Cambridge, Massachusetts

Michael T. Freehill, MD, FAOA
Associate Professor of Orthopaedic Surgery
Sports Medicine and Shoulder Surgery
Team Physician, Michigan Athletics
University of Michigan
Ann Arbor, Michigan

Nicholas B. Frisch, MD, MBA
Attending Orthopaedic Surgeon
Ascension Crittenton Hospital
Rochester, Michigan

Freddie H. Fu, MD, DSc (Hon), DPs (Hon)
Chair, Distinguished Service Professor, David Silver Professor
Department of Orthopaedic Surgery
University of Pittsburgh Medical Center
Pittsburgh, Pennsylvania

Daniel J. Fuchs, MD
Assistant Professor
Department of Orthopaedic Surgery
Sidney Kimmel Medical College at Thomas Jefferson University
Philadelphia, Pennsylvania

Michael J. Gardner, MD
Professor and Vice Chair
Department of Orthpaedic Surgery
Stanford University School of Medicine
Palo Alto, California

Joshua L. Gary, MD, FAOA
Associate Professor
Department of Orthopaedic Surgery
McGovern Medical Center at UTHealth Houston
Houston, Texas

Elizabeth B. Gausden, MD, MPH
Orthopaedic Adult Reconstruction Fellow
Department of Orthopaedic Surgery
Mayo Clinic
Rochester, Minnesota

Andrew G. Georgiadis, MD
Pediatric Orthopaedic Surgeon
Gillette Children's Specialty Healthcare
St. Paul, Minnesota
Assistant Professor
Department of Orthopedic Surgery
University of Minnesota
Minneapolis, Minnesota

Robert J. Gillespie, MD
Michael and Grace Drusinsky Chair in Orthopaedic Surgery and Sports Medicine
Chief, Division of Shoulder and Elbow
Orthopaedic Surgery Residency Program Director
Associate Professor
Department of Orthopaedic Surgery
Case Western Reserve University
University Hospitals Cleveland Medical Center
Cleveland, Ohio

Mary B. Goldring, PhD
Professor
Cell and Developmental Biology
Weill Cornell Medical College
Weill Cornell Graduate School of Medical Sciences Senior Scientist Emerita
Hospital for Special Surgery
New York, New York

Ranjan Gupta, MD
Professor and Chief of Shoulder Surgery
Department of Orthopaedic Surgery, Anatomy and Neurobiology, and Biomedical Engineering
University of California
Irvine, California

Jonathan A. Gustafson, PhD
Postdoctoral Fellow
Department of Orthopedic Surgery
Rush University Medical Center
Chicago, Illinois

Jacques H. Hacquebord, MD
Assistant Professor
Department of Orthopedic Surgery &
Hansjörg Wyss Department of Plastic Surgery
New York University School of Medicine
New York, New York

Andrew E. Hanselman, MD
Assistant Professor
Department of Orthopaedic Surgery
Duke University
Durham, North Carolina

Jonah Hebert-Davies, MD
Assistant Professor
Department of Orthopaedic Surgery and Sports Medicine
Harborview Medical Center, University of Washington
Seattle, Washington

MaCalus V. Hogan, MD, MBA
Associate Professor
Department of Orthopaedic Surgery
Department of Bioengineering
University of Pittsburgh Medical Center
Pittsburgh, Pennsylvania

Francis John Hornicek, MD, PhD
Professor and Chair
Department of Orthopaedic Surgery
David Geffen School of Medicine at UCLA
Los Angeles, California

Rudolph H. Houben, MD
Microvascular Research Fellow
Division of Hand Surgery
Department of Orthopedic Surgery
Mayo Clinic
Rochester, Minnesota

Elizabeth W. Hubbard, MD
Assistant Professor of Orthopaedic Surgery
Department of Orthopaedic Surgery
Duke University Medical Center
Durham, North Carolina

Aaron J. Huser, DO
Pediatric Orthopaedic Surgeon
Gillette Children's Specialty Healthcare
St. Paul, Minnesota

Izuchukwu Ibe, MD
Department of Orthopedics and Rehabilitation
Yale University School of Medicine & Yale University
New Haven, Connecticut

James N. Irvine, Jr, MD
Sports Medicine Fellow
Department of Orthopaedic Surgery
NYP/Columbia Irving University Medical Center
New York, New York

David S. Jevsevar, MD, MBA
Department of Orthopaedic Surgery
Dartmouth-Hitchcock Medical Center
The Geisel School of Medicine at Dartmouth
Lebanon, New Hampshire

Megan Johnson, MD
Assistant Professor
Department of Orthopaedic Surgery
Vanderbilt University Medical Center
Nashville, Tennessee

Brian A. Klatt, MD
Assistant Professor
Department of Orthopaedic Surgery
Chief, Adult Reconstruction
Fellowship Director
University of Pittsburgh
Pittsburgh, Pennsylvania

Jason S. Klein, MD
Orthopaedic Surgeon
Surgery of the Shoulder and Elbow
The Carrell Clinic
Dallas, Texas

Mitchell R. Klement, MD
Orthopedic Surgeon
Orthopaedic Associates of Wisconsin
Pewaukee, Wisconsin

Conor P. Kleweno, MD
Associate Professor
Department of Orthopaedic Surgery and Sports Medicine
Harborview Medical Center, University of Washington
Seattle, Washington

Jennifer C. Laine, MD
Pediatric Orthopaedic Surgeon and Director of Research
Gillette Children's Specialty Healthcare
St. Paul, Minnesota
Assistant Professor
Department of Orthopedic Surgery
University of Minnesota
Minneapolis, Minnesota

Jeffrey Lange, MD
Instructor
Department of Orthopedic Surgery
Harvard University
Cambridge, Massachusetts

A. Noelle Larson, MD
Associate Professor
Department of Orthopedic Surgery
Mayo Clinic
Rochester, Minnesota

Cato T. Laurencin, MD, PhD
University Professor
Albert and Wilda Van Dusen Distinguished Professor of Orthopaedic Surgery
Professor of Chemical and Biomolecular Engineering
Professor of Materials Science and Engineering
Professor of Biomedical Engineering
Director, The Raymond and Beverly Sackler Center for Biomedical, Biological, Physical and Engineering Sciences
Chief Executive Officer
The Connecticut Convergence Institute for Translation in Regenerative Engineering
The University of Connecticut
Farmington, Connecticut

Francis Y. Lee, MD, PhD
Professor with Tenure
Wayne O. Southwick Professor of Orthopedics and Rehabilitation, Pathology and Biomedical Engineering
Yale University School of Medicine & Yale University
New Haven, Connecticut

Yu-Po Lee, MD
Clinical Professor
Department of Orthopaedic Surgery
University of California
Irvine, California

Brett R. Levine, MD, MS
Associate Professor
Department of Orthopaedics
Rush University Medical Center
Chicago, Illinois

Ning Liu, MD
Clinical Researcher
Department of Orthopaedic Surgery
Stanford University
Redwood City, California

Dieter M. Lindskog, MD
Associate Professor
Department of Orthopaedics and Rehabilitation
Yale University
New Haven, Connecticut

Steven C. Ludwig, MD
Professor, Chief of Spine Surgery
Division of Spine Surgery
Department of Orthopaedics
University of Maryland School of Medicine
Baltimore, Maryland

C. Benjamin Ma, MD
Professor in Residence
Vice Chairman, Adult Clinical Operations
Department of Orthopaedic Surgery
University of California
San Francisco, California

Jorge Manrique, MD
Adult Joint Reconstruction
Orthopaedic Oncology
Cleveland Clinic Florida
Weston, Florida

Daniel Augusto Maranho, MD, MSc, PhD
Orthopaedic Surgeon
Division of Orthopaedic Surgery
Hospital Sírio-Libanês
Brasília, Federal District, Brazil
Post-Graduation Professor of Orthopaedic Surgery
Health Sciences Applied to the Locomotor System
RibeirãoPreto Medical School of University of São Paulo
RibeirãoPreto, São Paulo, Brazil
Postdoctorate Fellow in Pediatric Orthopaedics
Department of Orthopaedic Surgery
Boston Children's Hospital
Boston, Massachusetts

Kristofer S. Matullo, MD, MPH
Chief – Division of Hand Surgery
St. Luke's University Health Network
Bethlehem, Pennsylvania
Associate Clinical Professor of Orthopedic Surgery (Adjunct)
Temple University
Philadelphia, Pennsylvania

Sean V. McGarry, MD
Associate Professor
James R. Neff, MD Musculoskeletal Oncology Chair
Department of Orthopaedics
University of Nebraska Medical Center
Omaha, Nebraska

Amy L. McIntosh, MD
Associate Professor of Orthopedic Surgery
Texas Scottish Rite Hospital
Dallas, Texas

James McKenzie, MD
Resident Physician, Post-Graduate Year 5
Department of Orthopaedic Surgery
Rothman Institute at Thomas Jefferson University Hospital
Philadelphia, Pennsylvania

Alexander S. McLawhorn, MD, MBA
Assistant Professor
Department of Orthopedic Surgery
Hospital for Special Surgery
New York, New York

Adam G. Miller, MD
Beacon Orthopaedics and Sports Medicine
Cincinnati, Ohio

Daniel (Dan) J. Miller, MD
Pediatric Orthopaedic Surgeon
Gillette Children's Specialty Healthcare
St. Paul, Minnesota

Bryan S. Moon, MD
Professor
Department of Orthopaedic Oncology
University of Texas MD Anderson Cancer Center
Houston, Texas

Mark E. Morrey, MD, MSc
Associate Professor
Department of Orthopedic Surgery
Mayo Clinic
Rochester, Minnesota

William Morrison, MD
Professor
Department of Radiology
Thomas Jefferson University
Philadelphia, Pennsylvania

Wayne E. Moschetti, MD, MS
Assistant Professor
Department of Orthopaedic Surgery
Geisel School of Medicine, Dartmouth
Lebanon, New Hampshire

Naveen Nagiah, PhD
Postdoctoral Fellow
Connecticut Convergence Institute for Translation in Regenerative Engineering
University of Connecticut
Farmington, Connecticut

Jennifer Nance, DNP
Pediatric Nurse Practitioner
Orthopedics Institute
Children's Hospital Colorado
Aurora, Colorado

Eduardo Novais, MD
Assistant Professor of Orthopaedic Surgery
Department of Orthopaedic Surgery
Boston Children's Hospital
Boston, Massachusetts

Michael J. O'Malley, MD
Assistant Professor
Department of Orthopaedic Surgery
University of Pittsburgh
Pittsburgh, Pennsylvania

Sherayar Orakzai, BSc
Medical Student
Augusta University/University of Georgia Medical Partnership
Athens, Georgia

Alexander R. Orem, MD, MS
Assistant Professor of Orthopaedic Surgery
Dartmouth-Hitchcock Medical Center
The Geisel School of Medicine at Dartmouth
Lebanon, New Hampshire

Selene G. Parekh, MD, MBA, FAOA
Co-Chief Foot and Ankle Division
Professor, Department of Orthopaedic Surgery
Partner, North Carolina Orthopaedic Clinic
Adjunct Faculty, Fuqua Business School
Duke University
Durham, North Carolina

Don Young Park, MD
Assistant Professor
Department of Orthopaedic Surgery
University of California, Los Angeles
Los Angeles, California

Michael S. Pinzur, MD
Professor
Department of Orthopaedic Surgery
Loyola University Health System
Maywood, Illinois

Ashley Pistorio, MD
Plastic Surgery Resident
Department of Plastic Surgery
The University of Kansas Health System
Kansas City, Kansas

Robin Pourzal, PhD
Assistant Professor
Department of Orthopedic Surgery
Rush University Medical Center
Chicago, Illinois

Ross Puffer, MD
Peripheral Nerve Fellow
Department of Neurologic Surgery
Mayo Clinic
Rochester, Minnesota

Benjamin R. Pulley, MD
Orthopaedic Associates of Zanesville
Zanesville, Ohio

Nicholas Pulos, MD
Assistant Professor
Department of Orthopedic Surgery
Mayo Clinic
Rochester, Minnesota

Steven M. Raikin, MD
Chief of Foot and Ankle Service
Professor, Department of Orthopaedic Surgery
Sidney Kimmel Medical College at Thomas Jefferson University
Philadelphia, Pennsylvania

Matthew L. Ramsey, MD
Professor of Orthopaedic Surgery
Sidney Kimmel College of Medicine at Thomas Jefferson University
Philadelphia, Pennsylvania
Chief, Shoulder and Elbow Surgery
Rothman Institute
Philadelphia, Pennsylvania

Brandon J. Rebholz, MD
Orthopaedic Spine Surgery Division Chief
Assistant Professor of Orthopaedic Surgery and Neurosurgery
Medical College of Wisconsin
Milwaukee, Wisconsin

Mark C. Reilly, MD
Fracture Surgery, Hip and Pelvis Reconstruction
Chief, Orthopaedic Trauma Service
University Hospital Newark
Fred F. Behrens Endowed Chair, Orthopaedic Trauma
Professor, Department of Orthopaedic Surgery
Rutgers-New Jersey Medical School
Newark, New Jersey

Peter C. Rhee, DO, MSc
Associate Professor
Department of Orthopedic Surgery
Mayo Clinic
Rochester, Minnesota

Eric T. Ricchetti, MD
Staff, Associate Professor
Department of Orthopaedic Surgery
Cleveland Clinic
Cleveland, Ohio

Benjamin F. Ricciardi, MD
Assistant Professor
Center for Musculoskeletal Research
Department of Orthopaedic Surgery
University of Rochester School of Medicine
Rochester, New York

Jonathan C. Riboh, MD
Assistant Professor
Division of Sports Medicine
Department of Orthopaedic Surgery
Duke University
Durham, North Carolina

David Ring, MD, PhD
Associate Dean for Comprehensive Care
Professor of Surgery and Psychiatry
Department of Surgery and Perioperative Care
University of Texas - Dell Medical School
Austin, Texas

Claire B. Ryan, MD
Orthopedic Surgery Resident
Department of Surgery and Perioperative Care
University of Texas – Dell Medical School
Austin, Texas

Michael K. Ryan, MD
Orthopaedic Surgeon
Hip Preservation and Sports Medicine
Andrews Sports Medicine and Orthopaedic Center
The Hip Center at Andrews Sports Medicine
American Sports Medicine Institute
Birmingham, Alabama

Comron Saifi, MD
Assistant Professor
Director of Clinical Spine Research
Department of Orthopaedic Surgery
Perelman School of Medicine
University Of Pennsylvania
Philadelphia, Pennsylvania

Edward M. Schwarz, PhD
Professor and Director
Center for Musculoskeletal Research
Department of Orthopaedic Surgery
University of Rochester School of Medicine
Rochester, New York

Roshan P. Shah, MD, JD
Assistant Professor
Department of Orthopedic Surgery
Columbia University Irving Medical Center
New York, New York

Rachel J. Shakked, MD
Assistant Professor
Department of Orthopaedic Surgery
Sidney Kimmel Medical College at Thomas Jefferson University
Philadelphia, Pennsylvania

Arya Nick Shamie, MD
Professor & Chief
Orthopaedic Spine Surgery
Department of Orthopaedic Surgery
David Geffen School of Medicine at UCLA
Los Angeles, California

Sarah E. Sibbel, MD
Director of Pediatric Hand and Upper Extremity Program
Orthopedics Institute
Children's Hospital Colorado
Aurora, Colorado

Micah Sinclair, MD
Assistant Professor
Department of Orthopaedic Surgery
Children's Mercy Hospital
Kansas City, Missouri

Anshuman Singh, MD
Shoulder and Elbow Surgeon
Assistant Clinical Professor, UCSD Orthopaedics
Physician Director of Imaging Utilization and Quality
Kaiser Permanente, San Diego
San Diego, California

Andrew D. Sobel, MD
Clinical Assistant Professor
Lewis Katz School of Medicine at Temple University
Hand, Microvascular, and Trauma Surgery
Department of Orthopedic Surgery
St. Luke's University Health Network
Bethlehem, Pennsylvania

Samantha A. Spencer, MD
Immediate Past President, Massachusetts Orthopaedic Association
Assistant Professor of Orthopaedic Surgery
Department of Orthopaedic Surgery
Harvard Medical School
Staff Physician, Boston Children's Hospital
Boston, Massachusetts

Andre R.V. Spiguel, MD
Assistant Professor
Department of Orthopaedic Surgery
University of Florida
Gainesville, Florida

Robert J. Spinner, MD
Chair, Department of Neurologic Surgery
Burton M. Onofrio Professor of Neurosurgery
Professor of Orthopedics and Anatomy
Mayo Clinic
Rochester, Minnesota

Benjamin E. Stein, MD
Partner, Orthopaedic Surgeon
Centers for Advanced Orthopaedics
Washington, District of Columbia

Suzanne E. Steinman, MD
Clinical Associate Professor
Seattle Children's Hospital
Department of Orthopedics and Sports Medicine
University of Washington
Seattle, Washington

Justin Stull, MD
Resident
Department of Orthopaedic Surgery
Thomas Jefferson University
Philadelphia, Pennsylvania

Nina Suh, MD, FRCSC
Assistant Professor
Department of Surgery, Division of Orthopaedic Surgery
University of Western Ontario
London, Ontario, Canada

Linda I. Suleiman, MD
Assistant Professor of Orthopaedic Surgery
Northwestern University Feinberg School of Medicine
Chicago, Illinois

Rachel M. Thompson, MD
Assistant Professor-in-Residence
Associate Residency Program Director
Associate Director Center for Cerebral Palsy
Department of Orthopaedic Surgery
University of California Los Angeles/Orthopaedic Institute for Children
Los Angeles, California

Scott M. Tintle, MD
Department of Orthopaedic Surgery
Walter Reed National Military Medical Center
Bethesda, Maryland

Caroline Tougas, MD, FRCSC
Clinical Assistant Professor
Department of Orthopedic Surgery
UMKC School of Medicine
Children's Mercy Hospital
Kansas City, Missouri

Wakenda K. Tyler, MD, MPH, FAOA
Associate Professor
Department of Orthopaedic Surgery
Columbia University Medical Center
New York, New York

M. Farooq Usmani, MD, MSc
Research Fellow
Department of Orthopaedic Surgery
University of Maryland School of Medicine
Baltimore, Maryland

Alexander R. Vaccaro, MD, MPH, PhD
President of Rothman Orthopaedics at Jefferson Health
Chairman of Orthopaedics at Sidney Kimmel Medical College at Thomas Jefferson University
Philadelphia, Pennsylvania

Heather A. Vallier, MD
Professor of Orthopaedic Surgery
Clyde L. Nash MD Professor of Orthopaedic Education
Department of Orthopaedic Surgery
Case Western Reserve University
The MetroHealth System
Cleveland, Ohio

Carola F. van Eck, MD, PhD
Assistant Professor
Department of Orthopaedic Surgery
University of Pittsburgh Medical Center
Pittsburgh, Pennsylvania

Arya Varthi, MD
Assistant Professor
Department of Orthopedic Surgery
Yale University
New Haven, Connecticut

Jonathan M. Vigdorchik, MD
Assistant Professor
Department of Orthopaedic Surgery
Adult Reconstruction and Joint Replacement
Hospital for Special Surgery
New York, New York

Mark A. Vitale, MD, MPH
ONS Foundation for Clinical Research and Education
Active Staff, Greenwich Hospital
Yale-New Haven Heath
Greenwich, Connecticut

Derek Ward, MD
Assistant Professor
Medical Director of Surgical Patient Care Optimization
Department of Orthopaedic Surgery
University of California
San Francisco, California

Peter G. Whang, MD, FACS
Associate Professor
Department of Orthopaedics and Rehabilitation
Yale University School of Medicine
New Haven, Connecticut

Jennifer M. Weiss, MD
So. California Permanente Medical Group
Los Angeles, California

Klane K. White, MD, MSc
Professor, Director of Skeletal Health and Dysplasia
Department of Orthopedics and Sports Medicine
Seattle Children's Hospital
University of Washington
Seattle, Washington

Kirkham Wood, MD
Professor
Department of Orthopaedic Surgery
Stanford University
Redwood City, California

Elaine I. Yang, MD
Assistant Professor
Department of Anesthesiology
Critical Care & Pain Medicine
Hospital for Special Surgery
Weill Cornell Medicine
New York, New York

Antonia M. Zaferiou, PhD
Assistant Professor
Department of Biomedical Engineering
Stevens Institute of Technology
Hoboken, New Jersey

PREFACE

My first encounter with *OKU* was as a resident when I used this unique text to update myself prior to starting a rotation in a subspecialty or during preparation for the *Orthopaedic In-Training Examination*. It was my go-to text throughout the residency. A few attributes of the book drew me to it. First, I noted that the sections and chapters had been written by renowned experts whose name defined their subspecialty. Second, I found that the chapters were easy to read and truly contained the most up-to-date important material. The chapters were not intended to be comprehensive, a task that another publication from the American Academy of Orthopaedic Surgeons, the *AAOS Comprehensive Orthopaedic Review*, fulfills. The chapters were written to truly bring the reader up to date with the recent developments in the field, a task befitting of the name. Finally, I found the text easy to read and outlines to be well assembled. I have continued to purchase and read every volume of the *OKU* ever since and found it useful even as a full-time professor in orthopaedic surgery.

It is our pleasure to bring *OKU 13* to you. I hope you will find that this newest volume has kept up with the great tradition and exhibits the aforementioned attributes. This beautiful work has been written, edited, and assembled by section editors and authors who deserve all the accolades. They have worked diligently and meticulously to bring new and important material to you.

A work of this magnitude requires a well-functioning team. I want to convey my gratitude to the publication team at the AAOS, particularly Lisa Claxton Moore and the AAOS publications team, who organized the face-to-face meetings for the *OKU 13* editorial board and kept our feet to the fire to produce an on-time and high-quality product. In order for the material not to be "old" by the time of publication, this huge textbook was produced on an aggressive timeline. Lisa was always on top of things. I have had the pleasure of working with her as an author, section editor, and now an editor. She is amazing. Special thanks to the Wolters Kluwer team, who for the first time have taken the responsibility to produce the main OKU and have performed this task beautifully.

I wish to once again thank the section editors, who happen to be my wonderful friends, whom I respect and admire. They worked meticulously to assemble this great work together on time and with pride. My huge gratitude also goes to the authors, the front-line soldiers, who worked tirelessly to write the chapters and ensure that they contained NEW and important material for the readers. They were superb scholars who delivered high-quality work.

Finally, I want to thank my wife, Fariba, who is a source of sound advice and wisdom. She is always there to support my academic aspirations. I also want to thank my children, Niosha and Cyrus, who are the great joy in my life and from whom I steal time to pursue my academic activities.

I hope you will enjoy reading this great work, as I did.

Javad Parvizi, MD, FRCS
Editor

Section 11: Pediatrics

SECTION EDITOR:

AMY L. MCINTOSH, MD

Section 12: Oncology and Pathology

SECTION EDITOR:

MATTHEW R. DICAPRIO, MD, FAOA

Section 1

Principles of Orthopaedics

EDITOR

Yale A. Fillingham, MD

Chapter 1

Orthopaedic Research

Wayne E. Moschetti, MD, MS • Marcus P. Coe, MD, MS, FAOA

ABSTRACT

This chapter reviews the basics of orthopaedic research in regard to levels of evidence, tools for evaluating study quality, the use of clinical practice guidelines, grades of recommendations and ethical considerations. The chapter also covers the use of orthopaedic registries, their value and limitations.

Keywords: clinical practice guidelines; ethical considerations; grades of recommendations; levels of evidence; orthopaedic registries; orthopaedic research; tools for evaluating study quality

Introduction

Understanding the basics of conducting orthopaedic research is paramount when interpreting the literature, analyzing the results of studies, and applying orthopaedic research to clinical practice. There are several tools available to aid in determining the level of evidence and quality of research, which should affect how research influences one's clinical practice. Clinical practice guidelines are an attempt to synthesize the most valuable clinical evidence available for wide distribution. Registries capture large populations of patients with similar diagnoses or similar implants and are a powerful tool to follow longitudinal results. Finally, overarching all research must be a firm foundation in ethical study design and treatment of subjects.

Dr. Moschetti or an immediate family member is a member of a speakers' bureau or has made paid presentations on behalf of DePuy, A Johnson & Johnson Company; serves as a paid consultant to or is an employee of DePuy, A Johnson & Johnson Company; has received research or institutional support from DePuy, A Johnson & Johnson Company; has received nonincome support (such as equipment or services), commercially derived honoraria, or other non–research-related funding (such as paid travel) from Medacta and Omni Life Science; and serves as a board member, owner, officer, or committee member of the New England Orthopaedic Society. Dr. Coe or an immediate family member serves as a paid consultant to or is an employee of DePuy, A Johnson & Johnson Company and has received research or institutional support from Ferring Pharmaceuticals.

Levels of Evidence

Orthopaedic research—whether therapeutic, diagnostic, prognostic, or economic—aims to expand our knowledge about the field and inform clinical decision-making. To be most effective, research must reduce bias. Biases are systemic factors other than the intervention being studied that influence the results of a study. In other words, bias can deviate a study from the underlying truth it aims to reveal. The design of a study can help reduce bias, as can the quality of a study (discussed in the next section). As the level of evidence of a study becomes higher (with larger numbers representing poorer levels of evidence and "level 1" representing the highest level of evidence), so does the study's inherent ability to decrease bias.

The following represent the most common types of studies, listed in order from the generally accepted highest level of evidence (level 1) to the lowest (expert opinion) based on the Oxford Centre for Evidence-Based Medicine (OCEBM) Levels of Evidence Working Group[1] (**Figure 1**).

Systematic Reviews

Systematic reviews and meta-analyses aggregate the findings of multiple published works in a systematic way, while taking into account the quality of each individual study, to produce the highest level of evidence.[2] In a systematic review, an a priori detailed and comprehensive search strategy is executed with the goal of reducing bias by identifying, reviewing, and analyzing all relevant studies on a particular topic. A meta-analysis utilizes statistical methods to combine the data from multiple studies (commonly a systematic review) into a larger sample, which allows the creation of a single quantitative pooled estimate.[3-5] These studies are

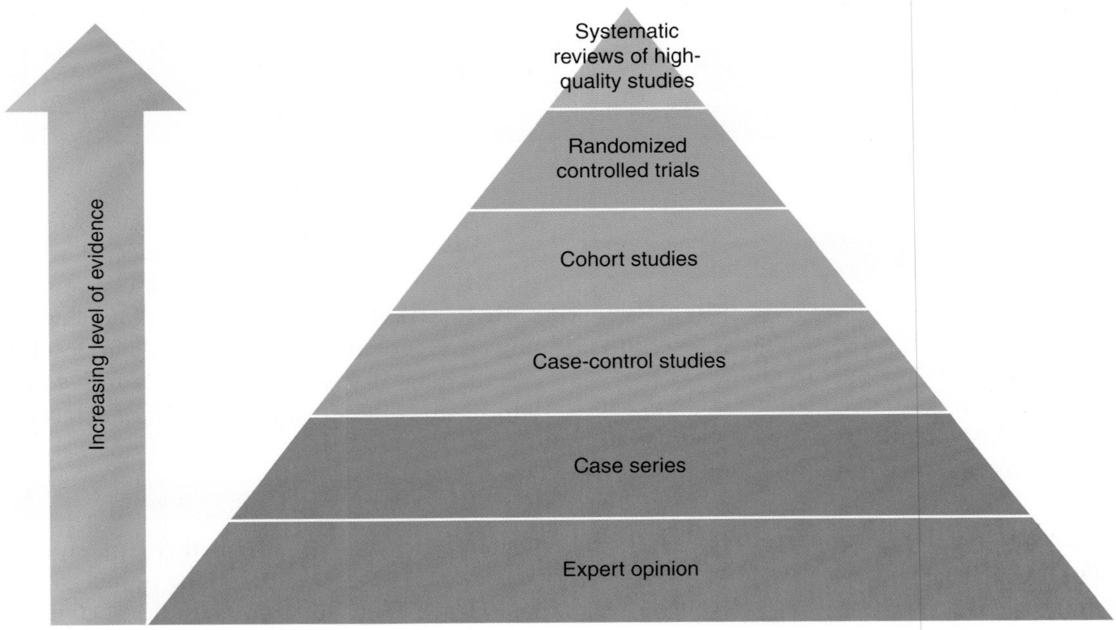

Figure 1 Level of evidence, with increasing levels of evidence from bottom to top, based on the Oxford Centre for Evidence-Based Medicine Levels of Evidence Working Group. (Data from the Oxford Centre for Evidence-Based Medicine Working Group.)

thus regarded as a fundamental source of the highest quality evidence and are frequently utilized for clinical practice guidelines and recommendations.[2,6] Systematic reviews of high-quality randomized controlled trials increase the level of evidence above high-quality randomized controlled trials alone, but are not without flaws and one must be careful when interpreting their findings.[7,8]

Randomized Controlled Trials

Considered the benchmark for therapeutic trials, randomized controlled trials aim to minimize bias by evenly distributing confounding factors across a study group and a control group. Confounding factors are prognostic variables that have the potential to affect the outcome of the study. Randomization evenly distributes subjects into either the study or control group based solely on chance, so that any factors not accounted for in the selection criteria, *even those that may be unknown*, affect the outcome evenly between both groups. In order for randomization to be most effective, the intervention (and at times the outcome) must be blinded to as many parties as practical. Ideally, neither the patient, the caregiver, nor anyone evaluating the patient or their outcomes should know whether the patient is in the intervention or the control group. In this manner, evaluation of outcomes is free from bias. Practically and ethically, blinding all parties is not always possible, particularly in studies involving a surgical intervention.

Cohort Studies

Cohort studies longitudinally compare a study group to a control group. Cohort studies can be either prospective (following patients from one point forward) or retrospective (looking back on previously treated patients on whom you have collected data). As patients are not randomized into the study and control groups, bias can affect how patients end up in one group or another and confounders are not evenly distributed. Oftentimes, randomization is not feasible or ethical and cohort studies are the best way to evaluate a specific intervention. Ideally, inclusion criteria should limit the effect of prognostic factors on the outcomes (eg, by including only nondiabetics, you remove the effect of diabetes on an outcome).

Case-Control Studies

Case-control studies retrospectively compare a group of patients with a condition to a group of patients without that particular condition. These are observational studies and not interventional studies. Usually these studies are designed to identify risk factors for a disease or outcome, though causality cannot be proven.

Case Series

Case series represent simple collections of patients who have undergone a specific intervention or have a specific condition. These are descriptive studies, and as there is no comparison group, it limits the conclusions that can be drawn from them. Case series can often identify venues for further study.

Expert Opinion

Expert opinions represent the thoughts and experiences of one or more person. Although anecdote and life experience can be useful "food for thought," they do not represent a high level of evidence unless systematically studied in one of the above ways.

In 2003, the *Journal of Bone and Joint Surgery* introduced a tool for determining the level of evidence based both on *the design of the study* and the *quality of the study*, which was again revised in 2015[9] (**Figure 2**).

Tools for Evaluation of Study Quality

While the design of a study influences its ability to determine the truth, so does the quality with which it is conducted. Quality can be a difficult thing to define when evaluating a clinical trial. There is a balance between limiting bias and study feasibility. Though there are numerous methods available to help assess study quality, studies are not routinely given a quality rating at the time of publication.[8] Randomized controlled clinical trials, thought to produce the highest level of clinical data, can be flawed in their execution, rendering them

Levels of Evidence for Primary Research Question[1,2]

Study Type	Question	Level I	Level II	Level III	Level IV	Level V
Diagnostic—Investigating a diagnostic test	Is this (early detection) test worthwhile? Is this diagnostic or monitoring test accurate?	• Randomized controlled trial • Testing of previously developed diagnostic criteria (consecutive patients with consistently applied reference standard and blinding)	• Prospective[3] cohort[4] study • Development of diagnostic criteria (consecutive patients with consistently applied reference standard and blinding)	• Retrospective[5] cohort[4] study • Case-control[6] study • Nonconsecutive patients • No consistently applied reference standard	• Case series • Poor or nonindependent reference standard	• Mechanism-based reasoning • Mechanism-based reasoning
Prognostic—Investigating the effect of a patient characteristic on the outcome of a disease	What is the natural history of the condition?	• Inception[3] cohort study (all patients enrolled at an early, uniform point in the course of their disease)	• Prospective[3] cohort[4] study (patients enrolled at different points in their disease) • Control arm of randomized trial	• Retrospective[5] cohort[4] study • Case-control[6] study	• Case series	• Mechanism-based reasoning
Therapeutic—Investigating the results of a treatment	Does this treatment help? What are the harms?[7]	• Randomized controlled trial	• Prospective[3] cohort[4] study • Observational study with dramatic effect	• Retrospective[5] cohort[4] study • Case-control[6] study	• Case series • Historically controlled study	• Mechanism-based reasoning
Economic	Does the intervention offer good value for dollars spent?	Computer simulation model (Monte Carlo simulation, Markov model) with inputs derived from Level-I studies, lifetime time duration, outcomes expressed in dollars per quality-adjusted life years (QALYs) and uncertainty examined using probabilistic sensitivity analyses	Computer simulation model (Monte Carlo simulation, Markov model) with inputs derived from Level-II studies, lifetime time duration, outcomes expressed in dollars per QALYs and uncertainty examined using probabilistic sensitivity analyses	Computer simulation model (Markov model) with inputs derived from Level-II studies, relevant time horizon, less than lifetime, outcomes expressed in dollars per QALYs and stochastic multilevel sensitivity analyses	Decision tree over the short time horizon with input data from original Level-II and III studies and uncertainty is examined by univariate sensitivity analyses	Decision tree over the short time horizon with input data informed by prior economic evaluation and uncertainty is examined by univariate sensitivity analyses

1. This chart was adapted from OCEBM Levels of Evidence Working Group, "The Oxford 2011 Levels of Evidence," Oxford Centre for Evidence-Based Medicine, http://www.cebm.net/ocebm-levels-of-evidence/. A glossary of terms can be found here: http://www.cebm.net/glossary/.

2. Level-I through IV studies may be graded downward on the basis of study quality, imprecision, indirectness, or inconsistency between studies or because the effect size is very small; these studies may be graded upward if there is a dramatic effect size. For example, a high-quality randomized controlled trial (RCT) should have ≥80% follow-up, blinding, and proper randomization. The Level of Evidence assigned to systematic reviews reflects the ranking of studies included in the review (i.e., a systematic review of Level-II studies is Level II). A complete assessment of the quality of individual studies requires critical appraisal of all aspects of study design.

3. Investigators formulated the study question before the first patient was enrolled.

4. In these studies, "cohort" refers to a nonrandomized comparative study. For therapeutic studies, patients treated one way (e.g., cemented hip prosthesis) are compared with those treated differently (e.g., cementless hip prosthesis).

5. Investigators formulated the study question after the first patient was enrolled.

6. Patients identified for the study on the basis of their outcome (e.g., failed total hip arthroplasty), called "cases," are compared with those who did not have the outcome (e.g., successful total hip arthroplasty), called "controls."

7. Sufficient numbers are required to rule out a common harm (affects >20% of participants). For long-term harms, follow-up duration must be sufficient.

Figure 2 Levels of evidence for the *Journal of Bone and Joint Surgery*. (Reproduced from Marx RG, Wilson, SM, Swiontkowski, MF: Updating the assignment of levels of evidence. *JBJS* 2015;97(1):1-2. doi:10.2106/JBJS.N.01112; Originally adapted from OCEBM Levels of Evidence Working Group, "The Oxce," Oford 2011 Levels of Evidenxford Centre for Evidence-Based Medicine, http://www.cebm.net/ocebm-levels-of-evidence/. A glossary of terms can be found here: http://www.cebm.net/glossary/. (CC BY 4.0).)

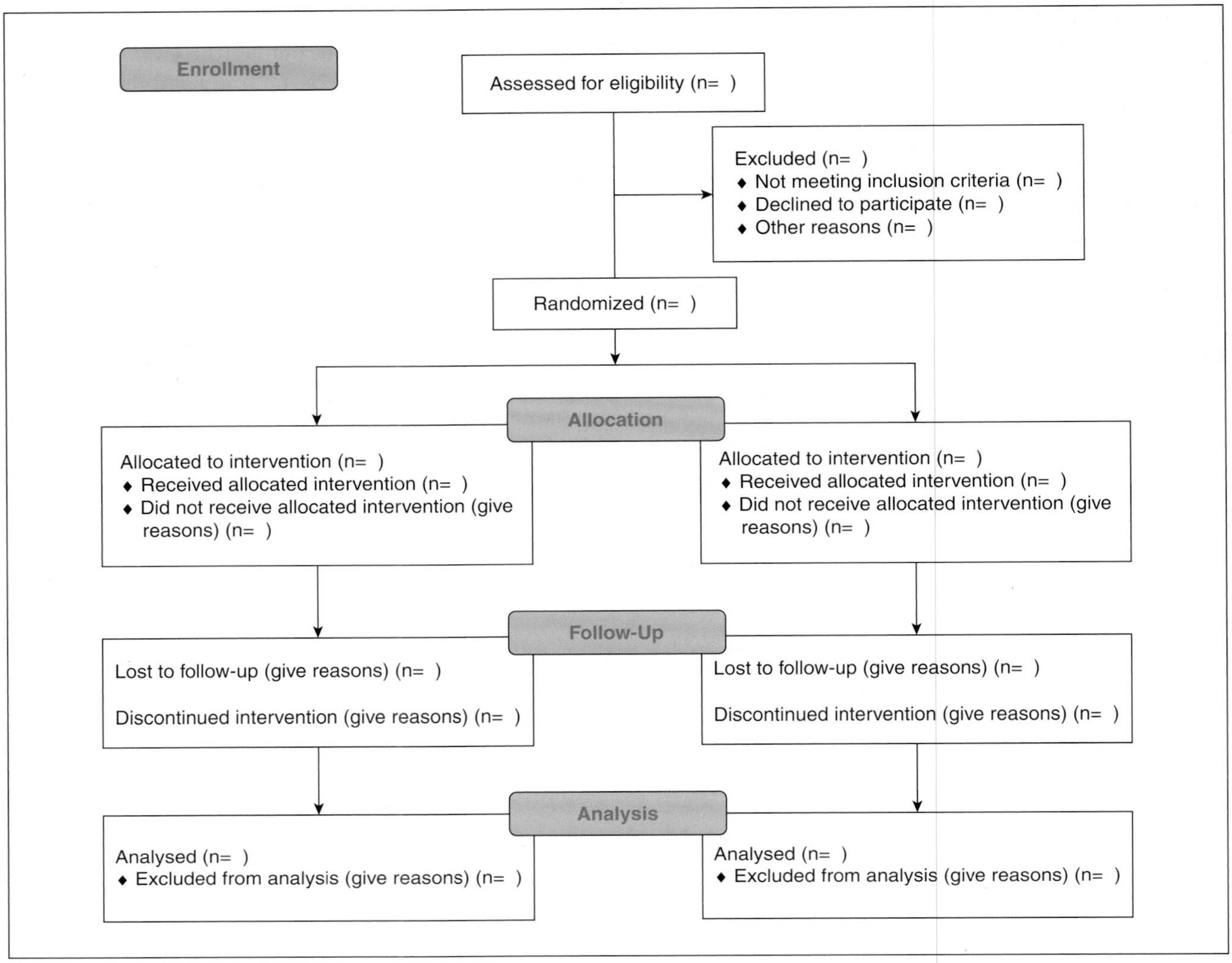

Figure 3 Consolidated Standards of Reporting Trials (CONSORT) 2010 flow diagram.

less useful than a more inherently flawed study design. A review paper may provide a compelling overview of a topic, but it can be driven by opinion and have the same potential for bias as expert opinion. A well-done cohort study may give more valuable clinical information than a randomized control with high crossover rates and high loss to follow up despite good study design. Thus, tools exist to evaluate the quality of various types of studies.

The Consolidated Standards of Reporting Trials (CONSORT) guidelines aim to improve the reporting of randomized controlled clinical trials.[10] These guidelines were created through consensus and collaboration between clinical trials experts with the goal of empowering readers to understand a trial's study design, analysis, and interpretation. Readers are thus better equipped to assess the validity of a trial's results. CONSORT achieves this using a checklist, which includes all the items deemed necessary to comply with the standard of reporting randomized clinical trials. Authors are expected to include a flow diagram outlining how the study population was recruited and handled throughout the course of the study[10] (**Figure 3**).

Systematic reviews collect and synthesize numerous studies, but as the phrase "garbage in, garbage out" illustrates, the strength of a systematic review is predicated on the strength of the studies that it synthesizes. Executing and completing a systematic review can be a challenging endeavor. The search strategy must include all relevant studies from all sources (common sources include Medline, Embase [Excerpta Medica database], CINAHL [Cumulative Index to Nursing and Allied Health Literature], Pubmed, abstracts, references, and the Cochrane Library databases). The systematic review should be registered on an international database, which attempts to catalog all systematic reviews and standardize their reporting (such as the International Prospective Register of Systematic Reviews—PROSPERO).[11] Finally, the studies themselves must be reviewed. More than one reviewer should assess each paper, applying predefined inclusion and exclusion criteria that assure appropriate study selection and data reporting. Methodologic and reporting quality is crucial to generate unbiased results and should be presented in accordance with the Preferred Reporting Items for Systematic Reviews and Meta-Analyses (PRISMA) statement[12] (**Figure 4**). For systematic reviews of observational studies, the use of the Meta-analysis of Observational Studies in Epidemiology (MOOSE) guideline is preferred.[13]

As the number of systematic reviews continues to increase, they are subject to a range of biases and it is important to distinguish high-quality systematic reviews from low-quality systematic reviews. The Assessment of Multiple Systematic Reviews (AMSTAR) index was developed to evaluate systematic reviews of randomized trials. This checklist of important attributes and practices has been adapted to the AMSTAR 2 index, which includes systematic reviews based on nonrandomized trials as well. As more weight is placed on these types of

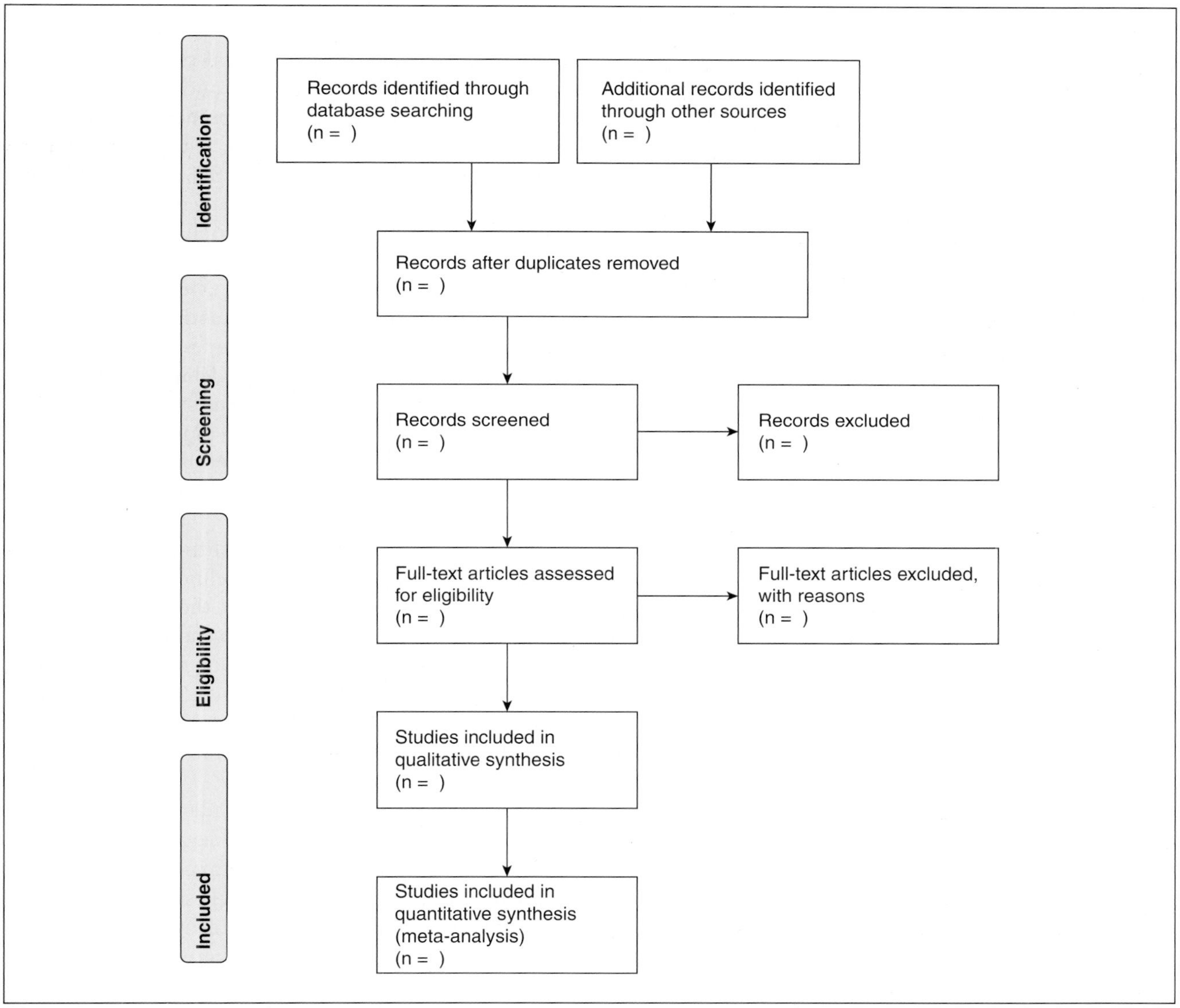

Figure 4 Generic PRISMA (Preferred Reporting Items for Systematic Reviews and Meta-Analyses) flow diagram. (Adapted from Moher D, Liberati A, Tetzlaff J, Altman DG; the PRISMA Group: Preferred reporting items for systematic reviews and meta-analyses: The PRISMA statement. *PLoS Med* 2009;6[7]:e1000097. doi:10.1371/journal.pmed1000097.)

studies for clinical and policy decisions, AMSTAR is a practical appraisal tool that allows for the reproducible assessments of the quality of systematic reviews.[14]

When evaluating individual studies, one must consider both the external and internal validity of the study. External validity can be thought of simply as whether or not the study is asking an appropriate research question that can generate applicable results. The internal validity of a study goes a step further and relates to whether the research question was answered correctly, that is, do the results represent what is "true" and were they obtained in a manner that minimizes bias?[15] High-quality studies are less prone to bias and thus more likely to have "true" results. Therefore, evaluation of study quality should always include an assessment of internal validity.

Regardless of study quality and methodological strategy, studies are always susceptible to bias, which, as discussed above, is a systematic deviation from true study results.[16] The most common forms of bias are selection bias, information bias, confounding bias, and publication bias. Selection bias can lead to a false association between exposure and outcome through a systematic error in patient enrollment.[16] Patients in both the treatment and control groups should be drawn from similar populations and efforts should be made to minimize loss to follow up. Information bias can result from flawed data collection. Patients may not remember an exposure or outcome (recall bias) and may be more likely to report complications if they have multiple medical comorbidities (reporting bias), and data collection may be inaccurately collected if the one collecting the data knows which treatment the study participant received (measurement bias). Standardized prospective data collection, as well as patient and provider blinding, can limit the predetermined beliefs of the patient and assessor and limit bias. When a third, commonly unmeasured variable leads to a potential outcome, a noncausal relationship between an exposure and the outcome may be inappropriately drawn, leading to confounding bias. For example, a study may demonstrate a higher infection rate in patients undergoing total hip replacement with metal femoral heads compared with those with ceramic femoral heads. If there are a greater number of diabetics in the metal head group and diabetics have higher rates of infection, then diabetes could act as a confounder, biasing the results. Lastly, studies with positive and favorable results are more likely to be published. Smaller studies, studies with negative results, or results perceived to be uninteresting are less likely to be published, have a delay in being published after several rejections, or get published in lower impact journals, leading to publication bias.

Use of Clinical Practice Guidelines

In 2012, it was estimated that there were approximately 28,100 active peer-reviewed journals which collectively published around 1.85 million articles a year; both these numbers continue to grow at roughly a rate of 3% per year.[17] It is impossible for a single individual to be aware of all the published literature. The goal of clinical practice guidelines is to improve the quality of care delivered to patients by consolidating and grading the current literature on important topics. Usually this falls to specialty societies, as they are most able to identify the topics of highest interest or debate in their field, collect and analyze data on a scale impractical for the independent practitioner, and then centralize and disseminate that information to the people most likely to use it. Specifically, clinical practice guidelines outline suggestions for diagnosis and treatment based on high-quality evidence. In the absence of high-quality evidence, and if the question is felt to be clinically important enough to warrant it, the group publishing the clinical practice guidelines may issue a consensus statement that amounts to expert opinion.[18]

It is important to realize that clinical practice guidelines do not represent mandates. Medical care is not delivered in a vacuum, and oftentimes, the patient population examined and/or the question that is being answered in a clinical practice guideline is not germane to the treatment of a specific patient by a specific orthopaedic provider at a specific time. Nonetheless, clinical practice guidelines aim to be generalizable and useful, providing a quick, condensed, and vetted resource for providers.

In accordance with the Institute of Medicines Guidelines, clinical practice guideline creation should involve the following: (1) defining the clinical problem and the patient population; (2) assembling a guideline-development group; (3) appraising the best evidence available; and (4) creating and disseminating the clinical practice guideline.[19] Since 2009, the American Academy of Orthopaedic Surgeons (AAOS) has produced clinical practice guidelines.[20]

The process that the AAOS undertakes to produce clinical practice guidelines is generally as follows.[21] After a general topic (for instance "compartment syndrome") is chosen, PICO questions are generated. PICO is an acronym that identifies the components of the question to be answered and stands for Patient or Population, Intervention, Comparison, and Outcome.[22] Numerous PICO questions are generated for each topic. **Table 1** demonstrates a typical PICO question for this example.

Table 1

PICO Guidelines as Defined by the American Academy of Orthopaedic Surgeons for a Clinical Practice Guideline Examining Compartment Syndrome

Question Components	Constructing Your Question
P—Patient or population Describe the most important characteristics of the patient (eg, age, disease/condition, gender)	Patients with extremity compartment syndrome (excluding chronic exertional)
I—Intervention; prognostic factor; exposure Describe the main intervention (eg, drug or other treatment, diagnostic/screening test)	Intramuscular pressure monitoring (intercompartmental pressure)
C—Comparison (if appropriate) Describe the main alternative being considered (eg, placebo, standard therapy, no treatment, the benchmark)	Absolute pressure vs. differential pressure/perfusion pressure, physical examination, timing of measurement
O—Outcome Describe what you are trying to accomplish, measure, improve, or affect. (eg, reduced mortality or morbidity, improved memory, accurate and timely diagnosis)	Sensitivity/specificity Likelihood ratios Secondary stratification: Timing to fasciotomy Need for fasciotomy Repeat surgeries

The PICO clinical question: For patients with suspected extremity compartment syndrome, does intramuscular pressure monitoring assist in diagnosing acute compartment syndrome?

After the guideline-development group has generated PICO questions, strict inclusion criteria are defined prior to a literature search. A research team then pulls all studies that meet the inclusion criteria taken from, at a minimum, a search of Pubmed, Embase, and hand searches of article bibliographies. At this point, excluded studies require an explanation of their exclusion. All included studies are then rated as high, moderate, low, or very low based on specific criteria that examine the number of flaws in a given study. Based on a critical appraisal of these studies, a recommendation, with an associated grade or strength, is made, followed by a period of peer and community review prior to publication.[23] Clinical practice guidelines thus provide a systematic review of the current scientific and clinical research leading to the creation of guidelines to help improve management of patients based on current best evidence.[24]

Grades of Recommendations

To help guide workgroups developing grades of recommendation for a clinical question, an international panel, including members of some of the premier evidence-based practice centers, created GRADE (Grading of Recommendations Assessment, Development and Evaluation). GRADE outlines a transparent and structured process that rates the quality of scientific evidence collected through the review process to develop guidelines that are as evidence-based as possible[23] (**Figure 5**). The steps involved in developing recommendations are specified by GRADE and provide clinicians a guide to using those recommendations in clinical practice.

Following the GRADE methodology helps the workgroup adhere to set parameters when evaluating the evidence. Once they complete their evidence-based literature review, the workgroup will summarize their findings as recommendations graded by the quality and number of studies included in the analysis using consistent language (**Table 2**). The summary findings and grade of recommendation may support or refute a certain intervention. There are typically four grades of recommendation.[21]

Treatments that receive an "A" or a "strong" level of recommendation are usually supported by level I studies such as randomized controlled clinical trials. Treatments with a "B" or a "moderate" level of recommendation are usually supported by fair evidence. These are commonly supported by level II or level III studies with consistent findings. Grade "C" or a "limited" recommendation is supported by poor-quality evidence with at times conflicting findings. This recommendation commonly includes level IV and level V studies. Treatments that receive an "I" level of recommendation do not have enough reliable information to allow

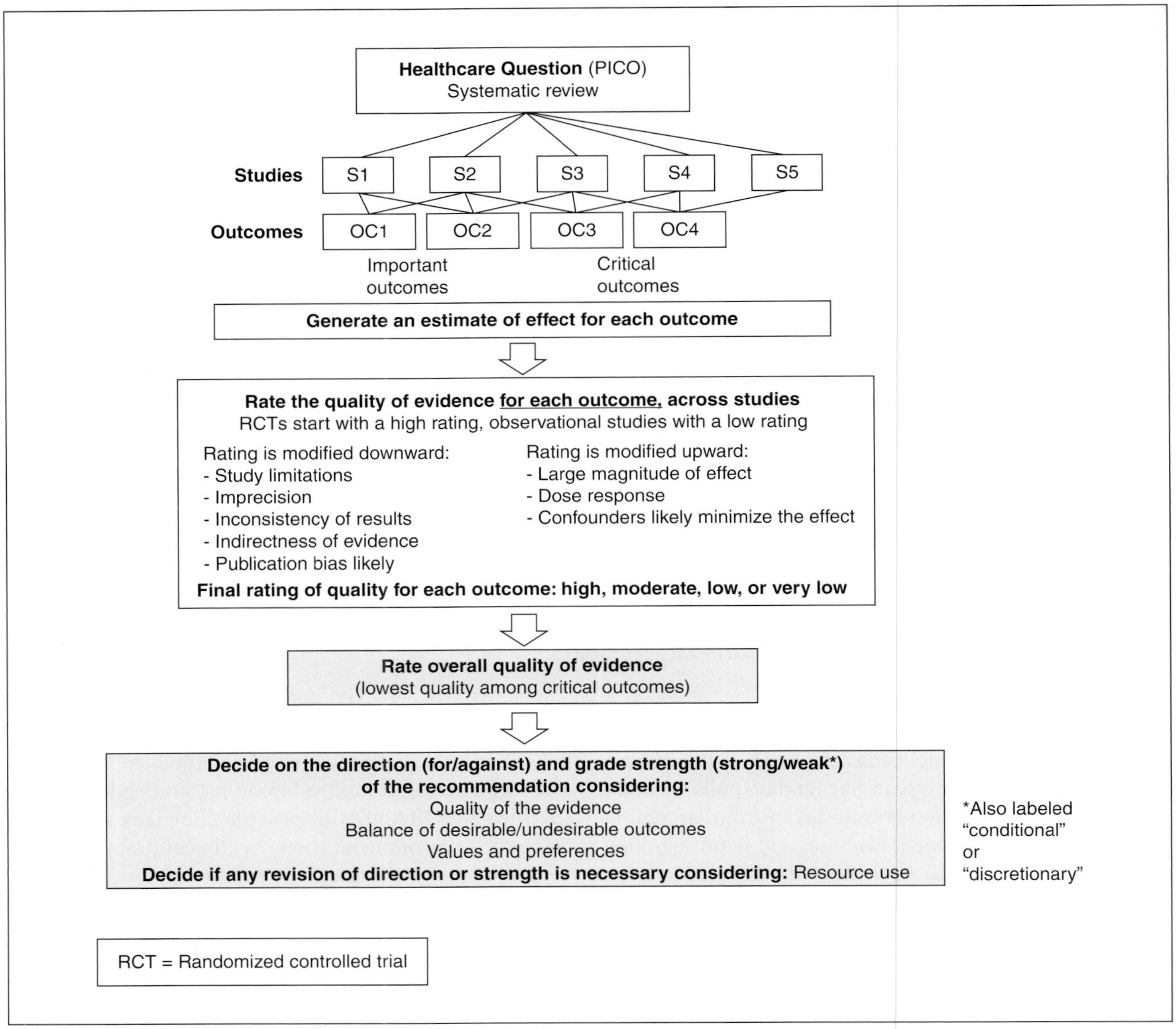

Figure 5 Overview of the GRADE (Grading of Recommendations Assessment, Development and Evaluation) process for developing evidence-based guidelines.

the workgroup to make an evidence-based statement, though they may elect to provide a consensus statement based on the expert opinion of the workgroup.[21,25]

Review of Commonly Used Registries and Databases

In 1975, the Swedish Knee Arthroplasty Registry was the first nationwide registry created to track outcomes after total knee arthroplasty (TKA). The goal was to track implants and identify early failures while reporting average results from the experience of an entire nation.[26] Individual institutions had started registries prior to this,[27] but the Swedish experience was the first foray into national data collection. This has led to the creation of national and regional arthroplasty registries in many other countries, including the United States, which established the American Joint Replacement Registry (AJRR) in 2009 (**Table 3**).

In addition to arthroplasty, there are orthopaedic registries for trauma and spine, yet these are few in number and primarily intended for epidemiological purposes. Orthopaedic registries are founded on the premise that patients with common characteristics (usually type of surgery) will be followed prospectively

Table 2

Strength of Recommendation Descriptions

Grade of Recommendations	Overall Strength of Evidence	Description of Evidence Quality	Guideline Recommendation
Strong	Strong	Evidence from two or more high-quality studies with consistent findings or evidence from a single high-quality study recommending for or against the intervention	There is moderate evidence against intervention X for patient Y to treat Z because...
Moderate	Moderate	Evidence from two or more moderate-quality studies with consistent findings or evidence from a single high-quality study recommending for or against the intervention	There is moderate evidence against intervention X for patient Y to treat Z because...
Limited	Low-strength evidence or conflicting evidence	Evidence from one or more low-quality studies with consistent findings or evidence from a single moderate-quality study recommending for or against the intervention or the evidence is insufficient or conflicting and does not allow a recommendation for or against the intervention	There is limited evidence to support intervention X for patient Y to treat Z because...
Inconclusive/ consensus	No evidence	There is no supporting evidence. In the absence of reliable evidence, the guideline workgroup is making a recommendation based on their clinical opinion. Consensus statements are published in a separate, complementary document	In the absence of clinical evidence, the opinion of the workgroup is...

Data from the American Academy of Orthopaedic Surgeons Clinical Practice Guidelines and Systemic Review Methodology.

after surgery without exclusion and regardless of the implant used. Data are collected about one or more health-related events in a geographically defined population to be used for research and public health.[28] The value of the information collected by the registry is predicated on completeness of the data entered and its quality. These data are collected longitudinally to assess the outcomes of patients and their implants. A unique identifier such as a social security number or national identity number is typically used to follow patients. This allows a revision surgery being performed at another institution to be linked to the primary procedure. Data are collected on all surgeons and patients, unlike the results of a clinical trial, which may have specific inclusion and exclusions criteria. The information in registries is thus likely a more pragmatic representation of the healthcare delivered to a population with a common condition.

As complications can be rare and revision rates low after orthopaedic surgery, specifically arthroplasty, registries provide an effective alternative to clinical trials that would require large numbers of patients and long-term follow-up to detect poorly performing devices.[28] Several examples of postmarket surveillance have led to recalls and voluntary withdrawal from the market of certain medical devices.[28,29] For instance, the articular surface replacement (ASR) metal-on-metal acetabular cup was noted to have higher than expected revision rates confirmed by several registries around the world, which led to the voluntary recall of this device.[29]

Creation and management of a registry require a significant amount of capital and resources. Some registries have been created by professional societies (such as in Sweden), while other large registries are supported by data from smaller, individual institutional registries reporting to a national data collection entity (such as in the United Kingdom). Despite the resources needed to fund a registry, there is the potential for cost savings if the rate of revision declines and inferior performing implants are removed from the market.[28]

Due to the heterogeneity of the data collected between registries, the International Consortium of Orthopaedic Registries (ICOR)[30] was established by the U.S. FDA in May 2011. The goal of this consortium was to pool data from orthopaedic registries around the world. Currently, there are over 30 registries sharing data worldwide. ICOR's goal is to improve collaboration between registries to allow for the sharing of data

Table 3

Common Registries for Total Hip and Total Knee Arthroplasty

Registry	Surgery	Year	Summary
Sweden	TKA THA	1975 1979	Created in 1975 (TKA) with the addition of THA in 1979. Began publically publishing results in 1989;73 nationwide registries
Finland	THA and TKA	1980	Initially voluntary reporting, now mandated since 1997
Norway	THA	1987	Small registry of a few thousand THAs annually
Denmark	THA	1995	Over 100,000 patients with ~ 9,000/yr
New Zealand	THA and TKA	1998	First English language arthroplasty registry. Limited data collection
Australia	THA and TKA	1999	Implant fees help fund registry. Started in 1999 but extended to the entire country in 2007. High volume of noncemented THA compared with European registries
Canada	THA and TKA	2001	Began as voluntary but now mandated in three provinces.
Romania	THA and TKA	2001	First Eastern European registry. Collects data on ankle, elbow, and shoulder joint replacements. Northern Ireland joined in 2013
England/Wales	THA and TKA	2003	Collects data on ankle, elbow, and shoulder joint replacements. Northern Ireland joined in 2013
The Netherlands	THA and TKA	1992 (failed) 2007	Netherlands Orthopaedic Association obtained public funding 15 yr after initial attempt at registry failed in 1992
American Joint Replacement Registry	TKA and THA	2009	Voluntary reporting with more than 1,000 participating institutions

THA = total hip arthroplasty; TKA = total knee arthroplasty

through infrastructure and data analytics.[30] This sort of partnership helps broaden the impact of data collection beyond individual registries.

Research Ethics

Ethics is inherently subjective, in as much as it attempts to understand the underpinnings of moral decision-making. However, a more objective framework can be constructed around moral decision-making to evaluate the ethics of scientific research. Adherence to certain principles can then be used as a means to examine whether research is ethical or not. The four principles guiding ethical research of human subjects are (1) beneficence; (2) nonmaleficence; (3) autonomy; and (4) distributive justice.

Beneficence is the concept that the patient's best interest should always be kept in mind. Thus, the purpose of any research study should be to improve the lives of patients. While arguably the most straightforward of the four guiding principles, it is also the most important, as it forms the backbone of any research study—to improve patient outcomes by better understanding a disease process, patient population, or treatment. It also places significant responsibility on the physician to be an advocate for patients, as a physician's knowledge and/or experience may give him or her insight into a patient's condition that the patient does not have.

Nonmaleficence is the idea that treatments should not harm patients. This is similar to, but separate from, beneficence, and again, at face value seems straightforward. Yet the balance between beneficence and nonmaleficence is affected by a patient's value system, their decision-making capacity, a physician's knowledge, and the fact that short-term harm may lead to long-term benefit (eg, chemotherapy decreases quality of life in the short term with the goal of increasing the length and quality of life in the future). Conversely, short-term benefit may lead to long-term harm (eg, an athlete may want to return to play after a concussion to gain the benefit of helping his or her team, though the long-term risk of another concussion is significant).

Autonomy refers to a patient's ability to choose his or her own treatment. The patient's right to decide his or her own treatment course is an inherent factor that must be respected in research and in practice. In research, it includes allowing patients to remove themselves from a study at any time, switch arms, or refuse to participate. In clinical practice, autonomy stands in contrast to paternalism or the concept that a physician should solely decide the best treatment for a patient because of his or her knowledge or expertise. Central to this concept in practice is the idea of shared decision-making—the practice of sharing all relevant information with a patient, so that they can make a well-informed decision that fits their value system and goals. In research, this concept is linked with consent and the idea that a patient should willfully participate in a study with full knowledge of the protocols, risks, and benefits of the study.

Finally, distributive justice is the concept that the potential benefits and harms of an intervention should not unfairly be focused on one sector of the population. For instance, if a new drug has the potential to help patients regardless of race or gender and is being tested only on white males, the remainder of the population is being unethically excluded. By contrast, if a new drug may have long-term benefits but also has known short-term harms and is being tested on prisoners, the risks are being unethically focused on an at-risk population with limited autonomy. Distributive justice requires the researcher to consider the population as a whole and not just the individual patient.

Clearly, these concepts are often at odds, and weighting these factors in a specific research setting must be considered on a case-by-case basis. As such, research ethics committees are charged with determining the ethicality of individual studies. As outlined by the World Health Organization (WHO), research ethics committees must determine that research (1) will be carried out with valid scientific methods and with adequate provisions for patients; (2) recruitment strategies do not unfairly target or exclude certain sectors of society, including at-risk populations who are prone to influence or neglect; (3) compensates patients for their time and effort if appropriate, though not in a way that influences their decision to enter a study; (4) protects patients' confidential health information; (5) follows an informed consent process that educates the patient prior to enrolling; and (6) factors in the effects of research on the community outside of the direct participants in the study.[31]

Summary

Certain basic fundamental knowledge is needed to conduct orthopaedic research. This foundation is necessary when interpreting the literature, analyzing the results of studies, and applying orthopaedic research to clinical practice. Several tools available to aid in determining the level of evidence and quality of research have been outlined. Clinical practice guidelines were reviewed which attempt to synthesize the most valuable clinical evidence available for wide distribution. An overview of registries and the benefit of data collection on large populations of patients with similar diagnoses or similar implants was outlined as a powerful tool to follow longitudinal results. Finally, overarching all research must be a firm foundation in ethical study design and treatment of subjects.

Key Study Points

- A basic understanding of conducting orthopaedic research, interpreting the literature, analyzing the results of studies, and applying research results are imperative to orthopaedic clinical practice.
- Several tools are available to determine the level of evidence and quality of research.
- Clinical practice guidelines synthesize the most valuable clinical evidence.
- Registries capture large populations of patients with similar diagnoses or similar implants and are a powerful tool to follow longitudinal results.
- All research must be a firm foundation in ethical study design and treatment of subjects.

Annotated References

1. CEBM Centre for Evidence-Based Medicine. Available at: https://www.cebm.net/index.aspx?o=5653.

   The Centre for Evidence-Based Medicine "levels of evidence" were created in 1998 to make the process of finding appropriate evidence more feasible and its results more clear. It aims to develop, teach, and promote evidence-based health care.

2. Bhandari M, Morrow F, Kulkarni AV, Tornetta P III: Meta-analyses in orthopaedic surgery. A systematic review of their methodologies. *J Bone Joint Surg Am* 2001;83-A(1):15-24.
3. DerSimonian R, Laird N: Meta-analysis in clinical trials. *Control Clin Trials* 1986;7(3):177-188.
4. Cohn LD, Becker BJ: How meta-analysis increases statistical power. *Psychol Methods* 2003;8(3):243.
5. Petticrew M, Roberts H: *Systematic Reviews in the Social Sciences: A Practical Guide*. Malden, MA, Blackwell Publishing, 2006.
6. Kuehn BM: IOM sets out "gold standard" practices for creating guidelines, systematic reviews. *JAMA* 2011;305(18):1846-1848.

7. Gagnier JJ, Kellam PJ: Reporting and methodological quality of systematic reviews in the orthopaedic literature. *J Bone Joint Surg Am* 2013;95(11):e771-e777.

8. Kunkel ST, Sabatino MJ, Moschetti WE, Jevsevar DS: Systematic reviews and meta-analyses in the orthopaedic literature: Assessment of the current state of quality and proposal of a new rating strategy. *Clin Res Orthop* 2018;1(1):1-7.

   This paper reviews methodologic quality for each of the 10 orthopaedic subspecialty journals using the PRISMA and AMSTAR guidelines. The overall quality of systematic reviews and meta-analyses in the orthopaedic literature was considered to be suboptimal.

9. Wright JG, Swiontkowski MF, Heckman JD: Introducing levels of evidence to the journal. *J Bone Joint Surg Am Vol* 2003;85A(1):1-3.

10. Schulz KF, Altman DG, Moher D; CONSORT Group: CONSORT 2010 statement: Updated guidelines for reporting parallel group randomised trials. *Int J Surg* 2011;9(8):672-677.

11. PROSPERO International Prospective Register of Systematic Reviews. Available at: https://www.crd.york.ac.uk/prospero/.

12. Moher D, Liberati A, Tetzlaff J, Altman DG; PRISMA Group: Preferred reporting items for systematic reviews and meta-analyses: The PRISMA statement. *Ann Intern Med* 2009;151(4):264-269, W64.

13. Stroup DF, Berlin JA, Morton SC, et al: Meta-analysis of observational studies in epidemiology: A proposal for reporting. Meta-analysis of Observational Studies in Epidemiology (MOOSE) group. *J Am Med Assoc* 2000;283(15):2008-2012.

14. Shea BJ, Reeves BC, Wells G, et al: AMSTAR 2: A critical appraisal tool for systematic reviews that include randomised or non-randomised studies of healthcare interventions, or both. *BMJ* 2017;358:j4008.

    The number of published systematic reviews of studies of healthcare interventions has increased, and these are used for clinical and policy decisions. AMSTAR is a popular instrument for critically appraising systematic reviews of randomized controlled clinical trials. This study developed AMSTAR 2 to enable critical appraisal of systematic reviews of randomized and nonrandomized studies of healthcare interventions.

15. Prictor M, Hill S: Cochrane consumers and communication review group: Leading the field on health communication evidence. *J Evid Based Med* 2013;6(4):216-220.

16. Szklo M, Nieto F: *Epidemiology: Beyond the Basics*, ed 2. Sudbury, MA, Jones and Bartlett Publishers, 2007.

17. Ware M: *The STM Report: An Overview of Scientific and Scholarly Journal Publishing*. The Hague, the Netherlands, International Association of Scientific, Technical and Medical Publishers, 2012.

18. American Academy of Orthopaedic Surgeons. Available at: aaos.org/guidelines.

19. Clinical Practice Guidelines We Can Trust. Available at: http://www.nationalacademies.org/hmd/Reports/2011/Clinical-Practice-Guidelines-We-Can-Trust.aspx.

20. AAOS OrthoGuidelines. Available at: www.orthoguidelines.org.

21. AAOS Clinical Practice Guideline and Systematic Review Methodology. Available at: https://www.aaos.org/uploadedFiles/PreProduction/Quality/Guidelines_and_Reviews/Guideline%20and%20Systematic%20Review%20Processes_v4.0_Final.pdf.

22. Bryant DM, Willits K, Hanson BP: Principles of designing a cohort study in orthopaedics. *J Bone Joint Surg Am* 2009;91(suppl 3):10-14.

23. Guyatt G, Oxman AD, Akl EA, et al: GRADE guidelines: 1. Introduction-GRADE evidence profiles and summary of findings tables. *J Clin Epidemiol* 2011;64(4):383-394.

24. McGrory BJ, Weber KL, Jevsevar DS, Sevarino K: Surgical management of osteoarthritis of the knee: Evidence-based guideline. *J Am Acad Orthop Surg* 2016;24(8):e87-e93.

    Guideline established from a systematic review of the current scientific and clinical research on surgical treatment of knee osteoarthritis. The guideline contains 38 recommendations pertaining to the preoperative, perioperative, and postoperative care of patients with osteoarthritis (OA) of the knee who are considering surgical treatment. The purpose of this clinical practice guideline is to help improve surgical management of patients with OA of the knee based on current best evidence. Level of evidence: I.

25. Wright J: *Levels of Evidence and Grades of Recommendations: An Evaluation of Literature*, 2005.

26. Robertsson O: Knee arthroplasty registers. *J Bone Joint Surg Br* 2007;89(1):1-4.

27. Berry DJ, Kessler M, Morrey BF: Maintaining a hip registry for 25 years. Mayo Clinic experience. *Clin Orthop Relat Res* 1997;(344):61-68.

28. Delaunay C: Registries in orthopaedics. *Orthop Traumatol Surg Res* 2015;101(1 suppl):S69-S75.

29. Hughes RE, Batra A, Hallstrom BR: Arthroplasty registries around the world: Valuable sources of hip implant revision risk data. *Curr Rev Musculoskelet Med* 2017;10(2):240-252.

    This paper describes the arthroplasty registries in general. It reviews international registries around the work and in the United States. It then provides a summary of total hip arthroplasty implant revision rates across registries at various time points.

30. International Consortium of Orthopaedic Registries. Available at: http://www.icor-initiative.org/.

31. *Standards and Operational Guidance for Ethics Review of Health-Related Research With Human Participants*. Geneva, WHO Document Production Services, 2011.

Chapter 2

Biostatistics

Linda I. Suleiman, MD • Chris Culvern, MS • Craig J. Della Valle, MD

ABSTRACT

Evidence-based medicine should be used by orthopaedic surgeons to inform clinical decisions. However, this requires the ability to critically review research with an emphasis on study design, statistical tests, and understanding of patient-reported outcomes. The purpose of this chapter is to provide a basic overview of biostatistics and research methodology to facilitate the interpretation of the published orthopaedic literature.

Keywords: common statistical tests; evidence-based medicine; patient-reported outcomes; study design

Introduction

Orthopaedic research investigators require knowledge of the published evidence to apply the appropriate interventions and address the healthcare needs of patients. Knowledge and comprehension of scientific research methodology requires a basic understanding of biostatistics. Biostatistics provides the scale in which information is reviewed and ultimately analyzed.[1] After reading this chapter, an orthopaedic surgeon should understand (1) the strengths and limitations of evidence-based medicine (EBM), meta-analysis, and systematic reviews; (2) the five Levels of Evidence by type of study; (3) the different tools used for commonly reported function scores; and (4) common statistical tests that are used and procedures that are required before conducting data analyses.

Dr. Della Valle or an immediate family member has received royalties from Smith & Nephew and Zimmer; serves as a paid consultant to or is an employee of DePuy, A Johnson & Johnson Company, Smith & Nephew, and Zimmer; has stock or stock options held in Parvizi Surgical Innovations; has received research or institutional support from Smith & Nephew, Stryker, and Zimmer; and serves as a board member, owner, officer, or committee member of the American Association of Hip and Knee Surgeons, the Arthritis Foundation, and the Hip Society. Neither of the following authors nor any immediate family member has received anything of value from or has stock or stock options held in a commercial company or institution related directly or indirectly to the subject of this chapter: Dr. Suleiman and Dr. Culvern.

Evidence-Based Medicine

Evidence-based medicine (EBM) was first defined by David Sackett in the *British Medical Journal* (*BMJ*) in 1996 and has drastically changed how orthopaedic surgeons practice medicine today. EBM is the process of utilizing and assessing scientific information and applying them to medical decisions.[2] This definition was adapted from Sackett's commonly quoted definition that "Evidence-based medicine is the conscientious, explicit and judicious use of current best evidence in making decisions about the care of individual patients."[3] He emphasized using individual clinical proficiency with the best externally validated research to guide clinical assessments. This emphasis has changed how orthopaedic research has been conducted.

To practice EBM, one must use the five steps (**Figure 1**) defined by Sackett: (1) formulate an answerable question, (2) gather evidence, (3) appraise the evidence, (4) implement the evidence, and (5) evaluate the process.[2,3] Formulating an answerable question requires the clinician to define the patient population, delineate the possible treatment modalities, and specify the outcomes of interest. After formulating an answerable question, the clinician must gather externally validated research by conducting a thorough review of the literature. Each study should be assessed for the level of evidence by asking the question, "how good is the evidence?" not "is this evidence perfect?"[2] To assess the evidence, understanding the levels of evidence based on the study design is critical (**Table 1**).

Although the EBM movement has held clinical studies to the highest level of evidence, it is not without limitations. The notion that clinical trial data have the highest level of reliability over clinical evidence and

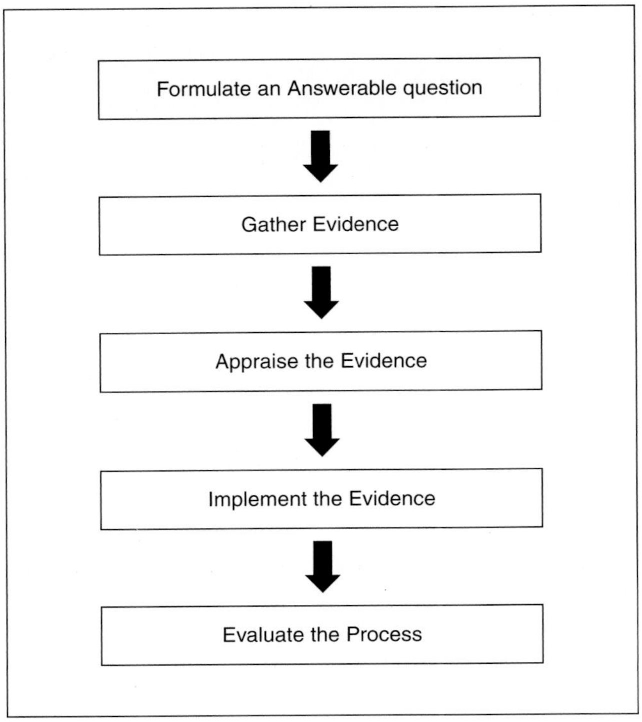

Figure 1 Illustration showing the five steps of evidence-based medicine.

mechanistic logic has been criticized.[4] In practice, as described in a 2016 study, mechanistic reasoning is used to deduce and apply large population studies to individual patients.[5] Additionally, the overreliance on the validity of clinical trials, underrepresentation of patients due to demographics, therapy, and comorbidities, and reliance on statistical significance over clinical significance have negatively impacted clinical medicine. As EBM continues to evolve with continued aims to demand reliable clinical research with a high level of external validity, systematic reviews and meta-analyses are being used to help formally synthesize research data and provide a conclusion when answering a specific clinical question.

Table 1

Levels of Evidence

Level	Type of Studies
I	Randomized controlled trials Systematic reviews of randomized controlled trials
II	Prospective cohort Randomized controlled trials with less than 80% follow-up
III	Case-control Retrospective cohort
IV	Case series
V	Expert opinion

Systematic Reviews and Meta-Analyses

Systematic reviews are high-level summarizations of primary research used to identify high-quality evidence related to a study question.[6] They account for individual study biases and combine patient outcomes from several distinct yet comparable clinical trials.[7,8] To perform a systematic review, the study purpose and a plausible and answerable question must be identified. Inclusion and exclusion criteria are determined based on the generation of a Preferred Reporting Items for Systematic Review and Meta-analysis (PRISMA) flowchart.[9] PRISMA enables the researcher to focus on relevant studies, reduces duplication of efforts, and prevents a researcher from conducting an arbitrary review of the literature. Search methodology must include several publically available electronic databases such as PubMED and the Cochrane Library and involve multiple reviewers. Extraction of data from these databases can be completed using a common published checklist provided by Spindler et al that allows the reporting of systematic reviews in orthopaedic surgery.[10] The strength of a systematic review in providing a recommendation relies on the quality of studies. Reviewers must evaluate the quality of the methodology and report the appropriate grading of evidence followed by the strength of the recommendation. Another similar, yet different approach to assessing information from multiple studies is the meta-analysis.

A meta-analysis differs from a systematic review by utilizing statistical methodology to assess collective data from individual studies.[6] The process used to collect the component studies is the same as a systematic review, and a good meta-analysis will be comprehensive and will explain the criteria for inclusion. While a systematic review may be more qualitative, a meta-analysis is an objective attempt to synthesize a collection of similar research studies. The goal is to combine many findings into one statistical analysis to determine if the overall effect is statistically present. This process involves combining the outcomes in a weighted-average fashion, so better studies, those that have larger samples or smaller variation, receive a higher weight[11,12] while newer methodologies have incorporated regression analysis.[13] A meta-analysis is helpful when studies offer conflicting results of varying strengths. When reviewing these types of meta-analysis, it is important to understand what studies were included and whether they are cohesive and consistent from a statistical standpoint. A growing trend is to incorporate some measure of this consistency in the analysis.[14]

While systematic reviews and meta-analysis allow for the assessment of multiple research studies, orthopaedic research investigators can be tasked with conducting their own studies. Planning research always begins with a clinical question and determining the appropriate study design. In orthopaedic literature, there are two main types of studies: analytic and descriptive.[15]

Analytic Studies

Analytic studies seek to answer a scientific hypothesis using inferential statistics (the use of sample data to make generalizations about a target population)[15] and fall into three main categories: randomized controlled trial (RCT), cohort, and retrospective case-control.

In the era of EBM, there are amplified demands for orthopaedic research to provide external validity such that the casual relationship discovered can be applied to patient populations. As such, the benchmark for a research study design is an RCT. Prior to 2000, RCTs encompassed approximately 5% of studies in the *Journal of Bone and Joint Surgery* (*JBJS*).[16] Since that time, the *JBJS* now includes 50% Level I, II, and III evidence, thus substantiating the importance of these studies to the field of orthopaedic medicine.[17,18]

One of the hallmarks of the RCT is the ability to eliminate selection bias and potentially regulating confounding variables, provided the appropriate level of power is achieved.[15] RCTs are ideal for evaluating adverse effects and effectiveness of new interventions. Study participants in an RCT are in a defined population and randomized into a treatment or control (placebo) group. The treatment group could be a new or existing treatment, and the control group could be an existing treatment or no treatment at all. Study participants are followed prospectively and results, by treatment group, are compared. Blinded RCTs provide the highest level of internal validity with randomization, providing balance between measured and unmeasured variables associated with outcome.[19] The primary advantage of an RCT is that they can provide evidence for causality by avoiding selection bias, selection by prognosis, and by ensuring balance between the treatment groups.[20]

Estimates suggest that over 18,000 RCTs are published each year. However, systematic reviews and clinical guidelines frequently conclude that there is limited evidence to support study findings.[19] While RCTs may provide internal validity, there is a potential for low external validity given limitations of identifying and enrolling enough patients. Additionally, depending upon resource constraints other circumstances, an RCT may not be economically feasible or ethical. As such, the use of other designs may be warranted.

Cohort studies compare groups with comparable demographics or exposure and follow them retrospectively or prospectively. These studies are suitable when approximating incidence, which represents the proportion of new cases of a disease within a specified time period. Typically, cohorts are described with specific risk factors and followed prospectively to observe outcomes. In orthopaedic studies, this design aids in determining prognosis of a given risk factor.

Retrospective case-control studies compare cases (patients with the disease of interest) and controls (patients without the disease) with respect to their level of exposure to a particular risk factor. While cohort studies select on exposure status, case-control studies select on disease status. Exposure differences between cases and controls are helpful in finding risk and protective factors associated with outcome. The most challenging part of this study design is defining the base population and selecting the appropriate, representative controls. This research design has been referred to as the "house red wine" of study design because it is more modest, has less risk, is inexpensive to conduct, and surprisingly good when compared with other designs.[21] These studies are typically longitudinal and observational. The odds ratio, the primary outcome measurement in case-control studies, is defined as the odds of disease in exposed individuals compared with the odds of disease in unexposed individuals.[22] The odds ratio is a good approximation of the relative risk when used in reporting rare diseases or events and can be determined from both case-control and cohort studies. However, the odds ratio should be used with some caution as it can overestimate the effect of events that occurs more than 10% of the time.[23]

Descriptive Studies

Descriptive studies include case report, case series, correlational (or ecological) studies, and cross-sectional studies. A case report is generally made by a clinician or group of clinicians on a seminal patient. They are used to document rare medical occurrences and highlight initial clues of an emerging disease or deleterious effect of a specific exposure. A case series is a larger version of the case report and describes a disease process or complication in a group of 10 or more patients.[15] Within the orthopaedic literature, case series (Level IV) evidence remains the most commonly reported research.[24]

Correlational studies, used to determine the potential relationship between two variables, use correlation data to represent average exposure levels within a particular population rather an actual individual levels. They are relatively easy to conduct (with the appropriate data), are low cost, and can help with hypothesis generation. However, the prevalence of correlation does not imply valid statistical association and relationships observed at the group level may not be applicable to individuals (ecological fallacy). Additionally, correlational studies also do not account for effect of potential confounding variables.[25]

Cross-sectional studies, used to examine the relationship between health outcomes and other variables, are often regarded as a "snap shot" of the health experience of a population at a given point in time. Because exposure and disease status are determined simultaneously, causality cannot be determined.[15] Cross-sectional studies are typically used to provide information on disease prevalence (proportion of cases at any given time point) and can be used for hypothesis generation about disease/exposure relationship.[1,26] The advantage of conducting this type of study is that they provide a general description and scope of a problem. Additionally, they are relatively low cost and can be completed within a short period of time. Results from cross-sectional studies are often used for health service evaluation, planning, and resource allocation. An example of a cross-sectional study is reviewing the incidence of prosthetic joint infections after a total knee arthroplasty. In all of the aforementioned study designs, orthopaedic research investigators use a variety of tools to collect important exposure and outcome data about their patients. Patient-reported outcome measures (PROMs) are commonly used in orthopaedic clinical practice and research to track patient response to management and guide clinical decision making.[27]

Commonly Reported Functional Scores

The evolution of value-based health care has garnered significant focus on PROMs as outcomes are now publicly reported and can impact physician reimbursement. As discussed in a 2016 study, the development of the Patient-Reported Outcome Measurement Information System (PROMIS) is an NIH (National Institutes of Health) initiative to obtain data on patient's mental, physical, and social health to develop valid and reportable outcome measures.[28] This system was constructed to validate and build item banks to quantify symptoms and apply them to a variety of chronic conditions allowing physicians to interpret patient-reported outcomes (PROs).[29] PROMIS was developed to overcome the limitations of the burdensome administration and narrow application to specific patient populations. A 2016 study reports that PROMIS overcomes this limitation by using item response theory, which uses underlying health traits in the item bank to assess function.[30] Using item response theory, PROMIS has less administrative burden and a wider scope compared with obstacles faced by legacy measures. In the orthopaedic outcome measures, PROMIS physical function has been validated in disorders of the foot and ankle, upper extremity, and spine with improvement in measurement characteristics.[30-32]

The most commonly used generic tools include the Medical Outcomes Study 36-item Short Form Health Survey (SF-36), the 12-item Short Form Health Survey (SF-12), the Short Form Six Dimensions (SF-6D), and the European Quality of Life-Five Dimensions questionnaire (EQ-5D). The SF-36 is the most commonly used tool and comprises 36 questions related to a patient's physical function, general health perceptions, social functioning, bodily pain, vitality, mental health, and emotional limitations.[33] SF-36 is significantly limited by the length of the survey with a high likelihood for deficient responses. The shortened version (SF-12) was developed to overcome the length and reporter reliability of the SF-36 but is limited to only providing an abbreviated summary of physical and mental data components. Further reducing the length of the SF-12, the SF-6D was developed to provide a cost utility assessment using a sample of multidimensional health states.[34] The EQ-5D uses five dimensions to evaluate patients: mobility, self-care, usual activities, pain or discomfort, and anxiety or depression.[33] The five dimensions are further categorized into three levels of severity, generating 243 possible responses, and provide an overall health profile with a weighted total value.[35] However, the EQ-5D has significant ceiling effect (**Table 2**) at the time of follow-up.[33] Condition-specific PROMs are self-administered pain, disability, and functional scores as it relates to the anatomic joint in question and not susceptible to the ceiling effect. These condition-specific PROMs have been validated, but there are limitations such as licensing fees on some of the instrument tools such as the Knee Injury and Osteoarthritis Outcome Score (KOOS) and the Hip Disability and Osteoarthritis Outcome Score (HOOS).[36,37]

The visual analog scale (VAS) applies to both generic and condition-specific outcomes and serves as a psychometric instrument.[33] The VAS can be applied to general health status, pain, and satisfaction by specifying how agreeable they are to a given statement and indicating

Table 2

Definition of Commonly Used Statistical Terms

Target population	The underlying group that the research intents to produce generalizations about
Sample	The specific collection of information used in the research to represent the population
Primary outcome measure	The one quantity that best answers the research objective
Minimal clinically important difference	The smallest change in the primary outcome measure that would be of clinical importance
Power	The probability that a test correctly rejects the null hypothesis
Null hypothesis	The assumption of no significant difference in hypothesis testing
Type I error	The rejection of a true null hypothesis (false-positive)
Type II error	Failing to reject a false null hypothesis (false-negative)
Ceiling effect	Occurs when data values exceed the measurement tool's maximum value resulting in measurement inaccuracy
Floor effect	Similar to a ceiling effect but pertains to a minimum value report inaccuracy
Confidence interval	The range of values computed from the observed data that contain the true population value
Independent observations	An important assumption in statistical testing ensuring the sample's observations are not linked to one another

their understanding on a continuous line with two end points.[38] However, the VAS can camouflage variation in the severity of pain, thus causing a ceiling effect.[39]

Power Analysis

A power analysis provides an estimate of the smallest number of observations needed to statistically support the primary outcome of a study. This is particularly important when an experiment may pose risks to the study participants and the fewest number enrollees that can answer the research question is desired. If the information is time or cost intensive to collect, determining the sample size also informs study feasibility. In studies that are designed to test equivalence among treatment groups, a power analysis is even more critical as they share a burden of the proof of equivalence.[40]

Power is the probability that a hypothesis test correctly rejects the null hypothesis and is affected by the magnitude of the effect size and the number of observations used to test the presence of that effect.[41] The larger the effect size being tested, or the larger the sample used to assess that effect, the greater the resulting power. The two major components of power are the alpha and beta (**Table 3**). Alpha is the chance of incorrectly rejecting a true null hypothesis (Type I error) and is commonly referred to as the significance level of a test. Beta is the chance of failing to reject a false null hypothesis (Type II error). Mathematically, power is $1 - \beta$. The levels of alpha and beta reflect how rigorously the hypothesis test will assess the effect in question.

Power Analysis Calculation

The first step in any a priori power analysis is to identify the primary outcome measure and the effect size of interest. The effect size is the difference expected, in means or a change in percent, that answers the main research question. To determine the appropriate effect size, the minimal clinically important difference (MCID) of the outcome measure must be identified. The MCID is the smallest difference that would be identified as important by the patient.[42] A review of the available literature on the primary outcome may reveal the medical community has already established the MCID for that particular outcome. This is the case for many common outcomes measures such as PROMs. If there is no established MCID, consider the results of similar studies and what effect might be clinically relevant.

Once the outcome measure and MCID are chosen, the test that will be used in the power analysis must be identified. Ideally the test used to support the power analysis is a reflection of the final analysis for the study. Two common tests to base a power analysis from are the chi-squared test for categorical variables and the *t*-test for continuous variables. These tests can incorporate data that are structured as one-sample, two-sample, or paired in nature. In addition, there are more rigorous tests used in power analysis such as those stemming from a regression, an analysis of variance, or a simulation-based approach.[41]

To estimate sample size, a few more assumptions must be made. Alpha is typically assumed to be 5% and power $(1 - \beta)$ is typically 80%. A more rigorous test that would result in a larger sample size would assume

Table 3

Types of Error

		Unknown Truth About Population	
		H_0[a] is True	H_0 is False
Research conclusion	Fail to reject H_0	Correct probability = $1 - \alpha$	Type II error probability = β
	Reject H_0	Type I error probability = α	Correct probability = $1 - \beta$ (Power)

[a]H_0: Null hypothesis.

90%. If Type II errors are really damaging to the research, a higher beta should be assumed. An assumption of the SD of the primary outcomes must also be made for numeric, measurement variables. Published research may help with this or a small pilot study can be done to better gauge this assumption. The larger the SD, the larger the resulting sample size. Ultimately a power analysis is an estimate whose accuracy depends on the quality of the assumptions used. If one of the inputs, like SD, is less known to the researcher then being conservative in that assumption may be wise. Also, it may be beneficial to perform several variations of the power analysis to understand the impact of these assumptions. Sometimes what is perceived as a small change in one of the inputs results in a substantial change in the required sample size.

Statistical Testing

The aim of analytic studies that involve inferential statistics is to generalize a relationship or property about the target population from a subset of data that was sampled to accurately reflect that population. This often includes testing research hypotheses concerning the presence of an effect through formal hypothesis testing and using estimation to report the effect size along with confidence intervals.[43] While the majority of medical research currently focuses on hypothesis testing, there is a growing trend to include more statistical estimation as it can better gauge the true effect size of interest instead of dichotomizing a study's results to an "effect"/"no effect" result.[44-46] Estimation methods involve reporting confidence intervals to present a range of plausible values of the effect in the underlying target population.[47] This range of values is better than a single value estimate of an effect as it incorporates the SD and sample size from the data to present the precision of certainty in that effect.

Hypothesis Testing

Common statistical techniques rely on the frequentist principle of hypothesis testing (as opposed to Bayesian methods).[48] Given a research question, hypothesis testing begins with stating the null (H_0) and alternative (H_a) hypothesis to reflect the goals of the research. The null hypothesis is the default statement in the statistical test and often reflects an absence of the effect in question. The alternate hypothesis is the presence of that effect. Consider a researcher testing two treatments. The null hypothesis would reflect that the two treatments produce the same results or that the difference in the outcome measure is zero, H_0:effect = 0. The alternative hypothesis would represent that a difference does exist in that outcome measure or that the difference does not equal zero. When the alternate hypothesis is not equal to zero, H_a:effect $\neq$ 0; this is called a two-sided alternative hypothesis or simply a two-sided test. Two-sided tests are common, and there are only few instances where a one-sided test is appropriate.[49]

The premise behind hypothesis testing is deciding whether any observed difference is beyond what is expected under random chance. The two bell-shaped curves represented in **Figure 2** represent the probability of every possible outcome under the null and alternate hypothesis. The *P*-value is the probability that the perceived difference would occur by random chance under the assumption of the null hypothesis, and it is calculated from the probability distribution and the critical value, the point on the distribution that determines the rejection region. Therefore, if the probability is small enough such as below 5%, then the difference is not likely due to random chance, the null hypothesis is rejected, and a statistically significant difference is claimed.

The null hypothesis is accepted only if there fails to be evidence to reject it. Statistically, equivalence cannot be proven with hypothesis testing, only that the effect in question is not present. In that way, the verbiage used is

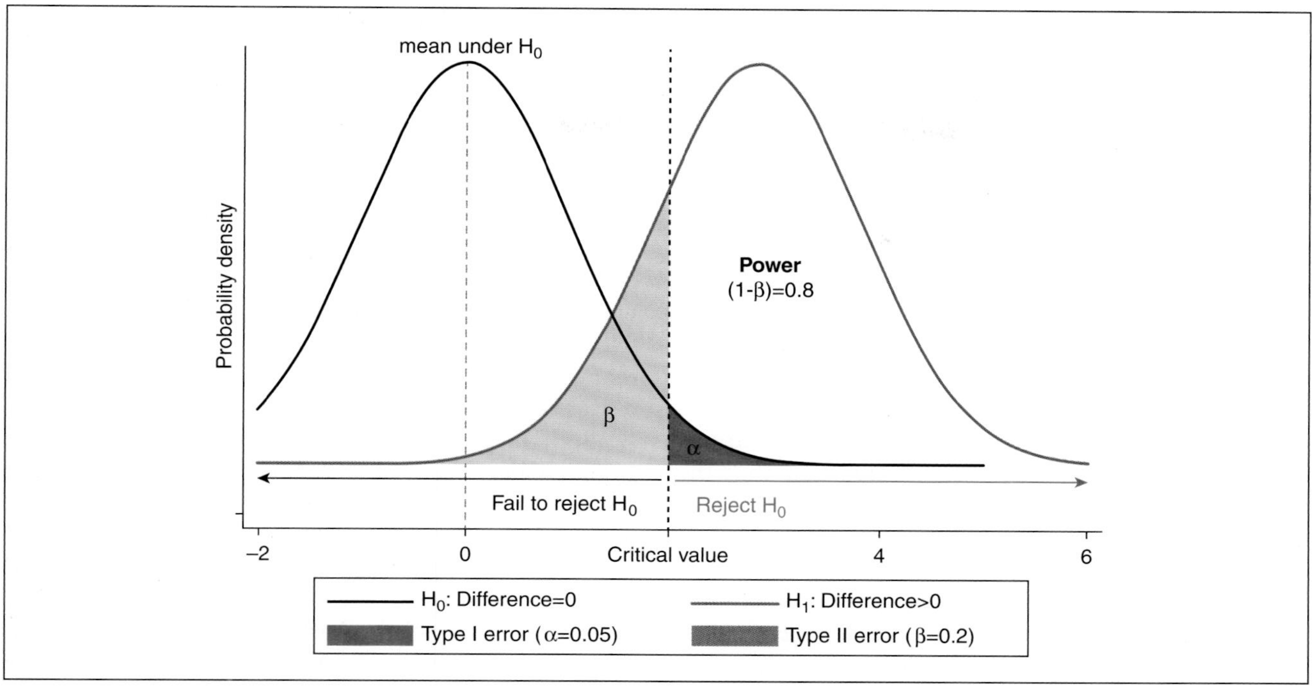

Figure 2 Illustration demonstrating hypothesis testing.

"fail to reject the null hypothesis" if the *P*-value is not sufficiently small enough to reject the null and accept the alternate hypothesis. The inability to prove equivalence is a common misconception in hypothesis testing, but given that understanding, there is a relatively new process that has been devised in an attempt to better support equivalence referred to as the two, one-sided tests (TOST) approach.[40]

Understanding hypothesis testing is often assumed in academic literature, and typically, the *P*-value and the specific test used to arrive at that value is all that gets reported. This process is commonly referred to as the statistical test, but the hypothesis testing conditions still apply. The specific test chosen should reflect the research question(s) of interest as well as attributes of the data, specifically the type of data being analyzed.

Data Types

In statistical analysis, data are typically either categorical or quantitative, and this format will dictate the appropriate statistical test. In general, the practice of dichotomizing information and turning numerical data into categorical should be avoided.[50] In addition to what is being measured, the test's distributional assumptions for the data should be assessed and nonparametric tests considered if there is a notable departure from the requisite distribution. Independence of observations should also be assessed for the analysis. Lack of independence occurs when observations are linked and one value is similar or related to other values. The validity of this assumption can be difficult to assess and care must be taken in designing the study and sampling the data to avoid this, as nonindependence often comes from observations being close in time or proximity in the sampling.

While nonindependent observations can be damaging when unintentional, it can also be the result of a proper study design. Longitudinal studies feature observations in the same subject at different time points. Repeated measures means the same data are measured several times, but instead of a change over time, there is another effect in place that changes the outcomes. Finally, clustered data feature a single observation per subject but the subjects are linked by some natural grouping that affects all subjects within that group such as subjects stemming from one of several hospitals or surgeons.[48] Maintaining independent observations is a critical assumption in most statistical models and must be accounted for in the analysis if present.

Testing Quantitative Data

Given that the variable of interest is a measurable quantity and a comparison of the mean is desired, a *t*-test may be the appropriate statistical test. A *t*-test can be used to assess the mean of a variable against a single number that is a known or an expected population mean. This is called a one-sample *t*-test. A two-sample *t*-test involves comparing the similarity of two independent variables. In biology, it is more common for the two-sample *t*-test to compare a measurement variable that is assessed across a nominal variable. An example of this would be comparing a measureable outcome in patients that received one of two treatment groups. A paired *t*-test is used to compare paired, longitudinal data across two time points such as a pre- and postintervention assessment.

To generate their *P*-values and have assumptions on the data that must be verified, *t*-tests rely on the Student's t-distribution. In addition to independent observations, the *t*-test requires that the observations in each group are normally distributed and that the variance in each group is the same, also known as homoscedasticity. These assumptions can be checked with statistical tests and are more likely to be correct in larger sample sizes due to the central-limit theorem.[51] In smaller sample sizes, these tests should receive some scrutiny. However, even in smaller samples or mild departures from the normality or equality of variance, the *t*-test is still appropriate and preferred over nonparametric tests that do not have distributional assumptions.[52] However, if the normality assumption is grossly violated, a Mann-Whitney test should be used instead of a two-sample *t*-test and a Wilcoxon signed-rank test instead of a paired *t*-test.

A *t*-test is used to compare means across exactly two treatment groups. When more than two treatment groups are being considered, an analysis of variance (ANOVA) can be used. A one-way ANOVA is ideal when one measurement variable is compared across a single nominal variable. A two-way ANOVA compares the measurement variables across two nominal variables, such as the primary outcome measure being tested across three treatment groups and gender. The assumptions for an ANOVA are similar to the *t*-test: independent observations, observations are normally distributed, and homoscedasticity.

The null hypothesis in an ANOVA is no difference across treatment groups, and the alternative hypothesis is the existence of a difference across treatment groups. Therefore, an ANOVA only shows if there is a difference among all the treatment groups combined and does not show which pair is different. To accomplish that, a post hoc test that makes pair-wise comparisons should be used. This can be accomplished with either a two-sample *t*-test or more commonly a Tukey-Kramer test. Whichever test is used, a correction for multiple comparison, such as a Bonferroni correction, should be considered.

Testing Categorical Data

Pearson's chi-squared test should be used when proportional equality is being tested across two categorical variables. An example of this would be testing the occurrence of treatment outcomes, such as number of successes in each treatment group, across another categorical variable. This type of information is often depicted in a 2 × 2 contingency table but bigger tables can also be assessed. Fisher's exact test is recommended when any cell in the contingency table contains less than five observations; however, there is evidence to suggest that even one observation is enough for the chi-squared test to be appropriate.[53]

Both Fisher's exact test and the chi-squared test assume independent observations. If this assumption is not valid and the data are longitudinal and paired in nature, a Cochran-Mantel-Haenszel test (a generalized McNemar test) should be considered. This test is used when there are three categorical variables to consider together that result in several 2 × 2 or larger contingency tables to compare. Often this results when there are two nominal variables being compared as in Fisher's exact test and chi-squared test and an additional third variable that identifies the repeated testing either in time or location.

Confounding Factors

A confounding factor is a third variable that affects the relationship of interest between two primary variables. Suppose the research explores the effect of a treatment as measured through an outcome variable. If a third factor, like age, is known to affect the outcome and age is not similar between treatment groups, age would be a confounding factor to the outcome of interest. Confounding factors are best controlled through good study design that minimizes sources of potential bias.[51] A proper randomization technique or a matched cohort design can also minimize several sources of confounding factors. However, if a confounding factor is identified, that effect may be controlled for by using multivariable regression analysis. These are difficult to perform and to interpret and should be left to biostatisticians.

Summary

Surgeons must understand biostatistics to truly appreciate the methodology and conclusions of orthopaedic clinical research. Practicing EBM has allowed orthopaedic surgeons to properly deduce information about their patient population and apply this knowledge to their everyday decision making. Reported outcomes and high-quality research designs should continue to be vetted and critically reviewed to advance the quality of medical care.

Key Study Points

- EBM is the process of utilizing and assessing scientific information and applying them to medical decisions.
- The effect size is the difference expected, in means or a change in percent, that answers the main research question.
- The premise behind hypothesis testing is deciding whether any observed difference is beyond what is expected under random chance.

Annotated References

1. Kocher MS, Zurakowski D: Clinical epidemiology and biostatistics: A primer for orthopaedic surgeons. *J Bone Joint Surg Am* 2004;86-A:607-620.
2. Bernstein J: Evidence-based medicine. *J Am Acad Orthop Surg* 2004;12:80-88.
3. Sackett DL, Rosenberg WM, Gray JA, Haynes RB, Richardson WS: Evidence based medicine: What it is and what it isn't. *BMJ* 1996;312:71-72.
4. Andersen H: Mechanisms: What are they evidence for in evidence-based medicine? *J Eval Clin Pract* 2012;18:992-999.
5. Sheridan DJ, Julian DG: Achievements and limitations of evidence-based medicine. *J Am Coll Cardiol* 2016;68:204-213.

   Overview of the history of evidence-based medicine and the movement to greater objectivity in medical decision making. Level of evidence: IV.
6. Harris JD, Quatman CE, Manring MM, Siston RA, Flanigan DC: How to write a systematic review. *Am J Sport Med* 2014;42:2761-2768.
7. Bhandari M, Morrow F, Kulkarni AV, Tornetta P: Meta-analyses in orthopaedic surgery. A systematic review of their methodologies. *J Bone Joint Surg Am* 2001;83-A:15-24.
8. Dijkman BG, Abouali JA, Kooistra BW, et al: Twenty years of meta-analyses in orthopaedic surgery: Has quality kept up with quantity? *J Bone Joint Surg Am* 2010;92:48-57.
9. Shamseer L, Moher D, Clarke M, et al: Preferred reporting items for systematic review and meta-analysis protocols (PRISMA-P) 2015: Elaboration and explanation. *BMJ* 2015;350:g7647.
10. Spindler KP, Kuhn JE, Dunn W, Matthews CE, Harrell FE Jr, Dittus RS: Reading and reviewing the orthopaedic literature: A systematic, evidence-based medicine approach. *J Am Acad Orthop Surg* 2005;13:220-229.
11. Hedges LV, Olkin I: *Statistical Methods for Meta-analysis.* Orlando, FL, Academic Press, 1985.
12. Hedges LV: *Statistical Methodology in Meta-Analysis.* Princeton, NJ, ERIC Clearinghouse on Tests, Measurement, and Evaluation, Educational Testing Service, 1982.
13. Brockwell SE, Gordon IR: A comparison of statistical methods for meta-analysis. *Stat Med* 2001;20:825-840.
14. Higgins JPT, Thompson SG, Deeks JJ, Altman DG: Measuring inconsistency in meta-analyses. *BMJ* 2003;327:557-560.
15. Jolles BM, Martin E: In brief: Statistics in brief. Study designs in Orthopaedic Clinical Research. *Clin Orthop Relat Res* 2011;469:909-913.
16. Bhandari M, Richards RR, Sprague S, Schemitsch EH: The quality of reporting of randomized trials in the *Journal of Bone and Joint Surgery* from 1988 through 2000. *J Bone Joint Surg Am* 2002;84-A:388-396.
17. Hanzlik S, Mahabir RC, Baynosa RC, Khiabani KT: Levels of evidence in research published in the *Journal of Bone and Joint Surgery (American Volume)* over the last thirty years. *J Bone Joint Surg Am* 2009;91:425-428.
18. Wright JG, Swiontkowski MF, Heckman JD: Introducing levels of evidence to the journal. *J Bone Joint Surg Am* 2003;85-A:1-3.
19. Castillo RC, Scharfstein DO, MacKenzie EJ: Observational studies in the era of randomized trials: Finding the balance. *J Bone Joint Surg Am* 2012;94(suppl 1):112-117.
20. Noordzij M, Dekker FW, Zoccali C, Jager KJ: Study designs in clinical research. *Nephron Clin Pract* 2009;113:c218-c221.
21. Hulley SB, Cummings SR, Browner WS, Grady D, Hearst N, Newman TB: *Designing Clinical Research: An Epidemiologic Approach*. Philadelphia, PA, Lippincott Williams & Wilkins, 2001.
22. Lui KJ: Estimation of sample sizes in case-control studies with multiple controls per case: Dichotomous data. *Am J Epidemiol* 1988;127:1064-1070.
23. Schmidt CO, Kohlmann T: When to use the odds ratio or the relative risk? *Int J Public Health* 2008;53:165-167.
24. Lefaivre KA, Shadgan B, O'Brien PJ: 100 most cited articles in orthopaedic surgery. *Clin Orthop* 2011;469:1487-1497.
25. Vavken P, Culen G, Dorotka R: Management of confounding in controlled orthopaedic trials: A cross-sectional study. *Clin Orthop* 2008;466:985-989.
26. Lim HJ, Hoffmann RG: Study design: The basics. *Methods Mol Biol* 2007;404:1-17.
27. Wright AA, Hensley CP, Gilbertson J, Leland JM, Jackson S: Defining patient acceptable symptom state thresholds for commonly used patient reported outcomes measures in general orthopedic practice. *Man Ther* 2015;20:814-819.
28. Baumhauer JF, Bozic KJ: Value-based healthcare: Patient-reported outcomes in clinical decision making. *Clin Orthop* 2016;474:1375-1378.

    The aim of PROMIS to develop valid, precise measurements of a patient's physical, mental, and social health. Level of evidence: III.

Principles of Orthopaedics

29. Cella D, Yount S, Rothrock N, et al: The patient-reported outcomes measurement information system (PROMIS): Progress of an NIH roadmap cooperative group during its first two years. *Med Care* 2007;45:S3-S11.

30. Brodke DJ, Saltzman CL, Brodke DS: PROMIS for orthopaedic outcomes measurement. *J Am Acad Orthop Surg* 2016;24:744-749.

Within Orthopaedic Surgery, PROMIS has been validated in foot and ankle, upper extremity, and spine. Level of evidence: V.

31. Hung M, Nickisch F, Beals TC, Greene T, Clegg DO, Saltzman CL: New paradigm for patient-reported outcomes assessment in foot & ankle research: Computerized adaptive testing. *Foot Ankle Int* 2012;33:621-626.

32. Döring A-C, Nota SPFT, Hageman MGJS, Ring DC: Measurement of upper extremity disability using the patient-reported outcomes measurement information system. *J Hand Surg* 2014;39:1160-1165.

33. Rolfson O, Rothwell A, Sedrakyan A, et al: Use of patient-reported outcomes in the context of different levels of data. *J Bone Joint Surg Am* 2011;93(suppl 3):66-71.

34. Brazier J, Usherwood T, Harper R, Thomas K: Deriving a preference-based single index from the UK SF-36 Health Survey. *J Clin Epidemiol* 1998;51:1115-1128.

35. EuroQol Group: EuroQol – A new facility for the measurement of health-related quality of life. *Health Policy* 1990;16:199-208.

36. Klässbo M, Larsson E, Mannevik E: Hip disability and osteoarthritis outcome score. An extension of the Western Ontario and McMaster Universities Osteoarthritis Index. *Scand J Rheumatol* 2003;32:46-51.

37. Roos EM, Roos HP, Lohmander LS, Ekdahl C, Beynnon BD: Knee Injury and Osteoarthritis Outcome Score (KOOS) – Development of a self-administered outcome measure. *J Orthop Sport Phys Ther* 1998;28:88-96.

38. Reips U-D, Funke F: Interval-level measurement with visual analogue scales in internet-based research: VAS generator. *Behav Res Methods* 2008;40:699-704.

39. González-Fernández M, Ghosh N, Ellison T, McLeod JC, Pelletier CA, Williams K: Moving beyond the limitations of the visual analog scale for measuring pain: Novel use of the general labeled magnitude scale in a clinical setting. *Am J Phys Med Rehabil* 2014;93:75-81.

40. Walker E, Nowacki AS: Understanding equivalence and non-inferiority testing. *J Gen Intern Med* 2011;26:192-196.

41. Cohen J: *Statistical Power Analysis for the Behavioral Sciences.* Hillsdale, NJ, Lawrence Erlbaum Associates, Inc., 1988.

42. Jaeschke R, Singer J, Guyatt GH: Measurement of health status: Ascertaining the minimal clinically important difference. *Control Clin Trials* 1989;10:407-415.

43. Altman DG, Bland JM: Measurement in medicine: The analysis of method comparison studies. *J R Stat Soc Ser Stat* 1983;32:307-317.

44. Gardner MJ, Altman DG: Confidence intervals rather than P values: Estimation rather than hypothesis testing. *Br Med J* 1986;292:746-750.

45. Goodman SN: Toward evidence-based medical statistics. 1: The P value fallacy. *Ann Intern Med* 1999;130:995-1004.

46. Sterne JA, Smith GD: Sifting the evidence – What's wrong with significance tests? *Phys Ther* 2001;81:1464-1469.

47. Altman D, Machin D, Bryant T, Gardner M: *Statistics With Confidence: Confidence Intervals and Statistical Guidelines.* John Wiley & Sons, 2013.

48. Bland JM, Altman DG: Bayesians and frequentists. *BMJ* 1998;317:1151-1160.

49. Moyé LA: *Statistical Reasoning in Medicine: The Intuitive P-value Primer.* Springer Science & Business Media, 2006.

50. MacCallum RC, Zhang S, Preacher KJ, Rucker DD: On the practice of dichotomization of quantitative variables. *Psychol Methods* 2002;7:19-40.

51. Bland M: *An Introduction to Medical Statistics.* UK, Oxford University Press, 2015.

52. Fagerland MW, Sandvik L, Mowinckel P: Parametric methods outperformed non-parametric methods in comparisons of discrete numerical variables. *BMC Med Res Methodol* 2011;11:44.

53. Campbell I: Chi-squared and Fisher–Irwin tests of two-by-two tables with small sample recommendations. *Stat Med* 2007;26:3661-3675.

Chapter 3

Patient Safety, Core Competencies, and Communication Skills

Jorge Manrique, MD • Scot A. Brown, MD

ABSTRACT

Many institutions are involved in supervising training to ensure surgeons are able to deliver safe, quality care. Others ensure patient safety and well-being throughout a surgeon's career via surgical and institutional protocols. Among the different institutions, the Accreditation Council for Graduate Medical Education (ACGME) ensures training quality and competency acquisition and the World Health Organization (WHO), as well as the Joint Commission, ensure patient safety. Different milestones for each training program are delineated by the ACGME, and institutional protocols have been defined by the WHO and Joint Commission. Additionally, to achieve patient-centered care, communication plays an essential role. Interactions of healthcare professionals with both patients and other team members are critical to avoid confusion and undesired errors. As orthopaedic surgeons, we must strive to provide excellent care while adhering to the available guidelines that have determined to be successful with a focus on effective communication and cultural competency to ensure patients are engaged in their care.

Keywords: patient satisfaction; person-centered care; shared decision making; surgical patient safety

Introduction

As part of patient-centered care, patient safety is a primary goal of orthopedic surgeons. High-quality patient-focused care not only ensures better outcomes but plays an important role in current healthcare policies. Core competencies at both the resident and attending level have been developed by various oversight bodies. A key component is clear effective communication and involvement of the patient in decision making along the course of their treatment. Ultimately, our responsibility can even extend beyond the office as we have a moral and often legal imperative to identify and report abusive behavior including child abuse, domestic abuse, and elder abuse. This chapter will cover different aspects of these topics.

Core Competencies and Patient-Centered Care

The Accreditation Council for Graduate Medical Education (ACGME) was created in 1981 to supervise and ensure the quality of postgraduate medical education and training in the United States. Many changes have taken place throughout the years in an attempt to ensure patient-centered care along with ensuring the well-being of training physicians. To standardize this effort, they developed the Clinical Learning Environment Review (CLER) Program.[1]

This program focuses on six competencies:

- Patient safety
- Quality improvement
- Transitions in care
- Supervision
- Duty hours oversight, fatigue management, and mitigation
- Professionalism

The CLER program has three areas or activities to accomplish its purpose: the site visit, the evaluation committee, and support for faculty and leadership development. The visit evaluates the sponsoring institution, focusing on the role of the residents and fellows in the six competencies described above. These are evaluated or assessed by five questions:

- Who and what form is the infrastructure of a Sponsoring Institution's (SI's) clinical learning environment?
- How integrated is the Graduate Medical Education (GME) leadership and faculty within the SI's current clinical learning environment infrastructure?

Dr. Manrique or an immediate family member serves as a paid consultant to or is an employee of Stryker. Neither Dr. Brown nor any immediate family member has received anything of value from or has stock or stock options held in a commercial company or institution related directly or indirectly to the subject of this chapter.

- How engaged are the residents and fellows in using the SI's current clinical learning environment infrastructure?
- How does the SI determine the success of its efforts to integrate GME into the quality infrastructure?
- What areas has the SI identified as opportunities for improvement?

The evaluation committee differs from the ACGME review committees, as it sets expectations for the six focus areas and provides institutions with feedback from the visit. Faculty and leadership development focuses on establishing resources to educate and support faculty and executive leadership across the six focus areas.

Core Competencies for Trainees

Different core competencies have been described in orthopaedic surgery throughout the years. Recently, the orthopaedic community has had special interest in determining the specific competencies of an orthopaedic surgeon to ensure the patient receives safe, timely, and adequate orthopaedic care. The ACGME, in conjunction with the American Board of Orthopaedic Surgery (ABOS), provides oversight and evaluation of trainees to ensure they have successfully completed their training. These institutions, as part of the above-mentioned efforts, promote strategies to ensure patient safety and quality of care.

A combined document has been developed by the ACGME and the ABOS.[2] This document has been created to define milestones for programs to be used in resident evaluation and training. The defined milestones are knowledge, skills, attitudes, and other attributes for each competency in a structured manner. This structure involves five different levels (**Table 1**).

Core Competencies for the Practicing Orthopaedic Surgeon

Core competencies for attending surgeons have also been defined to promote safe and appropriate care for patients. A recent consensus effort among orthopaedic surgeons aimed to identify these competencies was conducted.[3] The General Orthopaedic Competency Task Force (GOCTF) and the ABOS sent an e-mail–based questionnaire to written examination question writers. Core competencies of medical knowledge and patient care were combined into two major groups: assessment and management. It was considered that a practicing orthopaedic surgeon should have the following knowledge competencies (extracted form "The Core Competencies for General Orthopaedic Surgeons"[3]) (**Table 2**).

Table 1

Levels for Milestones Evaluation

Level 1	The resident demonstrates milestones expected of an incoming resident.
Level 2	The resident is advancing and demonstrates additional milestones but is not yet performing at a midresidency level.
Level 3	The resident continues to advance and demonstrate additional milestones, consistently including the majority of milestones targeted for residency.
Level 4	The resident has advanced so that he or she now substantially demonstrates the milestones targeted for residency. This level is designed as the graduation target.
Level 5	The resident has advanced beyond performance target set for residency and is demonstrating "aspirational" goals which might describe the performance of someone who has been in practice for several years. It is expected that only a few exceptional residents will reach this level.

Table 2

Knowledge Competencies

1. Understand bone and soft-tissue biology and pathophysiology including growth; development and aging; injury, disease, and repair of musculoskeletal tissues including rehabilitation; and assessment of return to vocational and recreational activities
2. Understand the relative effectiveness of various surgical and nonsurgical options
3. Understand the comorbidities of a patient that will impact the orthopaedic surgeon's care plan
4. Understand conditions that are expected to be cared for by other specialists or subspecialty orthopaedic surgeons, eg, metabolic bone disease in the adult including osteopenia and osteoporosis, crystalline arthropathy: gout and pseudogout, tumors of musculoskeletal system, diabetic foot ulcers, exercise-induced leg compartment syndrome, and stress fractures
5. Perform an assessment and management of postoperative complications for patients, even if referred
6. Perform an assessment of musculoskeletal conditions using a history, a physical examination, and an investigative plan to develop a differential diagnosis based on an understanding of the pathophysiology of musculoskeletal conditions

Communication Skills and cultural Competence

Communication with patients is one of the most important aspects of medicine. Successful communication with patients directly impacts care and quality.[4] When measured against our colleagues, orthopaedic surgeons have room for significant improvement in this area.[5] Levinson et al,[6] in their systematic review of surgeon-patient communication, saw that the main area of deficiency in communication skills among surgeons was empathy. They often did not adequately explore emotions or concerns of patients. Improving these skills can potentially lead to improved outcomes and greater patient satisfaction.

In the era of value-based care, excellent attention must be provided and this includes successful communication with both patients and team members. Epstein[7] states in her literature review that communication among healthcare workers and between healthcare workers and patients reduces the occurrence of adverse events, improves outcomes, decreased length of stay, and produced greater satisfaction among all. Furthermore, a study by Hwang et al,[8] which evaluated patients in the intensive care unit (ICU), saw that communication was directly correlated to satisfaction. In general, communication has been a common complain of patients throughout history. In a study by King et al,[9] 1,118 orthopedic patients' complaints were evaluated. They saw that the most common reason for complain was access and availability followed by communication. In a different study, Mehta et al[10] evaluated patients whose procedure had been canceled. Interestingly 29.3% had no communication regarding the reason for their cancelation. Eighty-three percent of patients stated their dissatisfaction and noted that they would have liked to talk to their doctor and discussed the cancellation. Patient satisfaction was significantly lower among those patients with inadequate communication by a physician.

Communication, as mentioned above, has been proposed to be a key component of physician training. The Royal College of Physicians and Surgeons of Canada (RCPSC) developed The CanMEDS 2005 Physician Competency Framework Project that emphasizes in communication skills.[11] In orthopaedic surgery, the American Academy of Orthopaedic Surgery (AAOS) has actively promoted communication skills through workshops and other activities.[12] They consider communication to improve satisfaction, adhere to treatments, improve outcomes, and reduce liability. Although multiple efforts have been made, it has been seen that residents lack communication skills training.[13]

Educational models have been created to develop successful communication skills. One of the most popular models describes the four E's model. The publication that mentions the four E's model also describes the useful techniques to implement the model.[11] This hypothesizes that the physician-patient relationship is a consequence of the understanding of the disease by the physician. The main problem has been described to derive from not separating the body from the mind. Therefore, to successfully address the mind, communication must be efficient and thorough to be able to address the body/pathology. The strategy for successful communication is based in four aspects that begin with the letter E and therefore called the four E's strategy. These four are engagement, empathize, educate, and enlist (**Table 3**).

Table 3

Four E's Strategy

1. Engagement: In a physician-patient relationship, engagement between the two actors must occur. Ideas, information, and feeling will only come across if a human connection exists. Initially the physician must support the patient to be able to express the situation in a logical way. Similarly, the physician must have the ability to understand and translate subsequent medical knowledge to simple words that the patient is capable of understanding. This way both will be talking in known terminology. Furthermore, the physician must have welcoming body language and attitudes such as listening without interruption.
2. Empathize: Understanding patients' feelings and concerns is crucial. It allows physicians to show their understanding and caring to the patient. It has been seen that empathy is a strong tool as it creates trust in the patient and allows them to express their concerns and allows for better understanding of the medical scenario.
3. Educate: When a patient understands the situation, their ability to make decisions is enhanced. Their anxiety secondary to uncertainty decreases, and their knowledge of risks and benefits reinforces communication between the physician and the patient. Educational conversations should not be one-sided. Physicians must allow for patients to formulate questions or concerns during this phase. Patients that do not exhibit concern or lack communication of the situation are often seen to complain of lack of provided information by the physician.[5]
4. Enlist: Allowing and motivating the patient to actively participate in decision making is crucial as it incorporates understanding and communication. Setting goals and making the patient part of the process generates patients' desire to work toward a goal that they desire. Patients that are not involved in the treatment plan have demonstrated lack of adherence.

Cultural Competency

Communication and culture are intimately related. To have successful communication, cultural competencies must be met and different cultural aspects must be discussed. Donahue[14] states that culture includes language, thoughts, ways of communication, actions, customs, beliefs, values, and institutions of racial, ethnic, religious, or social groups. He defines a culturally competent professional as one who is capable to understand that others have different needs based on the above-mentioned factors. This leads to the fact that all patients are not to be treated the same way.

According to Pedersen's Conceptual Framework for Developing Cultural and Cross-Cultural Competence published by the University of Colorado, there are four major components to cultural competence: awareness, attitude, knowledge, and skills.[15] Awareness is directly related to the notion of different values that different cultures have. Attitude is the feeling a subject has toward its own beliefs, and their strength, that could collide with others' if different. Knowledge is important because it allows us to understand and avoid judging and or "stepping on cross-cultural toes." Lastly, skills are crucial for interaction and put in practice the other competencies.

According to the Joint Commission, three main barriers exist that potentially harm physician-patient relationship.[16] Language, literacy, and cultural differences are a threat to accurate information exchange. According to the *Culturally Competent Care Guidebook* from the AAOS, being culturally competent is crucial as it enhances communication and allows a more accurate diagnosis, increases adherence to treatment, and ultimately leads to better patient care.[17] Patients from different cultural background might require a much more detailed understanding of their beliefs and norms to adequately guide treatment. Cultural competencies are crucial as US population is getting more diverse.

Shared Decision Making

Involving patients in decision making is crucial as this may impact different aspects of the treatment plan. As mentioned before, patients demonstrate higher adherence to treatment when they participate on deciding the course of action and they experience higher satisfaction with their care. This process requires excellent communication. Patients must be educated as to the different treatment options, including the benefits and potential complications of each option. Recently, given the potential for it to substantially improve patient outcomes and reduce costs, this has turned into a highly discussed topic.[18] Various efforts have also been made internationally to promote patients' engagement in decision making.[19]

Uncertainty is one of the most important scenarios where shared decision making is key and should be present. Medical evidence can be lacking in certain clinical decisions, and/or various options can be available. Patients should be aware of this and should take part while having an open dialogue to decide the course of action. For this matter, education and communication become crucial. The physician must recognize and overcome various limitations so that the patient is well educated. If, for instance, the patient has a different language and/or culture, other individuals must be incorporated into the dialogue such as interpreters, translators, and others.

Légaré et al[20] have described three elements/scenarios as to when shared decision making should take place:

1. Recognize and acknowledge that a decision is required.
2. Both must know and understand the best available evidence concerning the risks and benefits of each option.
3. The decision must consider both the provider's guidance and the patient's values and preferences.

The same authors have recognized several barriers to shared decision making. These were extracted from a systematic review that demonstrates when decision making would not take place or would not be possible. The three most common situations affecting shared decision making were identified as time constraint, patients' beliefs, and the clinical situation.[20,21]

As to why costs are positively impacted by shared decision making, a systematic review saw that patients usually prefer less invasive procedures.[22] These authors included seven studies, in which savings were seen to be ranging from $8 to $3068 per patient. However, studies predicting the highest savings had the highest risk of bias. These authors also state that evidence clearly shows that patients opt for less invasive and costly approaches; there is insufficient evidence that supports that implementation of patient decision support interventions leads to lower costs.

Shared decision making should always be implemented by the orthopaedic surgeon when appropriate. Patients should be well educated and informed in an effective way about their condition. Communication barriers should be overpassed, and two-way dialogue should be used. Benefits from shared decision making, such as patient satisfaction and reduced unnecessary costs, have been described in the literature.

Obtaining Informed Surgical Consent

The informed surgical consent is an essential part of any medical procedure. It involves many aspects of patient care including patient safety. It is a document that reflects the act of informing the patient about the procedure that will be performed and the included potential risks. The patient's acceptance is reflected with a signature, attesting to the fact that information was provided and has been fully understood. In the United States, Justice Benjamin Cardozo established the concept on which the informed consent is based. He stated in the case of Cardozo B. Schloendorff versus Society of New York Hospital in 1914 that "Every human being of adult years, and sound mind, has the right to determine what shall be done with his own body."[23]

According to the AAOS, the surgical consent provides three distinctive aspects: legal documentation, surgical facility documentation, and safety information such as site, side, level, implant, procedure, and patient confirmation.[23] Unfortunately, even though it is considered one of the most important elements in patient care, according to available data published in the Joint Commission Sentinel Events database, errors remain as one of the most frequent causes of preventable surgical harm.

When conducting a consent, communication must be as clear as possible. When special circumstances are encountered, these should be addressed appropriately. In a study by Gazmararian et al,[24] older and Spanish-speaking patients had inadequate or marginal health literacy. They also saw that the reading ability declined dramatically with age. Patients must understand everything that has been said in terms of risks and benefits. In the scenario of a patient with visual or hearing impairment, adequate strategies must be used including an interpreter. For patients that do not speak English, a translator must be provided if the person conducting the consent is not proficient in the patient's language. And those who are unable to read, a thorough explanation of the document must be provided. Furthermore, the language used by physicians should be the most simple and medical terminology should be avoided to avoid confusion.[25]

The patient should be in their full mental capacity to understand and freely consent or reject the proposed procedure. For patients who are not considered to be suitable to give an informed consent, a parent or guardian should be the one to give consent. Furthermore, the process of obtaining informed consent should be given in a prudential time frame in the clinic scenario. Studies have demonstrated that recollection of the discussed information is negatively affected by time.[24] A person can also designate someone to make medical decisions and provide informed consent if a durable power of attorney (POA) for health care exists. The POA allows the designated person, also referred to as the proxy, agent, or surrogate, to be legally responsible for making medical decisions on the patient's behalf. In the event that no family or healthcare POA is present and the procedure or treatment is needed, then a two-physician consent may be done or the treating physician can consult an ethics committee or other institutional resource.

"Informed consent: Agreement or permission accompanied by full notice about the care, treatment, or service that is the subject of the consent. A patient must be apprised of the nature, risks, and alternatives of a medical procedure or treatment before the physician or other health care professional begins any such course. After receiving this information, the patient then either consents to or refuses such a procedure or treatment."

Reprinted with permission from The Joint Commission. 2019. Comprehensive Accreditation Manual glossary.

Surgical Safety Checklists

Invasive procedures in the office and operating room are a key component of an orthopaedic practice. They are, however, prone to errors, which can adversely affect patient care. The use of checklists has been implemented with proven benefits of increased safety.[26] The goal of their use is to ensure that the entire care team is engaged proactively to prevent errors or complications such as medication errors, wrong side/site surgery, and inadequate equipment/blood/imaging needs.

The WHO, as part of patient safety, developed a checklist (**Figure 1**) to provide increased surgical safety. This is a 19-item checklist that has proven to reduce morbidity and mortality and has been used worldwide.[27] The checklist consists of three moments or sections. Section one is before anesthesia which involves verifying patient's identification and general information. The second section is before skin incision which involves the whole team in a conjoined effort to discuss what is going to happen; it is commonly known as the time-out. The last section is the closing statements before the patient leaves the operating room.

The Joint Commission (JC) developed the Universal Protocol[28] which is a safety surgical checklist required for hospitals to use to obtain accreditation. This protocol is intended to increase patient safety and assure quality of care. Similar to the WHO surgical checklist, this also contains three items: conduct a preprocedure verification process, mark the procedure site, and perform a time-out. Each of these includes of the following.

Surgical Safety Checklist — World Health Organization | Patient Safety — A World Alliance for Safer Health Care

Before induction of anaesthesia → **Before skin incision** → **Before patient leaves operating room**

Before induction of anaesthesia

(with at least nurse and anaesthetist)

Has the patient confirmed his/her identity, site, procedure, and consent?
- ☐ Yes

Is the site marked?
- ☐ Yes
- ☐ Not applicable

Is the anaesthesia machine and medication check complete?
- ☐ Yes

Is the pulse oximeter on the patient and functioning?
- ☐ Yes

Does the patient have a:

Known allergy?
- ☐ No
- ☐ Yes

Difficult airway or aspiration risk?
- ☐ No
- ☐ Yes, and equipment/assistance available

Risk of >500ml blood loss (7ml/kg in children)?
- ☐ No
- ☐ Yes, and two IVs/central access and fluids planned

Before skin incision

(with nurse, anaesthetist and surgeon)

- ☐ **Confirm all team members have introduced themselves by name and role.**
- ☐ **Confirm the patient's name, procedure, and where the incision will be made.**

Has antibiotic prophylaxis been given within the last 60 minutes?
- ☐ Yes
- ☐ Not applicable

Anticipated Critical Events

To Surgeon:
- ☐ What are the critical or non-routine steps?
- ☐ How long will the case take?
- ☐ What is the anticipated blood loss?

To Anaesthetist:
- ☐ Are there any patient-specific concerns?

To Nursing Team:
- ☐ Has sterility (including indicator results) been confirmed?
- ☐ Are there equipment issues or any concerns?

Is essential imaging displayed?
- ☐ Yes
- ☐ Not applicable

Before patient leaves operating room

(with nurse, anaesthetist and surgeon)

Nurse Verbally Confirms:
- ☐ The name of the procedure
- ☐ Completion of instrument, sponge and needle counts
- ☐ Specimen labelling (read specimen labels aloud, including patient name)
- ☐ Whether there are any equipment problems to be addressed

To Surgeon, Anaesthetist and Nurse:
- ☐ What are the key concerns for recovery and management of this patient?

This checklist is not intended to be comprehensive. Additions and modifications to fit local practice are encouraged. Revised 1 / 2009 ©WHO, 2009

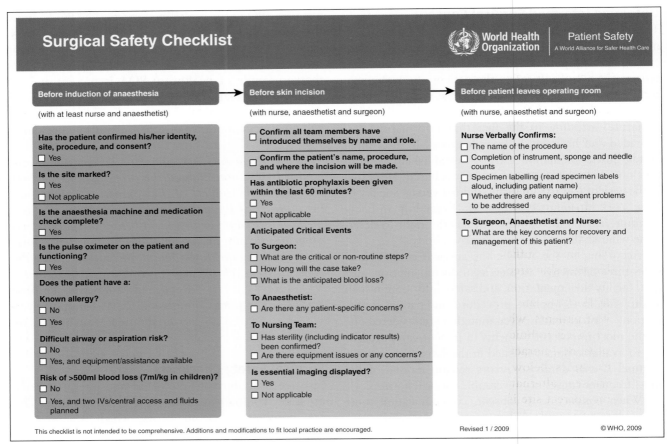

Figure 1 Surgical checklist based on the World Health Organization (WHO) Surgical Safety Checklist. (Reprinted with http://www.who.int/patientsafety/safesurgery/checklist/en/index.html. © World Health Organization 2009. All rights reserved. Accessed 9, 2019.)

The Universal Protocol—Developed by the Joint Commission

1. Conduct a preprocedure verification process
   a. Address missing information or discrepancies before starting the procedure.
      i. Verify the correct procedure, for the correct patient, at the correct site.
      ii. When possible, involve the patient in the verification process.
      iii. Identify the items that must be available for the procedure.
      iv. Use a standardized list to verify the availability of items for the procedure. (It is not necessary to document that the list was used for each patient.) At a minimum, these items include
         1. relevant documentation—examples include history and physical examination, signed consent form, preanesthesia assessment
         2. labeled diagnostic and radiology test results that are properly displayed—examples include radiology images and scans, pathology reports, biopsy reports
         3. any required blood products, implants, devices, special equipment
      v. Match the items that are to be available in the procedure area to the patient.
2. Mark the procedure site
   a. At a minimum, mark the site when there is more than one possible location for the procedure and when performing the procedure in a different location could harm the patient.
      i. For spinal procedures, mark the general spinal region on the skin. Special intraoperative imaging techniques may be used to locate and mark the exact vertebral level.
      ii. Mark the site before the procedure is performed.
      iii. If possible, involve the patient in the site marking process.

iv. The site is marked by a licensed independent practitioner who is ultimately accountable for the procedure and will be present when the procedure is performed.
v. In limited circumstances, site marking may be delegated to some medical residents, physician assistants (PA), or advanced practice registered nurses (APRN).
vi. Ultimately, the licensed independent practitioner is accountable for the procedure—even when delegating site marking.
vii. The mark is unambiguous and is used consistently throughout the organization.
viii. The mark is made at or near the procedure site.
ix. The mark is sufficiently permanent to be visible after skin preparation and draping.
x. Adhesive markers are not the sole means of marking the site.
xi. For patients who refuse site marking or when it is technically or anatomically impossible or impractical to mark the site (see examples below), use your organization's written, alternative process to ensure that the correct site is operated on. Examples of situations that involve alternative processes include
   1. mucosal surfaces or perineum
   2. minimal access procedures treating a lateralized internal organ, whether percutaneous or through a natural orifice
   3. teeth
   4. premature infants, for whom the mark may cause a permanent tattoo

3. Perform a time-out
   a. The procedure is not started until all questions or concerns are resolved.
      i. Conduct a time-out immediately before starting the invasive procedure or making the incision.
      ii. A designated member of the team starts the time-out.
      iii. The time-out is standardized.
      iv. The time-out involves the immediate members of the procedure team: the individual performing the procedure, anesthesia providers, circulating nurse, operating room technician, and other active participants who will be participating in the procedure from the beginning.
      v. All relevant members of the procedure team actively communicate during the time-out.
      vi. During the time-out, the team members agree, at a minimum, on the following:
         1. correct patient identity
         2. correct site
         3. procedure to be done
      vii. When the same patient has two or more procedures, if the person performing the procedure changes, another time-out needs to be performed before starting each procedure.
      viii. Document the completion of the time-out. The organization determines the amount and type of documentation.

Child/Spousal/Elder Abuse

As caregivers for our patients, we have a responsibility to identify and potentially report concerns for our patients' safety that arises from abusive situations. Abuse is not only physical, but also may be verbal or psychological. It is important to identify when it occurs as it can become repetitive and can often be confused with accidental injury. Elder abuse can occur up to 32 cases per 1,000, and it is an increasing public health problem.[29] Child abuse is also a very prevalent problem as it is estimated to occur at around 15 to 42 cases per 1,000.[30] Domestic, spousal, or intimate partner abuse also occurs at alarmingly high rates. It has been seen that as high as 35% of women seen in an emergency department for trauma are victims of domestic violence.[29]

Careful evaluation, clinical history, physical examination, and appropriate laboratories and imaging can help aid this diagnosis. Correctly identifying these cases often becomes a challenging situation for many different reasons. Many of the previously discussed topics are essential. Incorporating this into residency training creates increased sensibility for physicians to initially suspect and provide identification of these cases. Communication with the patient is essential, and allowing the patient to develop trust will allow them to express the truth of the situation. Different risk factors have been identified for victims as well as for caretakers, parents, and partners.

Orthopaedic surgeons often are involved with child abuse as fractures account for the second most common presentation behind soft-tissue injuries.[31] Physicians have an ethical and legal obligation to report suspected child abuse. Risk factors (**Table 4**) should be assessed when treating a child with suspected abuse. Among the most common clinical findings are multiple areas of ecchymosis in 62% of patients with noncorrelating history and clinical findings. Forty-five percent of victims of child abuse were diagnosed with a fracture. The battered child syndrome is a constellation of findings described by Kempe et al[32] that raise suspicion for child abuse. This included

Table 4

Risk Factors for Child Abuse

Patient risk factors: Unplanned single child, premature, concomitant disabilities.

Parent/guardian risk factors: Low socioeconomical conditions, drug dependency, single parent, step-child, unemployment, history of domestic abuse, stressful situations.

Table 5

Risk Factors for Elder Abuse

Patient risk factors: Dementia, poor health, aggressive behavior, history of violent behavior, history of abusive behavior to the caregiver, increasing age, race, and lower socioeconomic status.

Guardian/caregiver risk factors: Psychiatric illness, drug dependency, long-term responsibility for care, economic dependence of the elder patient, history of abuse, and stressful situations/life.

failure to thrive, subdural hematomas, multiple soft-tissue injuries, fractures/dislocations, and poor hygiene. Children with these associated diagnoses should raise concern and subsequent evaluation of child abuse. Furthermore, additional findings within fracture diagnosis such as multiple fractures in various states of healing, metaphyseal corner fractures, long bone fractures in the nonambulatory children, spine fractures, scapular fractures, rib fractures, and epiphyseal separations, should also increase concern.[33]

Elder abuse has been identified as a major source of morbidity and mortality in patients older than 65 years. Most states mandate the reporting of elder abuse, although many physicians are unaware, and thus, this is underreported. According to the American Medical Association,[34] the definition of elder abuse is *"the intentional infliction of physical or mental injury; sexual abuse; or withholding of necessary food, clothing, and medical care to meet the physical and mental needs of an elderly person by one having the care, custody, or responsibility of an elderly person."*

Patients are at risk for abuse both in their homes as well as in assisted living facilities. Similar to child abuse, in the setting of an elder patient abuse, the orthopaedic surgeon is often involved as fractures are often present. Other findings are also common such as inconsistent histories, dehydration, and malnutrition. Furthermore, delay in seeking medical assistance as well as implausible or nebulous explanations should also raise concern. In the setting of elder abuse, physicians should notify the authorities. Depending on the state and local laws, this could be a legal requirement; thus, physicians must be aware of local laws and regulations (**Table 5**).

Lastly, domestic or spousal abuse is a serious threat to patient safety. It has been estimated to occur from 8% up to 22% in a lifetime.[34] Thirty-five percent of women visiting an emergency department for trauma were identified as being victim of domestic/partner violence.[34] As with violence in other types of patient population, the way to diagnose this entity depends on the physician's ability to recognize it as such and that also depends on the index of suspicion. It is important to detect this as it conveys high mortality rates for victims of abuse. It has been reported by the U.S. Department of Justice and the Centre for Disease Control that around half of all murdered women were killed by a known person and 30% by their current or former partner. On the sex counterpart, only 3% of males were killed by a current or former partner[35,36] (**Table 6**).

Children, elder, and domestic violence are a public health concern. It has been seen that it conveys a high impact to society as it has a high morbidity and mortality. As orthopaedic surgeons, patients should be suspected of being victims of abuse when elements of concern are identified. As many of these patients have musculoskeletal trauma, educating orthopaedic surgeons in this matter is crucial. If uncertain of abuse, different support aids should be identified and used. A multidisciplinary approach with different support members should assess the patient when a diagnosis of abuse is established.

Table 6

Risk Factors and Characteristics for Domestic Abuse

Patient risk factors: Female gender, second or third decade of life, pregnancy.

Abuser risk factors and characteristics: Male sex, aggressive personality traits, avoid leaving patient alone, overly attentive, could adopt a hostile or aggressive behavior, over protective attitude, interferes with patient responses and responds for them.

Summary

A well-structured and planned education is crucial to achieve physician competency. Different entities have been designed to assure an appropriate balance between medical training and patient safety. All involved should be kept in good health to assure maximum performance. In the hospital and any patient care facility, overseeing and accrediting good practices is essential for patient safety.

Communication is one of the most important aspects of medicine and patient care. It is an essential element used in all the different clinical settings, from gathering a patients' history in the office to assuring patient safety in the operating room. Patients from different cultural backgrounds and ethnicities are encountered all over the United States and the world. Effective communication and understanding of every patient's unique cultural background makes a successful patient-physician relationship and contributes to a good outcome. All efforts should be made for the patient to understand and be aware of all procedures, risks, and benefits of medical actions. Finally, our responsibility to patient safety extends to identifying and reporting victims of abuse. Physicians and healthcare providers should be well aware of laws and policies to legally take action when these situations are encountered.

Study Facts/Key Study Points[3-5]

- Core competencies during orthopaedic postgraduate training are directed by the ACGME and ABOS which ensure patient-centered care along with well-being of training physicians.
- Physician-patient relationship is based on successful communication skills developed by physicians along with their understanding of patients' cultural background.
- Informed surgical consent is key to evaluate patients understanding of the procedure and its verification.
- Patient safety involves different verification steps throughout the hospital stay including a surgical safety checklist.

Annotated References

1. Weiss KB, Wagner R, Nasca TJ: Development, testing, and implementation of the ACGME clinical learning environment review (CLER) program. *J Grad Med Educ* 2012;4:396-398. doi:10.4300/JGME-04-03-31.
2. ACGME, ABOS: *The Orthopaedic Surgery Milestone Project*, 2015, pp i-48. https://www.acgme.org/Portals/0/PDFs/Milestones/OrthopaedicSurgeryMilestones.pdf.
3. Kellam JF, Archibald D, Barber JW, et al: The core competencies for general orthopaedic surgeons. *J Bone Joint Surg Am* 2017;99:175-181. doi:10.2106/JBJS.16.00761.

   This article provides a proposal for the knowledge and competencies needed for an orthopaedic surgeon to practice. Utilizing the Delphi method, the General Orthopaedic Competency Task Force proposed the core knowledge and competencies for an orthopaedic surgeon. The authors state that this document is the first step in defining a practice-based standard for training programs and certification groups. Level of evidence: NA.
4. Klein ER: Effective communication with patients. *Pa Nurse* 2005;60:14-15.
5. Tongue JR, Epps HR, Forese LL: Communication skills. *Instr Course Lect* 2005;54:3-9.
6. Levinson W, Hudak P, Tricco AC: A systematic review of surgeon-patient communication: Strengths and opportunities for improvement. *Patient Educ Couns* 2013;93:3-17. doi:10.1016/j.pec.2013.03.023.
7. Epstein NE: Multidisciplinary in-hospital teams improve patient outcomes: A review. *Surg Neurol Int* 2014;5:S295-S303. doi:10.4103/2152-7806.139612.
8. Hwang DY, Yagoda D, Perrey HM, et al: Assessment of satisfaction with care among family members of survivors in a neuroscience intensive care unit. *J Neurosci Nurs* 2014;46:106-116. doi:10.1097/JNN.0000000000000038.
9. King JD, van Dijk PAD, Overbeek CL, Hageman MGJS, Ring D: Patient complaints emphasize non-technical aspects of care at a tertiary referral hospital. *Arch Bone Joint Surg* 2017;5:74-81.

   This study evaluated the nature and prevalence of patient complaints regarding orthopaedic care. Patients between 40 and 60 years of age filed the most complaints. Half of concerns addressed interpersonal issues, and the largest category of it was related to access and availability. They concluded that quality improvement efforts can be used to improve access and availability as well as empathy and communication strategies. Level of evidence: III.
10. Mehta SS, Bryson DJ, Mangwani J, Cutler L: Communication after cancellations in orthopaedics: The patient perspective. *World J Orthop* 2014;5:45-50. doi:10.5312/wjo.v5.i1.45.
11. Keller VF, Carroll JG: A new model for physician-patient communication. *Patient Educ Couns* 1994;23:131-140.
12. The American Academy of Orthopaedic Surgeons, Institute for Health Care Communication: *Clinician-Patient Communication Workshop* n.d. https://www.aaos.org/communicationskills/.
13. Lundine K, Buckley R, Hutchison C, Lockyer J: Communication skills training in orthopaedics. *J Bone Joint Surg Am* 2008;90:1393-1400. doi:10.2106/JBJS.G.01037.
14. Donahue L: What Is Cultural Competence? PSJS 250 Soc Chang through Serv 2013. https://www.vanderbilt.edu/oacs/wp-content/uploads/sites/140/CulturalCompetence.pdf.

15. University of Colorado: *Center for Multicultural Affairs – Cultural Competence: The Next Step*, 1994, 3-4. https://cue.colorado.edu/sites/default/files/Cult Competence-the Next Step.pdf.
16. Schyve PM: Language differences as a barrier to quality and safety in health care: The Joint Commission perspective. *J Gen Intern Med* 2007;22(suppl 2):360-361. doi:10.1007/s11606-007-0365-3.
17. Jimenez R, Lewis VO: *Culturally Competent Care Guidebook*. Rosemont, IL, American Academy of Orthopaedic Surgeons, 2007.
18. Frosch DL, Moulton BW, Wexler RM, Holmes-Rovner M, Volk RJ, Levin CA: Shared decision making in the United States: Policy and implementation activity on multiple fronts. *Z Evid Fortbild Qual Gesundhwes* 2011;105:305-312. doi:10.1016/j.zefq.2011.04.004.
19. Härter M, van der Weijden T, Elwyn G: Policy and practice developments in the implementation of shared decision making: An international perspective. *Z Evid Fortbild Qual Gesundhwes* 2011;105:229-233. doi:10.1016/j.zefq.2011.04.018.
20. Légaré F, Witteman HO: Shared decision making: Examining key elements and barriers to adoption into routine clinical practice. *Health Aff* 2013;32:276-284. doi:10.1377/hlthaff.2012.1078.
21. Légaré F, Ratté S, Gravel K, Graham ID: Barriers and facilitators to implementing shared decision-making in clinical practice: Update of a systematic review of health professionals' perceptions. *Patient Educ Couns* 2008;73:526-535. doi:10.1016/j.pec.2008.07.018.
22. Walsh T, Barr PJ, Thompson R, Ozanne E, O'Neill C, Elwyn G: Undetermined impact of patient decision support interventions on healthcare costs and savings: Systematic review. *BMJ* 2014;348:g188.
23. AAOS: *Orthopaedic Surgical Consent – Information Statement*. American Academy of Orthopaedic Surgeons, 2014.
24. Gazmararian JA, Baker DW, Williams MV, et al: Health literacy among Medicare enrollees in a managed care organization. *J Am Med Assoc* 1999;281:545-551.
25. Gattellari M, Butow PN, Tattersall MH: Informed consent: What did the doctor say? *Lancet (London, England)* 1999;353:1713. doi:10.1016/S0140-6736(05)77027-6.
26. Kuo CC, Robb WJ: Critical roles of orthopaedic surgeon leadership in healthcare systems to improve orthopaedic surgical patient safety. *Clin Orthop Relat Res* 2013;471:1792-1800. doi:10.1007/s11999-012-2719-3.
27. Haynes AB, Weiser TG, Berry WR, et al: A surgical safety checklist to reduce morbidity and mortality in a global population. *N Engl J Med* 2009;360:491-499. doi:10.1056/NEJMsa0810119.
28. The Joint Commission: *Universal Protocol*. https://WwwJointcommissionOrg/Assets/1/18/UP_Poster1PDF 2012:1.
29. Chen AL, Koval KJ: Elder abuse: The role of the orthopaedic surgeon in diagnosis and management. *J Am Acad Orthop Surg* 2002;10:25-31.
30. Kocher MS, Kasser JR: Orthopaedic aspects of child abuse. *J Am Acad Orthop Surg* 2000;8:10-20.
31. McMahon P, Grossman W, Gaffney M, Stanitski C: Soft-tissue injury as an indication of child abuse. *J Bone Joint Surg Am* 1995;77:1179-1183.
32. Kempe CH, Silverman FN, Steele BF, Droegemueller W, Silver HK: The battered-child syndrome. *J Am Med Assoc* 1962;181:17-24.
33. Pandya NK, Baldwin K, Wolfgruber H, Christian CW, Drummond DS, Hosalkar HS: Child abuse and orthopaedic injury patterns: Analysis at a level I pediatric trauma center. *J Pediatr Orthop* 2009;29:618-625. doi:10.1097/BPO.0b013e3181b2b3ee.
34. Elder Abuse and Neglect: Council on scientific affairs. *J Am Med Assoc* 1987;257:966-971.
35. US Department of Justice Federal Bureau of Investigation: *Uniform Crime Reports: Crime in the United States*. Washington DC; 1997.
36. Paulozzi LJ, Saltzman LE, Thompson MP, Holmgreen P: Surveillance for homicide among intimate partners – United States, 1981-1998. *Surveilance Summ CDC MMWR* 2001;50:1-16.

Chapter 4

Regulation of Orthopaedic Devices

Elizabeth B. Gausden, MD, MPH • Michael B. Cross, MD

ABSTRACT

Medical devices used by orthopaedic surgeons must undergo approval through the FDA. Orthopaedic surgeons should familiarize themselves with the classification of devices, the different pathways for device approval, the classes of device recall, and their role in facilitating patient notification following a device recall.

Keywords: 510(k) pathway; device regulation; FDA; medical devices; premarket approval (PMA); premarket notification (PMN)

Introduction

In the past 50 years, the process of regulation of medical devices has continuously evolved. Today, there are multiple pathways in the United States through which medical devices are approved or cleared by the government. In this chapter, the history of the regulatory process in the United States as well as the status of the current pathways will be reviewed.

Dr. Cross or an immediate family member is a member of a speakers' bureau or has made paid presentations on behalf of Acelity and Flexion Therapeutics; serves as a paid consultant to or is an employee of Acelity, DePuy, A Johnson & Johnson Company, Exactech, Inc., Flexion Therapeutics, Intellijoint, Smith & Nephew, and Zimmer; has stock or stock options held in Imagen, Insight Medical, Intellijoint, and Parvizi Surgical Innovation; and has received research or institutional support from Acelity, Exactech, Inc., and Intellijoint. Neither Dr. Gausden nor any immediate family member has received anything of value from or has stock or stock options held in a commercial company or institution related directly or indirectly to the subject of this chapter.

Orthopaedic Implant Approval Pathways

Classes of Medical Devices

In the 1970s, the government issued the Cooper report, detailing over 10,000 injuries that occurred from medical devices.[1] This report prompted the Medical Device Amendment Act (MDAA) of 1976, which laid the foundation for medical device regulation in the United States. A timeline for the legislation that has followed since the 1970s is demonstrated in **Figure 1**.

The MDAA organized medical devices into three classes. Class I devices are low-risk devices that have substantial evidence supporting their safety. "General controls," such as maintenance of proper labeling and manufacturing processes, and reporting of adverse events are deemed sufficient regulation of Class I products. Class II devices are higher risk compared with Class I devices and require more regulation. Examples of Class II devices include sutures and bone wax,[2] as well as most orthopaedic implants including total knee arthroplasties, intramedullary nails, and most spinal implants. These are subject to a premarket process known as a 510(k) clearance that will be discussed in more detail in the next section. Following the premarket clearance, manufacturers of Class II devices must conduct postmarket surveillance. Class III devices are of substantial importance to sustaining or supporting human health but may present a "potential unreasonable risk of illness or injury," and these are the most highly regulated. Mobile bearing total knee replacements and spinal disk replacements are both examples of Class III devices.

The FDA organizes devices by 16 medical specialty "panels" and lists orthopaedic devices under Part 888 under the Code of Federal Regulations Title 21.[3] This is available online and helps delineate the classes of various orthopaedic implants.

Approval Process

Depending on the class of the device, the availability of a predicate device, and the target population characteristics of the device, there are four main pathways by which devices are approved. These four pathways are the premarket approval (PMA) pathway, the premarket

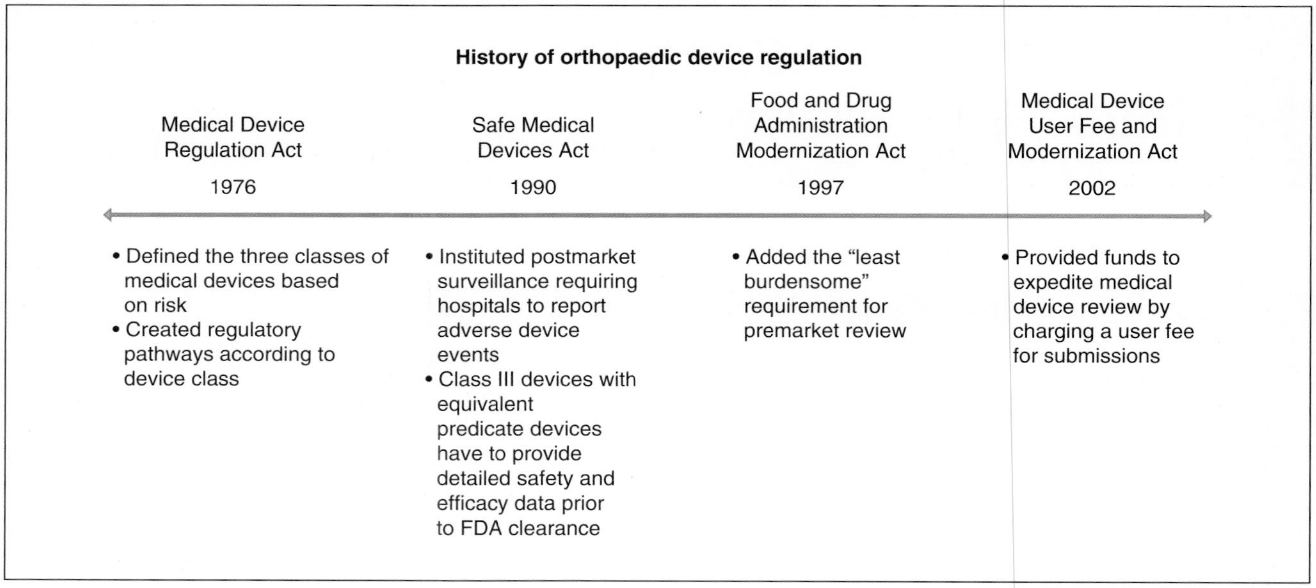

History of orthopaedic device regulation
Medical Device Regulation Act
1976
Safe Medical Devices Act
1990
Food and Drug Administration Modernization Act
1997
Medical Device User Fee and Modernization Act
2002
• Defined the three classes of medical devices based on risk
• Created regulatory pathways according to device class
• Instituted postmarket surveillance requiring hospitals to report adverse device events
• Class III devices with equivalent predicate devices have to provide detailed safety and efficacy data prior to FDA clearance
• Added the "least burdensome" requirement for premarket review
• Provided funds to expedite medical device review by charging a user fee for submissions

Figure 1 Illustration demonstrating the timeline of major US legislation regulating medical devices.

notification (PMN), which is also known as the 510(k) pathway, the product development protocol (PDP), and the humanitarian device exemption (HDE). Class III devices, those that potentially pose the highest risk to patients, are approved through a PMA, which is the most costly and arduous of the pathways.[4] The device manufacturers must complete an investigational new device (IND) application as well as provide results from a small safety trial.[2] A prospective trial that compares the IND to currently available devices, which is needed to demonstrate efficacy, often involves significant cost to the manufacturer. The PMA is reviewed by the Office of Device Evaluation, which is part of the Center for Devices and Radiological Health (CDRH), one of the six main branches of the FDA. Following PMA, devices may undergo significant postmarket modification, or "drift," and require monitoring via a PMA supplement review.[5]

Devices that have a "substantially equivalent" predicate device with which they compare may undergo a PMN pathway, which is also called the 510(k) process. Manufacturers must produce evidence that the proposed device has an equivalent predicate device. In 1990, a legislation was introduced that required "safety and efficacy" to also be demonstrated as part of the 510(k) pathway. The FDA typically reviews applications for devices under the 510(k) pathway, as described by the Federal Food, Drug, and Cosmetic Act within 90 days.

The average time for a manufacturer to recoup the cost of approval via the PMA process was 8.5 years compared with 2.4 years when the 510(k) pathway was used.[6] To avoid the cost of a prospective randomized controlled trial, many more devices are approved via the 510(k) pathway (over 4,000/yr) compared with the PMA pathway (<100/yr).[7] The 510(k) pathway results in FDA clearance rather than approval. This is an important distinction, as FDA approval provides immunity from litigation but clearance does not.[1] Day et al[8] found that orthopaedic devices are increasingly cleared through the 510(k) pathway over the use of PMA compared with nonorthopaedic devices. The same authors identified that devices cleared through the 510(k) pathway had 11.5 times the odds of having a subsequent recall compared with the PMA pathway.[8]

The use of the 510(k) pathway for clearance of Class III devices was not the long-term intention of lawmakers, and it is important to note that this pathway demands a lower burden of proof than typically required in evidence-based medicine. An example of a Class III device that was cleared perhaps inappropriately via the 510(k) pathway is the DePuy Articular Surface Replacement (ASR) XL Acetabular Cup System, a metal-on-metal total hip that combined metal-on-metal articulation with a large femoral head and a porous bone ingrowth surface. Ardaugh et al[9] traced the clearance of the ASR and found that those three characteristics were present in previous predicate devices, but not in combination. Also, clearance was based on the comparison to predicate devices that were used before 1976 and thus never underwent PMA. In this case, the use of 510(k) for clearance of the ASR allowed the manufacturer to avoid a costly clinical trial, but such a trial would have likely revealed the higher revision rate and avoided a later recall following implantation in over 93,000 patients.[10]

The HDE removes the regulatory burden for devices that are developed to treat conditions affecting fewer than 4,000 patients with no comparable device available. In 2016, the 21st Century Cures Act increased this to "no more than 8,000 patients" per year. This pathway was created to encourage developers to focus on producing devices for rare illnesses and injuries by lowering the burden of cost and time needed for approval. While the HDE process is similar to the PMA process, manufacturers do not need to demonstrate effectiveness of the device.

An alternative, and rarely used, approach for manufacturers is to pursue approval via a PDP. Under a PDP, the manufacturer and the FDA agree to a plan that includes preclinical and clinical evaluations and methods for assessment.[11] The Keramos ceramic-on-ceramic total hip arthroplasty (Encore, Austin, TX) was cleared through a PDP.

Custom Devices

The Custom Device Exemption was part of the 1976 legislation that was later modified by Section 617 of the 2012 Food and Drug Administration Safety and Innovation Act.[12] There are eight criteria that must be met to pursue this exemption.[13] These include the following: "(1) modified in order to comply with the order of an individual physician...(2) necessarily deviated from an otherwise applicable performance standard...(3) not generally available in the United States...(4) designed to treat a unique pathology or physiological condition that no other device is domestically available to treat...(5) intended to meet the special needs of such physician in the course of the professional practice of such a physician...(6) assembled from components or manufactured and finished on a case-by-case basis to accommodate the unique needs of individuals...(7) conducting clinical investigations on such a device would be impractical...(8) produced in quantities of 5 or less per year of a particular device type."[13] This can be used when a patient's condition warrants and allows the company to bypass the PMN pathway.

For circumstances and patients that do not qualify for a custom device exemption, a compassionate use request can be filed that can provide for timely approval of devices. The two criteria for compassionate use of devices are that a patient has a life-threatening or serious disease or condition and that no acceptable alternative treatment for the condition exists.[14]

Regulation of Orthopaedic Biologics

One of the six divisions within the FDA is the Center for Biologics Evaluation and Research (CBER), which is responsible for regulation of biologic products. This designation includes blood, blood components, vaccines, allergenic products or those that have the capacity to induce allergic sensitization, somatic cells and tissues, recombinant products, and gene therapy. Producers of biologics must submit a biologics license application to the CBER, which is regulated under 21 CFR 600-680 of the United States CFR for the FDA and the Department of Health and Human Services.[15]

Tissue banks are under the regulation of the FDA by the Public Health Services Act (PHSA) Section 361, and such tissues are referred to as "361 tissues." To qualify as a 361 tissue, the tissue has to be minimally manipulated, intended for homologous use only, and cannot be combined with anything other than water, crystalloids, or sterilizing agents.[16] Demineralized bone matrix (DBM), ligaments, tendons, and skin generally meet criteria and qualify as 361 tissues and do not require clearance via the 510(k) pathway.

Combination products are those that combine regulated devices or drugs with biologic products, and such products commonly must undergo clearance via the 510(k) pathway.

Reporting Adverse Events

The Safe Medical Devices Act of 1990 instituted postmarket surveillance measures for medical devices. The legislation mandates that healthcare facilities report serious device-related injuries or deaths to manufacturers as well as the FDA. Reporting, while mandatory from manufacturers, hospitals and surgical centers, is voluntary for providers and consumers. MedWatch is a system that allows both consumers and providers to report device issues to the FDA, but only 8% of reports are initiated by physicians.[1]

Surgeon's Responsibility Dealing With Recalled Implants

In response to adverse events, manufacturers can voluntarily recall devices, and in rare circumstances, the FDA mandates a device recall if the company refuses. Once the company identifies the issue and decides to recall a device, they must notify the FDA, and then the FDA defines the levels of device recall.[17] A class I recall occurs in response to the probability that use of a device may lead to a serious adverse health consequence or death. A class II recall is mandated when exposure to the device may cause temporary or reversible adverse health consequences. Finally, a class III recall occurs when a product or device is not likely to cause adverse health events. A market withdrawal is when the company voluntarily withdrawals a product or device for issues that would not warrant FDA legal action. Once the class of recall is established, the FDA lists the device on their Medical Device Recall Database.[17] The FDA monitors the company's recall strategy and helps determine the depth of the recall, whether it will be at the consumer level, the retail level, or the wholesale level. Although the FDA does not mandate physician or surgeon involvement in the process of patient notification or warning, the American Academy of Orthopaedic Surgeons (AAOS) has established guidelines for surgeons.[18] These guidelines encourage surgeons to be aware of device recalls and the health issues involved, to report adverse events via MedWatch, to cooperate with hospitals and manufacturers in notifying patients of the recall, to engage patients in a shared decision-making process following a recall, and to monitor the situation to inform future patient care.

Summary

Orthopaedic surgeons should understand the classification of orthopaedic devices and the various methods for FDA approval or clearance of devices, which include the 510(k) PMN process, the premarket approval process, the custom device exemption, and the HDE. Orthopaedic surgeons are responsible for maintaining awareness of device safety, efficacy, and the status of devices that have been recalled.

Key Study Points

- Medical devices have been regulated by the U.S. FDA since the Medical Device Regulation Act was passed in 1976. Prior to 1976, medical devices were largely unregulated.
- Medical devices are organized into three classes according to risk. The risk class also determines the pathway for device approval.
- The 510(k) pathway is most commonly used for clearance of orthopaedic devices and requires the manufacturer to prove that the device is "substantially equivalent" to a preexisting device.
- Hospitals and facilities are required to report adverse events related to medical devices to the FDA, but physicians are not mandated to do so. However, orthopaedic surgeons should be familiar with the resources available through which to report adverse events.

Annotated References

1. Lauer M, Barker JP, Solano M, Dubin J: FDA device regulation. *Mo Med* 2017;114:4.

   The Lauer article is a review of the US medical device legislation in terms of history as well as current pathways and controversies.

2. Maak TG, Wylie JD: Medical device regulation: A comparison of the United States and the European Union. *J Am Acad Orthop Surg* 2016;24:8.

   The Maak study is a review article that explains basic differences between device regulation in the United States compared with the European Union. The authors also discuss several high-profile medical device failures and recalls.

3. https://www.fda.gov/medicaldevices/deviceregulationandguidance/databases/ucm135680.htm.

   This website can be used to search the various "panel" designations used by the FDA to classify medical devices according to specialty.

4. Goodman SB, Mihalko WM, Anderson PA, Sale K, Bozic KJ: Introduction of new technologies in orthopaedic surgery. *JBJS Rev* 2016;4:5.

   This is another review article that discusses predominantly the 510(k) pathway as well as what surgeons' role in medical device regulation should ideally be.

5. Samuel AM, Rathi VK, Grauer JN, Ross JS: How do orthopaedic devices change after their initial FDA premarket approval? *Clin Orthop Relat Res* 2016;474:4.

   The Samuel et al study reviewed all orthopaedic medical devices approved from 1982 to 2014. They determined which pathways were used, the time to market of the device, and the incidence of postmarket changes or recalls. They found that the majority of orthopaedic devices do not undergo PMA and that those that do have substantial postmarket changes.

6. Yang BW, Iorio ML, Day CS: Orthopaedic device approval through the premarket approval process: A financial feasibility analysis for a single center. *J Bone Joint Surg Am* 2017;99:6.

   Yang et al used financial modeling to assess the feasibility of the PMA versus the 510(k) pathway and found that PMA would take considerably longer (>8 years) to recoup the investment compared with the 510(k) pathway (2.4 years).

7. Maisel WH: Medical device regulation: An introduction for the practicing physician. *Ann Intern Med* 2004;140:4.

8. Day CS, Park DJ, Rozenshteyn FS, Owusu-Sarpong N, Gonzalez A: Analysis of FDA-approved orthopaedic devices and their recalls. *J Bone Joint Surg Am* 2016;98:6.

   Day et al reviewed all orthopaedic devices that were recalled by the FDA and identified that those cleared from the 510(k) pathway were over 11 times more likely to be recalled compared with those who underwent PMA.

9. Ardaugh BM, Graves SE, Redberg RF: The 510(k) ancestry of a metal-on-metal hip implant. *N Engl J Med* 2013;368:2.

   Ardaugh does an in-depth review of how the ASR implant was cleared by the 510(k) pathway and the pitfalls in this specific case.

10. Kalra A: J and J to work with India on compensation for recalled hip implants. *Reuters Business News* 9/6/2018.

11. Kirkpatrick JS, Stevens T: The FDA process for the evaluation and approval of orthopaedic devices. *J Am Acad Orthop Surg* 2008;16:5.

12. US Food and Drug Administration Website: *A History of Medical Device Regulation and Oversight in the United States*. Available at: https://www.fda.gov/MedicalDevices/DeviceRegulationandGuidance/Overview/ucm618375.htm.

    The FDA website provided overview of the history of medical device regulation in the United States.

13. Mihalko WM: How do I get what I need? Navigating the FDA's custom, compassionate use, and HDE pathways for medical devices and implants. *J Arthroplast* 2015;30:6.

    Mihalko reviews the various pathways through which surgeons can obtain implants/devices for patients, specifically comparing the Custom Device Exemption (CDE) to the Compassionate Use pathway.

14. US Food and Drug Administration: *Expanded Access for Medical Devices*, 2018. Available at: https://www.fda.gov/medicaldevices/deviceregulationandguidance/howtomarketyourdevice/investigationaldeviceexemptionide/ucm051345.htm.

    FDA website provided review of special pathways for clearance of medical devices, including the "Emergent Use" pathway, the "Compassionate Use" pathway, and the "Treatment Use" pathway.

15. *FDA Regulation of Human Cells, Tissues, and Cellular and Tissue-Based Products (HCT/P's) Product List*, 2018. Available at: https://www.fda.gov/biologicsbloodvaccines/tissuetissueproducts/regulationoftissues/ucm150485.htm.

    FDA website provides a list of their regulation of human cells, tissues, and cellular and tissue-based products.

16. *Guidance for Industry and Food and Drug Administration Staff, Regulatory Considerations for Human Cells, Tissues, and Cellular and Tissue-Based Products: Minimal Manipulation and Homologous Use*, 2018. Available at: https://www.fda.gov/downloads/biologicsbloodvaccines/guidancecomplianceregulatoryinformation/guidances/cellularandgenetherapy/ucm585403.pdf.

    FDA website offers guidelines for interpretation of "minimal manipulation and homologous use" of cells, tissues and cell-based and tissue-based products.

17. US Food and Drug Administration: *What is a Medical Device Recall?*, 2018.

    FDA website offers a review of the process and implications of the medical device recall.

18. AAOS: *Information Statement: Implant Device Recalls*, 2016.

    AAOS (American Academy of Orthopaedic Surgeons) provides their own recommendations for orthopaedic surgeons regarding a medical device recall and how surgeons should participate in the process.

Chapter 5

Health Policy

Nicholas B. Frisch, MD, MBA • Roshan P. Shah, MD, JD • P. Maxwell Courtney, MD

ABSTRACT

With health policy at the forefront of national debate, orthopaedic surgeons must become familiar with the many recent regulatory and legislative changes affecting their ability to care for patients. This chapter provides a primer for the orthopaedic surgeon, helping understand the basics of Medicare and Medicaid and decipher the alphabet soup of acronyms including MACRA, MIPS, and BPCI. We will review reimbursement plans from both private and government payers, including several alternative payment models, which are becoming increasingly popular in adult reconstruction, spine, and shoulder. We also include a detailed discussion of the Affordable Care Act and its relevance to orthopaedic surgeons and their patients. We hope this chapter can help surgeons understand the current policy issues facing our field and continue to advocate for their patients.

Keywords: affordable care act; alternative payment models; bundled payments; medicaid; medicare

Introduction

National healthcare expenditures reached $3.3 trillion dollars in 2016, which accounts for 17.9% of gross domestic product (GDP).[1] Throughout the duration of health care in the United States a variety of approaches have taken shape in the form of payment protocols. These approaches have evolved over time, and the current system represents a blend of both past and new practices. When discussing these various practices, it is important to keep in mind the impact that each has on the parties involved: payer, provider, and patient. It is also important to remember, on a broader level, the implications each approach has to the healthcare system as a whole, in terms of cost, quality, and efficiency.

According to the 2016 census, the percentage of people with health insurance coverage was 91.2%.[2] Of those covered, 67.3% had private health insurance compared with 37.3% with government coverage. Major government programs include Medicare (16.7%), Medicaid (19.4%), and Military/Veterans' Administration (4.6%), as well as other programs such as the Indian Health Service system and Federal Employees Health Benefits Program. The Centers for Medicare and Medicaid Services (CMS) is a part of the U.S. Department of Health and Human Services (HHS). CMS tracks healthcare expenditures, and as of 2016, 32% went toward hospital care, 20% physician and clinical services, 10% prescription drugs, and 3% other professional services[3] (**Figure 1**). When comparing health spending by payer, CMS reports: 20% Medicare, 17% Medicaid, 34% private health insurance, and 11% out-of-pocket[3] (**Figure 2**).

Medicare

The Social Security Amendments of 1965 signed by President Lyndon B. Johnson established Medicare and Medicaid as the dominant public programs for health care in the United States. The programs have undergone significant modification over the years and represent a substantial portion of health care coverage. Medicare represents 20% of total national healthcare expenditures or roughly $672.1 billion.[1]

Medicare provides health insurance for (1) people aged 65 or older, (2) people younger than 65 years with certain disabilities, and (3) people of all ages with end-stage renal disease. It is estimated that as of 2016 there

Dr. Shah or an immediate family member serves as a paid consultant to or is an employee of Link Orthopaedics and serves as a board member, owner, officer, or committee member of the U.S. Food and Drug Administration. Dr. Courtney or an immediate family member is a member of a speakers' bureau or has made paid presentations on behalf of ConvaTec and serves as a paid consultant to or is an employee of Hip Innovation Technology. Neither Dr. Frisch nor any immediate family member has received anything of value from or has stock or stock options held in a commercial company or institution related directly or indirectly to the subject of this chapter.

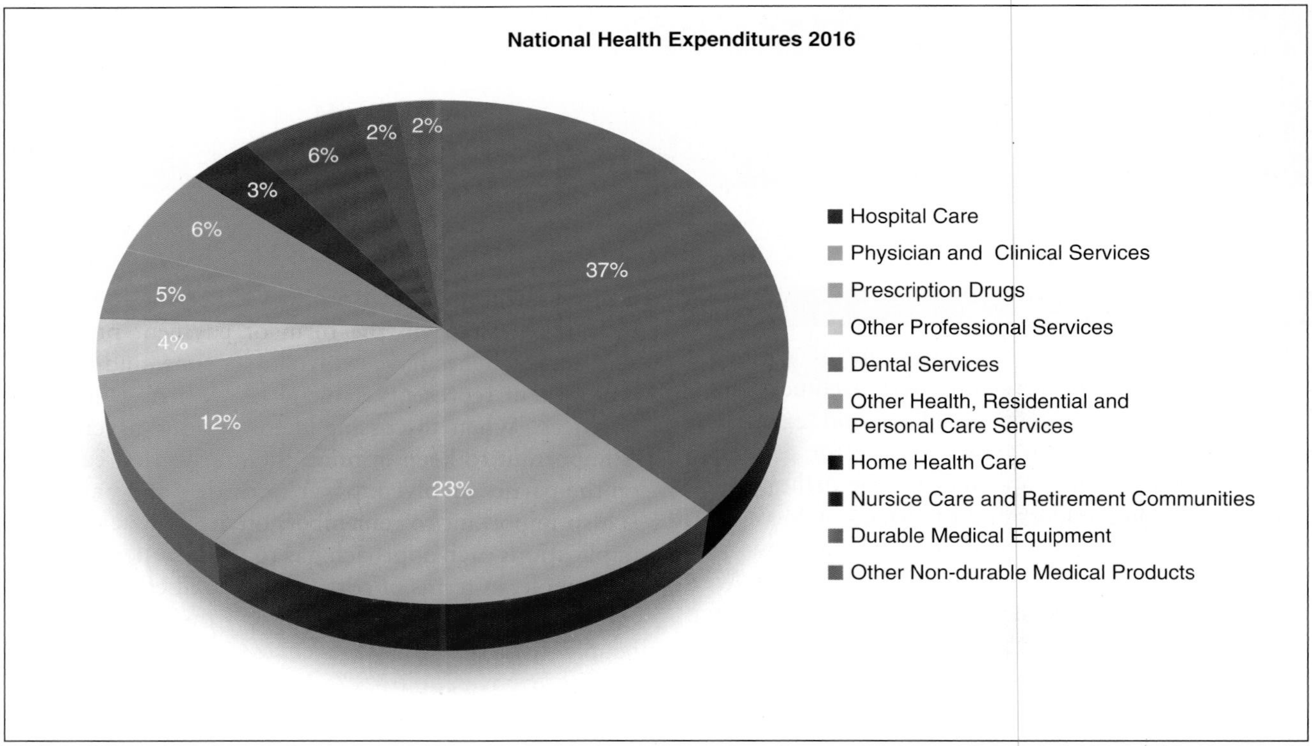

Figure 1 A breakdown of national health expenditures in 2016. Hospital care accounts for 37% of all health care spending in the United States, while physician services account for less than one-fourth of all spending. (From Centers for Medicare and Medicaid Services. *National Health Expenditures 2016 Highlights*. 2016. Available at: https://www.cms.gov/Research-Statistics-Data-and-Systems/Statistics-Trends-and-Reports/NationalHealthExpendData/NationalHealthAccountsHistorical.html. Accessed August 20, 2018.)

were 56.5 million people enrolled in Medicare programs in the United States. Medicare is composed of the following parts:

Medicare Part A is hospital insurance, which helps cover inpatient care in hospitals and skilled nursing facilities, as well as some hospice care and home health care for those beneficiaries who meet specified criteria. All individuals are automatically eligible if they paid into the Medicare trust fund for 10 or more years (40 quarters) and have reached the age of 65. It should be noted that skilled nursing facility coverage is only for posthospital coverage within 30 days of hospital stay of at least 3 days. Most people covered by Part A do not pay a premium because they, or their spouse, have paid for it through their payroll taxes while working. The US payroll tax, or the Federal Insurance Contributions Act (FICA) tax, requires employers and employees to pay a tax on their income to fund Social Security and Medicare. In general, employers and employees each pay 1.45% of worker's wages and self-employed workers pay 2.9% of net earnings. In 2017, Medicare covered 58.4 million people of which 49.5 million aged 65 and older and 8.9 million were disabled.[4]

Medicare Part B is medical insurance, which helps cover physician services, outpatient care, and various home health care, as well as some additional medical services not covered under Part A (ie, physical therapy and laboratory work). Part B is financed by a 25% beneficiary premium and annual federal appropriations for the rest. Most people pay a monthly premium for Part B. As of 2017, the Medicare Trustees reported enrollment of 53.4 million people for Part B.[4]

Medicare Part C, which is also referred to as Medicare Advantage Plan, provides all Part A and Part B coverage as well as additional coverage (ie, vision, hearing, dental, etc). These plans are purchased through Medicare-approved private companies and charge different out-of-pocket fees. Medicare Advantage enrollment has grown 71% since 2010 and as of 2017 roughly 33% of people with Medicare is enrolled in an Advantage plan.[5] The Kaiser Family Foundation reports that in 2017, 63% of Medicare

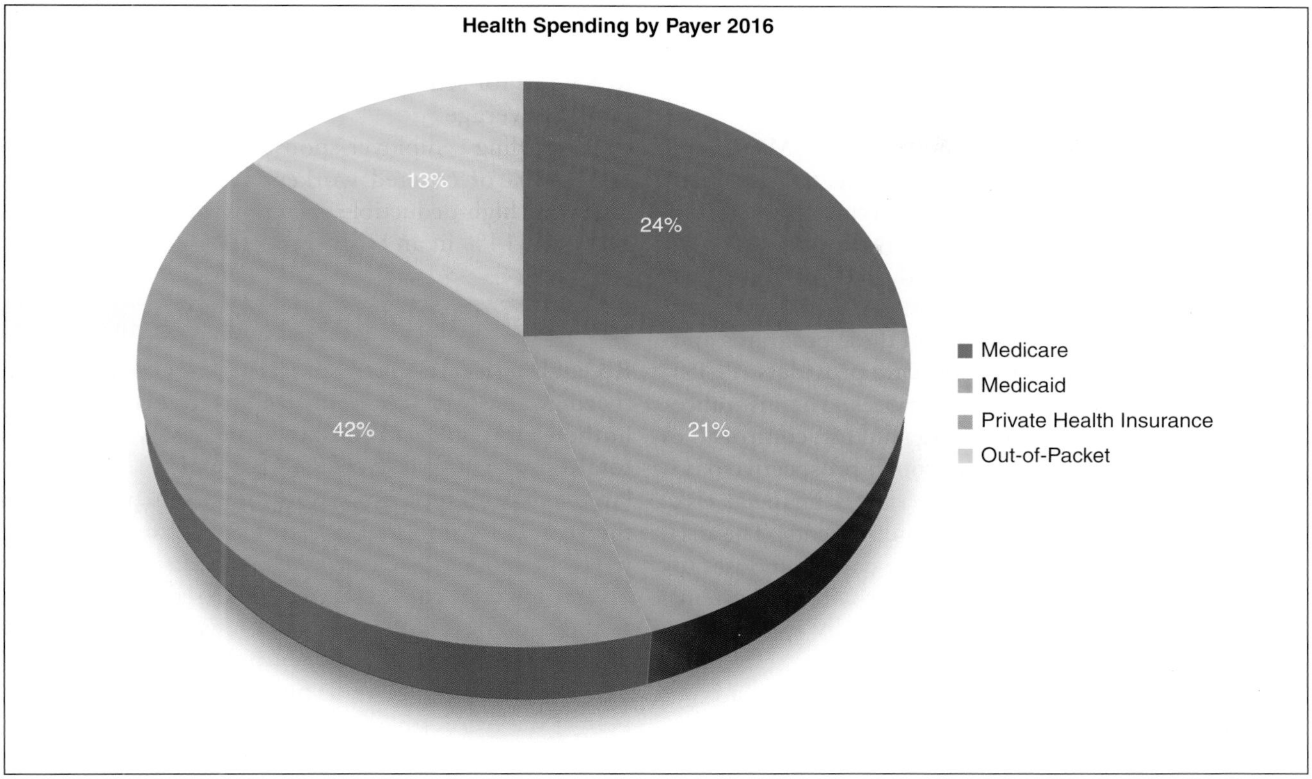

Figure 2 A breakdown of health spending by payer in 2016. While private insurers have the largest share of healthcare spending, nearly half of all healthcare spending in the United States comes from the government (Medicare and Medicaid). (From Centers for Medicare and Medicaid Services. *National Health Expenditures 2016 Highlights*. 2016. Available at: https://www.cms.gov/Research-Statistics-Data-and-Systems/Statistics-Trends-and-Reports/NationalHealthExpendData/NationalHealthAccountsHistorical.html. Accessed August 20, 2018.)

Advantage enrollees are in Health Maintenance Organizations (HMOs) compared with roughly one-third in Preferred Provider Organizations (PPOs).[5]

Medicare Part D, which was started in January 2006, provides prescription drug coverage to everyone with Medicare. This program is an insurance product, whereby Medicare beneficiaries may choose to purchase a drug plan through Medicare-approved private companies and pay a monthly premium. The purpose of the program is to lower prescription drug costs and help shield Medicare beneficiaries from higher costs in the future. As of 2017, the Medicare Trustees reported an enrollment of 44.5 million people for Part D.[4] In 2016 prescription drug spending reached $328.6 billion.[1]

Medicaid

Medicaid is a social program that is available to certain low-income individuals and families. It is a state-administered program, such that each state sets specific guidelines for utilization. Although eligibility requirements vary by state, in general, eligibility may be determined by age, pregnancy status, disability, or income. Children may also be eligible for Medicaid, independent of parent's eligibility. Unlike Medicare, which is funded at the federal level, Medicaid is funded partly by the federal government and partly by states. Medicaid represents 17% of total national healthcare expenditures or roughly $565.5 billion.[1]

The State Children's Health Insurance Program (SCHIP) is administered through the Centers for Medicare and Medicaid Service (CMS) to provide health care to millions of children across the country. The program is jointly funded by the federal and state governments and administered by states. As with Medicaid, states determine eligibility and benefits. In 2017, CMS reported enrollment in CHIP to be 9.4 million.[6]

Private Payer Reimbursement Models

Private health insurance can be purchased by individuals or through employers. There are many different commercial health insurance products available, which may include traditional fee-for-service, managed care, or consumer-directed health care programs. In 2014, it was estimated that 66% of nonelderly workers participated in employer-sponsored health coverage.[7]

Health Maintenance Organizations (HMOs) are managed care programs. These programs provide integrated coverage for patients that typically involves providers either employed by the HMO directly or in separate groups contracted with the HMO and often practicing in the HMO facilities. There is a strong emphasis on preventive medicine in these programs and it is not uncommon that primary care providers (PCPs) are required to access specialty services. The insurance company defines what services are paid for, controls the costs of those payments often through prospective payment models, and in many cases shares financial risk with physicians, health systems, and patients. The disadvantage of these plans is that if the patient chooses to receive care from an out-of-network provider or system, the individual cost may rise substantially (emergency medical care may be an exception).

Preferred Provider Organizations (PPOs) are a type of managed care program. The employer gives employees a list of physicians and health care facilities that they have selected. If the employee goes to one of those providers or facilities, they pay less. The providers and the facilities are independent. Patients typically do not need to choose a PCP to enlist other subspecialists for care, unlike in an HMO model.

Point-of-Service (POS) plans offer another alternative. The patient is a member of an HMO or PPO. If the patient receives medical care from a participating provider or system, the cost of that care is less. While encouraged to obtain medical services through those entities, they can get care from outside providers and plans albeit at a higher premium.

"Catastrophic" or "High-Deductible" health plans are available that provide insurance after a predefined amount of health care spending out-of-pocket. These plans are designed to have a higher deductible for those who may not routinely use significant medical resources, but provide coverage when those resources are needed at a greater level.

Health Savings Accounts allow individuals and employers to contribute resources dedicated to health care with certain tax advantages. These accounts were established as part of the Medicare Prescription Drug, Improvement and Modernization Act of 2003. As long as those dollars contributed are spent on health care, they are deductible to the individual and employer and may be carried over at the end of the year. These are generally reserved for patients covered by high-deductible plans. For 2018 an individual enrolled in a high-deductible plan can contribute up to $3,450 for self-only coverage and up to $6,900 for family coverage.[8]

Regarding employer-sponsored health plans, in 2017 48% of covered workers are enrolled in PPOs, 28% in high-deductible plans with health savings accounts, 14% in an HMO, and 10% in a POS.[9]

Alternative Payment Models

Recent health care reform efforts have focused on incentivizing value over volume in an effort to curb rising costs in the Unites States. Total hip arthroplasty (THA) and total knee arthroplasty (TKA) account for Medicare's largest expenditure, total $6.6 billion in payments in the year 2013 alone.[10] Under traditional fee-for-service payment models, each provider submits claims to the insurer for their role in services rendered to the patient. Both hospitals and providers are rewarded based upon the quantity of care that they provide, with minimal financial penalties for poor quality care. Authorized as part of the Affordable Care Act (ACA), the Centers for Medicare and Medicaid Services (CMS) began piloting the Bundled Payments for Care Improvement (BPCI) Initiative in 2013 to align incentives among providers to offer quality care at a lower cost. Under the BPCI program, CMS would provide one lump-sum payment for an entire episode of care across 48 different inpatient diagnosis-related groups (DRG), including THA and TKA, cervical fusion, lumbar decompression and fusion, and femur fracture fixation. The target payment price is based upon a historical average for that facility's Medicare beneficiaries and a National Trend Factor. Should the costs of caring for a patient during the episode of care come in below the target price, all BPCI participants could share in the profits. Conversely, participants are held financially accountable for higher-cost patients. While earlier models only included inpatient care, most BPCI participants assumed risk for a 90-day episode of care, but could choose from one of four models with varying episode length, and three tiers of risk (**Figure 3**).

Several centers have published early results from their BPCI programs in both total joint arthroplasty[11-14] and spine surgery.[15,16] Although some institutions report positive results with reduced postacute utilization, lower readmission rates, and decreased cost of care, concerns exist with regard to risk adjustment in these alternative payment models (APMs).[17-19] Patients with multiple medical comorbidities at increased risk for complications, lower socioeconomic status, and those

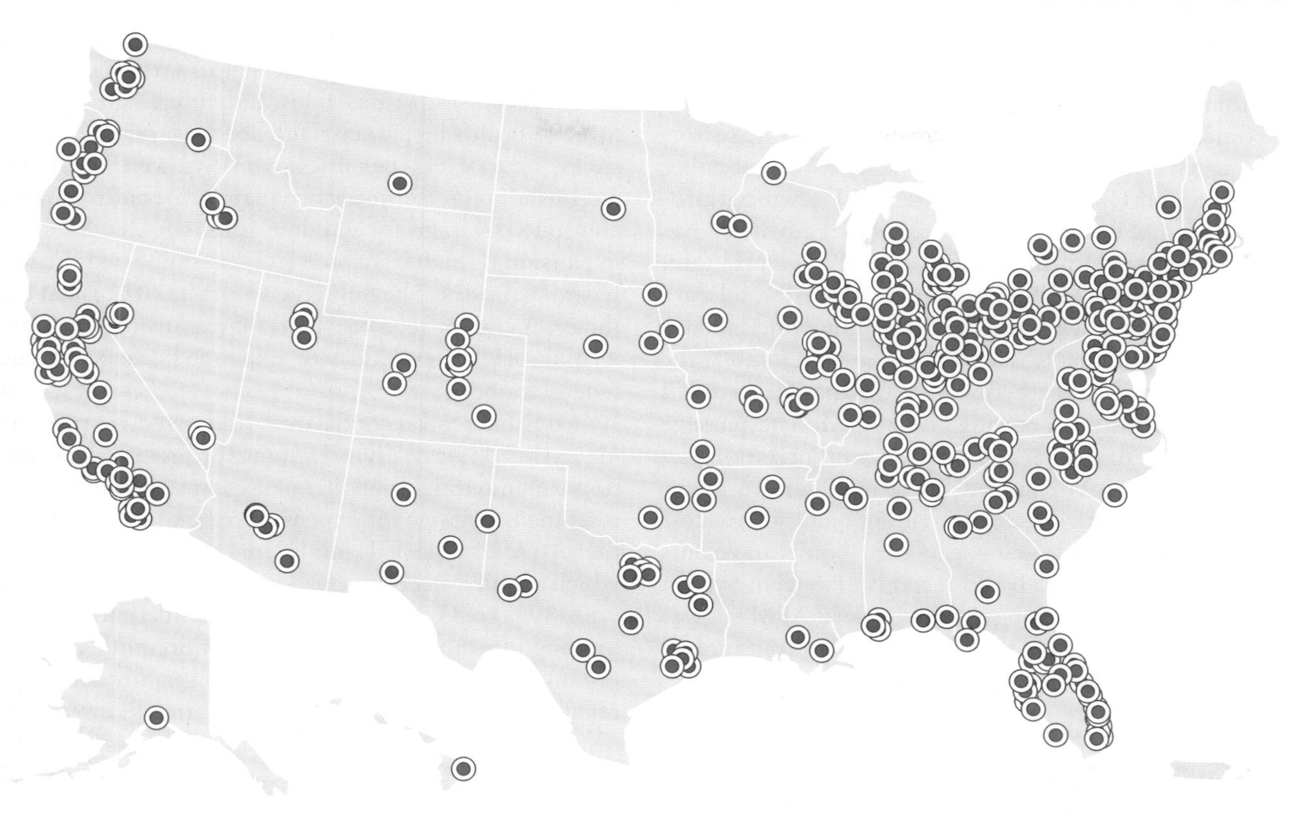

Figure 3 A map of current BPCI program participants. As of July 1, 2018, the BPCI program has 1,025 participants across the country (From Centers for Medicare and Medicaid Services. *Bundled Payments for Care Improvement (BPCI) initiative: General Information.* Available at: https://innovation.cms.gov/initiatives/bundled-payments/. Accessed August 26, 2018.)

social limitations precluding safe discharge to home may face access to care problems under current bundled payment models. Without appropriate risk adjustment, providers and hospitals may be disincentivized to care for patients who may be costly to their bundle. Further study is needed to determine what factors should be risk-adjusted and whether these high-risk patients are being denied care.

Beginning on April 1, 2016, CMS rolled out the Comprehensive Care for Joint Replacement (CJR) bundled payment program for THA and TKA. Despite the early success of the voluntary BPCI program, CMS mandated that the nearly 800 hospitals in 67 Metropolitan Statistical Areas (MSA) participate in this new value-based payment model. There are several differences in the programs. BPCI allowed for flexibility for participants, choosing between four different models for their bundle based upon episode length and level of risk. CJR provided only one option for providers. Instead of target pricing being set according to the hospital's historical performance under BPCI, the new CJR program has introduced regional pricing, which can foster competition among local facilities to provide the lowest cost care; however, some fear this may lead to access to care problems for patients who may use more resources. Orthopaedic surgeons raise concerns about physician input into these APMs. Only hospitals under CJR can act as bundle conveners; physician practices have the option of managing their own bundle with CMS through the BPCI program. CMS has heard some of these concerns and has made changes to the CJR program. As of 2018, participation is now voluntary for 33 of the 67 MSAs and for all rural and low-volume providers while CMS continues to collect data and evaluate this program.[20]

The success of the BPCI program in reducing CMS costs has led to an increase in other APMs as well. Several private insurers have partnered with hospitals and orthopaedic surgeon practices to align incentives and reduce episode-of-care costs. Because many reimbursement contracts with private payers are protected information, few studies have been published evaluating the outcomes of bundled payments in the private sector. The current BPCI program will conclude on September 30, 2018 and CMS will begin the BPCI advanced program which will run through 2023. BPCI advanced has many of the same features as the original BPCI program, but streamlined into one model incorporating all care from the day of discharge from the hospital and 90 days afterward. Participants will be at risk for up to 20% the final target price. Furthermore, participation in BPCI advanced qualifies as an advanced APM. The passage of the Medicare Access and CHIP Reauthorization Act of 2015 (MACRA) changed the way Medicare financially rewards clinicians for providing quality, low-cost care. Orthopaedic surgeons can earn bonus payments through the new Merit-based Incentive Payment System (MIPS) or by participating in an advanced APM such as CJR or BPCI advanced, the original BPCI program had not qualified in the past.

Patient Protection and Affordable Care Act of 2010

History and Controversy of the ACA

On March 23, 2010, President Barack Obama signed into law the ACA (Affordable Care Act), with the goal of reducing the number of uninsured patients, reducing costs, and improving quality of health care. This was the most significant overhaul of the healthcare system since the creation of Medicare and Medicaid in 1965. The original passage of the law was controversial and divided the country largely on party lines. While this achieved the goal of major healthcare overhaul legislation, the future of the law was built on shaky unipartisan ground, and therefore the law remains vulnerable to later Congresses with different party control.

Major Policy Changes of the ACA

The ACA encompasses over 900 pages of health care reform directed toward expanding access to insurance, increasing consumer protections, bolstering prevention and wellness programs, increasing the primary care workforce, improving quality, and most importantly, limiting federal health care costs. In general, shifting care from emergency department visits to preventive and primary care settings is seen as a major driver of cost savings; thus insurance coverage and access to care are primary goals of the ACA. Insurance coverage is expanded by several strategies. Employers are required to cover employees, with the help of tax credits for small businesses, or pay fines. Individuals are required to have health insurance, with the help of federal subsidies, or face tax penalties. Markets were created to aid in shopping for insurance plans. Parents are able to continue coverage for children until age 26. Medicaid expansion to higher income levels is supported through federal subsides. The Supreme Court in 2012 ruled that the ACA cannot require Medicaid expansion. As of this writing, 19 states have not expanded Medicaid with federal money.

Consumer protections were addressed by prohibiting exclusion or costly premiums for preexisting conditions, eliminating annual expense caps, and preventing rescinded coverage for expensive patients. Furthermore, the ACA established minimum medical loss ratios, which require a certain proportion of insurance premiums (80% to 85%) to be spent on medical care, thereby limiting insurance profit taking from premiums. If minimums are unmet, then insurance companies must send rebates to beneficiaries. Other programs like requiring restaurants with more than 20 locations to post nutrition information on menus are also designed to protect consumers and improve health.

The ACA was funded in part by an increase in Medicare taxes on individuals making $200,000 or joint filers making more than $250,000. Other taxes include the penalties levied on individuals for not buying insurance, taxes on insurance companies, and penalties paid by larger businesses who do not provide employee coverage. In 2016, this penalty was $695 per adult, $347.50 per child, and capped at $2,085 per family. Opposition to the mandate for individuals to buy insurance or face tax penalties was strong, and the legal fight reached the Supreme Court. In 2012, the court ruled that the mandate was constitutional, falling under Congressional powers to levy taxes. However, in 2017, Congress repealed the Individual Mandate provisions of the ACA in a tax bill. It remains to be seen what effect this will have on the risk pools, premium increases, and overall effect of the ACA, especially in light of pendulum swings in Congressional ideology with subsequent elections.

Impact of the ACA

Before the ACA, around 45 million Americans were uninsured. That number decreased considerably to around 27 million by 2016. By percentages, the rate of uninsured nonelderly Americans dropped from around 18% in 2010 to 10.9% in 2016.

With political efforts to undermine the ACA and uncertainty in the marketplace, as well as from rising premiums following the repeal of the individual mandate and decisions not to expand Medicaid, the rates of uninsured Americans have risen since the election of Donald Trump in 2016. Gallop polls found the rate of uninsured Americans to be around 12.3% by the end of 2017.[21] Medicaid expansion states on average had an uninsured rate of 9.1% and non-Medicaid expansion states had an uninsured rate of 15.9%. Primary and preventive services have generally improved in my published reports since the implementation of the ACA.

Access to Orthopaedic Care After ACA

With the expansion of Medicaid in over 30 states after passage of the ACA, the number of insured people has increased accordingly. However, the assumption that insurance increases access to care is one that has been tested, and it may not be true. Primary care and emergency services have improved for newly covered Americans, with the ACA requiring that primary care payments for Medicaid increase to Medicare levels. Access to specialty providers, however, may not have proportionally increased because of the relatively undervalued Medicaid provider rates and baseline disinclination to treat elective conditions below cost. This was the finding of a 2018 study examining the ease of making a simulated Medicaid appointment at 93 medical practices.[22] Only 18.3% of the practices offered an appointment, representing 13.3% of the orthopaedic surgeons in the study group. Removing safety-net facility surgeons, which are supported to take underinsured patients, only 7.1% of the practices studied offered a new appointment. Attaining Medicaid coverage removes lack of insurance as a barrier to care, but still places people in the less-than-desirable payment plans of Medicaid.

The impact on safety-net institutions may be significant despite an inequitable payment schedule with Medicaid. In a 2018 study examining the rates of uninsured patients before and after the ACA, the authors found a 36% absolute reduction in uninsured visits after implementation of the ACA.[23] Whether this was overall economically beneficial depends on whether state-support for safety-net institutions changed or will change in time and was not addressed by this paper. Furthermore, it is unclear whether fewer uninsured visits translated into more surgical interventions or improved orthopaedic outcomes.

In another 2018 study examining the effect of the ACA on hand surgery, the authors found a decrease in the uninsured rates (15% to 6.4%) and proportional increase in Medicaid (9.5% to 17.8%) and Medicare (15.4% to 20.3%).[24] There was a statistically insignificant drop in payment rate from 32.3% to 30.3%.

Future of the ACA

Core aspects of the original ACA have now been reversed, as discussed, including the individual mandate and required Medicaid expansion. There have been multiple effort by the current republican Congress to "repeal and replace," but no such overhaul or reversal has yet passed. The executive branch has equally whittled away the impact of the ACA through several mechanisms including discontinuing certain insurance company subsidies, not advertising exchanges or enrollment periods, shortening enrollment periods, and allowing work requirements and more stringent criteria on Medicaid eligibility.[25]

Ultimately the future of the ACA cannot be predicted. Potentially changing bicameral ideology with upcoming elections could lead to strengthening or dismantling the remaining provisions of the ACA.

Summary

With continued national debate regarding healthcare policy, orthopaedic surgeons should understand the issues facing their practices and their patients. While the ACA has reshaped the healthcare landscape, parts of the law continue to change. Both private payers and CMS continue to develop APMs to reduce costs while attempting to maintain quality, and physicians should continue to be a part of this conversation.

Key Study Points

- Healthcare reform will continue to play even a larger role for how orthopaedic surgeons in all subspecialties take care of patients.
- Medicare spending accounts for 20% of US national healthcare expenditures and consists of four parts.
- Private payor reimbursement models include point-of-service, high deductible, PPO and HMO, and plans
- Orthopaedic surgeons should understand CMS bundled payment programs including BPCI, CJR, and BPCI advanced.
- While the ACA has reduced the number of uninsured Americans, parts of the landmark health care law continue to change including the repeal of the individual mandate and required Medicaid expansion

Principles of Orthopaedics

Annotated References

1. CMS. *National Health Expenditures Fact Sheet*. April 17, 2018. Available at: https://www.cms.gov/Research-Statistics-Data-and-Systems/Statistics-Trends-and-Reports/NationalHealthExpendData/NHE-Fact-Sheet.html. Accessed August 15, 2018.

   This article discusses the breakdown of costs of health care in the United States.

2. Barnett JC, Berchick ER. *Health Insurance Coverage in the United States: 2016*. 2017. Available at: https://www.census.gov/library/publications/2017/demo/p60-260.html. Accessed August 15, 2018.

   This article discusses an overview of health insurance coverage in the United States.

3. Centers for Medicare & Medicaid Services. *National Health Expenditures 2016 Highlights*. 2016. Available at: https://www.cms.gov/Research-Statistics-Data-and-Systems/Statistics-Trends-and-Reports/NationalHealthExpendData/NationalHealthAccountsHistorical.html. Accessed August 20, 2018.

   This article discusses the breakdown of costs of health care in the United States and is detailed in Figure 1.

4. The Boards of Trustees, Federal Hospital Insurance and Federal Supplementary Medical Insurance Trust Funds. *The 2018 Annual Report of the Boards of Trustees of the Federal Hospital Insurance and Federal Supplementary Medical Insurance Trust Funds*. Washington, DC, 2018.

   This article discusses the Medicare program and details participants in Part B.

5. Jacobson G, Damico A, Neuman T, Gold M. *Medicare Advantage 2017 Spotlight: Enrollment Market Update*. 2017. Available at: https://www.kff.org/medicare/issue-brief/medicare-advantage-2017-spotlight-enrollment-market-update/. Accessed August 15, 2018.

   This article details the partnership between CMS and private insurers with the Medicare Advantage program.

6. Centers for Medicare & Medicaid Services. *Unduplicated Number of Children Ever Enrolled in CHIP and Medicaid*. 2018. Available at: https://www.medicaid.gov/chip/downloads/fy-2017-childrens-enrollment-report.pdf. Accessed August 20, 2018.

   This article discusses CHIP and the enrollment numbers of children in the program.

7. Long MRM, Claxton G, Damico A. *Trends in Employer-Sponsored Insurance Offer and Coverage Rates, 1999–2014*. 2016. Available at: https://www.kff.org/private-insurance/issue-brief/trends-in-employer-sponsored-insurance-offer-and-coverage-rates-1999-2014/. Accessed August 20, 2018.

   This article discusses employer-sponsored private health insurance plans.

8. Healthcare.gov. *Health Savings Account (HSA)*. 2018. Available at: https://www.healthcare.gov/glossary/health-savings-account-HSA/. Accessed August 20, 2018.

   This article details the benefits of the Health Savings Account program.

9. Claxton G Rae M, Long M, Damico A. *Employer Health Benefits 2017 Annual Survey*. 2017. Available at: http://files.kff.org/attachment/Report-Employer-Health-Benefits-Annual-Survey-2017. Accessed August 20, 2018.

   This article discusses benefits of private, employer-based, healthcare plans.

10. Centers for Medicare and Medicaid Services. New Medicare data available to increase transparency on hospital utilization. Available at: https://www.cms.gov/Newsroom/MediaReleaseDatabase/Fact-sheets/2015-Fact-sheets-items/2015-06-01.html.

11. Iorio R: Strategies and tactics for successful implementation of bundled payments: Bundled payment for care improvement at a large, Urban, Academic medical center. *J Arthroplasty* 2015;30(3):349-350.

12. Iorio R, Clair AJ, Slover J, Zuckerman JD: Early results of CMS bundled payment initiative for a 90 day total joint replacement episode of care. *J Arthroplasty* 2016;31(2):343-350.

    This study reported results of their CMS bundled payment program. Level of evidence: IV.

13. Mechanic RE: Mandatory Medicare bundled payments – it ready for prime time. *N Engl J Med* 2015;373(14):1291.

14. Courtney PM, Ashley BS, Hume EL, Kamath AF: Are bundled payments a viable reimbursement model for revision total joint arthroplasty? *Clin Orthop Relat Res* 2016;474(12):2714-2721.

    In a single institution review of revision TKA, the authors found no difference in costs with their BPCI program for revision arthroplasty. Level of evidence: III.

15. Martin BI, Lurie JD, Farrokhi FR, McGuire KJ, Mirza SK: Early effects of medicare's bundled payment for care improvement program for lumbar fusion. *Spine (Phila Pa 1976)* 2018;43(10):705-711.

    This study looked at outcomes following a bundled payment program for lumbar fusion. Level of evidence: III.

16. Bronson WH, Kingery MT, Hutzler L, et al: Lack of cost savings for lumbar spine fusions after bundled payments for care improvement initiative: A consequence of increased case complexity. *Spine (Phila Pa 1976)* 2019;44(4):298-304.

    This study found no cost savings in their institution's BPCI program for lumbar fusions. Level of evidence: III.

17. Courtney PM, Bohl DD, Lau EC, Ong KL, Jacobs JJ, Della Valle CJ: Risk adjustment is necessary in Medicare bundled payment models for total hip and knee arthroplasty. *J Arthroplasty* 2018;33(8):2368-2375.

    This CMS database study identified risk factors for increased episode of care costs. Level of evidence: IV.

18. Rozell JC, Courtney PM, Dattilo JR, Wu CH, Lee GC: Should all patients Be included in alternative payment models for primary total hip arthroplasty and total knee arthroplasty? *J Arthroplasty* 2016;31(9 suppl):45-49.

This was a retrospective review of a single institution's data on risk factors for increased resource utilization in THA and TKA. Level of evidence: III.

19. Courtney PM, Huddleston JI, Iorio R, Markel DC: Socioeconomic risk adjustment models for reimbursement are necessary in primary total joint arthroplasty. *J Arthroplasty* 2017;32(1):1-5.

    The authors report a review of the MARCQI registry and identified low socioeconomic status as a risk factor for increased resource utilization. Level of evidence: III.

20. Centers for Medicare and Medicaid Services. Comprehensive Care for Joint Replacement Model. Available at: https://innovation.cms.gov/initiatives/cjr. Accessed August 26, 2018.

    This article discusses the mandadory CJR bundled payment program for THA and TKA.

21. Gallup Poll on Insurance Coverage Rates. Available at: https://news.gallup.com/poll/233597/uninsured-rate-rises-states-2017.asp. Accessed August 31, 2018.

    This article discusses the rate of uninsured Americans in 2017.

22. Marrero CE, Igbokwe LI, Leonardi C: Access to orthopedic care post Medicaid expansion through the affordable care act. *J Natl Med Assoc* 2019;111(2):148-152.

    This simulated telephone survey attempted to make an appointment as a new Medicaid patient in January 2017 and found a low appointment rate.

23. Gil JA, Goodman AD, Kleiner J, Kamal RN, Baker LC, Akelman E: The affordable care act decreased the proportion of uninsured patients in a safety net orthopaedic clinic. *CORR* 2018;476:925-931.

    The authors found a significant reduction in uninsured patients following ACA implementation. Level of evidence: III.

24. Khansa I, Khansa L, Pearson GD, Jain SA: Effects of the affordable care act on payer mix and physician reimbursement in hand surgery. *J Hand Surg* 2018;43:511-515.

    Retrospective review of the effect of the ACA on a hand surgery practice. Level of evidence: IV.

25. Thompson FJ, Gusmano MK, Shinohara S: Trump and the affordable care act: Congressional repeal efforts, executive federalism, and program durability. *Publius J Federalism* 2018;48:396-424.

    Review of efforts to undercut the ACA.

26. Centers for Medicare and Medicaid Services. Bundled Payments for Care Improvement (BPCI) Initiative: General Information. Available at: https://innovation.cms.gov/initiatives/bundled-payments/. Accessed August 26, 2018.

    This article discusses the current BPCI program and its different models.

Chapter 6

Preoperative Evaluation and Postoperative Care of the Orthopaedic Patient

Elaine I. Yang, MD • Alexander S. McLawhorn, MD, MBA

ABSTRACT

Increasing patient complexity in the face of outcome-based cost-containment efforts necessitate a thorough but efficient preoperative assessment process. Unnecessary preoperative testing due to poor compliance with clinical guidelines can and often delay surgery while driving up health care costs. To avoid this, institutions should develop preoperative care pathways founded on sound and up-to-date evidence and ensure high compliance among its team members. In regard to orthopaedic trauma patients, proper evaluation should include appropriate triaging of care, timing of surgery, and utilization of resources; adherence to practice guidelines for geriatric trauma patients is of particular importance in these regards because of high associated morbidity and mortality. Postoperatively, optimal pain management should include the use of multimodal analgesia and a sensible and balanced approach to pharmacologic treatment with deterrence of opioid prescriptions whenever possible. Success requires collaboration between all the members of the perioperative team as well as organizational consistency.

Keywords: geriatric trauma; multimodal analgesia; presurgical testing; surgical risk stratification; trauma injury assessment

Dr. Yang or an immediate family member serves as a paid consultant to or is an employee of Intellijoint and Johnson & Johnson. Neither Dr. McLawhorn nor any immediate family member has received anything of value from or has stock or stock options held in a commercial company or institution related directly or indirectly to the subject of this chapter.

Introduction

The increasing population of aging Americans continues to drive the volume of orthopaedic procedures nationwide. Despite this, perioperative care of the orthopaedic patient remains inconsistent and contradictory. This has in turn led to two extremes—surgical delays as well as increased length of stay due to inadequate optimization. Sheffield et al estimated that over 56,000 Medicare patients underwent unnecessary cardiac workup before surgery, and Abbas et al demonstrated that even within a single institution, there was very little consistency in adherence to proposed guidelines for patients with acute proximal femur fractures.[1,2] With recent pressure from government-mandated cost-containment programs, proper risk stratification and efficient utilization of resources are imperative.

Preoperative Assessment

Revised Cardiac Risk Index

Cardiac risk stratification is an important part of shared surgical decision-making as it evaluates a patient's surgical candidacy and engenders appropriate risk/benefit discussions. The Revised Cardiac Risk Index (RCRI) proposed by Lee et al and modified by the ACC/AHA Task Force uses a 6-point scale[3] (**Table 1**). Patients with no positive predictors have a perioperative risk of 0.4% of a major cardiovascular complication (MCC). Those with predictors 1, 2, ≥3 have a 0.9%, 6.6%, and >11% risk of MCC, respectively. Despite its universality, recent studies suggest that the RCRI has low discriminative ability and has been inconsistent in predicting the rate of MCC.[4] In light of these findings, strides have been made to develop new propensity scales to improve the prediction of major adverse events.

American College of Surgeons NSQIP MICA

In 2011, Gupta et al devised a cardiac morbidity calculator to determine the risk of postoperative myocardial

Principles of Orthopaedics

Table 1

Revised Cardiac Risk Index and Risk of MCC

RCRI Criteria (1-6)	Predictors	Risk of MCC
1. History of ischemic heart disease	0	0.4%
2. History of congestive heart failure	1	0.9%
3. History of cerebrovascular disease	2	6.6%
4. History of diabetes	≥3	>11%
5. Chronic kidney disease (creatinine >2 mg/dL)		
6. Undergoing intermediate/high-risk surgery[a]		

[a]Refers to suprainguinal vascular surgery, intraperitoneal surgery, and intrathoracic surgery.

MCC = major cardiovascular complications, including death, myocardial infarction, and nonfatal cardiac arrest, RCRI = Revised cardiac risk index

Data from Lee TH, Marcantonio ER, Mangione CM, et al: Derivation and prospective validation of a simple index for prediction of cardiac risk of major noncardiac surgery. *Circulation* 1999;100(10):1043-1049.

infarction and cardiac arrests (MICA).[5] Gupta's study, which was validated on a cohort of 40,000 patients from the NSQIP database, showed that risk factors most predictive of MICA after surgery were American Society of Anesthesiologists (ASA) classification, dependent functional status, age, abnormal creatinine (>1.5), and type of surgery.

Total Joint Arthroplasty Cardiac Risk Index

Similarly in 2016, Waterman et al formulated and tested a cardiac risk index (Total Joint Arthroplasty Cardiac Risk Index, TJA CRI) specific to total joint arthroplasty patients. It is based on three primary predictors: age ≥80 years, history of hypertension, and a history of cardiac disease.[6] He was able to demonstrate not only that each factor independently predicted postoperative MCC more discriminately than the RCRI, but also that patients with all three predictors had the highest MCC risk.

Modified Frailty Index

Elderly patients pose a challenge to universal risk stratification because of the concept of frailty, defined as a decrease in physiologic reserves and accumulation of multisystem impairments separate from the normal process of aging. The Canadian Study of Health and Aging (CSHA) first introduced the Modified Frailty Index (mFI)[7] for all surgical patients; it was modified in 2016 and applied to approximately 40,000 NSQIP primary total joint arthroplasty patients.[8] Eleven variables from the CSHA-FI, matched to those from the NSQIP, were taken and each assigned one point (**Table 2**). The mFI score is calculated by dividing the total number of positive risk factors by 11, ranging from 0.0 to 1.0. Shin et al showed that an mFI score of ≥0.45 independently predicts major postoperative complications and is effective in guiding appropriate postoperative destination.

Table 2

Canadian Study of Health and Aging-Frailty Index Versus National Surgical Quality Improvement Program

CSHA-FI Variables	NSQIP
Congestive heart failure (1 point)	Congestive heart failure
Myocardial infarction (1 point)	Myocardial infarction
Cardiac problems (1 point)	Angina or cardiac stents
Arterial hypertension (1 point)	Hypertension requiring medication
Cerebrovascular problems (1 point)	Transient ischemic attack
History of stroke (1 point)	Cerebrovascular accident
Decreased peripheral pulses (1 point)	Peripheral vascular disease
Respiratory problems (1 point)	Chronic obstructive pulmonary disease
Diabetes mellitus (1 point)	Diabetes mellitus
Changes in ability to perform ADLs (1 point)	Nonindependent functional status
Clouding or delirium (1 point)	Impaired sensorium

ADLs = activities of daily living

Adapted from Shin JI, Keswani A, Lovy A, et al: Simplified frailty index as a predictor of adverse outcomes in total hip and knee arthroplasty. *J Arthroplasty* 2016;31[11]:2389-2394. Copyright 2016, with permission from Elsevier.

Presurgical Testing

Cardiac and pulmonary testing comprise most preoperative resources used and can be confounding because of ongoing updates. Below is a summary of the ACC/AHA approach to preoperative testing based on the 2014 Perioperative Guidelines and the 2016 focused update on the preoperative management of preexisting cardiac stents.[9,10]

Electrocardiogram

In any patient (with or without known cardiac comorbidities) undergoing low-risk surgery, the ACC/AHA does not currently recommend routine resting 12-lead electrocardiograms (ECG) before surgery. It is, however, recommended for all patients undergoing intermediate or high-risk surgery.

Echocardiogram

Asymptomatic patients without cardiac comorbidities need not undergo routine assessment of left ventricular (LV) function. The same applies for patients with known cardiac history who have undergone LV assessment within the last year. It is, however, reasonable to ascertain preoperative LV function in any patient without cardiac history with unexplained dyspnea, and in any patient with known cardiac structural abnormalities who has worsening symptoms of heart failure or who has not undergone reevaluation within the past year.

Exercise/Pharmacologic Stress Testing

Excellent functional status is a reliable predictor of perioperative success. As such, patients, regardless of medical risk factors, need not undergo preoperative stress testing if they can perform above 4 metabolic equivalents (METs). Functional capacity is divided into excellent (>10 METs), good (7 to 10 METs), moderate (4 to 6 METs), and poor (<4 METs) (**Table 3**). Conversely, in patients who cannot perform 4 METs or in whom the functional status is unknowable, it is reasonable to perform preoperative stress testing. The only exception is if the patient is undergoing low-risk surgery, in which case it is at the discretion of the perioperative physicians to decide if the results of the testing will alter intraoperative management, thereby justifying its use.

Table 3

Metabolic Equivalent (MET) Designations

MET	Examples	Stress Testing (Y/N)
Unknown	Unable to walk because of physical disability or pain	Yes
Poor (<4)	Walk 2-3 mph; can perform ADLs	Yes
Moderate (4-6)	Walk 4 mph, two flight of stairs	No
Good (7-10)	Run a short distance	No
Excellent (>10)	Run a long distance	No

ADLs = activities of daily living

Chest Radiograph

The value of preoperative testing to estimate postoperative pulmonary risk continues to be controversial. A thorough history and physical remains the most proven tool in identifying high-risk patients. As it stands, local institutional guidelines are what drive the routine use of screening chest radiographs before surgery. Limited evidence from multivariable risk factor studies does support the use of preoperative chest radiography for patients with known pulmonary disease as well as those older than 50 years undergoing intermediate or high-risk surgery.[11]

Advanced Pulmonary Testing

Spirometry may provide some risk stratification in vulnerable patients but, given the cost, does not add value as a routine tool to estimate postoperative pulmonary risk. Although there are currently no evidence-supported guidelines available, conventional practice advocates the use of spirometry in patients with known obstructive or restrictive lung disease to assess disease progression and to estimate risk. It is also not unreasonable to order preoperative spirometry on patients with no known disease but newly identified with abnormal chest radiograph or dyspnea of unclear etiology.[12]

Approach to Patients With Cardiac Stenting

Balloon Angioplasty and Bare Metal Stents

Patients with coronary angiography should wait a minimum of 2 weeks after balloon angioplasty before proceeding with elective surgery and should continue their aspirin perioperatively. If bare metal stents (BMSs) are placed, the patient should be observed for a minimum of 30 days before proceeding. Those needing nonelective surgery will require a consensus decision by perioperative physicians to decide on the timing of surgery in relation to the risk of coronary thrombosis.

Drug-Eluting Stents

Before 2016, patients who underwent placement of coronary drug-eluting stents (DESs) needed to wait a minimum of 1 year before proceeding with elective noncardiac surgery because of the theoretical risk of stent thrombosis in patients for whom dual antiplatelet therapy is prematurely discontinued. Several large studies have since suggested that the risk of thrombosis is less than previously thought.[13-15] Since the 2016 focused update, the ACC/AHA now states that patients can proceed with elective surgery 6 months after DES placement. Dual antiplatelet therapy should be continued perioperatively whenever possible, but in the event that it needs to be discontinued, the ACC/AHA advises continuing at least aspirin and restarting the $P2Y_{12}$ inhibitor as soon as possible.

Perioperative Surveillance

As of 2014, routine postoperative myocardial infarction screening with troponins and ECG in asymptomatic patients with cardiac risk factors remain controversial and without established benefits. Currently, the ACC/AHA recommends that postoperative troponins and ECG be primarily reserved for symptomatic patients. At many institutions it is at the discretion of the patient's cardiologist or intensivist whether postoperative screening ECGs and troponins are ascertained in selected patients.

Evaluation of the Orthopaedic Trauma Patient

Injury Severity Assessment

Comprehensive approach to the trauma patient should begin with an accurate assessment of injury severity. This is essential not only for appropriate triaging and allocation of resources but also for evaluating changes over time and outcome prognostication. To achieve this end, trauma scoring has undergone many alterations since its inception; despite the efforts of many, there is currently no universally accepted and applicable scoring system. We review the most widely used scoring systems below along with potential pitfalls involved in their use.

Glasgow Coma Scale

Described by neurosurgeons from the University of Glasgow in 1974, the Glasgow Coma Scale (GCS) was originally developed as a tool to assess consciousness after traumatic brain injury, but now has been incorporated into more complex scoring systems as a way to assess neurologic status after acute injury.[16] The scale comprises three graded components: (1) eye response (1 to 4 points), (2) verbal response (1 to 5 points), and (3) motor response (1 to 6 points). Higher points are awarded to responses indicative of advanced cortical function, whereas lower points signify the absence of even basic brain stem reflexes.

Injury Severity Score

Developed as a revision of the Abbreviated Injury Scale (AIS), which was one of the first injury-description systems ever developed but with many limitations, the Injury Severity Score (ISS) was created by Baker et al in 1974 to better assess injury severity in patients with polytrauma.[17] The ISS uses the AIS, which assigns points 1 to 5 in increasing severity for trauma to any of the nine regions of the body, as the basis for its scoring. The AIS scores for the three most severely injured areas of the body are squared and added together to yield the ISS score (1 to 75). Although this method predicts mortality better than the AIS and remained for many decades the most widely used model, its shortcoming is that it does not allow assessment of multiple injuries to the same body region. A revised version of the ISS, called the New Injury Severity Score (NISS), was developed in 1997 and addresses some of its previous deficiencies.

Trauma and Injury Severity Score

Historical trauma scoring systems primarily focused on anatomic variables, not taking into account that the physiologic course after injury is often highly dynamic and can profoundly affect outcomes. The Trauma and Injury Severity Score (TRISS) was developed to encompass both physiologic and anatomic data into the scoring system. A method that incorporates the (1) Trauma Score—a physiologic scale devised by Champion et al in 1981, (2) the ISS—primarily an anatomic survey of injury, and (3) patient age, TRISS has shown improved injury assessment and predictive abilities toward survival compared with its predecessors.[18] However, as it uses the ISS in its calculation, TRISS is limited by the same problems as the ISS.

Trauma Mortality Prediction Model

The Trauma Mortality Prediction Model (TMPM) was devised in 2008 as a mathematical model that employs severity values called model-average regression coefficients (MARC) derived from 1,322 AIS injury codes to predict mortality after trauma.[19] In 2009, the same model was applied to ICD-9 codes and found to have similar predictive abilities. These two methodologies have been compared with the ISS, the International Classification of Diseases-based ISS (ICISS), the NISS, and the Single-Worst Injury model (SWI) and have shown superior mortality prediction.[20,21] The downside of using such a model is its complexity in calculation as it uses large sets of trauma data.

Hospital Evaluation and Resuscitation

Advanced Trauma Life Support

In 1978, the American College of Surgeons developed an algorithm (Advanced Trauma Life Support, ATLS) to standardize evaluation and treatment of acute trauma patients.[22] It has since been adopted in more than 60 countries around the world and is considered standard of care in most trauma centers. The premise of ATLS is founded on a series of surveys targeted to recognize and treat first the most life-threatening and time-sensitive injuries.

The primary survey utilizes the mnemonic ABCDE: Airway, Breathing, Circulation, Disability, and Exposure. Airway includes cervical spine assessment and protection and Breathing encompasses the diagnoses of derangements within the thoracic cavity—such as flail chest, pneumothoraces, or cardiac tamponade. Circulation refers to the control of possible sources of hemorrhage, as this remains a common cause of death from trauma. Disability catalogs neurologic status through the GCS and any obvious injuries to the central nervous system. Exposure, or environmental control, brings attention to any elemental or toxic contact by fully exposing the patient.

Once the ABCDEs are accounted for and controlled, a secondary survey, which includes a thorough history and physical as well as review of any physiologic data, is conducted. Preliminary diagnostic testing such as chest radiography and CT scans are routinely obtained at this point. As many injuries are often missed even after a thorough primary and secondary survey, a tertiary survey is performed typically within the first 24 hours after admission to identify any previously overlooked injuries.

Resuscitation

Hemorrhagic shock is a predominant cause of avoidable trauma mortality. Consequently, many efforts have been dedicated to the prevention and treatment of uncontrolled bleeding. One such endeavor is the concept of damage control resuscitation, which underscores (1) rapid recognition of coagulopathy, (2) permissive hypotension, (3) surgical control of bleeding, (4) prevention of hypothermia, acidosis, hypocalcemia, (5) avoidance of dilutional coagulopathy from excessive crystalloid administration, (6) transfusions with balanced ratios of blood products, (7) early and appropriate use of factor concentrates, and (8) use of fresh red blood cells or whole blood whenever possible.[23] To achieve this end, American College of Surgeons Trauma Quality Improvement Program (ACS-TQIP) endorses massive transfusion protocols by trauma centers, thereby providing a standardized and efficient resuscitative approach to traumatic bleeding while giving guidance to the blood bank on blood product prioritization.[24]

In addition to timely blood replacement, the use of tranexamic acid (TXA) to control traumatic bleeding has also been debated. With evidence strongly supporting its administration in elective orthopaedic, cardiac, and liver transplant surgeries to reduce surgical bleeding, the CRASH-2 study was undertaken to assess its effects in trauma.[25] Published in 2010, the study found that although overall mortality was reduced in patients who received TXA, the amount of blood products transfused was not. Furthermore, the study was randomized based on the "uncertainty principle," meaning it excluded patients who would clearly benefit from TXA and instead enrolled only patients in whom the immediate providers could not decide if TXA was indicated. This and other limitations undermine the applicability of the study and makes universal utilization of TXA in trauma at this time difficult without further study.[26]

Triaging Care

Timing of Transfers

Appropriate and timely triage after trauma reduces morbidity and mortality by enabling efficient access to definitive care. The Emergency Medical Treatment and Active Labor Act of 1986 requires timely evaluation and stabilization of injured patients before swift transfer to a higher-level facility if the primary hospital lacks resources for further management. Proper primary triage is then critical as indiscretion can result in the transfer of severely injured patients to unprepared and ill-equipped facilities. To this end the National Expert Panel on Field Triage recommends that to minimize undertriage rates to 0% to 5%, an overtriage rate of 25% to 50% is acceptable.[27] Most argue, however, that those recommendations are intended for triage from the field and should not be applied to interfacility transfers. As shown in recent literature, overtriage of minimally injured patients to tertiary facilities increases overall health care costs and redirects limited resources from needed recipients.[28] Innovative solutions to combating overburdening of tertiary hospitals are being promoted, such as the diversion of lesser-acuity orthopaedic trauma patients to satellite operating rooms as a modus for increasing capacity.[29]

Timing of Operative Intervention

Polytrauma patients pose a unique challenge to physicians because of the consideration of concomitant injuries that require surgical intervention. As timing of treatment for specific injuries varies with institution, delays can lead to avoidable complications and greater costs of care. Protocols such as Early Appropriate Care (EAC) seek to minimize unnecessary delays through assembly of a multidisciplinary team led by the general trauma surgeon and using objective physiologic data such as improved acidosis and lack of vasopressor dependence to indicate stability and readiness for operative intervention. When adhered to, EAC decreases time to operating room and reduces complications, hospital length of stay, and costs.[30]

Acute Compartment Syndrome

Orthopaedic trauma emergencies such as acute compartment syndrome require urgent surgical decompression of affected compartments. As such, delayed diagnosis can lead to detrimental outcomes. Although there are many methods of assessing compartment syndrome, evidence supports continuous intracompartmental pressure monitoring with slit catheter technique in at-risk patients instead of relying on nonspecific symptoms such as pain or paresthesias.[31] Risk factors include young age and presence of an underlying fracture. Timing of fasciotomy is based on a differential pressure threshold of 30 mm Hg for greater than 2 hours.

Open Fractures

Traditionally, open fractures have been associated with high morbidity and were historically treated with surgical débridement and/or fixation within 6 hours after injury to minimize the risk of infection.[32] Débridement was repeated at intervals of 48 hours until definitive wound closure can occur. Recent studies, however, suggest that timing of surgical débridement has little association with development of wound infection[33]; instead, characteristics of fracture (typically Gustilo-Anderson grade IIIA or IIIB/C fracture)[34] and timing of antibiotics (>66 minutes) have a stronger association with infection risk.[35]

Geriatric Trauma and Hip Fracture Care

Geriatric Trauma

As previously discussed, elderly patients are at particular risk for poor outcomes after trauma because of frailty. In 2012, the Eastern Association for the Surgery of Trauma recommended the following for geriatric trauma patients (GTP) older than 65 years[36]: (1) lowering the threshold for trauma activation in patients with preexisting medical conditions, (2) patients with AIS scores ≥3 should be transferred to trauma centers for treatment, (3) consideration should be given to limiting aggressive therapy for those in whom the GCS does not improve after 72 hours, (4) patients on anticoagulation therapy with suspected head injury should be evaluated with CT as soon as possible, (5) coagulation profile should be obtained as soon as possible in those same patients and INR normalized (<1.6) within 2 hours, and (6) patients with metabolic acidosis (base deficit worse than −6) should be considered for an ICU admission. Despite their elevated risk, GTPs with ISS scores ≥30 treated at a level I trauma center had a survival to discharge of 66%, with a median "long-term" survival of approximately 3 years.[37]

Hip Fracture Care

Osteoporotic hip fracture care comprises a large percentage of orthopaedic care rendered to geriatric patients. Despite the high number of cases annually and advances in perioperative management of these patients, morbidity in this population remains high, often as a result of avoidable complications from delayed surgical intervention. ACS-TQIP best practice guidelines from 2015 recommend performing surgery for hip fracture patients within 24 to 48 hours of admission, as deferrals are associated with increased risk of complications and 30-day mortality.[38,39] Common causes of delays include excessive preoperative testing from poor adherence to ACC/AHA guidelines as well as prolonged wait times for normalization of coagulation profiles despite studies that show no difference in transfusion rates or complications between patients with INR <1.5 and those with INR of 1.5 to 3.1.[40,41] Emergence of institutional programs with standardized preoperative pathways shows promise, however, by decreasing unnecessary testing, increasing compliance with clinical practice guidelines, and expediting readiness for surgery.[42]

Postoperative Pain Management

Pain management for orthopaedic patients—trauma or elective—remains a challenge. Despite efforts to combat the national epidemic, opioids continue to be the mainstay of treatment for acute pain. In addition to effects such as CNS disturbance, cardiovascular/respiratory depression, gastrointestinal/genitourinary dysmotility, opioids facilitate upregulation of mu-receptors over time, leading to increased sensitivity to pain, tolerance, and propensity for addiction. Given the time required for bone healing, it is no surprise that orthopaedic surgeons are among the highest prescribers of opioids.[43] Furthermore, because of lack of pain management training, many find themselves ill-equipped to counsel patients who develop ongoing, protracted pain and are dependent on high doses of opioids. To this end, providing pain relief while safeguarding against abuse and addiction can be extremely difficult. Current literature recommends an interdisciplinary approach with use of multimodal analgesics.[44]

Multimodal Analgesia

A multimodal approach refers to the use of nonpharmacologic techniques to minimize surgical pain. To do so, a preemptive discussion with anesthesiologists to optimize opportunities for regional or local-based pain management is preferred. The ASA recommends neuraxial or peripheral nerve blocks and local anesthetic infiltration of incisions whenever possible.[45] These techniques (1) help delay the onset of surgical pain, thereby reducing opioid requirements at a time when acute pain is expected to be at its peak, (2) help reduce pain-induced inflammatory cytokines implicated in delayed wound healing, and (3) are hypothesized to downregulate pathophysiologic mechanisms associated with the development of chronic pain.

Although they can be an effective means of pain control, neuraxial and peripheral nerve blocks are associated with potential downsides. Minor disadvantages include ineffective or incomplete sensory blockade, delay of surgical start time, and undesired motor blockade, which has effects on postoperative mobility and function. Major effects include cardiotoxicity from intravascular injection of local, traumatic block placement causing spinal/epidural hematomas, and damage to peripheral nerves leading to prolonged or permanent numbness and weakness. Furthermore, recent use of anticoagulants or an abnormal bleeding profile, as well as active systemic infection—all common in orthopaedic and trauma patients—are contraindications to many regional techniques.

Novel and promising approaches to multimodal analgesia include extending the duration of local-mediated analgesia through the use of continuous peripheral nerve catheters, continuous periarticular catheters, ultrasound-guided peripheral nerve stimulation, and cryoneurolysis. In particular, cryoneurolysis of the infrapatellar branch of the saphenous nerve has shown promise in extending pain relief after total knee arthroplasty (TKA) for up to 5 months.[46] Similarly, a study comparing continuous femoral nerve catheters and indwelling periarticular catheters in patients undergoing TKA demonstrated improved pain relief and mobility in patients with periarticular catheters.[47]

In situations where chronic pain develops, early consultation with an outpatient pain management provider is recommended. Patients with preexisting chronic pain benefit from a preoperative discussion of inpatient pain management strategies and goals. Postoperatively, these physicians can perform interventional procedures while providing ongoing monitoring of pain symptoms and opioid consumption. Both reduce the likelihood of abuse. Many are also trained in pain addiction and can assist patients with detoxification from opioids.

"Balanced" Analgesia

In recent years, a "balanced" approach to postoperative pain has replaced the overuse of a single class of analgesics—primarily opioids. This approach integrates the use of nonopioid medications to target all the different receptors that activate the pain pathway.[48] It also cuts down on the severity of adverse events associated with repetitive and elevated exposure to a single medication.

Table 4 summarizes an interdisciplinary approach to pain management. Several trials suggest that patients receiving multimodal therapy benefited from improved analgesia while reporting a reduction in adverse effects and improved mobilization and rehabilitation.[49] These benefits in turn have led to shorter hospital lengths of stay. In light of this, efforts to eliminate opioids from the postoperative analgesic regimen while maintaining equivalent pain control are now underway through Enhanced Recovery After Surgery (ERAS) pathways at many institutions.

Table 4

Interdisciplinary Approach to Pain Management

Acute Pain	Chronic Pain

Multimodal Analgesia
• Neuraxial anesthesia
  • Spinals
  • Epidurals
• Peripheral nerve blocks
  • Single-shot blocks
  • Continuous nerve catheters
• Local infiltration
  • Wound infiltration
  • Periarticular injection
	Preoperative consultation
	• Pain history with outside provider
	• Verification of use with I-STOP and urine toxicology
	• Preemptive discussion of pain management strategy and goal
	• Patient education and delineation of expectations

Balanced Analgesia
• Preemptive Analgesia
  • Gabapentinoids
  • Acetaminophen
• Nonopioids
  • NSAIDs
  • NMDA-antagonists
  • α-2 antagonists
• Opioids
  • Intrathecal/epidural opioids
  • Long-acting opioids
	Postoperative follow-up
	• Outpatient monitoring of symptoms and prescription use
	• Assistance with taper and cessation of analgesics
	• Interventional procedures as applicable
	• Safe detoxification from opioids

I-STOP = Internet system for tracking overprescribing; NSAIDs = Nonsteroidal anti-inflammatory drugs

One of the drawbacks of balanced analgesia is the concurrent utilization of a multitude of medications, each with unique interactions, dosing schedules, and side-effect profiles, which confuse patients and lead to noncompliance. Nevertheless, providers believe that this risk is outweighed by the benefit of reduced life-threatening events from the use of high-dose opioids.

Preemptive Analgesia

One component of the multimodal pharmacologic approach to pain management is the use of medications preoperatively in an effort to delay or deter incipience of acute pain development.[50] This is known as preemptive analgesia and often includes the use of acetaminophen, gabapentinoids, alpha-2 receptor agonists, and long-acting opioids. In theory, preemptive analgesia prevents or minimizes production of inflammatory mediators early in the process by dampening hyperexcitable neurons in the CNS dorsal horn that convert acute pain into chronic pain. The most widely used and evidence-supported analgesics are reviewed below.

Nonsteroidal Antiinflammatories

Selective and nonselective cyclooxygenase-2 inhibitors are considered an important therapy in multimodal analgesia. They are exceedingly effective for orthopaedic pain and have no addictive potential.[48] Meta-analyses demonstrate decreased opioid consumption in patients on concurrent NSAID therapy.[49] Adverse effects include risk of gastrointestinal bleeding, inhibition of bone healing at high doses, and development of interstitial nephritis. Due to these effects, NSAIDs are not recommended at high doses for long durations.

Alpha-2 Agonists

Alpha-2 (α-2) receptor agonists have recognized antinociceptive and antihyperalgesic properties that are mediated through central and spinal cord α-2 receptor binding.[51] Clonidine and dexmedetomidine are common α-2 agonists used in acute pain management and can be administered through oral, intravenous, and epidural/intrathecal routes. These medications have opioid-sparing properties and can abate the development of opioid-induced hyperalgesia. Disadvantages include bradycardia and hypotension as well as depressed CNS at high doses.

NMDA Antagonists

N-methyl-D-aspartate (NMDA) receptors are known to mediate sensitivity and perception of pain. In "wind-up," repeated stimulation of NMDA/glutamate receptors leads to receptor upregulation and conversion of acute pain into chronic pain. Ketamine, an NMDA antagonist, inhibits this process.[52] Its activity on sigma opioid receptors also renders it an excellent analgesic. When administered intraoperatively, it decreases opioid requirements for up to 24 hours postoperatively.[53] Its effectiveness at subanesthetic levels reduces the likelihood of potential psychomimetic (hallucinatory), muscarinic (nausea/hypersecretory), and sympathomimetic (tachycardia, hypertension) effects seen at higher doses.

Gabapentinoids

Anticonvulsants such as gabapentin and pregabalin are not potent analgesics for acute pain when administered alone but decrease overall opioid use when used adjunctively with other medications. Their use derives from the theory that tissue injury causes both visceral and inflammatory pain as well as neuropathic pain through a sensitization process that is both peripheral and central in CNS origin. They are standard in the treatment of neuropathic pain but are less commonly prescribed for acute pain. A meta-analysis did not observe any differences between the efficacy of gabapentin and pregabalin but demonstrated analgesic efficacy and dose-dependent opioid-sparing effect with gabapentin when used after spine surgery.[54]

Opioids

Opioids continue to be used in the multimodal approach but are delivered whenever possible through different routes to minimize systemic absorption and activation of addiction pathways. These include intrathecal or epidural opioids as well as long-acting multireceptor opioids such as methadone.

The prolonged duration of action of intrathecal and epidural opioids can decrease systemic opioid consumption for up to 24 hours.[55] The downside of this route of administration includes central respiratory depression, which requires respiratory monitoring until past the peak effect of the medication (about 18 hours). Other clinically significant side effects include pruritus and nausea/vomiting.[56]

Methadone is well-established in treatment of opioid addiction but has only recently found favor with treatment of acute pain. It can be administered intraoperatively or as a scheduled medication postoperatively. Advantages include a long half-life without associated symptoms of "opioid euphoria," which decreases its addictive potential, as well as its multireceptor mechanism of action. Methadone has NMDA-antagonism activity similar to ketamine and also acts as a serotonin-reuptake inhibitor, which elevates mood and improves perception of pain.[57] At high doses methadone can cause prolongation of the QT-interval and even torsades de pointes; patients on chronic therapy require interval monitoring with electrocardiograms.

Summary

With an aging population and rapid advancements in medical care, increasingly complex patients are presenting for both elective and emergency orthopaedic surgery with alarming regularity. These patients require multifaceted perioperative care—from evaluation and optimization of preoperative conditions in elective procedures, to thorough assessment, resuscitation, and surgical intervention in acute traumas, to eventual postoperative mobilization and functional recovery. In the advent of cost-containment efforts and bundled payments, physicians are more than ever compelled to minimize utilization of hospital resources while reducing patient complications. These, in combination with the increasing importance of self-reported pain management quality and patient satisfaction scores, pose many challenges for the modern orthopaedic surgeon. Based on our review of the literature, we feel that a collaborative approach to the treatment of these patients—such as through the creation of multidisciplinary teams with dedicated institution-specific clinical care pathways—is likely to be the most successful.

Study Points

- Increasing patient complexity in the face of outcome-based cost-containment efforts necessitates a thorough but efficient preoperative assessment process.
- Institutions should develop preoperative care pathways founded on sound and up-to-date evidence and ensure high compliance among its team members.
- Appropriate evaluation of the orthopaedic trauma patient should include triaging of care, timing of surgery, and utilization of health care resources; adherence to practice guidelines for geriatric trauma patients is of particular importance in these regards.
- Optimal pain management includes the employment of multimodal analgesia and deterrence of opioid prescriptions whenever possible.
- Successful multimodal pain management requires collaboration between all the members of the perioperative team as well as organizational consistency. (eg, All minimally invasive spine surgeons agree to use the same ERAS pathway.)

Annotated References

1. Sheffield KM, McAdams PS, Benarroch-Gampel J, et al: Overuse of preoperative cardiac stress testing in medicare patients undergoing elective noncardiac surgery. *Ann Surg* 2013;257(1):73.
2. Abbas K, Umer M, Askari R: Preoperative cardiac evaluation in proximal femur fractures and its effects on the surgical outcome. *Acta Orthop Traumatol Ture* 2012;46(4):250-254.
3. Lee TH, Marcantonio ER, Mangione CM, et al: Derivation and prospective validation of a simple index for prediction of cardiac risk of major noncardiac surgery. *Circulation* 1999;100(10):1043-1049.
4. VISION Pilot Study Investigators, Devereaux PJ, Bradley D, Chan MT, et al: An international prospective cohort study evaluating major vascular complications among patients undergoing noncardiac surgery: The VISION pilot study. *Open Med* 2011;5(4):e193.
5. Gupta PK, Gupta H, Sundaram A, et al: Development of a risk calculator for prediction of cardiac risk after surgery. *Circulation* 2011;124:381-387.
6. Waterman BR, Belmont PJ, Bader JO, et al: The total joint arthroplasty cardiac risk index for predicting perioperative myocardial infarction and cardiac arrest after primary total knee and hip arthroplasty. *J Arthroplasty* 2016;31:1170-1174.

   TJA CRI predicted postoperative cardiac complications better than the RCRI.
7. Rockwood K, Mitnitski A: Frailty defined by deficit accumulation and geriatric medicine defined by frailty. *Clin Geriatr Med* 2011;27(1):17.
8. Shin JI, Keswani A, Lovy A, et al: Simplified frailty index as a predictor of adverse outcomes in total hip and knee arthroplasty. *J Arthroplasty* 2016;31:2389-2394.

   TJA-specific frailty index better predicts outcomes in elderly patients.
9. Fleisher LA, Fleischmann KE, Auerbach AD, et al: 2014 ACC/AHA Guideline on perioperative cardiovascular evaluation and management of patients undergoing noncardiac surgery. *Circulation* 2014;130(24):2215-2245.
10. Levine GN, Bates ER, Bittl JA, et al: 2016 ACC/AHA Guideline focused update on duration of dual antiplatelet therapy in patients with coronary artery disease. *Circulation* 2016;134(10):e123-55.

    Guidelines for perioperative approach to cardiac stents. Level of evidence: I.
11. Young EM, Farmer JD: Preoperative chest radiography in elective surgery: Review and update. *S D Med* 2017;70(2):81-87.

    Preoperative chest radiography is recommended only if indicated after a thorough history and physical and rarely adds additional information.
12. Smetana GW, Lawrence VA, Cornell JE: Preoperative pulmonary risk stratification for noncardiothoracic surgery: Systematic review for the American college of physicians. *Ann Intern Med* 2006;144:581-595.

13. Gwon H-C, Hahn J-Y, Park KW, et al: Six-month versus 12-month dual antiplatelet therapy after implantation of drug-eluting stents: The efficacy of xience/promus versus cypher to reduce late loss after stenting (EXCELLENT) randomized, multicenter study. *Circulation* 2012;125:505-513.
14. Schulz-Schüpke S, Byrne RA, Ten Berg JM, et al: ISAR-SAFE: A randomized, double-blind, placebo-controlled trial of 6 vs. 12 months of clopidogrel therapy after drug-eluting stenting. *Eur Heart J* 2015;36:1252-1263.
15. Giustino G, Baber U, Sartori S, et al: Duration of dual antiplatelet therapy after drug-eluting stent implantation: A systematic review and meta-analysis of randomized controlled trials. *J Am Coll Cardiol* 2015;65:1298-1310.
16. Teasdale G, Jennett B: Assessment of coma and impaired consciousness. A practical scale. *Lancet* 1974;2(7872):81-84.
17. Baker SP, O'Neill B, Haddon W, et al: The injury severity score: A method for describing patients with multiple injuries and evaluating emergency care. *J Trauma* 1974;14(3):187-196.
18. Boyd CR, Tolson MA, Copes WS: Evaluating trauma care: The TRISS method. *J Trauma* 1987;27(4):370-378.
19. Osler T, Glance L, Buzas JS, et al: A trauma mortality prediction model based on the anatomic injury scale. *Ann Surg* 2008;247:1041-1048.
20. Cook A, Weddle J, Baker S, et al: A comparison of the injury severity score and the trauma mortality prediction model. *J Trauma Acute Care Surg* 2013;76(1):47-53.
21. Haider AH, Villegas CV, Saleem T, et al: Should the ICD-9 Trauma Mortality Prediction Model become the new paradigm for benchmarking trauma outcomes? *J Trauma Acute Care Surg* 2012;72:1695-1701.
22. The ATLS Subcommittee: Advanced Trauma Life Support (ATLS): The ninth edition. *J Trauma Acute Care Surg* 2013;74(5):1363-1366.
23. Camazine MN, Hemmila MR, Leonard JC, et al: Massive transfusion policies at trauma centers participating in the American college of surgeons trauma quality improvement program. *J Trauma Acute Care Surg* 2015;78(6):S48-S53.
24. American College of Surgeons Trauma Quality Improvement Program: Best Practice Guidelines – Massive Transfusion in Trauma. https://www.facs.org/~/media/files/quality%20programs/trauma/tqip/massive%20transfusion%20in%20trauma%20guildelines.ashx.
25. Shakur H, Roberts I, Bautista R, et al: Effects of tranexamic acid on death, vascular occlusive events, and blood transfusion in trauma patients with significant hemorrhage (CRASH-2): A randomized, placebo-controlled trial. *Lancet* 2010;376(9734):23-32.
26. Binz S, McCollester J, Thomas S, et al: CRASH-2 study of tranexamic acid to treat bleeding in trauma patients: A controversy fueled by science and social media. *J Blood Transfusion* 2015;2015:1-12.
27. Sasser SM, Hunt RC, Sullivent EE, et al: Guidelines for field triage of injured patients: recommendations of the National Expert Panel on Field Triage 2008. http://www.cdc.gov/mmwr/preview/mmwrhtml/rr5801a1.htm.
28. Tang A, Hashmi A, Pandit V, et al: A critical analysis of secondary overtriage to a Level I trauma center. *J Trauma Acute Care Surg* 2014;77(6):969-973.
29. Waters PM, Yang BW, White D, et al: A dedicated satellite trauma orthopedic program operating room safely increases capacity. *JBJS* 2018;100:e70.

    Observational report of one institution's method to decrease overburdening of their trauma hospital.
30. Vallier HA, Como JJ, Wagner KG, et al: Team approach: Timing of operative intervention in multiply-injured patients. *JBJS* 2018;6(8):1-7.

    Observational report of one institution's method to facilitate early readiness to OR.
31. Duckworth A, McQueen MM: The diagnosis of acute compartment syndrome: A critical analysis review. *JBJS* 2017;5(12)e1-11.

    Review of evidence-based management of acute compartment syndrome.
32. Gustilo RB, Anderson JT: Prevention of infection in the treatment of one thousand and twenty-five open fractures of long bones: Retrospective and prospective analyses. *JBJS* 1976;58(4):453-458.
33. Schenker ML, Yannascoli S, Baldwin KD, et al: Does timing to operative debridement affect infectious complications in long-bone fractures? *JBJS* 2012;94(12):1057-1064.
34. Weber D, Dulai SK, Bergman J, et al: Time to initial operative treatment following open fracture does not impact development of deep infection: A prospective cohort study of 736 subjects. *J Orthop Trauma* 2014;28:613-619.
35. Lack WD, Karunakar MA, Angerame MR, et al: Type III open tibia fractures: Immediate antibiotic prophylaxis minimizes infection. *J Orthop Trauma* 2015;29:1-6.
36. Calland JF, Ingraham AM, Martin N, et al: Evaluation and management of geriatric trauma: An eastern association for the surgery of trauma practice management guidelines. *J Trauma Acute Care Surg* 2012;73:345-350.
37. Grossman MD, Ofurum U, Stehly CD, et al: Long-term survival after major trauma in geriatric trauma patients: The glass is half full. *J Trauma Acute Care Surg* 2012;72:1181-1185.
38. Anthony CA, Duchman KR, Bedard NA, et al: Hip factures: Appropriate timing to operative intervention. *J Arthroplasty* 2017;32:3314-3318.

    Retrospective study of hip fracture patients to compare timing to OR with risk of complications.
39. Pincus D, Ravi B, Wasserstein D, et al: Association between wait time and 30-day mortality in adults undergoing hip fracture surgery. *J Am Med Assoc* 2017;318(20):1994-2003.

    Retrospective study of hip fracture patients to compare timing to OR with risk of 30-day mortality.
40. Adair C, Swart E, Seymour R, et al: Clinical practice guidelines decrease unnecessary echocardiograms before hip fracture surgery. *JBJS* 2017;99:676-680.

    Retrospective review of preoperative echocardiogram utilization at one institution to determine extent of unnecessary testing.

41. Cohn MR, Levack AE, Trivedi NN, et al: The hip fracture patient on warfarin: Evaluating blood loss and time to surgery. *J Orthop Trauma* 2017;31(8):407-413.

    Retrospective study showing little association between INR and blood loss. Level of evidence: III.

42. Swart E, Kates S, McGee E, et al: The case for comanagement and care pathways for osteoporotic patients with a hip fracture. *JBJS* 2018;100:1343-1350.

    Case report of comanagement pathway at one institution to improve outcomes and reduce costs.

43. Volkow ND, McLellan TA, Cotto JH, et al: Characteristics of opioid prescriptions in 2009. *J Am Med Assoc* 2011;305(13):1299-1301.

44. Wiznia DH, Zaki T, Leslie MP, et al: Complexities of perioperative pain management in orthopedic trauma. *Curr Pain Headache Rep* 2018;22:58.

    Review of pain management in trauma.

45. American Society of Anesthesiologists Task Force on Acute Pain Management: Practice guidelines for acute pain management in the perioperative setting. *Anesthesiology* 2004;100(6):1573-1581.

46. Gabriel RA, Ilfeld BM: Novel methodologies in regional anesthesia for knee arthroplasty. *Anesthesiol Clin* 2018;36(3):387-401.

    Review of cryoablation and peripheral nerve stimulation for analgesia after knee arthroplasty.

47. Stathellis A, Fitz W, Schnurr C, et al: Periarticular injections with continuous perfusion of local anesthetics provide better pain relief and better function compared to femoral and sciatic blocks after TKA: A randomized clinical trial. *Knee Surg Sports Traumatol Arthrosc* 2017;25(9):2702-2707.

    Clinical trial comparing continuous femoral nerve blocks to continuous periarticular injections. Level of evidence: I.

48. Wick EC, Grant M, Wu C, et al: Postoperative multimodal analgesia with nonopioid analgesics and techniques. *JAMA Surg* 2017;152(7):691-697.

    Review of multimodal analgesia.

49. Elia N, Lysakowski C, Tramer MR: Does multimodal analgesia with acetaminophen, nonsteroidal anti-inflammatory drugs, or selective cyclooxygenase-2 inhibitors and patient-controlled analgesia morphine offer advantages over morphine alone? Meta-analyses of randomized trials. *Anesthesiology* 2005;103(6):1296-1304.

50. Kim SI, Ha KI, Oh IS, et al: Preemptive multimodal analgesia for postoperative pain management after lumbar fusion surgery. *Eur Spine J* 2016;25:1614-1619.

    RCT to evaluate preemptive multimodal analgesia at one institution.

51. Naik BI, Nemergut EC, Kazemi A, et al: The effect of dexmedetomidine on postoperative opioid consumption and pain after major spine surgery. *Anesth Analg* 2016;122:1646-1653.

    RCT to evaluate intraoperative dexmedetomidine as adjunctive analgesic in spine surgery.

52. Himmelseher S, Durieux ME: Ketamine for perioperative pain management. *Anesthesiology* 2005;102(1):211-220.

53. Jouguelet-Lacoste J, Colla LL, Schilling D, et al: The use of intravenous infusion or single dose of low-dose ketamine for post-operative analgesia: A review of the current literature. *Pain Med* 2015;16:385-403.

54. Liu B, Liu R, Wang L: A meta-analysis of the preoperative use of gabapentinoids for the treatment of acute postoperative pain following spinal surgery. *Medicine* 2017;96(37):1-11.

    Meta-analysis of 16 clinical trials to validate gabapentinoids for acute pain treatment.

55. Yen D, Turner K, Mark D, et al: Is a single low dose of intrathecal morphine a useful adjunct to patient-controlled analgesia for postoperative pain control following lumbar spine surgery? *Pain Res Manag* 2015;20(3):129-132.

56. Pendi A, Acosta F, Tuchmann A, et al: Intrathecal morphine in spine surgery. *Spine* 2017;42(12):E740-E747.

    Meta-analysis of eight RCTs showing intrathecal morphine decreases opioid consumption after spine surgery. Level of evidence: I.

57. Murphy GS, Szokol JW, Avram M, et al: Clinical effectiveness and safety of intraoperative methadone in patients undergoing posterior spinal fusion surgery. *Anesthesiology* 2017;126:822-833.

    RCT which validates methadone efficacy and safety in spine surgery

Chapter 7

Coagulation and Blood Management

Alexander R. Orem, MD, MS • David S. Jevsevar, MD, MBA

ABSTRACT

The prevention of venous thromboembolic disease is a challenge faced by virtually all orthopaedic surgeons. There is a wide spectrum of strategies for mechanical prophylaxis as well as chemical prophylactic agents available for use with varying levels of efficacy and risk of complication. In addition, achieving the goal of decreasing perioperative blood loss and minimizing the risk of allogeneic blood transfusion after many common orthopaedic procedures has been helped significantly by the use of tranexamic acid, but many questions continue to be investigated regarding its safety and most effective routes of administration. Multimodal approaches to decreasing the risk of perioperative venous thromboembolism and reducing the rate of allogeneic blood transfusions after orthopaedic procedures appear to be the most effective.

Keywords: allogeneic blood transfusion; anticoagulation; safety; tranexamic acid; venous thromboembolic disease

Introduction

Every orthopaedic surgeon will experience the related challenges of trying to prevent venous thromboembolic disease while simultaneously working to minimize perioperative blood loss and the risk of allogeneic blood transfusion. It is imperative that surgeons are aware of the most recent guidelines, recommendations, and research that can inform decisions to manage these conditions. To prevent venous thromboembolism (VTE), there are many mechanical and chemical strategies available with risks and benefits to each. For blood management, the use of tranexamic acid (TXA) has become the predominant strategy to minimize blood loss and decrease risk of blood transfusion after joint replacement surgery. Research continues to establish the most effective indications for TXA as well as to determine the appropriate safety guidelines for its use. In general, effective perioperative management of the risk of excess coagulation or bleeding requires a multimodal approach and careful examination of patient and surgical factors.

Dr. Jevsevar or an immediate family member is a member of a speakers' bureau or has made paid presentations on behalf of MedScape; has received research or institutional support from DePuy, A Johnson & Johnson Company; and serves as a board member, owner, officer, or committee member of the American Association of Hip and Knee Surgeons. Neither Dr. Orem nor any immediate family member has received anything of value from or has stock or stock options held in a commercial company or institution related directly or indirectly to the subject of this chapter.

Anticoagulation

Venous thromboembolism (VTE) is a spectrum of conditions ranging from asymptomatic deep vein thrombosis (DVT) to fatal pulmonary embolism (PE) that is a potential postoperative complication for most surgical procedures including orthopaedic surgeries. Orthopaedic surgeons should be aware of the surgical and patient-specific factors that contribute to VTE. Assessing these individual risk factors for VTE and weighing them against the possible risks associated with anticoagulation afford the orthopaedic surgeon a paradigm to effectively integrate the current mechanical and pharmacological treatments along with numerous published evidence-based clinical practice guidelines (CPGs) and utilize that information in limiting the risk of VTE in orthopaedic patient care.

Risk of Venous Thromboembolism

The historical rates of nonprophylaxis patients with postoperative (or nonsurgical) VTE are variable within orthopaedic surgery but have been reported as high as 65% to 80% in high-risk populations, with 2% to 7% incidence of fatal PE.[1] While much of the initial research

Principles of Orthopaedics

on VTE in orthopaedics was related to hip and knee surgery, VTE has been reported in most orthopaedic specialty patients. Pediatric orthopaedic patient risk for VTE is lower (0.058%) than adults, but at-risk patients should be assessed for VTE prophylaxis requirements. As the practice of orthopaedic surgery has moved in the direction of more ambulatory (outpatient) procedures, VTE risk assessment could have considerable impact on choice and duration of care for patients with higher risk profiles.

VTE prophylaxis is available in several forms ranging from mechanical prophylaxis using various compression devices to pharmacological prophylaxis including intravenous (IV) or subcutaneous heparin formulations and oral agents including aspirin (acetylsalicylic acid, ASA), warfarin, factor IIa direct thrombin inhibitors (dabigatran), and factor Xa inhibitors (low-molecular-weight heparins [LMWHs], fondaparinux, apixaban, and rivaroxaban). Familiarity with the mechanism of action of each modality, the potential risks of that modality for a specific patient and procedure, and the existing guideline recommendations are helpful in prescribing appropriate care.

Types of Venous Thromboembolism Prophylaxis

Mechanical

Mechanical VTE prophylaxis is used in many surgical specialties as the sole prophylactic treatment and has evidence for efficacy in orthopaedic spine procedures where the risks of bleeding associated with pharmacological therapy outweigh the benefits. Intermittent pneumatic compression (IPC) is a common form of DVT prophylaxis, and the antithrombotic effect of IPC is thought to be the result of increased venous velocity and stimulation of endogenous fibrinolysis. The American College of Chest Physicians (ACCP) guidelines recommend using battery-powered (portable) IPC devices because of greater patient acceptance and compliance.[2] The Surgical Care Improvement Project (SCIP) recommends use of either IPC or venous foot pumps. Compliance to the prescribed treatment protocol is of concern in the ambulatory setting. IPC can also be challenging to use in many orthopaedic conditions, where fracture, open wounds, and external fixators can limit applicability. Mechanical prophylaxis is routinely used intraoperatively where possible, and also commonly as an adjunct VTE prophylactic measure with other pharmacological therapies.

The rate of VTE in spine surgery has been reported between 0.3% and 31% and mechanical prophylaxis has been used as an isolated treatment in spine surgery.[3] The evidence base supporting this practice is limited, and further research into appropriate VTE prophylaxis in this population is warranted. VTE rates in shoulder surgery are not as well delineated, with smaller studies reporting incidences of PE of 0.6% to 3%.[4] Most authors recommend the use of mechanical VTE devices with pharmacological therapy based on patient risk factors.

Pharmacological

Aspirin

Aspirin inhibits the aggregation of newly produced platelets irreversibly and minimizes the risk of thrombosis via its inhibitory effect on cyclooxygenase (COX)-1. The antiplatelet effect of ASA lasts for the 7- to 10-day life of the platelets. The use of ASA has increased since its inclusion in the 2012 ACCP VTE Guidelines. It is attractive because of its efficacy, low cost, relative ease of use, lack of laboratory monitoring, and patient acceptance. Studies report using ASA in combination with other therapies, including mechanical prophylaxis. The additive effect of ASA plus mechanical prophylaxis has not been proven.[5] ASA has also been used post discharge in combination with LMWH with noninferior effect on VTE and a lower bleeding risk.[6] ASA has a documented lower incidence of bleeding complications, which may help to explain the observed decreased rate of periprosthetic joint infection of 0.4% compared with 1.5% with warfarin.[7]

The optimal dosage of ASA is unclear, but orthopaedic surgeons should consider using the minimal dosage of ASA needed to achieve VTE prophylaxis goals. In several trials, 160 mg of ASA has been shown to be an efficacious regimen.[8] Gastrointestinal bleeding remains a concern with the use of ASA, and a history of gastrointestinal bleeding should be factored into the decision for use by the orthopaedic surgeon.

Warfarin

Warfarin acts as a vitamin K-dependent clotting inhibitor affecting factors II, VII, IX, and X (**Figure 1**). Warfarin has a long history of clinical use for VTE prophylaxis in arthroplasty patients, and its efficacy and adverse effect profiles are generally understood by the orthopaedic community. It requires individualized patient dosing and close outpatient monitoring with laboratory testing for its duration of use. Because of the longer half-life of warfarin, initially achieving appropriate blood international normalized

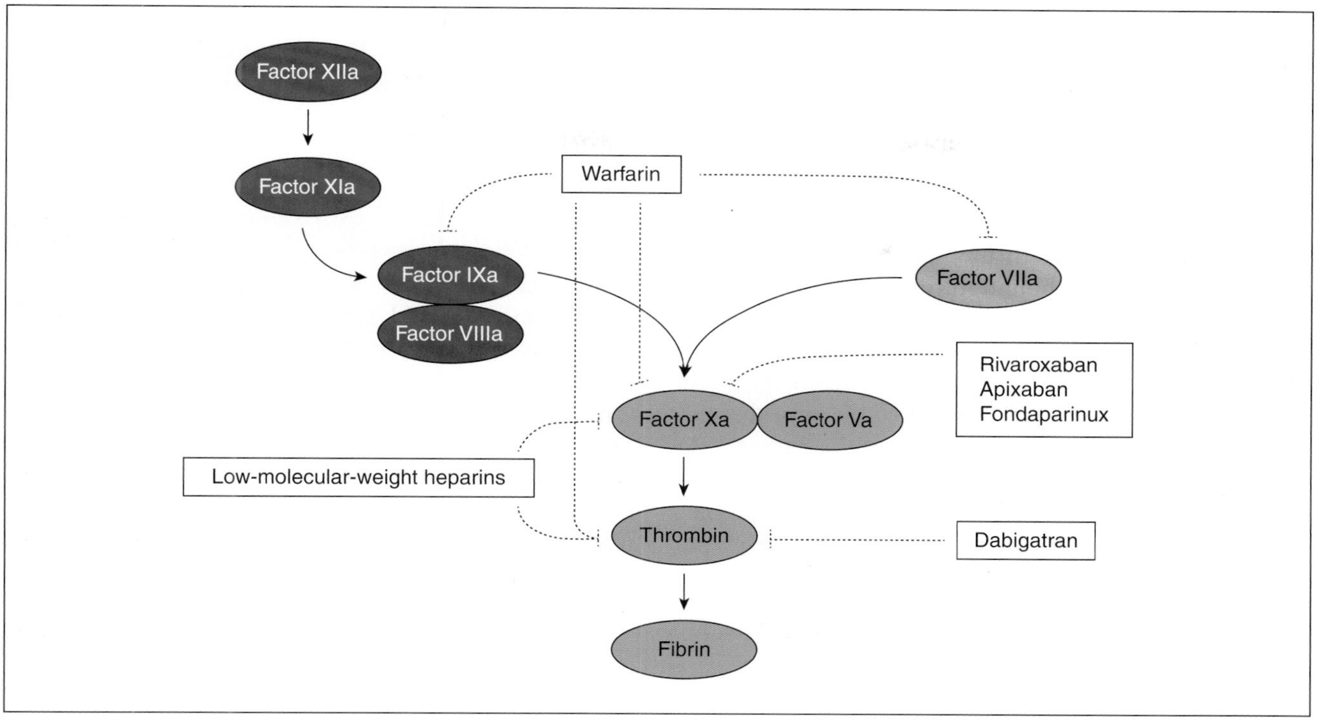

Figure 1 Diagram showing the coagulation cascade and pharmacologic targets. Aspirin, an antiplatelet agent, is not shown. (Reproduced with permission from Lieberman JR, Heckmann N: Venous thromboembolic disease prophylaxis after total hip arthroplasty, in Lieberman JR, Berry DJ, eds: *Advanced Reconstruction: Hip 2*. Rosemont, IL, American Academy of Orthopaedic Surgeons, 2017, pp 379-386.)

ratio (INR) levels can be challenging. Bridging therapy, where LMWH is used to anticoagulate the patient until a therapeutic INR is reached, has been shown to be efficacious for VTE prophylaxis but also with an increased risk for clinically important bleeding episodes.[9] Maintenance of adequate INR levels can be difficult to accomplish, and the effect of warfarin can be altered by a number of different foods. High INR levels associated with the use of warfarin can lead to life-threatening bleeding, hematoma formation, and wound problems.

Low-Molecular-Weight Heparins and Indirect Factor Xa Inhibitors

LMWHs bind antithrombin (AT) to inactivate factor Xa and prevent the conversion of prothrombin to thrombin, as well as prevent the conversion of fibrinogen to fibrin. Fondaparinux binds and enhances the anti-Xa activity of AT to a much greater extent but does not directly inhibit factor Xa. Both agents are approved by the U.S. FDA for VTE prophylaxis in both hip and knee arthroplasty patients. These agents do not require laboratory test monitoring but are given by subcutaneous injection. Because of the requirement for injection, patient compliance can be adversely affected. A study of trauma patients at a Level 1 Trauma Center showed that patients prefer the use of oral anticoagulants for VTE prophylaxis when indicated.[10] Several randomized controlled trials (RCTs) have compared LMWH with warfarin, finding similar VTE prophylaxis efficacy but increased bleeding risk.[11,12] RCTs comparing fondaparinux with LMWH found fondaparinux decreased VTE events but with increased risk for major bleeding complications.[13,14]

Direct Factor Xa Inhibitors

Apixaban and rivaroxaban are oral anticoagulants that work by directly inhibiting factor Xa. They are approved by the FDA for VTE prophylaxis in hip and knee arthroplasty patients. These anticoagulants also do not require routine laboratory monitoring. Multiple clinical trials have compared apixaban 2.5 mg twice daily with enoxaparin at enoxaparin dosages of 40 mg daily and 30 mg twice daily.[15,16] In these studies, apixaban reduced clinically relevant bleeding episodes by 16%. Multiple trials compared rivaroxaban 10 mg daily with enoxaparin dosing of 40 mg daily and one trial, with enoxaparin dosing of 30 mg twice daily.[17,18] Rivaroxaban significantly reduced the rate of VTE events by 45% but was also associated with an increase in clinically relevant bleeds of 27%. The dosing regimen used in most of these studies started these agents at 6 to 8 hours after surgery. Some have advocated for the delayed start of these agents until 18 to 24 hours postoperatively.[19]

Direct Thrombin Inhibitors

Dabigatran is a direct thrombin inhibitor, inhibiting both free and fibrin-bound thrombin. Dabigatran is FDA approved for hip arthroplasty only in the United States. Most clinical trials have compared dabigatran dosages of 150 mg or 220 mg daily with enoxaparin 30 mg twice daily, and one trial compared the same dosages of dabigatran with enoxaparin 30 mg twice daily.[20,21] At the 150 mg dosage, there was an increase in VTE events of 19% with no difference in bleeding complications. The 220 mg dosage showed no difference in VTE events or bleeding risk.

A recent meta-analysis of the newer oral anticoagulants for VTE prophylaxis graphically compared the relative risk of VTE with the relative risk of bleeding and is a helpful guide to the use of these agents.[22] (**Figure 2**).

Risk Stratification

More recent work on VTE prophylaxis has centered on the concept of risk stratification, specifically identifying those patient populations and patient comorbidities that create increased risk for VTE complications. One study retrospectively reviewed institutional data on more than 25,000 patients who had received either warfarin or ASA.[23] Independent risk factors for VTE in this patient population included total knee arthroplasty, elevated Charlson Comorbidity Index, atrial fibrillation, postoperative DVT, chronic obstructive

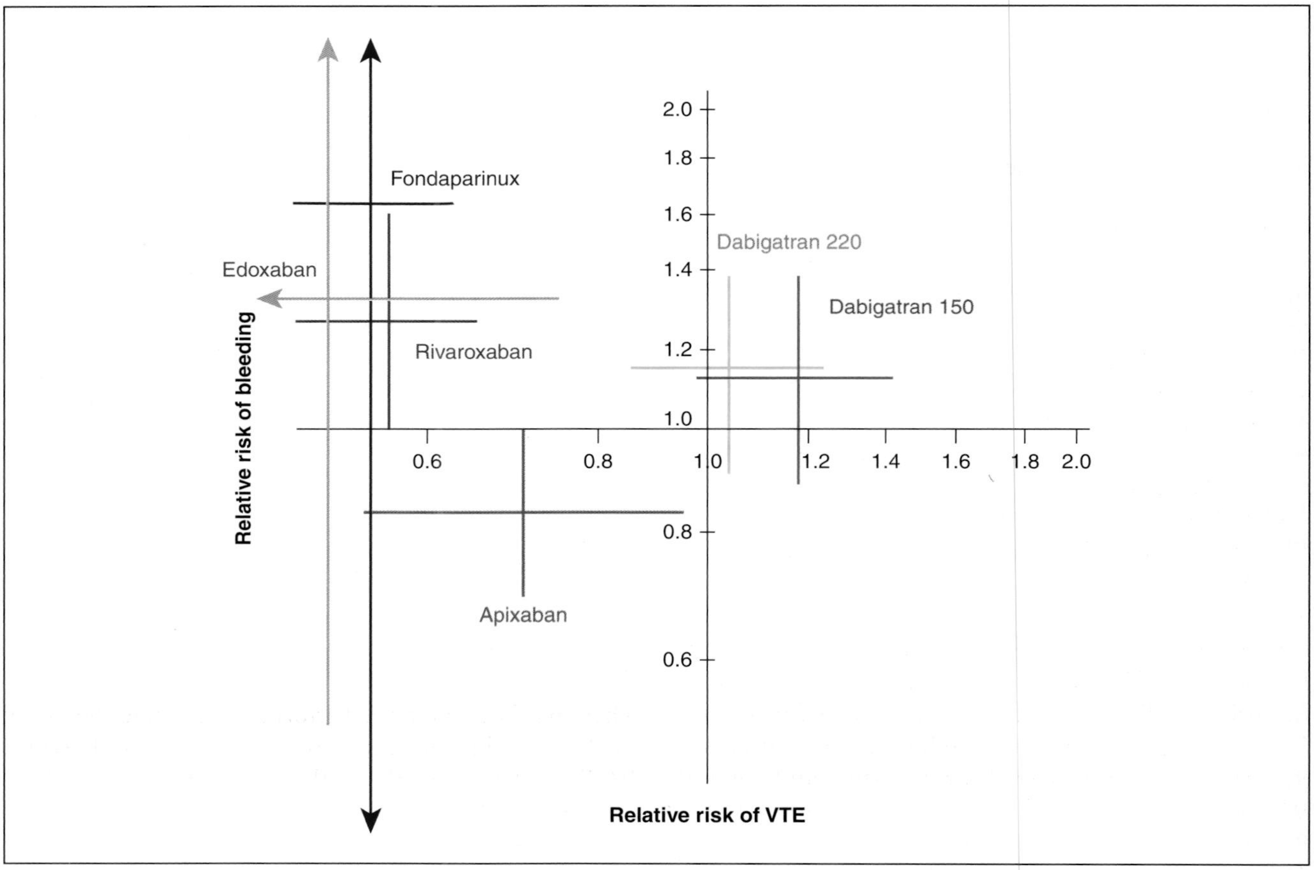

Figure 2 Illustration demonstrating relative risk (RR) of bleeding versus RR of venous thromboembolism (VTE). The black circle at the origin (1.0, 1.0) shows enoxaparin, the referent therapy. The RR of bleeding, either major or nonmajor clinically relevant bleeding, is represented in the vertical axis and the RR of VTE is represented in the horizontal axis. Each cross shows the 95% confidence intervals of the RR from a meta-analysis. (Reprinted from Venker BT, Ganti BR, Lin H, Lee ED, Nunley RM, Gage BF: Safety and efficacy of new anticoagulants for the prevention of venous thromboembolism after hip and knee arthroplasty: A meta-analysis. *J Arthroplasty* 2017;32:645-652, Copyright 2017, with permission of Elsevier.)

pulmonary disease, anemia, depression, and obesity. The authors created a risk nomogram of low- (PE rate 0.35%), medium- (PE rate 1.4%), and high-risk (PE rate of 9.3%) patients, but also found that anticoagulant choice was not predictive of symptomatic PE. Another group used the American College of Surgeons National Surgical Quality Improvement Program (NSQIP) database to analyze independent risk factors for symptomatic PE in 72,673 total hip arthroplasty (THA) and 45,800 total knee arthroplasty (TKA) patients.[24] Female sex, body mass index (BMI) of 25 to 30 kg/m^2, BMI ≥ 30 kg/m^2, age ≥ 70, and TKA were found to be independent risk factors, and the authors developed a risk stratification point system. This risk stratification scoring system was then validated at a single, high-volume institution. The observed symptomatic PE rate in this study was 0.44%, 1.51%, and 2.60% for low-, medium-, and high-risk patients, respectively, according to the scoring system.

Published Guidelines for Venous Thromboembolism Prevention

The publication of the ACCP 2012 Guidelines for Prevention of Venous Thromboembolism in Orthopaedic Surgery Patients provided a significant directional change from their previous guidelines.[2] In response to concern from the orthopaedic community and the release of the American Academy of Orthopaedic Surgeons 2011 Guidelines for Preventing Venous Thromboembolism Before Elective Hip or Knee Arthroplasty, the ACCP no longer used the screening for asymptomatic VTE events as their outcome of interest.[25] The ACCP also weighed the benefits of VTE prophylaxis against the risks of bleeding. With the convergence of guideline recommendations and the Surgical Care Improvement Project's (SCIP's) acceptance of ASA as an acceptable prophylaxis treatment, greater harmonization of VTE prophylaxis has occurred. The Orthopaedic Trauma Association recently published consensus recommendations on VTE prophylaxis in orthopaedic trauma patients.[26] Research continues into risk stratification and optimal VTE prophylaxis choice, including the Comparative Effectiveness of Pulmonary Embolism Prevention After Hip and Knee Replacement (PEPPER) Trial which is an open-label, randomized, parallel assignment trial in 25,000 patients comparing ASA, warfarin (target INR of 2.0), and rivaroxaban. Further study of VTE prevention in orthopaedic patients at risk is necessary.

Blood Management

Blood management is an important principle in orthopaedic surgery and significant effort has been made to reduce the risks associated with blood loss and subsequent blood transfusions. With significant costs associated with previously utilized predonation and intraoperative cell salvage and risks of transfusion being more clearly defined and understood, more recent efforts have focused on prevention of blood loss using medications such as TXA. TXA was used sporadically in orthopaedics beginning in the mid-1990s, and its use has become widespread over the past decade. TXA is an antifibrinolytic agent that works by competitively inhibiting lysine-binding sites on plasminogen, thereby preventing its conversion to plasmin and slowing the process of fibrinolysis.

Efficacy of Tranexamic Acid

The efficacy of TXA therapy at reducing perioperative blood loss and reducing the rate of postoperative blood transfusions after both TKA and THA has been well established.[27,28] A new CPG published in 2018 and endorsed by the American Academy of Orthopaedic Surgeons (AAOS), the American Association of Hip and Knee Surgeons (AAHKS), the American Society of Regional Anesthesia and Pain Medicine (ASRA), The Hip Society, and The Knee Society reports strong evidence supporting the use of TXA in appropriate total joint arthroplasty (TJA) patients to reduce perioperative blood loss and reduce the risk of postoperative transfusion.[29] Additionally, there are data supporting the efficacy of IV TXA at reducing postoperative blood loss and blood transfusion rates after bilateral TKA.[30] Other studies have demonstrated safe and effective use of IV TXA after revision of both THA and TKA.[31,32]

Safety of Tranexamic Acid

There has been continued effort at examining the safety of TXA in higher risk patient populations. Previous RCTs and meta-analyses that have demonstrated no difference in rates of VTE complications have specifically excluded high-risk patients with a history of DVT or PE.[27,33] Among studies that have included high-risk patients, a retrospective cohort study of 3,159 surgeries in 2,780 patients showed no difference in thromboembolic events after surgery on patients who received a bolus of 1 g of IV TXA prior to incision (n = 2,766) and surgery on high-risk patients who did not receive TXA (n = 393).[34] Patients in this study were contraindicated for TXA absolutely if they had experienced a DVT or other clotting complication in the three months prior to surgery, a history of severe kidney failure, previous allergy to TXA, or a history of disseminated intravascular coagulation. Relative contraindications for TXA included any history of DVT or PE and any family history of clotting disorder. Clinically suspected thrombotic complications were confirmed by venous Doppler ultrasonography for DVT and spiral chest CT for PE. The rate of confirmed thromboembolic events within 90 days of surgery (including myocardial infarction) was 1.0% in the TXA+ group and 1.0% in the TXA− group ($P = -0.55$). Another retrospective registry-level study of the Mayo Clinic Joint Replacement Database examined rates of VTE among 13,262 TJA surgeries in 11,175 patients.[35] The rate of VTE after TXA+ surgery was 1.3% and 1.5% after TXA− surgery (n = 10,477). The odds ratio for VTE after TXA was not statistically significant (OR = 0.98, CI = 0.67-1.45, P = 0.939). A second retrospective study also using the registry sought to specifically identify patients who had a history of previous VTE.[36] Patients with a documented history of DVT or PE were included with 1,620 arthroplasty surgeries. For 258 surgeries, the patient received a 1 g IV bolus of TXA at incision and another 1 g IV bolus at closure. For the remaining 1,362 surgeries, the patient did not receive any TXA. No topical TXA was used. The primary outcome for this study was evidence of VTE within 90 days of surgery. The rate of recurrent VTE in the TXA+ group was 2.3%, versus 1.8% in the TXA− group ($P = 0.599$). After a case-control matched analysis, the odds ratio for recurrent DVT in the group receiving TXA was 0.9 (CI = 0.29-2.75, $P = 0.85$). Another registry-level study involving more than 34,000 surgeries and more than 17,000 patients receiving TXA did not show an increase in VTE complications, including cardiovascular events, in patients receiving TXA.[37] In each of these previous studies, the authors concluded that TXA was likely safe to use in patients with prior history of VTE.

A recent direct meta-analysis of the safety of TXA was conducted to inform the 2018 CPG.[38] This meta-analysis included 77 high-level randomized clinical trials and concluded that the use of TXA did not increase the risk of VTE complication in TJA patients. In a subgroup analysis, patients with an American Society of Anesthesia score greater than 3 were used to represent patients at high risk for VTE complication such as a history of cardiac stents, previous DVT, or stroke. The study group concluded that moderate evidence exists that TXA can be safely administered in high-risk patients. They also conclude that these are the patients that are most likely to benefit from decreased blood loss and lower risk of transfusion, and they advocate for the use of TXA on a more regular basis while still taking individual patient factors into consideration. Ultimately, the CPG reported moderate evidence that TXA does not increase the risk of VTE complications in patients who are otherwise at higher risk. They reported that 983 patients in the TJA population would need to be treated with TXA to cause a VTE complication, but the number needed to treat with TXA to prevent a blood transfusion was three TKA patients and four THA patients.[29]

Alternative Routes of Tranexamic Acid Administration

Another focus of study on antifibrinolytic therapy involves the efficacy and cost of alternative routes of administration. Topical, or intra-articular (IA), TXA is directly applied to the tissue by the surgeon after fascial closure or tourniquet release. One recent RCT examined the effect of IA TXA versus IV TXA in TKA patients.[39] IA TXA was given as a 3,000-mg dose injected into the knee after wound closure. IV TXA was given as 3,000 mg in divided doses of 1,000 mg each, the first given prior to incision or prior to deflation of the tourniquet, with two additional 1,000 mg doses given every 8 hours after surgery. There were no differences between the IA and IV groups in either postoperative decrease in hemoglobin or in length of stay. There were no transfusions needed in either group. There was no statistically significant difference in postoperative complications between the groups. A similar RCT comparing IA and IV TXA in THA found similar effectiveness and safety using 2 g of IA or IV TXA.[40] Subsequent meta-analysis have confirmed the efficacy of IA TXA in reducing blood loss and risk of transfusion for both TKA and THA,[41,42] but no studies have shown clear superiority of either IA or IV formulations.

Several studies have looked at the effectiveness of combined dosing of both IA and IV formulations during surgery. One prospective RCT divided THA patients into three groups.[43] Group 1 received combined IV (15 mg/kg) plus topical (1 g) TXA, Group 2 received IV only (15 mg/kg), and Group 3 received placebo. There was a clear dose-response from placebo to combined dosing, with the combined group showing statistically improved hemoglobin and hematocrit levels on postoperative day 3, decreased intraoperative recorded blood loss and total blood loss, and decreased transfusion rates ($P < 0.05$). There was no difference between the three groups regarding postoperative VTE complications or hip function.

The 2018 CPG was informed by two network meta-analyses which sought to identify the most effective routes and timing of administration, as well as any differences in effectiveness between IV, IA, and oral formulations for THA and TKA patients.[44,45] For TKA patients, they compared TXA given IV high dose (>20 mg/kg or >1 g), IV low dose (<20 mg/kg or <1 g), topical high dose (>1.5 g), topical low dose (<1.5 g), oral (at least 2 g given 2 hours prior to incision), combined topical/IV, and combined IV/oral. There were not enough high-quality data for combined IV/oral dosing, and this was excluded from the final meta-analysis.[45] They reported no difference in efficacy between the various formulations of TXA at reducing blood loss and risk of transfusion, nor did they find any additional benefit to higher dosing or multiple dosing. They did report an apparent benefit of administration of TXA prior to skin incision for TKA.[45] The THA meta-analysis evaluated the same dosages and routes of administration.[44] They found similar results to the TKA analysis, with all formulations and dosing of TXA reducing the risk of blood loss and transfusion, with no significant difference between the various formulations.

Cost-Effectiveness and Alternatives to Tranexamic Acid

The cost-effectiveness of TXA is of interest because it will likely be administered in over one million arthroplasty procedures annually in the United States. One recent study seeking to evaluate the cost-effectiveness of routine TXA administration established a number-needed-to-treat of 9.3 patients to prevent one blood transfusion after THA and 8.0 patients after TKA.[46] By reducing their risk of transfusion by 54% and despite the cost of using IV TXA, they established that their use of IV TXA saved $34 per TKA and $59 per THA. Oral administration of TXA has also been an area of recent study, due to the decreased cost of oral TXA, with most oral formulations costing 70% to 90% less than IV formulations. One RCT found that an oral dose of 1,950 mg of TXA given 2 hours prior to THA surgery and 1 g of IV TXA given immediately prior to incision were equivalent in postoperative reduction of hemoglobin, total blood loss, and rate of postoperative blood transfusion.[47] At the authors' institution, the cost of oral TXA was $14 per dose compared with a range of $47 to $108. The savings of oral TXA would be even greater for institutions where multiple doses of IV or topical TXA are used. The same study group found similar efficacy for the same doses of oral and IV TXA prior to TKA with similar cost analysis.[48] Other options for cost reduction with antifibrinolytic therapy include using epsilon aminocaproic acid (EACA), which has been used extensively in cardiac surgery and may have a better safety profile with regard to seizure threshold. It has not been as extensively studied in the orthopaedic literature as TXA, but a retrospective review of its use at a Veterans Administration Medical Center found significant reductions in blood loss after TKA and THA, as well as a reduction in blood transfusion.[49] The contraindications for use in this study were similar to those of TXA in previous RCTs, except for including patients who had a history of seizures or epilepsy. This study did not comment on rates of postoperative VTE.

Allogeneic Blood Transfusion

Allogeneic blood transfusions increase the risk of several complications following elective joint arthroplasty, including infection and mortality. Preoperative anemia, defined as a serum hemoglobin level less than 13 g/dL in men and 12 g/dL in women, is a risk factor for requiring postoperative transfusion.[50] Other risks include female sex, older patients, and patients with lower BMI.[50] Evidence-based transfusion triggers are generally accepted at 7 g/dL in symptomatic patients without significant history of cardiac disease or decreased oxygen carrying capacity and 8 g/dL for patients with these comorbidities. Dedicated protocols for diagnosing and treating preoperative anemia, usually with oral or IV iron therapy and erythropoietin, combined with intraoperative blood loss mitigation strategy in the form of TXA, and adherence to restrictive postoperative transfusion triggers, have demonstrated effectiveness at lowering the transfusion rate even in higher risk patients.[51-53]

Summary

VTE is a common complication after orthopaedic surgery, especially in high-risk patients, and several strategies exist to mitigate this risk. Mechanical strategies include the use of intermittent pneumatic compression devices that can be worn both during and after surgery. Mechanical compression is frequently combined with chemical prophylaxis to prevent VTE. A wide spectrum of pharmacologic agents exists to decrease the risk of VTE. The risk of clotting must be balanced against the risks of bleeding complications with many of these medications. Aspirin has proven efficacy at VTE prevention and is frequently used in conjunction with mechanical compression. Aspirin has lower bleeding risks than many other pharmacologic strategies. Warfarin continues to be commonly used for VTE prevention but requires significant resources to maintain safety and efficacy. Other agents include both injectable and oral formulations and have variable efficacy and safety profiles. It is important to identify patients that may be at increased risk of VTE complications so that mitigation strategies can be customized.

Minimizing perioperative blood loss and reducing risk of allogeneic blood transfusion is another important aspect of blood management. The most commonly used agent in this regard is TXA, which has several different routes of administration. Oral and intra-articular formulations have similar efficacy at reducing blood loss and transfusion rates when compared with IV TXA. There has also been significant effort at establishing safety guidelines for the use of TXA, out of concern for causing VTE complications. Multiple RCT and meta-analysis have shown no increased risk of VTE complications with the use of TXA, even in patients considered high risk for VTE. There is still little evidence regarding its safety in patients who are known to have active DVT or are within 3 months of cardiac stenting. Multimodal blood management strategies including preoperative screening for anemia, the use of TXA, and using appropriate triggers for postoperative transfusion are effective at significantly decreasing the rate of allogeneic blood transfusion and their inherent risks.

Key Study Points

- Aspirin and mechanical compression are effective at reducing risk of VTE in normal-risk patients with minimal risk of bleeding.
- Warfarin and LMWH are both effective at VTE prevention, but both come with serious drawbacks. Several new oral agents such as factor Xa inhibitors and direct thrombin inhibitors have been developed to manage VTE risk. These oral agents may be effective for many patients, but concerns remain regarding their bleeding risk.
- TXA is effective at reducing blood loss and transfusion rate after TJA. IV, topical, and oral formulations exist and have similar effectiveness and safety profiles. Oral TXA may be the most cost-effective.
- TXA does not appear to increase the risk of VTE complications, even in patients considered high risk for VTE.
- Multimodal strategies for identifying patients at high risk for transfusion preoperatively, minimizing blood loss perioperatively with TXA, and following a restrictive transfusion strategy postoperatively is effective at reducing allogeneic blood transfusion.

Annotated References

1. Geerts WH, Pineo GF, Heit JA, et al: Prevention of venous thromboembolism: The seventh ACCP conference on antithrombotic and thrombolytic therapy. *Chest* 2004;126:338S-400S.
2. Falck-Ytter Y, Francis CW, Johanson NA, et al: Prevention of VTE in orthopedic surgery patients: Antithrombotic therapy and prevention of thrombosis, 9th ed: American College of Chest Physicians evidence-based clinical practice guidelines. *Chest* 2012;141:e278S-e325S.
3. Kepler CK, McKenzie J, Kreitz T, Vaccaro A: Venous thromboembolism prophylaxis in spine surgery. *J Am Acad Orthop Surg* 2018;26:489-500.

   Narrative review of the pathophysiology and treatments for VTE prophylxis in patients undergoing spine surgery. Level of evidence: V.
4. Aibinder WR, Sanchez-Sotelo J: Venous thromboembolism prophylaxis in shoulder surgery. *Orthop Clin North Am* 2018;49:257-263.

   Narrative review of the pathophysiology and treatments for VTE prophylxis in patients undergoing shoulder surgery. Level of evidence: V.
5. An VV, Phan K, Levy YD, Bruce WJ: Aspirin as thromboprophylaxis in hip and knee arthroplasty: A systematic review and meta-analysis. *J Arthroplasty* 2016;31:2608-2616.

   Systematic review and meta-analysis of the use of ASA for VTE prophylaxis in hip and knee arthroplasty patients. The analysis conlcudes that ASA is effective for VTE prophylaxis with low bleeding risk, but overall quality of studies is low. Level of evidence: I.
6. Anderson DR, Dunbar MJ, Bohm ER, et al: Aspirin versus low-molecular-weight heparin for extended venous thromboembolism prophylaxis after total hip arthroplasty: A randomized trial. *Ann Intern Med* 2013;158:800-806.
7. Huang R, Buckley PS, Scott B, Parvizi J, Purtill JJ: Administration of aspirin as a prophylaxis agent against venous thromboembolism results in lower incidence of periprosthetic joint infection. *J Arthroplasty* 2015;30:39-41.
8. Pulmonary Embolism Prevention Trial Collaborative Group. Prevention of pulmonary embolism and deep vein thrombosis with low dose aspirin: Pulmonary Embolism Prevention (PEP) trial. *Lancet* 2000;355:1295-1302.
9. Haighton M, Kempen DH, Wolterbeek N, Marting LN, van Dijk M, Veen RM: Bridging therapy for oral anticoagulation increases the risk for bleeding-related complications in total joint arthroplasty. *J Orthop Surg* 2015;10:145.
10. Haac BE, O'Hara NN, Mullins CD, et al: Patient preferences for venous thromboembolism prophylaxis after injury: A discrete choice experiment. *BMJ Open* 2017;7:e016676.

    Prospective discrete choice design in orthopaedic trauma patients at a Level 1 Trauma Center that found patients preferred oral anitcoagulants for VTE prophylaxis when indicated. Level of evidence: II.

11. Hull R, Raskob G, Pineo G, et al: A comparison of subcutaneous low-molecular-weight heparin with warfarin sodium for prophylaxis against deep-vein thrombosis after hip or knee implantation. *N Engl J Med* 1993;329:1370-1376.

12. Colwell CW Jr, Collis DK, Paulson R, et al: Comparison of enoxaparin and warfarin for the prevention of venous thromboembolic disease after total hip arthroplasty. Evaluation during hospitalization and three months after discharge. *J Bone Joint Surg Am* 1999;81:932-940.

13. Turpie AG, Bauer KA, Eriksson BI, Lassen MR, Committee PSS: Postoperative fondaparinux versus postoperative enoxaparin for prevention of venous thromboembolism after elective hip-replacement surgery: A randomised double-blind trial. *Lancet* 2002;359:1721-1726.

14. Lassen MR, Bauer KA, Eriksson BI, Turpie AG, European Pentasaccharide Elective Surgery Study Steering C: Postoperative fondaparinux versus preoperative enoxaparin for prevention of venous thromboembolism in elective hip-replacement surgery: A randomised double-blind comparison. *Lancet (London, England)* 2002;359:1715-1720.

15. Lassen MR, Gallus A, Raskob GE, et al: Apixaban versus enoxaparin for thromboprophylaxis after hip replacement. *N Engl J Med* 2010;363:2487-2498.

16. Lassen MR, Raskob GE, Gallus A, et al: Apixaban versus enoxaparin for thromboprophylaxis after knee replacement (ADVANCE-2): A randomised double-blind trial. *Lancet (London, England)* 2010;375:807-815.

17. Kakkar AK, Brenner B, Dahl OE, et al: Extended duration rivaroxaban versus short-term enoxaparin for the prevention of venous thromboembolism after total hip arthroplasty: A double-blind, randomised controlled trial. *Lancet (London, England)* 2008;372:31-39.

18. Eriksson BI, Borris LC, Friedman RJ, et al: Rivaroxaban versus enoxaparin for thromboprophylaxis after hip arthroplasty. *N Engl J Med* 2008;358:2765-2775.

19. Lieberman JR, Heckmann N: Venous thromboembolism prophylaxis in total hip arthroplasty and total knee arthroplasty patients: From guidelines to practice. *J Am Acad Orthop Surg* 2017;25:789-798.

    Narrative review of the pathophysiology and treatments for VTE prophylxis in patients undergoing hip and knee arthroplasty. Level of evidence: V.

20. Eriksson BI, Dahl OE, Rosencher N, et al: Dabigatran etexilate versus enoxaparin for prevention of venous thromboembolism after total hip replacement: A randomised, double-blind, non-inferiority trial. *Lancet* 2007;370:949-956.

21. Committee R-MW, Ginsberg JS, Davidson BL, et al: Oral thrombin inhibitor dabigatran etexilate vs North American enoxaparin regimen for prevention of venous thromboembolism after knee arthroplasty surgery. *J Arthroplasty* 2009;24:1-9.

22. Venker BT, Ganti BR, Lin H, Lee ED, Nunley RM, Gage BF: Safety and efficacy of new anticoagulants for the prevention of venous thromboembolism after hip and knee arthroplasty: A meta-analysis. *J Arthroplasty* 2017;32:645-652.

    Meta-analysis of the safety and efficacy of the newer anticoagulants in patients receiving VTE prophylaxis within 48 hours of surgery. This analysis found all of the newer anticoagulants to be efficacious, but with varying degrees of bleeding complications. Level of evidence: I.

23. Parvizi J, Huang R, Raphael IJ, Arnold WV, Rothman RH: Symptomatic pulmonary embolus after joint arthroplasty: Stratification of risk factors. *Clin Orthop Relat Res* 2014;472:903-912.

24. Bohl DD, Maltenfort MG, Huang R, Parvizi J, Lieberman JR, Della Valle CJ: Development and validation of a risk stratification system for pulmonary embolism after elective primary total joint arthroplasty. *J Arthroplasty* 2016;31:187-191.

    Retrospective analysis of 118,473 patients from the ACS NSQIP database identifying risk factors for symptomatic pulmonary embolism in patients undergoing hip and knee arthroplasty. A validated scoring system is presented. Level of evidence: III.

25. Mont MA, Jacobs JJ, Boggio LN, et al: Preventing venous thromboembolic disease in patients undergoing elective hip and knee arthroplasty. *J Am Acad Orthop Surg* 2011;19:768-776.

26. Sagi HC, Ahn J, Ciesla D, et al: Venous thromboembolism prophylaxis in orthopaedic trauma patients: A survey of OTA member practice patterns and OTA expert panel recommendations. *J Orthop Trauma* 2015;29:e355-e362.

27. Gandhi R, Evans HM, Mahomed SR, Mahomed NN: Tranexamic acid and the reduction of blood loss in total knee and hip arthroplasty: A meta-analysis. *BMC Res Notes* 2013;6:184.

28. Zhu J, Zhu Y, Lei P, Zeng M, Su W, Hu Y: Efficacy and safety of tranexamic acid in total hip replacement: A PRISMA-compliant meta-analysis of 25 randomized controlled trials. *Medicine (Baltim)* 2017;96:e9552.

    A meta-analysis of 25 randomized trials of IV TXA for hip replacement. The authors found significantly lower blood loss and transfusion rate. They did not find evidence of publication bias. Level of evidence: I.

29. Fillingham YA, Ramkumar DB, Jevsevar DS, et al: Tranexamic acid use in total joint arthroplasty: The clinical practice guidelines endorsed by the American Association of Hip and Knee Surgeons, American Society of Regional Anesthesia and Pain medicine, American Academy of Orthopaedic Surgeons, Hip Society, and Knee Society. *J Arthroplast* 2018;33:3065-3069.

    An updated clinical practice guideline for TXA use endorsed by AAOS, AAHKS, ASRA, The Hip Society, and The Knee Society. The guidelines were based on two network meta-analysis of efficacy and a direct meta-analysis of safety. Level of evidence: I.

30. Chen X, Cao X, Yang C, Guo K, Zhu Q, Zhu J: Effectiveness and safety of fixed-dose tranexamic acid in simultaneous bilateral total knee arthroplasty: A randomized double-blind controlled trial. *J Arthroplast* 2016;31:2471-2475.

31. Park KJ, Couch CG, Edwards PK, Siegel ER, Mears SC, Barnes CL: Tranexamic acid reduces blood transfusions in revision total hip arthroplasty. *J Arthroplast* 2016;31:2850-2855.e1.

This is a retrospective review of 161 consecutive revision THA patients that found patients that received IV TXA had less blood loss and lower transfusion rate than patients that did not receive TXA. There were no VTE complications in the TXA group. Level of evidence: III.

32. Tian P, Liu WB, Li ZJ, Xu GJ, Huang YT, Ma XL: The efficacy and safety of tranexamic acid in revision total knee arthroplasty: A meta-analysis. *BMC Musculoskelet Disord* 2017;18:273.

This meta-analysis of IV TXA in revision TKA found improved blood loss and transfusion rate in the TXA group with no increase in VTE complications. Level of evidence: III.

33. Alshryda S, Sarda P, Sukeik M, Nargol A, Blenkinsopp J, Mason JM: Tranexamic acid in total knee replacement: A systematic review and meta-analysis. *J Bone Joint Surg Br* 2011;93:1577-1585.

34. Madsen RV, Nielsen CS, Kallemose T, Husted H, Troelsen A: Low risk of thromboembolic events after routine administration of tranexamic acid in hip and knee arthroplasty. *J Arthroplast* 2017;32:1298-1303.

This registry study included 3,159 THA or TKA patients. The authors found no difference in VTE complications between groups that received IV TXA and those that did not. Level of evidence: III.

35. Duncan CM, Gillette BP, Jacob AK, Sierra RJ, Sanchez-Sotelo J, Smith HM: Venous thromboembolism and mortality associated with tranexamic acid use during total hip and knee arthroplasty. *J Arthroplast* 2015;30:272-276.

36. Sabbag OD, Abdel MP, Amundson AW, Larson DR, Pagnano MW: Tranexamic acid was safe in arthroplasty patients with a history of venous thromboembolism: A matched outcome study. *J Arthroplast* 2017;32:S246-S50.

This is a registry study including 1,620 patients with a history of VTE who underwent TJA. There was no difference in rate of VTE between patients who received TXA and those that did not. Level of evidence: III.

37. Hallstrom B, Singal B, Cowen ME, Roberts KC, Hughes RE: The Michigan experience with safety and effectiveness of tranexamic acid use in hip and knee arthroplasty. *J Bone Joint Surg Am Vol* 2016;98:1646-1655.

This is a registry study including 34,784 TJA patients. There was decreased blood loss and transfusion rate in the TXA group. There was no difference in the rate of VTE complications between groups. Level of evidence: III.

38. Fillingham YA, Ramkumar DB, Jevsevar DS, et al: The safety of tranexamic acid in total joint arthroplasty: A direct meta-analysis. *J Arthroplast* 2018;33:3070-3082.

This meta-analysis included 78 RCTs and 7,044 patients and was done to inform the safety recommendations for the combined clinical practice guidelines of the AAOS, AAHKS, The Hip Society, The Knee society, and ASRA. They determined that there was no increased risk of VTE complications with TXA, even in patients with ASA of 3 or greater. Level of evidence: I.

39. Goyal N, Chen DB, Harris IA, Rowden NJ, Kirsh G, MacDessi SJ: Intravenous vs intra-articular tranexamic acid in total knee arthroplasty: A randomized, double-blind trial. *J Arthroplast* 2017;32:28-32.

This is a randomized, double-blinded, noninferiority study of 168 unilateral TKA patients who received either topical or IV TXA. They determined that topical TXA was not inferior to IV TXA for hemoglobin decrease on postoperative day 1. No patients were transfused in either TXA group. Level of evidence: I.

40. North WT, Mehran N, Davis JJ, Silverton CD, Weir RM, Laker MW: Topical vs intravenous tranexamic acid in primary total hip arthroplasty: A double-blind, randomized controlled trial. *J Arthroplast* 2016;31:1022-1026.

This is a double-blinded, randomized, controlled trial comparing IV and topical TXA in THA patients. The authors report a trend favoring IV TXA for less Hgb drop. Both groups saw a decrease in transfusion rate compared with previous patients who had not received TXA. Level of evidence: I.

41. Xie J, Hu Q, Huang Q, Ma J, Lei Y, Pei F: Comparison of intravenous versus topical tranexamic acid in primary total hip and knee arthroplasty: An updated meta-analysis. *Thromb Res* 2017;153:28-36.

This meta-analysis included 18 RCTs involving TKA and 4 RCTs involving THA, which involved 2,260 total patients. The drop in Hgb was smaller in the IV TXA group, but there was no difference in transfusion rate between the IV and topical groups. Level of evidence: I.

42. Moskal JT, Capps SG: Intra-articular tranexamic acid in primary total knee arthroplasty: Meta-analysis. *J Knee Surg* 2018;31:56-67.

The authors of this meta-analysis found 41 articles, 3 of which had not been included in previous meta-analysis. They found that topical TXA was protective of blood loss and transfusion risk. They found no increased risk of VTE complications with topical TXA. Level of evidence: I.

43. Yi Z, Bin S, Jing Y, Zongke Z, Pengde K, Fuxing P: Tranexamic acid administration in primary total hip arthroplasty: A randomized controlled trial of intravenous combined with topical versus single-dose intravenous administration. *J Bone Joint Surg Am Vol* 2016;98:983-991.

A prospective, randomized trial of 150 consecutive THA patients. The authors found a dose-response with combined IV and topical TXA compared with monotherapy. There was no difference in VTE complications. Level of evidence: I.

44. Fillingham YA, Ramkumar DB, Jevsevar DS, et al: The efficacy of tranexamic acid in total hip arthroplasty: A network meta-analysis. *J Arthroplast* 2018;33:3083-3089.

This network meta-analysis was done to inform the combined clinical practice guidelines of the AAOS, AAHKS, The Hip Society, The Knee Society, and ASRA. Sixty-seven included studies examined the use of IV, oral, and topical TXA. All formulations provided benefit regarding blood loss and transfusion rate. No formulation or dosage provided clear benefit above others. Level of evidence: I.

45. Fillingham YA, Ramkumar DB, Jevsevar DS, et al: The efficacy of tranexamic acid in total knee arthroplasty: A network meta-analysis. *J Arthroplast* 2018;33:3090-3098.e1.

This network meta-analysis was done to inform the combined CPG of the AAOS, AAHKS, The Hip Society, The Knee society, and ASRA. Sixty-seven included studies examined the use of IV, oral, and topical TXA. All formulations provided clear benefit regarding blood loss and transfusion rate. No formulation or dosage provided clear benefit above others. There was benefit to dosing of TXA prior to incision. Level of evidence: I.

46. Evangelista PJ, Aversano MW, Koli E, et al: Effect of tranexamic acid on transfusion rates following total joint arthroplasty: A cost and comparative effectiveness analysis. *Orthop Clin N Am* 2017;48:109-115.

This is a retrospective review and cost analysis of IV TXA for TJA. The authors determined that IV TXA had improved blood loss and transfusion rates after TJA. They determined cost savings of almost $60 per case for THA and $35 per case for TKA with the use of IV TXA. Level of evidence: III.

47. Kayupov E, Fillingham YA, Okroj K, et al: Oral and intravenous tranexamic acid are equivalent at reducing blood loss following total hip arthroplasty: A randomized controlled trial. *J Bone Joint Surg Am Vol* 2017;99:373-378.

This prospective randomized controlled trial examined oral versus IV TXA. Both formulations were effective at reducing blood loss and transfusion. Oral TXA offered significant cost advantages from IV TXA. Level of evidence: I.

48. Fillingham YA, Kayupov E, Plummer DR, Moric M, Gerlinger TL, Della Valle CJ: The James A. Rand Young Investigator's Award: A randomized controlled trial of oral and intravenous tranexamic acid in total knee arthroplasty: The same efficacy at lower cost? *J Arthroplast* 2016;31:26-30.

The authors of this double-blinded, randomized, placebo-controlled trial determined that there was no difference in outcomes between patients receiving oral versus IV TXA. The authors determined that there was a significant cost savings with oral TXA versus IV with equivalent benefit. Level of evidence: I.

49. Hobbs JC, Welsby IJ, Green CL, Dhakal IB, Wellman SS: Epsilon aminocaproic acid to reduce blood loss and transfusion after total hip and total knee arthroplasty. *J Arthroplast* 2018;33:55-60.

This is a retrospective before and after study comparing blood loss and transfusion rate after initiation of standard administration of epsilon aminocaproic acid (EACA). The authors determined that EACA improved outcomes with less cost than TXA. Level of evidence: III.

50. Bini SA, Darbinian JA, Brox WT, Khatod M: Risk factors for reaching the post-operative transfusion trigger in a community primary total knee arthroplasty population. *J Arthroplast* 2018;33:711-717.

This retrospective cohort study examined 10,518 TKAs to establish risk factors for reaching an established blood transfusion trigger. The authors determined that not receiving TXA and having a preoperative hemoglobin less than 13 g/dL were independent risk factors for transfusion. Level of evidence: III.

51. Holt JB, Miller BJ, Callaghan JJ, Clark CR, Willenborg MD, Noiseux NO: Minimizing blood transfusion in total hip and knee arthroplasty through a multimodal approach. *J Arthroplast* 2016;31:378-382.

A registry of prospectively collected data was used to evaluate the effectiveness of a multimodal approach to minimizing blood transfusions. The authors determined that their algorithm was effective at reducing blood transfusion after primary TKA and THA. Level of evidence: III.

52. Loftus TJ, Spratling L, Stone BA, Xiao L, Jacofsky DJ: A patient blood management Program in prosthetic joint arthroplasty decreases blood use and improves outcomes. *J Arthroplast* 2016;31:11-14.

A retrospective cohort study of 12,590 patients was used to evaluate the effectiveness of a blood management program at reducing transfusion rates and improving several patient outcomes. The authors determined that the program benefited both outcomes. Level of evidence: III.

53. Markel DC, Allen MW, Hughes RE, Singal BM, Hallstrom BR: Quality initiative programs can decrease total joint arthroplasty transfusion rates-A multicenter study using the MARCQI total joint registry database. *J Arthroplast* 2017;32:3292-3297.

This is a registry review of prospectively collected data to examine the effectiveness of a multimodal program to decrease transfusion rates. The authors determined that the program was effective at reducing transfusion rates after primary THA and TKA. Level of evidence: III.

Principles of Orthopaedics

Chapter 8

Musculoskeletal Biomechanics

Antonia M. Zaferiou, PhD • Jonathan A. Gustafson, PhD • Robin Pourzal, PhD

ABSTRACT

Musculoskeletal biomechanics is an interdisciplinary field that utilizes principles of mechanics applied to the human body to prevent and to improve treatment of musculoskeletal injuries. Three basic topic areas of biomechanics will be explored in this chapter and include rigid body mechanics and free body analysis, mechanics of materials, and implant design considerations and mechanisms of wear.

Rigid body mechanics use basic laws of physics to analyze the effect of external loads on the body, whereas mechanics of materials further assess changes at the tissue level and quantify the properties of tissue that are vital to function. Lastly, considerations of material coupling in the implant field are vital to the function of the implant and potential for different wear mechanisms. This chapter will provide readers with a better understanding of biomechanics and an overview of the latest updates in the research field related to orthopaedics, with examples related to the clinical setting.

Keywords: biomechanics; joint replacement; materials; mechanics

Introduction

The musculoskeletal system accomplishes mechanically remarkable feats through structures and phenomena that are not yet fully understood or replicated. For instance, bipedal robots still struggle to perform pedestrian activities such as turning while walking, and tissue engineers are still unable to replicate the performance of native cartilage. Musculoskeletal biomechanics is intimately tied to the orthopaedics field because both nonsurgical and surgical interventions attempt to restore the remarkable feats of the native musculoskeletal system, with varied results. As both fields advance, opportunities remain to improve the results related to joint replacement because of the challenging demands of designing an implant to replicate native systems. Joint replacement materials have to fulfill several properties such as osseo-integration, wear and corrosion resistance, low friction, and biocompatibility. Lastly, the material must be chosen with a full understanding of the desired ranges and frequency of both motions and loads for optimal joint function. No material can fulfill all requirements; therefore most modern implants rely on modularity. Yet, as of today, no combination of materials is able to truly replace the complex mechanisms of the native musculoskeletal system.

Musculoskeletal biomechanics is the study of the relationship between forces and motion experienced by rigid and deformable musculoskeletal systems. Rigid body mechanics applies when examining the behavior of solid body systems, such as the forces acting on native joints and implants. Deformable mechanics applies when examining the effect of forces and motions on the internal stresses of the body or joint replacement components (eg, modular design). Both rigid body and deformable mechanics provide information about the behavior of the native and nonnative structures when exposed to loads. This is particularly important when these loads can contribute to injury.

As a field, musculoskeletal biomechanics focuses on understanding native joint behavior in order to improve movement mechanics through nonsurgical and, if necessary, surgical interventions. To appropriately understand and restore native joint behavior, knowledge of rigid body and deformable mechanics is required, discussed in Rigid Body Mechanics and Joint Kinetics

Dr. Gustafson or an immediate family member has stock or stock options held in Tetraphase. Dr. Pourzal or an immediate family member has received nonincome support (such as equipment or services), commercially derived honoraria, or other non–research-related funding (such as paid travel) from Zimmer. Neither Dr. Zaferiou nor any immediate family member has received anything of value from or has stock or stock options held in a commercial company or institution related directly or indirectly to the subject of this chapter.

and Deformable Mechanics sections, respectively. In Implant Materials for Joint Replacements section, the fundamental outcomes of rigid body and deformable mechanics are discussed via applications in joint replacement and implant behavior subspecialties.

Rigid Body Mechanics and Joint Kinetics

Rigid body mechanics assumes that any deformation caused by forces acting on a body is negligible. Although this assumption can aid in simplifying biomechanical analyses, it should be noted that no material in the human body can truly be a rigid body, as all tissues undergo some degree of deformation. Therefore, it is important to clearly understand when the rigid body assumption is applicable. If one material is much stiffer than the other or the deformations experienced by a body are much smaller than the translations or rotations of that body, then the rigid body assumption can be applied. For example, when analyzing gait, the translations and rotations of the lower extremity will be much greater than any deformations experienced by the segments of the lower extremity, allowing it to be treated as a rigid body. This assumption is also applicable when performing mechanical testing of a joint complex, such as the bone-ligament-bone complex, where the bones can be considered rigid bodies because they are much stiffer than the ligament tissue.

Joint kinetics—joint forces and torques—are typically determined using laws of rigid body dynamics and free body analysis. Specifically, the following two physical laws of rigid body dynamics are used, equating (Eqn. 1) the sum of forces to the rate of change in linear momentum and (Eqn. 2) the sum of torques to the rate of change in angular momentum. Joint kinetics provide useful clinical information about loading patterns and how multiple joints work together to coordinate body movement. This information can be used to advance our understanding of topics ranging from how surgery affects the distribution of load across a joint during activities of daily living,[1-3] to how each joint contributes to complex whole-body movement used during athletic maneuvers.[4-7]

$$\sum_{i=1}^{n} \vec{F_i} = m \times \vec{a} \qquad 1$$

where m is the free body's mass, $\vec{a}$ is the free body's linear acceleration vector, $\vec{F_i}$ is each force vector acting on the free body, and n is the number of forces acting on the free body.

$$\sum_{i=1}^{n} \vec{\tau_i} = [I] \times \vec{\alpha} \qquad 2$$

where [I] is the free body's moment of inertia (resistance to rotate) matrix, $\vec{a}$ is the free body's angular acceleration vector, $\vec{\tau_i}$ is each force vector acting on the free body, and n is the number of torques acting on the free body.

Example Clinical Application: Arm Elevation

In the example displayed in **Figure 1**, the upper extremity is moving free of an external contact force during an arm-elevation task performed by a preoperative reverse total shoulder arthroplasty (RTSA) patient. RTSA is being used increasingly to treat irreparable rotator cuff tears. However, RTSA and other shoulder replacements are revised at a rate of approximately 9% because of loosening or dislocation.[8,9] Loosening or dislocation of an implant could suggest that either implants are not fixated properly (eg, misaligned) or not designed adequately to withstand loading conditions in vivo. Therefore, it is of particular interest to calculate shoulder kinetics during activities of daily living in patients before versus after RTSA. To do so, mathematical models are developed of each patient's body segments and their 3D motion is measured to estimate joint kinetics throughout the duration of tasks of interest. However, for simplicity, in **Figure 1**, the analysis is executed at a single "quasi-static" time, which assumes that linear and angular accelerations are negligible. An additional useful simplification is conducting this analysis in 2D to align the determined net joint forces and torques with primary lines of action of certain muscles and ligaments (in **Figure 1**, the mediolateral axes of the hand, forearm, and upper arm are aligned with the X-Y coordinate system plane).

The first step in joint kinetics is to mathematically isolate each body segment of interest from the rest of the body or environment, as a "free body." In **Figure 1**, upper extremity joint kinetics are determined by treating the upper arm, forearm, and hand as free bodies that forces and torques act upon. A body segment or collection of body segments can be treated as free bodies (eg, whole-body, foot, leg-system). Known joint forces and torques include gravity and the contact with the environment. Unknown joint forces and torques are determined by using physical laws of rigid body dynamics (Eqn. 1,2). As demonstrated in this example, free body analysis is typically first applied to distal body segments and joints, and then toward proximal body segments and joints. If studying the lower extremity, joint kinetics are also calculated from

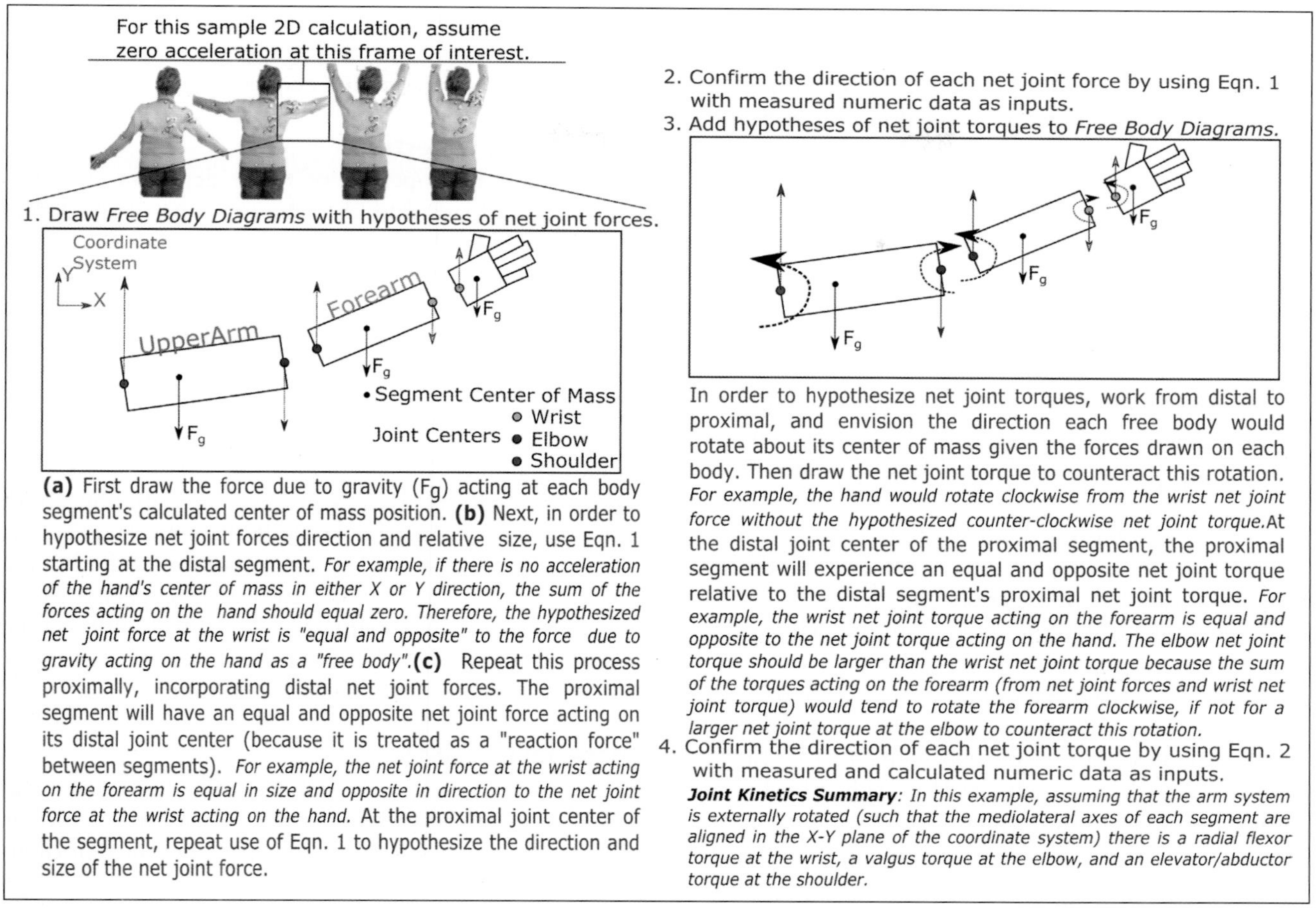
For this sample 2D calculation, assume zero acceleration at this frame of interest.
1. Draw *Free Body Diagrams* with hypotheses of net joint forces.
Coordinate System
Y
X
UpperArm
Forearm
F_g
• Segment Center of Mass
Joint Centers
Wrist
Elbow
Shoulder
(a) First draw the force due to gravity (F_g) acting at each body segment's calculated center of mass position. **(b)** Next, in order to hypothesize net joint forces direction and relative size, use Eqn. 1 starting at the distal segment. *For example, if there is no acceleration of the hand's center of mass in either X or Y direction, the sum of the forces acting on the hand should equal zero. Therefore, the hypothesized net joint force at the wrist is "equal and opposite" to the force due to gravity acting on the hand as a "free body".* **(c)** Repeat this process proximally, incorporating distal net joint forces. The proximal segment will have an equal and opposite net joint force acting on its distal joint center (because it is treated as a "reaction force" between segments). *For example, the net joint force at the wrist acting on the forearm is equal in size and opposite in direction to the net joint force at the wrist acting on the hand.* At the proximal joint center of the segment, repeat use of Eqn. 1 to hypothesize the direction and size of the net joint force.
2. Confirm the direction of each net joint force by using Eqn. 1 with measured numeric data as inputs.
3. Add hypotheses of net joint torques to *Free Body Diagrams.*
F_g
In order to hypothesize net joint torques, work from distal to proximal, and envision the direction each free body would rotate about its center of mass given the forces drawn on each body. Then draw the net joint torque to counteract this rotation. *For example, the hand would rotate clockwise from the wrist net joint force without the hypothesized counter-clockwise net joint torque.* At the distal joint center of the proximal segment, the proximal segment will experience an equal and opposite net joint torque relative to the distal segment's proximal net joint torque. *For example, the wrist net joint torque acting on the forearm is equal and opposite to the net joint torque acting on the hand. The elbow net joint torque should be larger than the wrist net joint torque because the sum of the torques acting on the forearm (from net joint forces and wrist net joint torque) would tend to rotate the forearm clockwise, if not for a larger net joint torque at the elbow to counteract this rotation.*
4. Confirm the direction of each net joint torque by using Eqn. 2 with measured and calculated numeric data as inputs.
Joint Kinetics Summary*: In this example, assuming that the arm system is externally rotated (such that the mediolateral axes of each segment are aligned in the X-Y plane of the coordinate system) there is a radial flexor torque at the wrist, a valgus torque at the elbow, and an elevator/abductor torque at the shoulder.*

Figure 1 Example step-by-step instructions to use free body analysis to determine joint kinetics to better understand shoulder joint kinetics during arm elevation in an orthopaedic population.

distal to proximal ("from the ground, up"). First, if the lower extremity is in contact with the ground at the time of interest, an external force known as the ground reaction force (often measured) is applied at a known location on the foot. This ground reaction force is included in the free body diagram of the foot to calculate ankle joint kinetics. Then, the ankle joint kinetics are used within the free body diagram of the shank to calculate knee joint kinetics. Finally, the free body diagram of the thigh is used to calculate hip joint kinetics. It is important to note that upper extremity joint kinetics can include an external force, depending on how the upper extremity interacts with the environment (eg, during push-ups, carrying a load, using an assistive device).

In the arm elevation example, it was determined that there was a radial flexor torque at the wrist, a valgus torque at the elbow, and an elevator/abductor torque at the shoulder. These types of joint torques generally make sense to describe upper extremity joint actions during an arm raise against gravity. This type of information contextualizes the muscle activation patterns or comparison of loading patterns (eg, within-patient before vs after surgery, or across patients). By using devices for measuring accelerations, the arm elevation analysis can be expanded to 3D, which can aid in comparing patients' kinetics before and after RTSA and significantly influence clinical practices. For instance, knowing the joint kinetics used during activities of daily living may eventually reduce the rate of RTSA revision by better informing the implant design process or implant centering procedures. Furthermore, the joint kinetics used by each patient during activities of daily living can help create a "functional profile" to personalize rehabilitation practices.

Current and Future Joint Kinetic Approaches

During joint kinetics analysis, body segments are typically assumed to be adequately represented using parameters (including mass and moment of inertia) from cadaver studies, scaled by the person's body weight and measured segment length.[10] However, other approaches can use personalized parameters from segment volume determined by optical motion capture[11,12] or image-based systems (eg, DXA-scans[13]). These techniques offer unique insights when studying populations whose segment parameters stray from the cadaveric study populations (eg, children, obese, athletes) or during experiments that push the boundary of rigid body assumptions (eg, high impact loading accompanied by excessive soft-tissue motion).

Joint kinetic analysis is used in other orthopaedic contexts and scales, including (but not limited to) studies of gait analysis with or without instrumented implants,[3] cadaveric studies of spine vertebrae,[14] fluoroscopy studies of knee loads during inclined gait,[15] wheelchair propulsion,[2] and in sport.[4-7] In addition to novel applications, emerging joint kinetics approaches attempt to understand aspects of human movement that traditional techniques fail to capture. This includes calculating and expressing joint kinetics using more functionally derived axes, for instance, relative to an "arm plane" or "leg plane" (or relative to the proximal segment to account for adjacent segments that may not be aligned with one another).[2,4,7] Further background information about joint kinetics can be found in other classic biomechanics resources.[16] The following section discusses deformable mechanics, when loads applied at the tissue level (ie, articular cartilage, ligaments, tendons, and bone) lead to deformations that describe tissue mechanical behavior and function.

Deformable Mechanics

Deformable mechanics is a subspecialty of mechanics of materials—the study of forces and their effects on motion within both rigid and deformable systems. Unlike rigid body mechanics, deformable mechanics examines the effect of forces and motions on the internal stresses of the body. Understanding the stress response of different "material" (both natural and synthetic) is vital to selecting appropriate replacement material and developing more advanced implant materials to replicate the native tissue function. In the context of musculoskeletal biomechanics, the field of deformable mechanics is focused on understanding the natural behavior of joint tissues, including soft (ie, tendon, ligament, cartilage, etc.) and hard (ie, bone) tissue types. When measuring the response of tissue to different forms of axial (ie, tension and compression) and rotational (ie, shear) loading, it is important to distinguish the intrinsic material properties, which is not influenced by tissue geometry, from the extrinsic structural properties, which take into account tissue material *and* geometry.

Structural Properties

The structural properties of tissue determine its ability to resist loads and deformation when considering the material and geometry. For example, the structural properties of a bone-ligament-bone complex can be determined in response to a tensile load to assess its load-elongation behavior. A tensile force is applied to the complex, causing the tissue to stretch until it ruptures. While loading is applied, the corresponding increase in length in the complex is measured. The resulting nonlinear load-elongation curve that is typical of biologic soft tissues provides information about the structural properties of the tissue complex, such as its stiffness—resistance to deformation—and ultimate load at failure—maximum load-bearing capacity. These parameters are important to define for healthy tissue because, clinically, they can factor into the decision for the replacement graft type used for surgery.

Material Properties

It is also important to understand the mechanical response of an individual tissue or material, which is independent of specimen geometry, by using normalized load and deformation parameters. Measuring the mechanical properties of tissues, such as ligaments, can be used to evaluate the quality of the tissue when making comparisons between normal, injured, and healing states and are represented by the stress-strain relationship. Stress is defined as the amount of force applied per unit area. Strain is considered is defined as the change in length per unit length. Similar to load-elongation measurements, stress-strain relationships are obtained experimentally during tensile, compressive, or shear loading of tissue.

A typical stress-strain curve for biologic tissues consists of four distinct regions (**Figure 2**):

- Toe region: Initial recruitment of the collagen fibers, where significant stretch of the material occurs with a minimal increase in stress. This is a direct result from stretching of the crimped collagen fibrils as the fibers are being drawn taut in the material and before significant tension occurs within the material.
- Linear region: Increased load-bearing through the ligament, where strain becomes linearly proportional to stress, and the slope of the curve in this region can be calculated to determine the tangent modulus of the tissue. The tangent modulus defines the threshold of the material beyond which permanent (plastic)

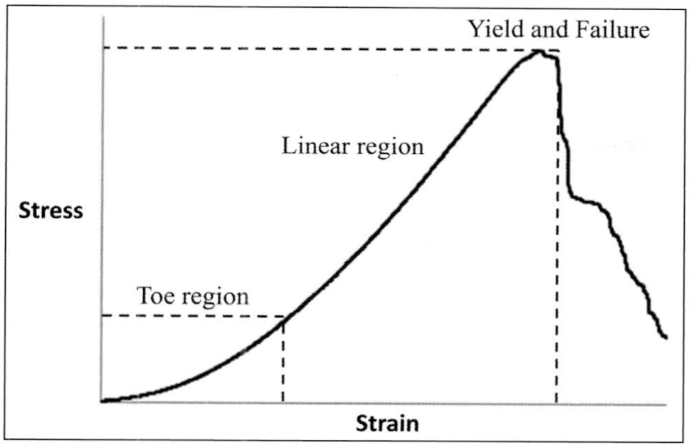

Figure 2 Stress-strain curve of a ligament substance during a load-to-failure test that characterizes the mechanical properties, defined by four distinct regions of loading: (1) Toe region: initial recruitment of the collagen fibers; (2) Linear region: increased load-bearing through the ligament; (3) Yield region: continued loading and deformation of the ligament, leading to permanent, nonrecoverable damage; (4) Failure region: ultimate rupture of the ligament.

deformation can begin to occur. This region is commonly reached during daily activities, where the tissue undergoes a form of "elastic" deformation, meaning the tissue will return to its original length or shape upon unloading.

- Yield region: Continued loading and deformation of the ligament, where abnormally large levels of strain occur in the tissue with only a marginal increase in corresponding stress. It is at this point that the tissue begins experiencing microscopic failures. Once the tissue undergoes this amount of deformation, the tissue does not recover and return to its original state in its entirety upon release of the deforming stress.
- Failure region: Lastly, if the tissue continues to deform, it will eventually experience ultimate rupture.

Common mechanical properties of tissues derived from mechanical tests include modulus, ultimate strength, ultimate strain, and strain energy density.

Clinical Applications

In the biomechanics field, it has been well established that factors such as age, injury, and healing can significantly affect the structural properties of a bone-ligament-bone complex as well as the failure mode of the complex.[17,18] Tensile failure tests in a rabbit femur–medial collateral ligament (MCL)–tibia complex demonstrated significant increases in tensile strength as a result of maturation. Additionally, failure modes in these models progressed from tibial avulsions in the younger tissue to failure in the midsubstance of ligament.[18] It has also been shown in a recovering femur-MCL-tibia complex that the recovering tissue complex exhibits significantly decreased stiffness (53%) and ultimate load (29%) compared with an uninjured joint state.[17] Clinically, the mechanical properties of tissue can be significantly influenced by injury and drastically change during recovery.[17,19] The detrimental effects of disuse injuries have been well documented. Specifically, immobilization of tendons and ligaments can significantly reduce the mechanical properties of the tissue as well as the mass of the structure.[19] Additionally, the long-term effects of disuse have been shown to require up to 12 months of time for complete recovery of ligament strength parameters.[20]

These classic studies have provided evidence as to how the structural and mechanical properties of tissue change as a result of aging, injury, and throughout recovery. The mechanical properties of tissue are vital to developing appropriate treatment solutions in the case of injuries and how introducing joint replacements within the body will affect the remaining native tissue. Recently, there have been significant advances in the measurement techniques of the mechanical behavior of different tissue types. One example is the use of shear wave elastography (SWE) to evaluate the mechanical properties of tendons and ligaments for determining disease status and follow-up to various treatments.[21,22] The potential of SWE is becoming more recognized, as the technique is possible with most current clinical scanners. Specifically, one study has attempted to characterize the heterogeneity within the tissue of heel pad using SWE.[23] Another promising technique for the noninvasive measurement of cartilage health is magnetic resonance imaging (MRI) T2 and T1ρ mapping.[24,25] One study in particular has been able to identify short-term T2 changes in cartilage mapping in individuals after ACL injury and reconstruction, potential indicators of risk for progressive cartilage degeneration.[25] These recent advances in noninvasive imaging of the mechanical properties of tissue require additional work for validating these metrics but show excellent promise for the future of the field.

Implant Materials for Joint Replacements

Rigid body and deformable mechanics are fundamental for the design of and material choice for total joint replacements (TJRs). From a materials point of view, implant component failure can occur in three different ways: fatigue, wear, and corrosion. The occurrence of fatigue failure of implant components (eg, femoral stem fracture) is rare, but catastrophic when it occurs.[21] Fatigue is usually due to crack formation and propagation under cyclic load and eventual fracture under overload. As described in previous Rigid Body Mechanics and Joint Kinetics and Deformable Mechanics sections, the mechanical conditions in different total joint arthroplasties—knee (TKA), hip (THA), and shoulder (TSA)—differ broadly and thus dictate the material consideration and design features of the implant. In contemporary TJA designs, implant fracture is rare, because its risk can be minimized early during the design phase.

Failure due to wear and corrosion are harder to control. Wear is a damage mode that is inherent to any bearing and cannot be entirely eliminated in systems with artificial materials. In most technical applications, wear leads to structural failure. However, joint arthroplasty failure is commonly caused by adverse reactions to nano- and micro-sized wear debris as opposed to structural failure of the implant.[26-28] In contrast to wear, corrosion is an entirely unintended occurrence, which usually affects modular junctions between two implant components.[29] Recent concepts and failure mechanisms on both the TJA bearing surfaces and modular junctions are described in the following sections.

Wear of Bearing Surfaces

The occurrence of bearing surface wear in TJRs of at least one of the two bearing surfaces cannot be avoided, only minimized. Different material options have been developed over time. The golden standard has been metal-on-polyethylene (MoP) in all three major bearing types (knee, hip, and shoulder). In this bearing couple, wear occurs primarily on the polyethylene (PE) component.[28,30] Historically, polyethylene wear has been linked to the occurrence of osteolysis and subsequent implant loosening.[26-28] However, PE as a material has undergone significant improvement in terms of the wear rate and subsequent decrease of wear particle generation.[31] Improvements have been made by sterilization of the implant in an inert atmosphere to prevent oxidation and in vivo delamination. Furthermore, modern materials undergo a cross-linking process, which leads to increased hardness and better wear behavior.[31-33] At its introduction, some surgeons and researchers were concerned that the increased hardness of cross-linked PE would go along with a more brittle material potentially more susceptible to fracture, especially in TKRs. However, an increase of failures due to fracture has not manifested clinically to date, but long-term clinical outcomes need to be continuously monitored. In general, the use of highly cross-linked PE in TJAs can be considered a success story. The material has been further improved by vitamin-E doping. Vitamin-E binds to free radicals within the PE chains and thus further prevents or at least prolongs the onset of oxidation and embrittlement in situ.[31] These developments have further solidified the status of PE as the benchmark bearing material.

The use of CoCrMo alloy has come under scrutiny because of adverse reactions to metal debris in some metal-on-metal (MoM) devices.[34-36] Certain hip implants with large femoral heads and low coverage angles between head and cup were associated with edge loading (**Figure 3**). This process shifts the acting wear mechanism from mild surface fatigue and tribochemical reactions to abrasion, resulting in elevated wear rates and larger CoCrMo alloy wear particles.[37] Such particles were shown to cause pseudo-tumors and other forms of adverse responses.[34,35] This development led to a fast decline of MoM THRs even though many MoM designs appeared to function without problems.[38] The current trend suggests that CoCrMo alloy is increasingly replaced with ceramic femoral heads in combination with a titanium alloy stem, even in MoP cases.[39] This trend has not occurred in TKRs because CoCrMo alloy remains the go-to material despite the availability of ceramic femoral components. Also, in shoulder replacements, MoP remains the most commonly used bearing couple even though one study suggests that the polyethylene component in anatomical total shoulder arthroplasties (ATSA) undergoes lower PE wear against ceramic compared with metals.[40] So far, clinical data and retrieval studies of the shoulder have not suggested any adverse reactions to metal debris or osteolysis; instead, implant failure appears mostly related to problems such as fixation, glenoid component seating, and humeral centering on the glenoid.[9] However, retrieval studies suggest that RTSA PE wear rate can lie within the osteolytic threshold reported for the hip.[41] Thus, it is possible that forthcoming TSA devices and tissue retrieval studies will establish a more clear correlation between implant debris and joint failure.

Ceramic-on-ceramic (CoC) articulation is mainly used in THRs. Even though CoC hips do report positive clinical outcomes, they occupy a smaller market share because of a potential risk of fracture followed by complicated revision surgery and higher expense. The use of ceramic-on-polyethylene (CoP) bearing over the traditional MoP bearing has gained favor because of reports of corrosion within modular junctions of MoP THRs,[42,43] which will be further discussed in the following section. However, it is important to note that when performing a revision procedure of a prior ceramic implant, it

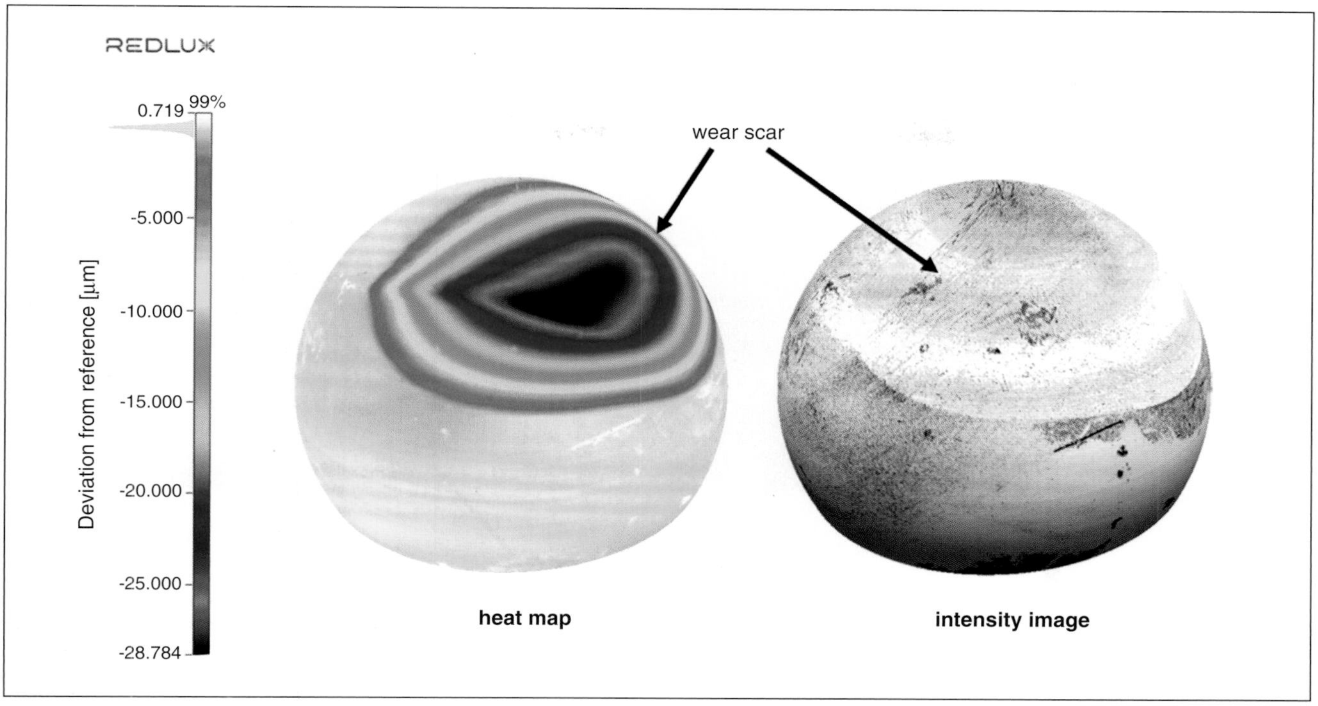

Figure 3 An optical coordinate measuring machine (CMM) (OrthoLux, RedLux, Southampton, UK) was used to quantify and image the damage on a CoCrMo alloy femoral head from a MoM total hip replacement. The heat map (left) illustrates a typical wear scar generated under edge loading conditions. The intensity image (right) shows a photorealistic representation of the surface without surface reflections. In this case a material loss of 11.6 mm³ was generated over 58 months in situ.

is crucial to employ a CoC bearing.[44,45] Any remaining ceramic particles from a fractured or severely worn ceramic component is harder than any other implant material and could cause excessive damage to any metal bearing surface because of abrasive wear.

Corrosion in Modular Interfaces

The most frequently used implant alloys in TJRs are cobalt base (wrought and cast CoCrMo) and titanium base (eg, Ti6Al4V, TMZF) alloys. Both alloys, in principle, exhibit excellent corrosion properties and biocompatibility. CoCrMo is protected by a thin, passive film of chromium oxide that is further enforced by molybdenum oxide, and titanium alloys are protected by a thick, stable titanium oxide passive film. Despite these protective passive films, corrosion-related implant failures have been reported with an increasing rate.[39,46] The material loss associated with modular junction corrosion is considerable (**Figure 4**) and leads to lymphocyte-dominated adverse local tissue reactions with similar histopathological patterns to those reported for MoM bearing surface failures.[43] The corrosion process has been summarized as mechanically assisted crevice corrosion (MACC).[26] The mechanical aspect of MACC is given by (1) cyclic stress applied during patient activities, which in itself may promote local corrosion, and (2) micromotion. Oscillating micromotion between two surfaces in contact leads to a damage mode known as fretting. Fretting can also cause disruption of the passive film and thus lead to a tribocorrrosive process called *fretting corrosion*.

The onset of micromotion—and therefore fretting—depends on a variety of factors such as implant design (taper angle, surface topography, contact length, flexural rigidity), patient factors (weight, activity, anatomy), and the surgeon (implant assembly force).[47-51] However, excessive material loss can be initiated by other mechanisms than fretting. For example, titanium stems have been reported to undergo oxide-induced stress corrosion cracking leading to fracture or gross trunnion failure due to abrasion.[52,53] CoCrMo alloys in particular appear to undergo different corrosion modes such as pitting, etching, and intergranular corrosion. Part of these corrosion processes are related to the microstructure of the implant alloy, which is defined by its grain size, hard phase content, and the homogeneity of alloying element distribution.[54] However, it is unclear how a chemical environment could be generated in vivo that would allow corrosion to occur on implant alloys. Some studies suggest that patient-specific joint

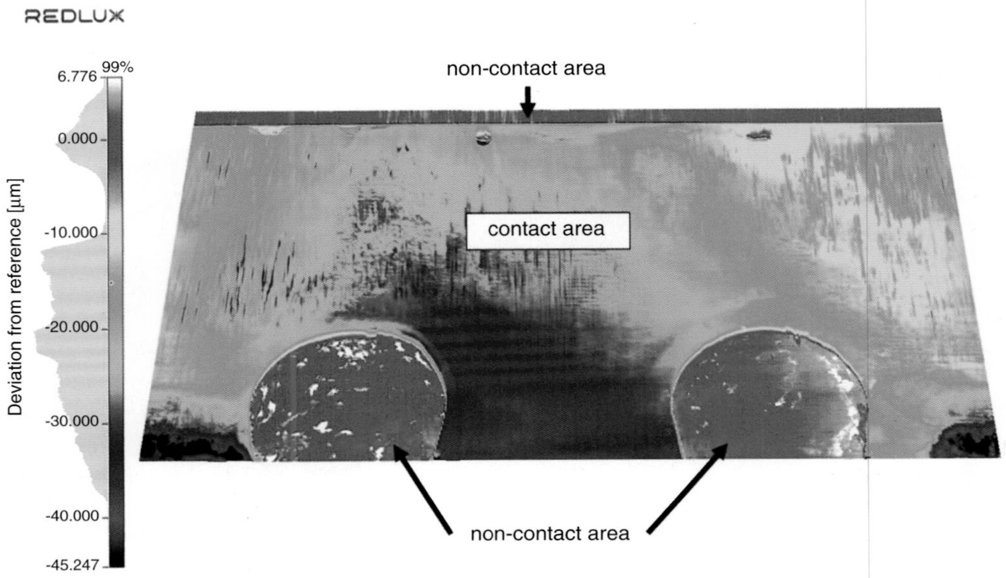

Figure 4 A taper surface of a femoral head surface from a MoP THR (81.7 months in situ) was imaged using an optical CMM. The heat map prominently illustrates areas that were in contact with the titanium alloy stem taper and subsequently underwent fretting and corrosion leading to a total material loss of 11.5 mm^3.

fluid chemistry could drive such corrosion processes,[55] whereas others point to the potential impact of changes of the local solution chemistry due to cell (eg, macrophages) activity.[42,56] Corrosion does not only occur within modular taper junctions of THRs but also within other implant components, such as the back side of metal acetabular liners, fixation screws, and TKR tibial stem extensions, among others.[38] It is important to note that corrosion processes usually need a mechanical trigger first, even though the actual corrosion process is chemically driven. Therefore, it is imperative to have an understanding of the biomechanical system of a specific joint to predict the initiation of mechanical damage processes such as fatigue and wear, but also chemical degradation processes such as corrosion.

Summary

To advance the field of musculoskeletal biomechanics, it is necessary to have a fundamental understanding of the concepts discussed in this chapter: rigid body mechanics, joint kinetics, deformable mechanics, implant material properties, and failure mechanisms. These principles are at the cornerstone of the field and vital for decision making in treating injuries. Applications of the principles of rigid body mechanics are demonstrated via joint kinetics analysis, using the relationships between forces and motion to understand joint loading patterns and how joints work together to coordinate body movement. The principles of deformable mechanics are used to create and identify new replacement tissue types with the goal of replicating the same function of the native tissue. These principles are also applied in the field of implant biomechanics and material behavior, where new iterations of TJRs must be evaluated for the highest probability of clinical success and restoration of function. Although the field is always changing, the fundamentals of musculoskeletal biomechanics will be a constant guide to inform decision making at the forefront of both the research and clinic.

Key Study Points

- Rigid body mechanics can apply when the deformation caused by load is considered negligible.
- Joint kinetics include calculations or measurements of joint forces and torques.
- Extrinsic structural properties differ from intrinsic material properties because structural properties are influenced by both geometry and material.
- Fatigue, wear, and corrosion are the three major types of failures that can occur in joint replacement components.

Annotated References

1. Mathiyakom W, McNitt-Gray JL, Requejo P, Costa K: Modifying center of mass trajectory during sit-to-stand tasks redistributes the mechanical demand across the lower extremity joints. *Clin Biomech Bristol Avon* 2005;20:105-111.
2. Russell IM, Raina S, Requejo PS, Wilcox RR, Mulroy S, McNitt-Gray JL: Modifications in wheelchair propulsion technique with speed. *Front Bioeng Biotechnol* 2015;3:1-11.
3. Lundberg HJ, Foucher KC, Wimmer MA: A parametric approach to numerical modeling of TKR contact forces. *J Biomech* 2009;42:541-545.
4. Peterson TJ, Mcnitt-gray JL: Coordination of lower extremity multi-joint control strategies during the golf swing. *J Biomech* 2018;77:26-33.

   This study compared how highly skilled golfers used each leg during the swing using different clubs. Despite player-specific joint kinetics, generally, during hitting with a driver, players increased target leg ankle, knee, and hip net joint torques versus during a 6-iron.
5. Havens KL, Sigward SM: Joint and segmental mechanics differ between cutting maneuvers in skilled athletes. *Gait Posture* 2015;41:33-38.
6. Fleisig GS, Andrews JR, Dillman CJ, Escamilla RF: Kinetics of baseball pitching with implications about injury mechanisms. *Am J Sports Med* 1995;23:233-239.
7. Zaferiou AM, Flashner H, Wilcox RR, McNitt-Gray JL: Lower extremity control during turns initiated with and without hip external rotation. *J Biomech* 2017;52:130-139.

   This study compared how highly skilled dancers used each leg during the initiation of turns initiated with versus without hip external rotation. Despite dancer-specific joint kinetics, dancers generally aligned the ground reaction force within the leg plane for both turn types.
8. Australian Orthopaedic Association National Joint Replacement Registry (AOANJRR): *Hip, Knee, & Shoulder Arthroplasty: 2017 Annual Report*, 2017.

   This annual report summarized joint replacements statistics in Australia in 2017.
9. Hsu JE, Hackett DJ, Vo KV, Matsen FA: What can be learned from an analysis of 215 glenoid component failures? *J Shoulder Elb Surg* 2018;27:478-486.

   This study analyzed 215 anatomic total shoulder replacements that needed revision because of glenoid component failure in order to elucidate if surgeon-controlled factors influenced the need for revision. The manuscript concludes with suggested ways for surgeons to reduce the risk of revision.
10. de Leva P: Adjustments to Zatsiorsky-Seluyanov's segment inertia parameters. *J Biomech* 1996;29:1223-1230.
11. Yeadon MR: The simulation of aerial movement–I. The determination of orientation angles from film data. *J Biomech* 1990;23:59-66.
12. Wilson C, King MA, Yeadon MR: Determination of subject-specific model parameters for visco-elastic elements. 2006;39:1883-1890.
13. Durkin JL, Dowling JJ, Andrews DM: The measurement of body segment inertial parameters using dual energy X-ray absorptiometry. *J Biomech* 2002;35:1575-1580.
14. Espinoza Orías AA, Malhotra NR, Elliott DM: Rat disc torsional mechanics: Effect of lumbar and caudal levels and axial compression load. *Spine J* 2009;9:204-209.
15. Farrokhi S, Voycheck CA, Klatt BA, Gustafson JA, Tashman S, Fitzgerald GK: Altered tibiofemoral joint contact mechanics and kinematics in patients with knee osteoarthritis and episodic complaints of joint instability. *Clin Biomech* 2014;29(6):629-635. doi:10.1016/j.clinbiomech.2014.04.014.
16. Zatsiorsky VM: *Kinetics of Human Motion*, Human Kinetics, 2002.
17. Abramowitch SD, Yagi M, Tsuda E, Woo SL-Y: The healing medial collateral ligament following a combined anterior cruciate and medial collateral ligament injury–a biomechanical study in a goat model. *J Orthop Res* 2003;21:1124-1130.
18. Woo SL, Orlando CA, Gomez MA, Frank CB, Akeson WH: Tensile properties of the medial collateral ligament as a function of age. *J Orthop Res* 1986;4:133-141.
19. Woo SL, Gomez MA, Woo YK, Akeson WH: Mechanical properties of tendons and ligaments. II. The relationships of immobilization and exercise on tissue remodeling. *Biorheology* 1982;19:397-408.
20. Noyes FR: Functional properties of knee ligaments and alterations induced by immobilization: A correlative biomechanical and histological study in primates. *Clin Orthop* 1977;(123):210-242.
21. Taljanovic MS, Gimber LH, Becker GW, et al: Shear-wave elastography: Basic physics and musculoskeletal applications. *Radiogr Rev Publ Radiol Soc N Am Inc* 2017;37:855-870.

    Basic ultrasound physics of shear wave elastography are discussed, along with applications in the evaluation of traumatic and pathologic conditions of the musculoskeletal system.
22. Suydam SM, Cortes DH, Axe MJ, Snyder-Mackler L, Buchanan TS: Semitendinosus tendon for ACL reconstruction: Regrowth and mechanical property recovery. *Orthop J Sports Med* 2017;5:2325967117712944.

    Continuous shear wave elastography (cSWE) was used to noninvasively measure elasticity and shear stiffness in the recovering hamstring tendon of individuals post anterior cruciate ligament reconstruction. Comparisons to contralateral tendon showed increased mechanical properties after 12 months.
23. Lin C-Y, Chen P-Y, Shau Y-W, Tai H-C, Wang C-L: Spatial-dependent mechanical properties of the heel pad by shear wave elastography. *J Biomech* 2017;53:191-195.

    Ultrasound-based shear wave elastography measurements made in 40 heel pads of 20 participants. Changes in shear wave stiffness through the depth of heel pad demonstrated heterogeneity of tissue. Noninvasive technique to measure mechanical properties and improve knowledge of heel biomechanics.

24. Monu UD, Jordan CD, Samuelson BL, Hargreaves BA, Gold GE, McWalter EJ: Cluster analysis of quantitative MRI T2 and T1ρ relaxation times of cartilage identifies differences between healthy and ACL-injured individuals at 3T. *Osteoarthr Cartil* 2017;25:513-520.

    Noninvasive quantitative magnetic resonance imaging (MRI) techniques evaluated cartilage health in ACL-injured individuals. Measures of T2 and T1ρ with a novel cluster analysis technique identified cartilage lesions and changes in cartilage quality between 6 months and 1 year.

25. Williams A, Winalski CS, Chu CR: Early articular cartilage MRI T2 changes after anterior cruciate ligament reconstruction correlate with later changes in T2 and cartilage thickness. *J Orthop Res* 2017;35:699-706.

    Quantitative magnetic resonance imaging (qMRI) evaluated changes in tibiofemoral cartilage health of patients post anterior cruciate ligament reconstructions. Changes in qMRI metrics (T2) between 6 months and 2 years showed strong correlations with changes in thickness.

26. Harris WH: The problem is osteolysis. *Clin Orthop* 1995:46-53.
27. Jacobs JJ, Hallab NJ, Urban RM, Wimmer MA: Wear particles. *J Bone Joint Surg Am* 2006;88(suppl 2):99-102.
28. Gallo J, Goodman SB, Konttinen YT, Wimmer MA, Holinka M: Osteolysis around total knee arthroplasty: A review of pathogenetic mechanisms. *Acta Biomater* 2013;9:8046-8058.
29. Gilbert JL, Buckley CA, Jacobs JJ: In vivo corrosion of modular hip prosthesis components in mixed and similar metal combinations. The effect of crevice, stress, motion, and alloy coupling. *J Biomed Mater Res* 1993;27:1533-1544.
30. Pourzal R, Knowlton CB, Hall DJ, Laurent MP, Urban RM, Wimmer MA: How does wear rate compare in well-functioning total hip and knee replacements? A postmortem polyethylene liner study. *Clin Orthop* 2016;474:1867-1875.

    This study compares the wear rate of postmortem-retrieved acetabular and tibial liners made from historic ultra-high-molecular-weight polyethylene. It was demonstrated that under the same conditions, tibial liners had a 50% lower wear rate than acetabular liners.

31. Kurtz SM, ed: *UHMWPE Handb*, Elsevier (Academic Press), 2009.
32. Brown TS, Citters Van, DW, Berry DJ & Abdel MP: The use of highly crosslinked polyethylene in total knee arthroplasty. *Bone Joint J* 2017;99-B:996-1002.

    This review paper provides the history of cross-linking in polyethylene (HXLPE) for total arthroplasties. The study points out the on-going clinical success of HXLPE, which is most evident in total hip replacements. In total knee replacements a similar trend can be observed, which is supported by good short-term clinical results.

33. Crowninshield RD, Wimmer MA, Jacobs JJ, Rosenberg AG: Clinical performance of contemporary tibial polyethylene components. *J Arthroplast* 2006;21:754-761.
34. Campbell P, Ebramzadeh E, Nelson S, Takamura K, Smet K, Amstutz HC: Histological features of pseudotumor-like tissues from metal-on-metal hips. *Clin Orthop Relat Res* 2010;468:2321-2327.
35. Kwon Y-M, Ostlere SJ, McLardy-Smith P, Athanasou NA, Gill HS, Murray DW: "Asymptomatic" pseudotumors after metal-on-metal hip resurfacing arthroplasty: Prevalence and metal ion study. *J Arthroplast* 2011;26:511-518.
36. Langton DJ, Joyce TJ, Jameson SS, et al: Adverse reaction to metal debris following hip resurfacing: The influence of component type, orientation and volumetric wear. *J Bone Joint Surg Br* 2011;93:164-171.
37. Callaghan JJ, Clohisy J, Beaule P, DellaValle C, Rosenberg AG, Rubash HE. *The Adult Hip 3-Volume Package: Arthroplasty and its Alternatives and Hip Preservation Surgery*, LWW, 2015.
38. Garbuz DS, Tanzer M, Greidanus NV, Masri BA, Duncan CP: The John Charnley Award: Metal-on-metal hip resurfacing versus large-diameter head metal-on-metal total hip arthroplasty: A randomized clinical trial. *Clin Orthop* 2009;468:318-325.
39. American Joint Replacement Registry: *Fifth AJJR Annual Report on Hip and Knee Arthroplasty*, 2019.
40. Mueller U, Braun S, Schroeder S, et al: Influence of humeral head material on wear performance in anatomic shoulder joint arthroplasty. *J Shoulder Elb Surg* 2017;26:1756-1764.

    This study investigated the polyethylene wear volume in anatomic total joint arthroplasties depending on the counter body—ceramic or metal. The results suggested that ceramic components caused a 26.7% lower polyethylene wear rate compared with metal components.

41. Lewicki KA, Bell J-E, Van Citters DW: Analysis of polyethylene wear of reverse shoulder components: A validated technique and initial clinical results. *J Orthop Res* 2017;35:980-987.

    In this study a method for the wear assessment of polyethylene in reverse total shoulder arthroplasties was developed. Measurements on retrieved components have shown that the overall wear volume was lower than in total hip replacements, but the volumetric wear rates were within the osteolytic threshold in the hip.

42. Hall DJ, Pourzal R, Lundberg HJ, Mathew MT, Jacobs JJ, Urban RM: Mechanical, chemical and biological damage modes within head-neck tapers of CoCrMo and Ti6Al4V contemporary hip replacements. *J Biomed Mater Res B Appl Biomater* 2018;106:1672-1685.

    This study determined different damage modes that occur within modular taper junctions of total hip replacements with metal femoral heads and either CoCrMo or Ti6Al4V alloy stems. The results demonstrated that damage can be either chemically or mechanically driven or a combination of both.

43. Cooper HJ, Urban RM, Wixson RI, Meneghini RM, Jacobs JJ: Adverse local tissue reactions Arising from corrosion at the neck-body junction in a dual taper stem with a CoCr modular neck. *J Bone Joint Surg AM* 2013;95:865-872.

44. Matziolis G, Perka C, Disch A: Massive metallosis after revision of a fractured ceramic head onto a metal head. *Arch Orthop Trauma Surg* 2003;123:48-50.

45. Traina F, Tassinari E, De Fine M, Bordini B, Toni A: Revision of ceramic hip replacements for fracture of a ceramic component: AAOS exhibit selection. *JBJS* 2011;93:e147.

46. McGrory BJ, MacKenzie J, Babikian G: A high prevalence of corrosion at the head–neck taper with contemporary Zimmer non-cemented femoral hip components. *J Arthroplast* 2015;30:1265-1268.

47. Porter DA, Urban RM, Jacobs JJ, Gilbert JL, Rodriguez JA, Cooper HJ: Modern trunnions are more flexible: A mechanical analysis of THA taper designs. *Clin Orthop* 2014;472:3963-3970.

48. Pourzal R, Hall DJ, Ha NQ, et al: Does surface topography play a role in taper damage in head-neck modular junctions? *Clin Orthop* 2016;474:2232-2242.

    This study investigated the impact of taper surface topography on subsequent in vivo damage. The results suggested that the femoral stem taper topography did impact the visual damage score, where a higher machining mark height correlated with lower damage scores.

49. Bishop N, Witt F, Pourzal R, et al: Wear patterns of taper connections in retrieved large diameter metal-on-metal bearings. *J Orthop Res* 2013;31:1116-1122.

50. Rehmer A, Bishop NE, Morlock MM: Influence of assembly procedure and material combination on the strength of the taper connection at the head-neck junction of modular hip endoprostheses. *Clin Biomech Bristol Avon* 2012;27:77-83.

51. Lundberg HJ, Ha NQ, Hall DJ, Urban RM, Levine BR, Pourzal R: in Greenwald AS, Kurtz SM, Lemons JE & Mihalko WM, eds: *Modul. Tapers Total Jt. Replace. Devices*. ASTM International, 2015, pp 59-82.

52. Gilbert JL, Mali S, Urban RM, Silverton CD, Jacobs JJ: In vivo oxide-induced stress corrosion cracking of Ti-6Al-4V in a neck-stem modular taper: Emergent behavior in a new mechanism of in vivo corrosion. *J Biomed Mater Res B Appl Biomater* 2011;100:584-594.

53. Martin AJ, Jenkins DR, Van Citters DW: Role of corrosion in taper failure and head disassociation in total hip arthroplasty of a single design. *J Orthop Res* 2018;36(11):2996-3003. doi:10.1002/jor.24107.

    This study analyzed the mechanism of gross trunnion failure occurring in THRs with TMZF alloy stems. The results suggest that corrosion of the CoCrMo femoral head triggers the eventual excessive wear of the titanium stem.

54. Pourzal R, Hall DJ, Ehrich J, et al: Alloy microstructure dictates corrosion modes in THR modular junctions. *Clin Orthop* 2017;475:3026-3043.

    This study describes the role of the implant alloy microstructure on corrosion. It was demonstrated that alloy segregation and hard phases can have a negative impact on the alloy's ability to withstand corrosion.

55. Igual Munoz A, Schwiesau J, Jolles BM, Mischler S: In vivo electrochemical corrosion study of a CoCrMo biomedical alloy in human synovial fluids. *Acta Biomater* 2015;21:228-236.

56. Gilbert JL, Sivan S, Liu Y, Kocagöz SB, Arnholt CM, Kurtz SM: Direct in vivo inflammatory cell-induced corrosion of CoCrMo alloy orthopedic implant surfaces. *J Biomed Mater Res A* 2015;103:211-223.

Chapter 9

Musculoskeletal Imaging Principles

Vishal Desai, MD • William Morrison, MD

ABSTRACT

Imaging plays an important role in the diagnosis of musculoskeletal pathologies, including trauma, arthropathies, tumors, and treatment follow-up. A working knowledge of the imaging modalities available is important in ensuring the correct study is performed to best answer the clinical question. Conventional radiography, CT, MRI, and ultrasonography are reviewed, including a basic background on each modality, advantages and limitations, and clinical applications for each. Multiple image-guided procedures are available for minimally invasive diagnostic and therapeutic interventions.

Keywords: CT; imaging; MRI; radiology; ultrasonography

Introduction

Imaging plays an important role in the evaluation of musculoskeletal symptoms, from evaluation of traumatic injury to tumor characterization to treatment follow-up. An understanding of the available imaging modalities and indications for each is critical to ensure that the correct study is performed and the clinical question is answered. Multiple image-guided interventions are available to aid in diagnosis and therapy.

Dr. Morrison or an immediate family member has received royalties from Apriomed, Inc.; is a member of a speakers' bureau or has made paid presentations on behalf of Zimmer; serves as a paid consultant to or is an employee of Samsung Medical and Zimmer; serves as an unpaid consultant to Apriomed, Inc.; and serves as a board member, owner, officer, or committee member of the American Board of Radiology, the American College of Radiology, and RSNA, ARRS, SSR. Neither Dr. Desai nor any immediate family member has received anything of value from or has stock or stock options held in a commercial company or institution related directly or indirectly to the subject of this chapter.

Conventional Radiography

Radiography is the most frequently used modality for evaluating bone and joint disorders. Despite the increased availability of more advanced imaging modalities, radiographs remain first line for diagnosing fractures, joint dislocations, suspected infection, tumors (benign and malignant); locating foreign objects; and guidance before, during, and after orthopedic procedures. Radiographs are complementary to all imaging modalities and should be routinely available for review when viewing CT, ultrasonography, or MRI.

Physics

Image formation for radiographs depends on the concept of differential absorption, where X-rays are absorbed nonhomogeneously depending on the density of each tissue. Bone, for instance, will absorb much more relative to soft tissue and even more so than fat. This leads to varying levels of radiolucency, such that bone appears white on a radiograph (radiopaque) whereas air, which absorbs the least, appears black (radiolucent). In addition, some X-rays are deflected or scattered as they pass through an object, which contributes to the ionizing radiation dose.

Technique

For optimal imaging technique, at least two views of the anatomy of interest at 90° angles are obtained. Generally, this includes standard AP and lateral views. Often, oblique views or other specialized views are obtained to help with evaluation of complex joints such as the wrist, elbow, and ankle, to inspect cortical margins in detail, and to assess for joint alignment such as the scapular Y-view for shoulder dislocation (**Figure 1**). In pediatric cases, views of the contralateral limb can be helpful to distinguish normal growth variation versus pathology.

Positional views can be helpful to define mechanical pathology that may not manifest at rest. The classic example is cervical flexion and extension views to diagnose instability. A weight-bearing view can offer dynamic evaluation of the joint space under body

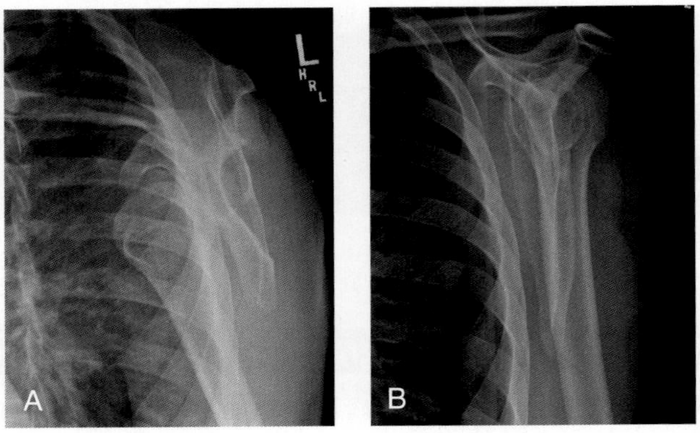

Figure 1 **A**, Scapular Y-view demonstrating an anterior shoulder dislocation. **B**, Postreduction scapular Y-view now shows the humeral head well-seated within the glenoid.

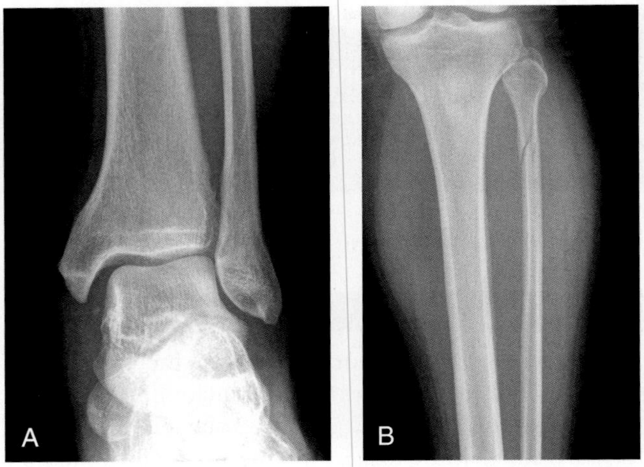

Figure 2 **A**, Mortise view of the ankle demonstrates widening of the medial clear space, suggesting ankle instability. **B**, AP view of the tibia and fibula proximally demonstrates a spiral fracture of the proximal fibular diaphysis, consistent with a Maisonneuve fracture.

weight. For instance, posterior tibialis tendon dysfunction in early stages may only be apparent radiographically on standing views with characteristic arch collapse, hindfoot valgus, and overpronation. On knee radiographs, the true severity of joint narrowing may only be seen when axial load is applied.

Trauma Evaluation

Radiographic examination serves as the best initial screening—and often diagnostic—imaging test for nearly all musculoskeletal pathology, as it is cost-effective and easy to obtain. Trauma is a common indication for plain radiographs, especially in the acute setting, to evaluate for fracture and joint alignment.[1] For fracture evaluation it is important to obtain orthogonal views, as this reduces the possibility of missing a fracture in a different plane. Additionally, imaging of the adjacent joints should be obtained to exclude an additional fracture (as in the setting of a Maisonneuve fracture) or to exclude a remote fracture which may be causing referred pain (**Figure 2**). Plain radiographs can provide quick, valuable information on joint alignment prereduction and postreduction in cases of dislocations. For more high-grade traumas, radiography offers the advantage of portable imaging. Although the imaging quality and positioning is less optimal, it can be extremely helpful for rapidly diagnosing fractures, dislocations, spinal trauma, foreign bodies, and line placements.

Atraumatic Evaluation

Radiography is also valuable for nontrauma evaluations. One of the most common indications for axial or appendicular radiographs is atraumatic pain, and plain radiographs can provide information regarding degenerative changes, impingement syndromes (such as femoroacetabular impingement), osseous lesions, arthropathies, osteomyelitis, insufficiency fractures, and osseous mineralization. For spinal imaging, radiographs can demonstrate degenerative disk disease and compression fractures of the spine; however, CT and MRI are better suited for spinal evaluation when indicated.

Imaging evaluation of arthritis usually requires plain radiographs only, with clinical and laboratory information helping to narrow the differential. The major findings for arthritides include distribution of disease, joint alignment, status of the joint space, osseous mineralization, erosive changes, and associated soft-tissue pathology—all of which can be adequately and quickly assessed by plain radiograph (**Figure 3**).[2,3] In complex cases, it may be necessary to use more advanced imaging such as MRI to look for synovitis, tenosynovitis, and other potential soft-tissue or subtle bone marrow changes.

Neoplasm

Radiographs are extremely useful and often necessary for adequate characterization of a musculoskeletal neoplasm—osseous or soft tissue.[4] For bony lesions, plain radiographs can evaluate if the lesion is lucent or sclerotic, the location of the lesion within the bone (ie, metaphyseal, eccentric), and if it has any features suggestive of malignancy such as cortical destruction, periosteal reaction, permeative pattern or wide zone of transition, and a soft-tissue component (**Figure 4**).[5] These features along with the patient's age and clinical history is usually enough information to narrow the differential

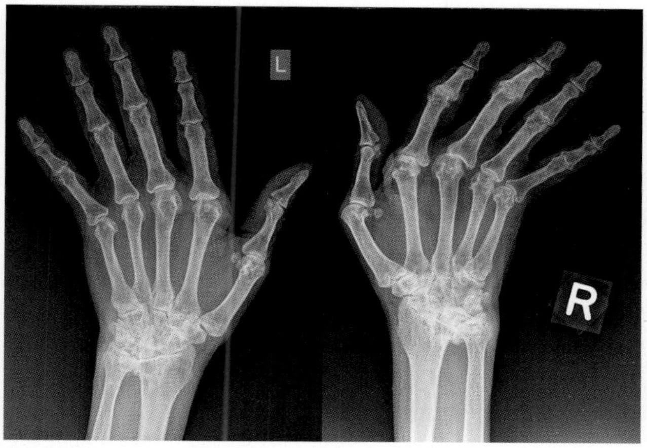

Figure 3 AP view of the hands demonstrates a proximal, bilateral symmetric arthritis with scattered marginal erosions, ulnar deviation at the MCP joints, and advanced degenerative change in the carpus, consistent with rheumatoid arthritis.

diagnosis. For purely soft-tissue lesions, radiography is less robust, but the pattern of calcification or ossification (if present) can still offer valuable diagnostic information, including differentiating between benign myositis ossificans and soft-tissue osteosarcoma.

Fluoroscopy

Fluoroscopy passes a continuous X-ray beam through the area of interest, providing real-time imaging evaluation. Although this can be valuable tool to assess anatomy in different positions and under stress, it is more commonly used for image-guided procedures. Fluoroscopy is especially useful for arthrograms, joint aspirations, therapeutic joint and bursal injections, and spine interventions. "Plain arthrography" is rarely performed, but injection for CT or MR arthrography is most commonly done under fluoroscopic or radiographic guidance.

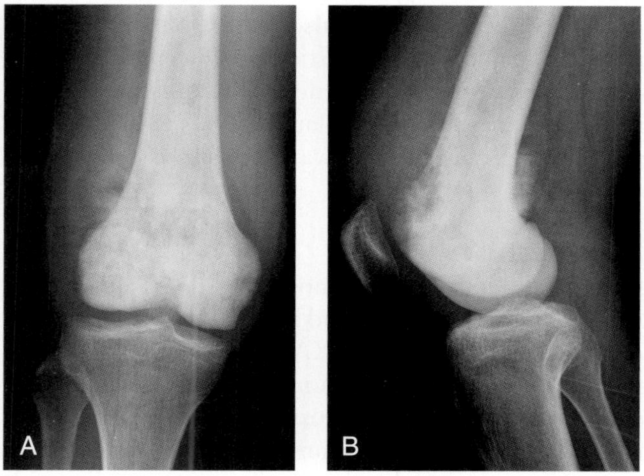

Figure 4 **A** and **B**, AP and lateral views of the right knee demonstrate a large sclerotic lesion within the distal femur with periosteal elevation (Codman's triangle) and sunburst periosteal reaction, characteristic of osteosarcoma.

Bone Health

X-ray-derived technologies are highly accurate in assessing bone density and predicting the risk of a future major osteoporotic fracture. Dual-energy X-ray absorptiometry (DXA) is the most widely used and remains the current benchmark. This involves passing two separate, low-dose source beams at distinct energies through the lumbar spine and/or hips, with soft tissue then subtracted and the resultant bone density calculated and scaled against reference values.[6] The World Health Organization Fracture Risk Assessment Tool (FRAX) is a useful adjunct that combines the DXA results with clinical factors and demographics to estimate the 10-year bone fracture risk.

Digital X-ray radiogrammetry (DXR) is a peripheral bone mineral density measurement method that uses a standard radiograph. Various measurements are used, frequently the bone width or cortical thickness of the nondominant second metacarpal to provide a computed bone mineral density equivalent. This predominantly automated, software-based method can also accurately predict hip fracture risk in both men and women.[7,8]

Computed Tomography

Unlike conventional radiography, CT utilizes a motorized X-ray source that rotates within a donut-shaped gantry around the patient. The beams travel through the patient with multiple detectors at the opposite end to acquire the data for that body region. The data are processed and a 2D cross-sectional image ("slice") created. The table then shifts and the process is repeated until the area of interest is fully imaged.

Advances in CT

With the advent of multidetector CT, which allows for multiple data streams to be acquired simultaneously, scan times have been cut down to seconds and motion artifact is substantially reduced, which is particularly helpful in the trauma setting.[9] After acquisition, the slices can be viewed in succession and can also be reconstructed in multiple planes (sagittal, coronal, obliques) as well as in 3D, providing a large amount of cross-sectional information about the osseous and soft-tissue structures in that region and serving as an invaluable tool for preoperative planning (**Figure 5**).[10,11]

Principles of Orthopaedics

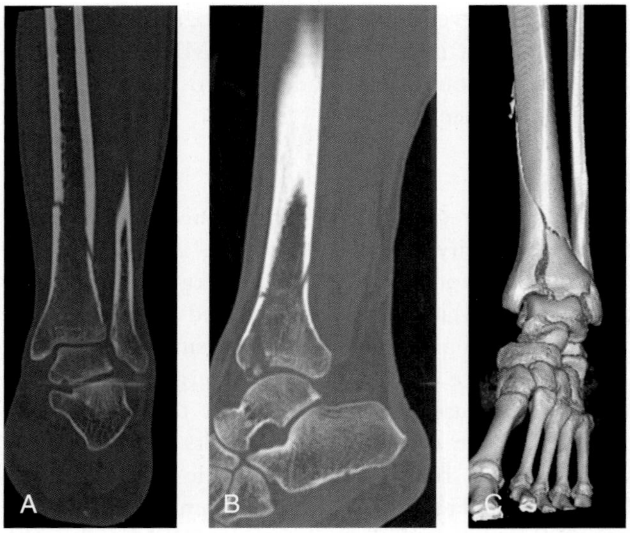

Figure 5 Sagittal (**A**) and coronal (**B**) CT reformats of the ankle demonstrate a comminuted fracture of the distal tibia with intra-articular extension. 3D reconstructions (**C**) can be helpful in assessing the fracture pattern and for preoperative planning.

Trauma CT

Given the rapid acquisition time and level of detail, CT is essential for evaluation of spinal fractures in the setting of trauma and has largely replaced radiography for this purpose.[12] MRI is superior in detecting acute fractures, particularly in osteopenic patients or radiographically-negative studies; however, CT can be used if MRI is contraindicated or not readily available.[13] CT is excellent for assessing the status of implanted hardware and possible complications such as osteolysis, loosening, or lack of osseous bridging.[14-16]

Operative Planning

Compared with radiography, the three-dimensional data offered by CT allows for better characterization of the fracture and joint alignment, particularly helpful for complex joints such as the elbow, ankle, and knee joints.[17] The CT data can be directly used by 3D printing software, which allows for modeling and preoperative planning for fixation hardware or prostheses.[18]

Neoplasm

For soft-tissue and osseous lesions, MRI is generally preferred because of the superior contrast resolution. However, CT may serve as a complementary tool to MRI particularly to evaluate for ossification and calcification. CT may be the study of choice in patients with contraindications to MRI (pacemakers, vascular clips, ocular implants, claustrophobia, etc).

Contrast

In cases where MRI is not available or contraindicated, intravenous iodinated contrast can be used with CT to improve detection and characterization of soft-tissue lesions. Intravenous contrast is generally not helpful in the evaluation of bone lesions, osteomyelitis (unless evaluating for fluid collections), or traumatic injuries.

Joint evaluation can be significantly enhanced with the administration of intra-articular contrast. CT arthrography can identify cartilage defects, intra-articular bodies, meniscal tears, and labral tears effectively in patients with contraindications to MRI or MR arthrography (**Figure 6**).[19]

Recent Advances

Newer techniques such as dual-energy CT have shown significant potential in musculoskeletal imaging. Dual-energy CT scanners allow simultaneous acquisition at two different energy levels. This can characterize the chemical composition of material according to the differential attenuation of the structures being examined at the two different energy levels, highly specific in detecting uric acid deposits in gout and in monitoring response to treatment. Other applications include minimizing metal prosthesis artifacts, detecting bone marrow edema, and visualizing pathologic tendons and ligaments.[20]

Image-Guided Interventions

CT guidance is now commonly used for both the diagnosis and treatment of numerous musculoskeletal conditions. CT-guided percutaneous biopsies of osseous and soft-tissue lesions provide increased safety, decreased cost, decreased time, and reduced pain compared with open biopsies with a high diagnostic accuracy.[21,22] CT guidance can also play a role in injections for pain management, particularly in patients with complex anatomy. Other safe and successful therapies included radiofrequency ablation for osteoid osteomas and radiofrequency/microwave ablations of tumors (**Figure 7**).

Bone Health

Quantitative computed tomography (QCT) uses low-dose imaging of the spine and hip to assess bone mineral density. Compared with DXA, QCT is less susceptible to artifact and miscalculation related to degenerative changes, osteophytes, scoliosis, and large body habitus.[23] Additionally, QCT can provide separate assessments of cortical and trabecular bone. Generally, with CT, ionizing radiation is a limiting factor but with QCT, low-dose techniques allow for each scan to be equivalent to a set of mammograms.

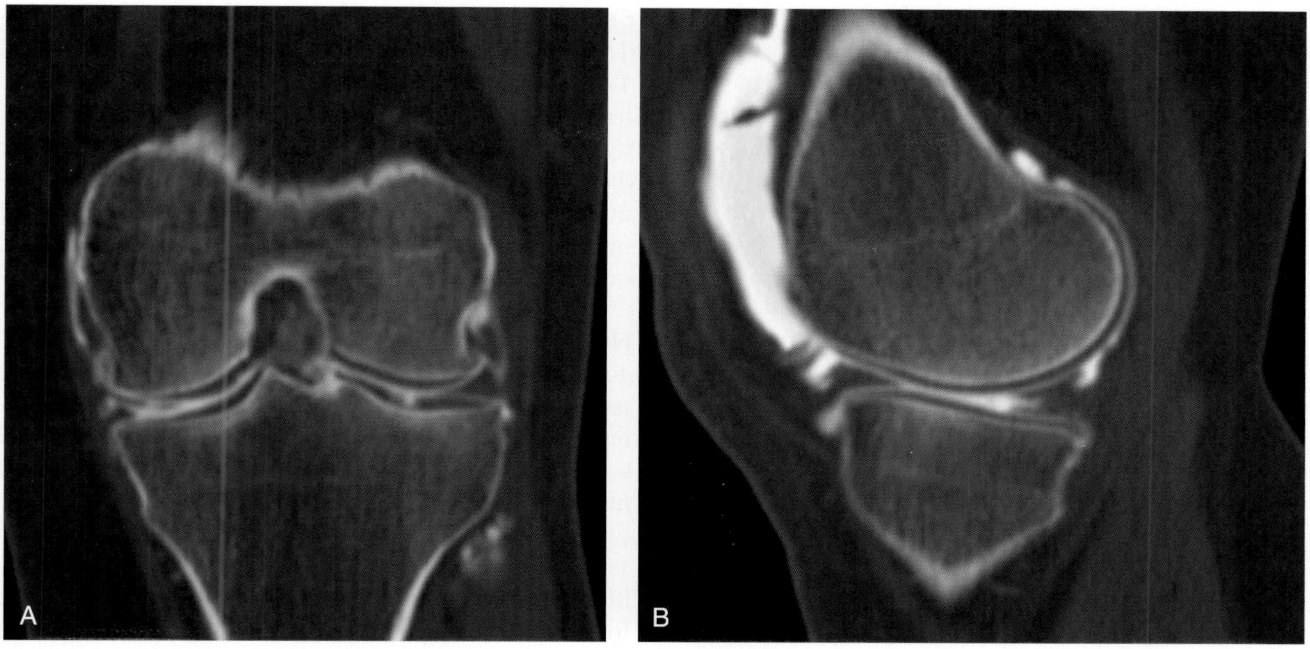

Figure 6 Coronal (**A**) and sagittal (**B**) CT arthrogram images of the knee show intra-articular contrast extending into the body and posterior horn of the medial meniscus, consistent with a meniscal tear.

Magnetic Resonance Imaging

As the mainstay in advanced musculoskeletal imaging, MRI provides a wealth of information on anatomy and tissue composition with unparalleled contrast resolution and no ionizing radiation.

Physics

MRI is based on the magnetization properties of atomic nuclei. A uniform magnetic field is applied, aligning the randomly oriented protons within the nuclei of tissues. Next, radiofrequency (RF) energy is used to disturb that alignment. The nuclei eventually return to their resting

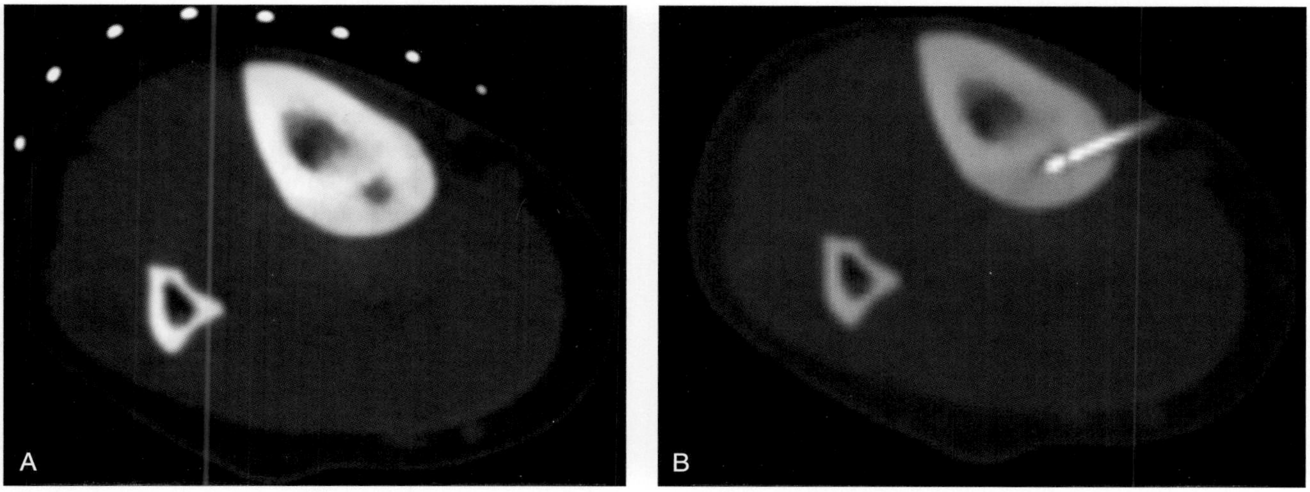

Figure 7 Planning axial CT image (**A**) demonstrates thickening and sclerosis along the posterior tibial cortex with a central lucency, which together with the clinical history is consistent with an osteoid osteoma. This lesion is readily accessed percutaneously for biopsy and ablation (**B**).

state while emitting a measurable amount of RF energy. That energy is converted into signal intensity for the matching location in the image.

Various changes to the RF pulse sequences and acquisitions—repetition time (TR) and echo time (TE)—create different images with additional information about the tissues of interest. Tissue can be characterized by two different relaxation times—T1 and T2, based on the rate at which protons return to equilibrium in the longitudinal and transverse planes, respectively. Image contrast is primarily based on the number of protons within each tissue.

Imaging Quality

In addition to the inherent tissue contrast, several external factors can play a role in the imaging information provided. Magnetic field strengths can vary from 0.2 to 3 T for clinical applications, with 1.5 T being the most common. In general, the higher the field strength, the higher the signal-to-noise ratio (more signal, less noise artifact), the better the contrast, and higher the resolution. This, in turn, improves overall image quality and diagnostic ability.

MR scanners are available in open and closed configurations, with the open scanners generally having a significantly lower field strength and multiple limitations, such as longer scan time (increasing susceptibility to motion artifact), wider field of view, and lack of adequate fat suppression. Evaluation of small joints and cartilage is often difficult on low-field-strength, open scanners. Open scanners should only be reserved for claustrophobic patients and obese patients who may not fit satisfactorily into a more robust closed MR scanner. Extremity scanners are available, which only require the patient's arm or leg to be within the bore, minimizing discomfort.

One of the most important and often overlooked decisions in musculoskeletal imaging is coil selection. Given the wide variation in configuration and quality of surface coils for extremities, there is significant potential to produce less than optimal images. In general, the smallest coil possible should be used for imaging to achieve the desired field of view, because the more closely the coil sits against the body part, the better the imaging quality. Regardless of coil choice, it should be positioned to optimally image the area of interest. When patients may not be able to hold a position because of discomfort, sometimes a more comfortable second option should be considered as the original position may cause patient motion and degraded images.

Sequences

The most commonly used MRI sequences are T1- and T2-weighted sequences. T1-weighted images are excellent for evaluating anatomy. Fat appears bright or hyperintense on T1-weighted imaging, and fluid appears dark or hypointense. Replacement of the normal fatty marrow on T1-weighted imaging is an indicator of underlying pathology, such as fracture, osteomyelitis, or malignancy.

Fluid-Sensitive Sequences

T2-weighted sequences are excellent for evaluating pathology, because edema or fluid appears hyperintense. Because fat is also hyperintense on T2-weighted sequences, fat saturation techniques can be used to make the edema and other pathology more apparent.

The most commonly used technique is frequency selective fat saturation, which uses an RF pulse to nullify signal from fat (**Figure 8**). In an MRI of the wrist, for instance, a T2-weighted fat-suppressed sequence provides high contrast resolution with fluid being hyperintense and the triangular fibrocartilage being hypointense. This technique can also be used in post-contrast T1-weighted imaging to assess enhancement patterns. The one pitfall is the possibility of heterogeneous fat suppression, particularly along curved surfaces and adjacent to hardware.

An alternative and also commonly used fat suppression technique in musculoskeletal imaging is a short tau inversion recovery, or STIR, sequence. Based on the varying relaxation times of fat and water, signal from fat can be markedly reduced. Fat suppression in STIR imaging is less susceptible to heterogeneity and appears more uniform. However, it should not be used for post-contrast imaging, as the relaxation properties of fat and contrast are similar and would cause signal loss of both.

Additional Sequences

Additional sequences relevant to musculoskeletal MRI include proton density (PD) and gradient echo (GRE). PD is an intermediate sequence with features of both T1- and T2-weighted sequences, which provides high signal-to-noise ratio and is particularly useful for joint imaging. GRE can be obtained with thin sections allowing for detailed evaluation of small structures and cartilage.

GRE sequences are highly sensitive to magnetic field homogeneities, leading to susceptibility artifact. However, this "artifact" can be used advantageously to locate displaced sutures or foreign bodies, identify the site of surgery if unknown, and evaluate for small

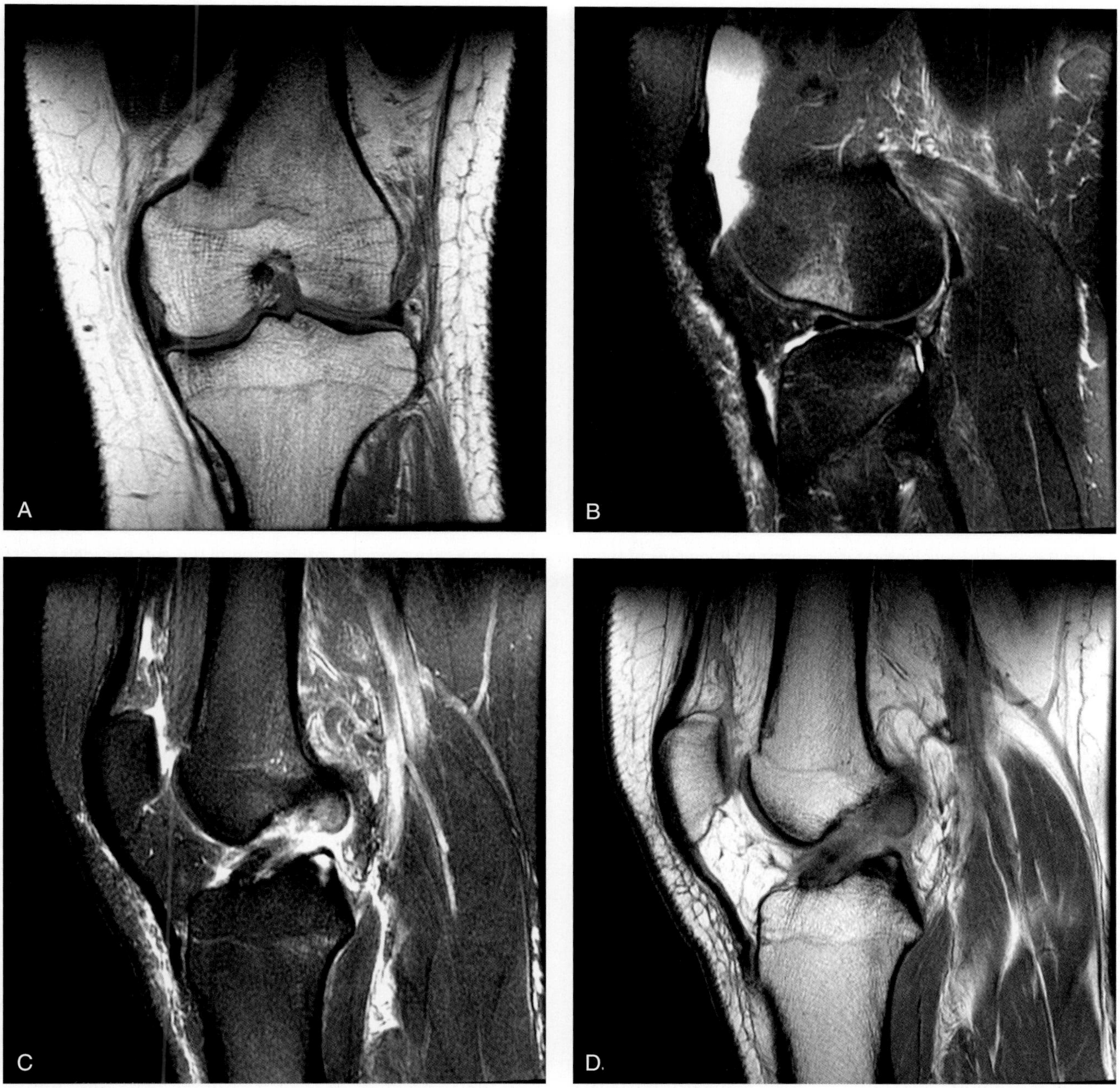

Figure 8 Coronal T1-weighted image of the knee (**A**) demonstrates normal fatty marrow signal. Sagittal T2-weighted fat-suppressed images (**B** and **C**) show a bone marrow edema pattern typical for pivot shift osseous contusions with an associated tear of the ACL. Sagittal PD image (**D**) offers increased signal and confirms the ACL (anterior cruciate ligament) tear.

avulsion fractures or loose bodies. This can also be helpful for characterizing lesions, as calcium deposits are accentuated and can aid in identifying enchondromas, osteosarcomas, synovial sarcoma, myositis ossificans, heterotopic bone, and calcific tendinosis. Hemosiderin deposits, as seen in pigmented villonodular synovitis, blooms on GRE sequences (**Figure 9**).

Metal Artifact Reduction Sequence

A variety of techniques exist to image bones and joints with hardware, making MRI useful in the evaluation of postoperative complications or hardware failure. A metal artifact reduction sequence (MARS) reduces the intensity of the hardware-related susceptibility artifact that results from the magnetic field

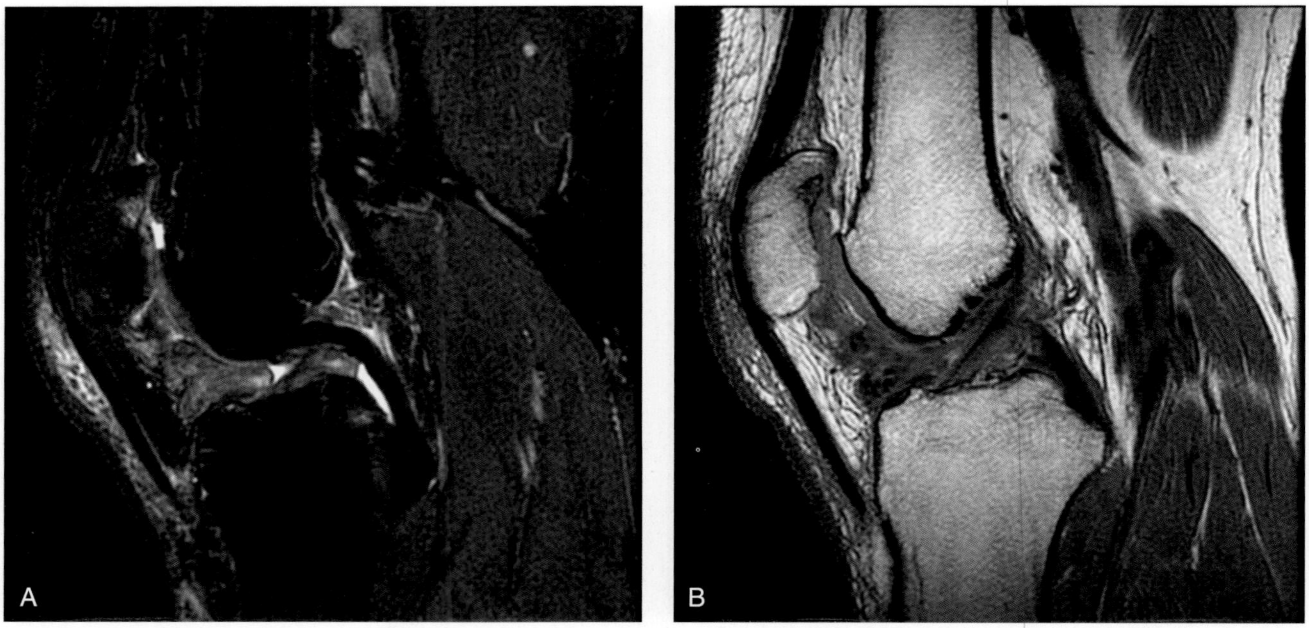

Figure 9 Sagittal T2-weighted fat-suppressed image (**A**) of the knee shows masslike synovial proliferation in the anterior joint recess. A T1-weighted gradient echo sequence (**B**) demonstrates low signal with slight blooming artifact within the lesion, consistent with pigmented villonodular synovitis.

distortion.[24,25] Such sequences allow for evaluation of osteolysis or adverse local tissue reaction with an implant in place.[26]

Contrast

MR arthrography (MRA) is an excellent tool for evaluation of intra-articular pathology.[27,28] Direct MRA is most common and involves injection of gadolinium-based contrast into the joint using either fluoroscopic or ultrasonographic guidance. Indirect MRA is less common and involves intravenous injection of contrast followed by delayed MR imaging. All compartments enhance with indirect MRA so abnormal communication of contrast material is absent. Typical imaging sequences include a combination of conventional MRI and fat-saturated T1-weighted sequences to highlight the intra-articular contrast.

The addition of intra-articular contrast causes distention of the joint to highlight structures more clearly and, in the presence of intra-articular pathology, T1 hyperintense contrast extends into the area involved (**Figure 10**). Direct MRA is ideal for evaluation of labral tears in the shoulder and hip with sensitivity of 92%.[29] MRA can also be used to evaluate for triangular fibrocartilage or scapholunate ligament tears in the wrist and ulnar collateral ligament tears in the elbow and for postoperative evaluation of meniscal re-tears in the knee.

Intravenous contrast for musculoskeletal imaging is generally reserved for problem-solving in noncharacteristic soft-tissue lesions and occasionally for osseous lesions. The enhancement pattern can be particularly helpful in discriminating benign versus more aggressive lesions, such as a nonenhancing myxoma versus an avidly enhancing sarcoma.

Clinical Applications

Given the very high contrast resolution, lack of ionizing radiation, and ability to assess soft tissues, osseous structures, ligaments, and tendons in detail, MRI is the workhorse of advanced musculoskeletal imaging. MRI is often the study of choice following initial radiography for assessment of joint pathology. The only limitations include longer scan time (relative to CT), potential incompatibilities with implanted nonorthopedic hardware, increased susceptibility to artifact, and cost.

Trauma and Degenerative Joint Disease

MRI is highly sensitive in the detection of traumatic injuries and degenerative joint disease. Bone contusions and subchondral fractures, easily missed or not visible on radiography or CT, are readily identified on MRI (**Figure 11**).[30] The bone marrow edema pattern and surrounding changes often allow for an estimation of the acuity and/or severity of the injury.

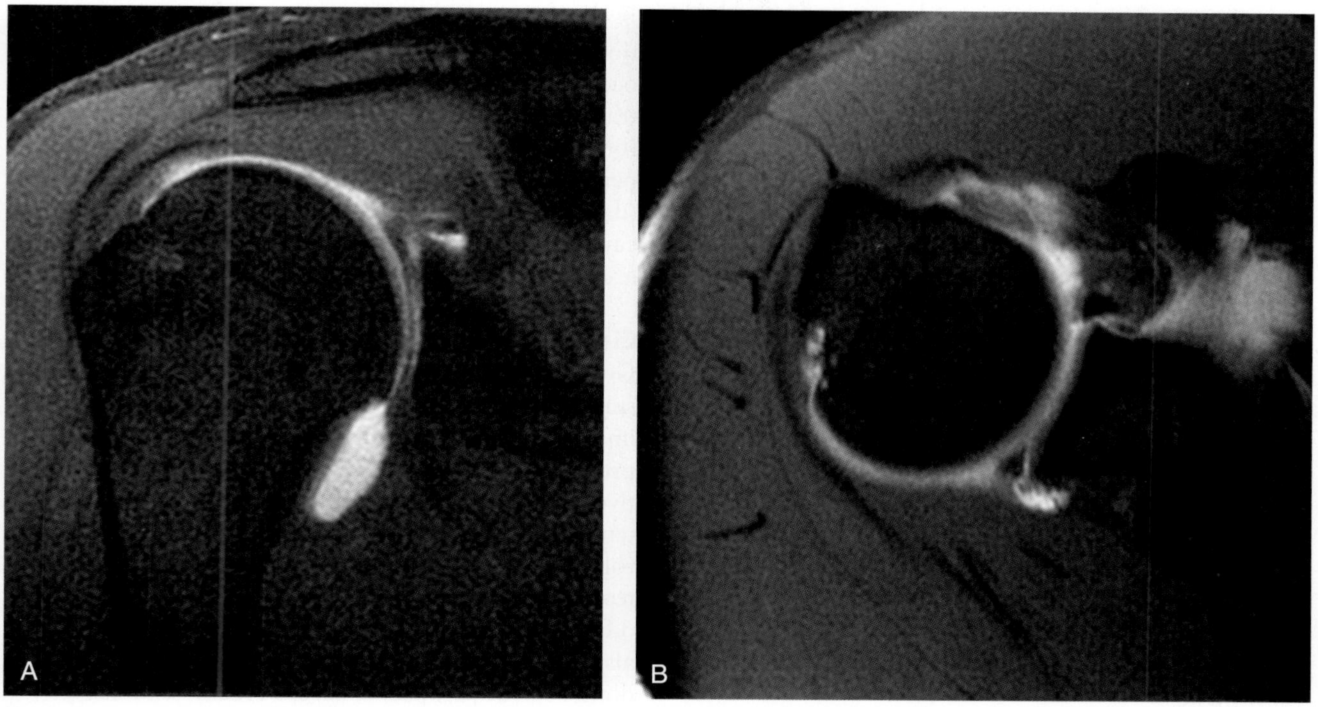

Figure 10 Coronal (**A**) and axial (**B**) T1-weighted fat-suppressed direct MR arthrogram images of the shoulder demonstrate intra-articular contrast extending into the posterior superior labrum with an adjacent paralabral cyst, consistent with a labral tear.

Generally, CT is the study of choice for suspected traumatic cervical spine injury. However, in the setting of a negative CT but abnormal neurologic examination, MRI of the cervical spine is warranted to evaluate for ligamentous injury or occult fracture.

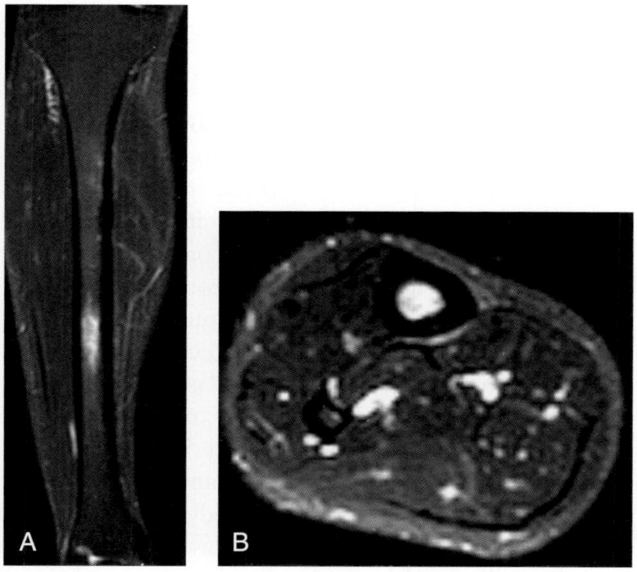

Figure 11 Coronal (**A**) and axial (**B**) T2-weighted fat-suppressed images of the lower extremity demonstrate bone marrow and intracortical signal abnormality consistent with a stress fracture, which was radiographically occult in this runner.

Ligamentous sprains, meniscal tears, and tendon or muscle strains are well visualized on T2-weighted imaging. Cartilage defects and osteochondral defects are also best seen by MRI. To evaluate for occult fractures, MRI is the best imaging test and an abbreviated protocol can be used for rapid evaluation, such as for femoral neck or scaphoid fractures.[31,32] This is especially true if the patient is osteopenic, as fractures can be missed on CT in that patient population.

Neoplasm

Similarly, osseous and soft-tissue lesions are most optimally characterized by MRI, ideally in conjunction with radiography for added information. For lesions, fat within a nonaggressive-appearing lesion is identified by MRI and can suggest a benign etiology such as enchondroma or vascular malformation. Hemosiderin, seen as dark signal with blooming on GRE sequences, can point toward pigmented villonodular synovitis or giant cell tumor of tendon sheath. Bone marrow replacement on T1-weighted sequences suggests an infiltrative process such as tumor or infection. The extent of marrow involvement, presence of pathologic fracture, muscle or vascular invasion, and soft-tissue components can be assessed by MRI for more aggressive lesions.[33,34]

Infection

MRI is the imaging modality of choice for suspected osteomyelitis, identified by hyperintense signal (bone marrow edema) on T2-weighted imaging and hypointense signal (bone marrow replacement) on T1-weighted imaging.[35-37] Intraosseous, subperiosteal, and soft-tissue abscesses are easily demonstrated by MRI. If MRI is contraindicated, alternative modalities such as triple phase bone scan can be used.

Musculoskeletal Ultrasonography

Ultrasonography has gained much popularity in musculoskeletal imaging in the past decade and is a powerful tool in the evaluation of musculoskeletal abnormalities. Ultrasonography is relatively low cost compared with MRI and CT, is fairly quick to perform, has no ionizing radiation, and lends itself to diagnostic evaluation and therapeutic interventions in one visit.[38-40]

Technique

Ultrasonography works by passing high frequency sound waves from the probe through the tissues of interest. The sound waves are then reflected back based on the tissue properties and the resultant echoes are collected by the transducer and processed into an image.

Proper ultrasonography evaluation in musculoskeletal imaging requires the use of a high-frequency linear transducer. Higher-frequency transducers produce higher-resolution images with the tradeoff of lower penetration. However, because most musculoskeletal structures of interest tend to be linear in configuration and superficial, higher-frequency transducers are ideal.

Curvilinear transducers can be used to evaluate deeper structures or for deep hip aspirations and soft-tissue biopsies. Smaller footprint linear transducers ("hockey stick transducers") are helpful in evaluation of the hands, wrist, and feet where the limited body surfaces prevent use of larger transducers. Correct focal zone location and minimizing depth to include only the region of interest are two additional easily selectable parameters to optimize imaging.

Color Doppler and power Doppler imaging are valuable adjuncts to assess for vascularity within lesions or synovium, with power Doppler being more sensitive and color Doppler having the ability to provide speed and flow direction. The use of Doppler imaging is very helpful in inflammatory arthropathies to evaluate for synovitis and response to therapy.

A common artifact during ultrasonography evaluation is anisotropy, or direction-dependence. Anisotropy occurs in tendon and ligaments when the angle of the transducer is changed. Tendon fibers have a hyperechoic (bright) fibrillar appearance when the transducer is perpendicular to the tendon, but can appear hypoechoic (dark) when the transducer is angled obliquely. This can cause interpretation error if areas that look tendinotic are not adequately evaluated at multiple angles.

Clinical Applications

Given its dynamic capability, ultrasonography is well suited for evaluating a patient's focal symptoms by imaging directly in the area of interest with and without provocative maneuvers. Ultrasonography is able to effectively assess the integrity of most ligaments, muscles, and tendons. It is especially well suited for evaluation of the rotator cuff with a sensitivity of 84% for partial-thickness tears and 96% for full-thickness tears, and no significant difference compared with MRI.[41] Ultrasonography can also confidently demonstrate active subluxation of tendons, such as peroneal or biceps brachii tendons.

Ultrasonography is limited in intra-articular evaluation particularly for meniscal tears, labral tears, and cartilage defects. Several studies have demonstrated the complementary nature of ultrasonography and MRI for detailed musculoskeletal assessment. Although ultrasonography is operator dependent, given its growth over the last several years, many sonographers and radiologists have been or are being trained in musculoskeletal ultrasonography with more standardized protocols for imaging and treatment.

Image-Guided Interventions

One of the major benefits of ultrasonography is the ability to treat at the time of diagnosis, in an outpatient setting with local anesthetic only. Numerous ultrasound-guided musculoskeletal interventions are available, including injections for pain management (joints, bursae, trigger points, neuromas), joint aspirations, arthrograms, biopsies, percutaneous needling/tenotomy to promote tendon healing, calcific tendinosis lavage and needling, platelet-rich plasma (PRP) injections, and carpal tunnel fenestration and release (**Figure 12**).[42-44] Multiple studies demonstrate improvement on follow-up imaging and more importantly improvement in patient symptomatology after needling interventions with and without corticosteroid or PRP injections. Direct visualization during needle placement and monitoring of injected/aspirated material makes ultrasonography ideal for these interventions.

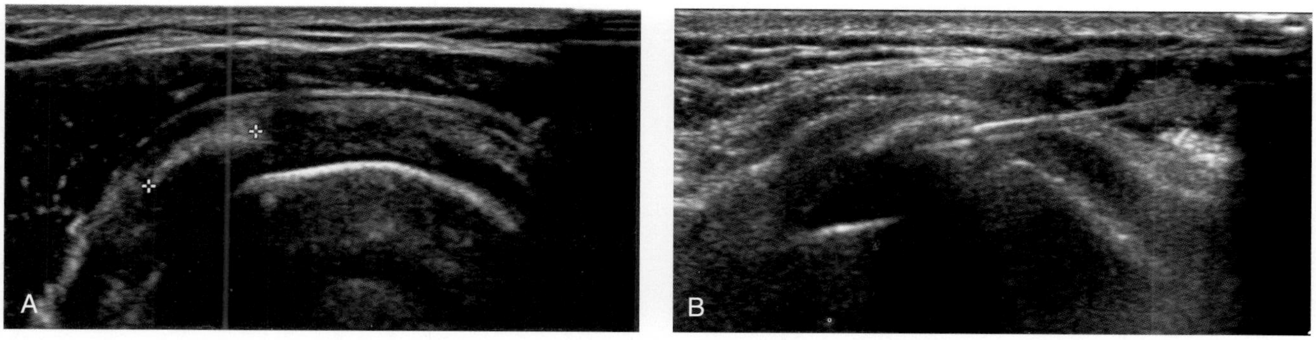

Figure 12 Short axis ultrasonography image (**A**) of the supraspinatus tendon demonstrate focal calcific tendinosis. This was successfully treated percutaneously with needling and lavage (**B**).

Summary

Imaging plays a large part in the diagnosis of musculoskeletal pathologies. Radiography is almost always the initial imaging test of choice for traumatic injuries, suspected arthropathies, and tumor evaluation. CT provides multiplanar and 3D imaging, which can be helpful in preoperative planning and can also serve as complementary study to MRI for lesion characterization. MRI has very high contrast resolution and is the study of choice to evaluate for internal derangement, characterizing soft-tissue and osseous lesions, and to assess for occult fractures. Ultrasonography provides dynamic evaluation, focused on the patient's symptoms and has high sensitivity for tendon, muscle, and several ligamentous injuries. Multiple image-guided diagnostic and therapeutic interventions are available with both CT and ultrasonography guidance.

Study Facts/Key Points

- Radiographs are the initial imaging test of choice for nearly all musculoskeletal complaints and should be available when interpreting CT, ultrasonography, and especially MRI.
- MRI is the workhorse for musculoskeletal imaging. Given the lack of ionizing radiation, high contrast resolution, and ability to assess nearly all tissues, MRI is the best study for detecting internal derangement, and occult fractures, osteomyelitis and for characterizing soft-tissue and osseous lesions.
- Ultrasonography provides dynamic evaluation, focused on the patient's symptoms, and has high sensitivity for tendon, muscle, and several ligamentous injuries.

Annotated References

1. Thomas J, Rideau AM, Paulson EK, Bisset GS: Emergency department imaging: Current practice. *J Am Coll Radiol* 2008;5(7):811-816.e2. doi:10.1016/j.jacr.2008.02.027.
2. Jacobson JA, Girish G, Jiang Y, Resnick D: Radiographic evaluation of arthritis: Inflammatory conditions. *Radiology* 2008;248(2):378-389. doi:10.1148/radiol.2482062110.
3. Jacobson JA, Girish G, Jiang Y, Sabb BJ: Radiographic evaluation of arthritis: Degenerative joint disease and variations. *Radiology* 2008;248(3):737-747. doi:10.1148/radiol.2483062112.
4. Costelloe CM, Madewell JE: Radiography in the initial diagnosis of primary bone tumors. *Am J Roentgenol* 2013;200(1):3-7. doi:10.2214/AJR.12.8488.
5. Plant J, Cannon S: Diagnostic work up and recognition of primary bone tumours: A review. *EFORT Open Rev* 2016;1(6):247-253. doi:10.1302/2058-5241.1.000035.

   Imaging of bone tumors is reviewed in multiple modalities with a focus on radiographic evaluation. Level of evidence: V.
6. Lorente-Ramos R, Azpeitia-Armán J, Muñoz-Hernández A, García-Gómez JM, Díez-Martínez P, Grande-Bárez M: Dual-energy X-ray absorptiometry in the diagnosis of osteoporosis: A practical guide. *Am J Roentgenol* 2011;196(4):897-904. doi:10.2214/AJR.10.5416.
7. Surrey D, Sharpe RE, Gorniak RJT, et al: QRSE: A novel metric for the evaluation of trainee radiologist reporting skills. *J Digit Imaging* 2013;26(4):678-682. doi:10.1007/s10278-013-9574-y.
8. Kälvesten J, Lui L-Y, Brismar T, Cummings S: Digital X-ray radiogrammetry in the study of osteoporotic fractures: Comparison to dual energy X-ray absorptiometry and FRAX. *Bone* 2016;86:30-35. doi:10.1016/j.bone.2016.02.011.

   The authors compare the DXR modality to the gold standard DXA in prediction of osteoporotic fractures. Level of evidence: III.

9. Ptak T, Rhea JT, Novelline RA: Radiation dose is reduced with a single-pass whole-body multi–detector row CT trauma protocol compared with a conventional segmented method: Initial experience. *Radiology* 2003;229(3):902-905. doi:10.1148/radiol.2293021651.
10. Calhoun PS, Kuszyk BS, Heath DG, Carley JC, Fishman EK: Three-dimensional volume rendering of spiral CT data: Theory and method. *RadioGraphics* 1999;19(3):745-764. doi:10.1148/radiographics.19.3.g99ma14745.
11. Wicky S, Blaser PF, Blanc CH, Leyvraz PF, Schnyder P, Meuli RA: Comparison between standard radiography and spiral CT with 3D reconstruction in the evaluation, classification and management of tibial plateau fractures. *Eur Radiol* 2000;10(8):1227-1232. doi:10.1007/s003300000326.
12. Inaba K, Byerly S, Bush LD, et al: Cervical spinal clearance: A prospective western trauma association multi-institutional trial. *J Trauma Acute Care Surg* 2016;81(6):1122-1130. doi:10.1097/TA.0000000000001194.

    The authors study the accuracy of CT for detection of clinically significant cervical spine injury. Level of evidence: I.
13. Sadozai Z, Davies R, Warner J: The sensitivity of ct scans in diagnosing occult femoral neck fractures. *Injury* 2016;47(12):2769-2771. doi:10.1016/j.injury.2016.10.019.

    The authors study the sensitivity of CT in detecting radiographically occult femoral neck fractures and overall recommend MRI over CT for fracture evaluation unless not available. Level of evidence: III.
14. Nam D, Barrack RL, Potter HG: What are the advantages and disadvantages of imaging modalities to diagnose wear-related corrosion problems? *Clin Orthop Relat Res* 2014;472(12):3665-3673. doi:10.1007/s11999-014-3579-9.

    The authors review the role of CT, MRI, and ultrasound in diagnosing adverse local tissue reaction. Level of evidence: III.
15. Ohashi K, El-Khoury GY, Bennett DL, Restrepo JM, Berbaum KS: Orthopedic hardware complications diagnosed with multi–detector row CT. *Radiology* 2005;237(2):570-577. doi:10.1148/radiol.2372041681.
16. Patel VV, Andersson GBJ, Garfin SR, Resnick DL, Block JE: Utilization of CT scanning associated with complex spine surgery. *BMC Musculoskelet Disord* 2017;18(1):52. doi:10.1186/s12891-017-1420-9.

    CT imaging of the postoperative spine is reviewed including indications and utilization patterns. Level of evidence: V.
17. Prat-Fabregat S, Camacho-Carrasco P: Treatment strategy for tibial plateau fractures: An update. *EFORT Open Rev* 2016;1(5):225-232. doi:10.1302/2058-5241.1.000031.

    The authors review tibial plateau fracture diagnosis, classification, and treatment strategies. Level of evidence: III.
18. Friedman T, Michalski M, Goodman TR, Brown JE: 3D printing from diagnostic images: A radiologist's primer with an emphasis on musculoskeletal imaging—putting the 3D printing of pathology into the hands of every physician. *Skeletal Radiol* 2016;45(3):307-321. doi:10.1007/s00256-015-2282-6.

    Various methods of 3D printing with a focus on musculoskeletal imaging are reviewed. Level of evidence: V.
19. Christie-Large M, Tapp MJF, Theivendran K, James SLJ: The role of multidetector CT arthrography in the investigation of suspected intra-articular hip pathology. *Br J Radiol* 2010;83(994):861-867. doi:10.1259/bjr/76751715.
20. Mallinson PI, Coupal TM, McLaughlin PD, Nicolaou S, Munk PL, Ouellette HA: Dual-energy CT for the musculoskeletal system. *Radiology* 2016;281(3):690-707. doi:10.1148/radiol.2016151109.

    Review of the principles behind dual-energy CT and clinical applications with a focus on musculoskeletal imaging. Level of evidence: V.
21. Pohlig F, Kirchhoff C, Lenze U, et al: Percutaneous core needle biopsy versus open biopsy in diagnostics of bone and soft tissue sarcoma: A retrospective study. *Eur J Med Res* 2012;17(1):29. doi:10.1186/2047-783X-17-29.
22. Omura MC, Motamedi K, UyBico S, Nelson SD, Seeger LL: Revisiting CT-guided percutaneous core needle biopsy of musculoskeletal lesions: Contributors to biopsy success. *Am J Roentgenol* 2011;197(2):457-461. doi:10.2214/AJR.10.6145.
23. Li N, Li X, Xu L, Sun W, Cheng X, Tian W: Comparison of QCT and DXA: Osteoporosis detection rates in postmenopausal women. *Int J Endocrinol* 2013;2013:895474. doi:10.1155/2013/895474.
24. Fritz J, Fritz B, Thawait GK, et al: Advanced metal artifact reduction MRI of metal-on-metal hip resurfacing arthroplasty implants: Compressed sensing acceleration enables the time-neutral use of SEMAC. *Skeletal Radiol* 2016;45(10):1345-1356. doi:10.1007/s00256-016-2437-0.

    Newer techniques for metal artifact reduction are evaluated in the setting of arthroplasties on MRI to improve imaging quality. Level of evidence: V.
25. Berkowitz JL, Potter HG: Advanced MRI techniques for the hip joint: Focus on the postoperative hip. *AJR Am J Roentgenol* 2017;209(3):534-543. doi:10.2214/AJR.16.17789.

    MRI sequences and metal artifact reduction techniques to improve diagnoses in postoperative hips are reviewed. Level of evidence: V.
26. Olsen RV, Munk PL, Lee MJ, et al: Metal artifact reduction sequence: Early clinical applications. *Radio Graphics* 2000;20(3):699-712. doi:10.1148/radiographics.20.3.g00ma10699.
27. Jbara M, Chen Q, Marten P, Morcos M, Beltran J: Shoulder MR arthrography: How, why, when. *Radiol Clin North Am* 2005;43(4):683-692. doi:10.1016/j.rcl.2005.01.004.
28. Major NM, Browne J, Domzalski T, Cothran RL, Helms CA: Evaluation of the glenoid labrum with 3-T MRI: Is intraarticular contrast necessary? *Am J Roentgenol* 2011;196(5):1139-1144. doi:10.2214/AJR.08.1734.
29. Toomayan GA, Holman WR, Major NM, Kozlowicz SM, Vail TP: Sensitivity of MR arthrography in the evaluation of acetabular labral tears. *Am J Roentgenol* 2006;186(2):449-453. doi:10.2214/AJR.04.1809.

30. Haramati N, Staron RB, Barax C, Feldman F: Magnetic resonance imaging of occult fractures of the proximal femur. *Skeletal Radiol* 1994;23(1):19-22.

31. Pejic A, Hansson S, Rogmark C: resonance imaging for verifying hip fracture diagnosis why, when and how? *Injury* 2017;48(3):687-691. doi:10.1016/j.injury.2017.01.025.

The authors assess the use of MRI to diagnose occult hip fracture and describe the outcomes of MRI-diagnosed hip fractures compared with radiography. Level of evidence: III.

32. Dorsay TA, Major NM, Helms CA: Cost-effectiveness of immediate MR imaging versus traditional follow-up for revealing radiographically occult scaphoid fractures. *Am J Roentgenol* 2001;177(6):1257-1263. doi:10.2214/ajr.177.6.1771257.

33. Raghavan M: Conventional modalities and novel, emerging imaging techniques for musculoskeletal tumors. *Cancer Control* 2017;24(2):161-171. doi:10.1177/107327481702400208.

A multimodality approach to musculoskeletal neoplasms is reviewed including advantages and limitations of each modality. Level of evidence: V.

34. Garner HW, Kransdorf MJ, Peterson JJ: Posttherapy imaging of musculoskeletal neoplasms. *Radiol Clin North Am* 2011;49(6):1307-1323. doi:10.1016/j.rcl.2011.07.011.

35. Lee YJ, Sadigh S, Mankad K, Kapse N, Rajeswaran G: The imaging of osteomyelitis. *Quant Imaging Med Surg* 2016;6(2):184-198. doi:10.21037/qims.2016.04.01.

The authors review the multiple modalities used for imaging osteomyelitis with an emphasis on MRI. Level of evidence: V.

36. Termaat MF, Raijmakers PGHM, Scholten HJ, Bakker FC, Patka P, Haarman HJTM: The accuracy of diagnostic imaging for the assessment of chronic osteomyelitis: A systematic review and meta-analysis. *J Bone Joint Surg* 2005;87(11):2464. doi:10.2106/JBJS.D.02691.

37. Modic MT, Pflanze W, Feiglin DH, Belhobek G: Magnetic resonance imaging of musculoskeletal infections. *Radiol Clin North Am* 1986;24(2):247-258.

38. Klauser AS, Peetrons P: Developments in musculoskeletal ultrasound and clinical applications. *Skeletal Radiol* 2010;39(11):1061-1071. doi:10.1007/s00256-009-0782-y.

39. Nazarian LN: The top 10 reasons musculoskeletal sonography is an important complementary or alternative technique to MRI. *Am J Roentgenol* 2008;190(6):1621-1626. doi:10.2214/AJR.07.3385.

40. Parker L, Nazarian LN, Carrino JA, et al: Musculoskeletal imaging: Medicare use, costs, and potential for cost substitution. *J Am Coll Radiol* 2008;5(3):182-188. doi:10.1016/j.jacr.2007.07.016.

41. Nazarian LN, Jacobson JA, Benson CB, et al: Imaging algorithms for evaluating suspected rotator cuff disease: Society of Radiologists in Ultrasound consensus conference statement. *Radiology* 2013;267(2):589-595. doi:10.1148/radiol.13121947.

42. Davidson J, Jayaraman S: Guided interventions in musculoskeletal ultrasound: what's the evidence? *Clin Radiol* 2011;66(2):140-152. doi:10.1016/j.crad.2010.09.006.

43. Louis LJ: Musculoskeletal ultrasound intervention: Principles and advances. *Radiol Clin North Am* 2008;46(3):515-533. doi:10.1016/j.rcl.2008.02.003.

44. Petrover D, Silvera J, De Baere T, Vigan M, Hakimé A: Percutaneous ultrasound-guided carpal tunnel release: Study upon clinical efficacy and safety. *Cardiovasc Intervent Radiol* 2017;40(4):568-575. doi:10.1007/s00270-016-1545-5.

The authors discuss the overall safety and efficacy of ultrasound-guided carpal tunnel release. Level of evidence: III.

Chapter 10

Patient Optimization

Mitchell R. Klement, MD • Andrew K. Battenberg, MD

ABSTRACT

The goal of all orthopedic surgery is to give the patient the best possible outcome. To achieve this goal, one must be technically proficient and minimize complications. Patient optimization involves the recognition of patient-specific risk factors for postoperative complications by the surgeon, and taking proactive measures to modify or reduce these risks before surgery. In general, these patient-specific risk factors are broken down into categories and those discussed herein are obesity, diabetes, malnutrition, smoking, alcohol and drug use, psychiatric disease, and rheumatologic conditions. Within each category this chapter will address the current literature, methods to identify those at increased risk, and steps to reduce these risks. Patient optimization involves a collaboration between family physicians, internal medicine specialists, infection disease specialists, anesthesiology, psychiatrists, and the ancillary staff. As a team, surgeons can ensure their patients are optimized before surgery and minimize complications.

Keywords: comorbidities; complications; patient optimization; perioperative management; risk factors

Introduction

In the era of value-based care, maximizing surgical outcomes, patient satisfaction, and minimizing perioperative complications are paramount. However, the key to surgical success starts not in the operating room but at the preoperative consultation. Optimization involves the recognition of patient-specific risk factors for complications and taking the appropriate steps to decrease, or modify, these risk factors. Postoperative complications directly affect patient outcomes, surgeon and hospital reimbursement, and increase costs to society. As orthopedic surgery becomes more common, and patients continue to live longer with more medical comorbidities, complications should be avoided whenever possible. Thus, a multidisciplinary, team-based approach to patient optimization should be used in the pre- and perioperative periods to provide the highest level of patient care.

Neither of the following authors nor any immediate family member has received anything of value from or has stock or stock options held in a commercial company or institution related directly or indirectly to the subject of this chapter: Dr. Klement and Dr. Battenberg.

Obesity

Obesity is defined as excessive fat accumulation and is commonly measured by the body mass index (BMI, weight in kg divided by meters squared, kg/m^2). By this measure, a person with a BMI above 25 kg/m^2 is considered overweight and a BMI above 30 kg/m^2 is considered obese (**Table 1**). The prevalence of obesity is increasing at alarming proportions. From 1998 to 2011, obesity prevalence has increased from 39% to 52% of patients undergoing total hip arthroplasty (THA) and from 57% to 70% of patients undergoing total knee arthroplasty (TKA).[1] Furthermore, obesity has been associated with an increased risk of complications and adverse events, including increased superficial and deep infection, greater revision surgery rate, and worse patient-reported outcomes.[2-4] In addition to higher rates of diabetes and vascular disease, worsening obesity has also been associated with greater rates of malnutrition, which may be a significant contributing factor to increased complications.[5]

Conventionally, body mass index has been studied as a categorical variable according to standard BMI classifications by the World Health Organization (WHO, **Table 1**). However, when treated as a continuous variable, increasing BMI remains associated with increased complication rates—most concerning is an 8% increased risk of infection for every unit of BMI greater than 25 kg/m^2.[4] In 2013, a workgroup was convened by the American Association of Hip and Knee Surgeons (AAHKS) to review the evidence on complications and obesity.[6] The authors concluded that in patients with a

Table 1

World Health Organization Classification of Underweight, Normal Weight, and Obesity

Description	Body Mass Index (BMI, Kg/m^2)
Underweight	<18.5
Normal Weight	18.5-24.9
Overweight	25.0-29.9
Obese	
Class I	30.0-34.9
Class II	35.0-39.9
Class III (ie, morbidly obese)	≥40.0

Kg = kilograms; m = meters

BMI >40 kg/m^2 the functional improvements become less and the complication profile increases. The authors argue that arthroplasty should be delayed above this threshold.[6]

Methods to lose weight preoperatively include dietary assistance, exercise, and surgical methods such as bariatric surgery. Although obesity is considered a modifiable risk factor for complications and adverse events, data regarding benefits of weight loss before orthopedic surgery are limited. Preoperative weight loss >5% was not associated with a decreased risk of SSI or readmission.[7] Additionally, the data regarding bariatric surgery is conflicting. Some studies demonstrate reduced complications[8] whereas others show no difference or even worse outcomes compared with morbidly obese nonbariatric surgical patients.[9,10] Dramatic weight loss or bariatric surgery without proper nutritional guidance may lead to malnutrition and a persistent catabolic state, which could explain the possibility of higher complications in the preoperative weight loss populations. Although further studies are needed demonstrating reduced weight reduces surgical complications, any loss of weight may make surgery technically easier and improve patient well-being.

Diabetes

In the United States, 29.1 million Americans (9.3%) are estimated to have diabetes, with projections to 48.3 million by 2050—nearly double the current number.[11] Diabetes has been associated with poor outcomes following orthopedic surgery, including more in-hospital complications,[12] greater readmission rates,[13] higher infection rates,[2,14] and worse patient-reported outcomes.[15] Patients who are insulin-dependent are at even greater risk of adverse events than those who are not insulin-dependent.[16] Alarmingly, when a recent study routinely screened arthroplasty patients for diabetes, 58.9% were found to be dysglycemic (prediabetic or diabetic),[17] and 20.6% were found to be diabetic, of which 40.9% were previously undiagnosed.[17] The rate is further elevated in patients older than 65 years.[17] Therefore, consideration should be made for routine preoperative screening for diabetes before elective orthopedic surgery, especially for patients older than 65 years, patients with medical comorbidities, patients with a family history of diabetes, and patients undergoing procedures with a higher risk of complications.

Hemoglobin A1c (HgbA1c) is most widely used and is the most widely studied measure of glycemic control. Preoperative recommendations for the prevention of surgical site infection (SSI) include HgbA1c less than 7% and glucose level less than 200 mg/dL from the 2013 International Consensus Meeting (ICM) on Periprosthetic Joint Infection, a glucose level less than 200 mg/dL from the Center for Disease Control, and a HgbA1c less than 7% from Society for Healthcare Epidemiology of America.[18] Preoperative glycemic control measured by HgbA1c correlates with postoperative blood glucose control, with HgbA1c greater than 7.45% associated with a significant risk of postoperative glucose levels greater than 200 mg/dL.[19] Regarding clinical outcomes, using a threshold of 7.7% appears to be more indicative of infection and may be a better cutoff than 7%.[20] However, there is controversy around its ability to predict surgical outcomes. Because HgbA1c depends on the life cycle of red blood cells, it may take up to 3 months to observe changes in perceived glycemic control. This can confound interpretation of varying HgbA1c values pre- and perioperatively and may lead to unnecessary delays in surgery.

Serum fructosamine levels measure glycated serum proteins and reflect mean glucose over shorter time periods, 14 to 21 days.[21] Patients with fructosamine levels greater than 292 μmol/L have a significantly higher risk for deep infection, readmission, and revision surgery.[21] This simple and inexpensive test can be an alternative to HgbA1c and give more information on recent glycemic control; however, further study is needed of whether correcting fructosamine preoperatively reduces adverse events.[21] Patients above this threshold should have further consultation with their internist or endocrinologist to improve their blood glucose control before elective surgery.

Malnutrition

Malnutrition is common in orthopedic patients and ranges from 4% to 45.9%.[22,23] Risk appears to increase with increasing age, particularly above 55 years.[24] Malnutrition is associated with greater risk of SSI, postoperative complication, readmission, and mortality.[22-24] Proposed mechanisms include lack of protein and other macronutrients needed for cellular proliferation, synthesis, and wound healing, as well as decreased immune function necessary to prevent and fight infection.[25]

Currently, there is no agreed upon definition of malnutrition and no single test is used to conclusively define it. Commonly used tests and their thresholds include serum albumin less than 3.5 mg/dL, serum prealbumin less than 15 mg/dL, and serum transferrin less than 200 mg/dL, with any one of these deficiencies indicating a possible malnourished state. Albumin is easy to measure, is inexpensive, and has the longest half-life (14 to 20 days). It is, therefore, most useful as an indicator of chronic malnutrition and is less sensitive to acute changes in nutritional status.[25] Transferrin has a 10-day half-life, but is less reliable in assessing mild malnutrition, and is more susceptible to derangement with liver disease or various forms of anemia. Prealbumin has the shortest half-life (2 to 3 days) and varies more widely in response to acute events or changes in protein intake. Further laboratory evidence of malnutrition is a total lymphocyte count <1,500 cells/mm. Additional methods to assess malnutrition include standardized scoring tools, such as the subjective global assessment, which combines patient responses on current weight, recent changes to weight, food intake, eating habits, and activity level with objective measures on physical examination.[25]

The efficacy of oral nutritional supplementation or correction of malnutrition in the nutritionally deficient patient has not been well studied, particularly in the orthopedic literature. Meta-analyses of nonsurgical patients have found significant reductions in complications, readmissions, and mortality with use of oral nutritional supplements, and further study in orthopedic surgical patients is needed.[26] Patients identified as malnourished should be counseled regarding their diet, and consultation with a nutritionist should be strongly considered. Supplementation with a high protein oral nutritional supplement may be beneficial, especially during the perioperative period.

Underweight Patients

Underweight patients are defined as having a BMI of less than 18.5 kg/m^2 (**Table 1**). These individuals have been shown to have a higher risk of infection, transfusion, readmission, and mortality.[27,28] There is contradictory evidence, however, with regard to wound complication and infection rates with some studies indicating lower rates for underweight patients.[29,30] Underweight patients have greater resource utilization as measured by length of stay, hospital charge, and need for skilled nursing.[29] The increases in length of stay and hospital charge postarthroplasty are likely related to greater rates of postoperative anemia and increased need for transfusion. Thus, identification, workup, and treatment of preoperative anemia should be performed in underweight patients for any procedure with a significant expected blood loss.

No studies have been performed that evaluate potential risk reduction with interventions that increase BMI of underweight patients. It is important to note that underweight status can have multiple causes and can be multifactorial, including genetic predisposition, age, eating disorders, or existence of a chronic disease state. Because of the heterogeneity of such patients, attempting to "optimize" underweight status can prove to be difficult. Most importantly, any nutritional deficiencies should be identified and treated, and underlying medical problems contributing to underweight status should be further evaluated and managed as part of multidisciplinary team with primary care, nutritionist, and the surgeon.

Vitamin D Deficiency

Vitamin D deficiency (VDD) is common, with rates reported to be up to 40% in orthopedic surgical patients.[31] VDD can be screened for by measuring serum 25-hydroxyvitamin D (25[OH]D) levels. VDD can be defined as normal (≥32 ng/mL), insufficient (<32 ng/mL), and deficient (<20 ng/mL) based on the serum measurement.[31] Vitamin D is well known for its role in calcium homeostasis, which impacts bone mineral density, fracture healing, and muscle function, but Vitamin D also plays an important role in immune function. Previous work has demonstrated vitamin-D's regulation and activation of the innate and adaptive immune responses.[32] Recent studies have shown a higher rate of VDD in periprosthetic joint infections and a higher rate of postoperative complications and infection in arthroplasty patients with VDD.[33,34] In a mouse model of periprosthetic infection, VDD mice were shown to have an increased bacterial burden when compared with VDD mice that received rescue vitamin D supplementation.[35] Bacterial burden was equivalent between normal mice and the VDD mice that received rescue supplementation, demonstrating vitamin D's importance in immune function and its potential as a modifiable risk factor.

Principles of Orthopaedics

Males, patients aged 51 to 75 years, patients with darker skin tones, and patients undergoing sports or trauma orthopedic surgery are most at risk of VDD.[31] Patients identified as having VDD should be treated perioperatively with a goal 25-hydroxyvitamin D level greater than 30 ng/mL. The recommended dietary allowance of vitamin D is between 200 and 2,000 international units (IU) per day for healthy adults,[36] but high-dose rapid-correction regimens have been described and can be implemented under the guidance of an internist or endocrinologist, particularly in cases of severe deficiency.

Smoking

Cigarette smoking remains the leading cause of preventable death in the United States and currently 15% of US adults still smoke.[37] Unlike the optimization of chronic medical conditions discussed herein, smoking is a preoperative habit that can be quit altogether. Cigarette smoke contains nearly 4,000 chemicals that result in vasoconstriction, displacement of oxygen on red blood cells, and deleterious effects on bone and soft tissues.[38] Smoking in orthopedic patients undergoing surgery ranges from 9% to 60%.[39,40] In addition to the known risks to general health and malignancy, smoking has been associated with increased nonsurgical and surgical readmissions,[39] increased bony nonunion (fractures, osteotomies, fusions),[41] and wound healing complications.[40] Screening can be performed by urine tobacco metabolites. For active smokers, a positive test is urine nicotine of greater than 200 ng/mL and urine anabasine greater than 10 ng/mL. For nonsmokers or former smokers using nicotine replacement, a negative test is urine nicotine of greater than 200 ng/mL and urine anabasine less than 2 ng/mL. Finally, for nonsmokers and those not using nicotine replacement, a negative test would be a urine nicotine of less than 17 ng/mL and urine anabasine less than 2 ng/mL.

Smoking cessation is strongly encouraged in all patients, and the orthopedic surgeon has a unique opportunity to counsel these patients either at the time of injury or during a preoperative consultation. Patients are often more likely to quit when they are made aware of the negative effects it may have on their surgical outcome.[42] A previous randomized controlled trial demonstrated that with preoperative counseling and nicotine replacement 4 weeks before surgery and continuing 4 weeks after, a reduction in overall complications was seen.[43] However, cessation for a period of shorter than 4 weeks before surgery may not decrease the complication rate.[44] Common methods to aid with smoking cessation preoperatively include brief behavior support therapy, nicotine replacement, intensive face-to-face intervention therapy, varenicline, and bupropion. Interventions that combine pharmacotherapy and behavioral support increase smoking cessation success compared with a minimal intervention or usual care.[45] Patients should be provided access to cessation materials and referral for treatment and pharmacotherapy in conjunction with their primary care physician.

Alcohol and Drug Use

Alcohol

Similar to smoking, alcohol and drug use are toxic habits that become dependencies leading to poor health and worse surgical outcomes. Alcohol abuse is a well-established cause of end-stage liver disease, cardiac disease, hemostatic dysregulation, immune incompetence, malnutrition, and osteonecrosis of the femoral head and is often associated with orthopedic trauma. Patients with alcohol abuse are more likely to leave against medical advice, have a prolonged hospital stay, and are at increased risk of postoperative medical and surgical complications after orthopedic surgery.[46,47] With this in mind, orthopedic surgeons should screen for alcohol use preoperatively. The CAGE questionnaire, Alcohol Use Disorder Identification Test (AUDIT), and Short Michigan Alcohol Screening Test (SMAST) are all effective tools (**Table 2**). Heavy drinking is defined as women who drink, on average, more than 7 drinks per week; men who drink, on average, more than 14 drinks per week.[47] When a heavy drinker is identified preoperatively based on screening tool scores (**Table 2**), initiation of withdrawal prophylaxis with benzodiazepines should begin postoperatively to prevent complications. The Clinical Institute Withdrawal Assessment for Alcohol (CIWA) scale can help guide duration and dosing of withdrawal-preventing medications.

Again, the risk of a worse postoperative outcome may provide an opportunity to counsel patients on cessation. Despite numerous reports regarding alcohol and other surgical specialties, the effect on orthopedics is just starting to be investigated. To date, no orthopedic study has examined alcohol cessation preoperatively. However, in other surgical specialties, complete alcohol cessation preoperatively has resulted in decreased postoperative complications.[48] Cessation methods include an intense 4- to 8-week intervention, group-based interventions, and pharmacological treatment (disulfiram, acamprosate, and opioid-antagonists). Complete cessation treatment is often intervention based with patient empowerment, information, and pharmacological

Table 2

Screening Questionnaires for Alcohol Abuse

Questions	Scoring and Significance
CAGE[a] Have you ever felt you should **C**ut down on your drinking? Have people **A**nnoyed you by criticizing your drinking? Have you ever felt bad or **G**uilty about your drinking? Have you ever had a drink first thing in the morning to steady your nerves or to get rid of a hangover (**E**ye opener)?	Physician-administered, four questions, each scored either 0 or 1, a score of 2 or more points is significant
AUDIT[b] How often do you have a drink containing alcohol? How many drinks containing alcohol do you have on a typical day when you are drinking? How often do you have six or more drinks on one occasion? How often during the last year have you found that you were not able to stop drinking once you had started? How often during the last year have you failed to do what was normally expected from you because of drinking? How often during the last year have you needed a first drink in the morning to get yourself going after a heavy drinking session? How often during the last year have you had a feeling of guilt or remorse after drinking? How often during the last year have you been unable to remember what happened the night before because you had been drinking? Have you or someone else been injured as a result of your drinking? Has a relative or friend or a doctor or another health worker been concerned about your drinking or suggested you cut down?	Physician-administered, 10-item screening tool, each scored 0-4, a score of 8 or more is considered to indicate significant or harmful alcohol use.
SMAST[c] Do you feel that you are a normal drinker? (By normal we mean do you drink less than or as much as most other people) Does your wife, husband, a parent, or other near relative ever worry or complain about your drinking? Do you ever feel guilty about your drinking? Do friends or relatives think you are a normal drinker? Are you able to stop drinking when you want to? Have you ever attended a meeting of Alcoholics Anonymous (AA)? Has your drinking ever created problems between you and your wife, husband, a parent, or other near relative? Have you ever gotten into trouble at work because of your drinking? Have you ever neglected your obligations, your family, or your work for two or more days in a row because you were drinking? Have you ever gone to anyone for help about your drinking? Have you ever been in a hospital because of drinking? Have you ever been arrested for drunken driving, driving while intoxicated, or driving under the influence of alcoholic beverages? Have you ever been arrested, even for a few hours, because of other drunken behaviors?	Self-administered, 13-item questionnaire, each scored 0 or 1, a score of 3 means borderline alcohol problem reported, a score of ≥4 means potential alcohol abuse reported

[a]Developed by Dr. John Ewing. Ewing JA. "Detecting Alcoholism: The CAGE Questionaire" *JAMA* 1984;252:1905-1907. These questions should not be preceded by questions about how much or how frequently the patient drinks. https://www.uspreventiveservicestaskforce.org/Home/GetFileByID/838.

[b]Alcohol Use Disorder Identification Test. Developed by the World Health Organization. Both a self-administered and clinician-administered version are available. Adapted from AUDIT: The Alcohol Use Disorders Identification Test: Guidelines for Use in Primary Care, 2nd ed., Babor TF, Higgins-Biddle JC, Saunders JB, Monteiro MG, p. 31, Copyright 2001. Available at: hhttps://apps.who.int/iris/bitstream/handle/10665/67205/WHO_MSD_MSB_01.6a.pdf?sequence=1&isAllowed=y.

[c]Short Michigan Alcohol Screening Test. Seltzer MA, Vinokur A, Van Rooijen LJ: A Self-Administered Short Michigan Alcohol Screening Test (SMAST). *J Stud Alcohol* 1975;36(1):117-126. Used with permission of Alcohol Research Documentation, Inc., publisher of the Journal of Studies on Alcohol, now the Journal of Studies on Alcohol and Drugs (www.jsad.com). https://hopequestgroup.org/wp-content/uploads/2011/09/SMAST-Short-Michigan-Alcohol-Screening-Test.pdf.

treatment to prevent relapse by addiction experts.[48] Preoperatively, these patients should undergo laboratory testing including nutritional workup, liver function tests, and coagulation studies.

Drug Use

In the United States alone, 8.2% of the population had reported using an illicit drug in the last month. Of the routes of administration, injection is the most harmful.[49] Poor injection technique, increased frequency, needle sharing, and dirty needles can predispose patients to increased systemic and soft-tissue infections.[49] These patients are at increased risk of pneumonia, endocarditis, and abscesses usually from the patients' commensal flora.[49] Not surprisingly, injection drug use in the setting of orthopedic implants places them at substantial risk of subsequent infection.[2] In a series of arthroplasty patients who injected drugs, the 10-year implant survival rate was 52.3%.[50] In addition, illicit drug use has been associated with increased rates of HIV and syphilis infection; greater consumption of intraoperative opioids, sedatives, and muscle relaxants; and increased postoperative complications compared with controls.[51] What is concerning, was that no patient admitted a history of drug use in a recent prospective study, but 7.5% of patients undergoing emergency surgery tested positive.[51] Although blood and urine testing can screen and identify illicit drug use, it is not routinely perfromed in orthopedic surgery. If a patient admits to a history of drug use before elective surgery orthopedic, counseling and drug testing may be warranted, only proceeding with surgery after testing is negative.

Psychiatric Disease

Psychiatric diseases, or mental health disorders, are defined as having a diagnosable mental, behavioral, or emotional disorder, other than a developmental or substance use disorder. The most common psychiatric diseases include depression, anxiety, bipolar disorder, and schizophrenia. The *Diagnostic and Statistical Manual of Mental Disorders* (*DSM-5*) is used by psychiatrists and mental health experts around the world for diagnosis and classification of these conditions. Prospective screening studies have demonstrated that an alarming 35% of patients undergoing elective orthopedic surgery may have some type of psychiatric disease,[52] putting it on par with other common risk factors such as diabetes and obesity. Psychiatric disease has been associated with worse outcomes and increased complications in spine, shoulder, arthroplasty, and trauma surgery.[53] Patients with psychiatric disease have a persistent inflammatory state and altered immune regulation. This chronic state of stress leads to measurable increases in cortisol, interleukin-6, tumor necrosis factor alpha, soluble interleukin-2 receptor, and other cytokines, which may explain the reported increase in infection.[54]

As the stigma toward mental health and psychiatric disease continues to change, orthopedic surgeons should be more aware of these conditions. Recent guidelines from the United States Preventive Services Task Force (USPSTF) recommend that all adults be screened for depression (grade B) by primary care physicians.[55] One such recommended screening tool is the Patient Health Questionnaire 9 (PHQ-9), which takes less than 5 minutes to complete. A positive screen should prompt referral for additional screening and treatment.[55] However, further evidence is needed in the orthopedic community if referral and pharmacologic treatment of psychiatric disease reduces their risk of complications and if this is indeed a "modifiable" comorbidity.[56,57]

Finally, the co-existence of psychiatric disease and a substance abuse disorder (smoking, alcohol, illicit drug use) is common and is often referred to as a "dual diagnosis." Up to 50% of patients with a psychiatric disease may also have a substance abuse disorder.[58] Patients with dual diagnosis have more symptoms, a higher prevalence of medical problems, more treatment noncompliance, more frequent relapses and hospitalizations, and more problems with self-care, violence, and homelessness than persons with psychiatric disorders alone.[58,59] Given the difficulty of identifying these patients, few studies in orthopedics have investigated this condition. In a study of THA patients, patients with dual diagnosis had increased infection, dislocation, and revision surgery compared with those with psychiatric disease alone.[58] Given the high association, when a psychiatric illness is identified preoperatively, one should inquire about co-existing substance abuse disorders.

Rheumatologic Disease

Rheumatologic diseases are immune-mediated disorders of the musculoskeletal system and commonly include rheumatoid arthritis (RA), ankylosing spondylitis, psoriatic arthritis, juvenile idiopathic arthritis, and systemic lupus erythematosus (SLE). The advent of disease-modifying antirheumatic drugs (DMARDS) and biologic medications have drastically reduced the need for orthopedic surgery and the incidence of joint replacement for RA in many countries.[60] Despite a reduction, these patients still suffer from disorders of the spine, hands, feet, shoulder, elbow, ankle, and large joints that may require orthopedic attention.[61] Not surprisingly,

DMARDs: CONTINUE these medications through surgery.	**Dosing Interval**	**Continue/Withhold**
Methotrexate	Weekly	Continue
Sulfasalazine	Once or twice daily	Continue
Hydroxychloroquine	Once or twice daily	Continue
Leflunomide (Arava)	Daily	Continue
Doxycycline	Daily	Continue
BIOLOGIC AGENTS: STOP these medications prior to surgery and schedule surgery at the end of the dosing cycle. RESUME medications at minimum 14 days after surgery in the absence of wound healing problems, surgical site infection, or systemic infection.	**Dosing Interval**	**Schedule Surgery (relative to last biologic agent dose administered) during**
Adalimumab (Humira)	Weekly or every 2 weeks	Week 2 or 3
Etanercept (Enbrel)	Weekly or twice weekly	Week 2
Golimumab (Simponi)	Every 4 weeks (SQ) or every 8 weeks (IV)	Week 5 Week 9
Infliximab (Remicade)	Every 4, 6, or 8 weeks	Week 5, 7, or 9
Abatacept (Orencia)	Monthly (IV) or weekly (SQ)	Week 5 Week 2
Certolizumab (Cimzia)	Every 2 or 4 weeks	Week 3 or 5
Rituximab (Rituxan)	2 doses 2 weeks apart every 4-6 months	Month 7
Tocilizumab (Actemra)	Every week (SQ) or every 4 weeks (IV)	Week 2 Week 5
Anakinra (Kineret)	Daily	Day 2
Secukinumab (Cosentyx)	Every 4 weeks	Week 5
Ustekinumab (Stelara)	Every 12 weeks	Week 13
Belimumab (Benlysta)	Every 4 weeks	Week 5
Tofacitinib (Xeljanz): STOP this medication 7 days prior to surgery.	Daily or twice daily	7 days after last dose
SEVERE SLE-SPECIFIC MEDICATIONS: CONTINUE these medications in the perioperative period.	**Dosing Interval**	**Continue/Withhold**
Mycophenolate mofetil	Twice daily	Continue
Azathioprine	Daily or twice daily	Continue
Cyclosporine	Twice daily	Continue
Tacrolimus	Twice daily (IV and PO)	Continue
NOT-SEVERE SLE: DISCONTINUE these medications 1 week prior to surgery	**Dosing Interval**	**Continue/Withhold**
Mycophenolate mofetil	Twice daily	Withhold
Azathioprine	Daily or twice daily	Withhold
Cyclosporine	Twice daily	Withhold
Tacrolimus	Twice daily (IV and PO)	Withhold

Figure 1 Image lists medications included in the 2017 American College of Rheumatology/American Association of Hip and Knee Surgeons Guideline for the Perioperative Management of Antirheumatic Medication in Patients with Rheumatic Diseases Undergoing Elective Total Hip or Total Knee Arthroplasty. Dosing intervals were obtained from prescribing information provided online by pharmaceutical companies. DMARDs = disease-modifying antirheumatic drugs; SQ = subcutaneous; IV = intravenous; SLE = systemic lupus erythematosus; PO = oral. (Reprinted with permission from Goodman SM, Springer B, Guyatt G, et al: 2017 American College of Rheumatology/American Association of Hip and Knee Surgeons guideline for the perioperative management of antirheumatic medication in patients with rheumatic diseases undergoing elective total hip or total knee arthroplasty. *J Arthroplast* 2017;32[9]:2628-2638, Copyright 2017, with permission from Elsevier.)

patients with rheumatologic diseases experience higher rates of complications compared with patients without these conditions. The underlying immune disorders and a higher comorbidity burden are frequently cited causes.[62]

While the underlying disease can be controlled with medications, there is little room for "optimization" of these patients. The most common issue with these patients before surgery is how to manage their medications.[63] To address this question, AAHKS and the American College of Rheumatology (ACR) recently collaborated to create a guideline for the perioperative management of antirheumatic medication in patients undergoing elective total joint arthroplasty (TJA). Experts from the fields of rheumatology and orthopedic surgery were included; in addition, patients with rheumatologic disorders who had a prior TJA were also asked for input. In summary, they recommended that DMARDs be continued through surgery with their usual dose and timing.[63] Biologic agents should be stopped before surgery at the end of their dosing cycle and resume at minimum 14 days depending on the appearance of the wound. Finally, for patients without severe SLE these medications should be stopped 1 week before surgery and patients with severe SLE (organ involvement) they should be continued (**Figure 1**).[63] Although these guidelines are specific to TJA, further research and guidelines in other orthopedic subspecialties will be important in the future.

Finally, some other preoperative considerations must be given to patients with rheumatologic conditions. These patients are at increased risk of cardiac complications including myocardial infarction (MI), and a preoperative cardiology evaluation should be considered to address management of potential risk factors.[64] RA involvement of the cervical spine is well known, and traditional teaching has recommended obtaining adequate cervical radiographs before anesthesia. However, there are no guidelines regarding radiographic imaging in RA patients before surgery, and previous literature has reported that a very small percentage of patients actually have adequate studies beforehand.[65] In fact, a recent series found that only 8% of RA patients had complete studies adequate enough to evaluate for subluxation.[66] In addition, only a difficult oropharyngeal class/glottic visualization grade (3 or 4) as determined by the anesthesiologist affected the type of anesthesia technique while radiographic findings did not.[66] With the increased use of neuraxial anesthesia for lower extremity orthopedic procedures, DMARDs, and the option of fiber-optic intubation, further studies will be needed to see if RA patients are still at risk of atlantoaxial instability and who would benefit from prior radiographic studies.

Summary

The implementation of global patient optimization program can lead to reduced readmissions and complications. Comorbidities such as obesity, diabetes, vitamin-D deficiency, and malnutrition are easier to screen and treat given the ease of measurement with a weight or laboratory test. However, conditions such as psychiatric disease, smoking, drug use, and alcohol abuse can be difficult to identify and treat given the high degree of interaction, the degree of dependence, and requirement for therapy. Patients with rheumatologic disease pose a greater risk of site-specific infection and cardiac complications, and appropriate management of their medications perioperatively is essential. However, these conditions have all been identified as risk factors for complications after orthopedic surgery and should be addressed in a multidisciplinary fashion before surgery. This will lead to the best outcomes for our patients.

Key Study Points

- Obesity, diabetes, malnutrition, smoking, alcohol and drug use, psychiatric disease, and rheumatological conditions all place patients at increased risk for complications after orthopedic surgery.
- Although some conditions are more easily modified preoperatively, the use of a multidisciplinary approach, screening tools, and evidence-based thresholds will assist the surgeon with patient optimization.
- Now that the literature has identified risk factors and treatment thresholds for complications, further work needs to be done investigating the outcomes of those patients who were successfully optimized.

Annotated References

1. George J, Klika AK, Navale SM, Newman JM, Barsoum WK, Higuera CA: Obesity epidemic: Is its impact on total joint arthroplasty underestimated? An analysis of national trends. *Clin Orthop Relat Res* 2017;475:1798-1806.

   Annual numbers of total joint arthroplasty were obtained from the Nationwide Inpatient Sample Database from 1998 to 2011, and national obesity prevalence was obtained from public health sources. The study showed that the prevalence of obesity has increased in patients undergoing primary, revision, and infected total joint arthroplasty in the United States. Level of evidence: II (Prognostic).

2. Tan TL, Maltenfort MG, Chen AF, et al: Development and evaluation of a preoperative risk calculator for periprosthetic joint infection following total joint arthroplasty. *J Bone Joint Surg Am Vol* 2018;100:777-785.

   This retrospective review of 27,717 patients (12,086 TKAs and 31,167 THAs, including 1,035 periprosthetic joint infections) analyzed 42 risk factors for infection, including patient characteristics and surgical variables. 25 of the 42 factors were not significant risk factors. The most influential were previous open surgical procedure, drug abuse, revision surgery, and HIV/AIDS. Level of evidence: IV (Prognostic).

3. Wagner ER, Houdek MT, Schleck C, et al: Increasing body mass index is associated with worse outcomes after shoulder arthroplasty. *J Bone Joint Surg Am Vol* 2017;99:929-937.

An institutional joint registry of 4,567 consecutive shoulder arthroplasty cases from 1970 to 2013 was studied and found that increasing BMI was associated with increased risk of revision surgery, reoperation, and superficial infection. Risk of revision increased in a linear fashion with 5% increased risk per 1 unit of BMI ($P = 0.03$). Level of evidence: IV (Prognostic).

4. Wagner ER, Kamath AF, Fruth KM, Harmsen WS, Berry DJ: Effect of body mass index on complications and reoperations after total hip arthroplasty. *J Bone Joint Surg Am Vol* 2016;98:169-179.

Using an institutional joint registry of 21,361 consecutive primary total hip arthroplasties between 1985 and 2012, BMI and its effect on complications and reoperations was studied as a continuous variable using smoothing spline parameterization. Reoperation, revision, early dislocation, wound infection, and deep periprosthetic infection rates increased with increasing BMI. Infection risk increased 8% for every unit of BMI >25 kg/m^2. Level of evidence: III (Prognostic).

5. Fu MC, D'Ambrosia C, McLawhorn AS, Schairer WW, Padgett DE, Cross MB: Malnutrition increases with obesity and is a stronger independent risk factor for postoperative complications: A propensity-adjusted analysis of total hip arthroplasty patients. *J Arthroplast* 2016;31:2415-2421.

The National Surgical Quality Improvement Program was queried from 2005 to 2013 for elective primary THA with 40,653 cases identified. Malnutrition was defined as albumin <3.5 g/dL. Malnutrition incidence increased from 2.8% in obese I to 5.7% in obese III patients. Malnutrition was also a greater predictor for postoperative complication than obesity class when using multivariable propensity-adjusted logistic regression. Level of evidence: III.

6. Workgroup of the American Association of Hip and Knee Surgeons Evidence Based Committee: Obesity and total joint arthroplasty: A literature based review. *J Arthroplast* 2013;28:714-721.

7. Inacio MC, Kritz-Silverstein D, Raman R, et al: The impact of pre-operative weight loss on incidence of surgical site infection and readmission rates after total joint arthroplasty. *J Arthroplast* 2014;29:458-464.e1.

8. Werner BC, Evans CL, Carothers JT, Browne JA: Primary total knee arthroplasty in super-obese patients: Dramatically higher postoperative complication rates even compared to revision surgery. *J Arthroplast* 2015;30:849-853.

9. Inacio MC, Paxton EW, Fisher D, Li RA, Barber TC, Singh JA: Bariatric surgery prior to total joint arthroplasty may not provide dramatic improvements in post-arthroplasty surgical outcomes. *J Arthroplast* 2014;29:1359-1364.

10. Martin JR, Watts CD, Taunton MJ: Bariatric surgery does not improve outcomes in patients undergoing primary total knee arthroplasty. *Bone Joint J* 2015;97-b:1501-1505.

11. Stryker LS: Modifying risk factors: Strategies that work diabetes mellitus. *J Arthroplast* 2016;31:1625-1627.

The increasing incidence as well as the burden of diabetes mellitus is discussed. Strategies for preoperative testing, perioperative management, and keys to implementation of a screening and management program are reviewed. Review article.

12. Martinez-Huedo MA, Jimenez-Garcia R, Jimenez-Trujillo I, Hernandez-Barrera V, Del Rio Lopez B, Lopez-de-Andres A: Effect of type 2 diabetes on in-hospital postoperative complications and mortality after primary total hip and knee arthroplasty. *J Arthroplast* 2017;32:3729-3734.e2.

The Spanish National Hospital Discharge Database was analyzed for patients undergoing total joint arthroplasty from 2010 to 2014. There were 115,234 THA and 195,355 TKA patients, 12.4% and 15.6% with type 2 diabetes, respectively. In-hospital postoperative complications were higher among diabetic THA patients (9.68% vs 8.98%, $P = 0.038$) and diabetic TKA patients (7.30% vs 6.76%, $P = 0.014$) when compared with nondiabetic patients. Level of evidence: III.

13. Mednick RE, Alvi HM, Krishnan V, Lovecchio F, Manning DW: Factors affecting readmission rates following primary total hip arthroplasty. *J Bone Joint Surg Am Vol* 2014;96:1201-1209.

14. Cancienne JM, Brockmeier SF, Werner BC: Association of perioperative glycemic control with deep postoperative infection after shoulder arthroplasty in patients with diabetes. *J Am Acad Orthop Surg* 2018;26:e238-e245.

The PearlDiver Patient Records Database was queried from 2007 to 2015 for patients with diabetes mellitus who underwent primary shoulder arthroplasty. 18,729 patients underwent shoulder arthroplasty, 8,068 of which had a diagnosis of diabetes. Diabetic patients had higher rates of wound complication (1.4% vs 0.9%, OR 1.22, $P = 0.028$) and deep infection (0.7% vs 0.4%, OR 1.47, $P = 0.001$). These rates also increased as HgbA1c level increased, with an inflection point of 8.0 mg/dL (sensitivity 50%, specificity 75%). Level of evidence: III (therapeutic, case-control, treatment study).

15. Armaghani SJ, Archer KR, Rolfe R, Demaio DN, Devin CJ: Diabetes is related to worse patient-reported outcomes at two years following spine surgery. *J Bone Joint Surg Am Vol* 2016;98:15-22.

This was a prospective cohort study of 1,005 elective spine surgery patients, 43% of whom were diabetic. At 2 years follow-up, patients with diabetes had lower SF-12 physical component scores, lower EQ-5D scores, higher ODI/NDI scores, and higher NRS scores ($P < 0.05$ for all). Diabetic patients had significant improvement, but did not improve to the extent that nondiabetic patients did postoperatively. Level of evidence: II (Prognostic).

16. Webb ML, Golinvaux NS, Ibe IK, Bovonratwet P, Ellman MS, Grauer JN: Comparison of perioperative adverse event rates after total knee arthroplasty in patients with diabetes: Insulin dependence makes a difference. *J Arthroplast* 2017;32:2947-2951.

Principles of Orthopaedics

A retrospective cohort study using the American College of Surgeons National Surgical Quality Improvement Program database analyzing TKA patients from 2005 to 2014. Of the 114,102 patients who underwent TKA, 82.2% were nondiabetic, 13.5% were noninsulin-dependent diabetics, and 4.3% were insulin-dependent diabetics. Noninsulin-dependent diabetic patients had greater risk for 2 of 17 adverse events, whereas insulin-dependent diabetic patients had greater risk for 12 of 17 adverse events compared with nondiabetic patients. Level of evidence: III.

17. Shohat N, Goswami K, Tarabichi M, Sterbis E, Tan TL, Parvizi J: All patients should Be screened for diabetes before total joint arthroplasty. *J Arthroplast* 2018;33:2057-2061.

    1,416 arthroplasty patients were screened prospectively for diabetes using HgbA1c and fasting blood glucose levels. Diabetes was determined by a history of diabetes, HgbA1c ≥ 6.5%, or fasting glucose ≥ 126 mg/dL. Prevalence of diabetes was 20.6%, 40.9% of which were previously undiagnosed. This led the authors to recommend universal glycemic screening for all elective arthroplasty patients. Level of evidence: II.

18. Parvizi J, Shohat N, Gehrke T: Prevention of periprosthetic joint infection: New guidelines. *Bone Joint J* 2017;99-b:3-10.

    A review of the strategies for prevention of surgical site infection and periprosthetic joint infection, including guidelines from the World Health Organization and Centre for Disease Control and Prevention. The review includes pre-, peri-, intra-, and postoperative measures for infection prevention. Review article.

19. Godshaw BM, Ojard CA, Adams TM, Chimento GF, Mohammed A, Waddell BS: Preoperative glycemic control predicts perioperative serum glucose levels in patients undergoing total joint arthroplasty. *J Arthroplast* 2018;33:S76-S80.

    A retrospective review of 773 diabetic patients undergoing total joint arthroplasty found that preoperative HgbA1c correlated with postoperative glucose levels, and HgbA1c >7.45% resulted in a greater chance of postoperative hyperglycemia >200 mg/dL. Patients with HgbA1c >8 had mean postoperative serum glucose of 276 mg/dL. Level of evidence: III.

20. Tarabichi M, Shohat N, Kheir MM, et al: Determining the threshold for HbA1c as a predictor for adverse outcomes after total joint arthroplasty: A multicenter, retrospective study. *J Arthroplast* 2017;32:S263-S267.e1.

    A multicenter retrospective study of 1645 diabetic patients undergoing primary total joint arthroplasty between 2001 and 2015 found that a HgbA1c threshold of 7.7 was distinct for predicting periprosthetic joint infection. HgbA1c below 7.7 had infection rate of 0.8% which increased to 5.4% above 7.7. Level of evidence: III.

21. Shohat N, Tarabichi M, Tischler EH, Jabbour S, Parvizi J: Serum fructosamine: A simple and inexpensive test for assessing preoperative glycemic control. *J Bone Joint Surg Am Vol* 2017;99:1900-1907.

    This study prospectively screened 829 total joint arthroplasty patients preoperatively using HgbA1c, fructosamine, and blood glucose levels. HgbA1c >7% was defined as poor glycemic control, and correlated to a fructosamine level of 292 µmol/L. Agreement between HgbA1c and fructosamine was not complete as 39.2% of patients with fructosamine >292 µmol/L had a HgbA1c <7. Patients with fructosamine >292 µmol/L had a significantly higher risk of deep infection (adjusted odds ratio 6.2, *P* = 0.009), readmission (adjusted OR 3.0, *P* = 0.03), and reoperation (adjusted OR 3.4, *P* = 0.02). Level of evidence: II (Prognostic).

22. Bohl DD, Shen MR, Hannon CP, Fillingham YA, Darrith B, Della Valle CJ: Serum albumin predicts survival and postoperative course following surgery for geriatric hip fracture. *J Bone Joint Surg Am Vol* 2017;99:2110-2118.

    This retrospective study of 29,377 patients ≥65 years old undergoing hip fracture surgery found that the prevalence of hypoalbuminemia was 45.9% in this cohort. Hypoalbuminemic patients had higher rates of death (9.94% vs 5.53%, relative risk 1.52, *P* <0.001), sepsis (1.19% vs 0.52%, RR 1.92, *P* <0.001), and intubation (2.64% vs 1.47%, RR 1.51, *P* <0.001). Length of stay was longer in hypoalbuminemic patients (5.67 vs 4.99, *P* <0.001). Readmission rates did not differ. The authors concluded that hypoalbuminemia was a powerful independent risk factor for mortality. Level of evidence: IV (Prognostic).

23. Bohl DD, Shen MR, Kayupov E, Della Valle CJ: Hypoalbuminemia independently predicts surgical site infection, pneumonia, length of stay, and readmission after total joint arthroplasty. *J Arthroplast* 2016;31:15-21.

    Using the American College of Surgeons National Surgical Quality Improvement Program database, 49,603 primary arthroplasty patients were identified. Prevalence of hypoalbuminemia was 4.0%. Hypoalbuminemic patients had a higher risk for surgical site infection, pneumonia, extended length of stay, and readmission compared with patient with normal serum albumin. Level of evidence: III.

24. Huang R, Greenky M, Kerr GJ, Austin MS, Parvizi J: The effect of malnutrition on patients undergoing elective joint arthroplasty. *J Arthroplast* 2013;28:21-24.

25. Messana J, Uhl RL, Aldyab M, Rosenbaum AJ: Orthopaedic primer of nutritional requirements for patients with musculoskeletal problems. *JBJS reviews* 2018;6:e2.

    This review article discusses nutritional requirements of both macro- and micronutrients, perioperative nutrition, malnutrition, and nutritional assessments for patients with musculoskeletal conditions. Review article.

26. Stratton RJ, Hebuterne X, Elia M: A systematic review and meta-analysis of the impact of oral nutritional supplements on hospital readmissions. *Ageing Res Rev* 2013;12:884-897.

27. Manrique J, Chen AF, Gomez MM, Maltenfort MG, Hozack WJ: Surgical site infection and transfusion rates are higher in underweight total knee arthroplasty patients. *Arthroplasty Today* 2017;3:57-60.

    A case-control study using a prospectively collected institutional database was performed on 27 underweight (BMI < 18.5) TKA patients matched and compared with 81 normal weight patients. Underweight patients were more likely to develop surgical site infections (11.1% vs 0%, *P* = 0.01) and were more likely to require transfusions (odds ratio 3.4, *P* = 0.02). Level of evidence: III.

28. Saucedo JM, Marecek GS, Wanke TR, Lee J, Stulberg SD, Puri L: Understanding readmission after primary total hip and knee arthroplasty: who's at risk?. *J Arthroplast* 2014;29:256-260.

29. Anoushiravani AA, Sayeed Z, Chambers MC, et al: Assessing in-hospital outcomes and resource utilization after primary total joint arthroplasty among underweight patients. *J Arthroplast* 2016;31:1407-1412.

Discharge data from the 2006 to 2012 National Inpatient Sample were used to study 4,865 arthroplasty patients. Underweight patients (BMI < 19) were at higher risk of developing postoperative anemia and sustaining cardiac complications, but had a decreased risk of postoperative infection. Length of stay and hospital charge were higher in the underweight cohort, and underweight patients were more likely to be discharged to a skilled nursing facility. Level of evidence: III.

30. Murgatroyd SE, Frampton CM, Wright MS: The effect of body mass index on outcome in total hip arthroplasty: Early analysis from the New Zealand joint registry. *J Arthroplast* 2014;29:1884-1888.

31. Bogunovic L, Kim AD, Beamer BS, Nguyen J, Lane JM: Hypovitaminosis D in patients scheduled to undergo orthopaedic surgery: A single-center analysis. *J Bone Joint Surg Am Vol* 2010;92:2300-2304.

32. Hewison M: Vitamin D and innate and adaptive immunity. *Vitam Horm* 2011;86:23-62.

33. Maier GS, Horas K, Seeger JB, Roth KE, Kurth AA, Maus U: Is there an association between periprosthetic joint infection and low vitamin D levels?. *Int Orthop* 2014;38:1499-1504.

34. Traven SA, Chiaramonti AM, Barfield WR, et al: Fewer complications following revision hip and knee arthroplasty in patients with normal vitamin D levels. *J Arthroplast* 2017;32:S193-S196.

In this retrospective review, 126 revision arthroplasty patients were studied. Prevalence of hypovitaminosis D was 55%. Low vitamin D was associated with increased risk of 90-day complications (37.7% vs 21.1%, $P = 0.043$) and greater likelihood that infection was the reason for revision surgery. Low vitamin D levels remained predictive when other nutritional factors were adjusted for. Level of evidence: III.

35. Hegde V, Dworsky EM, Stavrakis AI, et al: Single-dose, preoperative vitamin-D supplementation decreases infection in a mouse model of periprosthetic joint infection. *J Bone Joint Surg Am Vol* 2017;99:1737-1744.

This periprosthetic joint infection mouse model tested three groups of mice: (1) vitamin D sufficient, (2) vitamin D deficient, (3) vitamin D deficient mice given "rescue" vitamin D. Vitamin D deficiency resulted in increased bacterial burden, and rescue treatment for deficient mice significantly decreased bacterial burden and neutrophil infiltration to the levels of vitamin D sufficient mice. The effect was reversible. Level of evidence: III.

36. Bouillon R: Comparative analysis of nutritional guidelines for vitamin D. *Nat Rev Endocrinol* 2017;13:466-479.

An overview of nutritional guidelines for Vitamin D intake. Review article.

37. (CDC). CfDCaP: *Current Cigarette Smoking Among Adults in the United States*. https://wwwcdcgov/tobacco/data_statistics/fact_sheets/adult_data/cig_smoking/indexhtm. 2016. Accessed 13 July 2018.

38. Scolaro JA, Schenker ML, Yannascoli S, Baldwin K, Mehta S, Ahn J: Cigarette smoking increases complications following fracture: A systematic review. *J Bone Joint Surg Am Vol* 2014;96:674-681.

39. Tischler EH, Matsen Ko L, Chen AF, Maltenfort MG, Schroeder J, Austin MS: Smoking increases the rate of reoperation for infection within 90 Days after primary total joint arthroplasty. *J Bone Joint Surg Am Vol* 2017;99:295-304.

Retrospective review of an institutional database with 1,371 current smokers, 5,195 former smokers, and 8,698 nonsmokers included. Current smokers had an increased risk of reoperation for infection within 90 days of a surgical procedure compared with nonsmokers after controlling for confounding variables. Packs per decade smoked regardless of current status also increased 90-day nonsurgical readmissions. Level of evidence: III (prognostic).

40. Castillo RC, Bosse MJ, MacKenzie EJ, Patterson BM: Impact of smoking on fracture healing and risk of complications in limb-threatening open tibia fractures. *J Orthop Trauma* 2005;19:151-157.

41. Pearson RG, Clement RG, Edwards KL, Scammell BE: Do smokers have greater risk of delayed and non-union after fracture, osteotomy and arthrodesis? A systematic review with meta-analysis. *BMJ Open* 2016;6:e010303.

A systematic review and meta-analysis investigating the effect of smoking on fracture-healing, fractures, spinal fusion, osteotomy, arthrodesis, or established nonunions. The meta-analysis of 7516 procedures revealed that smoking is linked to an increased risk of delayed and/or nonunion. Compared with non-smokers, the risk of delayed or nonunion was 1.6 times in smokers. Level of evidence: III.

42. Matuszewski PE, Boulton CL, O'Toole RV: Orthopaedic trauma patients and smoking: Knowledge deficits and interest in quitting. *Injury* 2016;47:1206-1211.

A single-center, prospective cross-sectional cohort study where smokers and nonsmokers with a new fracture were given a survey on fractures in general and smoking. Compared with nonsmokers, smokers less fully understand the negative effects of smoking on fracture healing and general health. In 48% of patients, having a fracture in need of healing made them more likely to quit. Level of evidence: II.

43. Lindström D, Sadr Azodi O, Wladis A, et al: Effects of a perioperative smoking cessation intervention on postoperative complications: A randomized trial. *Ann Surg* 2008;248:739-745.

44. Wong J, Lam DP, Abrishami A, Chan MT, Chung F: Short-term preoperative smoking cessation and postoperative complications: A systematic review and meta-analysis. *Can J Anaesth* 2012;59:268-279.

45. Stead LF, Koilpillai P, Fanshawe TR, Lancaster T: Combined pharmacotherapy and behavioural interventions for smoking cessation. *Cochrane Database Syst Rev* 2016;3:Cd008286.

A Cochrane review that included 53 studies and more than 25,000 patients. They found that interventions that combined behavioral support with pharmacotherapy demonstrated increased cessation rates compared with usual care or minimal intervention. Level of evidence: II.

46. Best MJ, Buller LT, Gosthe RG, Klika AK, Barsoum WK: Alcohol misuse is an independent risk factor for poorer postoperative outcomes following primary total hip and total knee arthroplasty. *J Arthroplast* 2015;30:1293-1298.

47. Ponce BA, Oladeji LO, Raley JA, Menendez ME: Analysis of perioperative morbidity and mortality in shoulder arthroplasty patients with preexisting alcohol use disorders. *J Shoulder Elb Surg* 2015;24:167-173.

48. Oppedal K, Moller AM, Pedersen B, Tonnesen H: Preoperative alcohol cessation prior to elective surgery. *Cochrane Database Syst Rev* 2012;(7);CD008343.

49. Gordon RJ, Lowy FD: Bacterial infections in drug users. *N Engl J Med* 2005;353:1945-1954.

50. Wieser K, Zingg PO, Betz M, Neubauer G, Dora C: Total hip replacement in patients with history of illicit injecting drug use. *Arch Orthop Trauma Surg* 2012;132:1037-1044.

51. Li J, Ma H, Liao R, Huang Y, Chen G: Preoperative screening for illicit drug use in patients undergoing emergency surgery: A prospective observational study. *Sci Rep* 2018;8:7405.

    A prospective, observational study where 1007 patients undergoing emergency surgery were asked about intravenous drug use. No patient reported a history of drug use, but drug screening identified 7.5% as positive. Drug use was associated with increased rates of HIV and syphilis infection; greater consumption of intraoperative opioids, sedatives, and muscle relaxants; increased postoperative complications 30 days after surgery compared with nondrug users. Level of evidence: II (Prognostic).

52. Ellis HB, Howard KJ, Khaleel MA, Bucholz R: Effect of psychopathology on patient-perceived outcomes of total knee arthroplasty within an indigent population. *J Bone Joint Surg Am Vol* 2012;94:e84.

53. Weinberg DS, Narayanan AS, Boden KA, Breslin MA, Vallier HA: Psychiatric illness is common among patients with orthopaedic polytrauma and is linked with poor outcomes. *J Bone Joint Surg Am Vol* 2016;98:341-348.

    Retrospective study examining prevalence and effect on outcome of psychiatric illness in the orthopedic trauma population. Preexisting psychiatric disorders were identified in 39.2% of patients in addition to substance abuse in 16.9% of patients. Depression was independently associated with increased complications during hospitalization. Level of evidence: III (Prognostic).

54. Klement MR, Bala A, Blizzard DJ, Wellman SS, Bolognesi MP, Seyler TM: Should we think twice about psychiatric disease in total hip arthroplasty? *J Arthroplast* 2016;31: 221-226.

    Retrospective review using the Medicare database where 3,776 patients with depression, bipolar disorder, and schizophrenia were compared with 86,976 patients without psychiatric disease after total hip arthroplasty. A significant increase in infection, fracture, dislocation, and revision was seen in the psychiatric disease cohort. Level of evidence: III (Prognostic).

55. Siu AL, Bibbins-Domingo K, Grossman DC, et al: Screening for depression in adults: US preventive services task force recommendation statement. *JAMA* 2016;315:380-387.

56. Jorgensen CC, Knop J, Nordentoft M, Kehlet H: Psychiatric disorders and psychopharmacologic treatment as risk factors in elective fast-track total hip and knee arthroplasty. *Anesthesiology* 2015;123:1281-1291.

57. Greene ME, Rolfson O, Gordon M, Annerbrink K, Malchau H, Garellick G: Is the use of antidepressants associated with patient-reported outcomes following total hip replacement surgery? *Acta Orthop* 2016;87:444-451.

    Retrospective analysis of the Swedish Hip Arthroplasty Register examining the effect of antidepressant use on patient-reported outcomes. Overall, 10% of patients were on antidepressants and their usage before surgery was associated with reduced patient-reported outcomes after total hip arthroplasty. Level of evidence: III (Prognostic).

58. Klement MR, Nickel BT, Bala A, et al: Dual diagnosis and total hip arthroplasty. *Orthopedics* 2018;41:e321-e327.

    Retrospective review using the Medicare database where 2,000 patients with psychiatric disease plus a substance abuse disorder (dual diagnosis) were compared with 590,689 patients without these diseases after total hip arthroplasty. A significant increase in infection, dislocation, and revision was seen in the dual diagnosis cohort. Level of evidence: III (Prognostic).

59. Kessler RC: The epidemiology of dual diagnosis. *Biol Psychiatry* 2004;56:730-737.

60. Jamsen E, Virta LJ, Hakala M, Kauppi MJ, Malmivaara A, Lehto MU: The decline in joint replacement surgery in rheumatoid arthritis is associated with a concomitant increase in the intensity of anti-rheumatic therapy: A nationwide register-based study from 1995 through 2010. *Acta Orthop* 2013;84:331-337.

61. Richter M, Crowson CS, Matteson EL, Makol A: Orthopedic surgery among patients with rheumatoid arthritis: A population-based study to identify risk factors, sex differences, and time trends. *Arthritis Care Res* 2017;70(10):1546-1550.

    A retrospective study examining orthopedic surgery in 1077 patients with rheumatoid arthritis in a single county. Through the study time period of 23 years, there was a decline in the rate of small joint surgery but no decline in the rate of large joint surgery. Being rheumatoid factor positive and anti-CCP antibody positive were risk factors for subsequent orthopedic surgery. Level of evidence: IV (Prognostic).

62. Bernstein DN, Kurucan E, Menga EN, Molinari RW, Rubery PT, Mesfin A: Comparison of adult spinal deformity patients with and without rheumatoid arthritis undergoing primary non-cervical spinal fusion surgery: A nationwide analysis of 52,818 patients. *Spine J* 2018;18(10):1861-1866.

Retrospective study using the Nationwide Inpatient Sample examining the effect of rheumatoid arthritis in noncervical spine surgery. Overall, 1,814 patients with rheumatoid arthritis were compared with 51,004. The authors found that rheumatoid patients had increased risk of postoperative complications but not mortality. Level of evidence: III.

63. Goodman SM, Springer B, Guyatt G, et al: 2017 American College of Rheumatology/American Association of Hip and Knee Surgeons guideline for the perioperative management of antirheumatic medication in patients with rheumatic diseases undergoing elective total hip or total knee arthroplasty. *J Arthroplast* 2017;32:2628-2638.

A compilation of guidelines regarding the continuation, stoppage, and timing of antirheumatic drugs in patients undergoing total joint arthroplasty. Review article.

64. Schieir O, Tosevski C, Glazier RH, Hogg-Johnson S, Badley EM: Incident myocardial infarction associated with major types of arthritis in the general population: A systematic review and meta-analysis. *Ann Rheum Dis* 2017;76:1396-1404.

A systematic-review and meta-analysis investigating the myocardial infarction across the five major types of arthritis. Twenty-five studies were included for analysis and demonstrated that myocardial infarction was increased in all types of arthritis, with rheumatoid arthritis having the highest pooled relative risk. Level of evidence: III.

65. Krause ML, Matteson EL: Perioperative management of the patient with rheumatoid arthritis. *World J Orthop* 2014;5:283-291.

66. Lopez-Olivo MA, Andrabi TR, Palla SL, Suarez-Almazor ME: Cervical spine radiographs in patients with rheumatoid arthritis undergoing anesthesia. *J Clin Rheumatol* 2012;18:61-66.

Section 2

Basic Science

EDITOR

Hicham Drissi, PhD

Chapter 11

Orthopaedic Tissues

Sean V. Cahill, BA • Francis Y. Lee, MD, PhD

ABSTRACT

A sound understanding of musculoskeletal tissue biology and structure is fundamental to rapidly evolving orthopaedic practice. This chapter will begin by discussing the basic components of skeletal development and stem cell differentiation that underlie all orthopaedic tissues. We will summarize the pertinent elements of the cellular biology and structural organization of bone, joint, and connective tissue. Finally, we will discuss how physiologic and pathologic states such as advanced age, diabetes, and smoking affect the quality of these tissues.

Keywords: bone biology; cartilage; diabetes; mesenchymal stem cells; metastatic bone disease

Stem Cells, Differentiation, and Osteogenesis

Orthopaedic tissues are derived from pluripotent stem cells which become increasingly more specialized. Osteoblasts, chondrocytes, adipose cells, fibroblasts, and myocytes share the mesenchymal stem cell (MSC) as the common precursor, while osteoclasts are derived from the macrophage/monocyte lineage of hematopoietic stem cells.

Variable expression of transcription factors facilitates stem cell differentiation into terminal lineages to form orthopaedic tissues as cellular migration and ossification take place.[1] Runx2 and osterix are essential for differentiation of the osteoblast lineage. Sox5, 6, and 9 are markers of chondrocyte development, with Sox9 having been identified as an essential regulator[2] (**Figure 1**). The Wnt/β-catenin pathway is one of the most important signaling pathways for regulating bone formation, leading MSCs toward osteoblastic differentiation and suppressing adipose development.

During development, contact between mesenchymal cells and epithelial cells triggers preosteoblastic differentiation and intramembranous ossification, during which mesenchymal cells differentiate directly into periosteum and osteoblasts.[1] During endochondral ossification (**Figure 2**), mesenchymal tissue develops into bone from a cartilage template.[3] Chondrocytes proliferate and undergo hypertrophy and apoptosis, and the remaining matrix is mineralized and invaded by vasculature. Systemic factors, such as growth hormone and thyroid hormone, and local factors, such as Indian hedgehog and parathyroid hormone related peptide (PTHrP), promote and regulate these processes (**Figure 2**). Woven bone, secreted by osteoblasts, is eventually replaced by lamellar bone. After a rudimentary skeleton is formed, osteoblasts and chondrocytes undertake skeletal modeling to shape the skeleton and improve its strength and resilience.

Secondary ossification widens bones, with peripheral growth from the apophysis. In contrast to primary ossification, which begins in the embryonic stage and continues through adolescence, secondary ossification only begins during the postnatal period.

Although the classic, step-wise paradigm of mesenchymal differentiation marks the majority of skeletal formation from pluripotent stem cell to terminal tissue elements, recent research has identified that transdifferentiation, the process of one mature cell line becoming another, plays a role in the formation of bone.[4] It has been shown that osteocytes possess the ability to undergo transdifferentiation into chondrocytes either directly or through a pluripotent, intermediate form. There has also been evidence of hematopoietic transdifferentiation, with osteoclasts formed from immune cells such as macrophages and B lymphocytes. A current area of musculoskeletal investigation, signaling pathway manipulation may prevent depletion of chondrocyte precursors in osteoarthritis and may serve as a potential therapy for fracture nonunions.

Dr. Lee or an immediate family member has stock or stock options held in L&J BIO and has received research or institutional support from Musculoskeletal Transplant Foundation, National Institutes of Health (NIAMS & NICHD), and OREF. Neither Mr. Cahill nor any immediate family member has received anything of value from or has stock or stock options held in a commercial company or institution related directly or indirectly to the subject of this chapter.

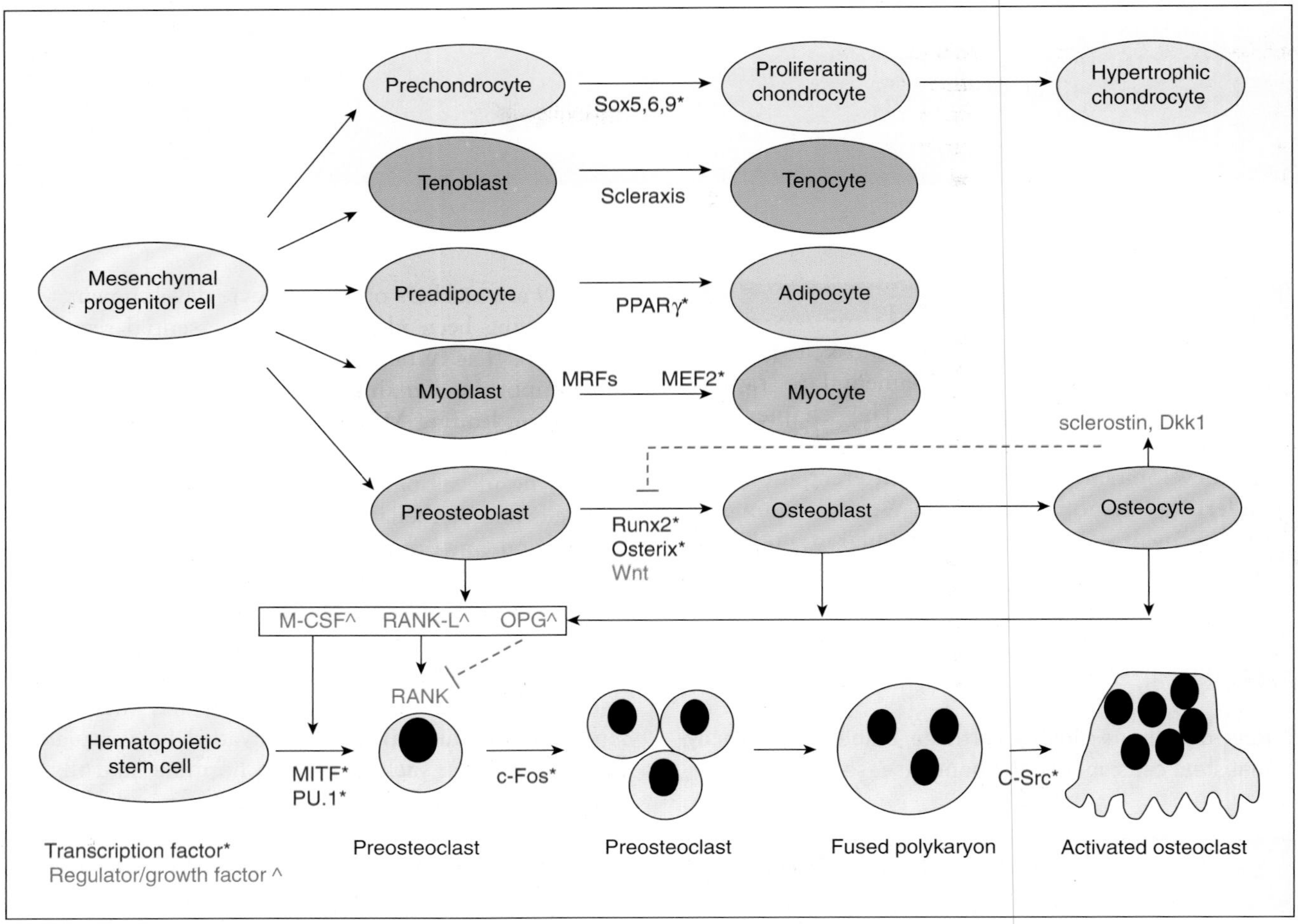

Figure 1 Illustration demonstrating the major transcription factors and regulators of bone cell differentiation. Mesenchymal stem cells differentiate via a stepwise progression into chondrocytes, adipocytes, osteoblasts, osteocytes, tenocytes, and myocytes. Osteoclasts arise from the monocyte lineage of hematopoietic stem cells. A host of transcription factors, genes, and growth factors regulate differentiation. Activation via RANK-L and inhibition by osteoprotegerin (OPG), both expressed by preosteoblasts, are major regulators for osteoclastogenesis. RANK = Receptor activator of nuclear factor kappa-B, RANK-L = Receptor activator of nuclear factor kappa-B ligand.

Bone, the Fundamental Orthopaedic Tissue

Cellular Biology

Bone is a rich, biologically active tissue. Osteoblasts, osteocytes, and osteoclasts maintain and renew the bony matrix and are involved in systemic processes such as mineral metabolism.

Mature osteoblasts contain abundant rough endoplasmic reticulum for collagen synthesis, as well as an extensive golgi apparatus. Osteoblasts synthesize bone through type I collagen secretion and production of osteoid (unmineralized matrix). Parathyroid hormone stimulation and Runx2 expression induce the expression of alkaline phosphatase, type 1 collagen, and bone sialoprotein II in the preosteoblast stage[5] (**Figure 1**). Transcriptional activation of RUNX2 and osterix results in osteoblast differentiation, allowing for matrix mineralization and expression of other proteins such as osteocalcin to occur. Osteoblasts create a basic environment with alkaline phosphate that helps catalyze calcium-phosphate crystal deposition.

Osteocytes, which comprise over 90% of all bone cells in adults, are differentiated from osteoblasts.[6] Our understanding of osteocytes has dramatically increased over the past decade, especially our understanding of the mechanisms of response to mechanical loading and their role in bone metabolism. The process of the osteoblast becoming embedded in bone lacunae induces changes in genetic expression to induce osteocyte differentiation, including participation in mineralization regulation and development of dendritic processes.[6] The expression of membrane type 1 matrix metalloproteinase is necessary for canaliculi formation, through which

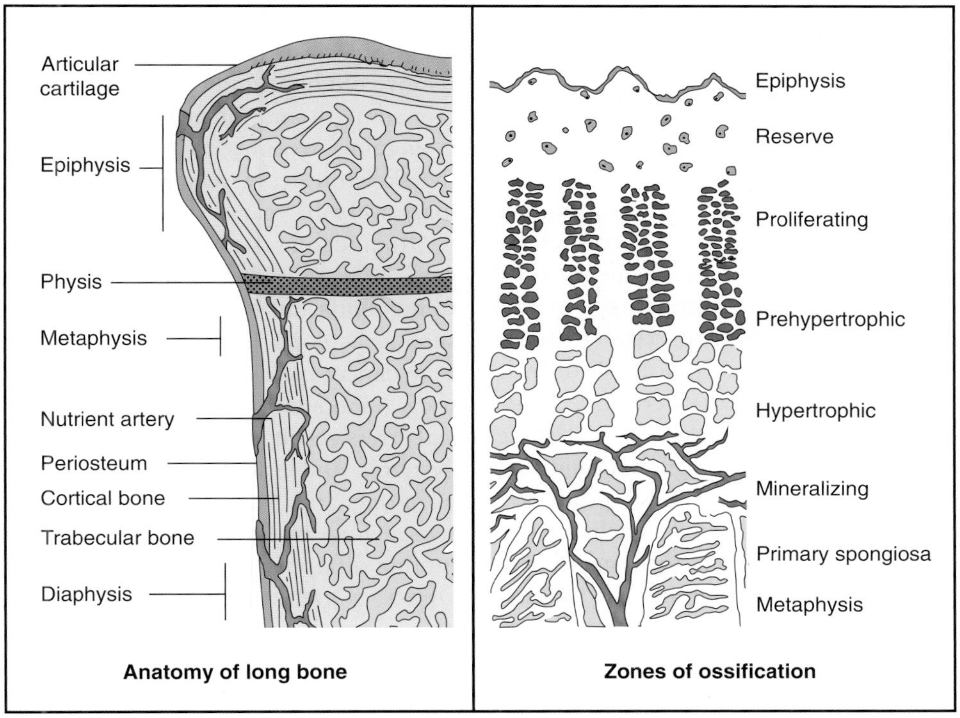

Figure 2 Illustration demonstrating the anatomy and ossification of long bone. The major regions of long bone include the epiphysis (nearest to the joint), physis, metaphysis, and diaphysis. Blood supply via nutrient arteries is derived from the periosteum. Endochondral ossification occurs at the physis, during which chondrocytes undergo proliferation, hypertrophy, and apoptosis. The matrix left behind is mineralized and invaded by blood vessels. Growth factors, including growth hormone, thyroid hormone, and fibroblast growth factor 3 (FGF3), promote osteogenesis. Indian hedgehog and PTHrP create a feedback loop to modulate and regulate chondrocyte proliferation and hypertrophy.

osteocytes form an extensive intercellular network of dendritic processes that directly communicate via gap junctions.[7] The lacunar-canalicular system contains circulating fluid that provides osteocytes with oxygen and nutrients and allows osteocytes to sense acute deformation of the bone matrix, inducing release of anabolic factors to increase bone mass in response to strain.

Osteocytes are the master regulators of bone metabolism. In addition to sensing fluid microcurrents and responding to bone matrix strain, osteocytes produce sclerostin and Dkk1, which are potent Wnt inhibitors and therefore key negative regulators of osteoblastogenesis.[6] Sclerostin and Dkk1 monoclonal antibodies are under investigation as a potential means of increasing bone mass and improving fracture healing, especially in osteoporosis and diabetes.[8]

Osteoclasts, derived from hematopoietic stem cells, appear as large, multinucleated cells housed in Howship lacunae, microscopic grooves on the bone surface. The ruffled border seals the bone surface, creating a closed microenvironment in which degradation products such as acid (produced by carbonic anhydrase and H^+-ATPase) and cathepsin K degrade the bone matrix.[9]

Osteoclast development and differentiation is tightly linked to the osteoblastic lineage, and dysregulation leads to bone pathology (**Figure 1**). Commitment to the osteoclastic lineage from hematopoietic precursors is induced by macrophage colony-stimulating factor (M-CSF), c-fos transcription factor, and RANK expression.[10] RANK-ligand (RANK-L), expressed by osteoblasts, is required for preosteoclast differentiation into osteoclasts. Osteoprotegerin (OPG), produced by cells of the osteoblast lineage as well as some hematopoietic cells, serves as a decoy receptor for RANK-L and competes with osteoclast RANK receptor; increased OPG decreases osteoclast differentiation and activation. Systemic factors help to regulate RANK-L and OPG production, including tumor necrosis factor-α (TNF-α), a catabolic factor, and parathyroid hormone (PTH) and estrogen, anabolic factors.

Although osteoclast differentiation is tightly regulated by the osteoblastic lineage, osteoclast activity is also influenced by hormones (**Figures 1 and 5**). Resorptive activity is increased by vitamin D, PTH, PTHrP, and prolactin and decreased by estrogen, calcitonin, and transforming growth factor beta (TGF-β). Cytokines also regulate osteoclast activity. Interleukin-17 (IL-17) has been shown to decrease bone resorption; IL-6 and TNF-α increase resorption.[10]

Marrow adipocytes have long considered inert place holders in the marrow space of long bone, ribs, sternum, and vertebrae. However, marrow fat has been increasingly recognized as an important, active element of the bone cell milieu and is considered a distinct type of adipocyte (as opposed to white, brown, or beige fat found elsewhere in the body). As discussed in a 2017 study, it has been shown that marrow adipocytes increase with age and are tightly correlated with reduced bone mass.[11] These regulatory effects on bone mass are thought to be induced through modulation of PPARγ and RUNx2 proteins.[12] Thus, marrow adipocytes and associated signaling pathways have become sought-after targets for bone disease therapies. In addition to bone metabolism, it is thought that marrow adipocytes influence other cell populations within the marrow and negatively affect hematopoiesis.[11]

Matrix Composition

The cellular components produce and maintain a mineralized bone matrix, which serves as the functional component of bone. The extracellular matrix is heterogeneous and structured. Mineral and organic components together impart strength and rigidity (**Tables 1** and **2**). The composition of bone varies with age, gender, and ethnicity. Health status can also affect matrix composition, and alterations of the matrix underlie diseases such as osteogenesis imperfecta and osteoporosis[13] (**Table 3**).

The mineral calcium hydroxyapatite, $Ca_{10}(PO_4)_6(OH)_2$, is the most abundant substance in bone, 60% to 70% of its mineral composition. Other abundant minerals include sodium, magnesium, and bicarbonate.[13] The organic component of bone, stabilizes the extracellular matrix, facilitates calcification and mineralization, and provides tensile strength. Type I collagen is the dominant organic substance of bone, comprising 90% of total protein and the second most abundant substance following hydroxyapatite. The collagen triple helix, characterized by glycine-X-Y repeating sequence, is highly cross-linked, providing elasticity. Fibronectin, another important structural protein of the bony matrix, helps develop and maintain the structure of the collagen network. Noncollagenous proteins, such as proteoglycans and osteocalcin, also play various roles[14] (**Table 1**).

Bone Metabolism

As forces from daily activity impart microscopic damage, osteoclasts and osteoblasts work in concert to remove old bone and replace it with new bone to maintain strength and integrity. This process of remodeling is ongoing, working to replace approximately 10% of the skeleton every year and replacing the entire bone mass every 10 years.[15]

Remodeling is a tightly regulated process, as osteogenesis is intimately coupled to osteoclastogenesis. Remodeling imbalances can result in systemic disease such as osteoporosis as well as local bone destruction as in cancer metastasis. Bone loading affects the rate of bone remodeling as stated by Wolff law that mechanical stress results in greater bone density and strength. Systemic and hormonal factors, such as parathyroid hormone and 1,25-dihydroxy vitamin D, modulate remodeling by inhibiting bone resorption and promoting differentiation of osteoblasts and osteoclasts.[16] Direct communication between osteoblasts and osteoclasts is also achieved through release of local factors from the bone matrix itself. As osteoblasts degrade the bony matrix, proteins including TGF-β, platelet-derived growth factor, and fibroblast growth factor are released to stimulate osteoblasts and thus enhance bone formation. Micro-RNA modulation has also been identified as a significant regulator of bone remodeling.[17]

Anatomy and Structure

Long bones allow for mechanical motion of the extremities and are formed by endochondral ossification (**Figure 2**). The epiphysis, covered by articular cartilage, forms joint surfaces. The physis, is the location of endochondral ossification, and is located between the epiphysis and the metaphysis. The apophysis, a feature of both long and flat bone, is an area of secondary ossification.

Periosteum is a thin, membranous tissue that surrounds both long and flat bones, and endosteum is the corresponding inner surface. The periosteum contains a rich vasculature that provides primary blood supply to bone, making it essential for fracture healing. It is also the site of muscle and tendon attachment.

Cortical bone is dense, compact tissue which functions to provide mechanical rigidity. Haversian canals run parallel to the diaphysis along the mechanical axis of bone. These spaces house nerves and microvasculature that supply the bone tissue. Laminae are discreet, concentric sheets of bone that surround the Haversian canal. Volkmann canals allow for communication between periosteal vessels and Haversian system.

Table 1

Bone and Cartilage Components and Associations With Orthopaedic Conditions

Tissue	Component	Substance	Character	Clinical Associations
Bone	Mineral 65% by weight	Hydroxyapatite, $Ca_{10}(PO_4)_6(OH)_2$	Provides hardness and compressive strength; functions as body's mineral reserve for calcium and phosphate	Osteoporosis, rickets, osteomalacia, chronic renal failure, osteogenesis imperfecta
		Trace minerals	Includes Mg, Na, K, H_2CO_3	
	Organic 35% by weight	Collagen type I	90%-95% of organic component; cross-linked lattice provides tensile strength, elasticity; scaffold for mineral deposition; serum hydroxyproline (byproduct) can be used as bone resorption assay	Osteogenesis imperfecta, Ehlers-Danlos, aging, osteoporosis
		Fibronectin	Glycoprotein; directs collagen arrangement; maintains integrity of collagen matrix; promotes osteoblast differentiation. Can be synthesized at distant (liver) or proximate sites	Osteoporosis, liver disease; high levels in intervertebral disk degeneration
		Osteocalcin	Unique to bone; serum marker of osteoblast activity and bone formation	
		Osteonectin	"Bone connector"; high affinity for mineral and collagen	
		Thrombospondin-2	Negative regulation of bone cell precursors	
		IGF-1, TGF-β, PDGF	Growth factors, promote bone synthesis; can be released with bone resorption	Diabetes mellitus (DM) (decreased IGF-1)
		SIBLINGS	Small, soluble, nonstructural integrin-binding proteins. Contribute to bone mineralization, modulate matrix metalloproteinase activity	Upregulated in cancer, plays role in tumor progression and metastasis to bone
Articular cartilage		Water	60% to 85% of total mass; trapping in matrix provides pressurization, weight-bearing ability	OA
		Collagen type II	20% of total mass; cross-linked with other collagen types to support joint movement and weight bearing; fibril arrangement varies based on depth from joint surface	Osteoarthritis (OA), achondrogenesis, skeletal dysplasia
		Glycosaminoglycans	Long, polar polysaccharides that trap water; includes hyaluronic acid, a joint lubricant in cartilage and synovial fluid	
		Proteoglycans	Proteins modified with carbohydrate groups attached; includes aggrecan, which combines with hyaluronan to resist compressive force, and lubricin, which lubricates the joint surface and plays a role in chondrocyte and extracellular matrix (ECM) maintenance	OA
		Collagen type IX	Cross-link with types II and XI collagen to form heteropolymer complex	OA, multiple epiphyseal dysplasia, lumbar disk disease
		Collagen type XI	Cross-link with types II and IX collagen to form heteropolymer complex	Stickler and Marshall syndrome
		Collagen type VI	Ubiquitous in most tissues; most concentrated in fibrocartilage	
		Collagen type III	Cross-links with type II collagen	

Table 2

Collagen Types and Associated Tissues

Type	Tissue
I	Tendon, bone, anulus fibrosus of intervertebral disk, skin
II	Articular cartilage, nucleus pulposus of intervertebral disk, vitreous humor
III	Skin, muscle, blood vessels
IV	Basement membrane, glomerulus, capillaries
V	Dermal-epidermal junction, placenta
IX	Articular cartilage
X	Hypertrophic cartilage, mineralization of cartilage in epiphyseal plate
XI	Articular cartilage
XII	Associates with type I collagen, modifies interactions with extracellular matrix (ECM)

Osteocytes are housed in lacunae and their dendritic processes communicate via small canaliculi. Cutting cones comprise the remodeling unit of cortical bone, with osteoclasts forming a canal along the longitudinal axis of bone and osteoblasts following to close the gaps.[18]

Trabecular (or cancellous) bone is a lower-density tissue. Trabecular bone has a porous, sponge-like structure which houses marrow elements, including hematopoietic stem cells and marrow fat. Remodeling occurs directly on the surface of the trabeculae, with osteoclasts forming lacunae which are subsequently filled by osteoblasts.[18]

The Synovial Joint: Cartilage and Synovium

Cartilage, synovial membrane, and synovial fluid compose synovial joints. Together, they provide lubrication and protection of joint surfaces and allow for movement along a virtually frictionless surface. Inflammation and degradation of these tissues underlie arthritic processes and result in debilitating pain and deformity.

The chondrocyte is the cellular component of cartilage and comprises only a small amount of its mass, approximately 5% of its dry weight. Cartilage is composed primarily of water and cross-linked type II cartilage, secreted by chondrocytes (**Table 1**). Proteoglycans, most abundant in the deep layer, trap fluid and contribute to pressurization and compressive tissue strength. SOX5 and SOX6 expression, along with interactions with CEBP/p300, stimulate chondrocytes to secrete type II collagen and proteoglycans.[19] In addition to secretion, chondrocytes regulate cartilage homeostasis by expression of metalloproteinases that break down the cartilage matrix. Components of the cartilage extracellular matrix, especially type XI collagen, have been identified in a 2017 study as playing a role in inducing chondrogenesis.[20]

Chondrocytes undergo terminal differentiation through the process of hypertrophy, marked by cellular swelling, decreased proliferation, and eventual apoptosis. While chondrocyte hypertrophy and death allow for bone formation in developing bone, a 2018 study reported that hypertrophy has been shown to be an essential step in the pathogenesis of osteoarthritis and marks the beginning of irreversible degradation to the cartilage matrix.[19]

Cartilage is avascular with limited healing capacity. Depth of articular cartilage injury determines its healing ability. The superficial (tangential) zone has the highest collagen concentration with limited metabolic and regenerative capacity activity (**Figure 3**). The tidemark, a separation of the deep zone and the calcified zone, marks the depth where injury must occur in order for healing to take place, with replacement by weaker fibrocartilage through an inflammatory process (**Figure 3**). A population of cartilage-derived progenitor cells have been identified which are thought to play a role in maintenance and may exhibit a limited respond to injury, which are housed in the superficial layer.[21]

The synovial membrane is contiguous with cartilage of synovial joints and forms the inner component of the joint capsule (**Figure 3**). Synovium also produces synovial fluid, essential in joint lubrication and nutrition delivery to cartilage. Synoviocytes comprise the cellular component of the synovium. Synoviocytes include macrophage-like (type A) cells, which have phagocytic and antigen-presenting functions; fibroblast-like (type B) cells, the predominant cell type, which produce synovial fluid and secrete hyaluronic acid, fibronectin, and collagen; and an intermediate cell type, type C cells, that have unknown function but are theorized to be precursors to the other cell types.[22] Unlike cartilage, synovium is highly vascularized. This allows for production of synovial fluid via serum ultrafiltration, through which nutrients can be delivered to chondrocytes. In conjunction with articular cartilage, synovial fluid creates a nearly frictionless gliding surface for joint mobility. Synovial fluid is thick and viscus, enriched with lubricant molecules such as hyaluronic acid, proteoglycans, and lubricin.

Table 3

Cellular Pathology of Orthopaedic Tissues

Cellular Origin	Disease	Genetics	Mechanism	Presentation
Osteoblast/bone synthesis	Osteogenesis imperfecta	Type I collagen (COL1A1 or COL1A2) genes	Decreased amount and poorer quality of collagen; poor bone mineralization	Fragile bone, low muscle tone, possible hearing loss, dentinogenesis imperfecta Type I: Most common and mildest form; blue sclera Type II: Most severe; respiratory failure at birth Type III: Significantly shorter stature, blue sclera Type IV: Normal sclera
	Fibrodysplasia ossificans progressiva	NOG gene, BMP-1 receptor	Heterotopic ossification	Heterotopic ossification and joint rigidity
	Osteoid osteoma		Benign, bone-forming tumor	<2 cm in diameter, young males in second and third decade. Severe nocturnal pain, relieved by NSAIDs. Femur, tibia most common sites
	Osteoblastoma		Benign, bone-forming tumor	Morphologically similar to osteoid osteoma; >2 cm, pain unresponsive to NSAIDs. Posterior spine most common site
	Osteosarcoma	Many mutations identified. RB, TP53, MDM2, CDK4 most common	Malignant, bone-forming tumor	Presents with painful mass, fracture, often at metaphysis of long bone/at knee. Occurs most frequently in patients younger than 20 yr, men more frequently. Mixed lytic/blastic lesion with Codman triangle (periosteal lifting) on imaging
Osteoclast/bone resorption	Osteopetrosis	Carbonic anhydrase type II; proton pump (human) c-src, M-CSF, CLCN7	Osteoclast dysfunction with poor resorption	Fragile bone, anemia, immune deficiencies secondary to bone marrow deficiency
Chondrocytes	Achondroplasia	FGF receptor 3 (loss-of-function mutation)	Inhibition of chondrocyte proliferation	Short stature (skeletal dysplasia), normal/large-sized head, shortened arms and legs (especially the upper arm and thigh), normal-sized trunk
	Multiple epiphyseal dysplasia	COMP or type IX collagen-encoding gene (COL9A2)	Abnormal cartilage formation	Short stature (skeletal dysplasia), early osteoarthritis
	Chondrosarcoma	Various mutations identified, inconsistent across tumors: EXT, IDH1, IDH2, CDKN2A	Malignant, cartilage-producing tumor	Painful, enlarging mass; adults >40 yr

(continued)

Basic Science

Table 3

Cellular Pathology of Orthopaedic Tissues (continued)

Cellular Origin	Disease	Genetics	Mechanism	Presentation
	Enchondroma	IDH1, IDH2	Benign, cartilage-producing tumor	Mostly asymptomatic; can cause pain, pathologic fracture
	Osteochondroma, hereditary exostoses	EXT1/EXT2 in hereditary exostoses	Benign, cartilage-capped bony outgrowth. Can progress to chondrosarcoma	Occurs at physis most frequently around the knee, can be painful. Men > women. In hereditary exostosis, multiple lesions diagnosed in childhood with shortened growth
Connective tissue	Ehlers-Danlos syndrome	Fibrillar collagen gene (collagen V or III)	Laxity and weakness of connective tissue	Joint laxity, hyperextensible skin
	Marfan syndrome	Fibrillin	Abnormality of connective tissue	Tall stature, scoliosis, myopia, lens dislocation, aortic aneurysm, mitral valve prolapse
Myocyte	Duchenne muscular dystrophy	Dystrophin	Absence of muscle dystrophin	Progressive weakness and degeneration of muscle, short life expectancy; Gower sign, calf pseudohypertrophy
Other/unknown origin	Ewing sarcoma	t(11;22): EWS of chromosome 22 fuses FLI of chromosome 11	Primitive neuroectodermal tumor in bone and soft tissue	Painful mass, young patients <20 yr, white race. Commonly occurs in diaphysis of long bone (femur), pelvis. Radiograph showing lytic tumor with margins extending into soft tissues, onion-skin periosteal reaction
	Giant cell tumor		Benign, locally aggressive, osteoclast-like giant cells, high RANKL expression	Pain, pathologic fracture, arthralgia. Arise at epiphysis, majority around knee
	Aneurismal bone cyst	USP6 rearrangement (primary tumor)	Benign tumor with blood-filled cysts. Primary or secondary to other bone tumors	Pain, swelling, lytic lesion on imaging. Arises at metaphysis, posterior vertebral bodies. Patients <20 yr
	Lipoma		Benign tumor of adipose cells	Painless, round, soft, mobile mass in superficial soft tissues
	Liposarcoma	12q13-q15 amplification, translocation of chromosomes 12 and 16	Sarcoma that can vary in severity from relatively benign to malignant	Affects deep soft tissues, most often in adults older than 50 years

The composition of lubricants, cytokines, and leukocytes in synovial fluid changes in response to injury and infection. Inflammation of the synovium, as seen in rheumatoid arthritis, decreases protein filtering and the synovial composition more closely resembles serum.[23] Additional molecular changes associated with synovial inflammation and injury include increased chimerin, increased citrullinated cellular fibronectin, and increased mesenchymal stem cells.[24,25]

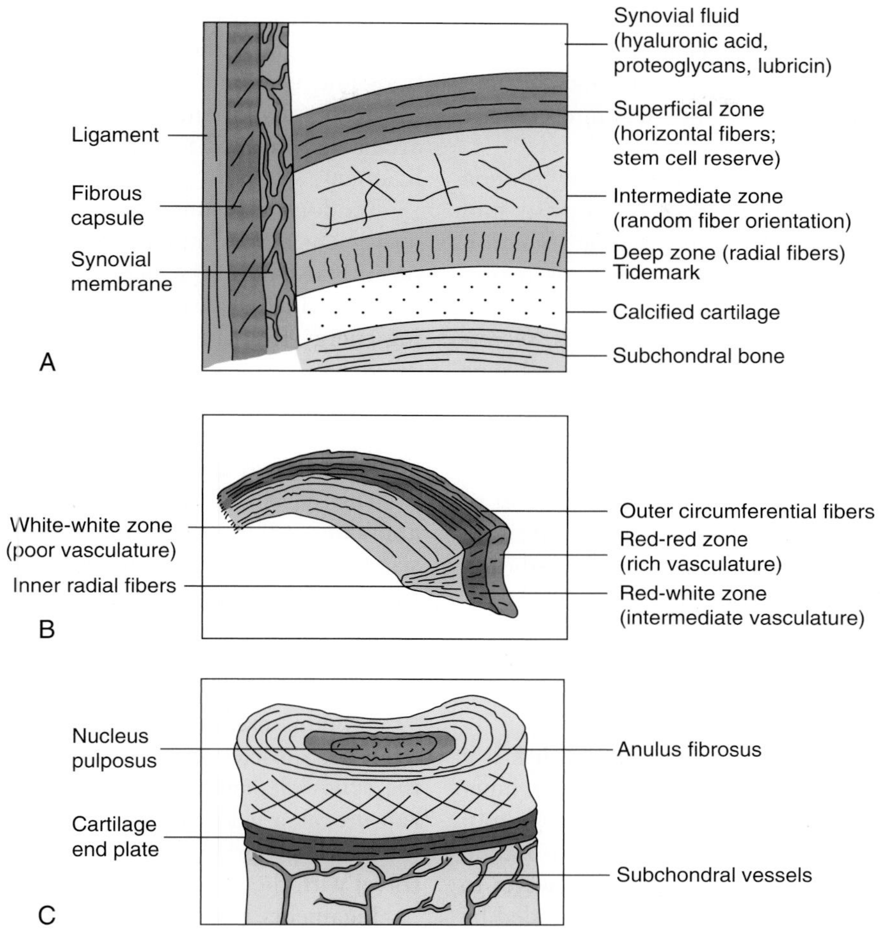

Figure 3 Illustrations demonstrating joint tissue structures: articular cartilage, meniscus, and intervertebral disk. **A**, Articular cartilage is comprised of distinct regions, each with distinct collagen type II fiber orientation patterns. Injuries above the tidemark are unable to heal. The synovium is vascularized and produces lubricating synovial fluid via ultrafiltration of blood plasma. **B**, The meniscus is composed of a meshwork of radial and circumferential fibers. Blood supply is limited, with the red-red zone (best vascularization) allowing the best healing potential. **C**, The intervertebral disk is composed of the central nucleus pulposus and the outer anulus fibrosus. Cartilage end plates separate the disk from the vertebral bodies above and below. As the disk is an avascular structure, the subchondral vessels are the main nutrient source.

Lubricin, a synovial fluid component secreted by synoviocytes as well as chondrocytes, has become increasingly investigated as a potential therapeutic target for osteoarthritis. Also known as superficial zone protein and expressed by the proteoglycan-4 gene (PRG-4), lubricin is a glycoprotein that lubricates cartilage and is thought to play a key role in biologic maintenance of cartilage structure and extracellular matrix. For this reason, a recent study discusses lubricin as a promising therapeutic target for cartilage regeneration in arthritis.[26]

Special Joint Elements: Meniscus and Intervertebral Disk

The meniscus and intervertebral disk share several common features: they are composed of fibrocartilage, aid in joint lubrication, and impart stability with load bearing and compressive forces.

The meniscus is composed of a meshwork of circumferential and radial fibrocartilaginous fibers, with circumferential fibers predominating on the outer component and radial fibers predominating on the inner.

The fibers become confluent and anchor to bone at the meniscal roots. The outer red-red region of the meniscus is vascular, allowing tears to heal after injury. The inner white-white region is avascular with poor healing potential. The middle red-white zone has intermediate vascularity and healing potential.

Cells of in the menisci have been variously termed (names include fibrochondrocytes, fibrocytes, and meniscus cells). Cells in the outer region function similarly to fibroblasts, and produce a fibrous region containing primarily type I collagen. Cells of the inner region behave more similarly to chondrocytes, secreting aggrecan and type II collagen.[27] A third cell type found in the meniscus is postulated to act as progenitor cells with the ability for regeneration.[27] Mechanical loading of the meniscus is a primary driver between anabolic and catabolic cellular physiology.[28] States of exercise, including loading following immobilization and compression of up to 10%, decrease degradation and inflammation and can lead to increased repair. Pathologic loading states, such as immobilization and extreme compression or strain greater than 20%, decrease cellular metabolism and lead to decreased tissue integrity.[28]

Similar to the meniscus, the intervertebral disk is a fibrocartilaginous structure. It is comprised an inner region of chondrocyte-like cells and an outer region of fibroblastic cells. The central nucleus pulposus is rich in type II collagen and proteoglycans that retain water to resist compressive forces. This region is surrounded by the annulus fibrosis, comprised of concentric layers of collagen. The inner layers of the annulus fibrosis contain primarily chondrocyte-like cells that produce type II collagen, while the outer layer contains fibroblastic cells that primarily secrete type I collagen. A thin layer of hyaline cartilage, the cartilage end plate, lies above and below each disk.

Unlike the meniscus, the intervertebral disk is entirely avascular, with its nutrient supply derived from the subchondral capillary network adjacent to each cartilage end plate. Alterations in blood delivery to these capillary beds due to factors such as atherosclerosis or sickle cell disease can result in poor nutrient supply and lactic acid buildup. The irreversible process of disk degeneration follows, marked by cell loss and reduced proteoglycan content.[29]

Connective Tissue: Tendons and Ligaments

Tendons and ligaments, which share similar composition, impart the skeleton with the stability and the ability to move. Both tissues are comprised primarily of water (50% to 60% of tendon weight, 65% to 70% of ligament weight) and type I collagen (70% to 80% of dry weight in both tissues).[30] The strength of tendons and ligaments is derived from highly organized, longitudinally oriented collagen fibrils that are hierarchically bundled to form the body of the tendon or ligament.

Tendons transmit forces from muscle to produce movement across joints. They can be characterized as positional tendons, which carry little load, or energy-storing, which drive movement while storing and releasing energy from high muscular forces. According to a 2016 biomechanical investigation, these two types of tendons have distinct compositions and biomechanical properties, with positional tendons actually exhibiting greater strength and stiffness.[30]

The tenoblast, a type of fibroblast, is the most abundant cellular component of tendons and synthesize tissue substances including collagen. Tenocytes are functionally similar to tenoblasts but exhibit lower metabolic activity. Tendons also contain smaller (<10%) populations of chondrocytes, as well as synovial cells if contained within a synovial sheath.

Tendons exhibit a limited vascular supply, arising from the muscle- and bone-tendon junction as well as the synovial membrane. There is an increased risk of rupture in areas with limited blood supply.[31] Nerves that sense proprioception, stretch, and pressure tend to travel with the vessels.

Ligaments provide joint stability and span from bone to bone. Although they do not directly transmit force, some ligaments ensure stable joint movement by tightening and relaxing during different phases of joint motion (eg, the ACL/PCL complex during knee flexion and extension). However, the exact composition of ligaments varies throughout the body, giving each ligament distinct biomechanical properties.[32]

Ligaments insert either directly or indirectly. With direct insertion, fibers attach directly onto the bone, with distinct zones containing ligament, fibrocartilage, mineralized fibrocartilage, and bone. With indirect insertion, superficial fibers are attached to periosteum, and deeper fibers attach to bone. Like other orthopaedic tissues, ligament integrity is dependent on mechanical activity. Animal models have shown that immobilization results in precipitous reduction of tissue strength and mass. Conversely, however, exercise only slightly increases ligament strength and does not increase size.[33]

The healing capabilities of ligaments are highly variable. For example, MCL tears can heal with conservative management alone, while the ACL demonstrates poor healing even with surgical repair. Tissue engineering methods have been investigated to promote ligamentous healing, such as growth factors, gene therapies, and biological scaffolding.[32] More recently, investigations into stem cells therapy have shown positive results in improving ligament healing and functional properties after injury.[34,35]

Determinants of Orthopaedic Tissue Quality: The Skeleton in Health and Disease

The quality of tissues including bone, cartilage, and ligaments plays a significant role in prevention and treatment of musculo skeletal disease. Physiologic causes, such as age, and pathologic states, such as diabetes mellitus and metastatic bone disease, can decrease the integrity of these tissues, resulting in increased fracture incidence and decreased surgical outcomes. A host of drugs, such as corticosteroids, can also affect bone quality.

Bone health and bone density can be affected by many physiologic, pharmacologic, and demographic factors that affect the balance of bone resorption and formation (**Figure 4**). While a comprehensive review of causes of impaired skeletal health are out of the scope of the chapter, a few key subjects, including aging, diabetes, malignancy, and smoking, are included here.

Aging

Aging bone is characterized by decreased bone mass due to progressively dysregulated remodeling. With increasing age, the amount of new bone formed with each remodeling cycle decreases slightly, while the amount of resorbed bone remains constant. This is associated with increased osteocyte apoptosis and decreased number of precursor cells. Other factors, such as decreased mechanical loading of bone and accumulation of reactive oxygen species, may also contribute to decreased osteocyte function. In addition to decreased bone mass, the bone quality changes with aging. As discussed in a 2017 study, collagen becomes increasingly cross-linked, resulting in bone that is more brittle with a disrupted mineralized matrix.[36] Bones become more slender with decreased trabecular bone mass, thinning cortices, and changes in center of gravity.[37] Overall, these changes contribute to greater risk of fracture in the elderly.

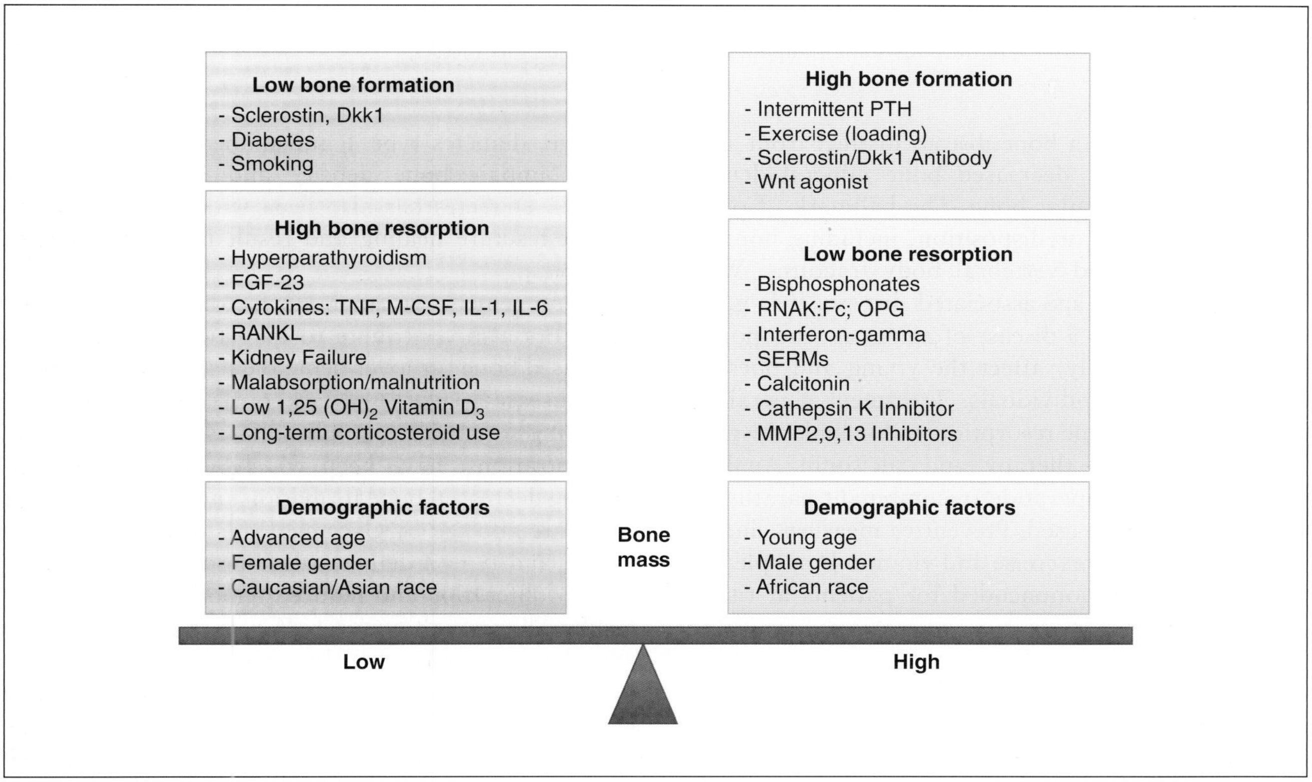

Figure 4 Illustration showing the bone mass determinants. Bone mass is determined by a balance between bone formation and resorption. Peak bone mass is achieved in early adulthood and slowly declines due to decreased bone synthesis during each remodeling cycle. FGF = fibroblast growth factor; IL = interleukin; M-CSF = macrophage colony-stimulating factor; MMP = matrix metalloproteinase; SERM = selective estrogen receptor modulator; TNF = tumor necrosis factor.

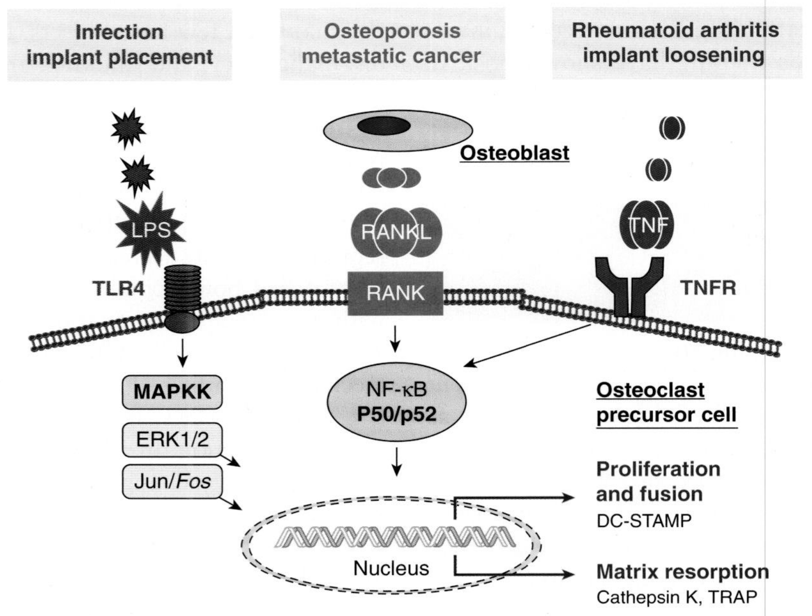

Figure 5 Illustration demonstrating osteoclastogenic pathways. Several insults can induce bone loss via increased osteoclast activity, with major mediators including toll-like receptors (TLR), increased RANK-L expression, and tumor necrosis factor (TNF). The MAP-kinase and nuclear factor-κ B (NF-κB) signaling pathways promote osteoclast proliferation, fusion (mediated by DC-STAMP), and matrix resorption (mediated by cathepsin K, tartrate-resistant acid phosphatase [TRAP] and other factors).

Osteoporosis is a bone disease distinct from aging that is marked by decreased bone mineral density, especially in trabecular bone. The hallmark of osteoporosis is fracture predisposition, including nontraumatic fractures and vertebral body fractures. While osteoporosis is an age-associated disease, it is generally not considered a disease of aging, as osteoporosis can (although rarely) affect the young and does not affect all elderly individuals. Treatment generally is targeted against bone resorption and includes bisphosphonates, hormone therapy, and calcitonin. Anabolic agents, such as teriparatide (recombinant parathyroid hormone), are also used. Preventive measures, including weight-bearing exercise and vitamin D supplementation, are also recommended for patients at risk of developing osteoporosis.

Diabetes

Diabetes is characterized either by absent insulin (type 1) or insulin resistance (type 2), which leads to elevated blood glucose levels, accumulated advanced glycosylated end products, increased inflammation, and microvascular compromise. In addition to end-organ damage, diabetes type 1 and diabetes type 2 significantly impair bone density and increase fracture risk.[38,39] Diabetes has also been widely recognized to impair fracture healing and result in higher rates of nonunion.[40]

Derangements in anabolic factors and osteoblast inhibitors also contribute to diabetic bone loss, with decreased bone turnover being the hallmark of diabetic bone disease[40] (**Figure 6**). Markers of osteoblast activity, including serum alkaline phosphatase and osteocalcin concentrations, have been widely observed, demonstrating decreased bone formation and turnover.[41] PTH levels are affected by glycemic loads decreased in both type 1 and type 2 diabetes, leading to reduced osteoblast proliferation and reduced remodeling. Decreased insulin-like growth factor 1 (IGF-1) levels, which also stimulate osteoblast proliferation, have also been observed in diabetic patients. Conversely, increased levels of sclerostin, a Wnt inhibitor that prevents osteocyte differentiation, have also been identified as playing a role in the pathophysiology of diabetic bone loss.[42]

Accumulation of advanced glycosylation end products (AGEs) and glycosylation of type 1 collagen

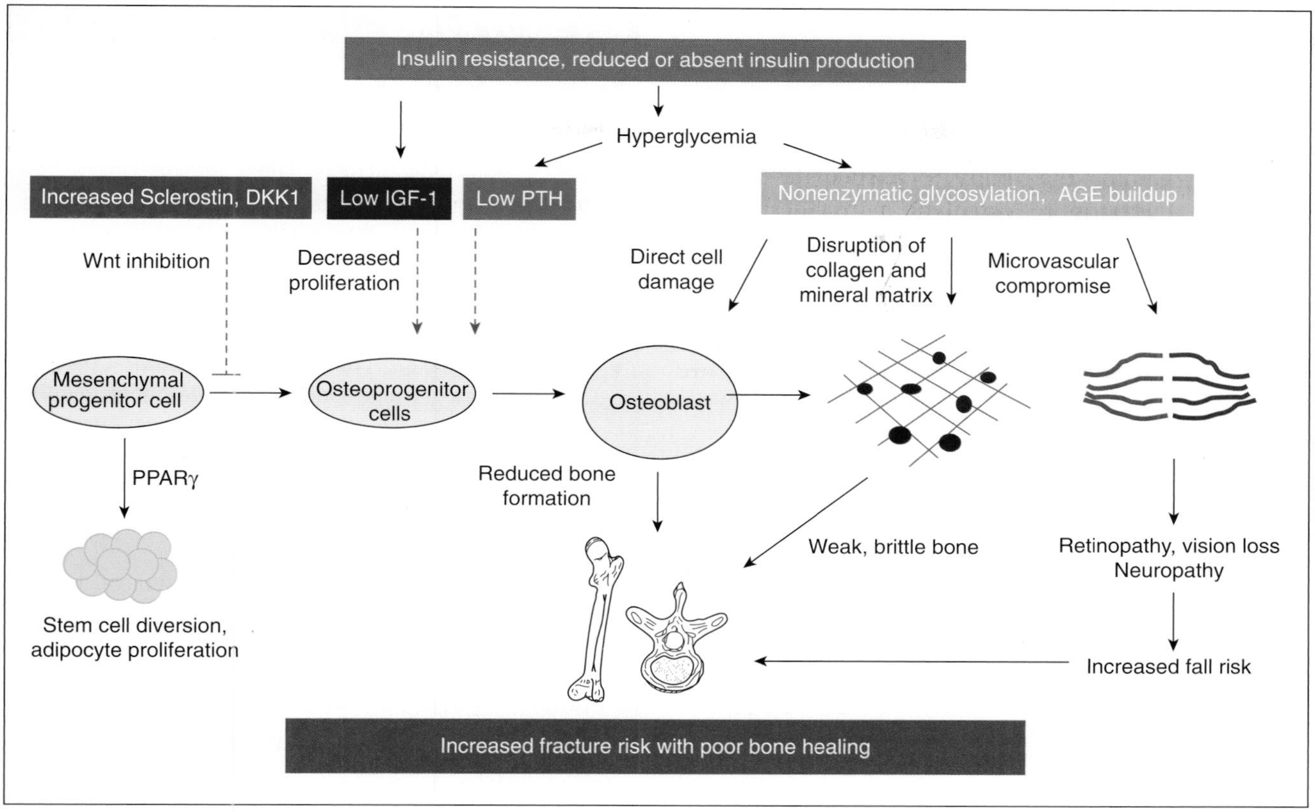

Figure 6 Illustration demonstrating the pathogenesis of diabetic bone disease. Diabetes results in increased fracture risk with poor healing. This is caused by osteoblast differentiation and proliferation, nonenzymatic glycosylation and advanced glycosylation end product (AGE) buildup, and microvascular disease.

interfere with osteoblast and osteocyte function and directly contribute to instability of the bone matrix.[43] AGEs also activate the nuclear factor-κ B (NF-κB) inflammatory pathway and contribute to bone resorption via cytokine production and osteoclastogenesis.[44] Diabetes has been associated with decreased levels of circulating osteoprogenitor cells, with diversion of mesenchymal stem cells into the adipocyte lineage.

Medical management for diabetes can also increase fracture risk in diabetic patients. Thiazolidinediones (Avandia, Actos), commonly used to treatment type 2 diabetes, can also promote mesenchymal stem cell differentiation into adipocytes rather than osteoblasts via PPAR-γ modulation. These drugs have been strongly implicated in contributing to increased fracture risk in diabetic patients.[45]

In addition to cellular and molecular causes, complications from diabetes, such as retinopathy and neuropathy, can directly contribute to falls and therefore also contribute to fracture in diabetic patients.[38] Microvascular disease, hyperglycemia, and impaired leukocyte function also contribute to high rates of orthopaedic infections among diabetic patients, leading to poorer clinical outcomes.

Malignancy

Bone destruction can be a devastating source of morbidity in cancer. Two major causes of bone destruction will be covered here: radiation therapy and metastasis to bone.

Radiation therapy, a common treatment for bone and soft-tissue tumors treatment, can cause inflammation, vascular fibrosis, and reduced tissue circulation. Bone necrosis can result from hypoxic and hypovascular conditions, tissue breakdown, and disrupted wound healing.[46] These conditions raise the risk for pathologic fracture and allow for development of chronic infections that are poorly responsive to systemic antibiotics.

Malignant bone metastases, an incurable progression of a primary tumor, can lead to pain, fracture, and hypercalcemia due to dysregulated bone remodeling.[47] Lung, breast, and renal cancer, as well as multiple myeloma, are best known for causing osteolysis. Several pathways contribute to tumor-driven bone destruction, including increased expression of RANK-L, matrix metalloproteinases, and PTHrP. Tumor cells can also undergo osteoclastic mimicry by fusing with osteoclast precursors, gaining the ability to participate in bone resorption. Furthermore, osteolytic matrix destruction facilitates cancer progression via TGF-β release, increase calcium, and hypoxia. Prostate cancer bone metastasis, on the other hand, is marked by pathologic production of immature, woven bone. Tumor cell epithelial-to-mesenchymal transdifferentiation and osteomimicry are the major osteoblastic pathways involved.

Smoking

Smoking is a leading cause of preventable morbidity and mortality worldwide and has significant, deleterious effects on bone health. Smoking generates reactive oxygen species, impairs mitochondrial activity, impairs fibroblast migration, and reduces blood flow to sites of injury.[48] Smoking is a risk factor for low bone density, with recent animal models demonstrating increased osteoclast numbers and impaired bone growth in response to long-term cigarette smoke exposure.[49] Smokers demonstrate greater time to union and impaired chondrogenesis following fracture, as well as higher rates of spinal fusion failure and pseudarthrosis compared with nonsmokers.[48,50] In addition to impaired bone integrity, smokers have been carry significantly increased risk of infection and osteomyelitis following trauma.[51]

Summary

Understanding the biology and structure of tissues such as bone, cartilage, tendons, and ligaments is crucial in orthopaedic practice, as these factors are directly related to disease pathogenesis and healing potential. The extracellular matrices of orthopaedic tissues impart function and mechanical support, while corresponding cell populations play key roles in tissue development, maintenance, repair, and metabolism. Stem cells and early progenitor cells are significant regulators of skeletal maintenance and development. Growth factors, cytokines, transcription factors, and gene expression also play important roles. Disease states such as diabetes, malignancy, and smoking adversely alter orthopedic cell populations and matrix composition, resulting in bone loss, poor fracture healing, and increased fracture risk.

Key Study Points

- Skeletal tissues are derived from stem cells. Osteoblasts, chondrocytes, tenocytes, myocytes, and adipocytes are derived from mesenchymal precursor cells, while osteoclasts are derived from the monocyte lineage of hematopoietic cells. The balance of osteoblast and osteoclast activity occurs at the level of precursor cells and plays a fundamental role in normal bone metabolism and the development of musculoskeletal disease.
- Synovial joints are composed of articular cartilage and synovium, while special joint elements include the intervertebral disk and meniscus. Variable vascularization across these elements results in variable healing capability, and currently, more research is focused on restoration of normal joint elements.
- Tendons and ligaments are composed of highly organized collagen fibers and allow for stability and movement of joints. The biomechanics and healing capabilities of these tissues varies, and disuse can dramatically diminish their integrity.
- Bone mass is determined by osteoblastic and osteoclastic factors. Age, diabetes, smoking, and malignancy affect the balance of these factors and can lead to pathologic bone loss and decreased quality of orthopaedic tissues.

Annotated References

1. Olsen BR, Reginato AM, Wang W: Bone development. *Annu Rev Cell Dev Biol* 2000;16:191-220.
2. Lefebvre V, Dvir-Ginzberg M: SOX9 and the many facets of its regulation of the chondrocyte lineage. *Connect Tissue Res* 2017;58(1):2-14.

   Reviews current understanding and research of SOX9 as the dominant regulator of chondrocyte differentiation. Level of evidence: V (Basic science).
3. Mackie EJ, Ahmed YA, Tatarczuch L, Chen KS, Mirams M: Endochondral ossification: How cartilage is converted into bone in the developing skeleton. *Int J Biochem Cell Biol* 2008;40(1):46-62.
4. Aghajanian P, Mohan S: The art of building bone. *Bone Res* 2018;6:19.

   Reviews current state of knowledge of mesenchymal stem cell differentiation and chondrocyte-to-osteoblast trans differentiation, as well as potential therapeutic applications and relationship to disease. Level of evidence: V (Basic science).

5. Titorencu I, Pruna V, Jinga VV: Osteoblast ontogeny and implications for bone pathology: An overview. *Cell Tissue Res* 2014;355:23-33.

6. Chen H, Senda T, Kubo K: The osteocyte plays multiple roles in bone remodeling and mineral homeostasis. *Med Mol Morphol* 2015;48:61-68.

7. Holmbeck K, Bianco P, Pidoux I, et al: The metalloproteinase MT1-MMP is required for normal development and maintenance of osteocyte processes in bone. *J Cell Sci* 2005;118:147-156.

8. Yee CS, Xie L, Hatsell S, et al: Sclerostin antibody treatment improves fracture outcomes in a type 1 diabetic mouse model. *Bone* 2016;82:122-134.

   Original investigation into the role of sclerostin in decreased bone healing in diabetes. Demonstrates application of a sclerostin antibody to improve fracture healing potential in diabetic mice. Level of evidence: V (Basic science).

9. Cappariello A, Maurizi A, Veeriah V, Teti A: *The Great Beauty* of the osteoclast. *Arch Biochem Biophys* 2014;558:70-78.

10. Boyle W, Simonet WS, Lacey DL: Osteoclast differentiation and activation. *Nature* 2003;423:337-342.

11. Horowitz MC, Berry R, Holtrup B, et al: Bone marrow adipocytes. *Adipocyte* 2017;6(3):193-204.

    Discusses recent developments in bone marrow adipocyte biology and understanding adipocyte relationship to orthopaedic disease. Level of evidence: V (Basic science).

12. Lecka-Czernik B, Baroi S, Stechschulte LA, Chougule AS: Marrow fat—A new target to treat bone diseases? *Curr Osteoporos Rep* 2018;16(2):123-129.

13. Boskey AL: Bone composition: Relationship to bone fragility and antiosteoporotic drug effects. *Bonekey Rep* 2013;2:447.

14. Young MF: Bone matrix proteins: Their function, regulation, and relationship to osteoporosis. *Osteoporos Int* 2003;14(suppl 3):S35-S42.

15. Cohen MM: The new bone biology: Pathologic, molecular, and clinical correlates. *Am J Med Genet A* 2006;140:2646-2706.

16. Raisz LG: Physiology and pathophysiology of bone remodeling. *Clin Chem* 1999;45:1353-1358.

17. Lian JB, Stein GS, van Wijnen AJ, et al: MicroRNA control of bone formation and homeostasis. *Nat Rev Endocrinol* 2012;8:212.

18. Eirksen EF: Cellular mechanisms of bone remodeling. *Rev Endocr Metab Disord* 2010;11:219-227.

19. Singh P, Marcu KB, Goldring MB, Otero M: Phenotypic instability of chondrocytes in osteoarthritis: On a path to hypertrophy. *Ann NY Acad Sci* 2019:17-34.

    Reviews hypertrophic differentiation of chondrocytes and discusses current understanding of the role of aberrant hypertrophy in osteoarthritis.

20. Li A, Wei Y, Hung C, Vunjak-Novakovic G: Chondrogenic properties of collagen type XI, a component of cartilage extracellular matrix. *Biomaterials* 2018;173:47-57.

    Original investigation identifying collagen type XI as an extracellular matrix component that has chondrogenic properties and supports matrix production and maintenance. Level of evidence: V (Basic science).

21. Jiang Y, Tuan R: Origin and function of cartilage stem/progenitor cells in osteoarthritis. *Nat Rev Rheumatol* 2015;11(4):206-212.

22. Smith MD: The normal synovium. *Open Rheumatol J* 2011;5:100-106.

23. Hui AY, McCarty WJ, Masuda K, Firestein GS, Sah RL: A systems biology approach to synovial joint lubrication in health, injury, and disease. *Wiley Interdiscip Rev Syst Biol Med* 2012;4(1):15-37.

24. Hampel U, Sesselmann S, Iserovich P, Sel S, Paulsen F, Sack R: Chemokine and cytokine levels in osteoarthritis and rheumatoid arthritis synovial fluid. *J Immunol Methods* 2013;396:134-139.

25. Matsukura Y, Muneta T, Tsuji K, Koga H, Sekiya I: Mesenchymal stem cells in synovial fluid increase after meniscus injury. *Clin Orthop Relat Res* 2014;472:1357-1364.

26. Lee Y, Choi J, Hwang NS: Regulation of lubricin for functional cartilage tissue regeneration: A review. *Biomater Res* 2018;22:9.

    Reviews current understanding of function and structure of lubricin, recent advances in understanding its biologic activity in regulating joint cells and tissues, and investigations into its potential role as a future therapy for arthritis. Level of evidence: V (Basic science).

27. Makris EA, Hadidi P, Athanasiou K: The knee meniscus: Structure-function, pathophysiology, current repair techniques, and prospects for regeneration. *Biomaterials* 2011;32(30):7411-7431.

28. McNulty AL, Guilak F: Mechanobiology of the meniscus. *J Biomech* 2015;48(8):1469-1478.

29. Chan WCW, Au TYK, Tam V, Cheah KSE, Chan D: Coming together is a beginning: The making of an intervertebral disc. *Birth Defects Res* 2014;102:83-100.

30. Herod T, Chambers N, Veres S: Collagen fibrils in functionally distinct tendons have differing structural responses to tendon rupture and fatigue loading. *Acta Biomater* 2016;42:296-307.

    Biomechanical investigation into the nature of collagen fibrils in various tendons, demonstrating tendon-specific patterns of strain and strength with loading. Level of evidence: V (Basic science).

31. Theobald P, Benjamin M, Nokes L, Pugh N: Review of the vascularization of the human Achilles tendon. *Injury* 2005;36:1267-1272.

32. Woo SLY, Abramowitch SD, Kilger R, Liang R: Biomechanics of knee ligaments: Injury, healing, and repair. *J Biomech* 2006;39:1-20.

33. Woo SLY, Inoue M, McGurk-Burleson E, Gomez MA: Treatment of the medial collateral ligament injury: II: Structure and function of canine knees in response to differing treatment regimens. *Am J Sports Med* 1987;15(1):22-29.

Basic Science

34. Jiang D, Yang S, Gao P, et al: Combined effect of ligament stem cells and umbilical-cord-blood-derived CD34+ cells on ligament healing. *Cell Tissue Res* 2015;362:587-595.

35. Saether EE, Chamberlain CS, Laiferman EM, et al: Enhanced medial collateral ligament healing using mesenchymal stem cells: Dosage effects on cellular response and cytokine profile. *Stem Cell Rev* 2014;10(1):86-96.

36. Boskey AL, Imbert L: Bone quality changes associated with aging and disease: A review. *Ann NY Acad Sci* 2017;1410:93-106.

 Discusses current state of knowledge of extracellular matrix changes associated with aging, osteoporosis, osteogenesis imperfecta, and other diseases. Level of evidence: V (Basic science).

37. Boskey AL, Coleman R: Aging and bone. *J Dent Res* 2010;89(12):1333-1348.

38. Vestergaard P: Discrepancies in bone mineral density and fracture risk in patients with type 1 and type 2 diabetes – A meta-analysis. *Osteoporos Int* 2007;18:427-444.

39. Janghorbani M, Van Dam RM, Willett WC, Hu FB: Systematic review of type 1 and type 2 diabetes mellitus and risk of fracture. *Am J Epidemiol* 2007;166:495-505.

40. Napoli N, Chandran M, Pierroz D, Abrahamsen B, Schwartz A, Ferrari S: Mechanisms of diabetes mellitus induced bone fragility. *Nat Rev Endocrinol* 2017;13:208-219.

41. Gaudio A, Privitera F, Battaglia K, et al: Sclerostin levels associated with inhibition of the Wnt/β-catenin signaling and reduced bone turnover in type 2 diabetes mellitus. *J Clin Endocrinol Metab* 2012;97(10):3744-3750.

42. Garcia-Martin A, Rozas-Moreno P, Reyes-Garcia R, et al: Circulating levels of sclerostin are increased in patients with type 2 diabetes mellitus. *J Clin Endocrinol Metab* 2012;97(1):234-241.

43. McCarthy AD, Uemura T, Etcheverry SB, Cortizo AM: Advanced glycation end products interfere with integrin-mediated osteoblastic attachment to a type-I collagen matrix. *Int J Biochem Cell Biol* 2004;36:840-848.

44. Hein GE: Glycation endproducts in osteoporosis—Is there a pathophysiologic importance? *Clin Chim Acta* 2006;371(1-2):32-36.

45. Schwartz AV, Chen H, Ambrosius WT, et al: Effects of TZD use and discontinuation on fracture rates in ACCORD bone study. *J Clin Endocrinol Metab* 2015;100(11):4059-4066.

46. Marx RE: Osteoradionecrosis: A new concept of its pathophysiology. *J Oral Maxillofac Surg* 1983;41(5):283-288.

47. Weilbaecher KN, Guise TA, McCauley LK: Cancer to bone: A fatal attraction. *Nature Rev* 2011;11:411-425.

48. Sloan A, Hussain I, Maqsood M, Eremin O, El-Sheemy M: The effects of smoking on fracture healing. *The Surgeon* 2010;8(2):111-116.

49. Sasaki M, Chubachi S, Kameyama N, et al: Effects of long-term cigarette smoke exposure on bone metabolism, structure, and quality in a mouse model of emphysema. *PLoS One* 2018;13:1.

 Original investigation using a long-term smoking mouse model, demonstrating increased osteoclast number, decreased bone growth, increased bone volume, and diminished quality of vertebral bone. Level of evidence: V (Basic science).

50. El-Zawawy HB, Gill CS, Wright RW, Sandell LJ: Smoking delays chondrogenesis in a mouse model of closed tibial fracture healing. *J Orthop Res* 2006;24:2150-2158.

51. Castillo RC, Bosse MJ, MacKenzie EJ, Patterson BM, LEAP Study Group: Impact of smoking on fracture healing and risk of complications in limb-threatening open tibia fractures. *J Orthop Trauma* 2005;19(3):151-157.

Chapter 12

Biomaterials and Implants: Regenerative Engineering Approaches for Orthopaedics

Cato T. Laurencin, MD, PhD • MaCalus V. Hogan, MD, MBA • Meng Deng, PhD • Naveen Nagiah, PhD

Basic Science

ABSTRACT

Musculoskeletal tissues are critical to the normal functioning of an individual, and following damage or degeneration they show extremely limited endogenous regenerative capacity. The future of regenerative medicine is the combination of advanced biomaterials, structures, and cues to reengineer/guide stem cells to yield the desired organ cells and tissues. Tissue engineering strategies were ideally suited to repair damaged tissues; however, the substitution and regeneration of large tissue volumes and multilevel tissues such as complex organ systems integrated into a single phase require more than optimal combinations of biomaterials and biologics. This chapter reviews advancements in novel regenerative scaffolds for musculoskeletal tissue repair and regeneration. Tissue and organ regeneration relies on the spatial and temporal control of biophysical and biochemical cues, including soluble molecules, cell-cell contacts, cell–extracellular matrix contacts, and physical forces. Strategies that recapitulate the complexity of the local microenvironment of the tissue and the stem cell niche play a crucial role in regulating cell self-renewal and differentiation. Biomaterials and scaffolds based on biomimicry of the native tissue will enable convergence of the advances in materials science, the advances in stem cell science, and our understanding of developmental biology.

"Regenerative Engineering" is the integration of advanced materials science, stem cell science, physics, developmental biology, and clinical translation to regenerate complex tissues and organ systems. Advanced biomaterials and stem cell science converge as mechanisms to guide regeneration and the development of prescribed cell lineages from undifferentiated stem cell populations. Studies on somite development and tissue specification have provided significant insight into pathways of biological regulation responsible for tissue determination, especially morphogen gradients, and paracrine and contact-dependent signaling. The understanding of developmental biology mechanisms is shifting the biomaterial design paradigm by the incorporation of molecules into scaffold design and biomaterial development that are specifically targeted to promote the regeneration of soft tissues. Successful regeneration of distinct and multiscale tissue systems necessitates development of advanced biomaterials that regulate cell function and phenotype development in a spatiotemporally controlled manner.

Keywords: 3D printing; biomaterials; electrospinning; regenerative engineering

Dr. Laurencin or an immediate family member has received royalties from Globus Medical; is a member of a speakers' bureau or has made paid presentations on behalf of DePuy, A Johnson & Johnson Company, Pfizer, and Zimmer; serves as a paid consultant to or is an employee of DePuy, A Johnson & Johnson Company, Soft Tissue Regeneration, and Zimmer; has stock or stock options held in Soft Tissue Regeneration, Inc.; and serves as a board member, owner, officer, or committee member of the W. Montague Cobb/NMA Institute. Dr. Hogan or an immediate family member is a member of a speakers' bureau or has made paid presentations on behalf of Miller Review Course and serves as a board member, owner, officer, or committee member of the American Academy of Orthopaedic Surgeons Board of Special Societies, the American Orthopaedic Foot and Ankle Society, the J. Robert Gladden Society, and the Nth Dimensions Education Solutions, Inc. Dr. Deng or an immediate family member has stock or stock options held in Adipo Therapeutics, LLC. Neither Dr. Nagiah nor any immediate family member has received anything of value from or has stock or stock options held in a commercial company or institution related directly or indirectly to the subject of this chapter.

Introduction

Bone injuries and defects caused by complex breaks and pathological fractures arising from malformation, osteoporosis, and tumors pose a significant clinical challenge for treatment and account for 60% to 67% of all unintentional injuries in the United States per annum.[1,2] It has been reported that more than 34 million musculoskeletal-related surgeries are performed each year in the United States.[3] Clinically, the main options available for the surgical treatment of musculoskeletal injuries include transplantation of autografts/allografts and utilization of synthetic substitutes composed of metals, ceramics, and/or polymers.[1] Surgical procedures to align and stabilize with metallic pins, screws, plates, and rods involve multiple procedures with associated risk of donor site morbidity.[1] Moreover, synthetic metal substitutes merely replace damaged tissues or organs rather than serve as a platform for repair and regeneration of tissue defects.[2] To overcome the drawbacks of current methods, regenerative engineering approaches provide an alternative for translational treatment. Regenerative engineering is an approach converging advanced materials science, stem cell science, physics, developmental biology, and clinical translation. Regenerative engineering will harness and expand these newly developed tools toward the regeneration of complex tissues.[4,5]

Native extracellular matrix (ECM) is majorly composed of nanoscale collagen fibers that offer structural integrity to tissues.[6,7] In bone, the basic building block of the ECM is the mineralized collagen I fibrils.[1] In addition to the nanofibrous architecture, high porosity is needed to allow for cell ingrowth and efficient mass transport of nutrients, oxygen, growth factors, and waste products to promote vascularization and avoid necrosis. Advanced biomaterial scaffolds are designed and developed through regenerative engineering techniques to mimic both the structure and function of the native ECM.[8] Different biomaterial cues are incorporated into scaffolds to promote cell-matrix interactions for desirable tissue regeneration (**Figure 1**).

Among the various processing techniques used in the recent years for the fabrication of nanofibrous scaffolds, the electrospinning process is the most promising and versatile technique.[3] Electrospinning is scalable and has been used to process a wide range of materials and composites with controllable mechanical properties through simple low-cost operation. Another emerging technique is 3D printing, which has the potential to serve as an essential fabrication process because of its ability to control bulk geometry and internal structure of tissue scaffolds.[9] The advancement of bioprinting methods and compatible ink materials for bone and other musculoskeletal tissue engineering has been a major focus in the development of optimal 3D scaffolds. Three general strategies have been adopted for the creation of tissue constructs: to use isolated cells or cell substitutes; to use acellular biomaterials/scaffolds that are capable of inducing tissue regeneration in vivo; and to use a combination of cells and materials typically in the form of scaffolds.[2] This chapter reviews recent advancements in the development of scaffolds for orthopaedic tissue repair and regeneration through regenerative engineering.

Electrospinning for Orthopaedics

Electrospinning and 3D printing of polymers and composites are two of the most important recent methods gaining widespread applications in orthopaedics. The term “electrospinning” derived from “electrostatic spinning,” first began to be used for tissue regeneration purposes in the late 1990s by Laurencin and his colleagues, with the first publication in the field in 2002.[10] The principle of electrospinning involves the application of a high electric field to a droplet of a fluid coming from the tip of a die, which acts as one of the electrodes. This leads to deformation of the droplet and finally to the ejection of a charged jet from the tip of the cone, accelerating toward the counter electrode and leading to the formation of continuous fibers.[11,12] Some of the major parameters influencing the formation of bead-free continuous fibers include polymer properties, solvent properties, solution flow rate, applied voltage, distance from needle to collector, and rheological properties of solution, among others.[1,3]

A wide variety of natural and synthetic polymers and their blends with composites and bioactive factors have been electrospun. Moreover, further modifications by posttreatment (ie, surface modification and thermal treatment) can be used to enhance the bioactivity of the electrospun scaffolds.[2] Multiaxial (coaxial/triaxial) structures with desired alignment (eg, uniaxially aligned, radially aligned, or wavy) can also be achieved through electrospinning.[13-15] The order of fibers or 3D architecture can be controlled by layer-by-layer stacking, 3D weaving, and template deposition.[2] These unique anisotropic structures and fibrous architectures of different musculoskeletal tissue can be recapitulated by scaffolds fabricated using electrospinning.[2] For example, biomimetic 3D scaffolds were created by orienting biocompatible polyphosphazene-polyester nanofiber matrices with fiber diameter of 50 to 500 nm in a concentric manner with an open central cavity to replicate bone

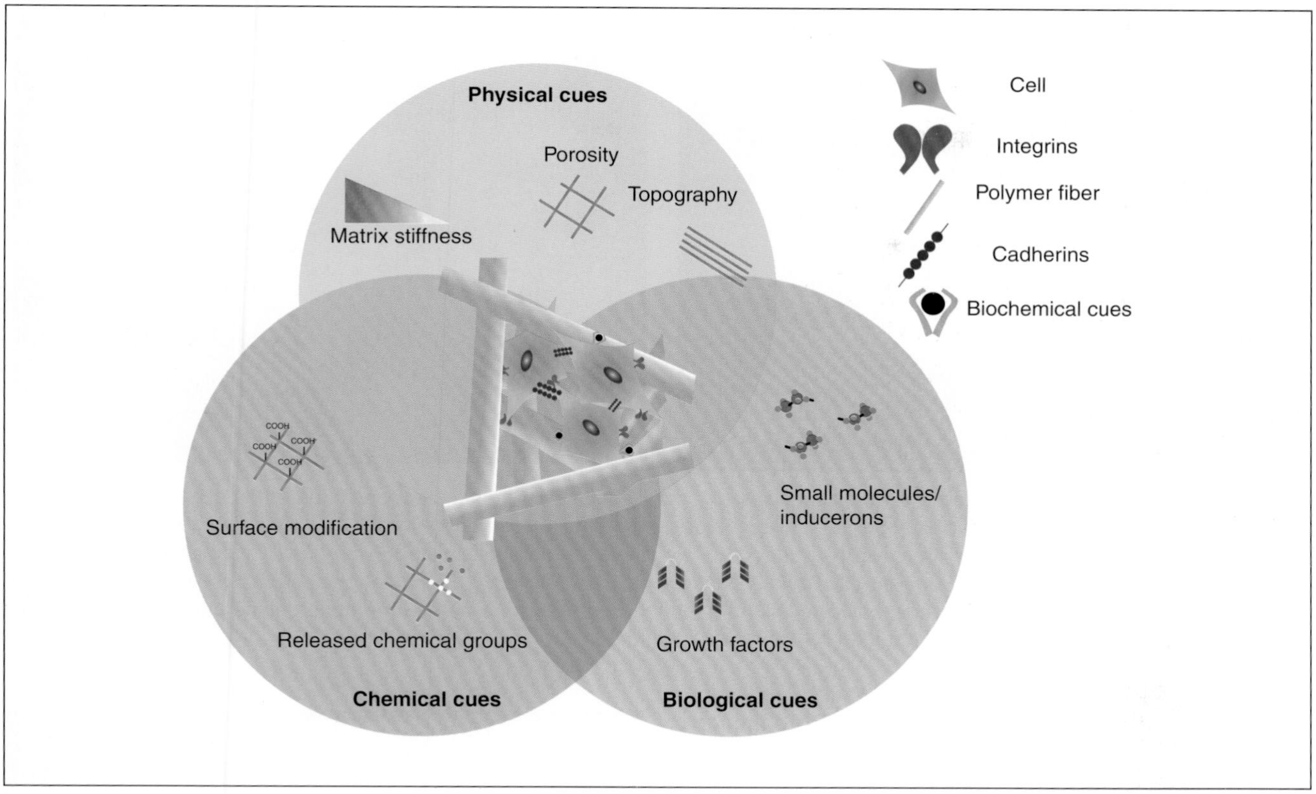

Figure 1 Design criteria for scaffold material cues on cell-material interactions. Physical cues, such as material topography, stiffness, and porosity, can dramatically affect cell fate and tissue development. Incorporation of chemical cues in the form of simple chemical groups into materials influences cell behavior. Additionally, material carrier presentation of various biological cues such as growth factors and small molecules/inducerons can lead to enhanced cellular responses. Integrating these cues is paramount in creating a synthetic matrix optimized for desirable cellular responses and inductive tissue regeneration (Reprinted by permission from Springer Nature Narayanan N, Jiang C, Uzunalli G, Thankappan SK, Laurencin CT, Deng M: Polymeric Electrospinning for Musculoskeletal Regenerative Engineering. *Regen Eng Transl Med* 2[2]:69-84, Copyright 2016.)

marrow cavity, as well as the lamellar structure of bone. In vitro culture with primary osteoblasts demonstrated that the biomimetic scaffolds promoted osteoblast proliferation and differentiation throughout the scaffold architecture, leading to a similar cell-matrix organization to that of native bone (**Figure 2**). The acellular biomaterials/scaffolds in electrospun materials may be divided into surface modified, blended, and composite scaffolds. Over the years, a combination of one or more types has been proved to be beneficial.

Blended–Surface Modified Electrospun Fibers

Electrospun submicron and nanofibrous scaffolds have been shown to support osteogenic differentiation of progenitor cells and stem cells in vitro.[2,14] The mechanical properties of the electrospun scaffolds play an important role in cellular behavior. Mechanically distinct scaffolds having identical microstructures and surface chemistries were produced using poly(ether sulfone) (core) and poly(ε-caprolactone) (sheath). The modulus of blended core–shell fibers were four times that of electrospun poly(ε-caprolactone) (PCL). Lower modulus PCL fibers provided more appropriate microenvironments for chondrogenesis, evident by upregulation of chondrocyte phenotypic marker gene expression (*Sox9*, *Type II collagen*, and *Aggrecan*) and chondrocyte-specific ECM glycosaminoglycan production. In contrast, the stiffer core–shell blended fibers supported enhanced osteogenesis by promoting osteogenic Runx2, alkaline phosphatase, and osteocalcin gene expression, as well as alkaline phosphatase activity. The findings demonstrate that the microstructural stiffness/modules of a scaffold and the pliability of electrospun fibers play a critical role in controlling stem cell differentiation. Electrospinning of blended natural and synthetic polymers prevents the downregulation of cell differentiation associated with the osteoblast linage.[16] Conventionally blended electrospun fibers are surface modified by the addition of extra polymer(s), thereby leading to the shift in mechanical and surface properties of the scaffolds. Blended poly-(L)-lactide acid

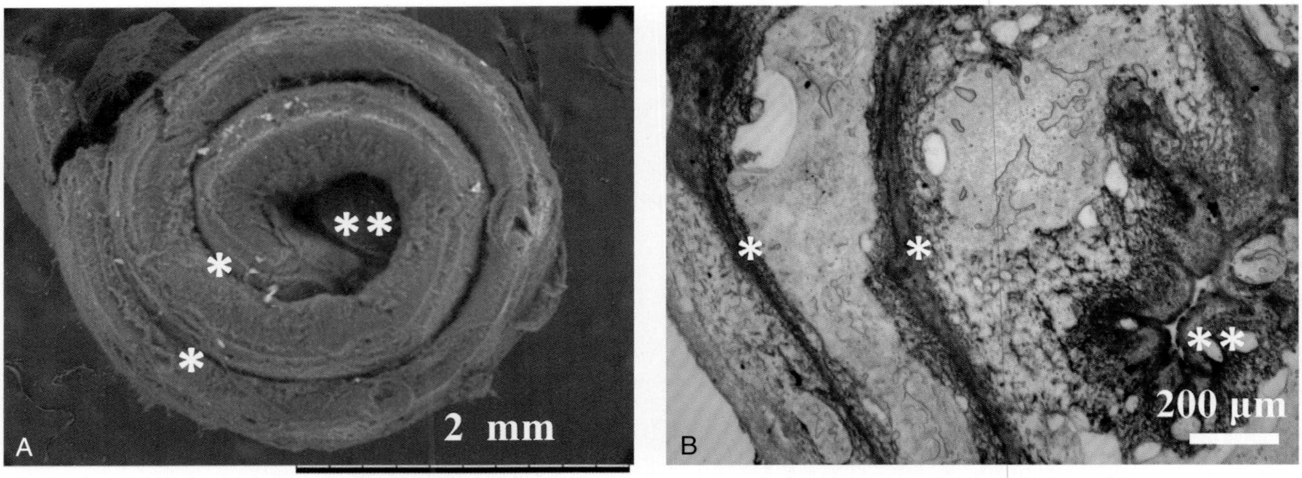

Figure 2 **A**, SEM image illustrating the morphologies of cell-seeded 3D biomimetic scaffolds after 28 days of culture. **B**, Immunohistochemical staining for osteopontin, a prominent component of the mineralized ECM, illustrating a homogenous ECM distribution throughout the scaffold architecture at day 28. (*) indicates interlamellar space, whereas (**) indicates central cavity. (Reproduced from Deng M, Kumbar SG, Nair LS, Weikel AL, Allcock HR, Laurencin CT: Biomimetic structures: Biological implications of dipeptide-substituted polyphosphazene–polyester blend nanofiber matrices for load-bearing bone regeneration *Adv Funct Mater* 2011;21[14]:2641-2651. © 2011 WILEY-VCH Verlag GmbH & Co. KGaA, Weinheim.)

with collagen and/or Bmp-2 demonstrated an enhanced osteoblast differentiation of hMSC by upregulation of different signal transduction pathways.[17]

Composite-Surface Modified Electrospun Fibers

Topical surface modified electrospun scaffolds also have similar effect. Electrospun nanohydroxyapatite-containing fibrous chitosan scaffolds subsequently cross-linked with genipin were used as potential substitutes for periosteum. Cross-linking with genipin resulted in fivefold increase in the Young's modulus approximating those of periosteum. The scaffolds were potential candidates for non–weight-bearing bone tissue engineering, for example, for cranial and maxillofacial reconstruction.[18] Calcium phosphate coating on electrospun scaffolds from a block copolymer-poly (ethylene oxide terephthalate)–poly(butylene terephthalate) improved their bioactivity in bone tissue engineering. The in vitro studies with human mesenchymal stem cells demonstrated cell proliferation on both uncoated and coated samples. Implantation of scaffold–goat mesenchymal stem cell constructs subcutaneously in nude mice resulted in bone formation in the calcium phosphate–coated samples, in contrast to the uncoated ones, where no new bone formation was observed. The results of this study showed that the biomimetic method can successfully be used to coat electrospun scaffolds with a calcium phosphate layer, which improved the in vivo bioactivity of the polymer.[19]

The Use of 3D Printed Scaffolds for Orthopaedic Applications

Three-dimensional (3D) bioprinting is an emerging technique derived from additive manufacturing technology and offers promising potential for orthopaedic applications.[20] It was first described by Charles W. Hull in 1986 as stereolithography.[20] The method has been diversified over the years and has been recently used to mimic the 3D architecture of the defective site for healing or regeneration.[21] Three-dimensional printing technologies involve building a well-defined 3D structure from a computer-aided design (CAD) model using layer-by-layer arrays with the information for a respective design model being collected by medical imaging technology, mainly CT and MRI. The acquired raw imaging data are processed and reconstructed as a volumetric model, which is transmitted to a 3D bioprinter system.[22] Computer-aided manufacturing (CAM) tools are used to produce 3D structures, based on the anatomical information of the tissue, to be regenerated or reconstructed.[10] Currently, biological materials are being explored to develop porous 3D printed custom-made structures with signaling biomolecules and seeded cells in several combinations. These frameworks behave as filling material and can be successfully transplanted into intended defects.[19,20] Extrusion-based bioprinting is commercially used for printing scaffolds because of its compatibility with a wide range of materials at high printing speed, which can facilitate scalable and rapid fabrication.[10,22] One of the major advantages of extrusion-based bioprinting is its ability to deposit materials that contain high cell densities at high cell viabilities. Metals, ceramics, and polymers have been 3D bioprinted for orthopaedic applications. Because of limited biodegradability of metals and binding properties of ceramics, polymers are often blended with ceramics to produce functional 3D bioprinted scaffolds.[10] Based on the polymer materials used for 3D bioprinting, they may be classified as natural, synthetic, natural-composite, and synthetic composite scaffolds.

Natural and Natural-Composite 3D Bioprinted Scaffolds

Natural polymers are biodegradable, and biofunctional molecules on their surface aid in attachment and differentiation of cells.[23] However, potential endotoxicity of the pathogenic impurities and poor mechanical properties are the primary limitations of natural polymers in the fabrication of tissue-engineered scaffolds.[24] Alginate is a commonly used bioink in 3D bioprinting. In 2017, a printability window for alginate of differing molecular weight (MW) by systematically varying the ratio of alginate to ionic cross-linker within the bioink was demonstrated. The molecular weight of alginate and choice of ionic cross-linker were tuned to control the mechanical properties (Young's modulus, degradation rate). These factors influence growth factor release from the bioinks, and spatial modulation directed the stiffness and MSCs' fate inside printed tissues. Spatially varying microenvironments were found to have a significant effect on the fate of MSCs within the alginate bioinks, with stiffer regions of the bioprinted construct preferentially supporting osteogenesis over adipogenesis.[24] Alginate/gelatin scaffolds with homogeneous nano-apatite coating using 3D printing and in situ mineralization were developed.[25] The thickness of nano-apatite coating was controlled by adjusting the amount of phosphate ions in the printing inks. The alginate/gelatin scaffolds with uniform nano-apatite coating had twofold higher Young's modulus compared with the scaffolds without apatite coating. Moreover, the coating significantly enhanced proliferation and osteogenic differentiation of rat bone marrow stem cells.

Synthetic and Synthetic-Composite 3D Bioprinted Scaffolds

Synthetic polymers can be tailored to site-specific applications because of which they are preferred over natural polymers for some regenerative engineering applications.[13] A series of custom-built 3D printed PCL scaffolds with anatomical shape and varying internal porosities were developed for the treatment of large craniomaxillofacial bone defects. These scaffolds supported the human adipose-derived stem cells to form vasculature and bone.[26] Similarly, 3D printed poly(propylene fumarate) scaffolds coated with calcium phosphate and rhBMP-2 were developed, and their mechanical and osseointegration performance in a critical-sized rabbit calvarial defect model was investigated. The scaffolds achieved a sustained rhBMP-2 release and persistent restoration of strength. After implantation, new bone formation around the scaffolds indicated that the composite scaffolds can be considered as promising bone substitutes for segmental bone defects.[27]

Combination Systems of Electrospun and 3D Printed Scaffolds for Orthopaedic Applications

In recent years, a combined use of the bioprinting and electrospinning techniques has been explored for large bone defects. A biphasic polycaprolactone–hyaluronic acid hydrogel loaded with recombinant human bone morphogenetic growth factor-2 (BMP-2) has been developed for vertical bone regeneration. The biphasic scaffold consisted of an outer shell mimicking native cortical bone for mechanical strength. A porous melt electrospun microfibrous mesh mimicking the architecture of cancellous bone was incorporated to facilitate hydrogel loading and subsequent osteogenesis and angiogenesis. A sustained release of BMP-2 over several weeks and high cell viability for over 21 days was maintained. qRT-PCR demonstrated the upregulation of bone markers such as osteopontin, osteocalcin, and collagen 1A1 at day 3 and 14 in the constructs loaded with BMP-2. In vivo assessment in a rabbit calvarial vertical bone augmentation model showed newly formed bone around the scaffolds.[28] Hierarchical 3D printed and aligned electrospun fibers of PCL with myoblast-laden scaffold with micro/nano-topological cues have been developed. The printed myoblasts were viable and were efficiently released from the cell-laden struts to neighboring nanofiber networks. The incorporation of micro/nanofibers in the hierarchical scaffold significantly affected myoblast proliferation and alignment, and even facilitated the formation of myotubes. Gene expression of myogenic genes (MyoD, myogenin, and troponin T) was significantly affected by the fiber alignment. The combination of cell-printing and a hierarchical scaffold that encourages fiber alignment is a highly promising technique for orthopaedic applications.[29]

Basic Science

Other Approaches for Orthopaedic Surgery

Braiding of polymer filaments of 15 μm in diameter into circular or rectangular configurations was found to mimic the mechanical and structural triphasic nature of the natural ligament. These synthetic scaffolds showed an initial low modulus followed by a linear region of increased modulus ending in a plateau region, suggesting plastic deformation and ultimate failure. Engineered ligaments can be designed to be matched to the ultimate tensile strengths seen in native ligaments by varying yarn density and braid shape.[30]

The use of MSC-seeded collagen sponge composites in rabbit patellar tendon defects resulted in improved histologic and biomechanical properties compared with normal tendon.[31] Many knowledge gaps remain in the clinical and preclinical aspects of tendon healing. Faster, more reliable healing is needed. The ultimate goal is tendon repair that leads to earlier and improved rehabilitation, minimal complications, and regeneration of tissue with characteristics that are as good as or better than those of normal tendon.[31]

Scaffolds for bone regenerative engineering applications are desired to have osteoconductive (promote osteoblast proliferation), osteoinductive (promote osteoblastic differentiation of progenitor cells), and osteointegrative (form an intimate contact and anchor into the surrounding bone) properties to promote bone regeneration. The scaffold is designed to maintain the structure of the defect and restore bone function and ideally should satisfy a number of design criteria to achieve properties comparable to autologous grafts: the scaffold should be (1) biocompatible so that it is integrated with host tissues without any immune response; (2) mechanically competent to tolerate the local mechanical forces; this is necessary to protect tissues and transmit the compressive and tensile cues to the regenerative cells; (3) biodegradable with nontoxic degradation products that can be metabolized and excreted by the body; and (4) osteoconductive with porous structure to allow cell infiltration, proliferation, neovascularization, and nutrient transport; (5) lastly, scaffolds should be able to integrate with the surrounding osseous tissue through the formation of bone bonding.

A heat sintering technique has been developed to fabricate sintered microsphere matrices with sufficient porosity for cellular migration and movement of fluids across the scaffolds.[32,33] These 3D heat sintered scaffolds were made using polymeric biomaterials such as poly(lactide-co-glycolide). By orderly packing and heating of PLAGA microspheres in a predefined mold, neighboring individual microspheres bind together resulting in scaffolds closely mimicking the mechanical properties of human trabecular bone. The pore structure is a negative template of trabecular bone in structure and volume, and the new bone would occupy the pores while the microsphere matrix slowly degraded leaving voids that will form the pore structure of newly formed trabecular bone. These scaffolds have approximately 30% pore volume with median pore sizes ranging from 100 to 300 μm, thus allowing bone cells and tissue ingrowth. When the polymer scaffold completely degrades, the regenerated bone tissue possesses approximately 70% void volume resembling that of human trabecular bone. These 3D porous scaffolds can act as a delivery vehicle for bioactive molecules, growth factors, and cells to the defect site for tissue morphogenesis and defect healing. Scaffolds derived from polymers of natural origin, namely, polysaccharides and proteins, are known to be bioactive and highly biocompatible, supporting cell attachment, proliferation, and differentiation in vitro and in vivo. Micro-nano structured biomimetic scaffolds composed of cellulose and fabricated using solvent/nonsolvent sintering techniques and surface functionalized with self-assembled collagen nanofibers exhibited superior mechanical properties suited for bone tissue engineering applications.[33,34] Scaffold mechanical and pore properties are inversely proportional and hence a balance between these two important parameters needs to be optimized. Microspheres in the diameter range of 300 to 425, 600 to 710, and 710 to 800 μm were fabricated into 3D porous structures via a solvent/nonsolvent sintering technique.[33,34] These microsphere scaffolds fabricated from natural polymers demonstrated compressive mechanical properties in the midrange of human trabecular bone, and functionalization with collagen nanofibers did not compromise mechanical and pore properties. Improved human osteoblast adhesion, proliferation, alkaline phosphatase expression, and mineralized matrix synthesis on these scaffolds were evidenced as compared with that on control tissue culture plastic and PLAGA scaffolds, confirming their potential for bone regeneration.

The field of cartilage bioengineering has advanced quickly over the last decade and a large number of novel approaches, exemplified by those described above, have been developed. However, while early results of these approaches have been promising, engineered cartilage with properties identical to those of native cartilage is currently unavailable. Significant obstacles remain, and the future of cartilage engineering lies in addressing issues such as ensuring optimal and stable chondrogenic cellular phenotype and cartilage matrix production, preventing matrix and cellular degradation, promoting appropriate cartilage integration, and delivering antioxidant and anti-inflammatory factors to provide durable cartilage constructs. Regulatory hurdles, as well as safety, viability, and potential immunogenicity of the engineered tissue are all outstanding challenges. Emerging technologies employing advanced materials have the potential to revolutionize the field of cartilage regeneration, which will continue to develop and flourish over the next decade.

Summary

In conclusion, technologies using electrospinning, 3D bioprinting, and its combination techniques for developing regenerative engineered scaffolds are an area of research undergoing rapid advances. These scaffolds may be the key to improving outcomes and quality of life for those suffering from musculoskeletal injury and the gateway to the next frontier of orthopaedic care.

Key Study Points

- Biomaterial-based approaches are gaining higher significance with improved understanding of biocompatible polymers and ceramics.
- Electrospinning and 3D printing techniques have gained considerable attention in recent years because of their ease and versatility in processing biomimetic structures.
- Combined scaffolds produced through electrospinning and 3D printing have great relevance in translational applications for the care of orthopaedic injuries.

Annotated References

1. Li WJ, Laurencin CT, Caterson EJ, Tuan RS, Ko F: Electrospun nanofibrous structure: A novel scaffold for tissue engineering. *J Biomed Mater Res* 2002;60(4):613-621.

   Review on various approaches for rotator cuff regeneration.

2. Narayanan N, Jiang C, Uzunalli G, Kottappally S, Laurencin CT, Deng M: Polymeric electrospinning for musculoskeletal regenerative engineering. *Regen Engg Transl Med* 2016;2(2):69-84.

   Review on development of electrospun polymeric structures to regenerate musculoskeletal tissues involving bone, tendon, skeletal muscle, and their interfaces.

3. Deng M, James R, Laurencin CT, Kumbar SG: Nanostructured polymeric scaffolds for orthopaedic regenerative engineering. *IEEE Trans Nanobiosci* 2012;11(1):3-14.
4. Laurencin CT, Khan Y: Regenerative engineering. *Sci Transl Med* 2012;4(160):160ed9.
5. Laurencin CT, Nagiah N: Regenerative engineering-the convergence quest. *MRS Adv* 2017;3(30):1665-1670.

   Review on Regenerative Engineering based on convergence of Advanced Materials Science, Stem Cell Science, Physics, Developmental Biology, and Clinical Translation.

6. Weiner S, Wagner HD: The material bone: Structure mechanical function relations. *Annu Rev Mater Sci* 1998;28:271-298.
7. Huang ZM, Zhang YZ, Ramakrishna S: Double-layered composite nanofibers and their mechanical performance. *J Polym Sci Polym Phys Ed* 2005;43(20):2852-2861.
8. Maretschek S, Greiner A, Kissel T: Electrospun biodegradable nanofiber nonwovens for controlled release of proteins. *J Control Release* 2007;127(2):180-187.
9. Sell S, Barnes C, Smith M, et al: Extracellular matrix regenerated: Tissue engineering via electrospun biomimetic nanofibers. *Polym Int* 2007;56(11):1349-1360.
10. Zhang L, Yang B, Johnson N: Three-dimensional (3D) printed scaffold and material selection for bone repair. *Acta Biomater* 2019;84:16-33.

    Review on biomaterials and tissue engineering scaffolds prepared by 3D printing in the repair of critical-sized bone defects.

11. Laurencin CT, Ko F: Hybrid nanofibril matrices for use as tissue engineering devices. U.S. Patent No. 6,689,166.
12. Nair LS, Bhattacharyya S, Laurencin CT: Development of novel tissue engineering scaffolds via electrospinning. *Expert Opin Biol Ther* 2004;4(5):659-668.
13. Xie J, Li X, Xia Y: Putting electrospun nanofibers to work for biomedical research. *Macromol Rapid Commun* 2008;19(22):1775-1792.
14. Arras MML, Grasl C, Bergmeister H, Schima H: Electrospinning of aligned fibers with adjustable orientation using auxiliary electrodes. *Sci Technol Adv Mater* 2012;13:035008.
15. Johnson R, Ding Y, Nagiah N, Monnet E, Tan W: Coaxially-structured fibres with tailored material properties for vascular graft implant. *Mat Sci Engg C* 2019;97:1-11.

    Coaxially electrospun structures with tunable mechanical properties for various regenerative engineering applications.

16. Nam J, Johnson J, Lannutti JJ, Agarwal S: Modulation of embryonic mesenchymal progenitor cell differentiation via control over pure mechanical modulus in electrospun nanofibers. *Acta Biomater* 2011;7:1516-1524.
17. Schofer MD, Veltum A, Theisen C: Functionalisation of PLLA nanofiber scaffolds using a possible cooperative effect between collagen type I and BMP-2: Impact on growth and osteogenic differentiation of human mesenchymal stem cells. *J Mater Sci Mater Med* 2011;22(7):1753-1762.
18. Frohhbergh ME, Katsman A, Botta GP: Electrospun hydroxyapatite-containing chitosan nanofibers crosslinked with genipin for bone tissue engineering. *Biomaterials* 2012;33(36):9167-9178.

19. Anandkumar N, Liang Y, Habibovic P, Blitterswijk C: Calcium phosphate coated electrospun fiber matrices as scaffolds for bone tissue engineering. *Langmuir* 2010;26(10):7380-7387.

20. Nyberg EL, Farris AL, Hung BP, et al: 3D-printing technologies for craniofacial rehabilitation, reconstruction, and regeneration. *Ann Biomed Eng* 2017;45(1):45-57.

Review on various 3D printing approaches for craniofacial defect repair.

21. Hull CW: Apparatus for production of three-dimensional objects by stereolithography, Google Patents (1986).

22. Maroulakos M: Applications of 3D printing on craniofacial bone repair: A systematic review. *J Dent* 2019;80:1-14.

Applications of 3D printing on craniofacial repair.

23. Ozbolat IT, Hospodiuk M: Current advances and future perspectives in extrusion-based bioprinting. *Biomaterials* 2016;76:321-343.

Applications of extrusion based 3D printing for orthopaedics.

24. Freeman F, Kelly D: Tuning alginate bioink stiffness and composition for controlled growth factor delivery and to spatially direct MSC fate within bioprinted tissues. *Sci Rep* 2017;7:17042.

Effect of 3D printed hydrogel stiffness, spatiotemporal alignment, and growth factor delivery on MSCs.

25. Luo Y, Li Y, Qin X, Wa Q: 3D printing of concentrated alginate/gelatin scaffolds with homogeneous nano apatite coating for bone tissue engineering. *Mater Des* 2018;146:12-19.

Effect of nanoapatite-coated 3D printed hydrogels for bone regeneration.

26. Temple JP, Hutton DL, Hung BP, et al: Engineering anatomically shaped vascularized bone grafts with hASCs and 3D-printed PCL scaffolds. *J Biomed Mater Res A* 2014;102(12):4317-4325.

27. Dadsetan M, Guda T, Runge MB, et al: Effect of calcium phosphate coating and rhBMP-2 on bone regeneration in rabbit calvaria using poly(propylene fumarate) scaffolds. *Acta Biomater* 2015;18, 9-20.

Recombinant BMP-2 release from polypropylene fumarate enhanced bone regeneration in rabbit calvaria.

28. Kumar S, Hashimi S, Saifzadeh S, Vaquette C: Additively manufactured biphasic construct loaded with BMP-2 for vertical bone regeneration: A pilot study in rabbit. *Mater Sci Eng C Mater Biol Appl* 2018;92:554-564.

Polycaprolactone and hyaluronic acid hydrogel with BMP-2 enhanced vertical bone growth.

29. Yeo M, Lee H,Kim GH: Combining a micro/nano-hierarchical scaffold with cell-printing of myoblasts induces cell alignment and differentiation favorable to skeletal muscle tissue regeneration. *Biofabrication* 2016;8:035021.

Combined 3D printed and electrospun polycaprolactone scaffolds aided skeletal muscle regeneration.

30. Lu H, Cooper J, Manuel S, et al: Anterior cruciate ligament regeneration using braided biodegradable scaffolds: In vitro optimization studies. *Biomaterials* 2005;26(23):4805-4816.

31. Hogan MV, Bagayoko N, James R, Starnes T, Katz A, Chhabra AB: Tissue engineering solutions for tendon repair. *J Am Acad Orthop Surg* 2011;19(3):134-142.

32. Borden M, Attawi M, Laurencin CT: The sintered microsphere matrix for bone tissue engineering: In vitro osteoconductivity studies. *J Biomed Mater Res* 2002;61(3):421-429.

33. Aravamudhan A, Ramos DM, Harmon MD, et al: Cellulose and collagen derived micro-nano structured scaffolds for bone tissue engineering. *J Biomed Nanotechnol* 2013;9(4):719-731.

34. Sobajima S, Vadala G, Shimer A, Kim JS, Gilbertson LG, Kang JD: Feasibility of a stem cell therapy for intervertebral disc degeneration. *Spine J* 2008;8(6):888-896.

Chapter 13

Fracture Healing

Benjamin A. Alman, MD

ABSTRACT

Bone is unique in its ability to regenerate following an injury, and most fractures will heal using currently available treatment approaches. Osseous repair progresses through three closely integrated and overlapping phases (initial, proliferative, and remodeling), during which multiple cell types and growth factors are activated in a coordinated manner. Despite this, a variety of situations are associated with poor repair. Advances in preclinical understanding of fracture repair have treatment implications for these situations. Work identifying the optimal mechanical factors, cells at the injury site, a role for inflammation and signaling molecules for optimal healing is being translated into patient care. Ultimately, well-designed clinical studies in patients are needed as promising preclinical studies do not always predict efficacy in the clinic.

Keywords: BMP; fracture repair; hemopoietic cells; platelets; ultrasound; Wnt

Introduction

Bone is one of the few tissues that can regenerate following an injury. Most others heal with scar. Although most fractures heal uneventfully following traditional therapy, systemic condition, poor fixation, and other local factors can lead to a delayed union or nonunion. Once the bone heals, it establishes its normal anatomic, structural, and mechanical properties. The outer layer of bone is surrounded by a thick nonbony connective tissue layer, the periosteum, which is itself surrounded in many locations by muscle. The outer cortex of bone is a well-organized structure on the gross and microscopic levels, providing much of the torsion and bending strength of the whole bone. There are relatively few cells in the cortex, primarily vascular and bone-forming cells. The inner region of the bone is the medullary canal, which is much more cellular, in which hematopoietic progenitor cells and their progeny also reside. The medullary bone provides much of the compressive strength of bone. Here we will review the basic biology of fracture repair, some of the methods to potentially improve repair based on recent preclinical work, and discuss the early phase clinical data that are available for some of these methods.

Dr. Alman or an immediate family member has stock or stock options held in ScarX and serves as a board member, owner, officer, or committee member of the Shrine Research Advisory Board.

Osseous Healing

Fracture healing is a complex regenerative process initiated in response to injury, in which bone can heal by primary or secondary mechanisms. In primary healing, new cortical bone is laid down without any intermediate. This type of healing occurs when a fracture is rigidly fixed usually through certain types of surgery. In the more common secondary healing, immature and disorganized bone forms between the fragments, which is termed the callus.[1] Osseous repair progresses through three closely integrated and overlapping phases, during which multiple cell types and growth factors are activated in a coordinated manner.

In the initial phase of fracture repair, bleeding from the damaged tissues causes a hematoma at the fracture site, stopping blood loss and liberating growth factors and cytokines. Endothelial cells respond and increase their vascular permeability, allowing leukocytes, monocytes, and macrophages to reach the fracture site.[2] The blood supply is temporarily disrupted for a few millimeters on the bone, on either side of the fracture, producing local necrosis and hypoxia. It is likely that necrosis also results in the release of sequestered growth factors (eg, bone morphogenetic proteins, BMPs), which promotes differentiation of the surrounding mesenchymal cells into bone-forming cells.[3] In the proliferative phase, undifferentiated mesenchymal cells aggregate at the site of injury, proliferate, and differentiate, presumably in response to growth factors produced by the response to injured tissues.[4] This process involves both intramembranous and endochondral ossification. Intramembranous ossification involves the formation of bone directly from committed osteoprogenitor cells and undifferentiated mesenchymal cells that reside in the periosteum, resulting in hard callus formation.[5] During endochondral ossification, mesenchymal cells differentiate into chondrocytes, producing cartilaginous matrix, which then undergoes calcification and eventually is replaced by bone. The formation of primary bone is followed by extensive remodeling until the damaged skeletal element regains original shape and size[1,5-7] (**Figure 1**).

Secondary healing shares many factors with endochondral ossification during development, but differs in that injury and activation of inflammatory cells initiate the healing response. Damage to the extracellular matrix, factors released by platelets, proteins in the initial blood clot at the injury site, and activation of hemopoietic cells initiate the repair process in fracture healing. Increasing evidence suggests that an appropriate inflammation response is critical to successful fracture repair. Macrophage cells are particularly important in the early stages of the repair process as without these cells, fractures will not heal.[8,9] Many cells can produce new osteoblasts, including periosteal cells, muscle derived cells, blood vessel cells (in particular pericytes), and undifferentiated mesenchymal cells in the bone marrow (MSCs). These cells can initially differentiate into

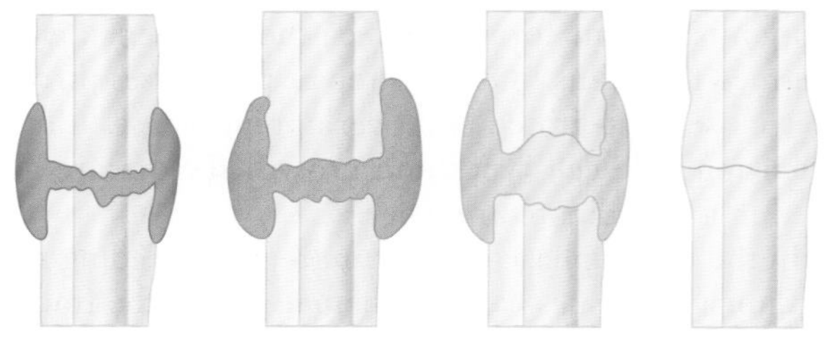

Figure 1 Illustration shows phases of fracture repair. Fracture healing proceeds through four distinct yet overlapping stages. The first stage is the initial or inflammatory phase, which is characterized by the formation of a hematoma at the site of fracture. The second stage is the proliferative phase when there is formation of a fibrocartilaginous callus phase, where the hematoma is invaded by fibroblasts and chondrocytes leading to the deposition of a fibrocartilaginous callus. The third stage is the formation of the bone callus. During this stage, osteoblasts produce a woven bone matrix leading to the deposition of a bony callus. This callus then undergoes the final remodeling phase in which the woven bone is replaced with compact bone, restoring the integrity of the bone. Undifferentiated mesenchymal cells differentiate into an osteochondral progenitor.

chondrocytes, or can differentiate directly into osteoblasts. Cartilage precedes bone formation in the initial or soft callus which bridges the bone gaps but lacks the degree of strength in a hard callous that is composed of bone. Blood vessels are critical to the repair process, and without appropriate vascularity, fractures also cannot heal. Osteoclasts are required for the remodeling phase, and these cells interact with bone-forming cells much like in physiologic bone homeostasis. Several growth factors and signaling proteins are activated in the early phases of repair, which stimulate new blood vessel formation, mesenchymal cell differentiation, and osteoblast formation. The mechanical environment also alters cell differentiation, with too little or too much mechanical stimulation of cells at the fracture site preventing bone healing. Many of these factors have the possibility to be modulated to improve poor bone headlining, but as the process is a coordinated response involving many factors and cells, no one protein or cell is completely responsible for the healing response.

When bone heals by secondary healing, a callus forms at the fracture site that is larger in diameter than the uninjured bone. The bone in the callus is initially weaker than the mature bone until it undergoes remodeling, a process that takes many months to complete. The larger diameter of the callus allows the bone as a unit to achieve strength similar to the uninjured bone. This is because having weaker material further from the center of the bone allows the bone as a unit to exhibit greater strength. This is a function of the moment of inertia, which is a measure of the distance of a material from the center of the bone, and predicts the torsional and bending strength of the bone.

When fracture healing is impaired, osteoblastic differentiation is inhibited, and undifferentiated mesenchymal tissue remains at the fracture site. In patients, this outcome results in delayed union, or nonunion, usually requiring additional surgery for successful fracture healing. Several risk factors have been associated with a delayed union. Patient-dependent risk factors include older age, diabetes, smoking, nutritional deficiencies, and the use of anti-inflammatory agents.[10,11] Other patient factors such as local infection and immune disorders can be deleterious to fracture healing. Local factors associated with a delayed union include the extent of soft-tissue injury, compartment syndrome, and certain anatomic locations, such as the tibia. Interestingly, bones with less muscle coverage are more apt to delayed union.[12] Because up to 5% of fractures go on to a delayed union, the development of therapies to reduce the rate of nonunion and to better treat nonunions is an area of intense investigation.

Mechanical Factors

The mechanical environment will alter the ability of fractures to heal. A gap in bone held rigidly, or too much motion at a fracture site will result in a delayed union. How the local mechanical environment influences cells to repair a fracture varies with different stages of healing. Loading during the early stages of repair may impede stabilization of the injury site, whereas loading during matrix deposition and remodeling are ongoing may enhance stabilization.[13] One method to mechanically stimulate cells during the repair process is through ultrasound. Low-intensity pulsed ultrasound will increase in cell proliferation, protein synthesis, collagen synthesis, membrane permeability, integrin expression, and increased cytosolic Ca(2+) levels as well as other increased indicators of bone repair in response to low-intensity pulsed ultrasound exposure.[14,15] Ultrasound also enhances angiogenesis mechanisms during bone healing.[16] These are all changes that should enhance fracture repair. Despite these preclinical findings, clinical studies have shown variable results. A recent large randomized trial showed no difference in acute fracture repair by adding ultrasound,[17] but a meta-analysis for nonunion showed a mild improved healing effect.[18] Despite the disparate reported clinical findings, preclinical data suggest that ultrasound may be effective in inducing bone healing when combined with other therapies.[19]

Cells and Cell Products

Platelets

Bleeding and the development of a blood clot is present when bone fractures. Contents in the clot, such as platelets, play a role in initiating the repair process. Several blood derivatives have been investigated to improve healing. Platelet-rich plasma (PRP) can effect inflammation, cytokines, growth factors, and angiogenic factors,[20] all factors which could improve bone headlining, and this has been investigated in fracture repair.[21] Data on animals show that adding PRP in controlled situations could enhance repair. However, despite these preclinical data, current clinical studies are limited by sample size and controls and provide little clinical support for the use of this modality.[22]

Mesenchymal Cells

The identification of skeletal stem cells in humans has been problematic because of the inability to trace cells the way one can in genetically modified animals. However, recently a self-renewing and multipotent human skeletal stem cell was identified that is present in adult bones.[23] Now that skeletal stem cells are more clearly identified, it is likely that there will be substantial future work identifying the role of these cells in repair and regeneration. In contrast, MSCs are a mixture of many cell types, and not all are stem cells. They can be derived from multiple sources including the bone marrow stromal cells, pericytes souring blood vessels, fat, and the periosteum. These cells can differentiate into bone-forming osteoblasts and can release factors that stimulate bone healing. Several animal studies show that adding MSCs will promote faster healing of bone defects, such as a recent study in rabbits showing that MSCs speed the healing of critical sized bone defects.[24] These data are supported by studies in genetically modified mice. Sclerostin domain-containing protein 1 (Sostdc1) maintains MSCs in the periosteum in a quiescence state, preventing them from participating in healing. Enhanced bone formation in fractures in *Sostdc1*deficient mice is consistent with the need for activation of MSCs to promote fracture repair.[25]

Interestingly, MSCs not only might contribute themselves to healing but also can secrete factors that enhance healing. Indeed, this later function seems to be the dominant mechanism by which MSCs enhance repair. Injecting MSCs to the fracture site is one way to use these cells as protein factories, allowing molecules to enhance repair to be liberated at the fracture site. An alternative approach has been developed in which MSC-derived exosomes are used instead. These are extracellular vesicles produced by cells that contain the protein contents of the cytoplasm. Investigations using exosomes isolated from MSC-conditioned medium can rescue slow fracture repair in mice known to have slow healing. This method exploits the factors produced by MSCs in a cell-free way to enhance fracture repair.[26]

Despite the preclinical work on MSCs, there is little high-quality clinical work showing efficacy. However, there are ongoing clinical trials,[27] which will provide information on which clinical decision making can be based.

Hematopoietic Cells

During the initial phase of fracture repair, hematopoietic cells are present at the repair site, and these cells produce factors that are critical to initiating the repair process.[8] Macrophage cells are present during the early phases of fracture repair, and in their absence, fractures cannot heal.[9] Investigators are beginning to study the possibility of using immune cells or the factors they produce to enhance fracture repair, for instance, targeting how macrophage cells and MSCs interact.[28] Osteoclasts also are present during fracture healing, although toward the later stages of the repair cascade. Osteoclasts are inhibited by diphosphonate drugs, and the continuous administration of bisphosphonates causes a delay in healing in certain animal studies, especially in the absence of rigid fixation.[29] However, overall patients on bisphosphonates seem to heal adequately,[30] although longer term use can cause osteopetrosis-like bone that is predisposed to atypical fractures.

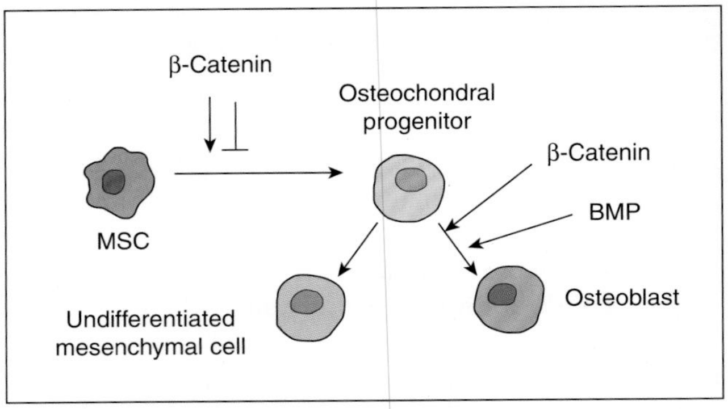

Figure 2 Illustration shows cell signaling pathways regulating mesenchymal differentiation in fracture repair. Mesenchymal progenitor cells (MSCs) differentiate into an osteochondral progenitor. β-Catenin needs to be precisely regulated for this differentiation: levels too high or too low prevent differentiation. Osteochondral progenitor cells can differentiate into osteoblast. β-Catenin or bone morphogenetic protein (BMP) will stimulate differentiation into osteoblasts.

Proteins and Pharmacologic Agents

Anabolic Agents

Agents that enhance osteoblast activity in bone homeostasis are termed anabolic. Parathyroid hormone (PTH) is an anabolic agent that is currently used in treating patients with osteoporosis. PTH and parathyroid hormone–related peptide activate a similar signaling system and lack of parathyroid hormone–related peptide in mice impairs bone fracture healing.[31] Thus, this anabolic effect PTH has on bone has led to research its use for bone regeneration and repair. Numerous animal studies found enhanced fracture healing as a result of PTH treatment. Although there are no large-scale studies, in a human case study, a nonunion that persisted despite treatment attempts with surgery, autograft, and BMP, healed when PTH was used. Use of a biomaterial scaffold to locally deliver PTH to a defect site is also being investigated. Taken together, this provides evidence that PTH may be used to promote bone regeneration.[32] Combination therapy is also being investigated in animal studies, and PTH along with MSCs in a bioengineered matrix may enhance repair better than either approach alone.[33]

Differentiation Agents

Several cell signaling pathways need to be activated in a sequential manner for undifferentiated mesenchymal progenitor cells to become osteoblasts. By understanding this process, it is possible that agents that modulate the signaling pathways can be used to enhance repair.

Wnt Signaling

Wnt signaling is one pathway that regulates the differentiation of mesenchymal cells into osteoblasts. In early phases of differentiation, it needs to be precisely regulated, or cells will persist in a fibroblastic state, but once cells become committed to a bone or cartilage lineage, Wnt activation will enhance bone formation.[34] Wnt can signal through the protein, β-catenin, and modulating this genetically in mice shows that its level cannot be too high or too low in the early phases of repair, but that higher levels are needed in later phases for normal healing[35] (**Figure 2**). One way to modulate β-catenin is with sclerostin antibody (SclAb), a pharmacologic approach that is being investigated for use in patients. Animal studies, however, suggest that although SclAb may help to increase bone formation early in the healing process it does not work as well in the later phases, illustrating the importance of understanding the timing of therapy to alter differentiation in the repair process.[36] An alternative approach is to use lithium to modulate β-catenin, and studies in animals show that appropriate dosing at the appropriate time frame can enhance fracture repair.[37]

BMP Signaling

BMPs are first commercialized growth factors approved for bone regeneration. BMP2 and BMP7 will induce osteoblast differentiation from a mesenchymal progenitor cells, but other important factors need to be present to induce regeneration, including inflammatory cells, mesenchymal progenitor cells that can differentiate into a bone or cartilage lineage, and an appropriate degree of vascularity.[38] Although BMP trials show effectiveness in healing,[39] these other necessary factors are important for successful use. The Cochrane review on the use of BMP continues to highlight a paucity of data on the use of BMP in fracture healing as well as considerable industry involvement in currently available evidence. Overall, they conclude that there is limited evidence to suggest that BMP may be more effective than controls for acute fracture healing.[40]

VEGF Signaling

Vascularity is critical for fracture repair, and vascular endothelial growth factor (VEGF) signaling is one factor important in the development and maintenance of blood vessels. Although blood vessels will not induce repair on their own, they are required for successful healing, and in situations where there is limited vascularity, VEGF might enhance repair. In animal fracture models, adding VEGF, such as the use of VEGF-loaded coated screws improved the quality of fracture repair.[41] Investigators have also studied the use of differentiating agents together, such as VEGF and BMP together, and such studies show synergistic effects, suggesting that a multipronged approach to enhance repair will have advantages over single agents.[42]

There are multiple other agents that play similar roles in altering cell differentiation that might improve fracture repair, such as platelet-derived growth factor (PDGF) or fibroblast growth factor (FGF), and while it is beyond the scope of this chapter to cover all, there are recent reviews that more comprehensively cover the topic[38] (**Table 1**).

Drug and Cell Delivery

The delivery of agents or cells to a fracture site, and maintaining them at that site, while preventing systemic effects is an important hurdle in translating some fracture therapies to clinical practice. For instance, daily injections of an agent into a fracture is not practical, and one would not want cells outside the bone, such as muscle tendon or cartilage cells to differentiate into bone. Drug delivery systems, including resorbable materials which slowly release compounds, implants coated with drugs or proteins, implantable drug delivery devices, and the development of methods to hone drugs delivered systemically to the site of fracture repair are all under investigation.[43] Furthermore, tissue-engineered strategies to mix appropriate cells and growth factors in a matrix that stimulates bone formation and has the appropriate mechanical properties are also under development.[44] Because fracture repair is a complex process involving multiple factors, it is likely that such multifactor approaches will provide effective methods to enhance the repair process.

Table 1

Possible Approaches to Improve Fracture Healing Based on Preclinical Investigations

Approach	Function	Clinical status
Mechanical Factors		
Ultrasound	Stimulates osteogenesis of mesenchymal cell	In use but lacking level 1 evidence
Cells and cell products		
Platelet-rich plasma	Provides factors normally produced in the initial phases of repair	In use but lacking level 1 evidence
MSCs	Provides cell produced factors and cells have the potential to differentiate into osteoblasts	In use but lacking level 1 evidence
Macrophages and other hematopoietic cells	Produce factors that stimulate bone healing	Preclinical development
Differentiation agents		
Anabolic agents (PTH)	Stimulates osteogenesis of mesenchymal cells	Off label use, lacking level 1 evidence
Wnt signaling	Regulates differentiation to bone- or cartilage-forming cells; stimulates osteogenesis in late phases	Most agents in preclinical development
BMP	Stimulates osteogenesis of mesenchymal cells	Approved for use
VEGF	Stimulates vascularity	Preclinical development

BMP = bone morphogenetic protein, MSCs = mesenchymal cells, PTH = parathyroid hormone, VEGF = vascular endothelial growth factor

Pathologic Healing

Understanding the mechanism by which certain conditions result in delayed healing will identify appropriate approaches to improve repair. There has been considerable preclinical work understanding why repair is delayed in certain conditions, and although it is well beyond the scope to include all such work, two examples of how preclinical is informing new treatments for such conditions are summarized here.

Fracture repair is delayed in diabetes, and there are many contributing factors, including poor vascularity, impaired neurogenetic function, and metabolic and cellular effects. Interestingly, studies in animals show that the reversal of blood glucose levels on its own will not improve repair, and treatment with metformin will actually slow healing in diabetic rats.[45] Macrophage function is abnormal in diabetes, and studies on mice suggest that correcting the abnormal function might improve bone repair.[46] Although lowering glucose levels on its own will not improve repair, insulin, which will lower glucose but also has glucose-independent effects on cells, could improve repair. Combination therapy with insulin and PTH[47] is one such approach.

Neurofibromatosis is associated with poor bone healing and pseudarthrosis of the tibia. Understanding how mesenchymal cell differentiation is altered in cells from patients or animals with neurofibromatosis can give clues into effective therapeutic approaches. In early phases of repair, mesenchymal cells do not differentiate into bone and cartilage cell precursors. Later in differentiation, cells do not maintain an osteoblastic phenotype, and there is osteoclastic activation. Thus, modulating differentiation early in the process by lowering an abnormally high β-catenin level, and enhancing osteoblastic differentiation and inhibiting osteoclasts later in the process using BMPs and bisphosphonates is an approach that is supported by studies in animals.[48-50]

Summary

Bone healing is a complex process by which multiple cells and proteins interact to reconstitute bone. Therapeutic approaches based on mechanical stimulation, cell therapy, or regulating signaling pathways are being investigated to improve repair. To date, only a few approaches have been translated to clinical care, but there are several promising approaches on the horizon.

Key Study Points

- Understand the biology of fracture repair.
- Review the role of various cell types and cell signaling pathways in fracture repair.
- Understand the connection between preclinical studies and the application to clinical care.

Annotated References

1. Einhorn TA: The cell and molecular biology of fracture healing. *Clin Orthop Relat Res* 1998:S7-S21.
2. Ozaki A, Tsunoda M, Kinoshita S, Saura R: Role of fracture hematoma and periosteum during fracture healing in rats: Interaction of fracture hematoma and the periosteum in the initial step of the healing process. *J Orthop Sci* 2000;5:64-70.
3. Onishi T, Ishidou Y, Nagamine T, et al: Distinct and overlapping patterns of localization of bone morphogenetic protein (BMP) family members and a BMP type II receptor during fracture healing in rats. *Bone* 1998;22:605-612.
4. Arnold IC: Bone development and repair. *Bioessays* 1987;6:171-175.
5. Rozalia D, Eleftherios T, Peter VG: Current concepts of molecular aspects of bone healing. *Injury* 2005;36:1392-1404.
6. McKibbin B: The biology of fracture healing in long bones. *J Bone Joint Surg Br* 1978;60-B:150-162.
7. Yu MD, Su BH, Zhang XX: Morphologic and molecular alteration during tibia fracture healing in rat. *Eur Rev Med Pharmacol Sci* 2018;22:1233-1240.

   This review summarizes the current knowledge about signaling pathways in fracture repair and suggests approaches to improve repair based on this information. Review Article.
8. Baht GS, Vi L, Alman BA: The role of the immune cells in fracture healing. *Curr Osteoporos Rep* 2018;16:138-145.

   This article summarizes the current understanding of the role of immune cells in the initiation of fracture healing. Review article.
9. Vi L, Baht GS, Whetstone H, et al: Macrophages promote osteoblastic differentiation in-vivo: Implications in fracture repair and bone homeostasis. *J Bone Miner Res* 2015;30:1090-1102.
10. Girgis FG, Pritchard JJ: Experimental production of cartilage during the repair of fractures of the skull vault in rats. *J Bone Joint Surg Br* 1958;40-B:274-281.
11. DeAngelis MP: Causes of delayed union and nonunion of fractures. *Vet Clin North Am* 1975;5:251-258.
12. Zura R, Xiong Z, Einhorn T, et al: Epidemiology of fracture nonunion in 18 human bones. *JAMA Surg* 2016;151:e162775.

   This study shows the location and incidence of nonunions in various bones. Level of evidence: III.

13. Liu C, Carrera R, Flamini V, et al: Effects of mechanical loading on cortical defect repair using a novel mechanobiological model of bone healing. *Bone* 2018;108:145-155.

    This study shows a method to predict the optimal mechanical loading for fracture repair. Level of evidence: III.

14. Khan Y, Laurencin CT: Fracture repair with ultrasound: Clinical and cell-based evaluation. *J Bone Joint Surg Am* 2008;90(suppl 1):138-144.

15. Harrison A, Lin S, Pounder N, Mikuni-Takagaki Y: Mode & mechanism of low intensity pulsed ultrasound (LIPUS) in fracture repair. *Ultrasonics* 2016;70:45-52.

    This study shows how ultrasound stimulates cells to possible improve fracture repair. Basic science article.

16. Vavva MG, Grivas KN, Carlier A, et al: Effect of ultrasound on bone fracture healing: A computational bioregulatory model. *Comput Biol Med* 2018;100:74-85.

    Using computer modeling, the investigators identify optimal signals to improve repair using ultrasound. Basic science article.

17. Busse JW, Bhandari M, Einhorn TA, et al: Re-evaluation of low intensity pulsed ultrasound in treatment of tibial fractures (TRUST): Randomized clinical trial. *BMJ* 2016;355:i5351.

    This level 1 randomized trial suggests that ultrasound does not speed fracture repair.

18. Leighton R, Watson JT, Giannoudis P, et al: Healing of fracture nonunions treated with low-intensity pulsed ultrasound (LIPUS): A systematic review and meta-analysis. *Injury* 2017;48:1339-1347.

    This meta-analysis of clinical studies shows little evidence for ultrasound improving fracture healing in patients. Level of evidence: II

19. Veronick JA, Assanah F, Piscopo N, et al: Mechanically loading cell/Hydrogel constructs with low-intensity pulsed ultrasound for bone repair. *Tissue Eng Part A* 2018;24:254-263.

    This investigation suggests that ultrasound can be used as part of a multimodality approach to fracture repair. Basic science article.

20. Zhang N, Wu YP, Qian SJ, et al: Research progress in the mechanism of effect of PRP in bone deficiency healing. *ScientificWorldJournal* 2013;2013:134582.

21. Gianakos A, Zambrana L, Savage-Elliott I, Lane JM, Kennedy JG: Platelet-rich plasma in the animal long-bone model: An analysis of basic science evidence. *Orthopedics* 2015;38:e1079-e1090.

22. Roffi A, Di Matteo B, Krishnakumar GS, Kon E, Filardo G: Platelet-rich plasma for the treatment of bone defects: From pre-clinical rational to evidence in the clinical practice. A systematic review. *Int Orthop* 2017;41:221-237.

    This review of clinical studies shows little evidence for platelet-rich plasma improving fracture healing in patients. Level of evidence: II

23. Chan CKF, Gulati GS, Sinha R, et al: Identification of the human skeletal stem cell. *Cell* 2018;175:43-56 e21.

    This is the first study to identify a skeletal stem cell in humans. This information can be used to develop new regenerative cell therapies for skeletal problems. Basic science article.

24. Ninu AR, Maiti SK, Kumar S, et al: Isolation, proliferation, characterization and in vivo osteogenic potential of bone-marrow derived mesenchymal stem cells (rBMSC) in rabbit model. *Indian J Exp Biol* 2017;55:79-87.

    This investigation shows the potential for bone marrow–derived MSCs to differentiate into bone. Basic science article.

25. Collette NM, Yee CS, Hum NR, et al: Sostdc1 deficiency accelerates fracture healing by promoting the expansion of periosteal mesenchymal stem cells. *Bone* 2016;88:20-30.

    This mouse study shows that mesenchymal progenitor cells from the periosteum are needed for fracture repair. Basic science article.

26. Furuta T, Miyaki S, Ishitobi H, et al: Mesenchymal stem cell-derived exosomes promote fracture healing in a mouse model. *Stem Cells Transl Med* 2016;5:1620-1630.

    This study shows that cell exosomes, which contain proteins produced by MSCs, stimulate fracture healing. It supports the notion that MSCs do not directly produce new bone, but provide proteins to stimulate other local cells to make bone. Basic science article.

27. Gomez-Barrena E, Padilla-Eguiluz NG, Avendaño-Solá C, et al: A multicentric, open-label, randomized, comparative clinical trial of two different doses of expanded hBM-MSCs plus biomaterial versus iliac crest autograft, for bone healing in nonunions after long bone fractures: Study protocol. *Stem Cells Int* 2018;2018:6025918.

    This reports the study design for an ongoing trial of MSCs in bone nonunion.

28. Pajarinen J, Lin T, Gibon E, et al: Mesenchymal stem cell-macrophage crosstalk and bone healing. *Biomaterials.* 2019;196:80-89.

    This study shows that macrophage cells can influence undifferentiated mesenchymal cells to become osteoblasts. Basic science article.

29. Hauser M, Siegrist M, Keller I, Hofstetter W: Healing of fractures in osteoporotic bones in mice treated with bisphosphonates - a transcriptome analysis. *Bone* 2018;112:107-119.

    This animal study found that bisphosphonate therapy would slow fracture repair. Basic science article.

30. Kates SL, Ackert-Bicknell CL: How do bisphosphonates affect fracture healing? *Injury* 2016;47 suppl 1:S65-S68.

    This is a literature review, suggesting that except in the case of atypical fractures, bisphosphonates do not influence facture healing. Level of evidence: II.

31. Wang YH, Qiu Y, Han X-D, et al: Haploinsufficiency of endogenous parathyroid hormone-related peptide impairs bone fracture healing. *Clin Exp Pharmacol Physiol* 2013;40:715-723.

32. Wojda SJ, Donahue SW: Parathyroid hormone for bone regeneration. *J Orthop Res* 2018;36(10):2586-2594.

    This article shows how PTH treatment will alter fracture repair. Basic science article.

33. Decambron A, Fournet A, Bensidhoum M, et al: Low-dose BMP-2 and MSC dual delivery onto coral scaffold for critical-size bone defect regeneration in sheep. *J Orthop Res* 2017;35:2637-2645.

This study shows how BMPs and MSCs might be used synergistically to improve bone repair. Basic science article.

34. Chen Y, Whetstone HC, Lin AC, et al: Beta-catenin signaling plays a disparate role in different phases of fracture repair: Implications for therapy to improve bone healing. *PLoS Med* 2007;4:e249.

35. Bao Q, Chen S, Qin H, et al: An appropriate Wnt/beta-catenin expression level during the remodeling phase is required for improved bone fracture healing in mice. *Sci Rep* 2017;7:2695.

    This study shows the importance of the appropriate regulation of signaling pathways, such as β-catenin, in fracture repair. Basic science article.

36. Kruck B, Zimmermann EA, Damerow S, et al: Sclerostin neutralizing antibody treatment enhances bone formation but does not rescue mechanically induced delayed healing. *J Bone Miner Res* 2018;33:1686-1697.

    This animal study suggests that sclerostin antibody will not improve fracture healing. Basic science article.

37. Bernick J, Wang Y, Sigal IA, et al: Parameters for lithium treatment are critical in its enhancement of fracture-healing in rodents. *J Bone Joint Surg Am* 2014;96:1990-1998.

38. Hankenson KD, Gagne K, Shaughnessy M: Extracellular signaling molecules to promote fracture healing and bone regeneration. *Adv Drug Deliv Rev* 2015;94:3-12.

39. Friedlaender GE, Perry CR, Cole JD, et al: Osteogenic protein-1 (bone morphogenetic protein-7) in the treatment of tibial nonunions. *J Bone Joint Surg Am* 2001;83-A(suppl 1):S151-S158.

40. Garrison KR, Shemilt I, Donell S, et al: Bone morphogenetic protein (BMP) for fracture healing in adults. *Cochrane Database Syst Rev* 2010:CD006950.

41. Li S, Yuan H, Pan J, et al: The treatment of femoral neck fracture using VEGF-loaded nanographene coated internal fixation screws. *PLoS One* 2017;12:e0187447.

    This manuscript shows that VEGF can enhance fracture repair in an animal model. Basic science article.

42. Hu K, Besschetnova TY, Olsen BR: Soluble VEGFR1 reverses BMP2 inhibition of intramembranous ossification during healing of cortical bone defects. *J Orthop Res* 2017;35:1461-1469.

    This study shows that BMP and VEGF together have a synergistic effect enhancing fracture healing. Basic science article.

43. Wang Y, Newman MR, Benoit DSW: Development of controlled drug delivery systems for bone fracture-targeted therapeutic delivery: A review. *Eur J Pharm Biopharm* 2018;127:223-236.

    This is a review of various drug-controlled delivery methods to enhance fracture repair. Basic science review article.

44. Ma J, Both SK, Yang F, et al: Concise review: Cell-based strategies in bone tissue engineering and regenerative medicine. *Stem Cells Transl Med* 2014;3:98-107.

45. La Fontaine J, Chen C, Hunt N, Jude E, Lavery L: Type 2 diabetes and metformin influence on fracture healing in an experimental rat model. *J Foot Ankle Surg* 2016;55:955-960.

    This study found that metformin had a negative effect on fracture healing in diabetic rats. Basic science article.

46. Shimoide T, Kawao N, Tamura Y, et al: Role of macrophages and plasminogen activator inhibitor-1 in delayed bone repair in diabetic female mice. *Endocrinology* 2018;159:1875-1885.

    This study shows how macrophage cells are impaired in fracture healing in diabetes. Basic science article.

47. Liu GY, Cao GL, Tian FM, et al: Parathyroid hormone (1-34) promotes fracture healing in ovariectomized rats with type 2 diabetes mellitus. *Osteoporos Int* 2017;28:3043-3053.

    This study shows how PTH will improve fracture healing in diabetes. Basic science article.

48. Govender S, Csimma C, Genant HK, Valentin-opran A: Recombinant human bone morphogenetic protein-2 for treatment of open tibial fractures: A prospective, controlled, randomized study of four hundred and fifty patients. *J Bone Joint Surg Am* 2002;84-A:2123-2134.

49. Ghadakzadeh S, Kannu P, Whetstone H, Howard A, Alman BA: beta-Catenin modulation in neurofibromatosis type 1 bone repair: therapeutic implications. *FASEB J* 2016;30:3227-3237.

    This study showed that the modulation of β-catenin can improve fracture repair in neurofibromatosis in mice. Basic science article.

50. Schindeler A, Ramachandran M, Godfrey C, et al: Modeling bone morphogenetic protein and bisphosphonate combination therapy in wild-type and Nf1 haploinsufficient mice. *J Orthop Res* 2008;26:65-74.

Chapter 14

Osteoarthritis, Cartilage Biology, and Stem Cell Therapy

Mary B. Goldring, PhD

ABSTRACT

Osteoarthritis (OA) is a destructive joint disease in which the initiation may be attributed to direct injury and mechanical disruption of joint tissues, but the progressive changes are dependent on active cell-mediated processes that occur during the long time-course of the disease. Recent clinical observations and experimental studies have identified OA phenotypes that allow subsetting of individual patients who exhibit common profiles of symptoms, structural abnormalities, and pathophysiological pathways that act independently or in combination within a background of genetic and epigenetic factors. Human adult articular cartilage is a complex tissue of matrix proteins with a resident population of chondrocytes that are normally quiescent and maintain the matrix in a low turnover state. During OA, these cells undergo phenotypic modulation, promoting matrix destruction and abnormal attempts at repair. Because cartilage has limited intrinsic capacity for regenerating new matrix with the same properties as that formed during development, research has focused on designing strategies for repairing cartilage using stem cell-based and other tissue engineering approaches.

Keywords: cartilage; extracellular matrix; osteoarthritis; regeneration; stem cell therapy

Introduction

The term arthritis is used to describe a variety of conditions affecting the joints. Generally, arthritis can be classified as autoimmune systemic disorders affecting joints and nonimmune, biomechanical joint disorders; the former is represented by rheumatoid arthritis (RA), which is an inflammatory disorder, in which the autoimmune state results in chronic progression of joint inflammation, synovitis, and destruction of cartilage and bone. Osteoarthritis (OA) is the prototypical nonimmune, and relatively noninflammatory, joint disorder, which is characterized by the progressive degeneration of articular cartilage.[1]

OA is the most common joint disorder and is a leading cause of disability in the adult population. Associated risk factors are age, prior joint injury, obesity, genetic predisposition, and mechanical factors, including malalignment and abnormal joint shape.[2,3] Although often regarded as a disease of articular cartilage, it is now appreciated that it is a disease of the whole joint as an organ with involvement of all joint components, including the articular and calcified cartilage, synovial joint lining, periarticular bone, and the ligaments and tendons, in pathological changes during the initiation and progression of OA[4] (**Figure 1**). The pathological changes in the composition, structural organization, and functional properties are generally attributed to direct injury and mechanical disruption of the tissues, but there is increasing recognition that the underlying destructive mechanisms are dependent on active cell-mediated processes. In addition to the impact of aging on cells and tissues, cartilage degeneration may occur in response to inappropriate mechanical stress and low-grade systemic inflammation associated with trauma, obesity, or metabolic syndrome (**Figure 2**). It is important to appreciate that OA is heterogeneous disorder in which multiple mechanisms can contribute to the initiation and progression of the joint pathology, giving rise to the concept of OA subtypes, or phenotypes.[5] Despite this heterogeneity, there are common underlying pathophysiological processes involved in the processes that destroy joint tissues.

Strong functional interactions among the cartilage, synovium, and subchondral bone impact on cartilage function in such a way that it is difficult to know where and when pathological changes begin. Notably, many of the mediators that are involved in the regulation of immune cell function also play important roles in

Neither Dr. Goldring nor any immediate family member has received anything of value from or has stock or stock options held in a commercial company or institution related directly or indirectly to the subject of this chapter.

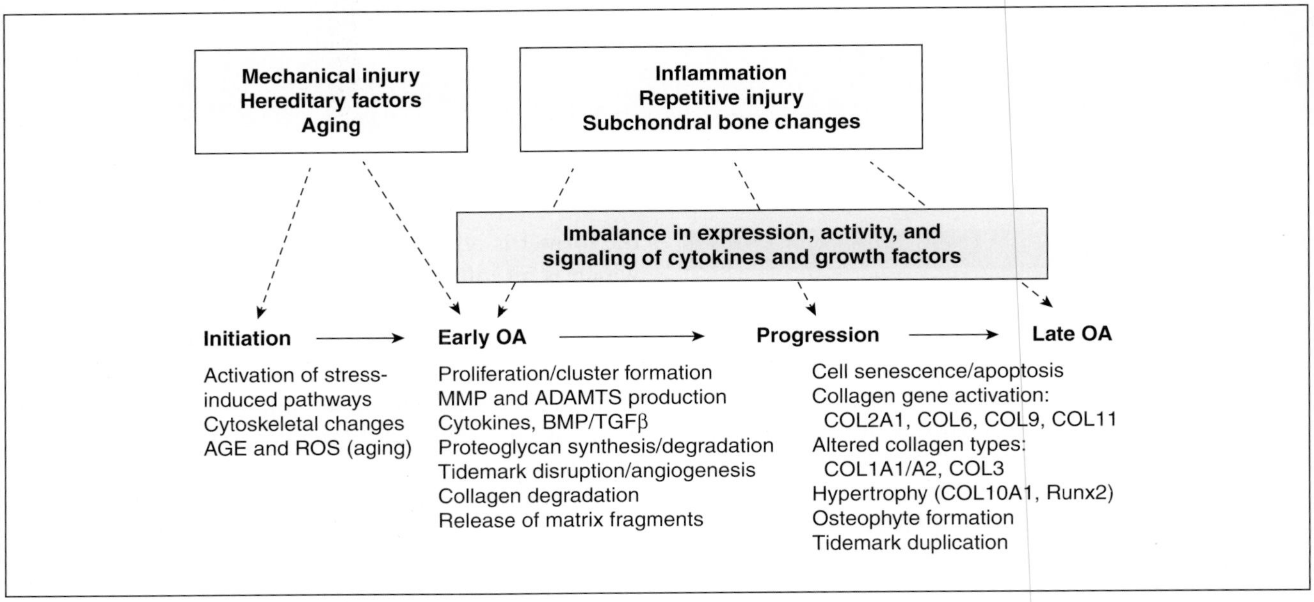

Figure 1 Scheme of events involved in the initiation of osteoarthritis (OA) and progression to late-stage OA. (Reproduced with permission from Goldring MB, Goldring SR: Osteoarthritis. *J Cell Physiol* 2007;213[3]:626-634.)

both physiological and pathological bone remodeling.[4] Nevertheless, the knowledge we have gained from studies of cartilage obtained from the clinic and from animal models has uncovered many important biological factors that impinge on chondrocytes, the cellular component of cartilage, in a temporal and spatial manner to produce pathological changes.

Cartilage Biology: Structure and Function

Articular cartilage is composed of a collagen network consisting mainly of type II collagen, which provides tensile strength to cartilage and restrains the swelling pressure created by the hydrophilic proteoglycans that fill the spaces within the network. The composition and cellular organization of the extracellular matrix (ECM) of human adult articular cartilage is complex with qualitative and quantitative differences in matrix constituents between the interterritorial region containing the collagen network of collagens II, IX, and XI and the pericellular matrix, containing collagen VI, fibromodulin, and matrilin 3, but little or no type II collagen. There are also zonal differences in the arrangement of the collagen fibrillar network ranging from the superficial, where they are parallel to the surface, becoming more random in the middle zone and then radial in the deep zone. Chondrocytes, which comprise the only cellular component of articular cartilage, have different morphologies ranging from more flattened at the surface to rounder and larger in the deeper zones. They exhibit distinct spatial patterns ranging from arrangement as single cells and pairs to clusters or strings depending upon the joint type.[6] Chondrocytes in the superficial zone uniquely produce lubricin, or superficial zone protein, a splice form of PRG4. Lubricin contributes to a boundary layer of lubrication, requiring complexes of lubricin and hyaluronic acid,[7] giving cartilage a smooth surface with a very low coefficient of friction that permits efficient gliding motion during joint movement. Chondrocytes in the middle zone synthesize relatively greater amounts of aggrecan and the relative amounts of small proteoglycans also differ.

Under normal, low turnover conditions, chondrocytes are resting in a nonstressed steady state and maintain synthesis of proteoglycans and other noncollagen molecules, whereas there is very little turnover of the type II collagen network, which has a half-life of 117 years unless it is damaged, and a recent study supports the view that a structurally permanent collagen matrix exists in human adult cartilage.[8]

The structural modifications of cartilage matrix proteins and their loss compromise the remarkable physical properties of cartilage, including its elasticity, compressive resistance, and tensile strength. Numerous investigations have aimed to identify mechanisms by which aging and mechanically driven stresses lead to fissuring, fibrillation, and wear of hyaline cartilage and

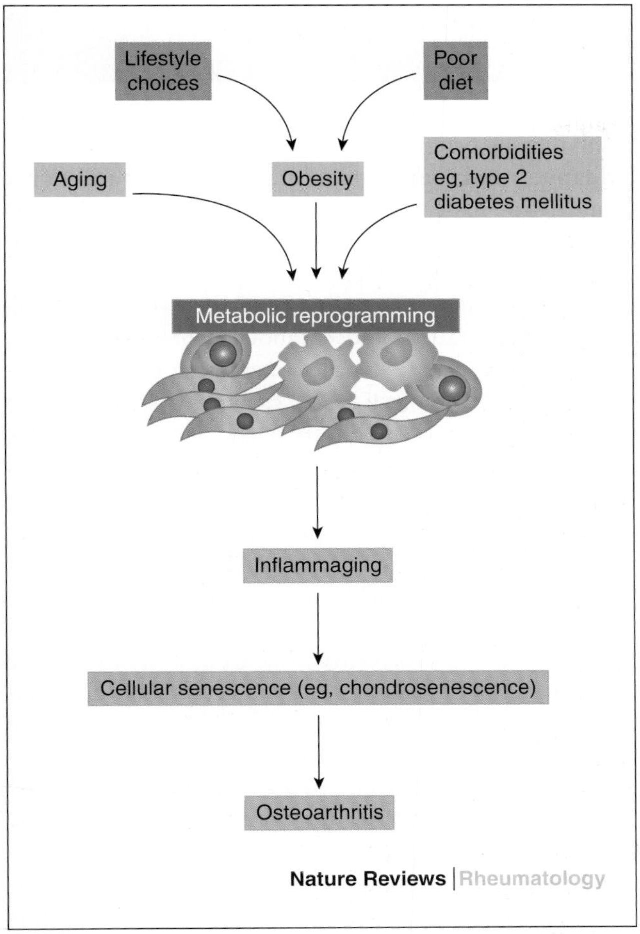

Figure 2 Illustration shows factors underlying metabolic alterations in osteoarthritis. (Reprinted by permission from Springer Nature Mobasheri A, Rayman MP, Gualillo O, Sellam J, van der Kraan P, Fearon U: The role of metabolism in the pathogenesis of osteoarthritis. *Nat Rev Rheumatol* 2017;13[5]:302-311, Copyright 2017. doi:10.1038/nrrheum.2017.50.)

fibrocartilage; however, a newer line of inquiry focuses on the roles of metabolically driven processes. Prolonged oxidative stress, which occurs during aging and chronic inflammation, and metabolic stress due to diabetes and metabolic syndrome can induce biochemical changes, including glycation, carbonylation, lipoxidation, and nitrosylation, in cartilage structural proteins. These posttranslational modifications induce aggregation and/or unfolding of cartilage matrix proteins, increasing their susceptibility to enzymatic cleavage and degradation.[9]

The calcified cartilage is the interface between the nonmineralized articular cartilage and the bone. The tidemark is a thin line revealed after hematoxylin staining that marks the mineralization front between the calcified and articular cartilage.[10] The calcified cartilage has unique matrix composition, with chondrocytes expressing markers of hypertrophy, as well as vascularization and innervation originating from the subchondral bone in association with advancing age.

Cartilage Changes in Osteoarthritis

The principal function of articular cartilage is to adjust to biomechanical forces during joint movement; a function mediated by the ECM. Cartilage homeostasis is defined by normal cartilage ECM compensating for mechanical stress without structural or cellular damage. Much work has been devoted to understanding how the homeostatic balance of healthy cartilage is perturbed and how this leads to disease. The common view is that cartilage degradation initiates at the joint surface in areas where mechanical forces such as shear stress are greatest.[3] Chondrocytes sense changes in their environment through integrins, syndecans, discoidin domain receptors, and other cell surface receptors (see for review Refs. 4,5). The subsequent loss of surface lubrication is associated with proteoglycan loss and collagen erosion. The receptors on the resting chondrocyte are protected from interacting with certain matrix components by the unique structure of the pericellular matrix. Among the earliest events may be the disruption of the pericellular matrix, associated with abnormal activation of cell surface receptors on chondrocytes in response to biomechanical stress and with induction and activation of matrix-degrading proteinases.[11]

Disruption of the normal resting state of chondrocytes may also be viewed as an injury response involving the recapitulation of developmental programs, leading to matrix remodeling, inappropriate hypertrophy-like maturation, and cartilage calcification.[12] The developmental process of endochondral ossification, involving TGFβ- and BMP-induced differentiation of osteochondroprogenitors, also drives osteophyte formation.[13] The increased cartilage calcification is associated with tidemark advancement or duplication, and vascular penetration from the subchondral bone.[14] The close relationship between the process of cartilage damage and subchondral bone changes is of increasing interest.[4]

Genomics studies have examined global gene expression profiles in cartilage and other joint tissues, comparing normal and OA-affected tissues.[15] Candidate gene studies and genome-wide linkage analyses have revealed polymorphisms or mutations in OA susceptibility genes encoding signaling and other regulatory molecules such as growth and differentiation factor 5 (GDF5), asporin (ASPN), secreted frizzled-related protein 3 (FRZB), deiodinase 2 (DIO2), Smad3, NCOA3, and ALDH1A2.[16] Many of these genes encode molecules associated with the TGFβ, BMP, and Wnt signaling pathways, which are involved in determining chondrocyte differentiation and maturation during skeletal development. Disruption of these pathways may induce chondrocytes to recapitulate a developmental molecular program with abnormal gene expression of hypertrophy markers such as type X collagen, matrix metalloproteinase (MMP) 13, and Runx2, resulting in cartilage calcification and matrix destruction. Gene defects associated with congenital cartilage dysplasias that affect the formation of cartilage matrix and patterning of skeletal elements may adversely affect joint alignment and congruity and thus contribute to early onset of OA in these individuals. However, these gene defects are rare, potentially defining subsets of OA patients; how gene polymorphisms contribute to OA susceptibility in the general population is a goal of ongoing large multicenter studies.

Epigenetic modifications are not associated with alterations in DNA sequences, but allow the cell to respond rapidly to alterations in the environment. These changes, including DNA methylation, histone modifications, and alterations in chromatin structure have been observed in OA cartilage.[17] Although there is no compelling evidence that DNA variation in inflammatory genes is an OA risk factor, epigenetic effects involving inflammatory genes are a component of OA, and alteration in the expression of these genes is also highly relevant to the disease process.[18,19] In aging and inflammatory models, OA chondrocytes exhibit prominent epigenomic alterations,[17] leading to deregulated gene expression, exacerbated and sustained NF-κB activation, and MMP production, all of which can be modeled in vitro by IL-1β stimulation. Specific microRNAs have been linked to alterations in gene expression in human OA. Indeed, miRNAs can exert positive or negative effects on multiple downstream targets affecting cartilage homeostasis and the OA disease state.[20]

Genomic analyses of joint tissues and proteomic analyses of synovial fluids collected at the time of arthroscopic evaluation or repair or joint replacement surgery have indicated that various cellular and molecular phenotypes can be defined along a spectrum from early through late stage. Interestingly, proteomic profiling of OA synovial fluid shows that a major proportion of the knee OA proteome contains acute phase response, coagulation, and complement proteins generated from the synovium, with a small proportion of synovial proteins generated by the cartilage.[21] Mitochondrial DNA variations may also define OA phenotypes related to metabolism, inflammation, and aging.[22] Profiling data, such as these, will likely enable phenotyping of OA populations for separating them into cohorts, but profiling single patients to guide individualized OA therapy is a long-term future goal.[23]

Mechanisms of Osteoarthritis Involving Chondrocytes

Chondrocyte-mediated processes become more prominent during progression of OA disease. Mechanical, oxidative, and inflammatory stresses activate signal transduction pathways in cartilage, which induce the phenotypic shift characterized by the release of the chondrocyte from growth arrest, imbalanced homeostasis, hypertrophic-like conversion, and aberrant expression of pro-inflammatory and catabolic genes. As a result, OA chondrocytes are unable to maintain tissue homeostasis and fail to replace ECM, especially collagen, once it is degraded by MMPs, in particular by MMP-13, the major MMP responsible for remodeling of type II collagen in cartilage tissue. The other major cartilage component, aggrecan, is degraded by the aggrecanases of the ADAMTS (A Disintegrin and Metalloproteinase with Thrombospondin Motifs) family, ADAMTS4 and 5 and other matrix-degrading enzymes found in the OA joint.[24] Until the proteoglycan coating is removed, the collagen network is somewhat protected from degradation by the collagenases, MMP-1 and MMP-13. Once the collagen network is degraded, this marks progression to irreversible cartilage degradation.

Inflammation can be observed at the macroscopic level as synovitis and synovial effusion during operative procedures such as arthroscopy or by MRI and is associated with more rapid progression to OA.[25-27] In patients with traumatic ACL or meniscal injury, but no radiographic evidence of OA, the synovium retrieved during arthroscopy is frequently inflamed and the inflammation scores are associated with increased pain and dysfunction, as well as unique cytokine and chemokine gene expression profiles.[25] Chronic low-grade inflammation, termed "microinflammation," associated with aging and the senescent secretory phenotype, can disrupt homeostasis in joint tissues and drive the degradative process.[2,28] This is an important consideration in OA joints, because mechanical stress may induce similar signaling responses in the absence of overt inflammation.

Oxidative stress, resulting from increased levels of reactive oxygen species (ROS) relative to antioxidants, may act together with inflammatory and/or mechanical stress to accentuate catabolic processes, depending upon the availability of signals and the state of the tissue damage. Mechanical injury, inflammatory cytokines, and matrix fragments, such as fibronectin fragments via integrins, can induce ROS, and the age-related decline in the responses of chondrocytes to anabolic growth factors may be attributable to altered cell signaling mediated by increased oxidative stress.[29] Because cartilage is an avascular tissue, the chondrocytes exist in a hypoxic environment, in which hypoxia inducible factor (HIF)-1α is important for the maintenance of homeostasis. During oxidative stress, NF-κB signaling is required for the induction of HIF-2α, which regulates both endochondral ossification and OA-related cartilage destruction, in part, by directly targeting HREs within the promoters of genes such as MMP13, COL10A1, and VEGFA, thereby inducing catabolic and inflammatory mediators in chondrocytes (for review, see Ref. 30).

Canonical NF-κB signaling, dependent on the IKKβ signaling kinase, is an integrating mechanism underlying most responses to inflammatory, mechanical, and oxidative stresses. In contrast, the noncanonical NF-κB signaling kinase, IKKα/CHUK, promotes the aberrant expression of genes involved in endochondral ossification and increased MMP-13 activity through increased gene expression of the MMP activator, MMP-10 (see for review Ref. 31). NF-κB signaling coordinates most of the inflammatory and catabolic events involved in OA pathogenesis, in addition to those mentioned above, including those involving alarmins via Toll-like receptors, sirtuins such as Sirt1, chemokines, and adipokines. The altered metabolism, cell death via apoptosis or senescence, and the compensating cell survival mechanisms such as autophagy are all subjects of investigation that may provide strategies for designing therapies for structure modification[5,32] (**Table 1**), or at least

Table 1

Pharmacological Targets Under Investigation for Structure Modification and Neuroinflammation-Driven Chronic Pain

Biological Process	Targets (Downstream Effectors)	Potential Therapeutics
Cartilage degradation	MMP-13, ADAMTS-5 DDR2 activated by TGFβ-induced HTRA1 serine proteinase Cathepsin K ADAM17 (via activating TNFα and EGFR ligands)	MMP inhibitors Tyrosine kinase inhibitors Serine proteinase inhibitors Nutraceuticals, eg, green tea polyphenol
Mechanical, inflammatory, and oxidative stress	Canonical NF-κB signaling JAK/STAT signaling Reactive oxygen species HIF-2α (proteinases and hypertrophy markers) Zinc-ZIP8-MTF1 axis (MMPs, ADAMTS5)	Curcumin, resveratrol, IKKβ inhibitor (SAR113945) Proteasome inhibitor (bortezomib) Tofacitinib SOCS Antioxidants, iNOS inhibitors; mitochondrial ROS scavengers
Innate immunity	TLRs Complement	6-Shogaol; boswellic acid; kaempferol; oleocanthal; quercetin CR2-fH
Chondrocyte hypertrophy	Hedgehog signaling IKKα (MMP10) ADAM10 (Notch signaling via RBPjk)	Small molecule inhibitors of Gli, Smo, etc
Angiogenesis and synovitis	VEGF	Bevacizumab
Subchondral bone	WNT/β-catenin Adenosine receptors	Sclerostin, DKK-1 antibodies A2AR antagonists
Pain	[a]Monocyte chemoattractant protein (MCP1)/CCR2 chemokine receptor [a]Peripheral calcitonin gene-related peptide (CGRP) receptor [a]Transient receptor potential vanilloid ion channels (eg, TRPV4) [a]Adenosine and purinergic receptors (via TRPV channels)	CCR2 receptor antagonist CGRP 8-37 receptor antagonist TRPV4 agonist (GSK1016790A) A3AR agonists; P2X and P2Y antagonists

[a]Both structure modification and pain relief have been demonstrated in animal models.

Adapted from Goldring MB, Berenbaum F: Emerging targets in osteoarthritis therapy. *Curr Opin Pharmacol* 2015;22:51-63, Copyright 2015, with permission from Elsevier.

Basic Science

biomarkers for diagnosis or monitoring therapies.[33] The overriding issue of how to alleviate pain in OA without causing more damage is beyond the scope of this review, but has been addressed extensively.[34] Many of the emerging targets for therapy, particularly those that promote anabolism, may be amenable for delivery to joints in cell-based approaches[5] (**Table 2**).

Cartilage Regeneration and Repair and Stem Cell Therapy

Cartilage represents a major clinical challenge because of its poor regenerative capacity after injury and the high prevalence of OA. Recently, radiocarbon dating was used to measure the life-long replacement rates of collagen in tibial plateau cartilage and showed that there is no significant turnover of collagen in adult cartilage in either healthy or OA cartilage.[8] These results indicate that OA pathogenesis involves primarily mechanical or biochemical breakdown of major cartilage structures without any new collagen matrix formation. The findings are in line with the relatively poor clinical success in cartilage repair approaches in OA-affected joints involving cartilage transplantation, pharmacological treatment with anabolic agents, or stem cell therapies (reviewed in Ref. 35). On the other hand, it is well known that physiological mechanical loading such as that gained in physical training can stimulate the production of proteoglycans, especially replenishing GAGs, thereby increasing the water content of the cartilage and the release of substances that are potentially chondroprotective.[36]

Understanding cartilage tissue turnover is the first step in determining regenerative therapies for OA. In the absence of effective strategies for cartilage repair, the

Table 2

Emerging Mediators and Molecular Therapies That Ameliorate OA and in Some Cases can Even Promote Regeneration

Biological Process	Mediators	Potential Therapeutics
Autophagy and cell survival	mTOR AKT/Fox03/mTOR PPARγ CXCR2	Rapamycin, polyamines, ω-6 polyunsaturated fatty acids; glucosamine Chemokine antagonists or blocking antibodies
Chondrogenesis and inhibition of endochondral ossification	Runx1 PTH receptor EGFR signaling	TD-198946 Kartogenin Recombinant human PTH(1-34) (teriparatide) Mitogen-inducible gene 6 (MIG6)
Calcification and crystals	NPP1 Transglutaminase inorganic pyrophosphate TLRs NLRP3	Phosphocitrates TLR and NLRP3 inhibitors
Subchondral bone	WNT/β-catenin BMPs BMP-7 TGFβ	Wnt antagonists (DKK1, SOST) BMP antagonists (Gremlin, follistatin) Recombinant BMP-7 (Eptotermin) TGFβ-specific antibody
Cartilage anabolism	IGF-1 FGF-18 PRG4 NFATc2/c2 Calcitonin	Humanized IGF-1-heparin-binding domain fusion protein Sprifermin Oral or intra-articular calcitonin
Circadian clock	Bmal1	REV-ERB agonists

Adapted from Goldring MB, Berenbaum F: Emerging targets in osteoarthritis therapy. *Curr Opin Pharmacol* 2015;22:51-63, Copyright 2015, with permission from Elsevier.

emphasis has been on defining risk factors leading to the development of cartilage disease and finding ways for assessing early OA with sensitive imaging approaches and biomarkers. However, once cartilage damage has occurred, the focus should be on counteracting further tissue damage by designing therapeutics that protect the remaining cartilage collagen structures and that target other, high-turnover components, such as GAGs, whose restorations can beneficially modify the mechanical properties of the remaining cartilage. These strategies and surgical approaches such as microfracture will likely delay the need for joint replacement. Thus, researchers are actively investigating tissue engineering approaches, including cell-based therapies for cartilage restoration[37-41] (**Figure 3**).

Mesenchymal Stem Cells

Mesenchymal stem cells (MSCs) are multipotent cells that have the ability to differentiate into a variety of cell precursors. They constitute a population of progenitor cells originally identified by Friedenstein and coworkers in bone marrow and other hematopoietic tissues for their capacity to form fibroblast-like colonies in vitro and to give rise to bone when transplanted heterotopically in vivo.[42] Later, Caplan proposed their potential for multilineage differentiation through the mesengenic process, in which a unique mesenchymal progenitor could give rise to multiple tissue phenotypes, including chondrocytes (see for review Ref. 43). More recently, the in vivo perivascular "niche" has been defined in multiple adult tissues.[44] Within the niche, MSCs interact with other local resident cells to maintain homeostasis by modulating cell proliferation and differentiation.

Several subpopulations of bone marrow perivascular MSCs can be distinguished by specific cell surface markers, including nestin (NES), NG2, leptin receptor (LepR), CD271, and CD146. These markers discriminate perisinusoidal, periarteriolar, and endosteal MSCs within the hematopoietic stem cell (HSC) niche at different stages of proliferation and differentiation.[44,45] HSCs, therefore, not only support hematopoiesis but also, depending upon their perivascular phenotype,[46] determine the site-specific physiological functions of MSCs in vivo during tissue repair following injury by orchestrating immunomodulatory and trophic responses through secretion of paracrine signaling factors. These potentially "therapeutic" features are common to MSCs throughout the body, complementing their originally defined roles as

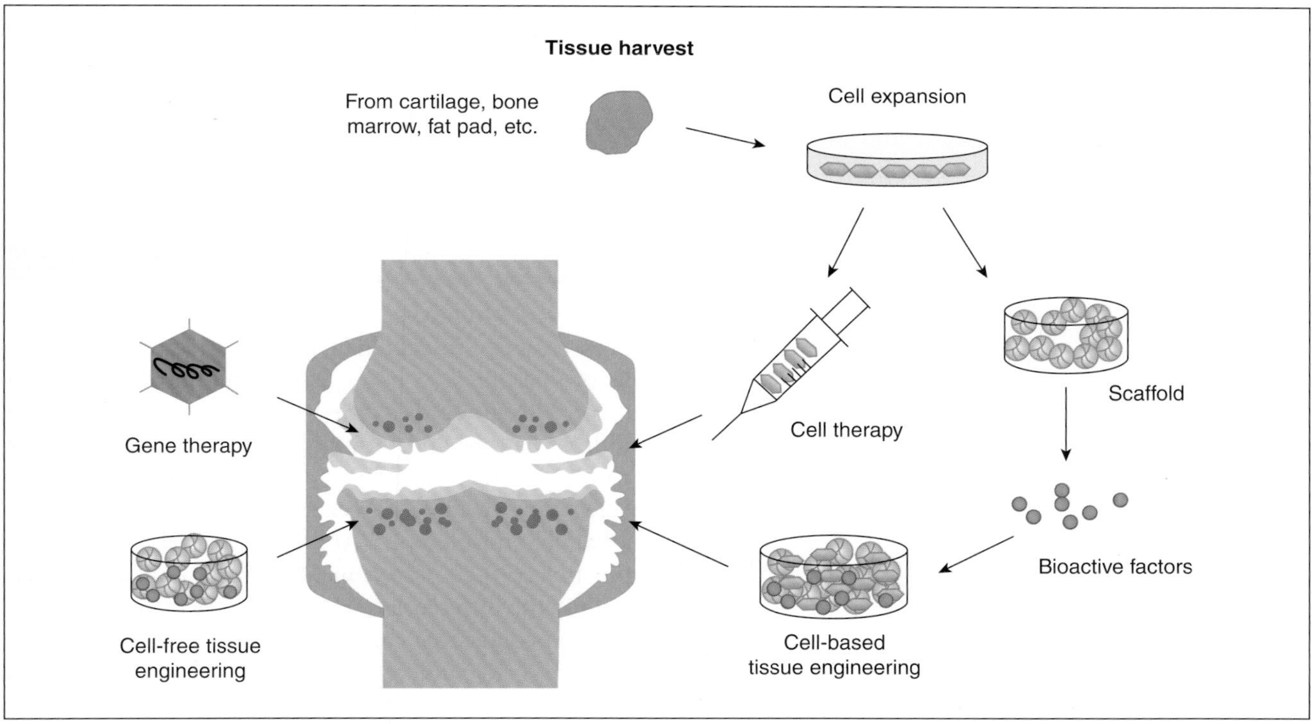

Figure 3 Scheme of cell-based strategies for regenerative treatment of osteoarthritis. (Reproduced with permission from Zhang W, Ouyang H, Dass CR, Xu J: Current research on pharmacologic and regenerative therapies for osteoarthritis. *Bone Res* 2016;4:15040. (CC BY 4.0).)

Basic Science

progenitors in the development of skeletal and other mesenchymal tissues. Consequently, studies performed in vitro and in vivo have exploited both the progenitor and therapeutic capabilities of MSCs for developing tissue engineering and cell therapy approaches to treat skeletal conditions.

MSCs for Cartilage Repair

Research on cell-based and tissue engineering applications for cartilage repair has focused on adult MSCs because they are accessible in high quantities with low donor site morbidity and are easy to manipulate to promote differentiation. There is evidence that cells with properties of MSCs exist in adult cartilage, including cartilage from OA patients, where there are cells with regenerative potential expressing mesenchymal progenitor cell markers, particularly in the chondrocyte clusters.[47-49] Indeed, OA chondrocytes exhibit "phenotypic plasticity" comparable to MSCs undergoing chondrogenesis by recapitulating aspects of chondrocyte hypertrophy.[12] Thus, promoting the intrinsic chondrogenic differentiation capacity of MSCs in cartilage with anabolic factors has been investigated extensively in both in vitro and in vivo models.

The preferred tissue sources for cartilage repair strategies using MSCs are the bone marrow and adipose tissue, but also MSCs have been isolated from periarticular tissues such as the synovium, periosteum, and infrapatellar fat pad, as well as from placenta, umbilical cord, amniotic fluid, muscle, and other adult tissues.[38,39] MSCs were first characterized in vitro by the multilineage (adipogenic, osteogenic, chondrogenic) differentiation capacity of MSC clones on plastic and their expression of specific cell surface markers such as CD105, CD106, CD90, and CD73.[48] The International Society of Cell Therapy (ISCT) added to the definition of MSCs as cells that must express CD105, CD73, and CD90, but they must also be negative for the hematopoietic markers CD11b or CD14, CD19 or CD79a, CD34, CD45, and HLA-DR. Additional markers are CD146 for the selection of MSCs with enhanced differentiation and colony-forming capacity and CD271, which identifies subpopulations with high chondrogenic potential (see for review Refs. 40,50).

Proliferation and Expansion of MSCs

Although MSCs can be expanded in vitro, their proliferative capacity is limited and related to their differentiation capacity. Therefore, to address this challenge, investigations of the influence of exogenous growth factors and 3D culture systems for tissue engineering approaches have been undertaken. Based on studies in limb development, FGF2 was the first additive used successfully to enhance both MSC expansion and differentiation capacity, and it is still the stimulus most used for the expansion of MSC in vitro,[51] although the in vitro response does not necessarily predict the activity in vivo.[44]

TGFβ has also been studied extensively with conflicting results. TGFβ signaling can promote cellular senescence of MSCs by inducing their cell cycle arrest through activation of p16, p21, and p53 proteins, but also stimulating proliferation of MSCs. PDGF, a potent stimulant of proliferation, which theoretically does not interfere with the differentiation potential of the cells,[52] is one of the main components of platelet-rich plasma (PRP) derivatives, which are of current interest for clinical use in the joint by orthopaedic surgeons because of their ostensible capacity of inducing proliferation and for sustaining differentiation of MSCs.[53,54] Thus, combinations of growth factors such as TGFβ, FGF2, and PDGF have been studied extensively in tissue engineering models and proposed as effective additives for expansion of MSCs.[50,55]

Recent work has shown that the combination of FGF2 with WNT3A further improves long-term expansion and chondrogenic capacity both in vitro and in vivo.[51] Interestingly, the administration of WNT protein alone can either stimulate or inhibit the proliferation of MSCs via the canonical Wnt pathway or the noncanonical pathway, respectively, but with remarkably different effects on differentiation capacity.[56]

Chondrogenic Differentiation of MSCs

Models of chondrogenic differentiation of MSCs have been designed in aggregate culture systems such as pellet or micromass to mimic embryonic cartilage development. This proceeds by three main stages: condensation, differentiation, and terminal differentiation, or hypertrophy, characterized by expression of N-cadherin, collagen type II, and aggrecan, and collagen type X and alkaline phosphatase (ALP), respectively. TGFβ was the first pro-chondrogenic factor described as essential for the differentiation of MSCs. A major limitation to achieving stable cartilage formation is the tendency of MSCs to undergo terminal differentiation, with subsequent mineralization. This has been addressed experimentally by interfering with signaling by parathyroid hormone (PTH), WNT, TGFβ, or different FGF ligands proteins during the different chondrogenic

21. Ritter SY, Subbaiah R, Bebek G, et al: Proteomic analysis of synovial fluid from the osteoarthritic knee: Comparison with transcriptome analyses of joint tissues. *Arthritis Rheum* 2013;65:981-992.

22. Blanco FJ, Valdes AM, Rego-Perez I: Mitochondrial DNA variation and the pathogenesis of osteoarthritis phenotypes. *Nat Rev Rheumatol* 2018;14:327-340.

    This review describes how mitochondrial (mtDNA) DNA variation influences OA phenotypes related to metabolism, inflammation, aging, and epigenetics, suggesting that specific mtDNA haplogroups could be used as diagnostic and prognostic biomarkers of OA.

23. Tonge DP, Pearson MJ, Jones SW: The hallmarks of osteoarthritis and the potential to develop personalised disease-modifying pharmacological therapeutics. *Osteoarthr Cartil* 2014;22:609-621.

24. Yang CY, Chanalaris A, Troeberg L: ADAMTS and ADAM metalloproteinases in osteoarthritis – looking beyond the "usual suspects". *Osteoarthr Cartil* 2017;25:1000-1009.

    This review provides the latest information indicating that, in addition to the well-characterized MMPs, ADAMTS-4 and ADAMTS-5, many other ADAMTSs and ADAMs are expressed in cartilage with altered expression in OA and may be considered for the design of targeted inhibitors of cartilage degradation while sparing cartilage repair pathways.

25. Scanzello CR, Goldring SR: The role of synovitis in osteoarthritis pathogenesis. *Bone* 2012;51:249-257.

26. Guermazi A, Roemer FW, Crema MD, Englund M, Hayashi D: Imaging of non-osteochondral tissues in osteoarthritis. *Osteoarthr Cartil* 2014;22:1590-1605.

27. de Lange-Brokaar BJ, Ioan-Facsinay A, Yusuf E, et al: Evolution of synovitis in osteoarthritic knees and its association with clinical features. *Osteoarthr Cartil* 2016;24:1867-1874.

    This investigation of the course of synovitis on contrast-enhanced magnetic resonance images (CE-MRI) in osteoarthritic knees over 2 years shows that synovitis in individual patients fluctuates during disease course associated with cartilage deterioration, but not with change in pain, suggesting a role for synovitis as a target for disease-modifying treatment.

28. Jeon OH, Kim C, Laberge RM, et al: Local clearance of senescent cells attenuates the development of post-traumatic osteoarthritis and creates a pro-regenerative environment. *Nat Med* 2017;23:775-781.

    This important study shows that selective removal of the senescent cells from OA chondrocytes may be beneficial for cartilage homeostasis.

29. Bolduc JA, Collins JA, Loeser RF: Reactive oxygen species, aging and articular cartilage homeostasis. *Free Radic Biol Med* 2019;132:73-82. doi:10.1016/j.freeradbiomed.2018.08.038.

    This review proposes that new therapeutic strategies targeting specific antioxidant systems including mitochondrial ROS may be of value in reducing the progression of age-related OA.

30. Fernandez-Torres J, Zamudio-Cuevas Y, Martinez-Nava GA, Lopez-Reyes AG: Hypoxia-inducible factors (HIFs) in the articular cartilage: A systematic review. *Eur Rev Med Pharmacol Sci* 2017;21:2800-2810.

    This review summarizes the roles of the three members of the human HIF-α family, HIF-1α as a protective factor in the hypoxic environment of articular cartilage, HIF-2α as a harmful factor in OA cartilage, and HIF-3α as a negative regulator of HIF-1α and HIF-2α.

31. Olivotto E, Otero M, Marcu KB, Goldring MB: Pathophysiology of osteoarthritis: Canonical NF-kappaB/IKKbeta-dependent and kinase-independent effects of IKKalpha in cartilage degradation and chondrocyte differentiation. *RMD Open* 2015;1:e000061.

    This review summarizes the different roles of NF-κB canonical and noncanonical signaling in chondrocyte function.

32. Vinatier C, Dominguez E, Guicheux J, Carames B: Role of the inflammation-autophagy-senescence integrative network in osteoarthritis. *Front Physiol* 2018;9:706.

    This review provides an excellent update on chondrocyte survival and inflammatory mechanisms examined in preclinical models and the potential for therapeutic intervention.

33. Bay-Jensen AC, Thudium CS, Mobasheri A: Development and use of biochemical markers in osteoarthritis: Current update. *Curr Opin Rheumatol* 2018;30:121-128.

    This is a useful update on OA biomarkers that highlights the possibility of distinguishing clinical subtypes and facilitating drug development for targeting early to late stage disease.

34. Syx D, Tran PB, Miller RE, Malfait AM: Peripheral mechanisms contributing to osteoarthritis pain. *Curr Rheumatol Rep* 2018;20:9.

    This review highlights how both peripheral and central mechanisms contribute to OA pain.

35. Huang BJ, Hu JC, Athanasiou KA: Cell-based tissue engineering strategies used in the clinical repair of articular cartilage. *Biomaterials* 2016;98:1-22.

    This review provides a critical discussion of the various tissue engineering strategies, including cell expansion, scaffold material, media formulations, and biomimetic stimuli, that have been used to develop products for cartilage repair in the clinic.

36. Allen KD, Golightly YM, White DK: Gaps in appropriate use of treatment strategies in osteoarthritis. *Best Pract Res Clin Rheumatol* 2017;31:746-759.

    This review critically discusses the evidence-based support for the major categories of treatment strategies for OA, including self-management, physical activity, weight management, physical therapy, and other rehabilitative therapies, as well as pharmacotherapies and joint replacement surgery.

37. Maia FR, Carvalho MR, Oliveira JM, Reis RL: Tissue engineering strategies for osteochondral repair. *Adv Exp Med Biol* 2018;1059:353-371.

    This review discusses the research on the design of the strategies for osteochondral regeneration, including cell-free, scaffold-free strategies, and combinatorial approaches.

38. Johnstone B, Alini M, Cucchiarini M, et al: Tissue engineering for articular cartilage repair–the state of the art. *Eur Cell Mater* 2013;25:248-267.

39. Van Osch GJVM, Barbero A, Brittberg M, et al: Cells for cartilage regeneration, in Gimble JM, Marolt D, Oreffo R, Redl H, Wolbank S, eds: *Cell Engineering and Regeneration*, Cham, Springer, 2018, pp 1-67.

This chapter is part of a volume on tissue engineering that covers the use of adipose tissue, tendon, ES cells, and peripheral blood monocytes in the repair and regeneration. This multi-author contribution focuses on tissue and cell sources for cartilage regeneration and repair, including chondrocytes from articular. Nasa, auricular, and cartilage meniscus, and mesenchymal stem cells.

40. Lv FJ, Tuan RS, Cheung KM, Leung VY: Concise review: The surface markers and identity of human mesenchymal stem cells. *Stem Cells* 2014;32:1408-1419.

41. Zhang W, Ouyang H, Dass CR, Xu J: Current research on pharmacologic and regenerative therapies for osteoarthritis. *Bone Res* 2016;4:15040.

This review highlights research on generative therapies, including new OA drugs, such as sprifermin/recombinant human FGF-18 and tanezumab/monoclonal antibody against NGF, as well as cell-based therapies using induced pluripotent stem cells that are emerging as promising alternatives for enhancing cartilage repair.

42. Kuznetsov SA, Friedenstein AJ, Robey PG: Factors required for bone marrow stromal fibroblast colony formation in vitro. *Br J Haematol* 1997;97:561-570.

43. Caplan AI: Cell-based therapies: The nonresponder. *Stem Cells Transl Med* 2018;7:762-766.

This recent review by the early pioneer who proposed the use of MSCs for cartilage repair discusses current challenges in the use of cell-based therapies in several phase III trials that are now being conducted.

44. Sacchetti B, Funari A, Michienzi S, et al: Self-renewing osteoprogenitors in bone marrow sinusoids can organize a hematopoietic microenvironment. *Cell* 2007;131:324-336.

45. Mendelson A, Frenette PS: Hematopoietic stem cell niche maintenance during homeostasis and regeneration. *Nat Med* 2014;20:833-846.

46. Butler JM, Kobayashi H, Rafii S: Instructive role of the vascular niche in promoting tumour growth and tissue repair by angiocrine factors. *Nat Rev Cancer* 2010;10:138-146.

47. Williams R, Khan IM, Richardson K, et al: Identification and clonal characterisation of a progenitor cell sub-population in normal human articular cartilage. *PLoS One* 2010;5:e13246.

48. Jiang Y, Tuan RS: Origin and function of cartilage stem/progenitor cells in osteoarthritis. *Nat Rev Rheumatol* 2015;11:206-212.

49. Mantripragada VP, Bova WA, Boehm C, et al: Primary cells isolated from human knee cartilage reveal decreased prevalence of progenitor cells but comparable biological potential during osteoarthritic disease progression. *J Bone Joint Surg Am* 2018;100:1771-1780.

This interesting report highlights the need to understand the biological implications of heterogeneity of chondrogenic connective-tissue progenitors in cartilage and characterize the quality and quantity of the cells in order to select appropriate subsets of populations and progenitors being administered to improve the efficacy of cartilage cell therapy procedures.

50. Samsonraj RM, Raghunath M, Nurcombe V, Hui JH, van Wijnen AJ, Cool SM: Concise review: Multifaceted characterization of human mesenchymal stem cells for use in regenerative medicine. *Stem Cells Transl Med* 2017;6:2173-2185.

This up-to-date review discusses the criteria for characterizing and selecting MSCs and proposes comprehensive and uniform guidelines for clinical-grade production to achieve predictably favorable treatment outcomes for stem cell therapy.

51. Narcisi R, Cleary MA, Brama PA, et al: Long-term expansion, enhanced chondrogenic potential, and suppression of endochondral ossification of adult human MSCs via WNT signaling modulation. *Stem Cell Reports* 2015;4:459-472.

52. Mizuno M, Katano H, Otabe K, et al: Platelet-derived growth factor (PDGF)-AA/AB in human serum are potential indicators of the proliferative capacity of human synovial mesenchymal stem cells. *Stem Cell Res Ther* 2015;6:243.

53. Fekete N, Rojewski MT, Lotfi R, Schrezenmeier H: Essential components for ex vivo proliferation of mesenchymal stromal cells. *Tissue Eng Part C Methods* 2014;20:129-139.

54. Muraglia A, Todeschi MR, Papait A, et al: Combined platelet and plasma derivatives enhance proliferation of stem/progenitor cells maintaining their differentiation potential. *Cytotherapy* 2015;17:1793-1806.

55. Reissis D, Tang QO, Cooper NC, et al: Current clinical evidence for the use of mesenchymal stem cells in articular cartilage repair. *Expert Opin Biol Ther* 2016;16:535-557.

This review discusses the robust clinical evidence that MSCs have significant potential for the regeneration of hyaline articular cartilage in patients.

56. Cleary MA, van Osch GJ, Brama PA, Hellingman CA, Narcisi R: FGF, TGFbeta and Wnt crosstalk: Embryonic to in vitro cartilage development from mesenchymal stem cells. *J Tissue Eng Regen Med* 2015;9:332-342.

57. Correa D, Somoza RA, Lin P, et al: Sequential exposure to fibroblast growth factors (FGF) 2, 9 and 18 enhances hMSC chondrogenic differentiation. *Osteoarthr Cartil* 2015;23:443-453.

58. Panadero JA, Lanceros-Mendez S, Ribelles JL: Differentiation of mesenchymal stem cells for cartilage tissue engineering: Individual and synergetic effects of three-dimensional environment and mechanical loading. *Acta Biomater* 2016;33:1-12.

This paper reviews the existing literature on the effect of mechanical stimulation on chondrogenic differentiation of MSCs and concludes that contradictory results using different modes of external loading can be explained by the different properties of the scaffolding system that influences adhesion, morphology, and spatial distribution of cells, as well as the stress experienced by the cells.

59. Leijten J, Georgi N, Moreira Teixeira L, van Blitterswijk CA, Post JN, Karperien M: Metabolic programming of mesenchymal stromal cells by oxygen tension directs chondrogenic cell fate. *Proc Natl Acad Sci USA* 2014;111:13954-13959.

60. de Vries-van Melle ML, Narcisi R, Kops N, et al: Chondrogenesis of mesenchymal stem cells in an osteochondral environment is mediated by the subchondral bone. *Tissue Eng Part A* 2014;20:23-33.

61. Barron V, Merghani K, Shaw G, et al: Evaluation of cartilage repair by mesenchymal stem cells seeded on a PEOT/PBT scaffold in an osteochondral defect. *Ann Biomed Eng* 2015;43:2069-2082.

62. Papadimitropoulos A, Piccinini E, Brachat S, et al: Expansion of human mesenchymal stromal cells from fresh bone marrow in a 3D scaffold-based system under direct perfusion. *PLoS One* 2014;9:e102359.

63. Ferlin KM, Prendergast ME, Miller ML, Kaplan DS, Fisher JP: Influence of 3D printed porous architecture on mesenchymal stem cell enrichment and differentiation. *Acta Biomater* 2016;32:161-169.

    The results reported in this study suggest that 3D printed scaffolds with ordered cubic pores are supportive of both MSC enrichment from unprocessed bone marrow as well as MSC differentiation.

64. Diaz-Gomez L, Alvarez-Lorenzo C, Concheiro A, et al: Biodegradable electrospun nanofibers coated with platelet-rich plasma for cell adhesion and proliferation. *Mater Sci Eng C Mater Biol Appl* 2014;40:180-188.

65. Dias IR, Viegas CA, Carvalho PP: Large animal models for osteochondral regeneration. *Adv Exp Med Biol* 2018;1059:441-501.

    This review of guidelines for use of large animal models in articular cartilage regeneration and repair studies highlights that the subchondral bone plate should always be taken into consideration and that generally a 6- to 12-month follow-up period is optimal for these types of studies.

66. da Silva Morais A, Oliveira JM, Reis RL: Small animal models. *Adv Exp Med Biol* 2018;1059:423-439.

    This review highlights the importance of considering the advantages and limitations of the various animal models, the different challenges in extrapolating data obtained for clinical translation, and the risks of misinterpretation.

67. Kon E, Roffi A, Filardo G, Tesei G, Marcacci M: Scaffold-based cartilage treatments: With or without cells? A systematic review of preclinical and clinical evidence. *Arthroscopy* 2015;31:767-775.

68. Cucchiarini M, Madry H: Biomaterial-guided delivery of gene vectors for targeted articular cartilage repair. *Nat Rev Rheumatol* 2019;15:18-29. doi:10.1038/s41584-018-0125-2.

    This article reviews the state-of-art on strategies for the delivery of gene vectors in biomaterial that can enable targeting to cartilage and protection from immune response.

69. Gadjanski I, Spiller K, Vunjak-Novakovic G: Time-dependent processes in stem cell-based tissue engineering of articular cartilage. *Stem Cell Rev* 2012;8:863-881.

70. Bornes TD, Adesida AB, Jomha NM: Mesenchymal stem cells in the treatment of traumatic articular cartilage defects: A comprehensive review. *Arthritis Res Ther* 2014;16:432.

71. Marquass B, Schulz R, Hepp P, et al: Matrix-associated implantation of predifferentiated mesenchymal stem cells versus articular chondrocytes: In vivo results of cartilage repair after 1 year. *Am J Sports Med* 2011;39:1401-1412.

72. Khozoee B, Mafi P, Mafi R, Khan WS: Mechanical stimulation protocols of human derived cells in articular cartilage tissue engineering – a systematic review. *Curr Stem Cell Res Ther* 2017;12:260-270.

    This review summarizes the available protocols for increasing the chondrogenic properties of human cells by mechanical stimulation with a focus on bioreactors used for articular cartilage tissue engineering.

73. Acharya C, Adesida A, Zajac P, et al: Enhanced chondrocyte proliferation and mesenchymal stromal cells chondrogenesis in coculture pellets mediate improved cartilage formation. *J Cell Physiol* 2012;227:88-97.

74. Bekkers JE, Tsuchida AI, van Rijen MH, et al: Single-stage cell-based cartilage regeneration using a combination of chondrons and mesenchymal stromal cells: Comparison with microfracture. *Am J Sports Med* 2013;41:2158-2166.

75. Diekman BO, Guilak F: Stem cell-based therapies for osteoarthritis: Challenges and opportunities. *Curr Opin Rheumatol* 2013;25:119-126.

76. Dimarino AM, Caplan AI, Bonfield TL: Mesenchymal stem cells in tissue repair. *Front Immunol* 2013;4:201.

77. de Windt TS, Vonk LA, Slaper-Cortenbach IC, et al: Allogeneic mesenchymal stem cells stimulate cartilage regeneration and are safe for single-stage cartilage repair in humans upon mixture with recycled autologous chondrons. *Stem Cells* 2017;35:256-264.

    This article reports a proof-of-principle, phase I (first-in-man) clinical trial applying allogeneic MSCs mixed with autologous cartilage-derived cells in chondrons for treatment of cartilage defects in the knees of symptomatic patients.

78. Burke J, Hunter M, Kolhe R, Isales C, Hamrick M, Fulzele S: Therapeutic potential of mesenchymal stem cell based therapy for osteoarthritis. *Clin Transl Med* 2016;5:27.

    This review details the cell-based therapies currently under investigation with focus on the sources and use of MSCs for cartilage regeneration in OA patients.

79. Orozco L, Munar A, Soler R, et al: Treatment of knee osteoarthritis with autologous mesenchymal stem cells: A pilot study. *Transplantation* 2013;95:1535-1541.

80. Soler R, Orozco L, Munar A, et al: Final results of a phase I-II trial using ex vivo expanded autologous Mesenchymal Stromal Cells for the treatment of osteoarthritis of the knee confirming safety and suggesting cartilage regeneration. *Knee* 2016;23:647-654.

This report of a phase I-II clinical trial shows the feasibility, safety, and efficacy of ex vivo expanded autologous bone marrow MSCs.

81. Koh YG, Choi YJ: Infrapatellar fat pad-derived mesenchymal stem cell therapy for knee osteoarthritis. *Knee* 2012;19:902-907.

82. Lamo-Espinosa JM, Mora G, Blanco JF, et al: Intra-articular injection of two different doses of autologous bone marrow mesenchymal stem cells versus hyaluronic acid in the treatment of knee osteoarthritis: Multicenter randomized controlled clinical trial (phase I/II). *J Transl Med* 2016;14:246.

This report suggests promising results in assessment of bone marrow–derived MSCs in combination with hyaluronic acid in a randomized clinical trial, showing feasibility and safety and clinical and functional improvement with some doses of BM-MSCs.

83. McCarrel TM, Mall NA, Lee AS, Cole BJ, Butty DC, Fortier LA: Considerations for the use of platelet-rich plasma in orthopedics. *Sports Med* 2014;44:1025-1036.

84. Jevasevar DS. *Treatment of Osteoarthritis of the Knee: Evidence-Based Guideline*. ed 2. Rosemont, IL: American Academy of Orthopaedic Surgeons; 2013.

85. Chu CR, Rodeo S, Bhutani N, et al: Optimizing clinical use of biologics in orthopaedic surgery: Consensus recommendations from the 2018 AAOS/NIH U-13 conference. *J Am Acad Orthop Surg* 2019;27(2):e50-e63.

This article is based on the concern that "biologic" treatments such as platelet-rich plasma and cell-based therapies are largely unproven, lack evidence-based medicine, and are currently being used because of misinformation from direct-to-consumer marketing. Recommendations are provided for design of clinical trials for knee OA.

86. Mobasheri A, Rayman MP, Gualillo O, Sellam J, van der Kraan P, Fearon U: The role of metabolism in the pathogenesis of osteoarthritis. *Nat Rev Rheumatol* 2017;13:302-311.

This is an excellent review of the metabolic pathways and mediators that can drive OA pathogenesis and that may serve as targets for therapy.

Chapter 15

Myopathies and Nerve Disorders

Ranjan Gupta, MD • Jacques H. Hacquebord, MD

ABSTRACT

Myopathies and nerve disorders continue to remain challenging diagnoses. The past several years, however, have seen significant progress in both elucidating the pathophysiology and advancing treatment particularly in muscle disorders. Investigation into muscle-derived stem cells (MDSCs), specifically MDSC transplantation, shows much potential for future use. Gene replacement therapy has also allowed for significant advancement in the treatment of muscular dystrophies along with medications such as eteplirsen and eculizumab, which have recently been approved for use in various muscle disorders. In the setting of nerve injury, understanding the difference in pathophysiology between acute and chronic nerve injuries is critical in directing treatment and further research.

Keywords: Becker muscular dystrophy; Duchenne muscular dystrophy; myopathy; nerve healing; nerve injury; neuropathy

Introduction

Myopathies and nerve disorders produce significant morbidity and remain challenging to treat. Advancements in our understanding of the pathophysiology have been made, but there remains significant need for a more complete understanding to develop meaningful therapies. This chapter includes our updated understanding of both the pathophysiology for common myopathies and nerve disorders and current therapeutic avenues.

Dr. Gupta or an immediate family member serves as a board member, owner, officer, or committee member of the American Shoulder and Elbow Surgeons and the American Society for Surgery of the Hand. Dr. Hacquebord or an immediate family member has received research or institutional support from Acumed, LLC.

Myopathies

Muscle Anatomy of Physiology

Human skeletal muscle develops force and allows for movement. Muscle comprises numerous muscle fibers arranged in a tubular structure, which function as the individual contractile units within muscles. Each muscle fiber consists of numerous tubular myofibrils. The myofibrils have repeating sections of sarcomeres. Sarcomeres give muscle its striated appearance and are the contractile subunit of muscle. Sarcomeres each contain rows of myosin overlapping with an actin framework. The length of the sarcomere where the myosin and actin framework overlap is directly related to the force capable to be generated by the muscle. This relationship between muscle length and active force is displayed in the Blix curve, which describes the relationships between the active force generated by muscle, passive force of muscle, and muscle length. The Blix curve identifies the sarcomere length(s) at which the muscle is biomechanically in the ideal position with optimal myosin and actin overlap to generate the maximum active force (**Figure 1**). Muscle phenotype is also controlled by several different signaling pathways. These include the Ras/MAP signaling pathway, calcineurin, Ca^{2+}/calmodulin-dependent protein kinase, and peroxisome proliferator γ coactivator 1. These pathways are exercise-induced and important in determining the specialized characteristics of slow-twitch and fast-twitch muscles. Skeletal muscle is often divided into slow-twitch (type 1) and fast-twitch (type 2). This distinction originates from the fact that chemical energy converted to mechanical work occurs either through anaerobic glycolysis or from oxidation of pyruvate or free fatty acids. The oxidative enzymes are localized inside mitochondria, whereas the enzymes of anaerobic glycolysis are not membrane-bound. The efficiency of anaerobic glycolysis is comparatively low; however, it has the advantage of not being impaired by lack of blood supply. Most skeletal muscle has the ability to shift between both metabolic pathways, and most muscle fibers are specialized and differ in their content of enzymes and substrates of metabolism. The

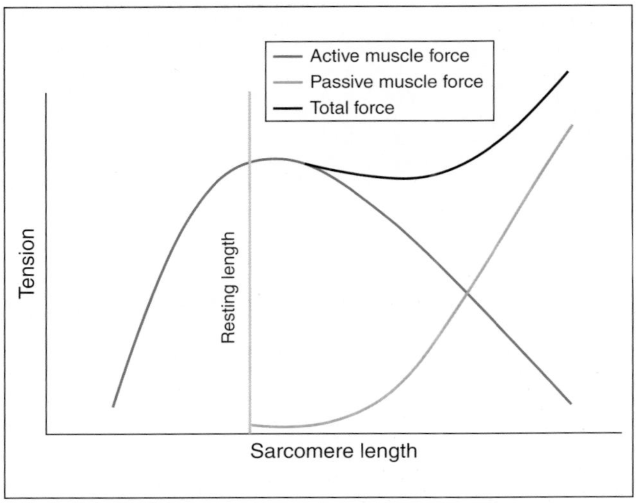

Figure 1 The Blix curve represents the relationship between sarcomere length and the muscle force—both active and passive.

muscles that are slower twitching tend to have high oxidative capacity, whereas the fast-twitch muscles rely on anaerobic glycolysis.

Muscle Injury Pathophysiology

Injuries to skeletal muscle involving degradation of myofibers and fibrosis and fatty cell infiltration of muscle can occur through (1) mechanical weakening of the sarcolemma, (2) inappropriate calcium influx, (3) aberrant cell signaling, (4) increased oxidative stress, and (5) recurrent muscle ischemia. The exact mechanisms by which this happens are quite complex but involve the dystrophin-glycoprotein complex. It was previously believed that there was one unifying mechanism, but it is now believed that the dystrophin-glycoprotein complex is involved in multiple different pathological pathways that result in skeletal muscle damage. Injury of skeletal muscle can also involve conversion of the muscle to bone. This can occur in myositis ossificans secondary to significant trauma or in fibrodysplasia ossificans secondary to a genetic mutation. The mechanism by which this occurs is debated; however, it is believed that most heterotopic bone originates through endothelial mesenchymal transition[1] and that smooth muscle cells do not contribute to any stage of heterotopic ossification.[2]

Another common degradation pathway for muscle is the loss of tendon attachment to bone, that is,, the enthesis with the ensuing changes in muscle physiology and structure. A common clinical scenario for these injuries includes rotator cuff tears. Tendon tears result in loss of muscle tensile forces, leading to decrease in muscle strength and atrophy both radially and longitudinally.[3] There is decreased sarcomere number and length, which results in an overall appearance of myofiber disorganization.[4,5] These changes result in increased fat content and fibrosis. The exact cause for fatty infiltration remains poorly understood.[6] The two primary progenitor cells that appear to be the source of fatty infiltration are adipose-derived mesenchymal stem cells (MSCs) and muscle-derived stem cells (MDSCs).[7-9] Muscular atrophy can recover, but it has been well demonstrated that fatty infiltration does not. Some studies support the theory that massive tear results in a neurologic injury through which fatty degeneration occurs as a result of denervation of the affected muscle. Other studies have postulated that the chronic unloading of the muscle-tendon unit leads to atrophy and fatty degeneration through infiltration of adipocytes. A final hypothesis is that the loss of tensile strength in muscle directly leads to phenotypic changes. This theory has been supported by molecular studies using animal models where loss of mechanical stretch in skeletal muscle results in the upregulation of specific adipogenic (PPARγ and C/EBPβ) and myogenic (Myf-5) transcription factors and the suppression of specific pathways (Wnt signaling) that then result in the upregulation of adipogenic transcription factors.[10,11]

Muscle-Derived Stem Cells

MDSCs were first discovered in 1961 when Alexander Mauro detected a clump of mononucleated cells in adult myofiber using electron microscopy.[12] Physically, MDSCs reside between the basal lamina and sarcolemma of adult muscle fibers.[13] Like typical adult stem cells, they possess the ability to proliferate and self-renew. The unique marker profile of MDSCs include Pax7/pax3, Myf5, CD56, and CD29.[14,15] Pax3 and Pax7 are transcription factors, which help to regulate myogenic differentiation by activating the expression of myogenic differentiation genes Myf5 and MyoD. CD56 is also expressed by myoblasts and neuronal-derived tissues, among others. CD29, also known as β1-integrin functions mainly as a collagen receptor but has been shown to be upregulated in MDSCs. Partly because of the ability to differentiate into adipocytes, osteocytes, myocytes, and chondrocytes, MDSCs have a high regenerative capacity in musculoskeletal tissue healing.[16] Transplanted MDSCs can vigorously self-renew, expanding and repopulating the host muscle. Collins et al confirmed that as few as seven MDSCs associated with one transplanted myofiber can generate over 100 new myofibers containing thousands of myonuclei. Injury or muscle damage is the most common stimulus for MDSCs to differentiate. They play a role in musculoskeletal tissue regeneration and can fuse with injured myofibers.[17] The fact that they are reversibly quiescent and are capable of self-renewal and differentiation after transplantation makes MDSCs very unique.[18] There is still much to learn regarding the role of MDSCs in muscle injury, but future avenues for the use of MDSCs include therapeutic treatment of neuromuscular diseases via transplantation and/or forced differentiation. Specifically, MDSC protein activators could be manipulated to aid in myofiber regeneration following massive rotator cuff tears. Although an alternative strategy is MDSC transplantation to improve postsurgical rotator cuff retear rates, there are currently no human data about what actually happens to MDSCs secondary to injury or aging.

Muscle Disorders

Duchenne and Becker Muscular Dystrophy

Duchenne and Becker muscular dystrophy (DMD and BMD) both occur because of a mutation affecting the DMD gene that encodes for the dystrophin protein. DMD is more severe and also three times more common than BMD. Because this gene is X-linked, it nearly always affects boys. The dystrophin protein has a unique three-dimensional structure that allows for binding to other proteins such as dystrobrevin and syntrophin and as such plays a critical role as a structural linker for other proteins. Because the deformational forces generated by muscle contraction are significant, dystrophin is essential to maintain the integrity of the muscle membrane. However, with translation of a dysfunctional dystrophin protein in the settings of both DMD and BMD, the muscle membrane is damaged, leading to elevations of creatine kinase in the serum and to calcium influx within the muscle fiber, which activates calcium-dependent proteases. In BMD, dystrophin protein is still partially functional due to "in-frame" mutations that allow for continuation of the open reading frame and translation of the protein. However, DMD causes an "out of frame" mutation that leads to ablation of the open reading frame and translation termination. Muscle biopsy was the mainstay of diagnosis for both DMD and BMD. However, molecular mutation analysis has improved and has increasingly become the primary means of diagnosis. Molecular therapies that allow for continued translation of the dystrophin gene are currently in clinical trials.

Many therapeutic interventions focus on modifying dystrophin DNA. Gene editing has potential as a more permanent treatment as permanent chromosomal DNA corrections can be made. Gene replacement therapy primarily utilizes a viral vector delivery system. Successful gene-replacement therapy for DMD requires widespread and efficient delivery of the therapeutic genes to all muscles. Because of the enormous size of the dystrophin gene (~11.5 kb) and the requirement to replace the gene distributed throughout the body, this has presented significant challenges for viral vector packaging. The adeno-associated virus (AAV) vectors have been found most appropriate to achieve this goal.[19,20] However, the dystrophin gene is too large to fit into a recombinant AAV (rAAV), which typically has packaging capacity of 5 kb. Therefore, a reduced-size dystrophin version that leads to a mild phenotype has been developed. One of the challenges has been to identify the appropriate microgene configurations along with AAV serotypes. Preclinical data show significant promise of intravascular AAV microdystrophin delivery in significantly ameliorating the pathology. Although underpowered to reliably evaluate efficacy, several early clinical trials evaluating the safety and tolerability of the gene therapy have shown significant clinical promise.[21,22] The continued advancements in animal trials to improve intravascular delivery have led to several current trials in the United States and Europe investigating specific AAV mircodystrophin therapy for DMD and spinal muscular atrophy patients. This is a very exciting development in the field.

Other than gene therapy, other therapies focus on transcription and translation of RNA. More specifically, these include nonsense-suppressing agents that induce translational machinery to "read-through" the premature stop codon, antisense oligonucleotides that "skip" over mutation-containing exons, and upregulation of proteins homologous to dystrophin. In 2016, eteplirsen was approved by the FDA for use in DMD. This medication treats DMD by splicing out one of the mutations, which then allows for correct downstream reading frame and translation. Based on the success of these trials, trials for other congenital muscle disorders including MTM and Pompe are under way.

Myasthenia Gravis

Myasthenia gravis (MG) is the most frequently acquired disorder affecting neuromuscular transmission. The most common etiology includes pathogenic antibodies against components of the postsynaptic muscle end plate membrane. MG is usually divided into subgroups based on clinical features and serum autoantibodies. Most patients have autoantibodies against the nicotinic acetylcholine receptor (AChR). Other common autoantibodies are against muscle-specific kinase and low-density lipoprotein-related protein 4. Knowing the serum autoantibodies is relevant to determine treatment. Traditionally, therapies have been divided into

(1) short-term symptom control (acetylcholinesterase inhibitors, ephedrine, and/or 3,4-diaminopyridine, which work to increase the amount of acetylcholine present at the neuromuscular junction [NMJ]) (2) immunosuppressive, and (3) immunomodulating and supportive, including thymectomy. More specific antigenic targets are emerging in MG but require greater study. Increasingly, immunological subclassification of the disease is important because future therapies will target cell-surface antigens with specific monoclonal antibodies. These targeted monoclonal antibody agents remain some of the more exciting potential emerging therapies. A recent phase 3 randomized double-blinded trial with eculizumab, a recombinant humanized monoclonal antibody to complement, has shown some promise. Although the MG-ADL score was not statistically different between the two groups, the eculizumab group had nearly a third of MG exacerbations as compared with the placebo group.[23] Eculizumab has recently been approved by the US FDA as an approved therapy for MG. Along with acetylcholinesterase inhibitor, they are the only therapies for MG that are not considered "off-label" by the US FDA.[24]

Nerve Disorders

Anatomy

Peripheral nerves are heterogeneous composite structures comprising multiple different components including neurons, Schwann cells, fibroblasts, and macrophages. The neuron forms the foundation of the nerve and is a polarized structure consisting of an axon, cell body, and dendrites. The axon projects toward the site of innervation to form a synapse with the target end-organ. The Schwann cells are glial cells that produce myelin to encapsulate the axon and allow for faster and more efficient conduction of the action potential down the axon. Neural blood supply is intricate and forms from anastomoses of epineural, perineural, and endoneural plexuses along with segmental supply from nutrient arteries.[25] This blood supply is fragile and is easily injured in the setting of trauma, compression, or with inappropriate repair.[26]

Trauma

Like other organs, the peripheral nervous system responds to injury through initiating an inflammatory response. Increased vascular permeability occurs through both epineurial vessel permeability through a signal cascade and endoneurial vessel permeability through direct trauma. Mast cells in the epineurium and endoneurium may also play an important role through the release of histamine and serotonin. The increase in pressure alters blood flow and consequently the supply of nutrients and disposal of waste products. This affects axonal transport and action potential conduction and further injury propagation. More specifically, nerve injuries vary depending on whether the injury is acute or chronic in nature.

Acute Nerve Injuries

Acute nerve injuries are axonal-mediated with Wallerian degeneration being initiated with granular disintegration of the axonal cytoskeleton. Within 48 hours of injury, Schwann cells break down myelin and phagocytose axonal debris. Macrophages are then recruited and release growth factors that encourage Schwann cell and fibroblast proliferation (**Figure 2**). Schwann cells form longitudinal bands of Büngner that function as growth-promoting conduits for regenerating axons.[27] The growth cone is the tip of the regenerating axon and is composed of cellular matrix with fingerlike projections called filopodia that explore the microenvironment. Proteases are released from the growth cone and clear a path toward the target organ. Concurrently, various neurotrophic factors are upregulated by the Schwann cells that play essential roles in the injury and regenerative response.[28]

Surgery remains the primary treatment for traumatic peripheral nerve injuries where discontinuity of the axons occur. The primary function of surgery is to align and approximate severed nerve segments. It is understood that immediate repair allows for improved results with the requirements of a clean wound, viable blood supply, adequate soft-tissue coverage, minimal tension at repair site, and skeletal stability. Although fascicular re-alignment is believed to be imperative, it remains debated whether an epineurial repair is sufficient or if a grouped fascicular repair with internal epineurial or perineurial sutures might improve fascicular re-alignment and outcomes or actually make them worse with increased fibrosis. Although microsurgical techniques and surgical repair have improved, outcomes after surgical repair remain unimpressive. Meaningful recovery has been defined in the literature as return of motor function of M3 or greater and sensory recovery of S3 or greater. As can be expected, this method of assessing recovery is subject to significant observer bias and variability and while it may be classified meaningful, it tends not to be functional. Although direct nerve coaptation is preferable, the use of a nerve graft is required when a segmental nerve gap persists so as to produce a tensionless repair. Processed nerve allografts contain the physical microarchitecture and

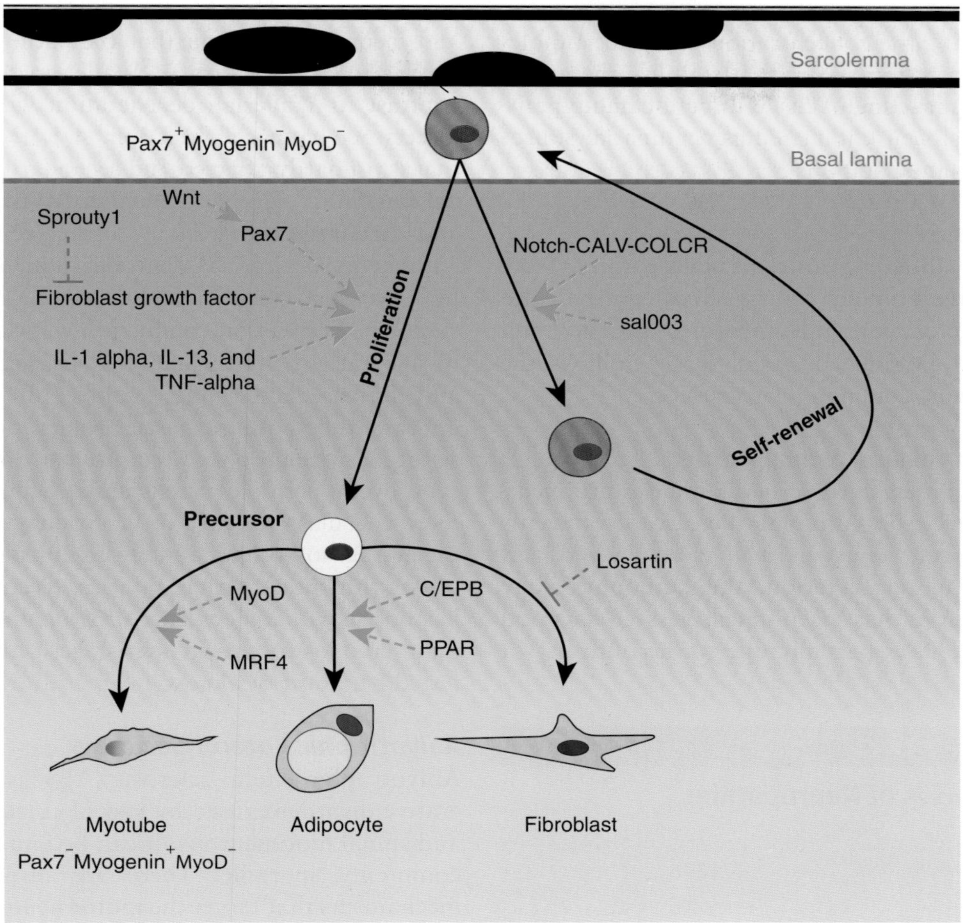

Figure 2 A schematic of muscle-derived stem cells and the factors that affect the proliferation and differentiation of the stem cells.

protein components inherent to nerve tissue.[29,30] Similar to autografts, they have the ability to revascularize and repopulate with host cells. The primary benefit over autograft is their ease of use and lack of donor site morbidity. Although there is evidence that processed nerve allografts provide some element of recovery, it remains controversial whether they are superior or even equivalent to autografts. Nerve conduits have long been an alternative to autografts. However, they are primarily limited to small diameter defects, small caliber nerves, and pure sensory nerves.[31] This limitation is likely a result of deficient Schwann cell migration, which has been shown to be important in the regeneration of long segmental defects in animal models.[32]

Peripheral nerve regeneration after acute injuries continues to be a challenge. Age of patient, location of injury, timing of presentation after injury, and timing of nerve repair are known factors that influence outcome. Inherent limitations also include rate of regeneration, specificity of regeneration, segmental nerve deficits, and degeneration of the target end-organ. A common teaching is that neural regeneration occurs at about 1 mm/d[33] This slow pace can be problematic because prolonged target deprivation reduces the ability of motor neurons to regenerate. This causes Schwann cells to lose their growth-supportive phenotypes.[34] Animal models have shown that following loss of innervation the AChRs located on end-organ muscle membranes degenerate. The degradation of motor endplates renders the target organ nonviable even if the nerve sufficiently regenerates. There is evidence that regenerating fibers can reinnervate distal muscles and reestablish structurally reformed NMJ even after several weeks of denervation.[35] As such, recent data have shown that preservation of the NMJ after traumatic nerve injury improves functional recovery after surgical repair[36] Preservation of the motor end plate is an active area of research. Areas of interest include increasing the concentration of Agrin, a molecule secreted by terminal SCs that stabilize the motor endplates, and targeting of the Wnt/beta-catenin pathway, which has been implicated as a potential source of motor end plate instability.[37]

Neuropathies

There are many different causes of neuropathies (**Table 1**). In general the etiology can be subcategorized into compressive, infectious, inflammatory, genetic, and associated with systemic diseases. Below follows the update of the most common neuropathies.

Chronic/Compression Neuropathies

Unlike acute injuries, chronic nerve injuries are mediated by Schwann cells. Although the cascade of events following an acute injury is well characterized and coined Wallerian degeneration, the pathophysiology of chronic injuries has been much less understood until recently. This is partially due to the difficulty of establishing a reliable animal model. Owing to the gradual nature of most chronic injuries, it was previously and incorrectly thought that the pathophysiology was similar to a mild form of Wallerian degeneration. In contrast to Wallerian degeneration where the neuron directs Schwann cell function, it is the Schwann cell that is primarily affected and secondarily affects neuronal function.[38] Mechanosensitivity of the Schwann cells and chronic ischemia likely further contributes to the pathogenesis. Gradual demyelination occurs followed by a wave of remyelination. In chronic nerve compressions, the decrease in conduction velocity is believed to be due to the remyelinated fibers having thinner myelin and decreased internodal lengths.[38] In addition, there appears to be both increased proliferation and apoptosis of SCs. Macrophage recruitment does occur, however, over a period of weeks unlike acute injuries where there is a massive wave of macrophage recruitment in the first 24 to 96 hours. Interestingly, despite demyelination with these chronic injuries, electron microscopy has not shown any evidence of axonal injury.[39] Axonal injury and loss occurs in later stages of disease as manifested by motor weakness.

Table 1

Common Causes of Neuropathies

Compressive neuropathies
- Carpal
- Cubital
- Pronator syndrome, etc

Genetic neurologic disorders
- Charcot-Marie-Tooth
- HNPP
- ALS

Infectious neuropathies
- Leprosy
- Lyme disease
- HIV polyneuropathy
- Hepatitis C
- Syphilis

Inflammatory neuropathies
- Guillain-Barré syndrome/acute inflammatory demyelinating polyneuropathy
- Chronic inflammatory demyelinating polyneuropathy
- Multifocal motor neuropathy

Neuropathy in systemic disease
- Endocrinopathies
- Rheumatologic disorders
- Malignancy

ALS = amyotrophic lateral sclerosis, HNPP = Hereditary neuropathy with predisposition/liability to pressure palsy

Amyotrophic Lateral Sclerosis

Amyotrophic lateral sclerosis (ALS) is a neurodegenerative disorder caused by loss of cortical, brain stem, and spinal motoneurons. It can be familial but is most commonly sporadic. There are several pathogenic mechanisms that target the motor neurons to cause the disease. These include oxidative stress, glutamate excitotoxicity, mitochondrial damage, protein aggregation, glia and neuroinflammation pathology, defective axonal transport, and aberrant RNA metabolism.[40] There currently is no cure for the disease with Riluzole being the only drug approved by the FDA that may prevent progression of the disease and increase lifespan. Fasciculations are a common finding in ALS and are often the first and only abnormality recorded in muscles. As such, identification of fasciculations can be very disconcerting to patients. It is important to remember that although fasciculations are a common feature in ALS, there are numerous other causes for fasciculations (**Table 2**). Fasciculations without weakness, muscle atrophy, or increased tendon reflexes suggest a benign etiology.[41] Although this is a disease of the upper and lower motor neurons, pain is a common and paradoxical problem in this disease. The etiology of pain can be primary in the form of cramps, spasticity, and neuropathy or secondary as nociceptive pain. It is important that physicians are aware of this and appropriately treat with sedatives and analgesics.[42]

Table 2

Causes of Fasciculations

Motor neuron disease
Spinal muscular atrophy and Kennedy syndrome
SCA 3 (Machado-Joseph disease)
Postpolio syndrome
Herpes virus one infection
Neuropathies
- Multifocal motor neuropathy with conduction block
- Chronic inflammatory demyelinating polyneuropathy
- Other immune-related neuropathies
- Charcot-Marie-Tooth syndromes
- Nerve entrapment syndromes and nerve injuries

Motor root and plexus lesions
- Inflammatory
- Radiation plexopathy

Spinal cord disorders
- Syringomyelia
- Cervical spondylosis with cord compression
- Radiation myelopathy
- Viral myelitis (herpes zoster, rabies)

Metabolic disease
- Hypocalcemia
- Hyperthyroidism
- Hypomagnesemia

Hyperexcitability of peripheral motor axons
- Benign fasciculation syndrome
- Cramp-fasciculation syndrome
- Postexercise fasciculation

Drug-related fasciculation
- Caffeine, cholinergic drugs, amphetamines, antihistamines, serotonin compounds, salbutamol, benzodiazepine withdrawal
- Organophosphate insecticide poisoning

Envenomization: bites by snakes, funnel-web spider, or scorpion
Pharmacological cholinergic block in anesthetic practice
Related autoimmune disorders
- Anti–voltage-gated potassium channels (VGKC) immune disease (encephalopathy with peripheral axonal disorder)
- Neuromyotonia

Inclusion body myositis

Charcot-Marie-Tooth

Charcot-Marie-Tooth (CMT) is the most common inherited neuropathy and is a genetically heterogeneous disorder of the peripheral nervous system but with a relatively homogenous clinical phenotype. The most common genetic mutations affect the production of myelin, either directly or indirectly. The disease affects up to 1 in 1,214 and involves progressive lower motor and sensory nerve dysfunction[43] and manifests as distal muscle weakness and atrophy, decreased reflexes, foot deformities, and sensory impairment. Therapies for the disease and other demyelinating neuropathies fall into one of two potential pathways: (1) targeting global signaling mechanisms of peripheral nerve biology and (2) addressing the underlying molecular pathogenesis of demyelination.[44] More specifically, although ascorbic acid initially showed promise, recent studies have been negative. Nonetheless, animal results have shown promising results for lonaprisan, curcumin, and histone deacetylase 6 inhibitors.[45]

Hereditary Neuropathy With Predisposition/Liability to Pressure Palsy

Hereditary neuropathy with predisposition/liability to pressure palsy (HNPP) is a rare autosomal dominant neuropathy characterized by recurrent mononeuropathies often exacerbated by compression or minor trauma. It is primarily caused by a mutation to the peripheral myelin protein-22 gene, the same gene affected by CMT type 1. This disease results in episodic, recurrent demyelinating neuropathy and commonly presents no sooner than adolescence.[45,46] The disease commonly has specific electrophysiological findings that can assist with diagnosis.[47] This is important to (1) differentiate it from other neuropathies and (2) to proceed with genetic testing if HNPP is suspected.

Multiple Sclerosis

Multiple sclerosis (MS) is a chronic disease of the central nervous system characterized by loss of motor and sensory function due to immune-mediated inflammation, demyelination, and subsequent axonal damage. It is widely accepted that the inflammatory process in MS is caused or propagated by an autoimmune cascade involving T-cells. However, more recent studies reveal it to be a heterogenous disease process involving both innate and adaptive immune-mediated inflammatory mechanisms. Several variants of MS have been identified and have been helpful to increase the diagnostic accuracy and identify the unique immunopathogenic profile to guide treatment.[48] There is also increasing evidence that environmental factors can play a substantive role in disease development. These include vitamin D deficiency, Epstein-Barr virus, smoking, western diet, and commensal microbiota.[49] Although there is no cure for MS, treatments serve to mitigate MS attacks, modify disease progression, and/or address the signs and symptoms of the disease.

Guillain-Barré Syndrome

Guillain-Barré syndrome (GBS) is the combination of rapidly progressive symmetrical weakness in the four limbs with or without sensory disturbances, hyporeflexia or areflexia, and in the absence of a cerebrospinal fluid cellular reaction. GBS can be divided into two major subtypes: acute inflammatory demyelinating polyneuropathy (AIDP) and the axonal subtypes: acute motor axonal neuropathy (AMAN) and acute motor and sensory axonal neuropathy (AMSAN).[50] A lumbar puncture is performed when GBS is suspected and typically shows increased protein with normal cell count. Electromyography can also be helpful, especially for subclassifying GBS into AMAN and AIDP. Although the diagnosis of GBS is typically not difficult, it is important to differentiate it from leptomeningeal malignancy, Lyme disease, West Nile virus infection, HIV-related GBS, or poliomyelitis when the presentation is not standard. Treatment consists of immunotherapy with plasmapheresis and intravenous immunoglobulin, corticosteroids, and supportive treatment.

Complex Regional Pain Syndrome

Complex regional pain syndrome (CRPS) is a chronic pain condition that is characterized by progressively worsening spontaneous regional pain without dermatomal distribution and that is out of proportion to the inciting event. Accompanying symptoms include skin changes, autonomic dysfunction, abnormal sensory and motor changes, and trophic changes that all can vary in severity. Diagnosis is based on clinical findings because no specific diagnostic test currently exists. The Budapest Criteria is used as the diagnostic criteria for CRPS to differentiate it from other causes of pain. CRPS can be divided into CRPS-1 or CRPS-2 and is based on the absence or presence of peripheral nerve damage, respectively. Extremity fracture is a common inciting event but the underlying pathophysiology remains controversial.[51] Treatment of CRPS typically is best with a multimodal approach. Mirror therapy does appear to be indicated and effective as part of a multidisciplinary approach to treat both CRPS-1 and CRPS-2.[52]

Parsonage Turner Syndrome

Parsonage Turner syndrome (PTS) is a rare disorder characterized by an acute onset of upper extremity pain with subsequent progressive neurologic deficits including weakness, atrophy, and sensory abnormalities. The distribution and severity of the nerves affected is variable and does not necessarily follow a specific pattern. The pathophysiology is also poorly understood. It is important to rule out other possible diagnoses that are more likely to have an injury pattern that can be explained by an identifiable and focal injury. As a result, electrodiagnostic studies and advanced imaging can be very helpful to rule out other causes. No specific treatments have been proven to reduce neurologic impairment or improve the prognosis of PTS. Overall, high-quality evidence for the treatment of PTS is lacking. There does exist some anecdotal evidence for corticosteroids that support its use to improve pain and accelerate recovery. For refractory cases, surgery can be considered and can include neurolysis, nerve grafting, and/or nerve transfer.[53]

Summary

Although there exist no curative treatments for many of the myopathies and neuropathies discussed above, early identification and diagnosis can be important to decrease the morbidity of the disease. It is important to continue with research in these areas to further improve understanding of the pathophysiology and identification of successful treatments.

Key Study Points

- The pathophysiology in acute nerve injuries is axonal-mediated, whereas chronic injuries are Schwann cell-mediated.
- Greater understanding and use of MDSCs hold promise to improve the healing of tendon ruptures, particularly rotator cuff tears.
- Understanding the surgical principles of nerve repair to treat an acute injury is essential for improving likelihood of meaningful recovery.

Annotated References

1. Medici D, Olsen BR: The role of endothelial-mesenchymal transition in heterotopic ossification. *J Bone Miner Res* 2012;27(8):1619-1622.
2. Lounev VY, Ramachandran R, Wosczyna MN, et al: Identification of progenitor cells that contribute to heterotopic skeletogenesis. *J Bone Joint Surg Am* 2009;91(3):652-663.
3. Ward SR, Sarver JJ, Eng CM, et al: Plasticity of muscle architecture after supraspinatus tears. *J Orthop Sports Phys Ther* 2010;40(11):729-735.
4. Baker JH, Hall-Craggs EC: Changes in sarcomere length following tenotomy in the rat. *Muscle Nerve* 1980;3(5):413-416.
5. Jamali AA, Afshar P, Abrams RA, Lieber RL: Skeletal muscle response to tenotomy. *Muscle Nerve* 2000;23(6):851-862.

6. Kang JR, Gupta R: Mechanisms of fatty degeneration in massive rotator cuff tears. *J Shoulder Elbow Surg* 2012;21(2):175-180.

7. Matsushita K, Dzau VJ: Mesenchymal stem cells in obesity: Insights for translational applications. *Lab Investig J Tech Methods Pathol* 2017;97(10):1158-1166.

   Mesenchymal stem cells (MSCs) are a major source of adipocyte generation and have potential roles in treating obesity.

8. Sohn J, Lu A, Tang Y, Wang B, Huard J: Activation of non-myogenic mesenchymal stem cells during the disease progression in dystrophic dystrophin/utrophin knockout mice. *Hum Mol Genet* 2015;24(13):3814-3829.

9. Uezumi A, Nakatani M, Ikemoto-Uezumi M, et al: Cell-surface protein profiling identifies distinctive markers of progenitor cells in human skeletal muscle. *Stem Cell Rep* 2016;7(2):263-278.

   Cell-surface proteins (CD82 and CD318 for satellite cells and CD201 for mesenchymal progenitors) are useful markers and functionally important molecules that provide valuable insight into human muscle biology and diseases.

10. Itoigawa Y, Kishimoto KN, Sano H, Kaneko K, Itoi E: Molecular mechanism of fatty degeneration in rotator cuff muscle with tendon rupture. *J Orthop Res* 2011;29(6):861-866.

11. Frey E, Regenfelder F, Sussmann P, et al: Adipogenic and myogenic gene expression in rotator cuff muscle of the sheep after tendon tear. *J Orthop Res* 2009;27(4):504-509.

12. Mauro A: Satellite cell of skeletal muscle fibers. *J Biophys Biochem Cytol* 1961;9:493-495.

13. Alway SE, Myers MJ, Mohamed JS: Regulation of satellite cell function in sarcopenia. *Front Aging Neurosci* 2014;6:246.

14. Kuang S, Kuroda K, Le Grand F, Rudnicki MA: Asymmetric self-renewal and commitment of satellite stem cells in muscle. *Cell* 2007;129(5):999-1010.

15. Boldrin L, Muntoni F, Morgan JE: Are human and mouse satellite cells really the same? *J Histochem Cytochem* 2010;58(11):941-955.

16. Collins CA, Olsen I, Zammit PS, et al: Stem cell function, self-renewal, and behavioral heterogeneity of cells from the adult muscle satellite cell niche. *Cell* 2005;122(2):289-301.

17. Sampath SC, Sampath SC, Ho ATV, et al: Induction of muscle stem cell quiescence by the secreted niche factor Oncostatin M. *Nat Commun* 2018;9(1):1531.

    The balance between stem cell quiescence and proliferation is a very important factor and perturbed in various disease states. This study better elucidates the factors that control muscle stem cell proliferation. Oncostatin M, a member of the interleukin-6 family of cytokines, is a potent inducer of muscle stem cell quiescence. It is produced by muscle fibers, induces reversible MuSC cell cycle exit, and maintains stem cell regenerative capacity.

18. Shea KL, Xiang W, LaPorta VS, et al: Sprouty1 regulates reversible quiescence of a self-renewing adult muscle stem cell pool during regeneration. *Cell Stem Cell* 2010;6(2):117-129.

19. Guiraud S, Chen H, Burns DT, Davies KE: Advances in genetic therapeutic strategies for Duchenne muscular dystrophy. *Exp Physiol* 2015;100(12):1458-1467.

20. Falzarano MS, Scotton C, Passarelli C, Ferlini A: Duchenne muscular dystrophy: From diagnosis to therapy. *Mol Basel Switz* 2015;20(10):18168-18184.

21. Duan D: Systemic AAV micro-dystrophin gene therapy for Duchenne muscular dystrophy. *Mol Ther J Am Soc Gene Ther* 2018;26(10):2337-2356.

    The highly abbreviated *micro-dystrophin* gene and body-wide systemic gene transfer with adeno-associated virus (AAV) allows to partly overcome the inherent challenges due to the enormous size of the gene and the distribution of muscle throughout the body.

22. Duan D: Micro-dystrophin gene therapy goes systemic in Duchenne muscular dystrophy patients. *Hum Gene Ther* 2018;29(7):733-736.

    Several human trials are currently in progress to advance AAV micro-dystrophin therapy to Duchenne muscular dystrophy patients. This has the potential to reshape the future of neuromuscular disease gene therapy.

23. Howard JF, Utsugisawa K, Benatar M, et al: Safety and efficacy of eculizumab in anti-acetylcholine receptor antibody-positive refractory generalised myasthenia gravis (REGAIN): A phase 3, randomised, double-blind, placebo-controlled, multicentre study. *Lancet Neurol* 2017;16(12):976-986.

    Although there was no statistically significant difference in the MG-ADL score between placebo and eculizumab group, the eculizumab group had a clearly decreased rate in myasthenia gravis exacerbation and need for rescue therapy.

24. Farmakidis C, Pasnoor M, Dimachkie MM, Barohn RJ: Treatment of myasthenia gravis. *Neurol Clin* 2018;36(2):311-337.

    Except for acetylcholinesterase inhibitors and complement inhibition with eculizumab, nearly all of the drugs used for MG are considered "off-label." There is good evidence that thymectomy is beneficial in both thymomatous and nonthymomatous disease.

25. Yegiyants S, Dayicioglu D, Kardashian G, Panthaki ZJ: Traumatic peripheral nerve injury: A wartime review. *J Craniofac Surg* 2010;21(4):998-1001.

26. Jung J, Hahn P, Choi B, Mozaffar T, Gupta R: Early surgical decompression restores neurovascular blood flow and ischemic parameters in an in vivo animal model of nerve compression injury. *J Bone Joint Surg Am* 2014;96(11):897-906.

27. Khuong HT, Kumar R, Senjaya F, et al: Skin derived precursor Schwann cells improve behavioral recovery for acute and delayed nerve repair. *Exp Neurol* 2014;254:168-179.

28. Scheib J, Höke A: Advances in peripheral nerve regeneration. *Nat Rev Neurol* 2013;9(12):668-676.

29. Brooks DN, Weber RV, Chao JD, et al: Processed nerve allografts for peripheral nerve reconstruction: A multicenter study of utilization and outcomes in sensory, mixed, and motor nerve reconstructions. *Microsurgery* 2012;32(1):1-14.

30. Cho MS, Rinker BD, Weber RV, et al: Functional outcome following nerve repair in the upper extremity using processed nerve allograft. *J Hand Surg* 2012;37(11):2340-2349.

31. Agnew SP, Dumanian GA: Technical use of synthetic conduits for nerve repair. *J Hand Surg* 2010;35(5):838-841.

32. Berrocal YA, Almeida VW, Gupta R, Levi AD: Transplantation of Schwann cells in a collagen tube for the repair of large, segmental peripheral nerve defects in rats. *J Neurosurg* 2013;119(3):720-732.

33. Sulaiman W, Gordon T: Neurobiology of peripheral nerve injury, regeneration, and functional recovery: From bench top research to bedside application. *Ochsner J* 2013;13(1):100-108.

34. Furey MJ, Midha R, Xu Q-G, Belkas J, Gordon T: Prolonged target deprivation reduces the capacity of injured motoneurons to regenerate. *Neurosurgery* 2007;60(4):723-732-733.

35. Sakuma M, Gorski G, Sheu S-H, et al: Lack of motor recovery after prolonged denervation of the neuromuscular junction is not due to regenerative failure. *Eur J Neurosci* 2016;43(3):451-462.

Evidence exists that there may be a time after nerve injury where, although regrowth to the muscle successfully occurs, there is a failure to reestablish motor function. This suggests a critical period for synapse reformation. Possible mechanisms for this are discussed.

36. Chao T, Frump D, Lin M, et al: Matrix metalloproteinase 3 deletion preserves denervated motor endplates after traumatic nerve injury. *Ann Neurol* 2013;73(2):210-223.

37. Kurimoto S, Jung J, Tapadia M, et al: Activation of the Wnt/β-catenin signaling cascade after traumatic nerve injury. *Neuroscience* 2015;294:101-108.

38. Pham K, Gupta R: Understanding the mechanisms of entrapment neuropathies. Review article. *Neurosurg Focus* 2009;26(2):E7.

39. Gupta R, Steward O: Chronic nerve compression induces concurrent apoptosis and proliferation of Schwann cells. *J Comp Neurol* 2003;461(2):174-186.

40. Harikrishnareddy D, Misra S, Upadhyay S, Modi M, Medhi B: Roots to start research in amyotrophic lateral sclerosis: Molecular pathways and novel therapeutics for future. *Rev Neurosci* 2015;26(2):161-181.

41. de Carvalho M, Kiernan MC, Swash M: Fasciculation in amyotrophic lateral sclerosis: Origin and pathophysiological relevance. *J Neurol Neurosurg Psychiatry* 2017;88(9):773-779.

Fasciculation commonly occurs in multiple different clinical scenarios. A benign fasciculation syndrome is suggested when no weakness, muscle atrophy, or increased tendon reflexes are present, even with a sudden onset. That being said, fasciculations often present as the initial abnormality in ALS.

42. Delpont B, Beauvais K, Jacquin-Piques A, et al: Clinical features of pain in amyotrophic lateral sclerosis: A clinical challenge. *Rev Neurol (Paris)* 2019;175(1-2):11-15.

Pain is a paradoxical problem in ALS, a disease of the upper and lower motor neurons. It can be in the form of cramps, spasticity, and neuropathy, or secondary as nociceptive pain. It may also present before any motor symptoms.

43. Mathis S, Goizet C, Tazir M, et al: Charcot-marie-tooth diseases: An update and some new proposals for the classification. *J Med Genet* 2015;52(10):681-690.

44. Zhou Y, Notterpek L: Promoting peripheral myelin repair. *Exp Neurol* 2016;283(pt B):573-580.

Facilitating remyelination in the setting of a peripheral nerve injury can significantly improve outcomes. There is evidence that Schwann cell function can be enhanced through interventions such as exercise, electrical stimulation, or pharmacology. Transplantation of healthy Schwann cells into the PNS enhanced by exercise and/or electrical stimulation, or the inclusion of engineered biomaterial shows promise.

45. Baets J, De Jonghe P, Timmerman V: Recent advances in Charcot-Marie-Tooth disease. *Curr Opin Neurol* 2014;27(5):532-540.

46. Chen B, Niu S, Wang X, Li W, Chen N, Zhang Z: Clinical, electrophysiological, genetic, and imaging features of six Chinese Han patients with hereditary neuropathy with liability to pressure palsies (HNPP). *J Clin Neurosci* 2018;48:133-137.

This article is a case series of 6 patients with HNPP and discusses the specific findings of their disease. There was significant variability between the patients with their specific clinical findings. Level of evidence: IV.

47. Potulska-Chromik A, Sinkiewicz-Darol E, Ryniewicz B, et al: Clinical, electrophysiological, and molecular findings in early onset hereditary neuropathy with liability to pressure palsy. *Muscle Nerve* 2014;50(6):914-918.

The diagnosis of HNPP can be challenging and this study summarizes the clinical, electrophysiological, genetic, and imaging features of six unrelated patients with HNPP.

48. Karussis D: The diagnosis of multiple sclerosis and the various related demyelinating syndromes: A critical review. *J Autoimmun* 2014;48-49:134-142.

49. Yadav SK, Mindur JE, Ito K, Dhib-Jalbut S: Advances in the immunopathogenesis of multiple sclerosis. *Curr Opin Neurol* 2015;28(3):206-219.

50. Fujimura H: The Guillain-Barré syndrome. *Handb Clin Neurol* 2013;115:383-402.

51. Urits I, Shen AH, Jones MR, Viswanath O, Kaye AD: Complex regional pain syndrome, current concepts and treatment options. *Curr Pain Headache Rep* 2018;22(2):10.

Pathophysiologic mechanisms of CRPS have recently been identified. This has led to significant improvements in understanding the disease process and bares promise for more effective and evidence-based therapies.

52. Sayegh SA, Filén T, Johansson M, Sandström S, Stiewe G, Butler S: Mirror therapy for Complex Regional Pain Syndrome (CRPS)-A literature review and an illustrative case report. *Scand J Pain* 2013;4(4):200-207.

53. Smith CC, Bevelaqua A-C: Challenging pain syndromes: Parsonage-Turner syndrome. *Phys Med Rehabil Clin N Am* 2014;25(2):265-277.

Chapter 16

Orthopaedic Infections and Microbiology

Benjamin F. Ricciardi, MD • Edward M. Schwarz, PhD

ABSTRACT

Infections of the musculoskeletal system are common and challenging to treat. In this chapter, we discuss the microbiology of the major classes of adult musculoskeletal infection. Advancements in our knowledge of the interaction of bacteria and the host immune system will be discussed including bacterial evasion of host immunity, formation of biofilm, bacterial resistance, and persistence within host cells and tissues. Finally, we will discuss therapeutic targets for treatment of musculoskeletal infection including novel antimicrobial agents, immunotherapy, local delivery systems, and dispersal agents.

Keywords: Biofilm; Musculoskeletal infection; Prosthetic joint infection; *Staphylococcus aureus*

Dr. Schwarz or an immediate family member is a member of a speakers' bureau or has made paid presentations on behalf of Asahi KASEI Pharma Corporation; serves as a paid consultant to or is an employee of Amedica, Asahi KASEI Pharma Corporation, DePuy, A Johnson & Johnson Company, MedImmune, Musculoskeletal Transplant Foundation, Regeneron, and Telephus Biomedical; has stock or stock options held in LAGeT Inc. and Telephus Biomedical; has received research or institutional support from DePuy, A Johnson & Johnson Company, Eli Lilly, LAGeT, and Telephus; and has received nonincome support (such as equipment or services), commercially derived honoraria, or other non–research-related funding (such as paid travel) from LAGeT and Telephus. Neither Dr. Ricciardi nor any immediate family member has received anything of value from or has stock or stock options held in a commercial company or institution related directly or indirectly to the subject of this chapter.

Introduction

Infections of the musculoskeletal system can involve bone, soft tissue, and implant-related material. The societal burden of musculoskeletal infection has been increasing over time because of higher rates of medical comorbidities in patients undergoing orthopaedic surgery and increasing bacterial antibiotic resistance. Novel insights into the mechanisms of musculoskeletal infection and immune system evasion will hopefully expand therapeutic opportunities to treat these challenging conditions.

Microbiology of Musculoskeletal Infection

Epidemiology

The overall incidence of infection at 1 year following orthopaedic surgery varies from 0.5% to 1% after total hip or knee replacement, 2% to 4% for instrumented lumbar fusion, and 5% to 10% after open reduction and internal fixation of open tibia fractures. The microbiological profile of musculoskeletal infection varies based on the anatomic site of infection, presence of an implant, involved tissues, and age of the patient (**Table 1**). The most common types of musculoskeletal infections are briefly discussed below.

Adult Septic Arthritis

There are over 10,000 adult in-patient admissions in the United States per year with a diagnosis of septic arthritis. Patient risk factors include older age, immunocompromised state (diabetes mellitus, chronic liver disease, chronic kidney disease, immunodeficiency, inflammatory arthritis), intravenous drug use, sexually transmitted disease, infection at other anatomic sites, and geographical exposures (Lyme disease). The knee remains the most commonly affected joint, however, followed by the hip, shoulder, and elbow in decreasing order (**Table 1**).

Adult Osteomyelitis

The most common cause of osteomyelitis outside of the foot and axial skeleton in adults is previous trauma with a high incidence of retained hardware. Vertebral

Basic Science

Table 1

Summary of the Epidemiology of Major Categories of Deep Musculoskeletal Infection

Common Classes of Deep Musculoskeletal Infection	Most Common Anatomic Sites	Most Common Isolated Organisms
Adult septic arthritis	Knee Hip Shoulder Elbow	*Staphylococcus aureus* (up to 50% of cases) *Streptococcus* sp. (group B strep most common) *Enterococcus* sp. Gram-negative sp. (*Neisseria gonorrhoeae* in young sexually active populations) *Mycobacteria* (immunocompromised, developing countries) *Propionibacterium acnes* (shoulder)
Adult osteomyelitis	Foot Spine/pelvis Sites of previous trauma with retained hardware	*Staphylococcus* sp. (up to 50% of cases) *Streptococcus* sp. *Enterococcus* sp. Gram-negative sp. (*Escherichia coli, Pseudomonas aeruginosa*)
Prosthetic joint infection	Knee Hip Shoulder	*Staphylococcus aureus* (up to 50% of cases) *Staphylococcus epidermidis* Other *Staphylococcus* sp. (Coagulase negative staphylococci) *Streptococcus* sp. *Enterococcus* sp. Gram-negative sp. *P acnes* (most commonly isolated organism in prosthetic shoulder infection)
Diabetic foot infection	—	Polymicrobial infection more common than monomicrobial isolates Gram-negative sp. (*P aeruginosa* most common) Gram-positive sp. (*Staphylococcus aureus* most common; streptococcal sp. [Group B Strep]) Anaerobic sp.

osteomyelitis is common in patients who are immunocompromised, those with indwelling catheters, previous spinal instrumentation or spine trauma, and systemic bacteremia from another site. Similar to septic arthritis, *Staphylococcus aureus* is the most common organism in both extremity and vertebral osteomyelitis and represents up to half of all cases with a high incidence of methicillin resistance in certain populations (**Table 1**).

Prosthetic Joint Infection

Prosthetic joint replacement is one of the most common procedures performed in the United States. Overall, the incidence of infection ranges from 0.5% to 2% depending on the anatomic site and study examined. The presence of an implant creates some changes to the microbiological profile from native joint infections. Similar to adult septic arthritis and osteomyelitis, *S aureus* is the most common cause of prosthetic joint infection (PJI) with resistant strains representing up to 50% of these cases depending on the underlying patient population. Unlike adult septic arthritis and osteomyelitis, *Staphylococcus epidermidis* also has a high prevalence in PJI with methicillin-resistant strains becoming more common in recent years. These two organisms represent over half of all cases of PJI (**Table 1**).

Diabetic Foot Infection

The incidence of diabetic foot ulcers has been increasing as the population of patients living with diabetes mellitus grows. Microvascular insufficiency, loss of protective sensation, and deformity from altered bony anatomy of the foot can lead to skin ulceration in these patients. Ulcerations create an opportunity for an infection to develop in the underlying soft tissue and bone. Infected diabetic ulcers increase the risk of lower extremity amputation and limb loss. Diabetic foot infections (DFIs) are more likely to be polymicrobial than the other types of infections discussed, and these are more common than monomicrobial isolates. Additionally, there is a higher incidence of gram-negative organisms isolated from DFI with *Pseudomonas aeruginosa* typically being the most common (**Table 1**).

Host Defense Mechanisms Against Infections

Innate Immune Response

Musculoskeletal infections begin with a breach in local host defenses most commonly involving the skin. This leads to both localized infection at the site of injury and systemic dissemination into other tissues via the circulatory or lymphatic systems. Evasion of host immunity by planktonic, or free floating, bacterial cells is the first step to establishing infection. Integral components of host immunity to acute bacterial infection include responses from cells of the innate immune system (neutrophils, macrophages) and complement. Neutrophils use several antimicrobial strategies to kill planktonic bacteria including phagocytosis, oxidative burst, release of proteases, and production of pro-inflammatory cytokines and chemokines.[1] Additionally, neutrophils produce neutrophil extracellular traps (NETs), which consist of nuclear contents expelled with several antimicrobial proteins deposited on chromatin that are released into the extracellular environment.[2] NETs help inactive virulence factors, immobilize bacteria, provide a favorable environment for complement activation, and promote phagocyte bacterial clearance.[3] Deficiencies in neutrophil number or function (eg, chronic granulomatous disease) result in a significant predisposition to invasive bacterial infection frequently with *S aureus*, further illustrating their primary importance to host defenses.

Macrophages, in particular classically activated (M1) macrophages, are important for bacterial clearance via phagocytosis in the setting of acute infection by direct recognition of bacterial surface targets through macrophage surface receptors or indirectly by recognizing immunoglobulin or complement on the bacterial surface. Macrophages also act as antigen presenting cells and can activate other components of the innate and adaptive immune system through the release of cytokines and chemokines.

Adaptive Immune Response

The importance of the adaptive immune system is less clear than the innate immune system particularly in the setting of staphylococcal infection. For example, results of a 2018 study show that almost half of patients with a previous *S aureus* skin infection experience a recurrence despite high titers of specific antibodies and memory T-cells.[4] Subsets of CD4+ T cells important in adaptive immunity include Th1, Th2, and Th17 cells. The role of Th1 cells (defined by production of interferon-γ (IFNγ)] in mediating protection against *S aureus* infection varies amongst studies including protective, detrimental, or noncontributory roles depending on the specific experimental conditions.[5] Th17 cells are defined by expression of Rorγt and cytokines IL-17A, IL-17F, and IL-22.[5] In the setting of infection, these cells are important in epithelial function and mucosal surface immunity to bacterial or fungal infection, and patients with hyper-IgE syndrome with an IL-17 deficiency have increased susceptibility to *S aureus* infection.[6] Undermining the appropriate development of Th17 cells may be another mechanism of *S aureus* pathogenesis and ability to reinfect hosts after previous infection.[7] Other T-cell subpopulations such as clonotypic TNF/IFNγ-producing γδ T cells may also play a role in cutaneous immunity against *S aureus* infection in preclinical models.[4]

B-cell–mediated humoral immunity has been successfully used in vaccine-mediated strategies to prevent bacterial infections such as *Haemophilus influenzae*. *S aureus* is unique because it is a commensal organism in humans with up to 30% of the population colonized, but also represents the major pathogenic species in many types of infections.[8] The immunodominant antigens in *S aureus* infection in humans and mice are the iron-sensing determinant (Isd) proteins IsdA and IsdB, and components of *S aureus* major autolysin (aminidase and glucosaminidase).[9] IgG titers against *S aureus*–associated proteins are common in healthy humans, and make them challenging for diagnostic purposes because of the high rates of colonization and previous *S aureus* infection.[9] Additionally, the presence of anti–*S aureus* antibodies appears to confer only limited protection against future infection, and vaccine strategies have not been effective in preventing deep *S aureus* infection (see Treatment section).

Evasion of Host Immunity

Bacterial species use different mechanisms to evade host immunity; however, some common patterns are seen. Using *S aureus* as a model organism given its propensity for musculoskeletal infection, we will illustrate the various ways bacteria evade host immunity. *S aureus* utilizes a number of cell-wall-anchored and secreted virulence factors and extracellular matrix binding proteins that promote immunoevasion and biofilm formation (**Table 2**). Biofilm is an aggregate of microorganisms contained within an extracellular matrix. Key steps in this process include counteracting host immune responses such as neutrophil-mediated killing and complement activation, binding to extracellular matrix components including collagen and fibrin, and scavenging nutrients such as iron in the form of heme via the Isd family of proteins.[10]

Table 2. *Staphylococcus aureus* virulence factors

Table 2

Summary of Selected Cell Wall–Anchored and Secreted Proteins Involved in *Staphylococcus aureus* Pathogenesis

Class of Protein	Examples	Function
MSCRAMM family proteins—cell wall anchored	Clumping factor A and B (ClfA and ClfB)	Binds host extracellular matrix components particularly fibrinogen. Degradation of complement (C3b)
	Fibronectin binding protein A and B (FnBpA, FnBpB)	Binds extracellular matrix (fibrinogen, fibrin, elastin)
	Collagen adhesion (CNA)	Binds extracellular matrix (collagen, complement protein C1q), inhibits complement activation
NEAT motif family—cell wall anchored	IsdA, IsdB, IsdH	Iron/heme uptake and transport, binds integrins/extracellular matrix components, provides resistance to neutrophil killing
Three helical bundle—cell wall anchored	Protein A	Binds Fc region of IgG to inhibit opsonophagocytosis; activates platelet aggregation via von Willebrand factor binding; B cell superantigenic activity by cross-linking Fab region of V_H3 bearing IgM; activates TNFR1
	Staphylococcal complement inhibitor (SCIN)	Inhibits complement activation by binding C3 convertases on bacterial surface
Hemolysins	α-Hemolysin (α-toxin, H1a), β-hemolysin, γ-hemolysin	Pore-forming toxin (α-, γ-hemolysin), sphingomyelinase (β-hemolysin). Lyse red blood cells, other leukocytes, epithelial/endothelial cells; alters immune cell signaling pathways involved in cell proliferation, immune response, cytokine expression
Leukocidins	LukAB, LukDE, PVL	Pore-forming toxins. Lyse neutrophils, monocytes, macrophages
Enzymes	Autolysin (AtlA)	Aminidase, glucosaminidase subunits. Peptidoglycan hydrolase. Cell separation, generates extracellular DNA in biofilm matrix
	Aureolysin	Protease. Inactivates PSMs, can activate other proteases
	Staphylokinase	Activates plasminogen to plasmin. Cleaves complement factor C3b
	Nuclease	Inactivate neutrophil extracellular traps (NETs)
Phenol-soluble modulins	δ-Hemolysin, PSMα1–α4	Small amphipathic peptides. Lyse neutrophils, break down biofilm matrix, critical for biofilm disassembly
Superantigenic exotoxins	Toxic shock syndrome toxin	Stimulate T cells nonspecifically without typical antigenic recognition. Can cause toxic shock syndrome. Activates bone resorption, inhibits host immunity in osteomyelitis.
	Staphylococcal enterotoxins (A-E, G)	Activate cytokine release, involved in gastroenteritis, sepsis, kidney injury
Chemotaxis inhibitory protein of *Staphylococcus aureus* (CHIPS)	—	Inhibits neutrophil migration and activation; prevents complement activation

MSCRAMM = microbial surface component recognizing adhesive matrix molecules, NEAT = NEAr-iron transporter (NEAT) domains, PSM = phenol-soluble modulin

Staphylococcal Abscess Communities

The formation of soft-tissue abscesses is one hallmark of musculoskeletal infection and promotes bacterial pathogenesis. For example, *S aureus* is able to form *Staphylococcal* abscess communities (SACs), which create a favorable environment for the organism to thrive while evading host immune responses. SAC formation is a pathogen-driven process characterized by the production of factors that recruit host immune cells to the vicinity of *S aureus* infection. A central, replicating group of bacteria develop and are surrounded by a protective pseudocapsule of fibrin that is created by *S aureus* coagulase cleavage of fibrinogen.[11] A peripheral ring of necrotic neutrophils then forms around the nidus, which are unable to effectively remove the *S aureus* and contribute to soft-tissue injury.[11] *Staphylococcal* virulence proteins such as nuclease and adenosine synthase A convert NETs into products that induce macrophage cytotoxicity, which may be a significant mechanism in protecting bacteria within the SAC.[12] Eventually, these SACs can rupture, releasing the bacterium into the surrounding tissue.[10]

Bacterial Biofilm

Another major mechanism of bacterial evasion of host immunity during musculoskeletal infections includes the formation of biofilm. Biofilms can be seen in many types of musculoskeletal infections including osteomyelitis, septic arthritis, PJIs, and soft-tissue infection. The formation of biofilms evolved as an adaptation to a hostile host environment, protecting bacterial cells from host immune responses such as leukocyte phagocytosis, opsonization, and complement deposition.[13] The first step in biofilm formation is bacterial cell attachment to a host or foreign surface. This is typically mediated by cell wall–anchored proteins that bind extracellular matrix components. Once adherence has occurred, this microcolony or small group of initial adherent cells proliferate and begin producing extracellular matrix. In a mature biofilm, the extracellular matrix comprises the largest proportion by mass and typically consists of polysaccharides (poly-N-acetylglucosamine [PNAG] or polysaccharide intercellular adhesion [PIA] being most well characterized), teichoic acids, proteins, and extracellular nucleic acids (eg, eDNA). This structure protects bacterial cells within the biofilm from immune cell invasion, antibiotic penetration, facilitate nutrient transport, cell-to-cell communication, and provide mechanical stability. Bacterial cells within a biofilm display slower growth rates, mutability, changes to pH, and altered nutritional requirements.[14-16] For example, *S aureus* biofilm contains slow growing persister cells and small colony variant (SCV) cells that display increased antibiotic resistance.[17,18] The final step in biofilm evolution is disassembly, which converts bacteria to their planktonic, or free floating, state. This allows bacterial migration into local and systemic sites. Biofilm disassembly in *S aureus* is regulated by the accessory gene regulator (*agr*) system, which is a well-characterized, two-component peptide quorum-sensing system present in all staphylococci.[19] The key step in this process is increased secretion of autoinducing peptide into the extracellular environment. At a certain threshold concentration, this triggers a cascade of downstream signaling events that leads to upregulation of protease, toxin, and phenol-soluble modulin (PSM) production that act against host defenses and break down biofilm matrix leading to disassembly.[20] In particular, PSMs are surfactant-like peptides that are critical components of the *agr* system and biofilm dispersal in *S aureus*.[21]

Novel Insights in Osteomyelitis

Adult osteomyelitis is characterized by a high rate of treatment failure despite extensive débridement of affected tissue, removal of any implants or foreign material, and intravenous antibiotic therapy. One possible explanation for these failures is the presence of previously unappreciated bacterial reservoirs. For example, *S aureus* has recently been shown in recent studies to colonize submicron cracks and canaliculi in both human and murine cases of chronic osteomyelitis, making it difficult for host immune cells to access the bacteria.[22,23] This challenges the historical dogma that *S aureus* is a nonmotile cocci ~1 µm in diameter, and the authors of a 2017 study showed that this canalicular colonization appears to be an active process involving bacterial deformation and replication.[22] Additionally, *S aureus* can persist within multiple cell types including neutrophils and macrophages after phagocytosis, which may serve as an additional reservoir of bacterial cells in chronic infections, in addition to colonizing other cell types such as osteoblasts, osteocytes, and epithelial cells.[24-26]

Bacterial Resistance Mechanisms

Bacterial resistance to antibiotic therapies has become a worldwide public health crisis. For instance, over 50% of *S aureus* bone and joint infections may be caused by methicillin-resistant strains in some geographic locations. Resistant genes in bacteria can be transferred through conjugation (direct transfer from one cell to another), transduction (gene transfer through a bacteriophage virus), and transformation (uptake of naked free DNA). Both conjugation and transduction play important roles in conferring *S aureus* resistance. *S aureus* carries its antibiotic resistant genes on its mobile genetic elements, which compose 15% to 20% of the genome and are highly variable in contrast to the core genome.[27] For example, staphylococcal chromosome cassettes (SCCs) are mobile genetic elements that insert into the *rlmH* gene.[27] The methicillin-resistance gene *mecA* is common in SCCs and provides resistance to β-lactams in MRSA stains.[27] Additionally, plasmids provide resistance to antibiotics such as erythromycin, chloramphenicol, tetracycline, β-lactams, aminoglycosides, and macrolides in staphylococcal species.[27]

Basic Science

Treatment of Musculoskeletal Infection: Novel Treatment Strategies and Therapeutic Targets

Systemic Antimicrobial Therapy

Antibiotics

Systemic antibiotic therapy is a critical component of curative treatment for musculoskeletal infection. Antibiotic resistance has increased across bacterial species and remains a significant treatment challenge. Additionally, the minimum inhibitory concentrations (MIC) used as susceptibility tests for cultured bacteria when selecting antibiotics for systemic treatment do not reflect the susceptibility of the bacteria within a biofilm, which can require many fold higher concentrations than the MIC to achieve the minimum biofilm eradication concentration (MBEC). Therefore, some novel antibiotic strategies and antimicrobial agents have been used to expand treatment options.

Optimal antibiotic selection should include activity against biofilm-embedded bacteria and metabolically quiescent SCVs. One current strategy that illustrates this principle is the addition of rifampicin to treat staphylococcal infections. Rifampicin has anti-staphylococcal biofilm activity; however, when given as a monotherapy, rapid resistance develops. In contrast, when used in combination with other anti-staphylococcal antibiotics such as beta-lactams, fluoroquinolones, and vancomycin improved in vivo and in vitro eradication is seen relative to monotherapy alone.[28,29] Another therapeutic strategy to combat antibiotic resistance is the development of novel therapeutic agents. Daptomycin, a cyclic lipopeptide, and linezolid, an oxazolidinone, are examples of novel antibiotics with broad-spectrum activity against resistant gram-positive organisms, and these have expanded treatment options in the setting of antibiotic resistance in the past decade. Next-generation oxazolidinones such as tedizolid and lipoglycopeptides like oritavancin or dalbavancin have been developed in recent years to further expand treatment options in the setting of antibiotic resistant gram-positive infections, as discussed in a 2016 review article.[30] Additionally, increased oral bioavailability (linezolid, tedizolid) or prolonged half-life (oritavancin, dalbavancin) may change the dosing strategies used relative to older-generation antibiotics, allowing for oral treatment regimens or less frequent dosing periods. Continued development of novel antimicrobial agents is necessary to keep pace with bacterial resistance profiles.

Silver

Improving the biofilm resistance of existing implant materials would both serve as primary prevention of PJI and reduce rates of treatment failure. Silver-based implant coatings have shown some promise in preclinical and limited clinical studies in orthopaedic trauma and limb reconstruction.[31-33] For example, a silver-coated megaprosthesis (Alguna) reduced rates of postoperative infection (11.8% vs 22.4%) and had improved success after débridement and implant retention relative to titanium implants in a small case-control study.[32] Concerns about local and systemic silver toxicity to surrounding tissues have led to alternative approaches such as additive manufacturing or nanoparticle-based delivery strategies to retain the antimicrobial efficacy while reducing potential off-target effects.[34]

Novel Local Delivery Mechanisms

The development of novel antibiotic or small molecule delivery systems may be a successful strategy to reduce biofilm formation on orthopaedic implants and treat local infection. Antibiotic eluting beads are one strategy that has been used clinically to treat confirmed or suspected osteomyelitis; however, strong clinical evidence regarding their use is scarce. The efficacy of absorbable antibiotic-containing beads in PJI remains controversial. According to a 2017 study, antibiotic-impregnated calcium sulfate beads did not improve outcomes after débridement and implant retention in acute hematogenous or acute postoperative PJI.[35]

Other strategies involving novel delivery systems have typically not progressed beyond the preclinical stages. One possibility is to increase the local concentration of antimicrobials without impairing host cell function or binding to the implant surface. Covalent bonding of an antibiotic to titanium may reduce biofilm formation on the implant without impairing osseointegration and host cell attachment.[36] Surface modifications that enhance osseointegration of titanium in combination with antibiotic coatings may be another strategy to increase biofilm resistance while promoting host cell adhesion to the exclusion of bacterial cell adhesion.[37] Use of antibiotic carriers such as hydrogels or phosphatidylcholine-based materials may allow the point-of-care application of implant coatings that elute antibiotics from the implant surface and provide local antibiotic delivery.[38-40]

Immunotherapy Strategies

Immunotherapy is another major area of interest as a complementary treatment in orthopaedic infection. Successful vaccines have been developed for certain strains of bacterial infections such as in *H influenzae* and *Streptococcus pneumoniae*. Active immunization strategies using vaccines have been attempted for common sources of musculoskeletal infection such as *S aureus*; however, these have not been successful beyond phase I clinical trials.[41-43] Vaccine strategies targeting components of the cell wall that are not universally expressed across strains such as poly-N-acetyl glucosamine, LTA acid, and capsular polysaccharides have failed.[41,44] Another vaccine from Merck (V710) showed preclinical promise by targeting IsdB; however, this strategy failed to reduce infection rates or mortality in a phase 2b/3 trial, which focused on prevention of *S aureus* infection after cardiothoracic surgery.[42] Interestingly, increased rates of mortality due to sepsis was found in patients who did get infected in the vaccine group, suggesting that this vaccine may have been detrimental to host immunity to *S aureus*.[42]

Passive immunization strategies may show more promise than vaccine-based approaches; however, these are mostly in preclinical stages of development. For example, to target biofilm, a monoclonal antibody (mAb) to DNA-binding proteins from the DNABII family was developed, which have conserved homologs across many bacterial species.[45] When used in combination with daptomycin systemic therapy, this reduced both planktonic and adherent bacteria in a murine implant-associated infection model relative to daptomycin monotherapy.[45] Alternatively, a combination of monoclonal antibodies to α-toxin and ClfA were used to target biofilm formation and resulted in decreased colony-forming units from bone/joint tissue, reduced propensity for infection, and less biofilm aggregates in a murine model of hematogenous MRSA infection.[46] Other passive immunotherapy strategies have targeted the glucosaminidase (Gmd) subunit of autolysin (Atl).[47,48] Other preclinical models have focused on intracellular reservoirs of *S aureus*. For example, one group used an antibody-antibiotic conjugate (AAC) that consists of a monoclonal antibody recognizing specific sugars on wall teichoic acids bound to rifamycin class derivative antibiotic.[49] This AAC binds to the surface of *S aureus*.[49] When opsonization occurs, the proteolytic environment of the phagolysosome of the host cell causes release of the active antibiotic form.[49] This AAC demonstrated improved results relative to systemic vancomycin alone in a murine MRSA hematogenous infection model.[49]

Dispersal Agents

Dispersal of biofilm is another major focus for antimicrobial therapeutics. Converting biofilm bacteria to planktonic form may increase bacterial cell susceptibility to common antibiotics. Enzymatic treatments such as trypsin, dispersin B, lysostaphin, and DNases can lead to dispersal of staphylococci from biofilm.[50] Studies have shown that fibrinolytics like streptokinase or nattokinase decrease the MBEC of available systemic antibiotics by breaking down biofilm-associated fibrin matrix.[50,51] Targeting the quorum-sensing system is another strategy to trigger biofilm dispersal, and autoinducing peptide type I treatment in vitro was able to trigger dispersal of MRSA on titanium disks.[51] One concern regarding dispersal agents is that bacterial cells disassembled from their biofilms are more capable of systemic infection in other locations in the body. Therefore, it is likely that dispersal agents must be used in combination with systemic therapies such as antibiotics.[50]

Summary

Musculoskeletal infections remain challenging to treat. Bacterial mechanisms to evade host immunity, formation of biofilm, and antibiotic resistance all contribute to difficulties in treating these infections. New antibiotics targeting resistant organisms and novel therapeutic strategies including immunotherapy and advancements in local delivery systems may all provide new therapeutic interventions in affected patients.

Key Study Points

- Staphylococcus species are most common organisms in adult musculoskeletal infections with the exception of diabetic foot ulcers, where polymicrobial and gram-negative infections are common, and prosthetic shoulder infection, where Propionibacterium acnes is most common.
- Multiple virulence factors contribute to bacterial pathogenesis in musculoskeletal infection including allowing adhesion and avoiding host immunity, particularly the innate immune system.
- Formation of biofilm is a pathogen-driven process with multiple virulence factors playing important roles. Key events include adhesion, formation of extracellular matrix, and dispersal.
- Possible therapeutic strategies in the future include novel antibiotics that act against resistant organisms or have improved pharmacokinetic properties, active or passive immunotherapy, improved local delivery mechanisms, and dispersal agents for biofilm.

Annotated References

1. Rigby KM, DeLeo FR: Neutrophils in innate host defense against *Staphylococcus aureus* infections. *Semin Immunopathol* 2012;34(2):237-259.
2. Brinkmann V, Reichard U, Goosmann C, et al: Neutrophil extracellular traps kill bacteria. *Science* 2004; 303(5663):1532-1535.
3. Yuen J, Pluthero FG, Douda DN, et al: NETosing neutrophils activate complement both on their own NETs and bacteria via alternative and non-alternative pathways. *Front Immunol* 2016;7:137.

   This was an in vitro study, which found that neutrophils deposit complement factor P onto NETs and *Pseudomonas aeruginosa*, that NET-mediated complement activation occurred by both the alternative pathway and nonalternative pathway mechanisms, and that complement activation by the alternative pathway only was dependent on complement factor P contributing to our knowledge about the interaction between neutrophils, complement cascade, and NETs.
4. Dillen CA, Pinsker BL, Marusina AI, et al: Clonally expanded γδ T cells protect against *Staphylococcus aureus* skin reinfection. *J Clin Invest* 2018;128(3):1026-1042.

   Using a mouse model of *Staphylococcus aureus* skin infection, the authors show that clonally expanded TNF- and IFN-γ-producing γδ T cells may represent a mechanism for long-lasting immunity against recurrent *S aureus* skin infections.
5. Karauzum H, Datta SK: Adaptive immunity against *Staphylococcus aureus*. *Curr Top Microbiol Immunol* 2017; 409:419-439.

   This is a review article focusing on the complex and sometimes contradictory role of the adaptive immune system in influencing host susceptibility and immunity against *S aureus*.
6. Milner JD, Brenchley JM, Laurence A, et al: Impaired T(H)17 cell differentiation in subjects with autosomal dominant hyper-IgE syndrome. *Nature* 2008;452(7188):773-776.
7. Sanchez M, Kolar SL, Muller S et al: O-acetylation of peptidoglycan limits helper T cell priming and permits *Staphylococcus aureus* reinfection. *Cell Host Microbe* 2017;22(4):543-551.e4.

   Impaired immunity to *S aureus* reinfection was associated with an impaired Th17 response and a robust IL-10 response in a murine model. The authors showed that O-acetylation of peptidoglycan by *S aureus* limits the induction of cytokines used for Th17 polarization. In this study, IL-10 deficiency restored protective immunity in a murine model. Adjuvancy with a staphylococcal peptidoglycan O-acetyltransferase mutant reduced IL-10 and promoted development of IL-17–dependent Th cell–transferable protective immunity.
8. Graham PL III, Lin SX, Larson EL: A U.S. population-based survey of *Staphylococcus aureus* colonization. *Ann Intern Med* 2006;144(5):318-325.
9. Nishitani K, Beck CA, Rosenberg AF, Kates SL, Schwarz EM, Daiss JL: A diagnostic serum antibody test for patients with *Staphylococcus aureus* osteomyelitis. *Clin Orthop Relat Res* 2015;473(9):2735-2749.
10. Cheng AG, DeDent AC, Schneewind O, Missiakas D: A play in four acts: Staphylococcus aureus abscess formation. *Trends Microbiol* 2011;19(5):225-232.
11. Cheng AG, Kim HK, Burts ML, Krausz T, Schneewind O, Missiakas DM: Genetic requirements for *Staphylococcus aureus* abscess formation and persistence in host tissues. *FASEB J* 2009;23(10):3393-3404.
12. Thammavongsa V, Missiakas DM, Schneewind O: *Staphylococcus aureus* degrades neutrophil extracellular traps to promote immune cell death. *Science* 2013;342(6160):863-866.
13. Hall-Stoodley L, Costerton JW, Stoodley P: Bacterial biofilms: From the natural environment to infectious diseases. *Nat Rev Microbiol* 2004;2(2):95-108.
14. Anderl JN, Franklin MJ, Stewart PS: Role of antibiotic penetration limitation in *Klebsiella pneumoniae* biofilm resistance to ampicillin and ciprofloxacin. *Antimicrob Agents Chemother* 2000;44(7):1818-1824.
15. Jefferson KK, Goldmann DA, Pier GB: Use of confocal microscopy to analyze the rate of vancomycin penetration through *Staphylococcus aureus* biofilms. *Antimicrob Agents Chemother* 2005;49(6):2467-2473.
16. Zheng Z, Stewart PS: Penetration of rifampin through *Staphylococcus epidermidis* biofilms. *Antimicrob Agents Chemother* 2002;46(3):900-903.
17. de la Fuente-Núñez C, Reffuveille F, Fernández L, Hancock RE: Bacterial biofilm development as a multicellular adaptation: Antibiotic resistance and new therapeutic strategies. *Curr Opin Microbiol* 2013;16(5):580-589.
18. Garcia LG, Lemaire S, Kahl BC, et al: Antibiotic activity against small-colony variants of Staphylococcus aureus: Review of in vitro, animal and clinical data. *J Antimicrob Chemother* 2013;68(7):1455-1464.
19. Novick RP, Geisinger E: Quorum sensing in staphylococci. *Annu Rev Genet* 2008;42:541-564.
20. Mann EE, Rice KC, Boles BR, et al: Modulation of eDNA release and degradation affects *Staphylococcus aureus* biofilm maturation. *PLoS One* 2009 ;4(6):e5822.
21. Periasamy S, Joo HS, Duong AC, et al: How *Staphylococcus aureus* biofilms develop their characteristic structure. *Proc Natl Acad Sci USA* 2012;109(4):1281-1286.
22. de Mesy Bentley KL, Trombetta R, Nishitani K, et al: Evidence of *Staphylococcus aureus* deformation, proliferation, and migration in canaliculi of live cortical bone in murine models of osteomyelitis. *J Bone Miner Res* 2017;32(5):985-990.

    Using a mouse model of *Staphylococcus aureus* osteomyelitis, the authors showed via transmission electron microscopy that *S aureus* can deform, enter the canalicular system, and migrate toward osteocyte lacunae via proliferation at the leading edge, creating a reservoir that is difficult to access by the immune system and providing new insight into why these infections may be so difficult to treat.

23. de Mesy Bentley KL, MacDonald A, Schwarz EM, Oh I: Chronic osteomyelitis with Staphylococcus aureus deformation in submicron canaliculi of osteocytes: A case report. *JBJS Case Connect* 2018;8(1):e8.

The authors showed in human chronic osteomyelitis resulting from a diabetic foot ulcer, there was evidence of *S aureus* colonization of the osteocytic-canalicular network using transmission electron microscopy. Level of evidence: IV.

24. Sinha B, Herrmann M, Krause KH: Is *Staphylococcus aureus* an intracellular pathogen? *Trends Microbiol* 2000;8(8):343-344.

25. Strobel M, Pförtner H, Tuchscherr L, et al: Post-invasion events after infection with *Staphylococcus aureus* are strongly dependent on both the host cell type and the infecting *S. aureus* strain. *Clin Microbiol Infect* 2016;22(9):799-809.

This study examined the response of different host cell types to multiple different strains of *S aureus*. Barrier cells took up high amounts of bacteria and were killed by aggressive strains. These strains expressed high levels of toxins and possessed the ability to escape from phagolysosomes. Osteoblasts and keratinocytes ingested less bacteria and were not killed, even though the primary osteoblasts were strongly activated by *S aureus*. In all cell types *S aureus* was able to persist.

26. Yang D, Wijenayaka AR, Solomon LB, et al: Novel insights into Staphylococcus aureus deep bone infections: The involvement of osteocytes. *mBio* 2018;9(2). pii:e00415-18.

The authors show that *S aureus* can infect and reside in human osteocytes without causing cell death both in vitro and ex vivo from patients with PJI. They also show that *S aureus* adapts during intracellular infection of osteocytes by becoming quasi-dormant small-colony variants (SCVs), which might contribute to persistent or silent infection.

27. Haaber J, Penadés JR, Ingmer H: Transfer of antibiotic resistance in *Staphylococcus aureus*. *Trends Microbiol* 2017;25(11):893-905.

This study is a review article illustrating the different mechanisms by which *S aureus* transfers antibiotic resistance.

28. Jørgensen NP, Skovdal SM, Meyer RL, Dagnæs-Hansen F, Fuursted K, Petersen E: Rifampicin-containing combinations are superior to combinations of vancomycin, linezolid and daptomycin against *Staphylococcus aureus* biofilm infection in vivo and in vitro. *Pathog Dis* 2016;74(4):ftw019.

In a mouse model of *S aureus* osteomyelitis, rifampicin-containing antibiotic combinations reduced bacterial load in the peri-implant bone most effectively.

29. Zimmerli W, Widmer AF, Blatter M, Frei R, Ochsner PE: Role of rifampin for treatment of orthopedic implant-related staphylococcal infections: A randomized controlled trial. Foreign-body infection (FBI) study group. *J Am Med Assoc* 1998;279(19):1537-1541.

30. Crotty MP, Krekel T, Burnham CA, Ritchie DJ: New gram-positive agents: The next generation of oxazolidinones and lipoglycopeptides. *J Clin Microbiol* 2016;54(9):2225-2232. Epub 2016 March 9.

The authors present a review article on the next generation of oxazolidinone and lipoglycopeptide antibiotic classes. These are active against resistant gram-positive infections.

31. Hardes J, von Eiff C, Streitbuerger A, et al: Reduction of periprosthetic infection with silver-coated megaprostheses in patients with bone sarcoma. *J Surg Oncol* 2010;101(5):389-395.

32. Wafa H, Grimer RJ, Reddy K, et al: Retrospective evaluation of the incidence of early periprosthetic infection with silver-treated endoprostheses in high-risk patients: Case-control study. *Bone Joint Lett J* 2015;97-B(2):252-257.

33. Alt V: Antimicrobial coated implants in trauma and orthopaedics-a clinical review and risk-benefit analysis. *Injury* 2017;48(3):599-607.

This was a systematic review article examining the use of antibiotic-coated implants in trauma and reconstructive orthopaedic procedures. The authors reviewed case series (7) and case control (2) studies looking at gentamicin poly(D, L-lactide) coating for tibial nails, silver coating for tumor endoprostheses, and a povidone-iodine coating for titanium implants. They conclude that the risk benefit ratio is favorable for the use of these technologies based on existing data. Level of evidence: IV.

34. van Hengel IAJ, Riool M, Fratila-Apachitei LE, et al: Selective laser melting porous metallic implants with immobilized silver nanoparticles kill and prevent biofilm formation by methicillin-resistant *Staphylococcus aureus*. *Biomaterials* 2017;140:1-15.

Silver nanoparticle–based treatment of a porous titanium implant resulted in strong antimicrobial activity without signs of cytotoxicity in a mouse model of methicillin-resistant *Staphylococcus aureus* infection.

35. Flierl MA, Culp BM, Okroj KT, Springer BD, Levine BR, Della Valle CJ: Poor outcomes of irrigation and debridement in acute periprosthetic joint infection with antibiotic-impregnated calcium sulfate beads. *J Arthroplasty* 2017;32(8):2505-2507.

In this case series, the authors examined the role of antibiotic-impregnated calcium sulfate beads in the setting of acute prosthetic joint infection of the hip and knee treated with irrigation, débridement with implant retention. At a mean 12.7 months, 16 of 33 (48%) patients failed this treatment despite the use of antibiotic-impregnated beads. This suggests that antibiotic-impregnated beads may not improve outcomes of DAIR. Level of evidence: IV.

36. Kucharíková S, Gerits E, De Brucker K, et al: Covalent immobilization of antimicrobial agents on titanium prevents *Staphylococcus aureus* and *Candida albicans* colonization and biofilm formation. *J Antimicrob Chemother* 2016;71(4):936-945.

The authors showed that covalent immobilization of vancomycin and caspofungin onto titanium substrates reduced in vivo and in vitro biofilm formation in the setting of *S aureus* and *C albicans* infection. The covalent immobilization of the antibiotics did not jeopardize osseointegration of the titanium.

Basic Science

37. Diefenbeck M, Schrader C, Gras F, et al: Gentamicin coating of plasma chemical oxidized titanium alloy prevents implant-related osteomyelitis in rats. *Biomaterials* 2016;101:156-164.

The authors showed that two types of gentamicin coating of a macroporous titanium oxide surface resulted in decreased rates of implant contamination with biofilm, reduced histological osteomyelitis scores, and reduced radiographic osteomyelitis scores in vivo.

38. Drago L, Boot W, Dimas K, et al: Does implant coating with antibacterial-loaded hydrogel reduce bacterial colonization and biofilm formation in vitro?. *Clin Orthop Relat Res* 2014;472(11):3311-3323.

39. Giavaresi G, Meani E, Sartori M, et al: Efficacy of antibacterial-loaded coating in an in vivo model of acutely highly contaminated implant. *Int Orthop* 2014;38(7):1505-1512.

40. Jennings JA, Carpenter DP, Troxel KS, et al: Novel antibiotic-loaded point-of-care implant coating inhibits biofilm. *Clin Orthop Relat Res* 2015;473(7):2270-2282.

41. Bhattacharya M, Wozniak DJ, Stoodley P, Hall-Stoodley L: Prevention and treatment of *Staphylococcus aureus* biofilms. *Expert Rev Anti Infect Ther* 2015;13(12):1499-1516.

42. Fowler VG, Allen KB, Moreira ED, et al: Effect of an investigational vaccine for preventing Staphylococcus aureus infections after cardiothoracic surgery: A randomized trial. *J Am Med Assoc* 2013;309(13):1368-1378.

43. McNeely TB, Shah NA, Fridman A, et al: Mortality among recipients of the Merck V710 Staphylococcus aureus vaccine after postoperative S. aureus infections: An analysis of possible contributing host factors. *Hum Vaccin Immunother* 2014;10(12):3513-3516.

44. Shinefield H, Black S, Fattom A, et al: Use of a *Staphylococcus aureus* conjugate vaccine in patients receiving hemodialysis. *N Engl J Med* 2002;346(7):491-496.

45. Estellés A, Woischnig AK, Liu K, et al: A high-affinity native human antibody disrupts biofilm from *Staphylococcus aureus* bacteria and potentiates antibiotic efficacy in a mouse implant infection model. *Antimicrob Agents Chemother* 2016;60(4):2292-2301.

The authors examine the use of human monoclonal antibody to DNABII homologs (a key component supporting eDNA in biofilm) from both gram-positive and gram-negative bacteria. This antibody showed efficacy in disrupting established biofilm in vitro. It reduced adherent bacterial cell counts in murine tissue cage infection model in combination with antibiotic treatment better than antibiotic treatment alone.

46. Wang Y, Cheng LI, Helfer DR, et al: Mouse model of hematogenous implant-related *Staphylococcus aureus* biofilm infection reveals therapeutic targets. *Proc Natl Acad Sci USA* 2017;114(26):E5094-E5102.

Using a murine hematogenous implant-related infection model, the authors demonstrated that a combination of neutralizing human monoclonal antibodies against α-toxin and ClfA inhibited in vitro biofilm formation, propensity for infection in vivo, and reduced bacterial burden in vivo.

47. Varrone JJ, de Mesy Bentley KL, Bello-Irizarry SN, et al: Passive immunization with anti-glucosaminidase monoclonal antibodies protects mice from implant-associated osteomyelitis by mediating opsonophagocytosis of *Staphylococcus aureus* megaclusters. *J Orthop Res* 2014;32(10):1389-1396.

48. Yokogawa N, Ishikawa M, Nishitani K, et al: Immunotherapy synergizes with debridement and antibiotic therapy in a murine 1-stage exchange model of MRSA implant-associated osteomyelitis. *J Orthop Res* 2018;36(6):1590-1598.

Using a murine implant–associated infection model, the authors found that immunotherapy with anti-Gmd monoclonal antibodies inhibited SACs while vancomycin reduced CFUs on the implant. Combination therapy provided the best results in soft tissue and implant infection control.

49. Lehar SM, Pillow T, Xu M, et al: Novel antibody-antibiotic conjugate eliminates intracellular *S. aureus*. *Nature* 2015;527(7578):323-328.

50. Hogan S, O'Gara JP, O'Neill E: Novel treatment of *Staphylococcus aureus* device-related infections using fibrinolytic agents. *Antimicrob Agents Chemother* 2018;62(2). pii:e02008-17.

The authors tested the use of multiple fibrinolytic agents against *S aureus* biofilms in vivo and in vitro. These fibrinolytic agents were able to disperse established biofilms and demonstrated no cytotoxicity, suggesting that they may be a valuable adjuvant treatment to device-related infections in addition to systemic antibiotics.

51. Jørgensen NP, Zobek N, Dreier C, et al: Streptokinase treatment reverses biofilm-associated antibiotic resistance in *Staphylococcus aureus*. *Microorganisms* 2016;4(3). pii:E36.

The authors show that streptokinase, which is a fibrinolytic agent, was able to disperse *S aureus* biofilm in vitro at physiologically relevant concentrations.

Section 3
Trauma

EDITOR

Robert V. O'Toole, MD

Chapter 17
Polytrauma Care

Heather A. Vallier, MD

ABSTRACT

Trauma algorithms using Advanced Trauma Life Support have improved care of injured persons. Specialty providers collaborate to optimize care, both in the case of an injured individual and in the case of iterative process improvements within trauma systems. Orthopaedic surgeons are key contributors, as reduction and stabilization of fractures and dislocations promote pain relief and facilitate mobility from bed. Fracture fixation can also reduce ongoing hemorrhage, thus contributing to resuscitation. Definitive fixation of most unstable axial, pelvic, and femoral fractures in resuscitated patients reduces pulmonary, thrombotic, and other complications and minimizes length of hospital stay. Patients in extremis may benefit from a damage control strategy, when possible, as this may provide bony stability without generating more hemorrhage and without contributing to systemic dysfunction. New practices including REBOA and TEG-based resuscitation are enhancing survival after massive hemorrhage from trauma.

Keywords: damage control; fixation; resuscitation; polytrauma

Introduction

Most trauma-related deaths are associated with closed head injuries or exsanguination, often at the scene of the injury. Survivors are at risk for various life-threatening complications, many of which are directly related to their musculoskeletal injuries. Trauma care has evolved to expedite assessment and resuscitation in the prehospital setting and within the minutes following arrival to a trauma center. Musculoskeletal injuries often play a large role in the initial burden of hemorrhage. Essential principles include multidisciplinary assessment, resuscitation, and provisional management of fractures and dislocations. Type and timing of orthopaedic treatment will vary depending on the response to resuscitation, and the scope and complexity of injuries to all systems.

Dr. Vallier or an immediate family member serves as a board member, owner, officer, or committee member of the Orthopaedic Trauma Association.

Initial Assessment of the Trauma Patient

The American College of Surgeons has developed advanced trauma life support (ATLS) algorithms for initial evaluation and resuscitation of the trauma patient.[1] These familiar protocols involve primary, secondary, and tertiary surveys of the patient. The primary survey is still a stepwise evaluation of **A**irway, **B**reathing, **C**irculation, **D**isability, and **E**xposure. This primary survey is followed by a secondary survey in which a detailed history and physical examination is completed. The tertiary survey involves serial evaluations during the initial hospital course.

The primary survey has changed little in recent years and is designed to identify the location and severity of most injuries, with an emphasis on life-threatening conditions. The airway is secured, using oral or nasal intubation as indicated. Severe head injuries and/or facial fractures are two conditions often necessitating emergent intubation. The cervical spine should remain immobilized during this time. Breathing is assessed by physical examination, and supplemental oxygen is delivered as needed. Patients with evolving chest or neck injuries may require emergent assistance, employing techniques such as mechanical ventilation, tube thoracostomy for pneumothorax, or pericardiocentesis for effusion. Continuous reassessment of circulation is critical including peripheral perfusion by palpating pulses and monitoring vital signs, as well as end-organ perfusion by monitoring hypo-oxygenation and resultant acidemia. The orthopaedic surgeon may play a key role in the initial assessment and care of the patient. Their presence will promote communication about injury severity and treatment goals. Initial wound management and reduction of fractures and dislocations should be undertaken.

Shock and Resuscitation: Assessment and Initial Management

Inadequate end-organ perfusion defines shock. There are four types of shock: hypovolemic, cardiogenic, obstructive, and septic.[1] Most musculoskeletal injuries are associated with hemorrhage (**Table 1**), and hypovolemic shock is most frequently encountered in trauma patients, especially those with pelvis and long bone fractures. Shock results in tissue hypoperfusion, hypoxemia, inflammation, and immune dysfunction.[2] It is displayed as tachycardia, then by hypotension[3]. Reduction and fixation of fractures is thought to promote control of hemorrhage and aids in resuscitation of a patient in hypovolemic shock. Cardiogenic shock is caused by inadequate heart function. Most often this results from myocardial infarction, due to preexisting disease; however, blunt cardiac injury may contribute. Presence of cardiogenic shock is manifested by hypotension, then bradycardia. Spinal cord injuries may cause neurogenic shock.[4] Loss of sympathetic tone results in hypotension and bradycardia, which can be confusing, as it is often concurrent with other injuries, which generate hemorrhage. Failure to respond to fluid resuscitation should be rapidly noted, and judicious usage of inotropic agents may be necessary.

Injuries to Other Systems: Assessment and Initial Management

Injury Severity Score

The Injury Severity Score (ISS) is an anatomic, validated scoring system that is used to predict mortality.[5] The ISS score is a value from 0 to 75. Each body area is graded for severity using the Abbreviated Injury Scale (AIS), and the sum of the squares of the scores of the three highest areas quantifies the overall injury (**Table 2**). Only the highest AIS score in each body region is used. Limitations of the ISS include difficulty calculating it during an initial evaluation, as the extent of injuries may not be appreciated. The ISS also does not take into account multiple injuries over a single body area. The New Injury Severity Score (NISS) was developed to include the three highest scores, regardless of anatomic area, and has been shown to be potentially more predictive of survival than ISS.[6]

Head Injury

Primary traumatic brain injury results directly from the traumatic event via tissue injury or hematoma formation. Secondary injuries, which are commonly iatrogenic, occur subsequently and include hypoxia, hypotension, seizures, fevers, and hypoglycemia, which impede recovery from the primary injury. Maintenance of euvolemia and normothermia will mitigate secondary injury.[7] Traumatic cerebral edema generates increased intracranial pressures (ICPs) that can further injure the brain. Hyperosmolar therapy, hyperventilation, and elevation of the head of bed, may all aid in reduction of ICP. Hypertension and bradycardia in this setting suggest impending herniation, and immediate interventions are required based on the specific injury.

Chest Injury

Chest injuries are very common in polytrauma patients. Chest injuries are painful and cause splinting and poor inspiratory effort in conscious patients. Recumbency results in poor ventilation, and narcotic medications suppress respiratory drive. Both increase the risk of pulmonary complications. Direct parenchymal lung damage

Table 1

Classification for Hemorrhagic Shock in a 70 kg Male[1]

	Class 1	Class 2	Class 3	Class 4
Blood loss (mL)	Up to 750	750-1,500	1,500-2000	>2000
Blood loss (% of volume)	Up to 15%	15%-40%	30%-50%	>40%
Heart rate	<100	>100	>129	>140
Blood pressure	Normal	Normal	Decreased	Decreased
Pulse pressure (mmHg)	Normal	Decreased	Decreased	Decreased
Respiratory rate	14-20	20-30	30-40	>40
Urine output (mL/hr)	>30	20-30	5-15	Negligible
Mental status	Slightly anxious	Mildly anxious	Confused	Lethargic

Table 2

Injury Severity Score (ISS) is Determined by Identifying the Three Most Injured Areas, Then Determining the Severity of Each as Defined by the Abbreviated Injury Scale (AIS) Designated as A, B, and C.[5] The ISS = $A^2 + B^2 + C^2$

AIS body areas
Soft tissue
Head and neck
Chest
Abdomen
Extremity and/or pelvis
AIS severity code
1 = Minor
2 = Moderate
3 = Severe (non–life-threatening)
4 = Severe (life-threatening)
5 = Critical (survival uncertain)
6 = Fatal

in patients with pulmonary contusions and other severe chest trauma will further diminish oxygenation within the days after injury. Tube thoracostomy will alleviate pneumothoraces and hemothoraces. Reduction and stabilization of axial and extremity fractures promote pain relief, upright posture, and mobility from bed, all of which reduce risks of pulmonary and other complications.

Rib fixation techniques have been recently described to provide mechanical support for ventilation and to relieve pain. Indications are evolving, but could include three or more ribs with severe bicortical displacement or within a flail segment.[8] A recent study indicates less mechanical ventilation time, shorter hospital stay, less pneumonia, and lower mortality after rib fixation.[8]

Abdominal Injury

Abdominal injuries occur commonly, and treatment over the past decade has become more nonsurgical.[9] Selective angiography and embolization for solid organ injury, such as the liver or spleen, is also more common.[10] Hepatic bleeding may be exacerbated by surgical exploration; however, some severe abdominal injuries may be better managed surgically. Persistent active bleeding within the spleen or kidney, pseudoaneurysms, or renovascular pedicle avulsions are surgical indications.

Pelvic Injury

Very large forces are required to disrupt the stability of the pelvis. Associated injuries and blood loss depend on the fracture pattern, based on the direction of impact. Certain pelvic fractures can be associated with blood loss of several liters, related to magnitude of displacement of the posterior pelvic ring. Anterior-posterior compression injuries with complete disruption of the posterior ring or vertical shear injuries may be associated with life-threatening hemorrhage. Emergent circumferential pelvic reduction with a sheet or binder reduces the pelvic ring diameter toward normal and promotes tamponade of venous bleeding.[11] Distal femoral skeletal traction can further improve ring alignment for patients with cephalad displacement of one hemipelvis. In up to 10% of mechanically unstable pelvic fractures major arterial bleeding is present.[12] Such a patient will typically not respond to pelvis reduction and fluid resuscitation. Emergent angiography and embolization or pelvic packing are lifesaving measures.[1] Early reports suggest utility of resuscitative endovascular balloon occlusion of the aorta (REBOA) in reducing mortality from exsanguination after major intrapelvic, abdominal, and/or proximal lower extremity injury.[13,14] It can be a temporizing measure until arterial embolization or surgical control of hemorrhage is possible. Adverse consequences related to REBOA have been infrequently reported, including distal tissue necrosis and renal failure.

Open fractures, urogenital trauma, and gastrointestinal injury in conjunction with pelvic fractures are infrequent and are also considered surgical emergencies. Mortality of open pelvic fractures has been up to 50% in some studies. Control of bleeding by emergently packing open wounds is likely the most important initial measure unique to open pelvis fractures. Patients with posterior or perineal wounds or rectal trauma can be treated with a diverting colostomy to eliminate fecal contamination.[15] Extraperitoneal bladder tears are often repaired if the patient receives open fixation of the anterior pelvic ring.[16] Urethral injuries are diagnosed with retrograde urethrogram before attempting Foley catheter insertion. Catheter realignment, with or without endoscopic guidance, is the preferred definitive management of urethral tears.

Emergent and Urgent Orthopaedic Management

Open Wounds

Open fractures are classified by their severity of soft-tissue injury and amount of contamination (see Chapter 18).[1] Despite controversy regarding risk associated with surgical delay, urgent débridement and irrigation in the operating room is still recommended and is generally combined with provisional or definitive fixation, as soon as is safely possible. Stabilization of an open fracture provides support to the surrounding soft tissues and decreases the risk of infection. Occasionally, provisional external fixation is preferred, because of massive contamination, surgical delay, or systemic instability, eg, severe hemorrhage or head injury.

Reduction of Fractures and Dislocations

Displaced fractures should be reduced and immobilized. Pelvic ring injuries with widening of the pelvic diameter and hemodynamic instability are reduced urgently via circumferential sheeting, but this treatment should also be considered for hemodynamically stable patients to reduce pain.[11] Femoral shaft fractures and some high-energy proximal femoral fractures benefit from application of skeletal traction to restore length and to provide relief of pain and spasm.[17] Dislocated joints cause pain and may result in neurologic and/or vascular compromise. Dislocations should be reduced urgently when possible and stabilized as indicated to prevent recurrence. Closed reductions are possible in most cases; however, some dislocations are most safely undertaken in the operating room under general anesthesia to provide muscular paralysis and to promote safe airway management.

Timing and Principles of Management of Orthopaedic Injury

Benefits of Early Care

Expeditious reduction and fixation of fractures may promote control of hemorrhage and further resuscitation of the patient. Initial provisional reduction of pelvis, acetabulum, and extremity injuries as described above is followed with timely definitive care. A stable fracture is typically less painful and is beneficial to patient physiology. Pain induces sympathetic discharge, which can contribute to the hyper-inflammatory response of injury. Pain can also lead to poor respiratory effort and impaired ventilation; atelectasis ensues and may progress to hypoxemia or pneumonia. Therefore, pain control is essential, especially in the care of the multiply injured patient. Fracture stabilization can provide pain relief. Early fracture fixation of certain fractures has been associated with reduced narcotic medication intake, and potentially less respiratory depression and other adverse effects.[18,19]

Fixation of certain fractures can also contribute to resuscitation. Reduction and fixation of pelvic ring injuries and long bone fractures reduces ongoing hemorrhage. There is evidence that fixation of these injuries as well as mechanically unstable thoracolumbar spine injuries and acetabulum fractures should also be expedited.[19-24] Each of these injuries otherwise relegates a patient to lie recumbent in bed, further increasing their pulmonary and thrombotic risks. In stable patients evidence has emerged that these fractures are best definitively managed within the first 36 hours after injury.[19-23] Even though some of the surgical approaches themselves may be associated with pain and bleeding, the net effect on patient physiology may be positive. Fixation is thought to promote mobility from bed, reducing risks of thrombotic complications, fat embolism, pneumonia, adult respiratory distress syndrome (ARDS), and sepsis. Multiple studies have documented the positive effects of early fracture management in general in diminishing morbidity and mortality.[19-31]

A historical review of practices illustrates the benefits of early fixation, but also denotes the risks of early definitive care in under-resuscitated patients. During the 1980s various surgeons described their experiences with early definitive care, generally referred to as within 24 hours, and with emphasis on intramedullary nailing of femoral shaft fractures.[19,20] Delay in definitive fixation was associated with more pneumonia, ARDS, fat embolism syndrome, and with longer hospital and ICU stays, ultimately generating much larger treatment costs.[20] The benefits of early femoral nailing were even more pronounced in patients with injury to multiple systems.[20] Several large retrospective and prospective studies have supported these concepts,[22,27-31] and more recent studies have additionally emphasized the need for team-based care in evaluating patients and developing treatment plans to expedite definitive fixation of axial, pelvic, and femoral fractures in adequately resuscitated and otherwise stable patients.[32,33] Fixation within 36 hours after injury in stable patients, so-called "Early Appropriate Care" has reduced complications, length of stay, and costs.[23,31,34] For patients with more than one axial or femoral fracture, treatment plans are developed jointly with all subspecialty physicians.[33] Mechanically unstable spinal fractures with neural elements at risk may be best served first in the sequence, to provide a stable spinal column before moving patients into various other positions to reduce and stabilize other fractures. Furthermore, femoral shaft fractures amenable to external fixation may be better treated last, since a suitable alternative to definitive fixation exists, unlike fractures of the spine, acetabulum, proximal femur, and most pelvis ring fractures.

Risks of Early Care

Any injury, especially a major fracture, represents a physiological burden to a patient, which must be evaluated and managed. Surgery to stabilize certain fractures may provide control of bony bleeding and provide pain relief and pulmonary benefits; however, surgery also causes further hemorrhage, referred to as the "second hit."[35-37] Severely injured patients with massive hemorrhage may enter a state of physiological decline, resulting in multiple organ failure and death.[36,37] Baseline cardiopulmonary function, location and magnitude of injury, and genetic profile all contribute to patients' responses to injury and to resuscitation. An adequate level of resuscitation, as measured by improvement of acidosis, is crucial to maintain tissue oxygenation and to minimize potential for adverse consequences.[38,39]

During the1990s the practice of early definitive fracture fixation, later referred to as "early total care," had resulted from recommendations for femur fracture fixation within 24 hours after injury.[19-21] This practice was called into question, because concurrent, sequential management of multiple injuries beyond the femoral shaft, within the same anesthetic setting may constitute a deleterious burden, even in a healthy patient when they are not adequately resuscitated. Pape et al corroborated the benefits of early femoral nailing in patients with no chest injury or only minor chest injury. However, ARDS was reported in 33% and mortality in 21% of patients with severe chest trauma who underwent femoral nailing within 24 hours.[40] The practices of early femoral fracture fixation and of performing medullary reaming in patients with severe chest trauma were considered potentially problematic and to be avoided.[41,42]

Indications for Damage Control

External fixation is an alternative to definitive femoral fixation in critically ill trauma patients who are considered not able to safely undergo more extensive surgery. Definitive internal fixation may be deferred for several days. External fixation requires minimal operating time and produces little surgical bleeding.[43] Indications may include severe head injury, hemodynamic instability, and cardiac insufficiency. Coagulopathy may also be present in patients who sustain massive hemorrhage.[44] Resuscitation with intravenous fluid and blood products will restore tissue oxygenation, normalizing acidosis. Massive resuscitation should consist of ratios for platelets and fresh frozen plasma to prevent dilution, with 1:1:1 administration of packed red blood cells, platelets, and fresh frozen plasma in extreme cases.[45-47] Recent literature also supports goal-directed resuscitation based on thromboelastography (TEG) or rotational thromboelastometry (ROTEM). These techniques promote early diagnosis of coagulopathy and may be predictive of transfusion requirements and mortality.

Recent literature has consistently shown that most patients with femoral shaft fractures may be resuscitated on arrival such that early definitive stabilization of femoral shaft fractures is safe and preferred to damage control. Definitive fixation in stable patients minimizes the risks and costs of staged fixation.[21,23,26-28,30,34] Early Appropriate Care consists of definitive fixation of pelvis, acetabulum, spine, proximal and diaphyseal femoral fractures within 36 hours of injury, as long as initial acidosis has improved to at least one of the following: lactate <4.0 mmol/L, pH ≥ 7.25, or base excess (BE) ≥−5.5 mmol/L, and the patient is otherwise stable. When these parameters are not met, provisional external fixation of femoral or pelvic fractures with amenable patterns is recommended[23,31,48] (**Table 3**).

Techniques of Damage Control

Provisional external fixation of the femur is performed by placing percutaneous pins on each side of the fracture. Two pins on each side of the fracture in a uniplanar configuration provide a stable construct and may be placed expeditiously. Distal femoral skeletal traction affords provisional restoration of fracture length and may be considered a reasonable alternative for femoral shaft fractures in patients not stable for surgery within the first days of hospitalization.[17] Many pelvic ring injuries are not patterns amenable to reduction and provisional external fixation, particularly those with complete disruption of the posterior ring, which is not adequately

Table 3

Early Appropriate Care Guidelines[23,31,48]

- On admission check ABG, lactate, CBC, platelets, INR
- Repeat labs every 8 hr until normal, then stop labs
- Recommend definitive stabilization within 36 hr of injury if:
  - pH ≥ 7.25
  - Base deficit ≥ −5.5 mmol/L
  - Lactate <4.0 mmol/L
- AND patient is responding to resuscitation without pressor support. This may require serial laboratory measurements in the presence of persistent bleeding and/or hypotension.
- If these criteria *are not met* within 12 hr of presentation, proceed with a damage control strategy such as external fixation of amenable femur and pelvis fractures. Continue to reassess until the patient meets above criteria before proceeding with definitive management.

controlled through anterior pins. Supra-acetabular iliac pins provide improved rotational control to the posterior ileum versus iliac crest pins. Damage control external fixation may be applied to anterior-posterior injuries and some vertical shear patterns. Skeletal traction provides reduction for vertical shear pelvic ring fractures and may maintain closed reduction of grossly unstable acetabulum fractures.

Controversies in Care

Fractures Associated With Severe Head Injury

Concurrent head injuries are common in orthopaedic trauma patients. Most head injuries are minor, with presenting Glasgow Coma Scale of 13 to 15. Less than 3% of patients with mild head injury will develop acute deterioration of mental status, and early fracture care is considered appropriate. However, the timing of fracture fixation in patients with severe head injury has been debated. Most prior studies have focused on femoral shaft fractures and support damage control orthopaedics for patients with elevated ICP and limited cerebral perfusion pressure (CPP). CPP is calculated as the mean arterial pressure minus the ICP, and it indicates sufficient blood flow to the brain. Ischemia with CPP <70 mm Hg for several hours can cause permanent brain damage. To perform definitive management of axial and femoral fractures, ICP should be ≤20 mm Hg and CPP should be >70 mm Hg.[7,49,50] When the CPP is <70 mm Hg, external fixation of femoral and pelvic fractures is appropriate, and various measures including ventriculostomy, craniotomy, mannitol infusion, and hypothermia may be undertaken to treat the head injury.

Fractures Associated With Vascular Injury

Limb ischemia due to disruption of major arterial flow is a surgical emergency. More than 75% of cases result from penetrating trauma, excepting knee dislocations, which carry an incidence of arterial injury up to 25%.[51,52] Dressings should be removed and fractures should be reduced, followed by rapid reassessment of limb perfusion. Vascular injury is suspected when a pulse is palpable or Dopplerable but asymmetrical.[52] Ankle brachial indices (ABI) should be obtained in the emergency department. The ABI is measured by placing a blood pressure cuff on the upper arm and inflating it to obtain a measurement of the systolic pressure. Subsequently, the procedure is repeated at the ankle of the affected leg. The ABI is the ratio of the systolic pressure of the ankle over the systolic pressure of the arm. If an ABI is less than 0.9, vascular consultation is indicated. In a pulseless extremity emergent surgical exploration and revascularization are essential. Within 6 hours of ischemia, death of nerve and muscle will occur. Reduction and stabilization of the injury are indicated before the vascular procedure.[52,53] This is to ensure safety of the vascular repair, that is, to avoid further arterial damage during fracture reduction and fixation. In many cases provisional external fixation may be the most appropriate method in maintaining limb alignment, without requiring extensive surgical time and dissection. After restoration of perfusion to the limb, distal fasciotomy is recommended to prevent compartment syndrome.

Limb Salvage Versus Amputation

Traumatic amputation and near-amputation are initially managed with direct pressure, then a tourniquet, in the field when possible, to control hemorrhage.[54,55] Antibiotics are administered on presentation and tetanus status is updated, because these injuries constitute open fractures.[56] Crush injuries, prolonged ischemia time, severe trauma elsewhere in the limb, serious systemic injury, advanced age, and underlying medical conditions are factors decreasing the likelihood of successful limb salvage. Emergent surgical débridement, skeletal stabilization, and control of hemorrhage are indicated. In some cases amputation is performed to contain massive hemorrhage in a mangled extremity and is considered a lifesaving intervention. Additionally, an expeditious amputation of a mangled limb in a multiply injured patient controls bleeding and reduces wound and injury burden, again contributing to the concept of saving life over limb.

More often salvage is attempted after initial surgical débridement and provisional or definitive stabilization of fractures. External fixation is a rapid means of stabilizing fractures in patients who are critically ill and under-resuscitated. Serial débridement and later definitive fixation (versus amputation) can be undertaken following discussions with the patient and other subspecialists.

Summary

Trauma algorithms promote continuous reassessment and have improved outcomes of trauma patients.[32,34] Orthopaedic surgeons perform expeditious reduction and stabilization of fractures and dislocations to provide pain relief and to facilitate mobility from bed. Fracture reduction and fixation can also reduce ongoing hemorrhage, thus contributing to resuscitation. Adequacy of resuscitation is most easily denoted by resolution of acidosis, as measured by lactate, base deficit, or pH. Definitive fixation of mechanically unstable axial, pelvic, and femoral fractures in resuscitated patients reduces pulmonary, thrombotic, and other complications and minimizes length of hospital stay. Early Appropriate Care has emerged as a treatment principle that promotes definitive fixation when acidosis has improved to a minimum of lactate <4.0, base excess ≥ −5.5, or pH ≥ 7.25. Others may benefit from a damage control strategy, if possible, to provide bony stability without generating more hemorrhage and without contributing to systemic dysfunction.

Key study points

- Damage control strategies are appropriate for patients in extremis to provide provisional bony stability without contributing to further hemorrhage and systemic dysfunction.
- Definitive management of axial, pelvis, and femoral fractures in resuscitated patients reduces pulmonary, thrombotic, and other complications and shortens length of hospital stay.
- Algorithm-based care using ATLS has developed over time, with iterative processes to promote consistency and optimal outcomes.
- Collaboration of specialty providers is essential in optimizing treatment of complex polytrauma.
- Reduction and stabilization of certain fractures and dislocations promotes resuscitation, provides pain relief, and facilitates mobility from bed.

Annotated References

1. American College of Surgeons: *Advanced Trauma Life Support: Student Course Manual*, ed 9. Chicago, IL, American College of Surgeons, 2012.
2. Paladino L, Sinert R, Wallace D, Anderson T, Yadav K, Zehtabchi S: The utility of base deficit and arterial lactate in differentiating major from minor injury in trauma patients with normal vital signs. *Resuscitation* 2008;77:363-368.
3. Heffernan DS, Thakkar RK, Monaghan SF, et al: Normal presenting vital signs are unreliable in geriatric blunt trauma victims. *J Trauma* 2010;69:813-820.
4. Summers RL, Baker SD, Sterling SA, Porter JM, Jones AE: Characterization of the spectrum of hemodynamic profiles in trauma patients with acute neurogenic shock. *J Crit Care* 2013;28:531.e1-5.
5. Baker SP, O'Neill B, Haddon W Jr, Long WB: The injury severity score: A method for describing patients with multiple injuries and evaluating emergency care. *J Trauma* 1974;14:187-196.
6. Osler T, Baker SP, Long W: A modification of the injury severity score that both improves accuracy and simplifies scoring. *J Trauma* 1997;43:922-925.
7. Flierl MA, Stoneback JW, Beauchamp KM, et al: Femur shaft fracture fixation in head-injured patients: When is the right time? *J Orthop Trauma* 2010;24:107-114.
8. Kasotakis G, Hasenboehler EA, Streib EW, et al: Operative fixation of rib fractures after blunt trauma: A practice management guideline from the Eastern Association for the surgery of trauma. *J Trauma Acute Care Surg* 2017;82:618-626.

   22 studies were reviewed, including 986 patients, 334 with rib ORIF. Rib ORIF for flail chest afforded lower pneumonia, shorter stay and ventilation time, fewer tracheostomies, and lower mortality. Level of evidence: III (Systematic review/meta-analysis).
9. Hurtuk M, Reed RL II, Esposito TJ, et al: Trauma surgeons practice what they preach: the NTDB story on solid organ injury management. *J Trauma* 2006;61(2):243-254.
10. Bhullar IS, Frykberg ER, Siragusa D, et al: Selective angiographic embolization of blunt splenic traumatic injuries in adults decreases failure rate of nonoperative management. *J Trauma Acute Care Surg* 2012;72:1127-1134.
11. Routt ML, Falicov A, Woodhouse E, Schildhauer TA: Circumferential pelvic antishock sheeting: A temporary resuscitation aid. *J Orthop Trauma* 2002;16:45-48.
12. Tai DK, Li WH, Lee KY, et al: Retroperitoneal pelvic packing in the management of hemodynamically unstable pelvic fractures: a level I trauma center experience. *J Trauma* 2011;71:79-86.
13. Morrison JJ, Galgon RE, Jansen JO, et al: A systematic review of the use of resuscitative endovascular balloon occlusion of the aorta in the management of hemorrhagic shock. *J Trauma Acute Care Surg* 2016;80:324-334.

    Systematic review of 41 studies evaluating REBOA for trauma and other indications showed an increase in mean systolic pressure by 53 mmHg. Despite an increase in central blood pressure in the setting of shock, no clear reduction in hemorrhage-related mortality has been demonstrated. Level of evidence: IV (Systematic review).
14. Pieper A, Thony F, Brun J, et al: Resuscitative endovascular balloon occlusion of the aorta for pelvic blunt trauma and life-threatening hemorrhage: A 20-year experience in a Level 1 trauma center. *J Trauma Acute Care Surg* 2018;84:449-453.

    Review of 32 REBOA patients showed improvement in mean systolic blood pressure, with only two technical failures and 5 vascular complications.
15. Woods RK, O'Keefe G, Rhee P, Routt ML Jr, Maier RV: Open pelvic fracture and fecal diversion. *Arch Surg* 1998;133:281-286.
16. Avey G, Blackmore CC, Wessells H, Wright JL, Talner LB: Radiographic and clinic predictors of bladder rupture in blunt trauma patients with pelvic fracture. *Acad Radiol* 2006;12:573-579.

Trauma

17. Scannell BP, Waldrop NE, Sasser HC, Sing RF, Bosse MJ: Skeletal traction versus external fixation in the initial temporization of femoral shaft fractures in severely injured patients. *J Trauma* 2010;68:633-640.

18. Barei DP, Shafer BL, Beingessner DM, Gardner MJ, Nork SE, Routt ML: The impact of open reduction internal fixation on acute pain management in unstable pelvic ring injuries. *J Trauma* 2010;68:949-953.

19. Johnson KD, Cadambi A, Seibert GB: Incidence of adult respiratory distress syndrome in patients with multiple musculoskeletal injuries: Effect of early operative stabilization of fractures. *J Trauma* 1985;25:375-384.

20. Bone LB, Johnson KD, Weigelt J, Scheinberg R: Early versus delayed stabilization of femoral fractures. A prospective randomized study. *J Bone Joint Surg Am* 1989;71:336-340.

21. Harvin JA, Harvin WH, Camp E, et al: Early femur fracture fixation is associated with a reduction in pulmonary complications and hospital charges: A decade of experience with 1376 diaphyseal femur fractures. *J Trauma* 2012;73:1440-1446.

22. Vallier HA, Cureton BA, Ekstein C, Oldenburg FP, Wilber JH: Early definitive stabilization of unstable pelvis and acetabulum fractures reduces morbidity. *J Trauma* 2010;69:677-684.

23. Vallier HA, Moore TA, Como JJ, et al: Complications are reduced with a protocol to standardize timing of fixation based on response to resuscitation. *J Orthop Surg Res* 2015;10:155-163.

24. Bliemel C, Lefering R, Buecking B, et al: Early or delayed stabilization in severely injured patients with spinal fractures? Current surgical objectivity according to the trauma registry of DGU: Treatment of spine injuries in polytrauma patients. *J Trauma Acute Care Surg* 2014;76:366-373.

25. Enninghorst N, Toth L, King KL, McDougall D, Mackenzie S, Balogh ZJ: Acute definitive internal fixation of pelvic ring fractures in polytrauma patients: A feasible option. *J Trauma* 2010;68:935-941.

26. Lefaivre KA, Starr AJ, Stahel PF, Elliott AC, Smith WR: Prediction of pulmonary morbidity and mortality in patients with femur fracture. *J Trauma* 2010;69:1527-1536.

27. McHenry TP, Mirza SK, Wang J, et al: Risk factors for respiratory failure following operative stabilization of thoracic and lumbar spine fractures. *J Bone Joint Surg Am* 2006;88:997-1005.

28. O'Toole RV, O'Brien M, Scalea TM, Habashi N, Pollak AN, Turen CH: Resuscitation before stabilization of femoral fractures limits acute respiratory distress syndrome in patients with multiple traumatic injuries despite low use of damage control orthopedics. *J Trauma* 2009;67:1013-1021.

29. Probst C, Probst T, Gaensslen A, Krettek C, Pape HC, Polytrauma Study Groups of the German Trauma Society: Timing and duration of the initial pelvic stabilization after multiple trauma in patients from the German Trauma Registry: Is there an influence on outcome? *J Trauma* 2007;62:370-377.

30. Stahel PF, Vanderheiden T, Flierl MA, et al: The impact of a standardized "spine damage-control" protocol for unstable thoracic and lumbar spine fractures in severely injured patients. *J Trauma Acute Care Surg* 2013;74(2):590-596.

31. Vallier HA, Wang X, Moore TA, Wilber JH, Como JJ: Timing of orthopaedic surgery in multiple trauma patients: Development of a protocol for Early Appropriate Care. *J Orthop Trauma* 2013;27(10):543-551.

32. Childs BR, Nahm NJ, Moore TA, Vallier HA: Multiple orthopaedic procedures in the initial surgical setting: When do the benefits outweigh the risks in patients with multiple system trauma? *J Orthop Trauma* 2016;30:420-425.

    Definitive fixation of femoral, pelvis, and axial fractures concurrent with other fracture management in resuscitated patients was associated with fewer complications, shorter stay, and less ventilation time, versus returning for a second surgical setting. Level of evidence: II (Therapeutic).

33. Vallier HA, Como JJ, Wagner KG, Moore TA: Team approach: Timing of operative intervention in multiply-injured patients. *JBJS Rev* 2018;6:e2.

    Team-based care involving the trauma critical care surgeon as the leader, and coordinating treatment planning with neurosurgery, orthopaedic surgery, and anesthesia facilitates safe and efficient management of the polytrauma patient.

34. Vallier HA, Dolenc AJ, Moore TA: Early appropriate care: A protocol to standardize resuscitation assessment and to expedite fracture care reduces hospital stay and enhances revenue. *J Orthop Trauma* 2016;30:306-311.

    Delay of definitive fixation of femoral, pelvis, and spine fractures in stable patients resulted in $6,380 loss per patient due to longer stay and more complications. Implementation of the EAC protocol resulted in more than $1.8 M additional revenue to the hospital per year. Level of evidence: IV (Economic).

35. Harwood PJ, Giannoudis PV, van Griensven M, Krettek C, Pape HC: Alterations in the systemic inflammatory response after early total care and damage control procedures for femoral shaft fracture in severely injured patients. *J Trauma* 2005;58:446-454.

36. Lasanianos NG, Kanakaris NK, Dimitriou R, Pape HC, Giannoudis PV: Second hit phenomenon: Existing evidence of clinical implications. *Injury* 2011;42:617-629.

37. Waydhas C, Nast-Kolb D, Trupka A, et al: Posttraumatic inflammatory response, secondary operations, and late multiple organ failure. *J Trauma* 1996;40:624-630.

38. Richards JE, Matuszewski PE, Griffen SM, et al: The role of elevated lactate as a risk factor for pulmonary morbidity after early fixation of femoral shaft fractures. *J Orthop Trauma* 2016;30:312-318.

    In patients undergoing femoral nail fixation within 24 hours of admission, median lactate of 2.8 mmol/L was not associated with prolonged mechanical ventilation. Level of evidence: III (Prognostic).

39. Weinberg DS, Narayanan AS, Moore TA, Vallier HA: Prolonged resuscitation of metabolic acidosis after trauma is associated with more complications. *J Orthop Surg Res* 2015;10:153-160.

40. Pape HC, Auf'm'Kolk M, Paffrath T, Regel G, Sturm JA, Tscherne H: Primary intramedullary femur fixation in multiple trauma pateints with associated lung contusion–a cause of posttraumatic ARDS?. *J Trauma* 1993;34:540-547.

41. Pape H-C, Rixen D, Morley J, et al: Impact of the method of initial stabilization for femoral shaft fractures in patients with multiple injuries at risk for complications (Borderline Patients). *Ann Surg* 2007;246:491-501.

42. Steinhausen E, Lefering R, Tjardes T, et al: A risk-adapted appropriate is beneficial in the management of bilateral femoral shaft fractures in multiple trauma patients: An analysis based on the trauma registry of the German trauma Society. *J Trauma Acute Care Surg* 2014;76:1288-1293.

43. Scalea TM, Boswell SA, Scott JD, Mitchell KA, Kramer ME, Pollak AN: External fixation as a bridge to intramedullary nailing for patients with multiple injuries and with femur fractures: Damage Control Orthopedics. *J Trauma* 2000;48(4):613-623.

44. Childs BR, Verhotz DR, Moore TA, Vallier HA: Presentation coagulopathy and persistent acidosis predict complications in orthopaedic trauma patients. *J Orthop Trauma* 2017;31:617-623.

Coagulopathy on presentation is a predictor of complications, sepsis, and death. Coagulopathy increased during the first 48 hours of hospitalization from 16% to 34% of all multiply injured orthopaedic patients. Level of evidence: I (Therapeutic).

45. Brakenridge SC, Phelan HA, Henley SS, et al: Early blood product and crystalloid volume resuscitation: Risk association with multiple organ dysfunction after severe blunt traumatic injury. *J Trauma* 2011;71(2):299-305.

46. Cotton BA, Faz G, Hatch QM, et al: Rapid thromboelastography delivers real-time results that predict transfusion within 1 hour of admission. *J Trauma* 2011;71:407-417.

47. Driessen A, Schafer N, Bauerfeind U, et al: Functional capacity of reconstituted blood in 1:1:1 versus 3:1:1 ratios: A thromboelastometry study. *Scand J Trauma Resusc Emerg Med* 2015;9:23-26.

48. Weinberg DS, Narayanan AS, Moore TA, Vallier HA: Assessment of resuscitation as measured by markers of metabolic acidosis and features of injury. *Bone Joint Lett J* 2017;99-B:122-127.

Markers of resuscitation indicate improvement of acidosis and are predictive of fewer complications (correction of pH to ≥7.25, base excess ≥−5.5, or lactate <4.0); however, incomplete resuscitation, defined as less than all three parameters met displayed a trend toward more complications versus full parameter resuscitation (all three met): 31.8% vs 22.6%, $P = 0.078$. Level of evidence: II (Prognostic).

49. Scalea TM, Scott JD, Brumback RJ, et al: Early fracture fixation may be "just fine" after head injury: No difference in central nervous system outcomes. *J Trauma* 1999;46:839-846.

50. Starr AJ, Hunt JL, Chason DP, Reinert CM, Walker J: Treatment of femur fracture with associated head injury. *J Orthop Trauma* 1998;12:38-45.

51. Wascher DC, Dvirnak PC, DeCoster TA: Knee dislocation: Initial management and implications for treatment. *J Orthop Trauma* 1997;11:525-529.

52. Weinberg DS, Scarcella NR, Napora JK, Vallier HA: Can vascular injury be appropriately assessed with physical examination after knee dislocation? *Clin Orthop Relat Res* 2016;474:1453-1456.

Obesity and open injuries were independently associated with vascular injury. Combination of palpable DP and PT pulses combined with ABI ≥ 0.9 was 100% sensitive for detection of vascular injury. Level of evidence: III (Diagnostic).

53. Franz RW, Shah KJ, Halaharvi D, Franz ET, Hartman JF, Wright ML: A 5-year review of management of lower extremity arterial injuries at an urban level 1 trauma center. *J Vasc Surg* 2011;53:1604-1610.

54. Inaba K, Siboni S, Resnick S, et al: Tourniquet use for civilian extremity trauma. *J Trauma Acute Care Surg* 2015;79:232-237.

55. Shlaifer A, Yitzhak A, Baruch EN, et al: Point of injury tourniquet application during Operation Protective Edge-What do we learn? *J Trauma Acute Care Surg* 2017;83:278-283.

90 patients were treated with 119 tourniquet applications, and 79 survived. Total complication rate attributed to tourniquet use was 11.7%; however, tourniquets were 70% successful, defined as survival, regardless of caregiver level or tourniquet type. Level of evidence: III and IV (Epidemiologic; therapeutic).

56. Lack WD, Karunakar MA, Angerame MR, et al: Type III open tibia fractures: Immediate antibiotic prophylaxis minimizes infection. *J Orthop Trauma* 2015;29:1-6.

Trauma

Chapter 18
Open Fractures Management

Conor P. Kleweno, MD • Jonah Hebert-Davies, MD

ABSTRACT

Management of open fractures continues to be challenging for the orthopaedic surgeon who takes call. These injuries are technically demanding to treat and continue to be associated with high morbidity, particularly open tibia fractures. Recent research has provided new guidance on surgical and medical management. This focus includes the early administration of antibiotics, timing and technique of surgical débridement, wound management, and timing of soft-tissue coverage.

Keywords: antibiotic prophylaxis; infection; open fracture; osteomyelitis

Introduction

The treatment of open extremity fractures continues to be challenging. Despite being an area of research and clinical emphasis, these injuries remain associated with substantial morbidity, high infection rates,[1] high cost,[2] and decreased quality of life[3] (**Figure 1**). Common mechanisms can range from low- to high-energy injuries with variation in severity. Recent literature has provided guidance for the practicing orthopaedic surgeon charged with caring for these injuries with certain historic dogma being replaced by newer evidence-based medicine. Although treatment strategies apply to all long bones, open tibia fractures are often the most problematic. The main topics of clinical and research focus include the early administration of antibiotics, timing and technique of surgical treatment including débridement, interval management of associated wounds, and timing of soft-tissue coverage.

Dr. Kleweno or an immediate family member serves as a paid consultant to or is an employee of Globus Medical and Stryker; serves as a board member, owner, officer, or committee member of the Western Orthopaedic Association. Dr. Hebert-Davies or an immediate family member serves as a paid consultant to or is an employee of Globus Medical and Synthes.

Classification

Gustilo and Anderson is still the most commonly used classification system to describe open fractures.[4] However, more recently the Orthopaedic Trauma Association (OTA) developed a novel classification for open fractures that is more descriptive in a variety of clinical domains (including skin injury, muscle injury, arterial injury, contamination level, and bone loss).[5] The OTA open fracture classification (OFC) has demonstrated high interobserver reliability[5] and high ability to predict treatment[6] and is more predictive of complications and outcomes, including amputation, when compared with the Gustilo-Anderson classification.[7] Further research and time will determine its value and utilization among practicing surgeons.

Antibiotic Prophylaxis

Open fractures are by definition contaminated. Multiple factors determine whether an open fracture will lead to a clinical infection including the amount of contamination and subsequent colonization, the virulence of the organism, the severity of soft-tissue injury, local tissue vascularity, and a host of medical comorbidities such as diabetes.

One area of clinical care focus is in the potential benefit of early administration of systemic antibiotics. The overall benefit of antibiotics in open fractures is not in question; the issue is whether giving it earlier in the process would be of additional benefit. The argument for earlier antibiotic delivery was initially based on early studies with small sample sizes and small effect sizes.[8] More recently, a highly influential study has supported early administration of antibiotics based upon an evaluation of timing of antibiotics and incidence of infection in type III open tibia fractures and suggested that early antibiotic administration decreases risk of infection.[9]

However, this is countered by a recent systematic review by Whitehouse et al[10] that concluded there was insufficient evidence based on current literature to determine the benefit of earlier administration. The authors evaluated eight studies addressing this topic.

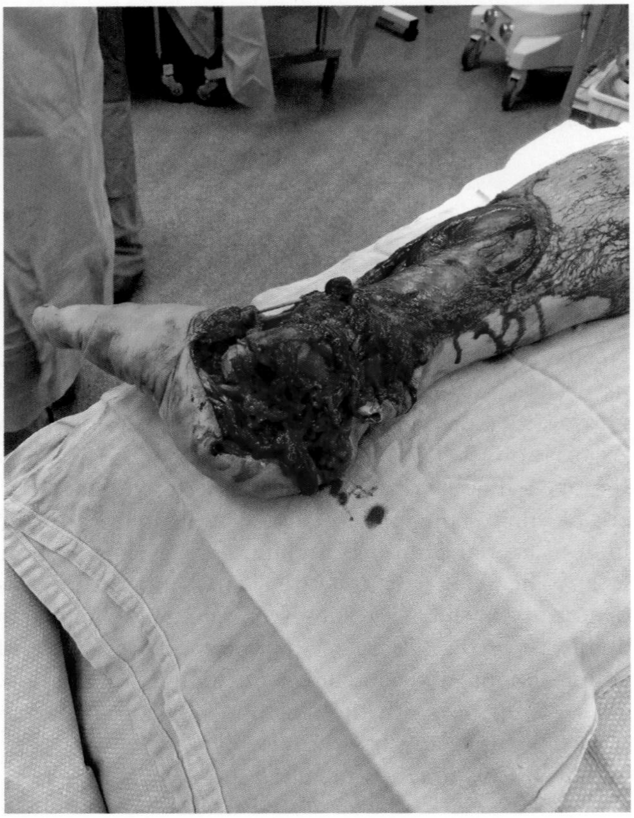

Figure 1 Clinical photograph of a 45-year-old male involved in a motorcycle crash with a severe type IIIC distal tibia fracture with associated severe fractures of the midfoot and hindfoot. The patient went on to have a below the knee amputation.

Seven of the eight studies showed no effect of early antibiotics[11-17]; only the one mentioned above by Lack et al reported a benefit.[9] None of the eight were randomized or nonrandomized controlled trials.

However, due to the perceived importance of timing, there has been expert opinion proposing early antibiotic delivery within one hour[18] and even via emergency medical services when available.[11,19] A recent 2017 study demonstrated a substantial reduction in time from admission to antibiotic administration (123 to 36 minutes) after institution of a formalized open fracture working group involving emergency medicine physicians and orthopaedic surgeons.[20] At this time, the data are conflicting as to the benefit of early antibiotic administration and further research is needed to quantify if there is a clinically meaningful effect.

Type of Antibiotic

Less severe (types I and II) open fractures can typically be treated with a first-generation cephalosporin as a single agent.[21] In severe (type III) open fractures some centers add coverage for both gram-positive and gram-negative pathogens. This is often provided by combination treatment with a first-generation cephalosporin, such as cefazolin, and by an aminoglycoside, such as gentamicin.[22] However, a thorough, meticulous guideline by Hauser et al[23] concluded that there is insufficient evidence to recommend the routine practice of adding additional antibiotic agents for gram-negative or clostridial species. On behalf of the Surgical Infection Society, the authors recommended large, randomized, controlled trials powered to demonstrate the efficacy and effect size of antibiotic interventions while also measuring the associated risks such as antibiotic resistance and opportunistic nosocomial infections.

Some trauma centers have transitioned to a single agent antibiotic for severe fractures. A 2014 study[24] looked at implementing a protocol using ceftriaxone 1 g IV for 48 hours for type III fractures instead of combination cephalosporin/aminoglycoside or vancomycin and found no significant difference in infection rate. The authors highlighted that the implementation of this protocol resulted in the significant decrease in use of aminoglycosides and glycopeptides (eg, vancomycin) for type III open fractures (54% vs 16%) as evidence of improved antibiotic stewardship. A 2016 retrospective cohort study of 72 patients with type III open fractures compared cefazolin plus gentamycin (37 patients) to piperacillin/tazobactam (35 patients) and found no difference in infection (12/37 vs 11/35, respectively), nonunion, mortality, and rehospitalization although of course a study of this size is only powered to detect very large differences.[25] The authors recommended limiting the utilization of the strong piperacillin/tazobactam antibiotic unnecessarily so as not to promote multidrug-resistant organisms.

There is a common concern regarding the risk of using gentamycin for gram-negative coverage in open fractures. A recent study found no difference in acute kidney injury when evaluating patients with open fractures who were treated either with cefazolin or with cefazolin and gentamicin.[26] However, a 2018 retrospective study evaluated the risk of kidney injury when gentamycin was used for open fractures and found that duration of gentamicin administration, lower baseline creatinine, female gender, age, and higher weight were independently associated with abnormal kidney function.[27] Furthermore, as noted above,[23] there is a lack of evidence for the routine use of this antibiotic.

Lastly, it is often recommended that anaerobic coverage (eg, penicillin) should be added in injuries potentially contaminated with clostridial organisms such as farm and barnyard injuries but without high-level evidence supporting this practice.[22]

There has been increasing interest in local application of antibiotics at the site of open fractures. A 2015 retrospective cohort study evaluated the effect of topical gentamicin and tobramycin on 168 open fractures and compared with 183 open fractures with standard systemic antibiotics only and reported lower deep infections (odds ratio, 3.0 [95% confidence interval, 1.1 to 8.5]).[28] Future research in animal models and human clinical trials are ongoing and may provide data to further support this practice; however, at this time there is not enough evidence for or against the use of topical antibiotics in open fractures.

Duration of Antibiotics

The duration of antibiotics in open fractures also remains a controversy. Clinical practice has changed with more emphasis on antibiotic stewardship and avoidance of prolonged courses that theoretically may lead to antibiotic resistance. In support of this trend, a recent meta-analysis of evidence regarding appropriate duration of antibiotic use in open fractures found no benefit of prolonged administration regardless of fracture severity, reporting short durations of 24 to 48 hours as equivalent to >72 hours.[29] The meta-analysis included all long bone fracture with specific subgroup analyses for tibial fractures as well as type III open fractures. Of note, there was no subgroup analysis done comparing fractures closed primarily versus those with delayed closure or flap coverage and no specific discussion regarding the various wound coverage scenarios. The authors' conclusions remained unchanged after subgroup analyses, recommending against durations >72 hours for all open fractures.

Timing of Débridement in Open Fractures

The true urgency and resultant recommendations for time to surgical débridement remain a controversy among orthopaedic traumatologists. Historic dogma mandated emergent débridement of open fractures regardless of classification and reference to a "6-hour rule" based on older animal model studies dating back to the time prior to the discovery of antibiotics. Clinical practice has shifted, and in general, most experts believe that the quality of surgical technique, soft-tissue handling, and appropriateness of débridement is potentially more important than a specific time delay threshold.

There is literature support for paradigm shift. In 2010, a seminal multicenter trial of 315 severe lower extremity open fractures showed no correlation of time to débridement and increased infection.[1] In addition, a 2012 meta-analysis concluded that the literature did not support the historic "6-hour rule" for timing of surgical débridement.[30] Interestingly, this held true even for type III fractures. Instead, the authors recommended surgery to be performed as early as possible without placing a polytraumatized patient at risk. Similarly, a 2014 prospective cohort study evaluated 736 open fractures and observed no association between time to surgery and infection.[14] Furthermore, a 2014 retrospective study evaluating timing of antibiotic administration in 137 type III tibia fractures (typically some of the highest risk) found time to surgical débridement not associated with development of infection.[9] A 2015 study stratified 315 open fractures into four groups based on the time of débridement (<6, 7 to 12, 13 to 18, and 19 to 24 hours after injury) and found no differences in infection rates.[31] Note that the study did include a high percentage of lower extremity (70%) and type III (48%) fractures, but did not include any patients with >24 hour delay in surgical débridement.

Clearly, if one waits long enough, the wound will become clinically infected and current guidelines tend to state 24 hours as a goal although there is not much data supporting this time point either. However, poorly performed and inadequate débridement done for the sake of urgency should be replaced with skilled, appropriate débridement in daylight hours. The importance of timing may vary based on the severity of the wound, and some clinicians place more time urgency for highly contaminated wounds than less severe open fractures with minimal contamination. The specific cutoff time points for each type of open fracture are unknown and remain an area of ongoing research.

Strategy and Technique at Initial Surgery

Appropriate surgical débridement is thought to be one of the most important aspects of treating open fractures. Perhaps the colloquialism "irrigation and débridement" should be better stated as "débridement then irrigation" with the understanding that the irrigation is useful to flush away contaminated and colonized clot, débrided material, and devitalized tissue, not merely to get the tissue wet. A systematic approach working superficial to deep, proceeding as skin, subcutaneous tissue, fascia, muscle, and finally bone is a recommended technique to optimize efficiency and quality. The first surgery is likely the best opportunity for thorough and meticulous débridement (**Figure 2**).

Classic teaching describes extension of the traumatic wound proximally and distally to the extent of periosteal stripping and zone of injury. However, this can be problematic for wound closure and lead to a larger

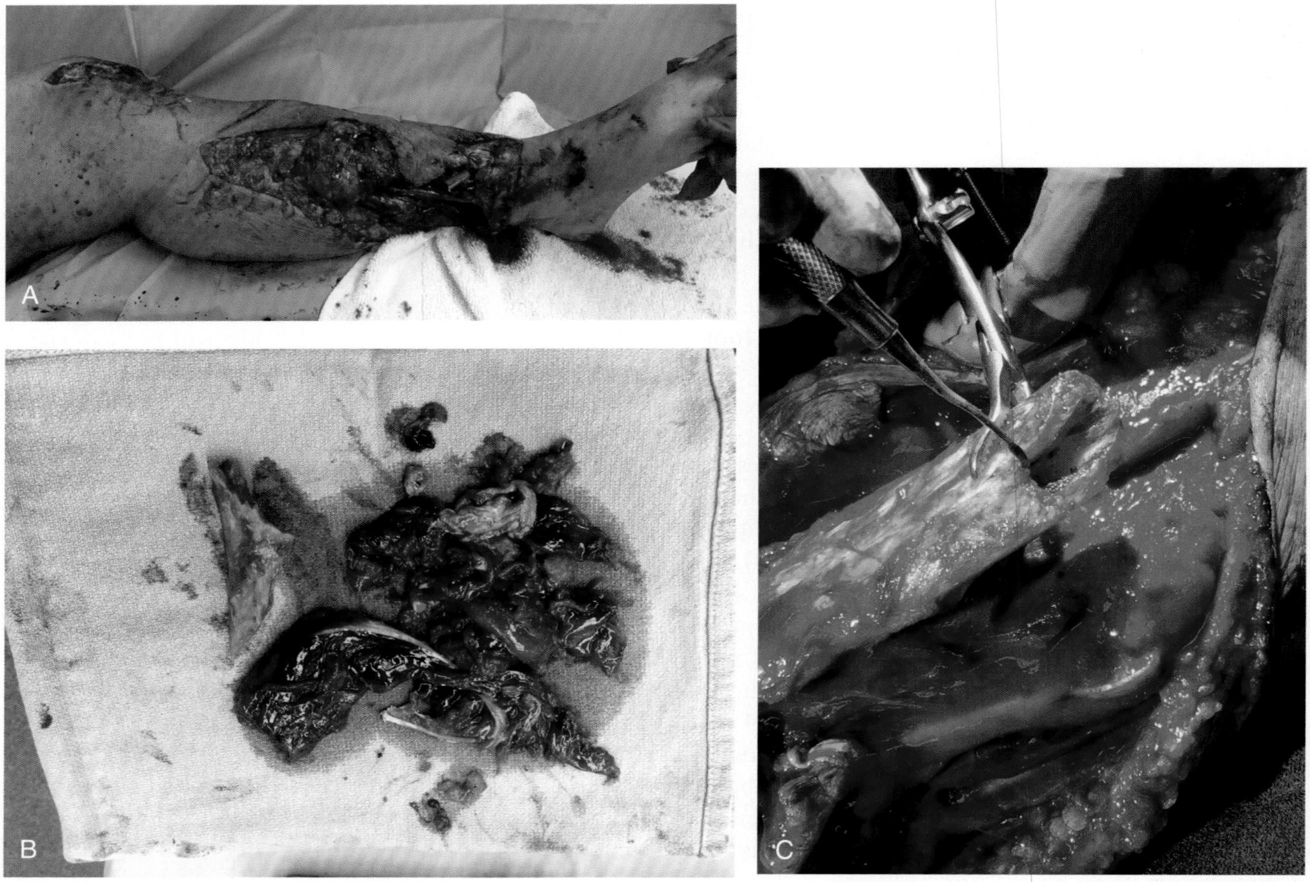

Figure 2 Thorough and meticulous surgical débridement of open fractures with respect of soft tissues is thought to be the key to preventing infection, although there are no clinical data supporting this firmly held belief. Many surgeons argue that a systematic approach working superficial to deep, proceeding with skin, subcutaneous tissue, fascia, muscle, and finally bone is a recommended technique to optimize efficiency and quality. **A**, Clinical photograph of a 30-year-old female involved in a motorcycle crash sustaining a severe type IIIB open segmental tibia fracture with substantial contamination of dirt and road debris. **B**, Photograph of débridement products including skin, subcutaneous fat, fascia, muscle, and devitalized segment of bone. **C**, A dental pick is shown in this intraoperative photograph as a useful instrument to débride the fracture edges and interstices of debris.

wound defect, particularly on the medial face of the tibia (a commonly challenging location). An alternative strategy is to use a counterincision in the line of a defined surgical approach.[32] For example, if a patient has a 2 cm wound on the anteromedial face of the tibia, the surgeon can make a larger anterolateral surgical incision and still provide sufficient débridement in the zone of injury and then close both wounds without extending the traumatic wound. A recent 2018 prospective cohort study evaluated this technique in 21 patients with an open tibia shaft fracture and compared them to 47 matched open tibia shaft fractures who underwent standard extension of the traumatic wound. The authors found a lower incidence of necessary flap coverage in the counterincision group (9/47 compared with 0/21; $P = 0.048$) although of course selection bias is a potential criticism of this particular nonrandomized study.[33]

Aggressiveness of débridement is also an area of debate and current dogma states that quality of débridement is the "most important" factor in reducing infection with no clinical data to support this opinion. Typical recommendation is for "aggressive" débridement to expose and include the entire zone of injury regardless of severity of injury or contamination. However, a 2013 retrospective study compared "aggressive" versus "less aggressive" débridement technique for open distal femur fractures between two separate trauma centers.[34] The authors reported no difference in infection rates and lower rate of revision surgery in the less aggressive cohort. Although there were several limitations in the study including being underpowered to detect a true difference in infection, less severe fractures may require less aggressive débridement and severely open and contaminated injuries will require substantial and aggressive débridement (**Figure 3**).

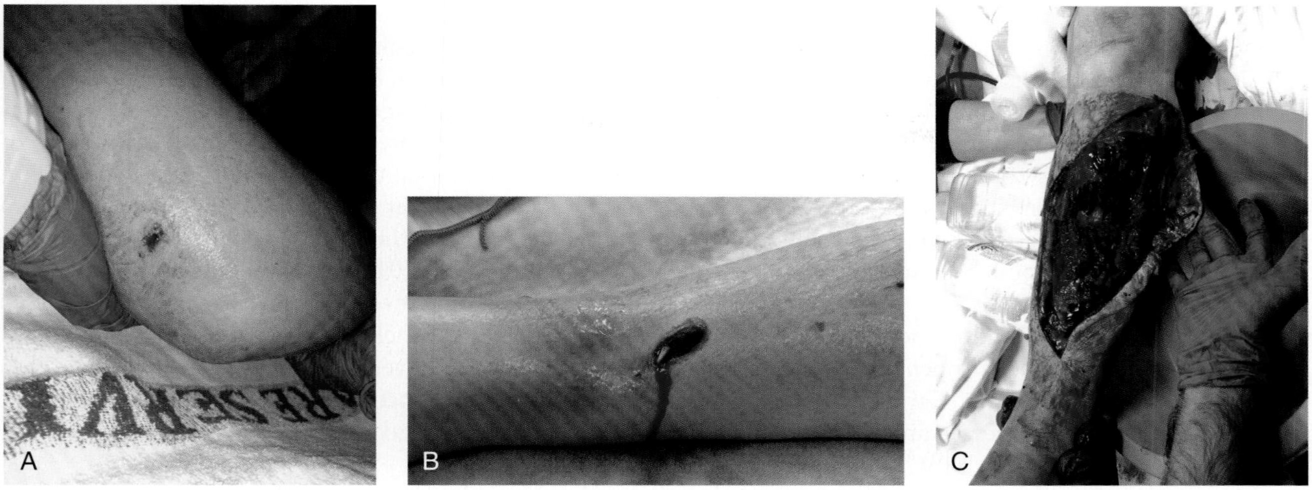

Figure 3 Clinical photographs of three open fractures of substantially varying severity. The surgical strategy of débridement will vary accordingly. **A**, A 14-year-old male fell while skateboarding with a type I open distal humerus fracture. Seen here is the posterior elbow with 5 mm wound caused by the distal humerus penetrating the triceps and then the posterior skin. No gross contamination is seen. **B**, A 25-year-old female who fell off of a bicycle. Type II open tibia fracture with minimal contamination. Note the small spike of a bone fragment protruding out of wound. **C**, A 53-year-old male pedestrian struck by motor vehicle with severe type IIIB open tibia fracture.

After débridement, irrigation of the open fracture wound bed is typically performed, which can be considered an aspect of débridement. Two variables in regard to irrigation have been debated: pressure of irrigation and use of soap. In 2015, a large multicenter randomized trial as part of the Fluid Lavage of Open Wounds (FLOW) study included 2,447 open fractures and evaluated the effects of using castile soap and the pressure of irrigation.[35] The authors report higher revision surgery rates with soap and no beneficial effect of higher pressure irrigation. They recommended against the use of soap in open fractures and for the use of low-pressure irrigation (given lower cost) compared with high pressure. On one-year follow-up including the same patient cohort, the authors report no difference in health-related quality of life regardless of irrigation solution type or pressure.[36]

Primary Closure of Open Fracture Wounds

Another area of debate is the consideration of closing open fracture wounds primarily. Older data reported on the effectiveness of repeated surgery. A 2010 study described a protocol of repeated débridement until culture data were negative on 346 upper and lower extremity open fractures and reported relatively low infection rates: 2.2% type IIIA lower extremity and 4.2% type IIIB lower extremity, 21% type IIIC lower extremity, and 4.3% overall upper and lower.[37]

However, this historic strategy of leaving all open fracture wounds open for repeated washouts has changed with a trend toward early closure whenever possible. A recent prospective cohort study concluded that immediate primary wound closure open fractures was safe; the authors analyzed 84 fractures (all type IIIA and less, upper and lower extremity) and reported 4% infection and 12% nonunion rates, both of which were significantly less than their historic matched series.[38] It is notable that this study included 38 (45%) upper extremity fractures, which are typically more forgiving in terms of wound management and lower expected infection rates. A larger, but retrospective, previous study of 297 open fractures where the authors attempted to close all type IIIA (and less) fractures and reported an overall low deep infection of 4.7% (9% for type IIIA).[39] This study also included both upper (29%) and lower extremity fractures. Utilizing the more rigorous study design of propensity-matching, Jenkinson et al[40] reported a lower infection rate in primary wound closure (4%) versus secondary wound closure (18%, $P = 0.0001$).

In general, it is recommended to close wounds related to open fractures as soon as adequate débridement is performed and not to leave wounds open unless severe contamination is present.

Interval Management of Open Wounds

After the initial surgical débridement, traumatic wounds and the surgical extensions are either closed primarily or left open. Wounds are left open either due to being true type IIIB injuries, in the setting of compartment syndrome and fasciotomies, or the surgical decision to return for repeated washout and secondary closures (secondary to severe contamination, eg,). In this situation, the ideal interval management of the wound before definitive closure remains a critical issue. Several options include traditional sterile gauze dressings (including wet-to-dry style), sterile sealed dressings, sealed adhesive dressings over antibiotic-eluting polymers ("antibiotic bead pouch"), and negative pressure wound therapy (NPWT).

Negative pressure wound therapy (NPWT) is commonly used in the setting of open extremity fractures that are not closed primarily. Early reports suggested a benefit to its use.[41-44] For example, a prospective, randomized trial evaluating NPWT for lower extremity open fracture found a significant difference in deep infection rate favoring the use of NPWT versus standard gauze dressing (5% vs 28%, respectively).[41] However, this was a relatively small study with 62 fractures total. Recently, a large multicenter randomized trial of 374 lower extremity open fractures (460 originally enrolled) observed no advantage of NPWT compared with standard sealed gauze dressing with respect to number of deep infections, fracture union, self-related disability, and quality of life at one-year follow-up; the authors thus concluded that their data do not support the routine use of NPWT.[45] A 2018 Cochrane systematic review of the topic including seven RCTs with over 1,300 patients was essentially inconclusive regarding infection, wound healing, cost-effectiveness, and quality of life.[46] That being said, some sort of sealed dressing (eg, NPWT, sealed antibiotic bead pouch) is recommended over an unsealed dressing.

Antibiotic bead pouches (**Figure 4**) offer the advantage of local antibiotic delivery and have shown some preliminary clinical efficacy.[47] This is often done by

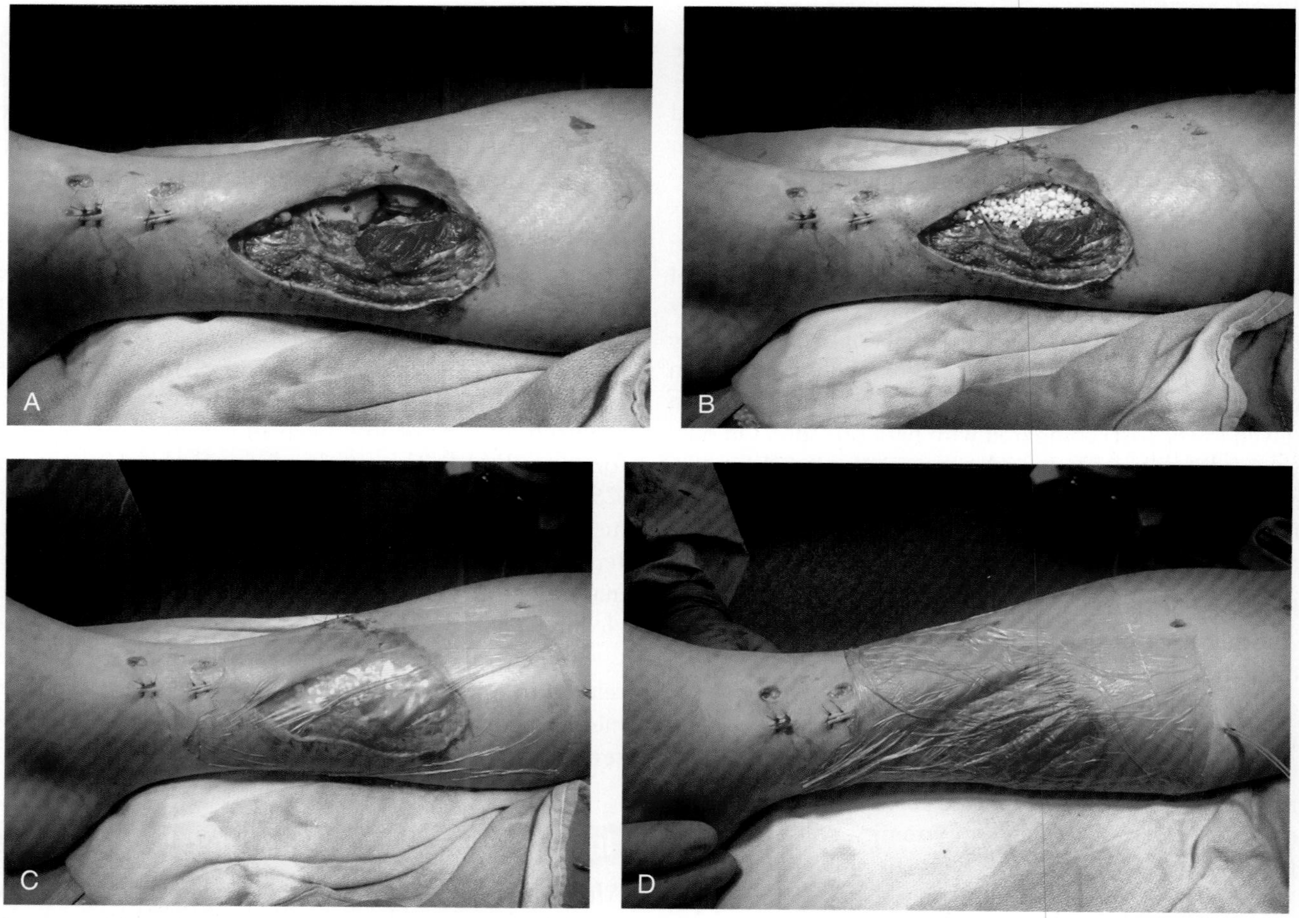

Figure 4 Clinical photographs of a type IIIB open tibia shaft fracture treated with a sealed antibiotic bead pouch. **A**, View of medial wound after thorough débridement and irrigation. **B**, Placement of polymethyl methacrylate (PMMA) beads mixed with vancomycin and tobramycin powder. **C**, Wound sealed with adhesive dressing; note the small drain exiting the skin distant to the wound. **D**, After application of suction via the drain.

mixing polymethyl methacrylate (PMMA) cement with antibiotic powders that have gram-positive and/or gram-negative coverage. There is currently a lack of data to guide type and dosing of antibiotics. Although there is ongoing clinical investigation, most of the previous research in topical antibiotics has been done in animal models.[48-50] Additional research is required to better evaluate the clinical benefit. Future clinical options for interval wound management include the use of biologics such as xenograft extracellular matrices[51] and bioengineered tissue for temporary or permanent application.

Timing to Definitive Coverage

The time delay to definitive coverage of soft-tissue defects in the setting of open fractures (eg, type III fractures) continues to be a challenge, even at level I trauma centers. The effect of time to coverage on complications remains controversial. Some surgeons argue that once a stable vascularized wound margin is established with appropriate control of contamination, the sooner the defect is covered the better. Typically, this issue is most prominently in the setting of open tibia fractures (**Figure 5**).

A 2014 study[52] evaluated the outcomes of soft-tissue flaps for open tibia fractures and contradicted prior work from the LEAP study,[1] finding that the time to flap coverage was a significant predictor of complications and infection, even when controlling for risk factors such as injury severity and fracture classification. The authors report no effect in delay less than 7 days, after which the odds of infection increased 16% per day of delay. As would be expected, residual wound size after final débridement partially determines short-term outcomes. A 2018 study performed secondary analysis on the FLOW trial data[35] and reported that wounds greater than 200 cm^2 resulted in higher rates of wound complications but no difference in revision surgery rates.[53]

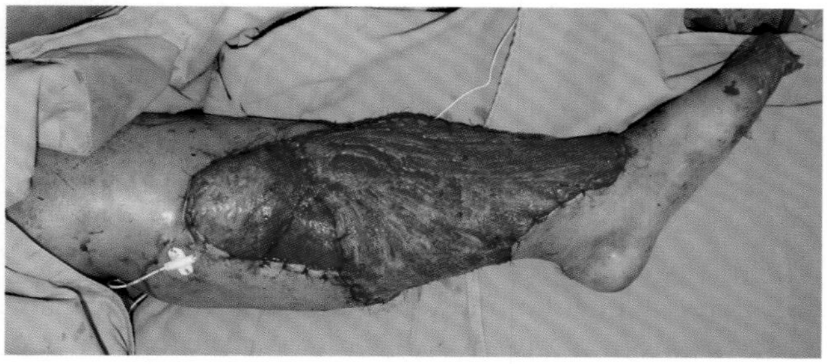

Figure 5 Clinical photograph of free latissimus transfer to medial tibia wound (same patient injury from **Figure 2**).

Summary

Treatment of open fractures remains a common clinical challenge. However, recent research has challenged some long-held clinical paradigms in treatment in terms of timing of débridement, surgical strategy, and wound management. Future research with a focus on large randomized controlled trials is needed to decrease rates of infection and improve long-term function and patient-reported outcomes.

Key Study Points

- Thorough and meticulous surgical débridement of open fractures with respect of soft tissues remains key to preventing infection.
- Although open fractures can be severe injuries requiring urgent treatment, specific time threshold to surgical débridement is less important than quality of surgical technique. Multiple studies have demonstrated no difference in infection rates between early and delayed time to débridement.
- Recent literature recommends the use of low-pressure saline irrigation without soap during the débridement and irrigation of open fractures.

Trauma

Annotated References

1. Pollak AN, Jones AL, Castillo RC, et al: The relationship between time to surgical debridement and incidence of infection after open high-energy lower extremity trauma. *J Bone Joint Surg Am* 2010;92(1):7-15.
2. MacKenzie EJ, Jones AS, Bosse MJ, et al: Health-care costs associated with amputation or reconstruction of a limb-threatening injury. *J Bone Joint Surg Am* 2007;89(8):1685-1692.
3. Sprague S, Petrisor BA, Jeray KJ, et al: Factors associated with health-related quality of life in patients with open fractures. *J Orthop Trauma* 2018;32(1):e5-e11.

   The authors evaluated health-related quality of life in patients with open fracture using the data from the FLOW trial. They observed that only the presence of a lower extremity fracture reached clinical significance for effect. Level of evidence: II.
4. Gustilo RB, Anderson JT: Prevention of infection in the treatment of one thousand and twenty-five open fractures of long bones: Retrospective and prospective analyses. *J Bone Joint Surg Am* 1976;58(4):453-458.
5. Agel J, Evans AR, Marsh JL, et al: The OTA open fracture classification: A study of reliability and agreement. *J Orthop Trauma* 2013;27(7):379-384; discussion 384-5.
6. Agel J, Rockwood T, Barber R, Marsh JL: Potential predictive ability of the orthopaedic trauma association open fracture classification. *J Orthop Trauma* 2014;28(5):300-306.

7. Hao J, Cuellar DO, Herbert B, et al: Does the OTA open fracture classification predict the need for limb amputation? A retrospective observational cohort study on 512 patients. *J Orthop Trauma* 2016;30(4):194-198.

   Authors found that the OTA-OFC was better than the Gustilo-Anderson system for predicting outcomes and complications after open fracture although they acknowledge the limitations of a retrospective study. Level of evidence: IV.

8. Patzakis MJ, Wilkins J: Factors influencing infection rate in open fracture wounds. *Clin Orthop Relat Res* 1989(243):36-40.

9. Lack WD, Karunakar MA, Angerame MR, et al: Type III open tibia fractures: Immediate antibiotic prophylaxis minimizes infection. *J Orthop Trauma* 2015;29(1):1-6.

10. Whitehouse MR, McDaid C, Kelly MB, et al: The effect of timing of antibiotic delivery on infection rates related to open limb fractures: A systematic review. *Emerg Med J* 2017;34(9):613-620.

    The authors present an expansive literature review on the effect of timing of antibiotic delivery on infection rates and found insufficient compelling evidence to determine the effect of timing. They thus recommended future prospective data to be obtained to help address this lack of evidence.

11. Thomas SH, Arthur AO, Howard Z, et al: Helicopter emergency medical services crew administration of antibiotics for open fractures. *Air Med J* 2013;32(2):74-79.

12. Dellinger EP, Miller SD, Wertz MJ, et al: Risk of infection after open fracture of the arm or leg. *Arch Surg* 1988;123(11):1320-1327.

13. Zumsteg JW, Molina CS, Lee DH, Pappas ND: Factors influencing infection rates after open fractures of the radius and/or ulna. *J Hand Surg Am* 2014;39(5):956-961.

14. Weber D, Dulai SK, Bergman J, et al: Time to initial operative treatment following open fracture does not impact development of deep infection: A prospective cohort study of 736 subjects. *J Orthop Trauma* 2014;28(11):613-619.

15. Leonidou A, Kiraly Z, Gality H, et al: The effect of the timing of antibiotics and surgical treatment on infection rates in open long-bone fractures: A 6-year prospective study after a change in policy. *Strategies Trauma Limb Reconstr* 2014;9(3):167-171.

16. Enninghorst N, McDougall D, Hunt JJ, Balogh ZJ: Open tibia fractures: Timely debridement leaves injury severity as the only determinant of poor outcome. *J Trauma* 2011;70(2):352-356; discussion 356-7.

17. Al-Arabi YB, Nader M, Hamidian-Jahromi AR, Woods DA: The effect of the timing of antibiotics and surgical treatment on infection rates in open long-bone fractures: A 9-year prospective study from a district general hospital. *Injury* 2007;38(8):900-905.

18. Obremskey W, Molina C, Collinge C, et al: Current practice in the management of open fractures among orthopaedic trauma surgeons. Part A: Initial management. A survey of orthopaedic trauma surgeons. *J Orthop Trauma* 2014;28(8):e198-202.

19. Jones CB, Wenke JC: Open fractures, in Browner B, Jupiter J, Krettek C, Anderson P, eds: *Skeletal Trauma: Basic Science, Management, and Reconstruction*. ed 5. Philadelphia, PA: Elsevier Saunders; 2015.

20. Johnson JP, Goodman AD, Haag AM, Hayda RA: Decreased time to antibiotic prophylaxis for open fractures at a level one trauma center. *J Orthop Trauma* 2017;31(11): 596-599.

    Retrospective cohort study demonstrating reduced time to antibiotic administration after implementation of a focused multidisciplinary working group. Level of evidence: III.

21. Hoff WS, Bonadies JA, Cachecho R, Dorlac WC: East practice management guidelines work group: Update to practice management guidelines for prophylactic antibiotic use in open fractures. *J Trauma* 2011;70(3):751-754.

22. Zalavras CG: Prevention of infection in open fractures. *Infect Dis Clin North Am* 2017;31(2):339-352.

    Review of key techniques and strategies in the treatment of open fractures.

23. Hauser CJ, Adams CA, Eachempati SR: Surgical infection society guideline: Prophylactic antibiotic use in open fractures: An evidence-based guideline. *Surg Infect* 2006;7(4):379-405.

24. Rodriguez L, Jung HS, Goulet JA, et al: Evidence-based protocol for prophylactic antibiotics in open fractures: Improved antibiotic stewardship with no increase in infection rates. *J Trauma Acute Care Surg* 2014;77(3):400-407; discussion 407-8; quiz 524.

25. Redfern J, Wasilko SM, Groth ME, et al: Surgical site infections in patients with type 3 open fractures: Comparing antibiotic prophylaxis with cefazolin plus gentamicin versus piperacillin/tazobactam. *J Orthop Trauma* 2016;30(8): 415-419.

    A retrospective cohort study comparing the two antibiotic regimens for type III open fractures was performed and demonstrated no difference in infection, nonunion, and rehospitalization. Level of evidence: III.

26. Pannell WC, Banks K, Hahn J, et al: Antibiotic related acute kidney injury in patients treated for open fractures. *Injury* 2016;47(3):653-657.

    The authors conducted a retrospective cohort study and reported no difference in incidence of acute kidney injury when giving gentamicin compared with cefazolin for open fractures

27. Folse J, Hill CE, Graves ML, et al: Risk factors for kidney dysfunction with the use of gentamicin in open fracture antibiotic treatment. *J Orthop Trauma* 2018;32(11):573-578.

    This was a retrospective case control study evaluating the use of gentamicin in open fractures. The authors observed several independent risk factors contributed to kidney dysfunction after gentamicin administration including female gender, obesity, concomitant CT contrast, and ICU admission. Level of evidence: IV.

28. Lawing CR, Lin FC, Dahners LE: Local injection of aminoglycosides for prophylaxis Against infection in open fractures. *J Bone Joint Surg Am* 2015;97(22):1844-1851.

29. Messner J, Papakostidis C, Giannoudis PV, et al: Duration of administration of antibiotic agents for open fractures: Meta-analysis of the existing evidence. *Surg Infect* 2017;18(8): 854-867.

This was a systematic review of the literature specifically evaluating the duration of antibiotics in the setting of open fractures. The authors determined there was insufficient evidence to support prolonged duration.

30. Schenker ML, Yannascoli S, Baldwin KD, et al: Does timing to operative debridement affect infectious complications in open long-bone fractures? A systematic review. *J Bone Joint Surg Am* 2012;94(12):1057-1064.

31. Srour M, Inaba K, Okoye O, et al: Prospective evaluation of treatment of open fractures: Effect of time to irrigation and debridement. *JAMA Surg* 2015;150(4):332-336.

32. Evans AR, Henley B: Tibial shaft fractures, in Gardner M, Henley B, eds: *Harborview Illustrated Tips and Tricks in Fracture Surgery*. Philadelphia, PA, Lippincott, Williams, and Wilkens, 2010.

33. Marecek GS, Nicholson LT, Auran RT, et al: Use of a defined surgical approach for the debridement of open tibia fractures. *J Orthop Trauma* 2018;32(1):e1-e4.

This was a prospective cohort study comparing the use of a counter incision ("defined surgical approach") versus extending the traumatic wound for the formal debridement of open fractures. The author found that the use of the counter incision was safe and led to fewer required flaps. Level of evidence: III.

34. Ricci WM, Collinge C, Streubel PN, et al: A comparison of more and less aggressive bone debridement protocols for the treatment of open supracondylar femur fractures. *J Orthop Trauma* 2013;27(12):722-725.

35. Flow Investigators, Bhandari M, Jeray KJ, Petrisor BA, et al: A trial of wound irrigation in the initial management of open fracture wounds. *N Engl J Med* 2015;373(27):2629-2641.

36. Sprague S, Petrisor B, Jeray K, et al: Wound irrigation does not affect health-related quality of life after open fractures: Results of a randomized controlled trial. *Bone Joint Lett J* 2018;100-B(1):88-94.

The authors analyzed data from the FLOW trial regarding quality of life after open fractures and observed no effect of irrigation solution composition or pressure. Overall decreased health-related quality of life was demonstrated after open fracture. Level of evidence: I.

37. Lenarz CJ, Watson JT, Moed BR, et al: Timing of wound closure in open fractures based on cultures obtained after debridement. *J Bone Joint Surg Am* 2010;92(10):1921-1926.

38. Scharfenberger AV, Alabassi K, Smith S, et al: Primary wound closure after open fracture: A prospective cohort study examining nonunion and deep infection. *J Orthop Trauma* 2017;31(3):121-126.

Prospective cohort study demonstrating that the practice of acute primary closure of open fracture wounds for those that are 3A and lower is safe and effective. Level of evidence: II.

39. Moola FO, Carli A, Berry G, et al: Attempting primary closure for all open fractures: The effectiveness of an institutional protocol. *Can J Surg* 2014;57(3):E82-E88.

40. Jenkinson RJ, Kiss A, Johnson S, et al: Delayed wound closure increases deep-infection rate associated with lower-grade open fractures: A propensity-matched cohort study. *J Bone Joint Surg Am* 2014;96(5):380-386.

41. Stannard JP, Volgas DA, Stewart R, et al: Negative pressure wound therapy after severe open fractures: A prospective randomized study. *J Orthop Trauma* 2009;23(8):552-557.

42. Blum ML, Esser M, Richardson M, et al: Negative pressure wound therapy reduces deep infection rate in open tibial fractures. *J Orthop Trauma* 2012;26(9):499-505.

43. Liu DS, Sofiadellis F, Ashton M, et al: Early soft tissue coverage and negative pressure wound therapy optimises patient outcomes in lower limb trauma. *Injury* 2012;43(6): 772-778.

44. Virani SR, Dahapute AA, Bava SS, Muni SR: Impact of negative pressure wound therapy on open diaphyseal tibial fractures: A prospective randomized trial. *J Clin Orthop Trauma* 2016;7(4):256-259.

The authors present a randomized trial demonstrating decreased infection when using negative pressure wound therapy in the setting of open tibia fractures. Level of evidence: I.

45. Costa ML, Achten J, Bruce J, et al: Effect of negative pressure wound therapy vs standard wound management on 12-month disability among adults with severe open fracture of the lower limb: The WOLLF randomized clinical trial. *J Am Med Assoc* 2018;319(22):2280-2288.

A multicenter randomized trial comparing negative pressure wound dressing versus standard dressing in the setting of severe open fracture. The authors found no difference in disability, infection, or quality of life between the two and concluded that their study did not support the use of negative pressure wound dressings in severe open fractures. Level of evidence: I.

46. Iheozor-Ejiofor Z, Newton K, Dumville JC, et al: Negative pressure wound therapy for open traumatic wounds. *Cochrane Database Syst Rev* 2018;7:CD012522.

The authors conducted a Cochrane Database systematic review on the use of negative pressure wound therapy (NPWT) for open traumatic wounds and conclude that there is no difference for wound healing at 6 weeks, it is not cost-effective, and there is insufficient evidence to support it overall when considering wound infection, adverse events, time to closure, pain, or health-related quality of life.

47. Warner M, Henderson C, Kadrmas W, et al: Comparison of vacuum-assisted closure to the antibiotic bead pouch for the treatment of blast injury of the extremity. *Orthopedics* 2010;33(2):77-82.

48. Tennent DJ, Shiels SM, Sanchez CJ, et al: Time-dependent effectiveness of locally applied vancomycin powder in a contaminated traumatic orthopaedic wound model. *J Orthop Trauma* 2016;30(10):531-537.

This was an animal model study of rat femur fractures inoculated with staph aureus. Vancomycin applied topically showed a time-dependent benefit of decreased bacterial colonization suggesting its potential benefit in open fractures.

49. Rand BC, Penn-Barwell JG, Wenke JC: Combined local and systemic antibiotic delivery improves eradication of wound contamination: An animal experimental model of contaminated fracture. *Bone Joint Lett J* 2015;97-B(10):1423-1427.

50. Penn-Barwell JG, Murray CK, Wenke JC: Local antibiotic delivery by a bioabsorbable gel is superior to PMMA bead depot in reducing infection in an open fracture model. *J Orthop Trauma* 2014;28(6):370-375.

A retrospective review of 55 patients compared transarticular screws, dorsal bridge plating, or a combination of the two in Lisfranc injuries. They found no significant difference in implant failure, need for removal, or functional outcomes in the three groups. Only anatomic reduction was predictive of improved functional outcomes. Level of evidence: III (Therapeutic).

51. Fokin AA, Puente I, Hus N, et al: Extracellular matrix applications in the treatment of open fractures with complex wounds and large soft tissue defects. *J Orthop Trauma* 2018;32(2):e76-e80.

The authors describe a technique of applying porcine urinary bladder extracellular matrix to open fractures with large soft-tissue defects and report on successful achievement of a stable soft-tissue envelope.

52. D'Alleyrand JC, Manson TT, Dancy L, et al: Is time to flap coverage of open tibial fractures an independent predictor of flap-related complications? *J Orthop Trauma* 2014;28(5):288-293.

53. Shea P, O'Hara NN, Sprague SA, et al: Wound surface area as a risk factor for flap complications among patients with open fractures. *Plast Reconstr Surg* 2018;142(1):228-236.

The authors performed a secondary analysis of FLOW trial data demonstrating that wound surface area of >200 cm2 was an independent risk factor for wound complications but not for flap-related reoperation. Level of evidence: III.

Trauma

Chapter 19
Upper Extremity Trauma

Benjamin R. Pulley, MD • Claire B. Ryan, MD • David Ring, MD, PhD • Michael J. Gardner, MD

ABSTRACT

Many of the principles of upper extremity trauma have remained unchanged for some time, but the role of surgical treatment and methods of fixation are subjects of debate for acromioclavicular dislocation, displaced diaphyseal clavicle fractures, and diaphyseal humerus fractures. There are even advocates for fixation of a subset of displaced fractures of the scapula. The mainstays of discussion regarding proximal humerus fractures revolve around patient selection for nonsurgical management, methods of surgical fixation, and the growing role of reverse total shoulder arthroplasty. Recent research regarding periarticular fractures of the elbow addressed the biomechanics of plate fixation for supracondylar humerus fractures, the management of elbow joint instability, the role and design of radial head arthroplasty, the treatment of olecranon fractures, and the outcomes of total elbow arthroplasty after distal humerus fractures. There are still advocates for intramedullary nail fixation of diaphyseal fractures of the forearm. Distal radioulnar joint instability, compartment syndrome, and forearm fracture nonunion are also highlighted in recent reports. Diagnostic strategies, treatment modalities, and cost-effectiveness are areas of investigation for fractures of the distal radius and scaphoid.

Keywords: acromioclavicular joint injury; clavicle fracture; forearm fracture; hand fracture; humeral shaft fracture; periarticular elbow fracture; proximal humerus fracture; wrist fracture

Dr. Ring or an immediate family member has received royalties from Skeletal Dynamics and Wright Medical Technology, Inc. and serves as a board member, owner, officer, or committee member of the American Academy of Orthopaedic Surgeons and the Orthopaedic Trauma Association. Dr. Gardner or an immediate family member has received royalties from Synthes; is a member of a speakers' bureau or has made paid presentations on behalf of KCI; serves as a paid consultant to or is an employee of Conventus, Globus Medical, KCI, OsteoCentric, SI-Bone, StabilizOrtho, StabilizOrtho, and Synthes; has stock or stock options held in Conventus, Genesis Innovations Group, Imagen Technologies, and Intelligent Implants; has received research or institutional support from Medtronic, OsteoCentric, SmartMedical Devices, and Zimmer; and serves as a board member, owner, officer, or committee member of the American Academy of Orthopaedic Surgeons, the American Orthopaedic Association, the Orthopaedic Research Society, and the Orthopaedic Trauma Association. Neither of the following authors nor any immediate family member has received anything of value from or has stock or stock options held in a commercial company or institution related directly or indirectly to the subject of this chapter: Dr. Pulley and Dr. Ryan.

Introduction

This chapter reviews evidence published in the last 5 years that might help guide decision making for patients regarding upper limb trauma. High-level data have raised questions about common treatment strategies and additional data are needed.

Acromioclavicular Joint Injury

The role of surgical treatment of acute acromioclavicular (AC) dislocation is debated. Only complete dislocations (100% loss of apposition of the joint) are considered for surgery. Some people believe that dislocations with muscle interposition merit surgery, but that can only be discerned at surgery, and it is not clear that the degree of displacement correlates with muscle interposition. Guesses based on radiographs may not be helpful.

A recent meta-analysis of 19 studies (954 patients)[1] favored nonsurgical treatment of complete AC joint dislocations. There were five randomized controlled trials comparing a variety of surgical interventions (ie, K-wire, screw, nonrigid reconstruction, hook plate, etc) with nonsurgical treatment. The surgical fixation group had better aesthetic and radiographic outcomes. The nonsurgical treatment group had quicker return to activity and avoided implant removal and other adverse events related to surgery. The Constant-Murley score (CMS) was slightly better in the surgical group, a difference that may not be meaningful to people with this injury. The Disabilities of the Arm, Shoulder, and Hand (DASH) score, return to sport, and subsequent surgery were comparable.

A prospective randomized trial involving 83 patients found that hook plate fixation of acute complete AC joint dislocation and nonsurgical treatment had comparable patient-reported outcomes.[2] A smaller retrospective cohort study found comparable Short Form-36 (SF-36) scores after hook plate fixation or nonsurgical treatment.[3]

Two meta-analyses[4,5] found loop suspensory fixation was associated with better CMS and lower Visual Analog Scale (VAS) for pain at the cost of longer surgical time[4] and higher complication rates when compared with a hook plate.[5] Additionally, a retrospective cohort study found a better SF-36, VAS for pain, DASH, CMS, and global satisfaction after arthroscopic-assisted coracoclavicular fixation versus hook plate fixation.[6]

Clavicle Fracture

Clavicle shaft fractures have transitioned from no surgery to frequent surgery in the last three decades, because the benefit of surgical treatment of completely diaphyseal fractures of the clavicle (more than 100% loss of apposition of the fracture surfaces) is unclear. In three recent prospective randomized controlled trials comparing surgical versus nonsurgical management for displaced midshaft clavicle fractures,[7–9] there were more nonunions, but comparable patient-reported outcomes with nonsurgical treatment.

In a prospective randomized trial involving 160 patients evaluated for 1 year[7] in the Netherlands, there were no differences in Constant or Disabilities of the Arm, Shoulder, and Hand (DASH) scores at any time point, but the rate of nonunion was significantly greater in the nonsurgical group (23% vs 2.4%). Only about half the patients chose to have surgery to treat the nonunion (13% in the nonsurgical group and 1.2% in the surgical group).

In a trial of 117 patients evaluated for a year[8] in Brazil, DASH scores were comparable at all time points. The rate of nonunion was 15% with nonsurgical treatment compared with no nonunions with surgical treatment.

A multicenter trial from the United Kingdom with a total of 301 patients[9] found that CMS and DASH scores were better in the surgical group 6 weeks and 3 months after fracture, but comparable at 9 months. Nine months after injury there were fewer nonunions in the surgical group (0.8%) than the nonsurgical group (11%).

The weight of evidence to date (including these three trials) is that nonunions are more common with nonsurgical treatment, but—on average—symptoms and limitations are similar a year after injury.[10,11] Recent meta-analyses compared fracture healing and functional outcomes after surgical and nonsurgical treatment of displaced diaphyseal clavicle fractures. Most recently, a systematic review of 1,352 patients treated in 14 randomized trials found a lower risk of nonunion with surgical treatment. Three of 14 studies included analyzed DASH scores at short-term follow-up and found significantly better scores in patients treated with surgery. Seven studies found a higher DASH score at 9-month follow-up in the surgical group. These results are limited, however, by the fact that no studies included in the meta-analysis blinded patients to the treatment they received. It should also be noted that seven other studies in the meta-analysis found no significant difference in long-term functional outcomes in patients treated with surgery as compared with those treated nonsurgically.[10]

A systematic review that included both randomized control trials and well-designed observational studies comparing surgical and nonsurgical treatment of displaced midshaft clavicle fractures found lower rates of nonunion with surgical treatment, but no clinically significant difference in symptoms and limitations measured using DASH and Constant-Murley scores.[11] In other words, nonunions are more common without surgery, but clinical outcomes are similar over the long term, suggesting that many nonunions can be accommodated.

A retrospective cohort study of 1,215 patients found a higher rate of total complications in patients who had surgery for midshaft clavicle fracture nonunion compared with surgical fixation of acute midshaft clavicle fracture. The most common complications were wound infections, but no individual type of complication was significantly more common in nonunions.[12] When interpreting studies that compare surgery for acute fracture with surgery for nonunion, readers should be mindful that many patients with nonunion do not request surgery. Furthermore, both patients with nonunion as well as patients who request surgery for nonunion may have important differences from the average patient with a completely displaced midshaft clavicle fracture that are not adequately accounted for in these types of studies. It would be helpful to determine the number needed to treat, number needed to harm, and similar numbers.

When surgical treatment of midshaft clavicle fractures is selected, there is debate about the best method of fixation. A prospective randomized trial of 123 patients compared elastic nailing (2.0 to 3.5 mm titanium) versus plate fixation and found that plate fixation had a lower rate of implant removal and yielded quicker functional recovery (based on CMS and DASH score at time points up to 6 months after surgery) especially in comminuted fractures. However, elastic nailing had shorter surgical time (53 vs 70 minutes) and lower rate of infection.[13]

One downside of surgical fixation of a midshaft clavicle fracture is the prominence of implants placed on a subcutaneous bone in a prominent aesthetic location and an area of straps that may bear weight. A retrospective cohort study involving 81 patients reported that their technique of dual mini-fragment plating for midshaft clavicle fractures yielded good union and functional recovery and a low rate of implant removal for soft-tissue irritation (3.7%).[14] It is difficult to interpret the advantages and disadvantages of specific techniques in terms of implant prominence without randomization and controls.

Scapula Fracture

Scapula fractures are usually treated nonsurgically with good success and most surgeons see little role for surgery in the absence of a glenoid rim fracture contributing to glenohumeral instability. Nevertheless, several recent reports from advocates of surgical treatment suggest a subset of fractures might benefit from surgery.

An uncontrolled retrospective cohort study reported good functional outcomes in 61 patients with extra-articular fractures of the scapula that were treated surgically[15] based on specific displacement criteria: medial or lateral displacement ≥20 mm, angulation ≥45°, medial or lateral displacement ≥15 mm plus angulation ≥30°, double disruptions of the superior shoulder suspensory complex with both displaced ≥10 mm, glenopolar angle ≤22°, and open fractures.

A retrospective cohort study from the same group described[16] patients aged 65 and older with scapula fractures treated surgically based on the same extra-articular criteria as well as more than 4 mm of articular step or gap. They reported low complication rates (three patients had temporary postoperative delirium, one patient had a urinary tract infection, one patient had removal of an intra-articular screw, and one patient had a second surgery to remove postoperative heterotopic ossification) and good functional outcomes (mean range of motion and strength of the affected shoulder was >70% of that of the contralateral shoulder and DASH and SF-36 were comparable to normal populations).[16]

Another retrospective case series of 24 patients with fractures of the glenoid fossa treated nonsurgically found that those with intra-articular displacement 3 mm or less had better CMS than those with displacement 5 mm or greater.[17] A study in cadavers found that measurement of glenopolar angles is more reliable on 3D CT reconstructions of the scapula than radiographs.[18] In another cadaveric study the modified Judet approach allowed access to the same key anatomic landmarks despite exposing only 20% of the surface area as the classic Judet approach.[19]

Proximal Humerus Fractures

Fractures of the proximal humerus are common, particularly in older patients with osteoporosis. Deformity is relatively well adapted, particularly for low-demand or infirm individuals. There was optimism that locking plates had improved the results of surgical treatment, but there is no fixation method that is not prone to technical adverse events such as implant migration or prominence and loss of reduction. Hemiarthroplasty is less used and inverse total shoulder arthroplasty more used for complex fractures in infirm, less active patients. Given the success of nonsurgical treatment, there is increasing interest in starting nonsurgical and moving to inverse arthroplasty when merited.

The 5-year results of the PROximal Fracture of the Humerus Evaluation by Randomisation (PROFHER) trial, a prospective randomized trial involving 164 patients, were consistent with the original report. There was no difference in function based on the Oxford Shoulder Score (OSS), quality of life based on EuroQol 5D-3L (EQ-5D-3L), or subsequent surgery between nonsurgical and surgical treatment groups.[20]

A prospective randomized trial involving 72 patients compared intramedullary nail versus locking plate fixation in patients with two- or three-part surgical neck fractures of the proximal humerus and found no differences in functional scores, range of motion, or humeral neck-shaft angle 12 months after surgery but reported more complications and reoperations in patients receiving intramedullary nails.[21]

A prospective cohort study looked at 60 patients with osteoporotic four-part proximal humerus fractures treated either with open reduction and internal fixation (ORIF) incorporating a fibular strut allograft and a plate or with hemiarthroplasty and found better motion and functional recovery (CMS and DASH) in the surgical fixation group.[22]

Reverse total shoulder arthroplasty (rTSA) has become a preferred method of treatment for proximal humerus fractures in older, more infirm, and less active adults, particularly those with more complex fracture, bad bone quality, and large rotator cuff defects. When comparing rTSA versus hemiarthroplasty, a meta-analysis of seven studies involving 255 patients found superior forward elevation, abduction, tuberosity healing, and outcome scores after rTSA; only external rotation was better after hemiarthroplasty.[23]

Given the difficulty demonstrating a benefit—on average—to surgical treatment of acute fractures, one idea is to treat fractures in older, infirm, and inactive patients nonsurgically to start and then address major problems with later rTSA. Three separate retrospective cohort studies recently compared patients treated with acute rTSA for fracture with those who underwent delayed rTSA, either after loosened or broken ORIF or after nonunion or malunion after nonsurgical treatment. It is important to note these studies have the important drawbacks of comparing people with surgery for an acute fracture with people who choose surgery because they are not happy with the results of the treatment of the acute fracture.

One study involving 44 patients found that rTSA after loss of fixation of a proximal humerus fracture was associated with slightly higher complication rates compared with acute rTSA for an acute fracture, but there was no difference in revision surgery rate or American Shoulder and Elbow Surgeons (ASES) score.[24]

A second study involving 60 patients found that patients with loose proximal humerus locking plate fixation who had a second surgery for rTSA had marginally worse CMS and DASH scores and experienced more complications than patients treated with immediate rTSA.[25]

A third study of 49 patients found comparable outcome scores (Shoulder Pain and Disability Index [SPADI], Simple Shoulder Test-12 [SST-12], ASES score, University of California-Los Angeles [UCLA] shoulder rating scale, CMS, and Short Form-12 [SF-12]) and motion in patients who underwent rTSA as the initial treatment for fracture and those who had rTSA for later nonunion or malunion. They also reported that acute rTSA for fracture is marginally better than salvage rTSA for problems after hemiarthroplasty or plate fixation.[26]

Humeral Shaft Fracture

The role of surgical treatment and the optimal method of fixation of diaphyseal humerus fractures are still being debated. A large meta-analysis involving 832 patients (16 of 17 studies were prospective randomized controlled trials) compared open reduction and plate and screw fixation, intramedullary nail fixation, and MIPO and found no differences in rates of nonunion or infection, but more shoulder pain with intramedullary fixation and more radial nerve palsy in the open reduction plate fixation group.[27]

Another meta-analysis comparing the same treatment groups included eight prospective randomized controlled trials involving a total of 376 patients and concluded that MIPO resulted in a superior functional outcome compared with ORIF or intramedullary nailing and also reported that ORIF had the highest complication rate of the three groups.[28] Most reports of MIPO to date are introductory and promotional, so the data may not be representative.

A retrospective study compared MIPO versus intramedullary nailing in 30 patients with humeral shaft fractures and found a higher rate of major complications (radial nerve palsy, nonunion, infection, and revision surgery) in the intramedullary nailing group (53%) compared with the MIPO group (7%).[29]

A recent prospective randomized controlled trial involving 110 patients compared MIPO and nonsurgical treatment with a functional brace. There were 15% nonunions with nonsurgical treatment and none with surgical treatment. At 6 months postoperatively, before treatment of the nonunions in the nonsurgical group, the functional brace group had worse DASH scores on average.[30]

Intramedullary nailing of humeral shaft fractures raises concern about injury to the rotator cuff and subacromial impingement of implants. A prospective, randomized controlled trial involving 40 patients compared the use of an arthroscope to ensure proper nail placement with standard technique. Patients in the scope-assisted group were found to have better outcome scores and shorter fluoroscopy time as compared with the standard technique, although total surgical time was not reported.[31]

Distal Humerus Fractures

Researchers continue to measure the mechanics of surgical fixation of fractures of the distal humerus, perhaps because they can be problematic, particularly with low quality bone. A sawbones study comparing parallel versus orthogonal plating for ORIF of intra-articular distal humerus fractures found similar mechanics, but parallel plating was stiffer during axial loading of the radial column.[32] A similar study in simulated extra-articular distal humerus fractures in cadavers found parallel plating to be stiffer in torsion and bending, and to have a higher extension load to failure.[33] Given that parallel plating uses longer screws in the articular segment (more metal), these conclusions seem to reflect common sense.

Total elbow arthroplasty does better than ORIF of distal humerus fractures in people older than 65 years in the short-term, but there are concerns about long-term outcomes and management of infection, loosening within a few years of surgery, and periprosthetic fracture. A retrospective cohort study described 44 patients treated with total elbow arthroplasty for distal humerus fractures 10 years after surgery and noted 92% survivorship in patients without rheumatoid arthritis (76% survivorship in patients with rheumatoid arthritis), but a relatively high rate of major complications, including 11% deep infection, 18% revision or resection, and 11% periprosthetic fracture.[34]

Radial Head Fracture

Radial head arthroplasty is an alternative to ORIF for restoring radiocapitellar contact in the setting of a comminuted, displaced fractures of the radial head associated with other ligament injuries or fractures. A meta-analysis involving 319 patients with unstable displaced fractures of the radial head found that arthroplasty yielded higher satisfaction, better elbow scores, shorter surgical time, and lower incidence of recurrent instability compared with ORIF.[35]

Radial head arthroplasty varies by modularity, movement (some have an articulation between head and neck), and stem (smooth loose vs porous fixed). A retrospective cohort study involving 57 patients found that DASH scores and Mayo Elbow Performance Index scores were the same between patients treated with radial head arthroplasties with either a smooth or porous stem design, but the porous stem group had higher rates of unintended loosening (64% vs 24%), greater loss of elbow flexion, and higher rates of overstuffing of the radiocapitellar joint.[36]

Olecranon Fracture

Olecranon fractures tend to occur from a direct blow to the elbow. Displaced fractures are generally treated surgically, with the exception of infirm and low-demand patients.

A prospective randomized controlled trial involving 19 patients greater than 75 years old compared nonsurgical treatment with tension band fixation for management of geriatric olecranon fractures and found that there was no difference in functional outcome scores 1 year after injury. The trial was stopped after 19 enrollments because of an unacceptably high rate of complications in the surgical treatment group (82%).[37]

The same investigators also compared plate and screw fixation with tension band wire fixation for treatment of olecranon fractures in a level I study involving 67 patients and found a higher rate of implant removal with tension band wires (50% vs 22%), but both of these rates are relatively high and may reflect local preferences and habits for implant removal. The rate of infection was higher in the plate group (13% vs 0%).[38]

Persistent or recurrent instability of the elbow joint after fracture or dislocation is a challenging problem. A recent prospective cohort of 24 patients treated with an internal elbow joint stabilizer that allows a function range of motion of the elbow while the ligaments and fractures heal reported maintenance of concentric reduction of the elbow joint in 23 of 24 patients, as well as good final motion (mean elbow flexion arc 119° and mean forearm rotation 151°) and functional scores (Broberg-Morrey and DASH scores) after healing and device removal.[39]

Forearm Fracture

Modern plate and screw fixation solved the problem of diaphyseal forearm fractures with no notable improvements since the introduction of 3.5 mm dynamic compression plates. Nevertheless, intramedullary nails are often attempted. A prospective randomized trial involving 87 patients compared four different methods of fixation for both bone forearm fractures: both bone plating, both bone intramedullary nailing, plate fixation of the radius with intramedullary nailing of the ulna, and plate fixation of the ulna with intramedullary nailing of the radius. The group that underwent plating of the radius with intramedullary nailing of the ulna had the lowest rate of complications and the best functional recovery. Among 21 patients treated with plate and screw fixation of both bones, 3 had infections and 3 had nonunions—much higher rates than typical for this surgery. We therefore feel these data should be interpreted with great caution. They also performed a biomechanical analysis of the four different fixation constructs that found both bone plating and plate fixation of the radius with intramedullary nailing of the ulna were comparable and stronger than the other two options.[40]

A retrospective study published in a relatively low tier journal and involving 90 patients with single bone diaphyseal forearm fractures compared plate fixation to intramedullary nailing and found that the intramedullary nailing group had a shorter surgical time and roughly a 2-week shorter time to fracture union, as well as comparable functional scores (DASH score and Grace-Eversmann rating) and range of motion compared with plate fixation.[41] It can be risky to rely on intramedullary fixation when anatomical alignment is important, which is the case with Monteggia and Galeazzi fractures. Avoiding shortening can also be more difficult with intramedullary fixation, which could lead to distal radioulnar joint incongruity.

Distal radioulnar joint (DRUJ) instability in the setting of isolated radial shaft fractures—the Galeazzi fracture—is incompletely understood. A retrospective study involving 66 patients looked at radiographic factors previously associated with DRUJ instability (radial shaft fracture within 7.5 cm of the wrist, >5 mm of positive ulnar variance, or associated ulnar styloid fracture) and found that these parameters are only moderately accurate. Only 11% of the entire cohort ultimately were diagnosed with DRUJ instability (based on unclear criteria), but 39% of the fractures were within 7.5 cm of the wrist, 32% had >5 mm positive ulnar variance, and 11% had associated ulnar styloid fractures. Of note four of seven patients with ulnar styloid fractures were diagnosed with DRUJ instability. Routine assessment of the DRUJ after fixation of the radius is advisable.[42]

Compartment syndrome of the forearm after both bone forearm fractures is predominantly a clinical diagnosis and the treatment is urgent forearm fasciotomy. A retrospective cohort study involving 151 patients evaluated the Orthopaedic Trauma Association (OTA)/ Arbeitsgemeinschaft für Osteosynthesefragen (AO) classification of both bone forearm fractures for association with fasciotomy. They reported that overall, 15% of both bone forearm fractures had fasciotomy; 7.5% of type 22-A3, 18% of type 22-B3, and 33% of type 22-C3.[43] Since many of these were likely prophylactic, these data do not inform the true risk of forearm compartment syndrome.

Nonunion of surgically treated diaphyseal forearm fractures is associated with technical deficiencies or infection. Adequate plate fixation and either cancellous or corticocancellous bone grafting usually gains union. A recent prospective randomized trial of 49 patients looked at treating diaphyseal radius and ulna nonunions with plate fixation and corticocancellous iliac crest autograft either with or without augmentation using bone morphogenetic protein (BMP)-2 or BMP-7. The choice between using BMP-2 or BMP-7 was not specified or randomized, but they reported that they found that the addition of the BMP did not improve healing or function.[44]

Distal Radius Fractures

Fractures of the distal radius nearly always heal, and deformity is often well adapted, particularly in less active or infirm people. There are several surgical techniques to try to improve alignment, each with specific advantages and disadvantages. It is still not clear who benefits from surgery and how to select a surgical technique. And there is notable surgeon-to-surgeon variation in how patients are treated, which suggests the patient may not be adequately involved in choosing treatment strategies.

Diagnosis

Arthroscopy was used to evaluate the triangular fibrocartilage complex (TFCC) during ORIF of 85 fractures of the distal radius and found that 50 were abnormal, but this did not correlate with fracture displacement/ angulation and TFCC injury.[45] The authors did not focus on foveal detachment of the origin of the distal radioulnar ligaments and they did not exclude fractures of the ulnar styloid and neck (considered an alternative to detachment of the ligaments). They included likely degenerative lesions (central perforations of the articular disk) and likely unrelated or unimportant lesions (triquetrolunate ligament abnormalities). The vast majority of the abnormalities they diagnosed (26) were on the radial side. It is not clear if radial side lesions are clinically meaningful and they may simply be related to the articular component of the fracture. There were only 9 fovea (ulnar) detachments, but there were 54 ulna fractures (64%)—which seems to confirm that ulna fracture is an alternative to foveal detachment. It might have been even more interesting to study factors associated with foveal detachment or fracture of the ulnar styloid at its base because these are more closely related to trauma and the potential for distal radioulnar instability.

Twenty-three patients in whom handheld ultrasound was used in addition to radiographs to diagnose fracture of the distal radius and assess adequacy of reduction were compared with 20 control patients in whom only radiographs were used. Ultrasound was 100% sensitive but only 90% to 95% specific using radiographs as the reference standard for diagnosis of fracture depending on the observer. The diagnostic performance characteristics of categorized adequacy of reduction included 76% to 93% sensitivity and 93% to 94% specificity. There was good interrater reliability between the two observers for both diagnosis of fracture ($K = 0.86$) and categorized adequacy of reduction ($K = 0.82$).[46]

Treatment

There continues to be controversy regarding fixation methods and patient selection for surgical treatment of distal radius fractures. Extra-articular distal radius fractures with well-maintained radiocarpal alignment are traditionally treated nonsurgically, sometimes with a closed reduction if necessary. Current indications for surgical treatment include significant intra-articular displacement or comminution and/or significant radial angulation or shortening. However, recent literature suggests that older, low-demand patients may not benefit from surgical intervention, even in the setting of significant deformity.

A randomized controlled trial of 140 patients aged 50 to 74 with dorsally displaced fractures of the distal radius compared volar locking plate fixation with external fixation. There was no significant difference in patient-reported outcomes at any time point during the study period. Volar locking plate fixation was found to be associated with more accurate restoration of volar radial tilt. Patients treated with volar locking plate had better grip strength at 3 months, but not at 1 year.[47]

A retrospective review of 359 patients compared patients with intra-articular distal radius fractures treated with either closed reduction and percutaneous Kirschner wire fixation or ORIF with a volar locking plate. The volar locking plate group was less likely to have a residual intra-articular step of ≥1 mm after initial reduction. Initial intra-articular displacement was associated with persistent intra-articular step at final union, but no difference in persistent step-off found at final union between the two treatment groups. Similarly, there was no significant difference between the two groups in terms of change in persistent step size (ie, settling of a step that results in an increased step-off).[48]

A prospective evaluation of radiographic alignment 1 year after volar plate fixation of an intra-articular distal radius fracture found a statistically significant change in fracture alignment, but the mean change was clinically unimportant (less than 1 mm or 1°) and within measurement error. There was also no difference in maintenance of reduction or grip strength/range of motion between patients who had one row of distal screws and those with two rows.[49]

A prospective study of 129 highly functioning patients aged 55 and older with fracture of the distal radius found no significant difference in patient-reported outcomes between patients who were treated surgically or nonsurgically. The fractures treated surgically had significantly worse radiographic deformity. Persistent articular step, persistent articular gap, and ulnar positivity of >2 mm were associated with lower functional outcome scores regardless of treatment modality. It is not clear how to interpret this study. Does operating on displaced fractures help them get to outcomes comparable to less displaced fractures or is surgical treatment unhelpful?[50]

Cost-effectiveness

A randomized controlled trial of 40 unstable fractures of the distal radius compared open reduction and volar locking plate with closed reduction and pinning with K-wires found better DASH scores at 6, 9, and 12 weeks postoperatively and better wrist motion, supination, and grip strength at 6 and 9 weeks postoperatively with plating, but there were no differences 1 year after surgery. ORIF was associated with significantly higher costs perioperatively (CR = 2.7/1.0) and at 90 days (CR = 2.03/1.0), but by the 1 year time point, ORIF was only 60% more expensive than CRPP (CR = 1.6/1.0), mostly because of the high cost of postoperative clinic visits for patients treated with CRPP. CRPP required additional office visits for pin removal and additional appointments with a therapist to help with exercises, accounting for the increase in cost in this group at the 1 year time point. This increase in postoperative costs in the CRPP group narrowed the overall cost gap between the two groups at 1 year follow-up.[51]

Carpal Fractures

Scaphoid

Current best evidence suggests that scaphoid waist fractures verified as nondisplaced on CT heal with adequate protection. There are some studies that adequate protection may not need to include prolonged cast immobilization. Displaced fractures are prone to nonunion and best treated surgically. Diagnosis of displacement and union are not reliable or accurate with radiographs, but it is not clear that CT is meaningfully better or that it improves healing rates, motion, symptoms, and limitations.

A systematic review comparing surgical and nonsurgical treatment of nondisplaced fractures of the scaphoid found no differences in return to work, subsequent surgery, or time to radiographic union.[52] A systematic review of five studies including 166 patients with a scaphoid nonunion treated with low-intensity pulsed ultrasound (LIPUS) found 79% healed in an average of 4.2 months, but there was no control group.[53] These types of studies tend to mistakenly include fractures that are radiographically visible, but on their way to healing. Only randomized trials comparing enhancement with simulated enhancement with adequate blinding of patient and surgeon should be considered when evaluating these types of treatments.

A prospective study of 28 patients with unstable, displaced scaphoid waist fractures examined outcomes of percutaneous screw placement as a treatment modality.

Manual closed reduction with percutaneous pinning was attempted for all patients. Ultimately, 14 patients had an open reduction. The remaining 14 patients were followed up to assess time to union and functional outcomes. Thirteen out of 14 fractures treated healed.[54]

Hook of Hamate

The hook of the hamate has trouble healing, even though most fractures are nondisplaced. We do not know the incidence and healing rate of these fractures because we tend to meet people when they have continued tenderness long after the injury. Hook of hamate nonunion can be an incidental finding on wrist CT, suggesting it may be well adapted for some people. People with symptoms from a nonunion can be offered surgery to excise the hook of the hamate.

Some people consider surgery for hamate hook fracture. In a retrospective review of 51 patients with a hook of hamate fracture (14 treated surgically, 10 with fragment excision, and 4 with ORIF), there were no differences in pain, grip, motion, or satisfaction between patients treated surgically and those treated without surgery. Twenty nine patients in the study were assessed for fracture union via CT scan: the 4 patients who underwent ORIF and 25 who underwent nonsurgical treatment. All four patients treated with ORIF achieved union. Of the 25 patients treated nonsurgically, 6 experienced delayed union as defined by no evidence of healing on CT scan at least 93 days after injury.[55]

One study noted that hamate hook fractures are often noted incidentally on CT of fractures of the distal radius or scaphoid. One can assume that with radiographs alone these fractures go undiagnosed. And they seem to give few problems. Based on these data, patients can be informed that most acute fractures of the hook of hamate heal. Those that do not may cause few problems.[56]

Lunate

The lunate is known as the carpal key stone for its strong ligamentous attachments to the radius and adjacent carpal bones. Injuries to the lunate are, as a result, usually the result of a high-energy mechanism and almost universally require surgical intervention. Thus, recent literature focuses on outcomes of surgical treatment. In a prospective series of 16 patients treated surgically for perilunate dislocations, patients had a mean grip strength of 59% as compared with the unaffected side 2 years after surgery. Fourteen of sixteen patients returned to work within 6 months, and 10 returned to sports within 1 year. The authors also found that a delay in time to surgery significantly decreased patients' DASH and VAS satisfaction scores.[57]

Extra-articular Hand Fractures

Hand fractures comprise a significant percentage of all fractures treated each year and are a common cause of ED visits. As a result, much current research focuses on costs of treatment and patient-reported outcomes for various types of hand injuries. There is debate about early active range of motion after hand fractures versus traditional immobilization in those treated both surgically and nonsurgically.

Cost-effectiveness

A Canadian cost analysis study comparing closed reduction and percutaneous pinning of hand fractures done in a hospital operating room versus those done in office setting found that treatment in the OR was three times as expensive. Office surgery avoids the costs of nursing and anesthesia personnel, anesthesia and regional block, and a greater number of opened supplies. In a survey of hand surgeons, lack of in-office fluoroscopy was the most common impediment to office surgery.[58]

Outcomes

A systematic review of 22 studies assessed the relationship between psychological factors and patient-reported outcomes in patients with upper extremity injury. Symptoms of depression were addressed in 17 of the 22 studies. Catastrophic thinking in response to nociception and anxiety were also addressed in several studies. The review was limited in its ability to detect trends in the data given the heterogeneity of the literature included in the study.[59]

A prospective cohort study examined postoperative opioid consumption after upper extremity surgery in patients of a single private practice. Over a 6-month period, surgeons prescribed a mean of 24 pills to 1,416 patients who underwent outpatient upper extremity surgery. Patients used a mean of only 8.1 pills. Opioid consumption varied based on type of procedure and anatomical location; patients who underwent soft-tissue procedures used the least number of opioids (5.1 pills) and those who underwent upper arm/shoulder procedures used the most with a mean of 22 pills used over 6 days. Only 5.3% of patients in the study were given information about excess opioid disposal. From the data, the authors suggest a standardized opioid prescription regimen for upper extremity surgery: ≤10 pills for hand/wrist soft-tissue procedures, ≤20 pills for hand/wrist fracture or joint procedures, ≤15 pills for elbow and forearm soft-tissue procedures, ≤20 pills for elbow and forearm fracture/joint procedures, and ≤30 pills for upper arm or shoulder procedures.[60]

One study randomized patients with little finger metacarpal neck fractures to treatment with either a soft wrap and buddy taping or treatment with closed reduction and casting. Sixty seven patients with isolated little finger metacarpal neck fractures angulated ≤70° were randomized between the two groups. There was no significant difference in DASH scores between the two treatment groups at 4-month follow-up. There was also no difference between the two groups in the secondary outcomes in the study which included pain, aesthetic appearance, range of motion of the metacarpophalangeal joints, and grip strength.[61]

A prospective, single-center study evaluated the treatment of metacarpal diaphyseal fractures with buddy strapping and early functional range of motion. Patients included in the study were those who had a metacarpal diaphyseal fracture with less than 35° angulation, less than 5 mm shortening, and no rotation deformity. Patients were treated with 1 month of buddy taping that allowed PIP and DIP range of motion. Six out of 51 patients included in the study were found to have additional displacement on subsequent radiographs. One hundred percent of fractures healed by the two-month follow-up appointment. Active range of motion and passive range of motion were similar to the contralateral finger at two-month follow-up in 90% of patients included in the study.[62]

A prospective cohort study of 22 patients demonstrated good patient satisfaction and functional outcomes after treatment of proximal phalanx fractures with open reduction, internal fixation, and subsequent early active range of motion. Patients with displaced spiral, oblique, or comminuted midshaft proximal phalanx fractures were included in the study. All participants were treated with ORIF and early active range of motion with formal hand therapy starting on postoperative day 5. All patients in the study had complete fracture healing based on follow-up radiographs. Nineteen patients reported an excellent outcome according to the digital functional assessment. Extensor lag of the PIP joint occurred in seven patients, which is a point of concern and a known disadvantage of open treatment of phalanx fractures. At final evaluation, mean total active range of motion was 242°.[63] If surgeons want to promote open treatment of phalanx fractures that could be pinned, we need a randomized trial.

A retrospective study of 49 patients with proximal phalanx fractures found that the only factor associated with total active range of motion at 6-week follow-up was time to commencement of active exercises. Patients treated with open reduction, internal fixation were able to start range of motion exercises sooner.[64] This study more or less proves the obvious: immobilized joints are initially stiffer. What we need to know is the final motion, particularly given the association of open treatment with extensor lag.

Fracture-Dislocations of the Digits

Fracture-dislocations of the digits are high-energy injuries that can sometimes be missed on initial presentation. If addressed in a timely manner, these injuries can often be treated with closed reduction and immobilization. However, they can be irreducible secondary to soft-tissue interposition, requiring surgical intervention. Recent studies focuses on surgical techniques for treating missed fracture-dislocations as well as new imaging modalities to improve diagnosis.

A case series of 12 patients examined functional outcomes after augmented hamate replacement arthroplasty for treatment of chronic PIP joint fracture-dislocation. The augment seems to be routine volar plate repair and temporary blocking pin fixation. The surgeries were performed by the same surgeon at a single center. Hamate grafting was used to augment the unstable PIP joint. And, trans-osseous sutures were then used to repair the volar plate and ligamentous structure of the PIP joint. A trans-articular K-wire was placed to fix the joint at 20° of flexion and prevent hyperextension, which is relatively unconventional and should not be necessary with this technique. Patients were treated with a standard postoperative protocol that included dorsal/volar splinting for 3 weeks with transition to another 3 weeks of aluminum finger splint that restricted 20° of terminal extension. Patients in the study were found to have increased range of motion from a mean of 14° preoperatively to a mean of 77° postoperatively. Grip strength improved from a mean of 69% preoperatively to a mean of 81% of the contralateral side postoperatively. Two patients in the small series had complications. One had collapse and resorption of the hamate graft; the other patient had ankylosis of the PIP joint as 2-year follow-up.[65]

A retrospective review of 30 cases of ring and little finger carpometacarpal fracture-dislocations used three dimensional CT images to develop a novel classification system for ring and little finger carpometacarpal joint fracture subluxations. The intra- and interobserver reliability of the new classification system using 3D CT were compared with a classification system using traditional, two-dimensional CT. The study found that the classification system using 3D CT reconstruction was significantly more reliable in both intra- and interobserver

Trauma

reliability as compared with the classification system using 2D CT images (interclass correlation coefficient of 0.98 for 3D CT as compared with 0.85 for 2D CT).[66]

Open Finger Fractures

Traditionally, an open hand fracture has been considered an indication for surgery. But recent evidence suggests that antibiotic timing—not surgical debridement—is the most important factor in preventing infection in open hand fracture treatment.

A systematic review of several studies on antibiotic management and time to débridement after open fracture in the upper extremity found lower infection rates with the use of antibiotics. Though varying antibiotic regimens are used in the literature, oral antibiotics are likely sufficient as prophylaxis in open hand fractures, specifically. Similarly, patients with open distal radius fractures should receive antibiotics, but time to administration of treatment was not found to affect outcome. Time to débridement was also not found to be significantly associated with decreased risk of infection for open upper extremity fractures based on the authors' analyses.[67]

In another meta-analysis of 12 studies of open hand fractures, the use of antibiotic prophylaxis did correlate with a lower risk of infection. There was no association between time to débridement and rate of infection in the authors' review of the relevant literature. The authors conclude that open fractures of the phalanges and metacarpals that are not significantly contaminated can be safely débrided in the emergency department. Three studies within the review investigated whether degree of soft-tissue injury impacted infection risk in hand fractures. These studies found that patients with a higher Gustilo Anderson grade had a higher risk of infection, suggesting that soft-tissue compromise also impacts development of complications.[68]

Summary

Recent evidence should draw surgeon's attention to the importance of offering nonsurgical options to patients and ensuring they make a treatment choice consistent with what matters most to them and not based on misconceptions, because a lot of these recent findings are counterintuitive. For instance, complete acromioclavicular joint dislocations and displaced clavicle fractures create deformity and some movement (when the clavicle does not heal), but symptom intensity and magnitude of limitations on average comparable to surgical treatment that corrects deformity and limits movement. Proximal humerus and humeral shaft fractures that heal are likewise associated with comparable symptoms and limitations, whereas nonunions in this region are more problematic. Displaced distal humerus fractures and olecranon fractures can be treated nonsurgically in less active or infirm patients. The possibility of salvaging problems related to proximal and distal humerus fracture with arthroplasty increase the appeal of initial nonsurgical treatment. Nonsurgical treatment is also a good option for most isolated radial head partial articular and neck fractures, many if not most distal radius fractures, and scaphoid waist fractures that are nondisplaced. Most of the technical surgical developments in recent years have not had a substantial influence on outcomes, and people are starting to study optimal stewardship of resources. For instance, should we use pins that cost a few dollars or plates that cost hundreds or thousands of dollars if we can not demonstrate a benefit?

Key Study Points

- Nonsurgical management of high-grade acromioclavicular joint injuries is supported by level I data.
- The nonunion rate for displaced midshaft clavicle fractures treated nonsurgically is between 11% and 23% compared with 0% to 2% with surgical fixation, but there are no differences in patient-reported outcomes.
- The role of surgical treatment of proximal humerus needs better definition.
- Nonsurgical management is an option for olecranon fractures in older, less active, and more infirm patients.
- The advantages of plate fixation for distal radius fractures need additional study.

Annotated References

1. Chang N, Furey A, Kurdin A: Operative versus nonoperative management of acute high-grade acromioclavicular dislocations: A systematic review and meta-analysis. *J Orthop Trauma* 2018;32:1-9.

   Meta-analysis involving a total of 954 patients with high grade AC joint injury. Comparison of surgical versus nonsurgical intervention. Level of evidence: III.

2. Mah JM, Canadian Orthopaedic Trauma Society: Treatment for acute, complete acromioclavicular joint dislocation: Results of a multicenter randomized clinical trial. *J Orthop Trauma* 2017;31:485-490.

Prospective randomized controlled trial involving 83 patients with high grade AC joint injury. Comparison of hook plate fixation versus nonsurgical treatment. Level of evidence: I.

3. Natera Cisneros L, Sarasquete Reiriz J: Acute high-grade acromioclavicular joint injuries: Quality of life comparison between patients managed operatively with a hook plate versus patients managed non-operatively. *Eur J Orthop Surg Traumatol* 2017;27:341-350.

   Retrospective cohort study involving 32 patients with high grade AC joint injury. Comparison of hook plate fixation versus nonsurgical treatment. Level of evidence: IV.

4. Arirachakaran A, Boonard M, Piyapittayanun P, et al: Comparison of surgical outcomes between fixation with hook plate and loop suspensory fixation for acute unstable acromioclavicular joint dislocation: A systematic review and meta-analysis. *Eur J Orthop Surg Traumatol* 2016;26:565-574.

   Meta-analysis involving a total of 112 patients with high grade AC joint injury. Comparison of loop suspensory coracoclavicular fixation versus hook plate fixation. Level of evidence: IV.

5. Arirachakaran A, Boonard M, Piyapittayanun P, et al: Post-operative outcomes and complications of suspensory loop fixation device versus hook plate in acute unstable acromioclavicular joint dislocation: A systematic review and meta-analysis. *J Orthop Traumatol* 2017;18:293-304.

   Meta-analysis involving a total of 1389 patients with high grade AC joint injury. Comparison of loop suspensory coracoclavicular fixation versus hook plate fixation. Level of evidence: IV.

6. Natera Cisneros L, Sarasquete Reiriz J, Escola-Benet A, et al: Acute high-grade acromioclavicular joint injuries treatment: Arthroscopic non-rigid coracoclavicular fixation provides better quality of life outcomes than hook plate ORIF. *Ortho Traumatol Surg Res* 2016;102:31-39.

   Retrospective cohort study involving 31 patients with high grade AC joint injury. Comparison between arthroscopic nonrigid coracoclavicular fixation versus hook plate. Level of evidence: IV.

7. Woltz S, Stegeman SA, Krijnen P, et al: Plate Fixation compared with nonoperative treatment for displaced midshaft clavicular fractures: A multicenter randomized controlled trial. *J Bone Joint Surg* 2017;99:106-112.

   Prospective randomized controlled trial involving 160 patients with displaced midshaft clavicle fracture. Comparison of surgical fixation with a plate versus nonsurgical treatment. Level of evidence: I.

8. Sugawara Tamaoki MJ, Matsunaga FT, Ferreira da Costa AR, et al: Treatment of displaced midshaft clavicle fractures: Figure-of-eight harness versus anterior plate osteosynthesis: A randomized controlled trial. *J Bone Joint Surg* 2017;99:1159-1165.

   Prospective randomized controlled trial involving 117 patients with displaced midshaft clavicle fracture. Comparison of surgical fixation with a plate versus nonsurgical treatment. Level of evidence: I.

9. Ahrens PM, Garlick NI, Barber J, et al: The clavicle trial: A multicenter randomized controlled trial comparing operative with nonoperative treatment of displaced midshaft clavicle fractures. *J Bone Joint Surg* 2017;99:1345-1354.

   Prospective randomized controlled trial involving 301 patients with displaced midshaft clavicle fracture. Comparison of surgical fixation with a plate versus nonsurgical treatment. Level of evidence: I.

10. Guerra E, Previtali D, Tamborini S, Filardo G, Zaffagnini S, Candrian C: Midshaft clavicle fractures: Surgery provides better results as compared with nonoperative treatment: A meta-analysis. *Am J Sports Med* 2019. doi:10.1177/0363546519826961.

    Meta-analysis of randomized controlled trials comparing surgery versus nonsurgical treatment for displaced midshaft clavicle fractures. Level of evidence: IV.

11. Smeeing DPJ, van der Ven DJC, Hietbrink F, et al: Surgical versus nonsurgical treatment for midshaft clavicle fractures in patients aged 16 years and older: A systematic review, meta-analysis, and comparison of randomized controlled trials and observational studies. *Am J Sports Med* 2017;45(8):1937-1945.

    Systematic review of randomized controlled trials and well-designed observational studies comparing surgical versus nonsurgical treatment for displaced midshaft clavicle fractures. Level of evidence: IV.

12. McKnight B, Heckmann N, Hill JR, et al: Surgical management of midshaft clavicle nonunions is associated with a higher rate of short-term complications compared with acute fractures. *J Shoulder Elbow Surg* 2016;25:1412-1417.

    Retrospective cohort study involving 1215 patients with midshaft clavicle fracture. Comparison between surgical fixation acutely versus surgical fixation of those that went on to nonunion. Level of evidence: III.

13. Fuglesang HFS, Flugsrud GB, Randsborg PH, et al: Plate fixation versus intramedullary nailing of completely displaced midshaft fractures of the clavicle: A prospective randomised controlled trial. *Bone Joint Lett J* 2017;99-B:1095-1101.

    Prospective randomized controlled trial involving 123 patients with displaced midshaft clavicle fracture. Comparison of plate fixation versus elastic nailing. Level of evidence: I.

14. Czajka CM, Kay A, Gary JL, et al: Symptomatic implant removal following dual mini-fragment plating for clavicular shaft fractures. *J Orthop Trauma* 2017;31:236-240.

    Retrospective cohort study describing outcomes in 81 patients with midshaft clavicle fractures treated with dual mini-fragment plating technique. Level of evidence: IV.

15. Schroder LK, Gauger EM, Gilbertson JA, et al: Functional outcomes after operative management of extra-articular glenoid neck and scapular body fractures. *J Bone Joint Surg* 2016;98:1623-1630.

    Retrospective cohort study describing outcomes in 61 patients with displaced extra-articular scapula fractures treated surgically. Level of evidence: IV.

16. Cole PA Jr, Gilbertson JA, Cole PA Sr: Functional outcomes of operative management of scapula fractures in a geriatric cohort. *J Orthop Trauma* 2017;31:e1-e8.

Retrospective cohort study describing outcomes in 16 elderly patients with displaced scapula fractures treated surgically. Level of evidence: IV.

17. Konigshausen M, Coulibaly MO, Nicolas V, et al: Results of non-operative treatment of fractures of the glenoid fossa. *Bone Joint Lett J* 2016;98-B:1074-1079.

Retrospective cohort study involving 24 patients with intra-articular glenoid fractures treated surgically. Comparison of outcomes based on amount of articular displacement prior to fixation. Level of evidence: IV.

18. Suter T, Henninger HB, Zhang Y, et al: Comparison of measurements of the glenopolar angle in 3D CT reconstructions of the scapula and 2D plain radiographic views. *Bone Joint Lett J* 2016;98-B:1510-1516.

Cadaveric study involving 68 specimens to compare utility of 3D CT reconstructions versus plain radiograph of the scapula to assess the glenopolar angle. Level of evidence: V.

19. Harmer LS, Phelps KD, Crickard CV, et al: A comparison of exposure between the classic and modified Judet approaches to the scapula. *J Orthop Trauma* 2016;30:235-3239.

Cadaveric study involving 10 specimens to compare surgical exposure of the scapula by modified Judet approach versus classic Judet approach. Level of evidence: V.

20. Handoll HH, Keding A, Corbacho B, et al: Five-year follow-up results of the PROFHER trial comparing operative and non-operative treatment of adults with a displaced fracture of the proximal humerus. *Bone Joint Lett J* 2017;99-B:383-392.

Prospective randomized controlled trial involving 164 patients with displaced proximal humerus fractures involving the surgical neck. Comparison of surgical versus nonsurgical treatment at 5-year follow-up. Level of evidence: I.

21. Gracitelli MEC, Malvolta EA, Assuncao JH, et al: Locking intramedullary nails compared with locking plates for two- and three-part proximal humeral surgical neck fractures: A randomized controlled trial. *J Shoulder Elbow Surg* 2016;25:695-703.

Prospective randomized controlled trial involving 72 patients with two- or three-part surgical neck fractures of the proximal humerus. Comparison between intramedullary nail fixation and locking plate fixation. Level of evidence: I.

22. Chen H, Ji X, Gao Y, et al: Comparison of intramedullary fibular allograft with locking compression plate versus shoulder hemi-arthroplasty for repair of osteoporotic four-part proximal humerus fracture: Consecutive, prospective, controlled, and comparative study. *Orthop Traumatol Surg Res* 2016;102:287-292.

Prospective cohort study involving 60 patients with osteoporotic four-part proximal humerus fractures. Comparison between plate fixation including a fibular strut versus hemiarthroplasty. Level of evidence: II.

23. Shukla DR, McAnany S, Kim J, et al: Hemiarthroplasty versus reverse shoulder arthroplasty for treatment of proximal humeral fractures: A meta-analysis. *J Shoulder Elbow Surg* 2016;25:330-340.

Meta-analysis involving 255 patients with proximal humerus fractures treated with either reverse total shoulder arthroplasty or hemiarthroplasty. Level of evidence: IV.

24. Shannon SF, Wagner ER, Houdek MT, et al: Reverse shoulder arthroplasty for proximal humeral fractures: Outcomes comparing primary reverse arthroplasty for fracture versus reverse arthroplasty after failed osteosynthesis. *J Shoulder Elbow Surg* 2016;25:1655-1660.

Retrospective case-controlled study involving 44 patients with proximal humerus fractures treated with reverse total shoulder arthroplasty. Comparison between patients treated with acute reverse total shoulder arthroplasty for fracture versus those treated with reverse total shoulder arthroplasty after failed open reduction internal fixation. Level of evidence: III.

25. Sebastia-Forcada E, Lizaur-Ultrilla A, Cebrian-Gomez R, et al: Outcomes of reverse total shoulder arthroplasty for proximal humeral fractures: Primary arthroplasty versus secondary arthroplasty after failed proximal humeral locking plate fixation. *J Orthop Trauma* 2017;31:e236-e240.

Retrospective cohort study involving 60 patients with proximal humerus fractures treated with reverse total shoulder arthroplasty. Comparison between patients treated with acute reverse total shoulder arthroplasty for fracture versus those treated with reverse total shoulder arthroplasty after failed open reduction internal fixation. Level of evidence: IV.

26. Dezfuli B, King JJ, Farmer KW, et al: Outcomes of reverse total shoulder arthroplasty as primary versus revision procedure for proximal humerus fractures. *J Shoulder Elbow Surg* 2016;25:1133-1137.

Retrospective cohort study involving 49 patients with proximal humerus fractures treated with reverse total shoulder arthroplasty. Comparison between patients treated with acute reverse total shoulder arthroplasty for fracture versus those treated with reverse total shoulder arthroplasty after failed open reduction internal fixation versus those treated with reverse total shoulder arthroplasty for nonunion or malunion. Level of evidence: III.

27. Zhao J, Wang J, Meng X, et al: Surgical interventions to treat humerus shaft fractures: A network meta-analysis of randomized controlled trials. *PLoS One* 2017;12:1-12.

Meta-analysis involving a total of 832 patients with humeral shaft fractures. Comparison between open reduction internal fixation, minimally invasive plate osteosynthesis, and intramedullary nailing. Level of evidence: II.

28. Hohmann E, Glatt V, Tetsworth K: Minimally invasive plating versus either open reduction and plate fixation or intramedullary nailing of humeral shaft fractures: A systematic review and meta-analysis of randomized controlled trials. *J Shoulder Elbow Surg* 2016;25:1634-1642.

Meta-analysis involving a total of 376 patients with humeral shaft fractures. Comparison between open reduction internal fixation, minimally invasive plate osteosynthesis, and intramedullary nailing. Level of evidence: II.

29. Davies G, Yeo G, Meta M, et al: Case-match controlled comparison of minimally invasive plate osteosynthesis and intramedullary nailing for the stabilization of humeral shaft fractures. *J Orthop Trauma* 2016;30:612-617.

    Retrospective case-controlled study involving 30 patients with humeral shaft fractures. Comparison between intramedullary nailing and minimally invasive plate osteosynthesis. Level of evidence: III.

30. Matsunaga FT, Tamaoki MJS, Matsumoto MH, et al: Minimally invasive osteosynthesis with a bridge plate versus a functional brace for humeral shaft fractures: A randomized controlled trial. *J Bone Joint Surg* 2017;99:583-592.

    Prospective randomized controlled trail involving 110 patients with humeral shaft fractures. Comparison between minimally invasive plate osteosynthesis and functional bracing. Level of evidence: I.

31. Dedeoglu SS, Imren Y, Cabuk H, et al: Arthroscopy-assisted versus standard intramedullary nail fixation in diaphyseal fractures of the humerus. *J Orthop Surg* 2017;25:1-6.

    Prospective randomized controlled trial involving 40 patients with humeral shaft fractures. Comparison of intramedullary nailing versus arthroscopic-assisted intramedullary nailing. Level of evidence: I.

32. Kudo T, Hara A, Iwase H, et al: Biomechanical properties of orthogonal plate configuration versus parallel plate configuration using the same locking plate system for intra-articular distal humeral fractures under radial or ulnar column axial load. *Injury* 2016;47:2071-2076.

    Biomechanical sawbones study in six specimens comparing parallel versus orthogonal plating for fixation of intra-articular supracondylar humerus fractures. Level of evidence: V.

33. Taylor PA, Owens JR, Benfield CP, et al: Parallel plating of simulated distal humerus fractures demonstrates increased stiffness relative to orthogonal plating with a distal humerus locking plate system. *J Orthop Trauma* 2016;30:e118-e122.

    Biomechanical cadaveric study in 18 specimens comparing parallel versus orthogonal plating for fixation of intra-articular supracondylar humerus fractures. Level of evidence: V.

34. Barco R, Streubel PN, Morrey BF, et al: Total elbow arthroplasty for distal humeral fractures: A ten-year minimum follow-up study. *J Bone Joint Surg* 2017;99:1524-1531.

    Retrospective cohort study reporting outcomes in 44 patients treated with total elbow arthroplasty after distal humerus fracture. Level of evidence: IV.

35. Sun H, Duan J, Li F: Comparison between radial head arthroplasty and open reduction and internal fixation in patients with radial head fractures (modified mason type III and IV): A meta-analysis. *Eur J Orthop Surg Traumatol* 2016;26:283-291.

    Meta-analysis involving a total of 319 patients with modified Mason III or IV fractures of the radial head. Comparison of surgical fixation versus arthroplasty. Level of evidence: III.

36. Laflamme M, Grenier-Gauthier P-P, Leclerc A, et al: Retrospective cohort study on radial head replacements comparing results between smooth and porous stem designs. *J Shoulder Elbow Surg* 2017;26:1316-1324.

    Retrospective cohort study involving 57 patients who underwent radial head replacement. Comparison of smooth verus porous stem designs. Level of evidence: III.

37. Duckworth AD, Clement ND, McEachan JE, et al: Prospective randomised trial of non-operative versus operative management of olecranon fractures in the elderly. *Bone Joint Lett J* 2017;99-B:964-972.

    Prospective randomized controlled trial involving 19 geriatric patients with olecranon fractures. Comparison of tension band fixation versus nonsurgical treatment. Level of evidence: I.

38. Duckworth AD, Clement ND, White TO, et al: Plate versus tension-band wire fixation for olecranon fractures: A prospective randomized trial. *J Bone Joint Surg* 2017;99:1261-1273.

    Prospective randomized controlled trial involving 67 patients with olecranon fractures. Comparison of plate verus tension band wire fixation. Level of evidence: I.

39. Orbay JL, Ring D, Kachooei AR, et al: Multicenter trial of an internal joint stabilizer for the elbow. *J Shoulder Elbow Surg* 2017;26:125-132.

    Prospective case series reporting outcomes in 24 patients with elbow joint instability treated with a novel internal device. Level of evidence: IV.

40. Zhang XF, Huang JW, Mao HX, et al: Adult diaphyseal both-bone forearm fractures: A clinical and biomechanical comparison of four different fixations. *Orthop Traumatol Surg Res* 2016;102:319-325.

    Prospective randomized controlled trial involving 87 patients with both bone forearm fractures. Comparison of surgical fixation by both bone plating, both bone intramedullary nailing, plate fixation of the radius with intramedullary nailing of the ulna, and plate fixation of the ulna with intramedullary nailing of the radius. Level of evidence: II.

41. Kose A, Aydin A, Ezirmik N, et al: A comparison of the treatment results of open reduction internal fixation and intramedullary nailing in adult forearm diaphyseal fractures. *Turk J Trauma Emerg Surg* 2017;23:235-244.

    Retrospective comparative cohort study involving 90 patients with diaphyseal forearm fractures. Comparison of plate fixation versus intramedullary nailing. Level of evidence: IV.

42. Tsismenakis T, Tornetta P: Galeazzi fractures: Is DRUJ instability predicted by current guidelines? *Injury* 2016;47:1472-1477.

    Retrospective cohort study involving 66 patients with radial fractures. Accuracy of current radiographic guidelines to predict instability of the distal radioulnar joint was assessed by evaluation of the cohort. Level of evidence: IV.

43. Auld TS, Hwang JS, Stekas N, et al: The correlation between the OTA/AO classification system and compartment syndrome in both bone forearm fractures. *J Orthop Trauma* 2017;31:606-609.

Retrospective cohort study involving 151 patients with both bone forearm fractures. A relationship between OTA/AO fracture classification and the need for forearm fasciotomies was evaluated. Level of evidence: III.

44. von Ruden C, Morgenstern M, Hierholzer C, et al: The missing effect of human recombinant Bone Morphogenetic Proteins BMP-2 and BMP-7 in surgical treatment of aseptic forearm nonunion. *Injury* 2016;47:919-924.

Prospective randomized controlled trail involving 49 patients with diaphyseal forearm nonunions. Comparison between compression plating nonunion repair using just iliac crest autograft or also including either BMP-2 or BMP-7. Level of evidence: I.

45. Kasapinova K, Kamiloski V: The correlation of initial radiographic characteristics of distal radius fractures and injuries of the triangular fibrocartilage complex. *J Hand Surg Eur Vol* 2016;41(5):516-520. doi:10.1177/1753193415624669.

Prospective study of 85 patients with distal radius fractures to determine the prevalence of concomitant TFCC tears using wrist arthroscopy at the time of surgical intervention. Level of evidence: III.

46. Lau BC, Robertson A, Motamedi D, Lee N: The validity and reliability of a pocket-sized ultrasound to diagnose distal radius fracture and assess quality of closed reduction. *J Hand Surg Am* 2017;42(6):420-427. doi:10.1016/J.JHSA.2017.03.012.

Prospective study of the use of ultrasound to diagnose and assess reduction of distal radius fractures as compared with traditional radiographs. Twenty-three patients were assessed with ultrasound as well as radiographs and compared with 20 controls assessed with radiographs alone. Level of evidence: II.

47. Mellstrand Navarro C, Ahrengart L, Törnqvist H, Ponzer S: Volar locking plate or external fixation with optional addition of K-wires for dorsally displaced distal radius fractures. *J Orthop Trauma* 2016;30(4):217-224. doi:10.1097/BOT.0000000000000519.

Randomized trial comparing the use of volar plating to external fixation with Kirschner wire placement for treatment of dorsally displaced distal radius fractures in 140 patients. Level of evidence: I.

48. Johnson NA, Dias JJ, Wildin CJ, Cutler L, Bhowal B, Ullah AS: Comparison of distal radius fracture intra-articular step reduction with volar locking plates and K wires: A retrospective review of quality and maintenance of fracture reduction. *J Hand Surg Eur Vol* 2017;42(2):144-150. doi:10.1177/1753193416669502.

Retrospective study of 359 patients with intra-articular distal radius fractures comparing maintenance of reduction in those treated with closed reduction percutaneous pinning to those treated with open reduction internal fixation. Level of evidence: IV.

49. Teunis T, Jupiter J, Schaser KD, et al: Evaluation of radiographic fracture position 1 year after variable angle locking volar distal radius plating: A prospective multicentre case series. *J Hand Surg Eur Vol* 2017;42(5):493-500. doi:10.1177/1753193417690478.

Prospective case series of 73 patients with distal radius fractures treated with volar locking plate. Computed tomography was used to assess maintenance of fracture reduction at one year postoperatively. Level of evidence: IV.

50. Larouche J, Pike J, Slobogean GP, et al: Determinants of functional outcome in distal radius fractures in high-functioning patients older than 55 years. *J Orthop Trauma* 2016;30(8):445-449. doi:10.1097/BOT.0000000000000566.

Prospective cohort study of patients aged 55 years and older with distal radius fractures comparing patient-reported outcomes in patients treated nonsurgically with those treated with surgical intervention. Level of evidence: I.

51. Nandyala SV, Giladi AM, Parker AM, Rozental TD: Comparison of direct perioperative costs in treatment of unstable distal radial fractures. *J Bone Jt Surg* 2018;100(9):786-792. doi:10.2106/JBJS.17.00688.

Cost analysis study of 40 patients with unstable distal radius fractures randomized to undergo ORIF or CRPP. Level of evidence: II.

52. Alnaeem H, Aldekhayel S, Kanevsky J, Neel OF: A systematic review and meta-analysis examining the differences between nonsurgical management and percutaneous fixation of minimally and nondisplaced scaphoid fractures. *J Hand Surg Am* 2016;41(12):1135-1144.e1. doi:10.1016/J.JHSA.2016.08.023.

Systematic review involving 10 studies of patients with nondisplaced scaphoid fractures. Comparison of outcomes in nonsurgical management with percutaneous fixation. Level of evidence: II.

53. Seger EW, Jauregui JJ, Horton SA, Davalos G, Kuehn E, Stracher MA. Low-intensity pulsed ultrasound for nonoperative treatment of scaphoid nonunions: A meta-analysis. *Hand (N Y)* 2018;13(3):275-280. doi:10.1177/1558944717702470.

Meta-analysis of five studies of the use of low-intensity pulse ultrasound as treatment for scaphoid nonunion. Mean time to union and healing index reported across the included studies. Level of evidence: II.

54. Matson AP, Garcia RM, Richard MJ, Leversedge FJ, Aldridge JM, Ruch DS: Percutaneous treatment of unstable scaphoid waist fractures. *Hand (N Y)* 2017;12(4):362-368. doi:10.1177/1558944716681948.

Case series of 28 patients with closed, unstable scaphoid waist fractures. Comparison of outcomes of patients treated with open reduction and those treated with percutaneous fixation. Level of evidence: III.

55. Kadar A, Bishop AT, Suchyta MA, Moran SL: Diagnosis and management of hook of hamate fractures. *J Hand Surg Eur Vol* 2018;43(5):539-545. doi:10.1177/1753193417729603.

Retrospective study of 51 paitents with hook of hamate fractures examining time to diagnosis, method of treatment, time to union, and patient-reported outcomes. Level of evidence: IV.

56. Spit SA, Becker SJE, Hageman MGJS, Ring D: The prevalence of unanticipated hamate hook abnormalities in computed tomography scans: A retrospective study. *Arch bone Jt Surg* 2017;5(3):133-138.

Retrospective review of 2489 CT scans of the hand to determine the prevalence of undiagnosed hook of hamate injuries. Level of evidence: IV.

57. Griffin M, Roushdi I, Osagie L, Cerovac S, Umarji S: Patient-reported outcomes following surgically managed perilunate dislocation. *Hand (N Y)* 2016;11(1):22-28. doi:10.1177/1558944715617222.

Prospective study of 16 patients with perilunate injuries examining patient-reported outcomes, grip strength, and return to work. All patients in the study were treated surgically. Level of evidence: IV.

58. Gillis JA, Williams JG: Cost analysis of percutaneous fixation of hand fractures in the main operating room versus the ambulatory setting. *J Plast Reconstr Aesthetic Surg* 2017;70(8):1044-1050. doi:10.1016/j.bjps.2017.05.011.

Cost analysis study of closed reduction internal fixation as a treatment modality for distal radius fractures. Comparison between costs of CRIF in the operating room versus the ambulatory setting. Level of evidence: III.

59. MacDermid JC, Valdes K, Szekeres M, Naughton N, Algar L: The assessment of psychological factors on upper extremity disability: A scoping review. *J Hand Ther* 2018;31(4):511-523. doi:10.1016/J.JHT.2017.05.017.

Systematic review of 22 studies assessing the relationship between psychological factors and patient-reported outcomes. Level of evidence: II.

60. Kim N, Matzon JL, Abboudi J, et al: A prospective evaluation of opioid utilization after upper-extremity surgical procedures: Identifying consumption patterns and determining prescribing guidelines. *J Bone Joint Surg Am Vol* 2016;98(20):e89. doi:10.2106/JBJS.15.00614.

Prospective cohort study of 1,416 patients examining opioid prescription behaviors and utilization rates based on upper extremity surgical procedures. The authors stratified opioid use among different procedures in the upper extremity including soft-tissue procedures, fracture procedures, and joint procedures. Level of evidence: III.

61. van Aaken J, Fusetti C, Luchina S, et al: Fifth metacarpal neck fractures treated with soft wrap/buddy taping compared to reduction and casting: Results of a prospective, multicenter, randomized trial. *Arch Orthop Trauma Surg* 2016;136(1):135-142. doi:10.1007/s00402-015-2361-0.

Randomized controlled trial of 68 patients with fifth metacarpal neck fractures comparing buddy taping with reduction and casting. Outcomes include quickDASH scores, pain, function, and radiographic measures. Level of evidence: I.

62. Rey P-B, Obert L, Jardin E, Pechin C, Rey P-B, Uhring J: Functional treatment of metacarpal diaphyseal fractures by buddy taping: A prospective single-center study functional treatment of metacarpal diaphyseal fractures by buddy taping: A prospective single-center study. *Hand Surg Rehabil* 2016;35(1):34-39. doi:10.1016/j.hansur.2015.12.001.

Prospective case series of 51 patients with minimally displaced metacarpal diaphyseal fractures. Patients were treated nonsurgically with early active range of motion and buddying taping and assessed at several time points for radiographic healing and functional outcomes. Level of evidence: II.

63. Ataker Y, Uludag S, Ece SC, Gudemez E: Early active motion after rigid internal fixation of unstable extra-articular fractures of the proximal phalanx. *J Hand Surg Eur Vol* 2017;42(8):803-809. doi:10.1177/1753193417709949.

Prospective case series of 22 patients with extra-articular proximal phalanx fractures treated with surgical intervention and given early active range of motion rehab protocols postoperatively. Outcomes include functional range of motion, DASH scores, and pain. Level of evidence: IV.

64. Miller LG, Ada L, Crosbie J, Wajon A: Time to commencement of active exercise predicts total active range of motion 6 weeks after proximal phalanx fracture fixation: A retrospective review. *Hand Ther* 2017;22(2):73-78. doi:10.1177/1758998316679386.

Retrospective study of 49 patients with proximal phalanx fractures treated postoperatively. Comparison of functional outcomes between patients who began early active range of motion and those who had delayed rehabilitation. Level of evidence: IV.

65. Thomas BP, Raveendran S, Pallapati SR, Anderson GA: Augmented hamate replacement arthroplasty for fracture-dislocations of the proximal interphalangeal joints in 12 patients. *J Hand Surg Eur Vol* 2017;42(8):799-802. doi:10.1177/1753193417707381.

Prospective case series of 12 patients undergoing hemi-hamate replacement arthroplasty with combined volar plate arthroplasty. Outcomes include grip strength and patient-rated hand and wrist scores. Level of evidence: IV.

66. Kim JH, Kwon S-S, Moon SJ, et al: Reliability of classification of ring and little finger carpometacarpal joint fracture subluxations: A comparison between two-dimensional computed tomography and three-dimensional computed tomography classifications. *J Hand Surg Eur Vol* 2016;41(4):448-452. doi:10.1177/1753193415602589.

Retrospective review of 30 patients with fifth CMC fracture-dislocations. Authors used three observers to validate a new three-dimensional classification system. Level of evidence: IV.

67. Warrender WJ, Lucasti CJ, Chapman TR, Ilyas AM: Antibiotic management and operative debridement in open fractures of the hand and upper extremity. *Hand Clin* 2018;34(1):9-16. doi:10.1016/j.hcl.2017.09.001.

Systematic review of literature regarding open fractures in the upper extremity. Authors synthesized recommendations based on results of various studies' assessments of infection rates based on time to antibiotics, time to debridement, etc. Level of evidence: II.

68. Ketonis C, Dwyer J, Ilyas AM: Timing of debridement and infection rates in open fractures of the hand: A systematic review. *Hand (N Y)* 2017;12(2):119-126. doi:10.1177/1558944716643294.

Systematic review of 12 articles on open hand fractures comparing treatment outcomes, infection rates, and timing of antibiotics/debridement. Level of evidence: II.

Chapter 20

Pelvic Trauma

Mark R. Adams, MD • Mark C. Reilly, MD

ABSTRACT

Pelvic ring injuries and acetabular fractures can be challenging to treat, especially in elderly patients. Accurate assessment of any associated imaging studies is important to identify the severity of injury. Determination of the degree of instability of the pelvic ring or hip is required to determine the best course of treatment.

Keywords: acetabular fracture; acetabulum; pelvic ring injury; pelvis

Introduction

It is important to be aware of the recent trends in the literature as it pertains to pelvic ring injuries and acetabular fractures in adult patients. The general principles of care of these injuries are well established, and these recent trends represent the evolution in care of patients with these complex injuries.

Pelvic Ring Injuries

The typical goals for the care of an adult patient with a pelvic ring injury are for union in a well-aligned position while avoiding serious complications. Although the goals are constant from patient to patient, the spectrum of injury to the pelvic ring, as it relates to severity and instability, is wide ranging. Assessing the degree of mechanical instability and developing an individualized treatment plan based on that instability as well as other associated patient-related factors can be challenging.

Dr. Reilly or an immediate family member is a member of a speakers' bureau or has made paid presentations on behalf of Stryker. Neither Dr. Adams nor any immediate family member has received anything of value from or has stock or stock options held in a commercial company or institution related directly or indirectly to the subject of this chapter.

The recent literature has documented issues with revision surgery of pelvic injuries due to failure of fixation, residual instability, and loss of alignment.[1-5] Failure of fixation is most commonly attributed to inferior reduction quality, inadequate fixation stability for the level of mechanical instability or a combination thereof, and the majority of the recent literature is dedicated toward improving understanding of these issues.

Surgical Indications

The typical indication for surgery for a pelvic ring injury is primarily based on the amount of mechanical instability thought to be present. Although the available classifications do not specifically direct treatment, they can help the surgeon better understand instability of the pelvic ring. An unstable pelvic ring is unlikely to heal in an acceptable position and is therefore indicated for reduction and fixation, whereas a stable pelvic ring injury may be managed nonsurgically.

Determining the correct procedure for each patient who requires pelvic ring surgery may be challenging. Injuries to the same anatomic structures but with differing degrees of instability may require different techniques to obtain and maintain a reduction. However, as radiographs and CT scans are static tests, the true degree of instability can often be difficult to determine. Recent articles have highlighted situations in which the preoperative workup and treatment can result in the surgeon underestimating the degree of instability present. The presence of a pelvic binder, a common emergency department resuscitative tool, has been noted to decrease clinicians' ability to properly diagnose pelvic ring injuries.[6] Furthermore, a recent case series of 72 patients with symphyseal injuries evaluated without binders noted that the circumferential wrap of the CT scanner consistently reduced the diastasis at the symphysis. In both of these studies, an AP radiograph of the pelvis prior to binder placement was more predictive of the degree of instability present.[6,7]

In a 2011 study, a fluoroscopic examination of the pelvis under anesthesia consistently demonstrated a greater magnitude of instability than the initial radiographs revealed.[8] The examination of the pelvis under anesthesia is a powerful test because of its dynamic nature, and it was considered the benchmark for diagnosis of a pelvic ring injury in the pelvic binder study mentioned previously.[6] This test has also been verified for its negative predictive value, as patients with a negative stress examination consistently obtain fracture union with appropriate alignment with closed treatment.[9] The natural history of patients who have instability present only on stress examination is still unknown.

Reduction and Fixation

Posterior Pelvic Ring

A variety of reduction and fixation options exist for an unstable posterior pelvic ring injury, but irrespective of the treatment strategy, the surgical goal is obtaining and maintaining an accurate reduction and creating a stable fixation construct in a well-aligned pelvis. Reductions can be performed closed, percutaneously, or open.

Percutaneous reduction and fixation techniques for the posterior pelvic ring have increased in frequency over time. Between 2003 and 2015, the number of pelvic ring injuries treated by candidates sitting for Part II of the ABOS examination was constant from year to year. Percutaneous treatment of the posterior pelvic ring increased from 49% in 2003 to 79% in 2015, with a corresponding decrease in the percentage of open procedures.[10] This trend toward more percutaneous fixation techniques has not necessarily been accompanied by a change in the reduction quality, however. A retrospective review of 113 patients at two trauma centers compared open reduction and internal fixation (ORIF) and closed reduction and percutaneous fixation of unstable pelvic ring injuries, and the reduction quality was considered slightly better in the closed reduction and percutaneous fixation group.[11]

Recent literature has seen an increase in the number of publications related to the use of transiliac-transsacral screws, the accurate insertion of percutaneous posterior pelvic ring fixation, and novel methods of increasing stability of the posterior ring percutaneously.[12-16] Transiliac-transsacral screws have been demonstrated to have a clear biomechanical advantage when compared with the use or shorter iliosacral screws.[17] Furthermore, transiliac-transsacral screw fixation is capable of stabilizing bilateral injuries with a single implant.[18]

Execution of proper placement of transiliac-transsacral screws has been noted to be technically demanding. As a result, several articles have been recently dedicated to describing the anatomical variations in the pelvis, as well as the fluoroscopic imaging utilized for the procedure.[12,13,18] Planning includes using the trauma CT scan of the pelvis and involves evaluation of the size and trajectory of the available osseous fixation pathways, measurements of planned screws for expected length, and assessment of the space available for multiple screw insertions.[12]

Iliosacral screws are most commonly inserted with conventional fluoroscopic guidance. Certain centers have fluoroscopically guided computer navigated surgery capability, and a comparative multicenter cohort study at two trauma centers in the Netherlands compared the two methods. Although there was no difference between the two groups in terms of their accuracy, the postoperative CT scan showed 17% of the screws placed to be inaccurate; 5 of the 80 patients underwent revision procedures as a result.[19] This finding highlights the need for improved understanding of fluoroscopic images. A 2016 study noted that surgeons may perceive the position of iliosacral screws incorrectly with certain positions of misplaced screws. Surgeons consistently did not recognize the inaccuracy of iliosacral screws that penetrated the anterior border of S1, the superior sacral ala, and the S1 foramen when standard inlet and outlet views were obtained. They described variations on these views that improved the surgeons' accuracy in identifying malpositioned screws.[20]

In addition to malpositioned fixation, another potential complication is related to the proximity of the starting point for iliosacral screws to the superior gluteal artery. A CT arteriography study from 2017 measured 12.4 mm between the transsacral S1 screw and the superior gluteal neurovascular bundle.[21]

As a transiliac-transsacral screw used for a unilateral injury crosses the contralateral sacroiliac joint, concerns about the effect of the screw on that uninjured joint exist among surgeons. A recent retrospective comparative study of 62 patients treated with either unilateral iliosacral screws or transiliac-transsacral screws did not support those concerns, however. Majeed Pelvic Scores and side-specific Numeric Rating Scale pain scores demonstrated no difference between the two groups at 3-year follow up.[14]

Other strategies regarding posterior pelvic ring fixation have also been explored in the recent literature. Two recent studies have explored the possibility of using the third sacral segment as an osseous fixation pathway for a 7.0 mm diameter transiliac-transsacral screw. Interestingly, patients with dysmorphic sacra commonly had a pathway of sufficient diameter to accommodate a transiliac-transsacral screw in the third sacral segment. This corridor could potentially supplement the fixation performed at the higher sacral levels, when additional stability is desired[15,16] (**Figure 1**).

An alternate strategy that has recently been proposed focused on increasing the density of the bone in the osteoporotic patient being treated with an iliosacral

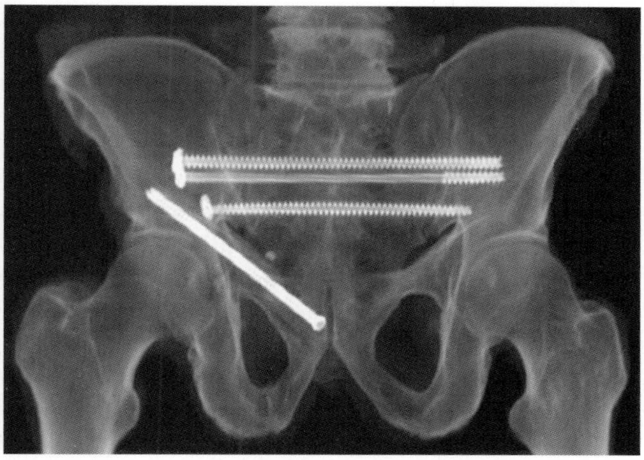

Figure 1 Outlet view of the pelvis reformatted from the postoperative CT scan. Transiliac-transsacral screws cross the second and third sacral segments.

screw. A 2016 study described a technique of percutaneously injecting calcium phosphate into the sacrum, prior to the full insertion of the screw.[22] Ideally, this would supplement the fixation of the screw in the sacrum as prior biomechanical study demonstrated a significant improvement in both stiffness and screw pull-out strength in a human cadaveric iliosacral screw model.[23]

Anterior Pelvic Ring

The anterior pelvic ring has comparatively received less attention in the recent literature than the posterior pelvic ring. Anterior ring injury typically involves fractures of the rami, disruption of the symphysis, or a combination thereof. There are open and percutaneous methods of treatment, similar to posterior ring; both methods have been studied in the past few years.

Open treatment of a pubic symphysis disruption commonly involves a direct clamp reduction of the symphysis dislocation, followed by plate stabilization. Two studies have questioned this typical process in the recent literature.[5,24]

The clamp is traditionally applied anteriorly, in close proximity to the pubic tubercles. Although sexual dysfunction after a pelvic ring injury is common, this has generally been attributed to the trauma, and not to the surgical treatment of the injury. However, the spermatic cord lies immediately adjacent to the pubic tubercles, and can easily be penetrated with a clamp applied in this location during the surgery.[24]

It is well established that plate fixation can fail after ORIF of the symphysis pubis.[25-28] Although it is also established that failure of the plate does not necessarily correlate with a loss of alignment or a change in outcome, a 2015 study investigated whether symphyseal fusion at the time of ORIF would make a difference in terms of alignment and implant failure rate.[2,5,29] In this study, patients in the symphyseal fusion arm had lower rates of implant failure and revision surgery than patients in the standard ORIF group.[5]

Implant failure and malunion can also be affected by the addition of posterior fixation in patients with APC 2 pelvic ring injuries. When compared with patients treated with a symphyseal plate alone, those with combined anterior and posterior pelvic ring fixation had substantially lower rates of malunion and implant failure.[4]

Percutaneous treatment of the anterior pelvic ring generally comes in two forms: intramedullary screw fixation and external fixation. Modifications to the standard external fixator have been made to avoid issues with pin care and patient mobilization that occur because of the prominent pins; this is termed anterior subcutaneous internal pelvic fixator.[30-32]

Anterior subcutaneous internal pelvic fixator, when compared with plate fixation, is associated with an inferior reduction of the symphysis in those patients with a symphyseal injury. This implant is used with a planned second anesthetic for removal; plates typically do not require removal. In a retrospective review of 83 patients treated with this device, patients treated with this fixator appear to score well overall on validated functional outcome measures. However, issues with the lateral femoral cutaneous nerve and heterotopic ossification are frequent. The authors also highlight that there is a learning curve to the procedure.[31,33]

Perhaps this learning curve is responsible for some of the other complications associated with this device reported in the literature. Femoral nerve palsies were noted in eight femoral nerves in six patients treated with this device; resolution of the issue was noted to be variable after the removal of the fixator. A persistent femoral nerve palsy was noted to significantly affect patient function.[34]

Spinopelvic Dissociation

Patients with a spinopelvic dissociation are a subset within patients with pelvis injuries, even though several types can involve the pelvic ring. Although these injuries have certain things in common with pelvic ring injuries, there are several issues that are particular to spinopelvic dissociation. Lumbopelvic instability is primarily a sagittal plane issue; flexion of the pelvis and lower sacral fragment on the body of the upper sacrum result in kyphosis of the sacrum and compromise of the cauda

Trauma

equina within the sacral spinal canal. ORIF, classically done through a vertical midline approach, typically involves spinal instrumentation from the lumbar spine to the pelvis for patients with significant instability and may also include a neural decompression.[35,36]

Because of these significant issues in patients with lumbopelvic instability, it behooves the provider to correctly assess patients for this injury. The axial and sagittal cross-sectional imaging from the patient's CT scan can be used as a screening evaluation for this injury. A unilateral sacral fracture has a high negative predictive value for lumbopelvic instability. Conversely, bilateral sacral fractures noted on the axial CT images are highly predictive of finding a transverse fracture component on the sagittal images. In one study, no patients with unilateral sacral fractures had associated lumbopelvic instability, but 87% of bilateral sacral fractures were associated with lumbopelvic issues.[37]

With lumbopelvic instability, a kyphotic deformity typically develops. This sagittal imbalance can persist despite an attempt at a surgical correction and is associated with higher degrees of pain and disability. As this deformity is commonly inadequately reduced, this is a potential area for improvement in surgical care.[38]

Similar to the pelvic ring, there is increasing research interest in percutaneous treatment for these injuries. This is likely for similar reasons; percutaneous treatment should theoretically decrease the established problems with open treatment, such as blood loss and wound complications.[39] Although percutaneous treatment of a spinopelvic injury has been described with iliosacral screws in the past, only recently has percutaneous lumbopelvic fixation been described as a technique.[40,41] This represents an area for further development.

Outcomes

Patients with pelvic ring injuries frequently qualify as polytrauma patients on the basis of their Injury Severity Score. The outcome measure of primary importance for these critical patients is survival; functional outcomes, although important, are often of secondary concern as they may be influenced significantly by the severity of other associated injuries. Survival appears to be improving because of changes in care over the years, as there has been a significant decrease in adjusted pelvic fracture mortality rates. Healthy patients with unstable pelvic ring injuries currently have the same mortality rate as healthy patients with stable pelvic ring injuries.[42]

At the other end of the spectrum are patients with noncompressible torso hemorrhage and associated pelvic ring injuries. These patients have potentially preventable deaths, but outcomes from resuscitative thoracotomy have been traditionally poor. Resuscitative endovascular balloon occlusion of the aorta (REBOA) was first described in the Korean War and has recently gained popularity as a hemorrhage control agent for various situations involving exsanguination (ruptured aortic aneurysm, postpartum uterus, gastrointestinal tract, trauma to abdominal viscera, pelvic trauma, etc). Although it does appear that its use positively affects the systolic blood pressure in these patients, it is questionable thus far as to whether there is a demonstrable change in mortality rates.[43-45] The literature specific to the pelvic ring for this application is so far sparse, but a recent study from the United Kingdom had positive results. The REBOA was attempted in 19 patients and was successfully delivered in 13. All 13 survived, 4 of the 6 failed attempts expired. Cardiac arrest was lower in the REBOA group and systolic blood pressure was improved. Ten of the 13 REBOA patients required a thrombectomy for a distal arterial thrombus.[46] This complication highlights one of the limitations of the procedure; ideally, its risk profile will improve and the true benefit of its utility will become clear over the coming years.[47]

It has been demonstrated that for anterior-posterior compression–type injuries, patients with higher ISS scores tend to have worse functional outcomes. Patients with more severe pelvic injury types (ie, anteroposterior compression type 3 [APC-3]) do not appear to have worse functional outcomes as a result; however, those patients who experience a major loss of reduction and are not revised properly are more likely to experience a poor functional outcome.[3]

Fractures of the Acetabulum

The goals of surgical treatment for an acetabular fracture are well established; the principles include an anatomic reduction of the fracture, a concentric relationship between the femoral head and the acetabulum, and a proper realignment of the acetabulum within the pelvis. Emile Letournel is credited with the establishment of these principles and also the demonstration that an accurate reduction of the acetabulum with an acceptably low complication rate was possible. Later studies, by other surgeons, verified the relationship between these principles and hip durability.[48] However, certain studies show that surgeons are still having difficulty meeting that standard. Issues with hip durability persist in the literature, as do high complication rates.[49,50]

Surgical Indications

One of the classic indications for surgery is a nonconcentric relationship between the femoral head and acetabulum. A nonconcentric hip has resultant increased contact pressures and a significantly increased incidence of posttraumatic arthritis.[48] There is increased interest in trying to discern the stability of the hip joint in the setting of a posterior wall fracture. The concentricity of the joint is first evaluated with radiographs and CT scans, which are static measures that may not reveal dynamic instability between the head and acetabulum. The size of the posterior wall, as well as the location of the displaced fragment, may not provide the surgeon with enough information to determine whether the potential for hip instability exists. Although small posterior wall fragment size is less frequently associated with hip instability, patients with small posterior wall fragments can still have dynamic hip instability on a stress exam under anesthesia.[51] An exit point that is closer to the dome for the posterior wall fracture is also associated with a greater incidence of hip instability.[51,52] As an independent risk factor, however, no one determinant is universally reliable and the exam under anesthesia is currently the benchmark in diagnosing hip instability.[52] Those patients with negative exams under anesthesia reliably do well with closed treatment; therefore the test has excellent negative predictive value.[53] The natural history of patients with small wall fractures and a positive stress exams is unknown as these patients typically undergo surgery.

Surgical Approaches

Certain acetabular fracture patterns are indicated for an anterior surgical approach; and the ilioinguinal is the classic anterior acetabular approach. Matta[54] used this approach with successful outcomes and an acceptably low complication rate. Alternate anterior acetabular approaches have been developed, and there is a great deal of commonality between them and the traditional ilioinguinal. All the approaches have the same surgical goals, and many of the reduction and fixation maneuvers are the same. The ilioinguinal is a technically demanding operation and is in close proximity to the external iliac vessels and femoral nerve. Surgeons have looked for alternative approaches that provide adequate visualization, but are less technically demanding and perhaps safer as a result. The anterior intrapelvic approach (AIP), when compared to the traditional ilioinguinal, also provides the surgeon with access to the anterior elements of the pelvis, with the exception of the iliac fossa. Surgeons who utilize the AIP typically add a secondary lateral window in order to reduce and fix fractures that involve the internal iliac fossa.[55] In order to further expand the access provided from the AIP with a lateral window, some surgeons recommend an osteotomy of the ASIS, which allows for further distal and medial access through the lateral window.[56] The middle window of the ilioinguinal, with its dissection between the femoral nerve and the external iliac vessels, is not performed in the AIP with a lateral window.[55]

Reduction and Fixation (Developing Surgical Techniques)

The goal of surgical treatment of acetabular fractures is to obtain and maintain an anatomic reduction of the articular surface of the hip. Recent literature has focused on improved construct biomechanics, and improved understanding of anatomy and imaging as it relates to screw placement. As the amount of knowledge in these areas expands, surgeons should improve in their ability to safely access the various fracture components, perform accurate reductions, and utilize fixation constructs of optimal stability.

For the acetabular fractures traditionally treated through an ilioinguinal approach, the femoral head frequently displaces the quadrilateral surface in a medial direction. Mechanically, a buttress plate for the quadrilateral surface to prevent this medial displacement has obvious appeal. Two biomechanical studies were recently done to examine this, but these studies had conflicting results.

In a 2018 study, a Sawbones fracture model with a simulated anterior column posterior hemitransverse pattern and four different fixation constructs was mechanically tested. The medial infrapectineal buttress plate did not perform differently than the models fixed without it.[57] However, a clear advantage was demonstrated with the addition of this plate in a 2017 cadaver study.[58] This plate has also been studied in the clinical setting. In Germany, a recent study showed that patients had 40% anatomic and 33% imperfect reductions after treatment with a plate that covered the quadrilateral surface.[59]

Screw placement for acetabular fractures can be difficult because of the complexity of the bony anatomy

Trauma

and the understanding of the associated imaging. Percutaneous techniques of screw insertion require a thorough understanding of both in order to be effective. For the acetabulum, anterior column screw fixation is commonly placed under fluoroscopic guidance. Proper imaging of the anterior column has been previously described.[60,61] Additional methods described in the recent literature deepens the understanding of imaging and anatomy. Furthermore, it is important to confirm all screws to be extra-articular prior to leaving the operating room when treating an acetabular fracture. Modifications on the five commonly used views of the pelvis (AP, inlet, outlet, iliac oblique, obturator oblique) can be used for these purposes. An iliac oblique-outlet view can provide the surgeon with additional information when placing an anterior column screw.[62] An inlet-obturator oblique view can help confirm that screws used for fixation of a posterior wall fracture are extra-articular.[63]

Postoperative Assessment of Reduction and Fixation

Historically the postoperative assessment was done with plain radiographs. However, currently there is no standard way of performing radiographic measurements.[64] As the durability of the hip is thought to be directly related to the quality of the reduction, it is natural to investigate the reduction quality further. CT scans have been validated as superior in identifying malreductions when compared with radiographs, and the accuracy of the reduction noted on CT correlates with outcomes.[65,66] Besides its use as a scientific tool in multiple recent studies, it has the potential to change management in a small percentage of patients.[59,65-67] In a 2015 study, surgeons revised only 2.5% of their patients because of intra-articular hardware, intra-articular osteochondral fragments, and/or malreduction found on the postoperative CT scan.[67]

Outcomes

Functional outcome after acetabular fracture hinges on hip durability and the patient's ability to return to activities. Patients with a low Injury Severity Score and a high preinjury fitness level are the most likely to return to activities; conversely, the more severely injured patients with low preinjury fitness levels are the least likely to return to activities.[68]

Durability of the hip is affected by several factors. In a cohort study, patients after an acetabular ORIF were 25 times more likely to undergo total hip arthroplasty (THA) than age-matched control patients from the general population. The overall rate of THA was 13.9%; interestingly, those patients who did not require a THA in the first 10 years trended toward the general population in terms of risk. Surgeons who performed a low volume of acetabular ORIF had patients go on to THA at a higher rate.[50] This may have to do with reduction quality, as an inadequate reduction is a risk factor for future THA.[66]

Geriatric Patients With Acetabular Fractures

It is generally accepted that among patients with acetabular fractures, the elderly represent a particularly challenging subset of patients. When compared with younger patients, these patients are different for several reasons. Because of decreased bone mineral density, the fractures in the elderly frequently have characteristics that are not present in young patients. These different fracture patterns have their own treatment challenges. Also, the elderly patients frequently have associated comorbidities, and their functional demands are less.

Surgical Indications for the Elderly Patient

Indications for surgery are unclear at this time and there is no consensus on this issue. In a 2016 study, extensive variability in the treatment currently rendered between different surgeons at 15 Level I Trauma Centers for the elderly population was observed.[69] It is apparent that the criteria for surgery in the young do not apply as well to the elderly population, as there is a much higher rate of conversion to THA from ORIF in the elderly when compared with the young.[50,70] Furthermore, elderly patients can have good functional outcomes with acetabular fractures treated nonsurgically that would typically be indicated for surgery in younger patients with higher functional demands.[71]

Surgical Treatment Options

The role for arthroplasty in the elderly patient is continuing to evolve. As acute ORIF has a higher rate of subsequent arthroplasty than in the young patient, interest in THA as a part of the acute treatment has increased.[70,72,73] However, when the patients with ORIF were compared with those treated with THA, the rate of complications and revision surgery were no different between the two groups, although pain scores were better in the THA group.[72] A combination of ORIF and THA is another surgical option, but there are no comparative studies on this subject[73] (**Figure 2**).

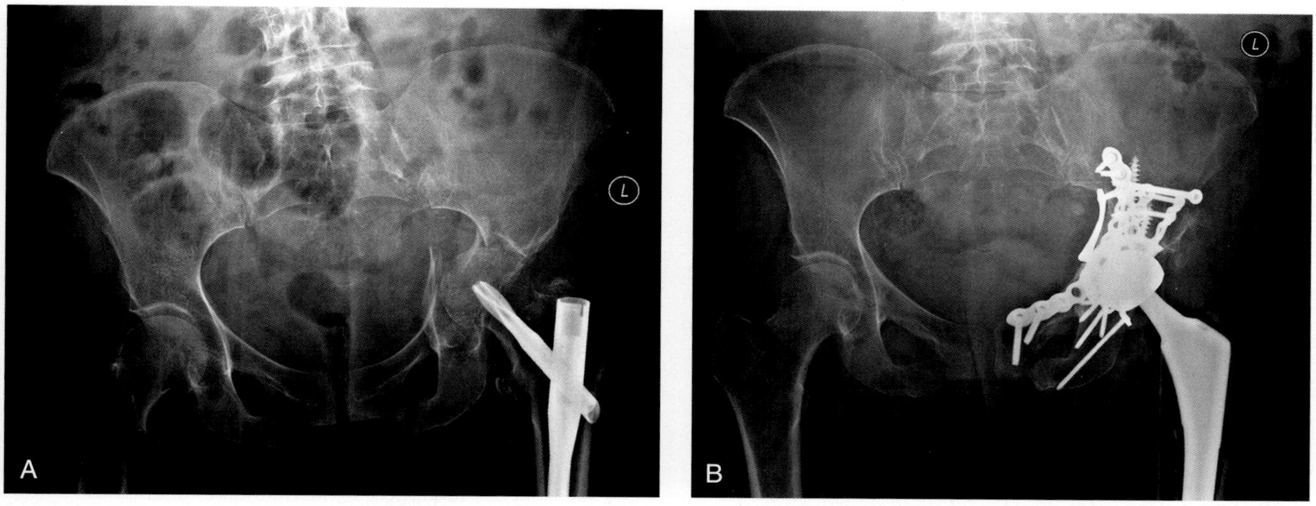

Figure 2 **A** and **B**, Complex associated both-column fracture in an elderly patient. Treatment with anterior intrapelvic reduction and fixation of the anterior column, wall, and quadrilateral surface followed by removal of hip nail, fixation of the segmental posterior column, and insertion of arthroplasty.

Outcomes

Given the advanced age and comorbidities, and the issues with prolonged recumbency, mortality is the primary concern in elderly patients. However, in a study of 454 patients older than 60 years between 2002 and 2009 with an acetabular fracture, the mortality rate was 16% at 1 year.[74] Risk for mortality was affected by comorbidities, increased age, and associated fracture patterns (as opposed to elementary patterns). Surgical treatment was not an independent risk factor for mortality.

The difference in functional outcomes between the available treatment options is difficult to ascertain currently. This is due to the variability in treatment options utilized for similar injuries as well as the use of different validated outcome scores in the available studies.[69,71,72]

Summary

Pelvic and acetabular trauma management continues to be an area of significant investigation and interest. Determination of mechanical pelvic stability after injury is facilitated by an understanding of the mechanism and severity of injury, complete radiographic evaluation, and dynamic stress evaluation. Improvements in implant selection and insertion techniques continue to evolve and allow for safer and more effective stabilization of complex pelvic injuries. Fractures of the acetabulum are best treated by accurate articular reduction and internal fixation. Understanding the utility and the limitations of the surgical approaches to the acetabulum allows the surgeon to minimize surgical complications while still striving to achieve a perfect articular reduction and optimizing the patient's likelihood of retaining a well-functioning, durable, pain-free hip joint.

Key Study Points

- Understanding pelvic stability following injury is key to determining if that fracture requires surgical intervention or may be managed with progressive mobilization and close radiographic and clinical follow-up.
- Obtaining and correctly interpreting appropriate imaging intraoperatively is the key to safely inserting posterior pelvic ring internal fixation.
- Percutaneous internal fixators for stabilization of anterior pelvic ring injuries have had a higher complication rate than that of standard open reduction and internal fixation techniques.
- Use of the anterior intrapelvic approach and implantation of anatomically shaped infrapectineal implants continues to increase in popularity for the treatment of certain acetabular fracture patterns. Achieving an anatomic articular reduction remains the primary goal of acetabular fracture surgery and is most closely associated with improved outcomes.
- The role for acute arthroplasty, with or without internal fixation, following acetabular fracture in the geriatric patient continues to evolve.

Annotated References

1. Ochenjele G, Reid KR, Castillo RC, et al: Predictors of unplanned reoperation after operative treatment of pelvic ring injuries. *J Orthop Trauma* 2018;32:e245-e250.

   Unplanned revision surgeries, typically for infection and failure of fixation, were common issues. The factors most commonly associated with revision surgery were related to the severity of the visceral pelvic and abdominal injuries.

2. Frietman B, Verbeek J, Biert J, Frölke J-P: The effect of implant failure after symphyseal plating on functional outcome and general health. *J Orthop Trauma* 2016;30:336-339.

   No difference in outcome scores was discerned between patients with implant failure and those with intact implants after a symphyseal plating.

3. Lybrand K, Bell A, Rodericks D, Templeman D, Tornetta P: APC injuries with symphyseal fixation: What affects outcome? *J Orthop Trauma* 2017;31:27-30.

   Patients with higher ISS and those who experienced a major loss of reduction had worse outcomes among patients with APC pelvic injuries.

4. Avilucea FR, Whiting PS, Mir H: Posterior fixation of APC-2 pelvic ring injuries decreases rates of anterior plate failure and malunion. *J Bone Joint Surg Am* 2016;98:944-951.

   In APC-2 pelvic ring injuries, a supplemental posterior screw significantly decreased the rate of symphyseal plate failure and loss of reduction with resultant malunion.

5. Lybrand K, Kurylo J, Gross J, Templeman D, Tornetta P: Does removal of the symphyseal cartilage in symphyseal dislocations have any effect on final alignment and implant failure?. *J Orthop Trauma* 2015;29:470-474.

   Lower rates of implant failure and revision surgery were noted in patients with symphyseal dislocations treated with excision of the symphyseal cartilage and plate fixation.

6. Swartz J, Vaidya R, Hudson I, Oliphant B, Tonnos F: Effect of pelvic binder placement on OTA classification of pelvic ring injuries using computed tomography. Does it mask the injury? *J Orthop Trauma* 2016;30:325-330.

   A fluoroscopic stress examination under anesthesia was used as the preferred diagnostic test in this study of patients with pelvic ring injuries. Prebinder radiographs were diagnostic in 69.4% of the patients; a CT scan in patients with pelvic binders was diagnostic in 50% of the patients.

7. Gibson PD, Adams MR, Koury KL, Shaath MK, Sirkin MS, Reilly MC: Inadvertent reduction of symphyseal diastasis during computed tomography. *J Orthop Trauma* 2016;30:474-478.

   When compared with the measurement done on a screening AP radiograph, 97% of patients had a reduction of their symphyseal diastasis on the CT scan. 19.2% had a reduction from greater than 25 mm on the AP radiograph to less than 25 mm on the CT scan.

8. Sagi HC, Coniglione FM, Stanford JH: Examination under anesthetic for occult pelvic ring instability. *J Orthop Trauma* 2011;25:529-536.

9. Whiting PS, Auston D, Avilucea FR, et al: Negative stress examination under anesthesia reliably predicts pelvic ring union without displacement. *J Orthop Trauma* 2017;31:189-193.

   Patients with pelvic ring injuries who were deemed stable after a negative stress examination under fluoroscopy were made weight bearing as tolerated and went on to union without displacement.

10. Gire JD, Jiang SY, Gardner MJ, Bishop JA: Percutaneous versus open treatment of posterior pelvic ring injuries: Changes in practice patterns over time. *J Orthop Trauma* 2018;32(9): 457-460. doi:10.1097/BOT.0000000000001236.

    Candidates for Part II of the ABOS examination between 2003 and 2015 have done a similar number of posterior pelvic ring surgeries from year to year. The incidence of percutaneous posterior pelvic ring fixation shifted from 49% of the surgeries submitted by the candidates in 2003 to 79% in 2015, with a corresponding decrease in the incidence of open posterior pelvic ring surgery.

11. Lindsay A, Tornetta P, Diwan A, Templeman D: Is closed reduction and percutaneous fixation of unstable posterior ring injuries as accurate as open reduction and internal fixation? *J Orthop Trauma* 2016;30:29-33.

    Posterior pelvic ring injuries were treated at two centers; one center performed ORIF and the other center performed a closed reduction with percutaneous fixation. In a retrospective review, closed reduction and percutaneous fixation had slightly better reduction quality than open reduction internal fixation.

12. Lucas JF, Routt MLC, Eastman JG: A useful preoperative planning technique for transiliac-transsacral screws. *J Orthop Trauma* 2017;31:e25-e31.

    A description of a preoperative planning technique based on the CT scan of the pelvis for percutaneous iliosacral screw placement is provided.

13. Blum LE, Hake ME: Preoperative planning for percutaneous transsacral, transiliac screws. *J Orthop Trauma* 2018;32 suppl 1:S22-S23.

    Preoperative planning for iliosacral screws involves scrutinizing the preoperative imaging and provides the surgeon with an understanding of the relationship between the intended implants and the nearby neurovascular, muscular, and bony structures.

14. Mardam-Bey SW, Beebe MJ, Black JC, et al: The effect of transiliac-transsacral screw fixation for pelvic ring injuries on the uninjured sacroiliac joint. *J Orthop Trauma* 2016;30:463-468.

    The outcome scores and pain scores were no different in patients treated with transiliac-transsacral screws when compared with those treated with unilateral iliosacral screws.

15. Eastman JG, Adams MR, Frisoli K, Chip Routt ML: Is S3 a viable osseous fixation pathway?. *J Orthop Trauma* 2018;32:93-99.

    15.2% of patients have an osseous fixation pathway at the third sacral segment that will accept a 7.0 mm transiliac-transsacral screw.

Trauma

16. Hwang JS, Reilly MC, Shaath MK, et al: Safe zone quantification of the third sacral segment in normal and dysmorphic sacra. *J Orthop Trauma* 2018;32:178-182.

This CT study measured the third sacral segment osseous fixation pathway and compared normal with dysmorphic sacra. Dysmorphic sacra have a larger third sacral segment osseous fixation pathway than the third sacral segment pathway in normal sacra.

17. Tabaie SA, Bledsoe JG, Moed BR: Biomechanical comparison of standard iliosacral screw fixation to transsacral locked screw fixation in a type C zone II pelvic fracture model. *J Orthop Trauma* 2013;27:521-526.

18. Eastman JG, Kuehn RJ, Chip Routt ML: Useful intraoperative technique for percutaneous stabilization of bilateral posterior pelvic ring injuries. *J Orthop Trauma* 2018;32:e191-e197.

Transiliac-transsacral screws can be utilized to care for bilateral posterior pelvic ring injuries. The details of the reduction and fixation technique are described in this manuscript.

19. Verbeek J, Hermans E, van Vugt A, Frölke J-P: Correct positioning of percutaneous iliosacral screws with computer-navigated versus fluoroscopically guided surgery in traumatic pelvic ring fractures. *J Orthop Trauma* 2016;30:331-335.

83% of percutaneous iliosacral screws were placed correctly with computer navigation; 82% of screws were accurately positioned with conventional fluoroscopy.

20. Kim JW, Quispe JC, Hao J, Herbert B, Hake M, Mauffrey C: Fluoroscopic views for a more accurate placement of iliosacral screws: An experimental study. *J Orthop Trauma* 2016;30:34-40.

Surgeons had difficulty fluoroscopically identifying three different types of errant screws in plastic pelvic models with standard inlet and outlet views. These three errant screws were penetration of the anterior edge of S1 body, penetration of the cranial sacral ala, and partial penetration of the S1 foramen. Variant views were described to identify these errant screws.

21. Maslow J, Collinge CA: Risks to the superior gluteal neurovascular bundle during iliosacral and transsacral screw fixation: A computed tomogram arteriography study. *J Orthop Trauma* 2017;31:640-643.

Transsacral S1 screws have a starting point that, on average, is closer to the superior gluteal neurovascular bundle than iliosacral S1 and transsacral S2 screws.

22. Collinge CA, Crist BD: Combined percutaneous iliosacral screw fixation with sacroplasty using resorbable calcium phosphate cement for osteoporotic pelvic fractures requiring surgery. *J Orthop Trauma* 2016;30:e217-e222.

Calcium phosphate can be used as a potential augment to iliosacral screw fixation of the posterior pelvic ring. The technique for percutaneous application of the calcium phosphate is described.

23. Grechenig S, Gansslen A, Gueorguiev B, et al: PMMA-augmented SI screw: A biomechanical analysis of stiffness and pull-out force in a matched paired human cadaveric model. *Injury* 2015;46 suppl 4:S125-S128.

24. Collinge CA, Beltran MJ: Anatomic relationship between the spermatic cord and the pubic tubercle: Are our clamps injuring the cord during symphyseal repair? *J Orthop Trauma* 2015;29:290-294.

25. Sagi HC, Papp S: Comparative radiographic and clinical outcome of two-hole and multi-hole symphyseal plating. *J Orthop Trauma* 2008;22:373-378.

26. Morris SAC, Loveridge J, Smart DKA, Ward AJ, Chesser TJS: Is fixation failure after plate fixation of the symphysis pubis clinically important? *Clin Orthop Relat Res* 2012;470:2154-2160.

27. Collinge C, Archdeacon MT, Dulaney-Cripe E, Moed BR: Radiographic changes of implant failure after plating for pubic symphysis diastasis: An underappreciated reality? *Clin Orthop Relat Res* 2012;470:2148-2153.

28. Moed BR, Grimshaw CS, Segina DN: Failure of locked design-specific plate fixation of the pubic symphysis: A report of six cases. *J Orthop Trauma* 2012;26:e71-e75.

29. Eastman JG, Krieg JC, Routt MLC: Early failure of symphysis pubis plating. *Injury* 2016;47:1707-1712.

11.1% of 126 patients had a failure of the symphyseal plate at an average of 29 days. Two of the 126 patients had a loss of reduction that warranted revision surgery.

30. Vaidya R, Woodbury D, Nasr K: Anterior subcutaneous internal pelvic fixation/INFIX: A systemic review. *J Orthop Trauma* 2018;32 suppl 6:S24-S30.

This meta-analysis identified 25 articles on the subject. 99.5% of patients went on to union. Complications included lateral femoral cutaneous nerve irritation (26.3%), heterotopic ossification (36%), infection (3%), and femoral nerve palsy (1%).

31. Vaidya R, Martin AJ, Roth M, Tonnos F, Oliphant B, Carlson J: Midterm radiographic and functional outcomes of the anterior subcutaneous internal pelvic fixator (INFIX) for pelvic ring injuries. *J Orthop Trauma* 2017;31:252-259.

Eighty-three patients treated with the anterior subcutaneous internal pelvic fixator were reviewed. The average Majeed score was categorized as "good." All patients required a removal of the device, and frequently there were issues with the lateral femoral cutaneous nerve and heterotopic ossification.

32. Vaidya R, Tonnos F, Nasr K, Kanneganti P, Curtis G: The anterior subcutaneous pelvic fixator (INFIX) in an anterior posterior compression type 3 pelvic fracture. *J Orthop Trauma* 2016;30 suppl 2:S21-S22.

The surgical technique is described in this manuscript and the accompanying video.

33. Vaidya R, Martin AJ, Roth M, Nasr K, Gheraibeh P, Tonnos F: INFIX versus plating for pelvic fractures with disruption of the symphysis pubis. *Int Orthop* 2017;41:1671-1678.

Patients treated with plates had better alignment than those treated with the anterior subcutaneous pelvic fixator and did not require a second operation. No difference was noted in outcome scores.

Trauma

34. Hesse D, Kandmir U, Solberg B, et al: Femoral nerve palsy after pelvic fracture treated with INFIX: A case series. *J Orthop Trauma* 2015;29:138-143.

Eight cases of femoral palsy in six patients treated with the anterior subcutaneous pelvic fixator were described in this retrospective chart review.

35. Schildhauer TA, Bellabarba C, Nork SE, Barei DP, Routt MLC, Chapman JR: Decompression and lumbopelvic fixation for sacral fracture-dislocations with spino-pelvic dissociation. *J Orthop Trauma* 2006;20:447-457.

36. Yi C, Hak DJ: Traumatic spinopelvic dissociation or U-shaped sacral fracture: A review of the literature. *Injury* 2012;43:402-408.

37. Bishop JA, Dangelmajer S, Corcoran-Schwartz I, Gardner MJ, Routt MLC, Castillo TN: Bilateral sacral ala fractures are strongly associated with lumbopelvic instability. *J Orthop Trauma* 2017;31:636-639.

87% of patients with bilateral sacral fractures had an associated transverse component, which indicated lumbopelvic instability. No patients with unilateral sacral fractures had an associated transverse component.

38. Lee H-D, Jeon C-H, Won S-H, Chung N-S: Global sagittal imbalance due to change in pelvic incidence after traumatic spinopelvic dissociation. *J Orthop Trauma* 2017; 31:e195-e199.

A spinopelvic dissociation causes lumbosacral kyphosis and a resultant sagittal imbalance, which affects pain and function.

39. Bellabarba C, Schildhauer TA, Vaccaro AR, Chapman JR: Complications associated with surgical stabilization of high-grade sacral fracture dislocations with spino-pelvic instability. *Spine* 2006;31:S80-S88, discussion S104.

40. Nork SE, Jones CB, Harding SP, Mirza SK, Routt ML: Percutaneous stabilization of U-shaped sacral fractures using iliosacral screws: Technique and early results. *J Orthop Trauma* 2001;15:238-246.

41. Williams SK, Quinnan SM: Percutaneous lumbopelvic fixation for reduction and stabilization of sacral fractures with spinopelvic dissociation patterns. *J Orthop Trauma* 2016;30:e318-e324.

Lumbopelvic fixation is commonly applied open, and there are complications related to the procedure's open nature. A technique for percutaneous application is described here.

42. Black SR, Sathy AK, Jo C, Wiley MR, Minei JP, Starr AJ: Improved survival after pelvic fracture: 13-year experience at a single trauma center using a multidisciplinary institutional protocol. *J Orthop Trauma* 2016;30:22-28.

There was a significant decrease in adjusted pelvic mortality rates over a 13-year period.

43. Gamberini E, Coccolini F, Tamagnini B, et al: Resuscitative endovascular balloon occlusion of the aorta in trauma: a systematic review of the literature. *World J Emerg Surg* 2017;12:42.

The authors evaluated preliminary results or REBOA in 1,355 patients.

44. Manzano-Nunez R, Naranjo MP, Foianini E, et al: A meta-analysis of resuscitative endovascular balloon occlusion of the aorta (REBOA) or open aortic cross-clamping by resuscitative thoracotomy in non-compressible torso hemorrhage patients. *World J Emerg Surg* 2017;12:30.

REBOA was suggested to have a positive effect on mortality in patients experiencing noncompressible torso hemorrhage.

45. Morrison JJ, Galgon RE, Jansen JO, Cannon JW, Rasmussen TE, Eliason JL: A systematic review of the use of resuscitative endovascular balloon occlusion of the aorta in the management of hemorrhagic shock. *J Trauma Acute Care Surg* 2016;80(3):554.

The authors performed a systematic review to assess clinical use of REBOA and the effect on hemodynamic profle and mortality; no clear reduction in hemorrhage-related mortality was shown. Level of evidence: IV.

46. Lendrum R, Perkins Z, Chana M, et al: Pre-hospital resuscitative endovascular balloon occlusion of the Aorta (REBOA) for exsanguinating pelvic haemorrhage. *Resuscitation* 2019;135:6-13.

The authors determined that REBOA is an acceptable prehospital resuscitation method for patients with exanguinating pelvic hemorrhage.

47. Rasmussen TE, Franklin CJ, Eliason JL: Resuscitative endovascular balloon occlusion of the aorta for hemorrhagic shock. *JAMA Surg* 2017;152(11):1072-1073.

48. Tannast M, Najibi S, Matta JM: Two to twenty-year survivorship of the hip in 810 patients with operatively treated acetabular fractures. *J Bone Joint Surg Am* 2012;94: 1559-1567.

49. Ding A, O'Toole RV, Castillo R, et al: Risk factors for early reoperation after operative treatment of acetabular fractures. *J Orthop Trauma* 2018;32:e251-e257.

Seven hundred and ninety-one patients who were treated with an ORIF for a displaced acetabular fracture were reviewed retrospectively. The infection/wound complication rate was 7%. Early revision surgery occurred in 8% of patients; risk factors identified for revision surgery were hip dislocation, articular comminution, femoral head fracture, femoral neck fracture, and advanced age.

50. Henry PDG, Si-Hyeong Park S, Paterson JM, Kreder HJ, Jenkinson R, Wasserstein D: Risk of hip arthroplasty after open reduction internal fixation of a fracture of the acetabulum: A matched cohort study. *J Orthop Trauma* 2018;32:134-140.

A total hip arthroplasty was 25 times more likely in an acetabular fracture patient than matched controls. The rate of THA increased for female gender, advanced age, and patients treated by low-volume surgeons.

51. Firoozabadi R, Spitler C, Schlepp C, et al: Determining stability in posterior wall acetabular fractures. *J Orthop Trauma* 2015;29:465-469.

52. Patel JH, Moed BR: Instability of the hip joint after posterior acetabular wall fracture. *J Bone Joint Surg* 2017;99: e126-e127.

This study was unable to identify independent risk factors for instability of the hip after a posterior wall fracture.

53. McNamara AR, Boudreau JA, Moed BR: Nonoperative treatment of posterior wall acetabular fractures after dynamic stress examination under anesthesia: Revisited. *J Orthop Trauma* 2015;29:359-364.

54. Matta JM: Operative treatment of acetabular fractures through the ilioinguinal approach: A 10-year perspective. *J Orthop Trauma* 2006;20:S20-S29.

55. Archdeacon MT: Comparison of the ilioinguinal approach and the anterior intrapelvic approaches for open reduction and internal fixation of the acetabulum. *J Orthop Trauma* 2015;29 suppl 2:S6-S9.

56. Sagi HC, Bolhofner B: Osteotomy of the anterior superior iliac spine as an adjunct to improve access and visualization through the lateral window. *J Orthop Trauma* 2015;29:e266-e269.

57. May C, Egloff M, Butscher A, et al: Comparison of fixation techniques for acetabular fractures involving the anterior column with disruption of the quadrilateral plate. *J Bone Joint Surg* 2018;100:1047-1054.

Synthetic bone models were used to evaluate different fracture fixation constructs biomechanically. Periarticular long screws from the plate applied superior to the pelvic brim performed better than the infrapectineal buttress plate.

58. Gillispie GJ, Babcock SN, McNamara KP, et al: Biomechanical comparison of intrapelvic and extrapelvic fixation for acetabular fractures involving the quadrilateral plate. *J Orthop Trauma* 2017;31:570-576.

Cadaver pelves were osteotomized to create an anterior column fracture with quadrilateral plate involvement; the various fracture fixation constructs were then biomechanically tested. The addition of an intrapelvic plate substantially improved stability at the fracture site.

59. Gras F, Marintschev I, Grossterlinden L, et al: The anterior intrapelvic approach for acetabular fractures using approach-specific instruments and an anatomical-preshaped 3-dimensional suprapectineal plate. *J Orthop Trauma* 2017;31:e210-e216.

Patients treated with an anterior intrapelvic approach and a preshaped suprapectineal plate had 75% good to excellent Matta grades and 53% good to excellent modified Merle d'Aubigne scores.

60. Routt ML, Simonian PT, Grujic L: The retrograde medullary superior pubic ramus screw for the treatment of anterior pelvic ring disruptions: A new technique. *J Orthop Trauma* 1995;9:35-44.

61. Routt ML, Nork SE, Mills WJ: Percutaneous fixation of pelvic ring disruptions. *Clin Orthop Relat Res* 2000;(375):15-29.

62. Cunningham BA, Ficco RP, Swafford RE, Nowotarski PJ: Modified iliac oblique-outlet view: A novel radiographic technique for antegrade anterior column screw placement. *J Orthop Trauma* 2016;30:e325-e330.

An alternative radiographic view for the evaluation of an anterior column screw is described.

63. TosounidisGiannoudis THPV: Use of inlet-obturator oblique view (leeds view) for placement of posterior wall screws in acetabular fracture surgery. *J Orthop Trauma* 2017;31:e133-e136.

An alternative radiographic view for the evaluation of posterior wall fixation is described.

64. Dodd A, Osterhoff G, Guy P, Lefaivre KA: Radiographic measurement of displacement in acetabular fractures: A systematic review of the literature. *J Orthop Trauma* 2016;30:285-293.

In the current literature, there is no standard method for measurement of displacement on radiographs for acetabular fractures.

65. Verbeek DO, van der List JP, Moloney GB, Wellman DS, Helfet DL: Assessing postoperative reduction after acetabular fracture surgery: A standardized digital computed tomography-based method. *J Orthop Trauma* 2018;32:e284-e288.

A CT-based method for measuring displacement after acetabular ORIF is described.

66. Verbeek DO, van der List JP, Villa JC, Wellman DS, Helfet DL: Postoperative CT is superior for acetabular fracture reduction assessment and reliably predicts hip survivorship. *J Bone Joint Surg Am* 2017;99:1745-1752.

Radiographs were not as accurate as CT scans for the identification of residual displacement. The quality of the reduction on CT scan correlated with hip durability.

67. Archdeacon MT, Dailey SK: Efficacy of routine postoperative CT scan after open reduction and internal fixation of the acetabulum. *J Orthop Trauma* 2015;29:354-358.

68. Phruetthiphat O-A, Koehler DM, Karam MD, Rungprai C, Gao Y, Marsh JL: Preinjury aerobic fitness predicts postoperative outcome and activity level after acetabular fracture fixation. *J Orthop Trauma* 2016;30:e267-e272.

Functional outcome was most affected by preinjury aerobic fitness as a risk factor.

69. Manson TT, Reider L, O'Toole RV, et al: Variation in treatment of displaced geriatric acetabular fractures among 15 level-I trauma centers. *J Orthop Trauma* 2016;30:457-462.

Site varied significantly for the choice of treatment for a geriatric acetabular fracture.

70. Butterwick D, Papp S, Gofton W, Liew A, Beaulé PE: Acetabular fractures in the elderly: Evaluation and management. *J Bone Joint Surg Am* 2015;97:758-768.

71. Ryan SP, Manson TT, Sciadini MF, et al: Functional outcomes of elderly patients with nonoperatively treated acetabular fractures that meet operative criteria. *J Orthop Trauma* 2017;31:644-649.

Functional outcome scores were good for elderly patients treated nonsurgically for acetabular fractures that would meet criteria for an operation in a younger patient.

72. Weaver MJ, Smith RM, Lhowe DW, Vrahas MS: Does total hip arthroplasty reduce the risk of secondary surgery following the treatment of displaced acetabular fractures in the elderly compared to open reduction internal fixation? A pilot study. *J Orthop Trauma* 2018;32 suppl 1:S40-S45.

No difference was identified in the rate of revision surgery or Harris hip scores between patients treated with an ORIF and those treated with a THA. Pain scores were improved in the THA group.

73. Lin C, Caron J, Schmidt AH, Torchia M, Templeman D: Functional outcomes after total hip arthroplasty for the acute management of acetabular fractures: 1- to 14-year follow-up. *J Orthop Trauma* 2015;29:151-159.

74. Gary JL, Paryavi E, Gibbons SD, et al: Effect of surgical treatment on mortality after acetabular fracture in the elderly: a multicenter study of 454 patients. *J Orthop Trauma* 2015;29(4):202–208.

The surgical treatment of acetabular fractures does not affect increase or decrease in mortality.

Chapter 21

Lower Extremity Trauma

Joshua L. Gary, MD, FAOA • Marschall B. Berkes, MD • Christopher Doro, MD

ABSTRACT

Musculoskeletal injury to the lower limb is common and can greatly impact a patient's ability to ambulate and function. The evidence for or against specific treatments remains imperfect but continues to grow and improve in quality. A summary of the highest quality evidence from the past half-decade follows.

Keywords: external fixation; fractures; injury; internal fixation; lower extremity

Introduction

Injury is a leading cause of morbidity and mortality worldwide. Lower extremity trauma can have great impact on an individual's ability to function as articular injuries may lead to posttraumatic osteoarthritis and metaphyseal or diaphyseal injuries can lead to malunion with limb shortening, angulation, or malrotation if not properly reduced and stabilized until bony union occurs. Arthroplasty is considered for older patients with certain articular injuries, especially about the hip, to allow for early mobilization with a goal of decreasing rates of secondary surgeries. Open fractures are commonly encountered with lower extremity trauma and are discussed in a separate chapter. Recent evidence and treatment recommendations vary by specific anatomic locations as described below.

Dr. Gary or an immediate family member is a member of a speakers' bureau or has made paid presentations on behalf of Smith & Nephew; has stock or stock options held in Summitt Medventures; has received research or institutional support from AO North America and Microbion; and serves as a board member, owner, officer, or committee member of the AO North America and Orthopaedic Trauma Association. Neither of the following authors nor any immediate family member has received anything of value from or has stock or stock options held in a commercial company or institution related directly or indirectly to the subject of this chapter: Dr. Berkes and Dr. Doro.

Femoral Head

Femoral head fractures are rare injuries most frequently seen after a high-energy traumatic mechanism. Associated injuries include hip dislocations and their associated soft-tissue injury, acetabular fractures, femoral neck fractures, and ligamentous knee injuries seen with "dashboard" mechanisms. While the acetabulum acts like a "splint" for concentrically reduced injuries,[1] a stress examination under anesthesia may be warranted to ensure a concentric reduction is not unstable, as is common with posterior wall acetabular fractures.

Almost 90% of fractures treated with ORIF using a Smith-Peterson approach united without complication in a large single-center series.[1] However, in the same series, all five patients with Pipkin III injuries proceeded to catastrophic failure or osteonecrosis within 6 months of their index procedure,[1] suggesting that primary arthroplasty should be considered in any patient with an associated femoral neck fracture. A series of 17 consecutive Pipkin I, II, and IV injuries treated with surgical hip dislocation, as described by Ganz, with only one patient (6%) developing osteonecrosis and converting to arthroplasty. Heterotopic ossification was reported in both series, but was rarely symptomatic.[1,2]

Femoral Neck

Femoral neck fractures continue to fall into two broad categories: low-energy mechanisms in osteopenic patients and high-energy mechanisms in younger patients with different treatment options and considerations in each of the groups. Treatment decisions are usually made based upon the patient's age, bone quality, and degree of displacement at injury.

The blood supply to the femoral head plays an important role in surgical decision making. The superior retinacular artery (SRA) derives from the deep branches of the medical femoral circumflex artery (MFCA) and has long been thought to be the dominant blood supply to the dome of the femoral head.[3] However, recent attention has been given to the contributions of the inferior retinacular (IRA) (transverse branch of MFCA) and anterior retinacular arteries (ARA) (from the ascending branch of the lateral femoral circumflex artery) that form an anastomotic network of blood supply within the femoral head.[3,4] These are less frequently injured than the SRA in femoral neck fractures and may be much more important to the viability of the femoral head than previously thought.[4]

For physiologically younger patients with a femoral neck fracture, complications after reduction and fixation remain common. A meta-analysis of open or closed reduction techniques for fractures resulting from high-energy mechanisms in younger patients showed no differences in rates of nonunion (11.6% vs 14.9%) or osteonecrosis (17.2% vs 17.7%) in the closed versus open reduction groups.[5] Another meta-analysis found no association between timing of fixation and development of osteonecrosis, but surgical delay from injury greater than 24 hours tripled the rate of nonunion.[6] However, selection bias may play a role in these retrospective results. Newer implants that include multiple telescoping screws with a side-plate have been introduced with nonunion and osteonecrosis rates of 1.2% and 13.8%, respectively, for treatment of 29 displaced fractures in a single-center series.[7] The generalizability of the results remains unknown.

The Fixation using Alternative Implants for the Treatment of Hip fractures (FAITH) study has provided a large body of prospective randomized evidence regarding fixation choice for patients with low-energy osteopenic femoral neck fractures.[8] Both stable and unstable fractures were included if the operating surgeon felt the patient older than 50 years with a femoral neck fracture was suitable for internal fixation as treatment, and patients were randomized to surgical fixation with a sliding hip screw or at least two cancellous screws of diameter 6.5 mm or greater.[9] Across the entire cohort of more than 1,100 patients, there were no differences in revision surgery rates within 24 months between either fixation construct; however, cancellous screws had significantly higher revision surgery rates for implant removal and sliding hip screws had significantly higher rates of conversion to total hip arthroplasty and osteonecrosis.[8] Certain subgroups of patients, including those who were current smokers or who had displaced fractures, had less revision surgery at 24 months when treated with a sliding hip screw compared with treatment with cancellous screws.[8] Risk factors for revision surgery within 24 months include female sex, increased body mass index, initially displaced fracture, unacceptable quality of implant placement, and smokers treated with cancellous screws, and consideration for primary arthroplasty should be strongly given to these patients with low-energy femoral neck fractures.[10] Health-related quality of life (HRQL) after these fractures is worse with older age, female gender, increasing body mass index, increased American Society for Anesthesiologists (ASA) class, and displaced fracture.[11]

When arthroplasty is chosen as treatment, meta-analysis of multiple studies suggests total hip arthroplasty is favored when compared with hemiarthroplasty for patients with longer life expectancies and higher activity levels because of risk of acetabular erosion.[12] For hemiarthroplasty, meta-analysis of available data favors direct lateral approach over a posterior approach to lower postoperative dislocation risk[12] and cemented over press-fit femoral stems to decrease risk of periprosthetic fracture and improve functional outcomes.[12,13]

Intertrochanteric Femur

Unlike femoral neck fractures, reduction and fixation is the primary treatment in patients of any age. For standard obliquity fracture patterns with posteromedial comminution (AO/OTA 31-A2), a randomized, controlled trial (RCT) comparing sliding hip screws and cephalomedullary (CM) nails demonstrated no differences in functional outcomes, but less femoral neck shortening with CM nails, at 12 months after surgery.[14] Although failure rates remain low with either treatment, later conversion to hip arthroplasty does not appear to favor one implant over the other for operative time, hospital length of stay, Trendelenburg gait, postoperative complication rates, or 5-year survivorship of the arthroplasty.[15]

A retrospective, comparative clinical study between patients treated with a CM implant with two integrated screws versus a CM implant with a single screw demonstrated 2.5 times more varus collapse and 2 times more femoral neck shortening at 12 months for a single screw CM nail when compared with one with two integrated screws.[16] The choice for long or short CM nails continues to remain controversial with proponents of short nails citing lower blood losses, transfusion rates, operative times, similar rates of periprosthetic fractures, and similar rates of revision surgery.[17] One retrospective study comparing long and short CM nails in 256 patients demonstrated a trend approaching significance toward increased periprosthetic fractures with short nails (3%) compared with long nails (0%).[18]

Subtrochanteric Femur

Recent research has focused on atypical femur fractures found in association with diphosphonate use. Two large series of complete atypical femur fractures both found an approximately 70% union rate with many fractures failing to unite until 6 to 12 months after the index procedure. Supra-isthmic location, anterolateral bowing greater than 10°, and the presence of a lateral endosteal beak were predictive of delayed healing with modifiable risk factors including iatrogenic cortical breakage and varus/flexion malreduction.[19,20]

Femoral Shaft

The ideal treatment for adult femoral shaft fractures remains a reamed, statically locked intramedullary nail. Identifying associated pathologies including knee injuries and femoral neck fractures is critical. In a series of 429 femoral shaft fractures, 131 cases of ipsilateral knee injury were seen, 87 (20% overall) of which were ligamentous knee injuries with frequent delay in diagnosis and risk factors including C-type fracture patterns, male gender, and motor vehicle accidents.[21] Although nonunion is rare after intramedullary nailing, a series of 211 femoral shaft fractures where 23 developed a hypertrophic nonunion identified poor reduction, C-type fracture pattern, and nail fit less than 70% of the canal diameter as risk factors.[22] Pulmonary insult remains a consideration in femoral reaming, and recent data demonstrated that femoral nails performed in the lateral position were associated with less ICU days and without increased risk of pulmonary complications compared with supine femoral nailing.[23]

Distal Femur

After their introduction in the early 2000s, lateral locking plating became the predominant construct for distal femur fracture fixation. A series of 241 fractures treated with lateral locked plating demonstrated a 13% nonunion rate; however, stainless steel plates had a 41% rate compared with 10% rate with titanium plates,[24] but selection bias may be present. Plate characteristics such as thickness, screw density and geometry, and modulus of elasticity may play a role in the development of nonunion. Variable angle locking plate constructs have been recently introduced with a 22% failure rate in a single-center series of 36 cases with metaphyseal comminution as a risk factor.[25] These results have prompted other techniques for acute fixation. A nail-plate combination construct (**Figure 1**) has shown promising results, with seven of eight acute fractures and eight of eight nonunions healing without additional operations.[26] Distal femur fractures in the elderly can represent the beginning of a life-threatening process as is observed with geriatric hip fractures with 1 year mortality at 13.4% and increased risk for those with greater than 2-day delay to surgical treatment and higher Charlson Comorbidity index.[27]

Patella

Patella fractures are associated with high complication rates and persistent symptoms despite appropriate treatment. Attention has recently turned toward ventral plating, especially for comminuted fractures. Precontoured plates as well as generic plates that can be customized to patellar anatomy have been described, with or without the use of locking technology. In 20 fractures treated with a precontoured plate, there was

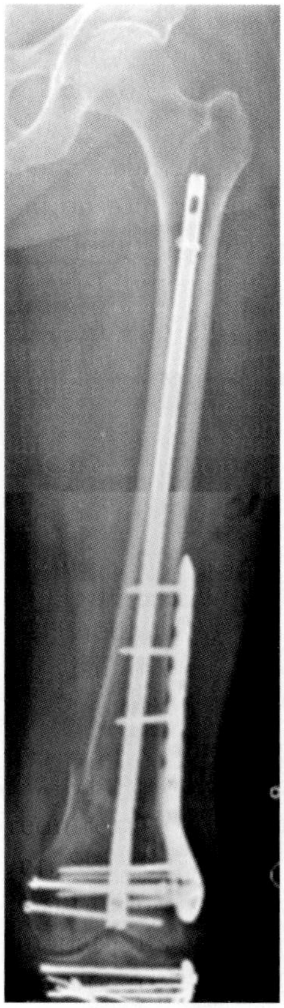

Figure 1 Postoperative AP view of a distal femur fracture in an 87-year-old man treated with a combination of retrograde nail and lateral distal femoral precontoured plate. The patient was allowed immediate weight bearing as tolerated postoperatively.

Trauma

one implant failure and one infection with all fractures healed at an average of 3 months and good to excellent results were reported.[28] Lorich used a of 2.4/2.7 mm mesh plate application for patella fractures with its use dating back to 2012 and has reported excellent clinical results in 25 cases.[29] The key portions of his technique include a lateral parapatellar arthrotomy to directly visualize the fracture and articular reduction to allow for plate application in a subchondral fashion with multiplanar screw fixation (**Figure 2**). Moore et al presented follow-up data on 20 of 36 comminuted patella fractures and found median knee range of motion to be 0° to 130° and only one instance of fixation failure and no symptomatic hardware removal reported.[30]

Tibial Plateau

Newer classification systems now specifically characterize the posterior column of plateau fractures, which was traditionally overlooked. In a prospective cohort of 65 patients, surgical tibial plateau fractures were studied with postoperative CT, and the malreduction (articular step or gap >2 mm) rate was 32.5%, with 77% of these located in the posterior quadrants.[31] A retrospective study of 138 patients who underwent ORIF for tibial plateau fractures evaluated loss of reduction, and the presence of a coronal or posterior column fracture was associated with a loss of reduction (odds ratio 9.2) in 41B and 4.8 in 41C fractures.[32] Although these studies do not represent level I evidence, the literature indicated surgeons should carefully scrutinize the involvement, reduction, and fixation of the posterior column (**Figure 3**).

Soft-tissue injuries about the knee are associated with tibial plateau fractures, yet the utility of MRI is unclear. A cohort of 82 patients with surgically treated tibial plateau fractures and preoperative MRI in a prospective database found 73% of the patients with soft-tissue injuries; however, only lateral meniscal injuries were repaired acutely and there were only two delayed procedures for the other soft tissues injuries with no differences in patient-reported outcomes or range of motion at final follow-up.[33]

Although early external fixation for complex injuries is common to protect soft-tissue integrity, a single-center, retrospective cohort with 101 Patients sustaining AO/OTA 41C fractures treated definitively in less than 72 hours from injury has questioned that practice with reports of similar infection rates (8.8%) and functional outcomes to historical controls.[34]

Tibial Shaft

Semi-extended versions of intramedullary nailing for tibia fractures continue to grow in popularity. A recent meta-analysis of four RCTs that included 293 patients was conducted comparing supra- and infrapatellar nailing. The authors found suprapatellar nailing superior with regard to total blood loss, VAS scores, Lysholm knee scores, and fluoroscopy time, and there were no

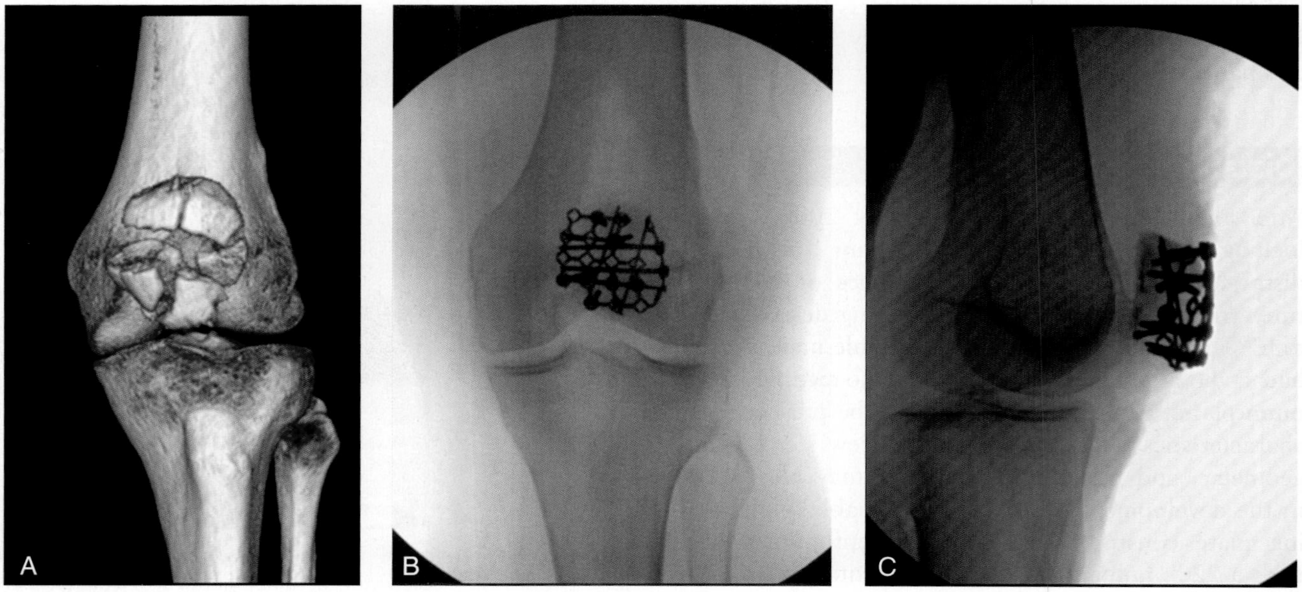

Figure 2 **A**, 3D surface rendered CT scan of a comminuted patella fracture managed with (**B** and **C**) ORIF with a 2.4/2.7 mm mesh plate on its ventral surface.

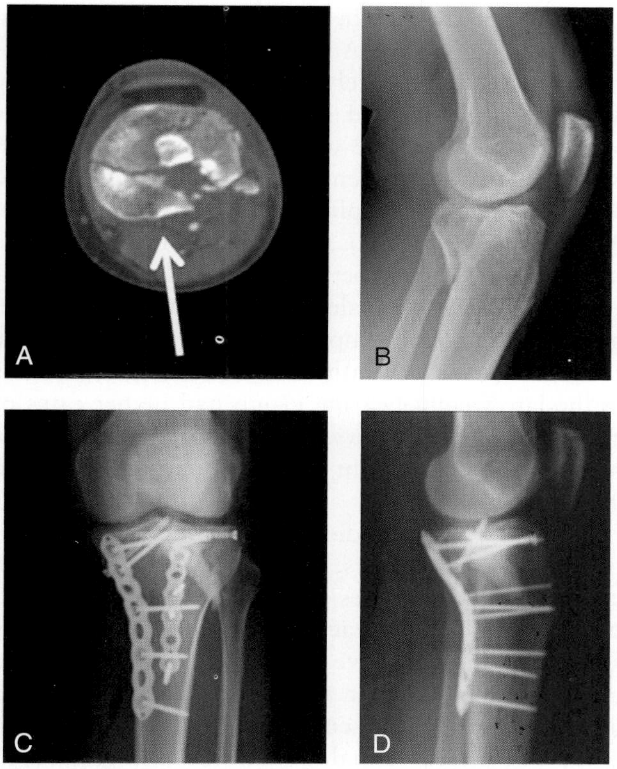

Figure 3 **A**, Axial CT scan of a complex tibial plateau fracture with posterior column involvement (white arrow). **B**, Lateral view of injury radiograph. **C** and **D**, Postoperative AP and lateral views after staged prone Lobenhoffer approach followed by a lateral parapatellar arthrotomy.

differences seen in range of motion, length of hospital stay, or postoperative hospitalization.[35] A retrospective cohort of 266 patients with distal third tibia fractures was evaluated for alignment after suprapatellar or infrapatellar intramedullary nailing. The authors found ≥5° malalignment, statistically significant, in 26% patients with infrapatellar nailing compared with only 4% patients who underwent suprapatellar nailing.[36]

Plate fixation remains an excellent option for the distal tibia, and a multicenter trial of 321 patients with extraarticular distal tibia fractures randomized the injuries to an intramedullary nail or a fixed angle plate. Early functional outcomes favored nailing; however, by 6 and 12 months there was no significant differences between the groups, and complication rates were similar.[37]

A retrospective matched cohort of 340 patients with tibia and fibula shaft fractures with and without fibular fixation found no difference between infection rates, time to union, postoperative complications, or rates of nonunion supporting either treatment in association with fixation of a tibial shaft fracture.[38]

A recent RCT with 90 diaphyseal tibia fractures treated with intramedullary nails was randomized to either weight-bearing-as-tolerated (WBAT) or non-weight bearing (NWB) for the first 6 weeks, including all open fractures except Gustilo-Anderson type IIIC. The mean time to union in each group was 22 weeks with no differences in infection, loss of reduction, malunion, or patient-reported outcomes.[39]

Pilon

Pilon fractures have traditionally had poor long-term functional results despite appropriate management. Preoperative planning and soft-tissue management are critical for the treating surgeon. 200 CT scans in patients with AO/OTA 43A-C fractures were reviewed for peroneal tendon dislocation or entrapment of posteromedial structures on soft-tissue windows with an 11% rate of peroneal displacement and 19% rate of posteromedial structure entrapment.[40] These findings were much more likely to be found in complete articular patterns.

Tibial plating on the compression side of the injury provides a biomechanical advantage compared with tension sided plating (**Figures 4** and **5**). In a retrospective study of 103 patients with pilon fractures, varus failures (with a transverse fibula fracture) demonstrated statistically significant increased complication rates with a lateral tibial plate (80%) compared with medial tibial plating (14%), and valgus failures (with a comminuted fibula fracture) demonstrated a nonsignificant and underpowered increase in complication rates with medial plates (36%) versus lateral plates (17%).[41]

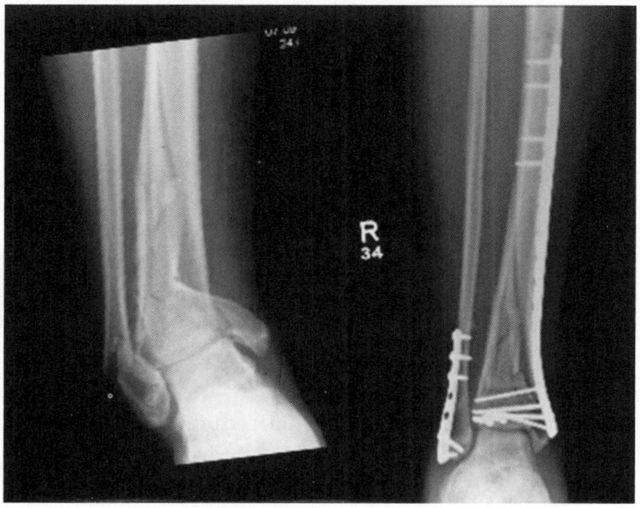

Figure 4 Injury and postoperative AP views of a comminuted pilon fracture with varus failure pattern treated with open reduction and internal fixation with primary medial tibial plating.

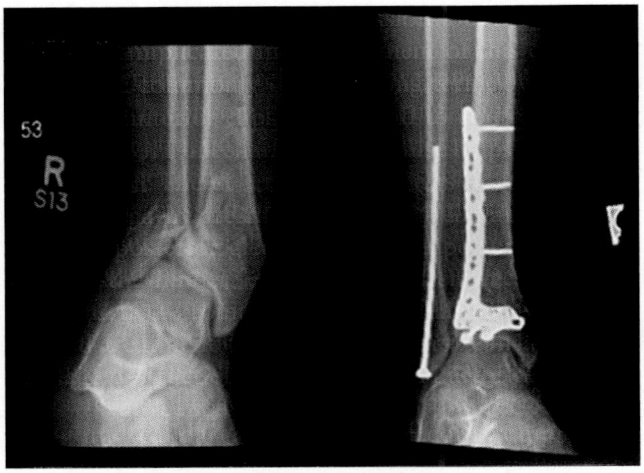

Figure 5 Injury and postoperative AP views of a comminuted pilon fracture with valgus failure pattern treated with open reduction and internal fixation with primary lateral tibial plating.

Recent interest in fragment-specific approaches has grown with sequential posterior, followed by an anterior approach to reduce and stabilize complete articular injuries. A retrospective review of 166 patients with AO/OTA 43-C injuries compared 35 patients who underwent a posterior and anterior approach to 81 patients who had an anterior approach only. Higher nonunion rates were seen with a dual approach (40%) with no difference in infection rates, whereas statistically insignificant rates of articular malreduction > 2 mm were seen in patients treated with an anterior-only approach.[42]

Ankle and Foot

Techniques for syndesmotic reduction and fixation lack consensus. A systemic review of 21 studies evaluated diagnosis, treatment indications, assessment of malreduction, implant, postoperative implant removal, and outcomes.[43] Based upon meta-analysis of available data, no evidence exists that fixation of a nondisplaced, but "stress-test" positive, syndesmosis injury results in improved outcomes and that subtle malrotation of the fibula that has been found to be present in up to 50% of patients has a detrimental clinical impact. Suture fixation in general has been associated with a lower rate of implant removal, implant failure, and subtle malreduction. The meta-analysis also demonstrated that rotational ankle fractures with associated syndesmotic injury have worse clinical outcomes when compared with bimalleolar ankle fractures.[43]

Timing of weight bearing after surgical fixation also lacks consensus. An RCT with 110 ankle fractures treated operatively was randomized to early weight bearing (placed in a boot at 2 weeks postoperative visit) or late weight bearing (casted for 6 weeks) with no difference at 12 months for return to work, wound complications, or loss of fixation. Ankle range-of-motion and Olerud-Molander ankle function scores were better in the early group; however, these were equivalent at 12 months. The SF-36 physical component improved score persisted in the early group at 12 months and interestingly, patients in the late weight-bearing group had higher rates of hardware removal. Given these findings the authors recommend early weight bearing and range of motion in these patients.[44]

Several recent studies have evaluated interventions in elderly patients. 620 patients >60 years with unstable ankle fractures were randomized to surgical treatment or close contact casting under anesthesia by a surgeon for definitive treatment. Patient-reported outcomes were similar at 6 months with increased infection and wound complications in the surgical group and increased malunion in the casting group.[45] Another prospective RCT of 100 patients >65 years randomized to ORIF or locked fibular nailing found significantly fewer infections and lower total cost of treatment (despite a higher implant cost) in the nail group and no difference in patient-reported outcomes.[46] Finally, a prospective, randomized, controlled study compared tibio-talo-calcaneal (TTC) nailing (with no casting and immediate weight bearing) versus ORIF (with casting and 6 weeks non–weight bearing) in unstable elderly ankle fractures in 87 patients with lower complication rates and shorter hospital stay in the TTC nail group at more than 1 year; however, no difference in patient-reported outcomes was seen between the groups.[47]

Calcaneus fractures are relatively common high-energy foot injuries. A meta-analysis comparing the clinical outcomes of surgical and nonsurgical treatment for displaced intra-articular calcaneal fractures with 908 patients from seven RCTs found that if surgery was "successful," the patients had improved shoe wear and walking ability; however, there were no differences in patient-reported outcomes, return to work, need for subsequent subtalar fusion, and complex regional pain syndrome between the groups and higher infection rates in the surgical group.[48]

Less extensile approaches to minimize infection are gaining in popularity. A prospective study of 30 patients with displaced intra-articular calcaneal fractures treated with lateral extensile or sinus tarsi approaches, based upon hospital of treatment, showed similar complication rates, clinical and radiographic outcomes between approaches with the sinus tarsi group having shorter surgical time, time to surgery, and possibly lower soft tissue complication rate.[49]

For Lisfranc injuries, a retrospective review of 55 patients compared transarticular screws to dorsal plating, or a combination of the two, and found no significant difference in implant failure, need for removal, or functional outcomes in the three groups with anatomic reduction predictive of improved outcomes in any of the groups.[50]

Summary

Lower extremity trauma is common and presents many challenges to the orthopaedic surgeon to restore function and limit long-term disability. The surgeon must evaluate each patient and injury individually to provide appropriate care according to injury and patient characteristics. Although fracture reduction often plays a pivotal role in functional recovery, the surgeon should understand published evidence that helps to guide care and appropriate treatment interventions for specific injuries.

Study Facts/Key Study Points

- Blood supply to the femoral head derives from an anastomotic ring formed primarily by the superior and inferior retinacular arteries, both terminal branches of the medial circumflex femoral artery.
- For femoral neck fractures resulting from low-energy mechanisms, cancellous screws were more likely to have secondary operation within 24 months for implant removal, whereas sliding hip screws were more likely to be converted to total hip arthroplasty and/or sustain osteonecrosis.
- Nonunion rates between 10% and 25% are seen for distal femur fractures treated with an isolated laterally based distal femur locking plate, and retrospective data suggest plate characteristics may play a role in the development of nonunion.
- Syndesmotic injury associated with ankle fractures remains challenging to properly reduce and stabilize, and early literature shows promising results for suture fixation between the tibia and fibula when compared with standard screw fixation.

Annotated References

1. Scolaro JA, Marecek G, Firoozabadi R, Krieg JC, Routt MLC: Management and radiographic outcomes of femoral head fractures. *J Orthop Traumatol* 2017;18(3):235-241.

   Single- center retrospective study of femoral head fractures with at least 6 months follow-up with 90% of fractures went to uneventful union; however, Pipkin III fractures (femoral head and femoral neck) had a 100% catastrophic failure rate by 6 months of follow-up. Level of evidence: IV (Prognostic).

2. Masse A, Aprato A, Alluto C, Favuto M, Ganz R: Surgical hip dislocation is a reliable approach for treatment of femoral head fractures. *Clin Orthop Relat Res* 2015;473(12):3744-3751.
3. Lazaro LE, Klinger CE, Sculco PK, Helfet DL, Lorich DG: The terminal branches of the medial femoral circumflex artery: The arterial supply of the femoral head. *Bone Joint Lett J* 2015;97-B(9):1204-1213.
4. Zhao D, Qiu X, Wang B, et al: Epiphyseal arterial network and inferior retinacular artery seem critical to femoral head perfusion in adults with femoral neck fractures. *Clin Orthop Relat Res* 2017;475(8):2011-2023.

   Using CT data in 30 uninjured patients, the intraosseous blood supply to the femoral head was evaluated and demonstrated the relevance of the inferior retinacular artery. 27 patients with femoral neck fractures were evaluated with similar methods demonstrating the integrity of the IRA in 100% of Garden I and II fractures and 60% of Garden III fractures. Level of evidence: IV (Prognostic).

5. Ghayoumi P, Kandemir U, Morshed S: Evidence based update: Open versus closed reduction. *Injury* 2015;46(3):467-473.
6. Papakostidis C, Panagiotopoulos A, Piccioli A, Giannoudis PV: Timing of internal fixation of femoral neck fractures. A systematic review and meta-analysis of the final outcome. *Injury* 2015;46(3):459-466.
7. Takigawa N, Yasui K, Eshiro H, et al: Clinical results of surgical treatment for femoral neck fractures with the Targon((R)) FN. *Injury* 2016;47(suppl 7):S44-S48.

   Single-center series of displaced femoral neck fractures treated with a side-plate that incorporates multiple telescoping screws into the femoral head and neck demonstrating nonunion rate <2% and AVN rates of 14%. Level of evidence: IV (Therapeutic).

8. The FAITH Investigators: Fracture fixation in the operative management of hip fractures (FAITH): An international, multicentre, randomised controlled trial. *Lancet* 2017;389(10078):1519-1527.

   Prospective, randomized, multinational controlled trial of fixation for femoral neck fracture with a sliding hip screw or cancellous screws that showed no difference in reoperation rates between either treatment arm. Level of evidence: I (Therapeutic).

9. The FAITH Investigators: Fixation using alternative implants for the treatment of hip fractures (FAITH): Design and rationale for a multi-centre randomized trial comparing sliding hip screws and cancellous screws on revision surgery rates and quality of life in the treatment of femoral neck fractures. *BMC Muscoskelet Disord* 2014; 15(1):219.

10. Sprague S, Schemitsch EH, Swiontkowski M, et al: Factors associated with revision surgery after internal fixation of hip fractures. *J Orthop Trauma* 2018;32(5):223-230.

    Secondary analysis from the FAITH study that identifies risk factors for revision surgery following operating fixation of femoral neck fractures with increased risk associated with female sex, elevated BMI, displaced fractures, poor reduction quality, and smokers treated with cancellous screws. Level of evidence: II (Prognostic).

11. Sprague S, Bhandari M, Heetveld MJ, et al: Factors associated with health-related quality of life, hip function, and health utility after operative management of femoral neck fractures. *Bone Joint Lett J* 2018;100-B(3):361-369.

    Secondary analysis from the FAITH trial showing worse HRQL for patients with older age, female gender, higher BMI, ASA class III or IV, and displaced fracture. Level of evidence: II (Prognostic).

12. Rogmark C, Leonardsson O: Hip arthroplasty for the treatment of displaced fractures of the femoral neck in elderly patients. *Bone Joint Lett J* 2016;98-B(3):291-297.

    Meta-analysis of multiple studies suggest total hip arthroplasty is favored when compared with hemiarthroplasty for patients with longer life expectancies and higher activity levels because of risk of acetabular erosion and that cemented stems have superior outcomes to uncemented stems. Level of evidence: II (Prognostic).

13. Inngul C, Blomfeldt R, Ponzer S, Enocson A: Cemented versus uncemented arthroplasty in patients with a displaced fracture of the femoral neck: A randomised controlled trial. *Bone Joint Lett J* 2015;97-B(11):1475-1480.

14. Reindl R, Harvey EJ, Berry GK, Rahme E, Canadian Orthopaedic Trauma S: Intramedullary versus extramedullary fixation for unstable intertrochanteric fractures: A prospective randomized controlled trial. *J Bone Joint Surg Am* 2015;97(23):1905-1912.

15. Yuan BJ, Abdel MP, Cross WW, Berry DJ: Hip arthroplasty after surgical treatment of intertrochanteric hip fractures. *J Arthroplasty* 2017;32(11):3438-3444.

    Conversion to hip arthroplasty after treatment of intertrochanteric femur fracture with sliding hip screw on cephalomedullary nail does not appear to favor one implant over the other for surgical time, hospital length of stay, Trendelenberg gait at final follow-up, postoperative complication rates, or five-year survivorship of the arthroplasty. Level of evidence: IV (Therapeutic).

16. Serrano R, Blair JA, Watson DT, et al: Cephalomedullary nail fixation of intertrochanteric femur fractures: Are two proximal screws better than one?. *J Orthop Trauma* 2017;31(11): 577-582.

    Retrospective comparative study between Gamma 3 and InterTAN cephalomedullary nails for treatment of intertrochanteric femur fracture demonstrated less shortening and varus collapse with the InterTAN device. Level of evidence: III (Therapeutic).

17. Kleweno C, Morgan J, Redshaw J, et al: Short versus long cephalomedullary nails for the treatment of intertrochanteric hip fractures in patients older than 65 years. *J Orthop Trauma* 2014;28(7):391-397.

18. Vaughn J, Cohen E, Vopat BG, Kane P, Abbood E, Born C: Complications of short versus long cephalomedullary nail for intertrochanteric femur fractures, minimum 1 year follow-up. *Eur J Orthop Surg Traumatol* 2015;25(4):665-670.

19. Cho JW, Oh CW, Leung F, et al: Healing of atypical subtrochanteric femur fractures after cephalomedullary nailing: Which factors predict union? *J Orthop Trauma* 2017;31(3):138-145.

    Forty-eight displaced atypical subtrochanteric femur fractures underwent cephalomedullary nailing. 68.7% healed without further intervention with a mean time to union of 10.7 months. Malalignment in coronal and sagittal plate significantly correlated with failure and delayed healing. Thus, quality of reduction was seen as the most important factor for timely union. Level of evidence: IV (Therapeutic).

20. Lim H-S, Kim C-K, Park Y-S, Moon Y-W, Lim S-J, Kim S-M: Factors associated with increased healing time in complete femoral fractures after long-term bisphosphonate therapy. *J Bone Joint Surg Am Vol* 2016;98(23):1978-1987.

    One hundred nine atypical femur fractures were followed postoperatively; there was a 30% rate of delayed or nonunion. Supraisthmic fracture location, bowing more than 10°, and lateral endosteal beaking were predictive of problematic healing, as well as modifiable factors including iatrogenic factors including iatrogenic cortical breakage and malreduction. Level of evidence: IV (Therapeutic).

21. Byun SE, Shon HC, Park JH, et al: Incidence and risk factors of knee injuries associated with ipsilateral femoral shaft fractures: A multicentre retrospective analysis of 429 femoral shaft injuries. *Injury* 2018;49(8):1602-1606.

    A series of 429 femoral shaft fractures reported 113 cases involving ipsilateral knee injuries, most commonly ligamentous knee injury. Risk factors identified for ipsilateral knee injury included male gender, C-type fractures, and motor vehicle accident. Level of evidence: II (Prognostic).

22. Millar MJ, Wilkinson A, Navarre P, et al: Nail fit: Does nail diameter to canal ratio predict the need for exchange nailing in the setting of aseptic, hypertrophic femoral nonunions? *J Orthop Trauma* 2018;32(5):245-250.

    Two hundred eleven femoral shaft fractures without risk factors for nonunion were retrospectively reviewed; 23/211 developed hypertrophic nonunion requiring exchange nailing. Risk factors for nonunion included poor reduction, Winquist 4, and poor nail fit. Nail fit <70% of canal was noted as risk factor for nonunion; therefore, the authors recommend a nail/canal fit >70%. Level of evidence: III (Prognostic).

23. Reahl GB, O'Hara NN, Coale M, et al: Is lateral femoral nailing associated with increased intensive care unit days? A propensity-matched analysis of 848 cases. *J Orthop Trauma* 2018;32(1):39-42.

Femoral nailing in the lateral position was associated with a shorter ICU length of stay. The conclusions were that lateral position was likely not associated with an increased risk of pulmonary complications. Level of evidence: III (Therapeutic).

24. Rodriguez EK, Zurakowski D, Herder L, et al: Mechanical construct characteristics predisposing to non-union after locked lateral plating of distal femur fractures. *J Orthop Trauma* 2016;30(8):403-408.

Two hundred forty one supracondylar femur fractures treated with either stainless steel or titanium plates were reviewed retrospectively. The rate of nonunion with titanium was 13.3%; however, nonunion rates with stainless steel plates were reported at 41%. It is possible that stiffer stainless steel constructs may not create the ideal healing environment at the distal femur. Level of evidence: III (Therapeutic).

25. Tank JC, Schneider PS, Davis E, et al: Early mechanical failures of the synthes variable angle locking distal femur plate. *J Orthop Trauma* 2016;30(1):e7-e11.

Thirty-six distal femur fractures were treated with a variable angle stainless steel plate with an associated failure rate of 22%. This was significantly higher than patients treated with standard laterally based locking plates. This was most commonly seen in cases with metaphyseal comminution. Level of evidence: III (Therapuetic).

26. Spitler CA, Bergin PF, Russell GV, Graves ML: Endosteal substitution with an intramedullary rod in fractures of the femur. *J Orthop Trauma* 2018;32:S25-S29.

This paper demonstrates the technique of nail plate combination fixation in the setting of obese patients or in those patients where prolonged healing time is expected. 15/16 fractures healed without further intervention. Level of evidence: IV (Therapeutic).

27. Myers P, Laboe P, Johnson KJ, et al: Patient mortality in geriatric distal femur fractures. *J Orthop Trauma* 2018;32(3):111-115.

Retrospective evaluation of 283 elderly distal femur fractures. 1 year mortality was reported at 13.4%. Delay to surgery greater than 48 hours was associated with an increased risk of mortality; a lower Charlson comorbidity index was noted among survivors. Level of evidence: III (Prognostic).

28. Wild M, Fischer K, Hilsenbeck F, Hakimi M, Betsch M: Treating patella fractures with a fixed-angle patella plate—a prospective observational study. *Injury* 2016;47(8):1737-1743.

This paper describes the use of a proprietary ventral plate construct for patella fracture fixation. There was one case of implant failure reported, with all 20 patients reporting good/excellent results. Level of evidence: IV (Therapeutic).

29. Lorich DG, Fabricant PD, Sauro G, et al: Superior outcomes after operative fixation of patella fractures using a novel plating technique: A prospective cohort study. *J Orthop Trauma* 2017;31(5):241-247.

Thirty-three patients with comminuted patella fractures were treated with mesh plate fixation. Compared with tension band fixation, plated patients reported improved subjective outcomes (KOS-ADL), increased thigh circumference, and decreased anterior knee pain. Level of evidence: IV (Therapeutic).

30. Moore TB, Sampathi BR, Zamorano DP, Tynan MC, Scolaro JA: Fixed angle plate fixation of comminuted patellar fractures. *Injury* 2018;49(6):1203-1207.

A clinical retrospective series of 36 comminuted patella fractures treated with lockign plate fixation. 4/20 cases reported symptomatic implants although none were removed. One fixation failure was reported, and generally good to excellent outcomes were reported. Level of evidence: IV (Therapeutic).

31. Meulenkamp B, Martin R, Desy NM, et al: Incidence, risk factors, and location of articular malreductions of the tibial plateau. *J Orthop Trauma* 2017;31(3):146-150.

Prospective cohort of 65 patients after plateau ORIF underwent CT evaluation. The malreduction rate was 32.5%. (77% of these were located in the posterior quadrants.) Malreduction was 16% in patients who had a submeniscal arthrotomy and 41% in patients who only had a fluoroscopic reduction ($P = 0.0021$). Level of evidence: II (Therapeutic).

32. Kim CW, Lee CR, An KC, et al: Predictors of reduction loss in tibial plateau fracture surgery: Focusing on posterior coronal fractures. *Injury* 2016;47(7):1483-1487.

Retrospective study in which 138 patients who underwent ORIF for tibial plateau were analyzed for loss of reduction postoperatively. Coronal fractures and comminution were the only two significant variables associated with a loss of reduction. Level of evidence: IV (Therapeutic).

33. Warner SJ, Garner MR, Schottel PC, et al: The effect of soft tissue injuries on clinical outcomes after tibial plateau fracture fixation. *J Orthop Trauma* 2018;32(3):141-147.

Prospective database cohort of 82 patents with surgically treated tibial plateau fractures and preoperative MRIs were evaluated. Of the patients, 73% had soft-tissue injuries on MR. Only the lateral meniscal injuries were repaired acutely, while 99% of the other soft tissue injuries seen on MR were not. The authors were unable to show any clinical difference between the patients at final follow-up. This suggests that preoperative MR does not alter the surgical treatment and most likely is not necessary in typical cases. Level of evidence: III (Prognostic).

34. Unno F, Lefaivre KA, Osterhoff G, et al: Is early definitive fixation of Bicondylar tibial plateau fractures safe? An observational cohort study. *J Orthop Trauma* 2017;31(3):151-157.

Retrospective cohort identifying 101 patients with AO/OTA 41C fractures that were treated definitively in less than 72 hours from injury. Their revision surgery rate at 12 months was 12.7%, if hardware removal was excluded. The physical component of the SF-36 was comparable to values reported in previous studies for surgical treatment of bicondylar plateau fractures. Level of evidence: IV (Therapeutic).

35. Yang L, Sun Y, Li G: Comparison of suprapatellar and infrapatellar intramedullary nailing for tibial shaft fractures: A systematic review and meta-analysis. *J Orthop Surg Res* 2018;13(1):146.

Meta-analysis of four RCT included 293 patients comparing supra- and infrapatellar nailing. Improved outcomes found regarding total blood loss (WMD = 7.92, $P = 0.022$), VAS scores (WMD = 0.70, $P < 0.0001$), Lysholm knee scores (WMD = −5.58, $P < 0.0001$), and fluoroscopy time (WMD = 26.70, $P = 0.026$). There were no differences seen in range of motion, length of hospital stay, or postoperative hospitalization. Level of evidence: III (Therapeutic).

36. Avilucea FR, Triantafillou K, Whiting PS, Perez EA, Mir HR: Suprapatellar intramedullary nail technique lowers rate of malalignment of distal tibia fractures. *J Orthop Trauma* 2016;30(10):557-560.

Retrospective cohort of 266 patients with distal tibia fractures was evaluated for alignment after suprapatellar or infrapatellar intramedullary nailing. The authors found ≥ 5° malalignment in 35 (26.1%) patients with infrapatellar nailing compared with only five (3.8%) patients who underwent suprapatellar nailing ($P < 0.0001$)

37. Costa ML, Achten J, Griffin J, et al: Effect of locking plate fixation vs intramedullary nail fixation on 6-month disability among adults with displaced fracture of the distal tibia: The UK FixDT randomized clinical trial. *JAMA* 2017;318(18):1767-1776.

An RCT of 321 patients with distal tibia fractures treated with an intramedullary nail or a fixed angle plate. There were no differences in outcomes or complications between the groups. Level of evidence: I (Therapeutic).

38. Githens M, Haller J, Agel J, Firoozabadi R: Does concurrent tibial intramedullary nailing and fibular fixation increase rates of tibial nonunion? A matched cohort study. *J Orthop Trauma* 2017;31(6):316-320.

Retrospective matched cohort of 160 tibia fractures treated with IMN and fibular fixation. A matched cohort of 174 patients with tibia fractures, without fibular fixation. No difference was found between infection rates, time to union, postoperative complications, or rates of nonunion (8% tibia only vs 12% tibia and fibula, $P = 0.28$). Fibular fixation does not impact the nonunion rate; the study did not, however, demonstrate any benefits of concomitant fibular fixation. Level of evidence: II (Therapeutic).

39. Gross SC, Galos DK, Taormina DP, Crespo A, Egol KA, Tejwani NC: Can tibial shaft fractures bear weight after intramedullary nailing? A randomized controlled trial. *J Orthop Trauma* 2016;30(7):370-375.

An RCT with 88 patients with 90 diaphyseal tibia fractures treated with intramedullary nails was randomized to either weight-bearing-as-tolerated or non–weight bearing for the first 6 weeks. There was no difference in mean time until union or in the secondary outcome variables. The authors concluded that for 42A and B fractures patients should be able to WBAT. Level of evidence: I (Therapeutic).

40. Fokin A Jr, Huntley SR, Summers SH, et al: Computed tomography assessment of peroneal tendon displacement and posteromedial structure entrapment in pilon fractures. *J Orthop Trauma* 2016;30(11):627-633.

Retrospective cohort study of 200 CT scans in AO/OTA 43A-C fractures. Only 50% of “final radiologist read” recognized posteromedial entrapment or displaced peroneal tendons. The rate of these soft-tissue problems in their study was 11% for peroneal displacement and 19% for posteromedial structure entrapment. In 43C fractures, 91% for peroneal displacement and 82% for posteromedial structure entrapment. The presence of a fibular fracture seemed to be protective for peroneal displacement. Level of evidence: III (Prognostic).

41. Busel GA, Watson JT, Israel H: Evaluation of fibular fracture type vs location of tibial fixation of pilon fractures. *Foot Ankle Int* 2017;38(6):650-655.

Retrospective case study of 103 patients with AO/OTA 43A-C fractures were grouped based on the fibular fracture pattern. The authors evaluated the type of fibula fracture, location of the primary tibial fixation (medial or lateral), and evidence of mechanical failure. The transverse fibula group showed mechanical complications in 14.3% of medially placed plate versus 80% for lateral plating ($P = 0.006$). In the comminuted fibular group, they noted 36.4% of medially placed plates demonstrated mechanical complications versus 16.7% for laterally based plates ($P = 0.156$). Level of evidence: III (Therapeutic).

42. Chan DS, Balthrop PM, White B, Glassman D, Sanders RW: Does a staged posterior approach have a negative effect on OTA 43C fracture outcomes? *J Orthop Trauma* 2017;31(2):90-94.

43. Michelson JD, Wright M, Blankstein M: Syndesmotic ankle fractures. *J Orthop Trauma* 2018;32(1):10-14.

Retrospective review of 166 patients with AO/OTA 43C fractures who were treated surgically; 35 underwent staged fixation of the posterior tibia first followed by an anterior procedure, and 81 had an anterior procedure only. A higher nonunion rate was seen in the staged a posterior approach group (40%) versus the anterior only approach (19%, $P = 0.015$). The infection rates were similar. Postoperative CT analysis for articular reduction demonstrated a 6% >2mm malreduction in the staged group versus 17% in the anterior only group, but this was nonsignificant. Level of evidence: III (Therapeutic).

44. Dehghan N, McKee MD, Jenkinson RJ, et al: Early weightbearing and range of motion versus non-weightbearing and immobilization after open reduction and internal fixation of unstable ankle fractures: A randomized controlled trial. *J Orthop Trauma* 2016;30(7):345-352.

An RCT of 110 Patients who underwent open reduction and internal fixation for ankle fractures was randomized to early weight bearing or late weight bearing. No difference in return to work, wound complications, ROM, OMAS, or loss of fixation between the two groups. Level of evidence: I (Therapeutic).

45. Willett K, Keene DJ, Mistry D, et al: Close contact casting vs surgery for initial treatment of unstable ankle fractures in older adults: A randomized clinical trial. *JAMA* 2016;316(14):1455-1463.

An RCT of 620 patients 60 years old or greater with unstable ankle fractures to undergo surgical treatment or to receive close contact casting with no difference in functional outcomes at 6 months. There were increased infections in the surgical group and increased malunion in the casting group. Level of evidence: I (Therapeutic).

46. White TO, Bugler KE, Appleton P, Will E, McQueen MM, Court-Brown CM: A prospective randomised controlled trial of the fibular nail versus standard open reduction and internal fixation for fixation of ankle fractures in elderly patients. *Bone Joint Lett J* 2016;98-B(9):1248-1252.

RCT of 100 patients older than 65 years randomized to ORIF or locked fibular nailing. Fewer wound infections occurred in the fibular nail group ($P = 0.002$), while there was no evidence of difference in Olerud-Molander ankle scores. Additionally, the overall cost of treatment in the fibular nail group was less than in the ORIF group despite the higher initial cost of the implant. Level of evidence: I (Therapeutic).

47. Georgiannos D, Lampridis V, Bisbinas I: Fragility fractures of the ankle in the elderly: Open reduction and internal fixation versus tibio-talo-calcaneal nailing: Short-term results of a prospective randomized-controlled study. *Injury* 2017;48(2):519-524.

RCT was performed to compare tibio-talo-calcaneal nailing (TTC nail) versus ORIF in 87 unstable elderly ankle fractures. At greater than one year, lower complication rate in the TTC nail group (8% vs 33%, $P < 0.05$) and shorter hospital stay (5.2 vs 8.4 days, $P < 0.001$) when compared with the ORIF group was found. No difference in Olerud-Molander ankle scores was found. Level of evidence: I (Therapeutic).

48. Zhang W, Lin F, Chen E, Xue D, Pan Z: Operative versus nonoperative treatment of displaced intra-articular calcaneal fractures: A meta-analysis of randomized controlled trials. *J Orthop Trauma* 2016;30(3):e75-81.

A meta-analysis in 908 Patients from seven RCTs that compared the clinical outcomes of operative and nonoperative treatment for displaced intra-articular calcaneal fractures. If surgery was successful, patients had improved shoe wear and walking ability. No differences were found in functional outcomes. The surgical group had higher overall complications with infection as the largest complication subgroup. Level of evidence: II (Therapeutic).

49. Basile A, Albo F, Via AG: Comparison between sinus tarsi approach and extensile lateral approach for treatment of closed displaced intra-articular calcaneal fractures: A multicenter prospective study. *J Foot Ankle Surg* 2016;55(3):513-521.

Prospective cohort of 30 patients with displaced intra-articular calcaneal fractures were compared after differing the approach, extensile or sinus tarsi, based on the hospital they were treated at. Their results showed similar clinical and radiographic outcomes and overall complication rate between the two groups; however, the sinus tarsi group had a faster surgical procedure (122 vs 187 minutes, $P < 0.0001$), a shorter waiting time to surgery (7 vs 19 days, $P < 0.0001$), and possibly lower soft-tissue complication rate (0 vs 7.9%, $P > 0.05$). Level of evidence: IV (Therapeutic).

50. Lau S, Guest C, Hall M, Tacey M, Joseph S, Oppy A: Functional outcomes post lisfranc injury-transarticular screws, dorsal bridge plating or combination treatment? *J Orthop Trauma* 2017;31(8):447-452.

A retrospective review of 55 patients compared transarticular screws, dorsal bridge plating, or a combination of the two in Lisfranc injuries. They found no significant difference in implant failure, need for removal, or functional outcomes in the three groups. Only anatomic reduction was predictive of improved functional outcomes. Level of evidence: III (Therapeutic).

Chapter 22

Spinal Trauma

Sherayar Orakzai, BSc • M. Farooq Usmani, MD, MSc • Steven C. Ludwig, MD

ABSTRACT

Traumatic injuries to the spine can present with a range of neurological deficits. The initial emergency department management of spine trauma depends on the severity and level of the injury and could range from discharge with follow-up to immediate intubation. For evaluation of trauma, utilization of imaging modalities varies based on the injury type. The types and details of imaging recommended are discussed here. The management of spine fractures depends on the severity of the neurological deficits, patient characteristics, and treatment goals. The chapter discusses surgical and nonsurgical management strategies with a focus on long-term outcomes. Early management and treatment of spine fractures can reduce morbidity and mortality associated with spinal trauma. In addition to standard surgical treatment, new treatment strategies for patients with spinal cord injuries are also discussed. The latest guidelines for the management of cervical, thoracic, and lumbar fractures are presented here.

Dr. Ludwig or an immediate family member has received royalties from DePuy, A Johnson & Johnson Company, and Globus Medical; is a member of a speakers' bureau or has made paid presentations on behalf of DePuy, A Johnson & Johnson Company, and Synthes; serves as a paid consultant to or is an employee of DePuy, A Johnson & Johnson Company, Globus Medical, K2Medical, and Synthes; has stock or stock options held in ASIP, ISD; has received research or institutional support from AO Spine North America Spine Fellowship Support, Globus Medical, K2M spine, OMEGA, and Pacira; and serves as a board member, owner, officer, or committee member of the American Board of Orthopaedic Surgery, Inc., the American Orthopaedic Association, Cervical Spine Research Society, and the Society for Minimally Invasive Spine Surgery. Neither of the following authors nor any immediate family member has received anything of value from or has stock or stock options held in a commercial company or institution related directly or indirectly to the subject of this chapter: Mr. Orakzai and Mr. Usmani.

Keywords: cervical spine fracture; management of spine injuries; spinal cord injury; spine trauma; thoracolumbar fractures; Thoracolumbar Injury Classification and Severity (TLICS) score

Introduction

Traumatic injuries to the spine require immediate attention. Spinal injuries usually involve high-energy trauma and can have serious deleterious consequences for patients. One of the rare but devastating sequelae of spinal trauma is spinal cord injury (SCI). SCI often results in irreversible sensory, motor, and autonomic dysfunction, and is associated with high morbidity and mortality.[1] The incidence of SCI is approximately 54 cases per one million people in the United States. Depending on the severity of trauma, the average healthcare costs and living expenses can range from about $350,000 to $1.1 million in the first year.[2] The management of spinal trauma has evolved over time, and with the development of new implants and techniques, more management options are becoming available. Additionally, the development of new classification systems helps guide surgeons with decision making. This chapter will provide background on spinal trauma and highlight the recent developments in management of these conditions.

Epidemiology

The incidence and prevalence of traumatic spine fractures varies based on geographical region, population density, and level of urbanization. In the United States and Canada region, the incidence rate is about 6 patients (95% CI: 3 to 9) per 100,000 people.[3] Cervical fractures are more common (50%) than thoracic (24%) and lumbosacral fractures (24%).[3] The average age at time of spinal injury is 29 years, and males are three times more likely to be injured than females.[3] In patients suffering from blunt trauma, the rate of thoracolumbar (TL) fractures is 7% (95% CI: 3% to 11%).[4] The most common fractures are burst fracture (40%), closely followed by compression fractures (34%).[4] Of the patients who sustain TL trauma, 11% (95% CI: 6% to 17%) also sustained noncontiguous cervical spine fractures. The incidence of neurologic injury depends on fracture morphology and extent of spinal canal narrowing.

Spinal Cord Injury

SCI is rare but devastating sequelae of spinal trauma. There are about 17,700 new cases per year, and an estimated 288,000 patients are currently living with SCI in the United States. The average age of patients with SCI has increased from 29 years in 1970s to 43 years in 2018, and 78% of patients are male.[2] In a longitudinal study evaluating outcomes in 5,500 patients with SCI, 1.4% were ventilated, 6.3% had C1-C4 injury, 23.4% had C5-C8 injury, and 41.2% were paraplegic. Cumulative 25-year survival rate for those with a C1-C4 injury was 40% compared with 70% for those with paraplegia.[5]

Injury to the spinal cord occurs by two different mechanisms. The primary injury occurs at the moment of impact and may involve laceration, compression, distraction, and shearing forces exerted directly to the cord. The secondary injury occurs after the initial trauma and can continue for days to weeks. Disruption of blood supply, cord edema, and activation of inflammatory and apoptotic pathways significantly contributes to the secondary injury mechanism.[6]

Acute management of SCI is critical to optimal recovery. Surgical decompression, and medical management such as use of steroids, and mean arterial pressure ≥ 85 mm Hg are central to management of SCI.[6] The role of neuroprotective agents is of increasing importance. In phase I/II clinical trials, riluzole has shown potential neuroprotective role against glutamate excitotoxicity in SCI patients.[7] Minocycline, a tetracycline antibiotic, and therapeutic hypothermia (32°C to 34°C) have also demonstrated a protective role by reducing CNS energy requirements and inflammatory cell activity. Phase III clinical trials are currently underway for minocycline, riluzole, and granulocyte-colony stimulating factor.[7] Additionally, ganglioside 1 (GM-1), naloxone, thyrotropin-releasing hormones, and tirilazad, a steroid derivative, have also been evaluated in randomized controlled trials for treatment of SCI.[8] For patients with complete SCI, a phase I clinical trial evaluating the use of Neuro-Spinal Scaffold is also underway.[7]

Initial Management of Spinal Trauma

Evaluation and Prehospital Transport

Initial evaluation of trauma patients has been standardized by the American College of Surgeons according to the Advanced Trauma Life Support (ATLS) protocol. An algorithmic approach to rapid initial evaluation of patients includes the well-known ABCDE: airway, breathing, circulation, disability, and exposure. Once the airway, breathing, and circulation are secured, less acute components of injury should be considered, namely assessment of sensory and motor function. Neurogenic shock should be given specific consideration in patients with SCI because loss of sympathetic tone may cause hypotension without tachycardia.

The spine should be immobilized with the patient in a supine, in-line position, usually on a rigid long backboard. The use of rigid cervical collars on a hard-padded backboard with abdominal straps provides the greatest degree of immobilization and can reduce the risk for pressure necrosis.[1] Spinal immobilization follows the common principle of fracture management: immobilizing the joint above and below, namely the head and pelvis.[1]

Stabilization and Resuscitation

The level of SCI determines the acute management of patients in the emergency setting. Early elective intubation of patients with complete lesions above C5 has been recommended even though ventilatory failure generally occurs about 5 days after complete SCI.[8] Furthermore, patients with incomplete injuries and evidence of respiratory failure should also be intubated early because this leads to fewer days on ventilators and shorter intensive care unit (ICU) stays.[8] For those with hemodynamic instability, ICU placement is recommended for continuous monitoring of cardiovascular and respiratory function for the first 7 to 14 days after injury.[9] Hypotension should be managed with aggressive fluid resuscitation and vasopressors to counteract autonomic dysfunction from neurogenic shock. In patients with cervical or thoracic injuries, adrenergic agents with alpha and beta activity are recommended to maintain MAP, while patients with lower thoracic injuries should be managed with alpha adrenergic agents only.[1,8] Guidelines from the American Association of Neurological Surgeons and the Congress of Neurological Surgeons for cervical spine injury management recommend MAP > 85 mm Hg and avoidance of systolic blood pressure < 90 mm Hg for the first 5 to 7 days after SCI, as this may improve spinal cord perfusion and clinical outcomes.[8]

Diagnostic Imaging

Imaging evaluation is important to determine all osseous and soft-tissue injuries in patients with spinal trauma. The Joint Section on Disorders of the Spine and Peripheral Nerve has provided updated imaging recommendations in spinal trauma. In alert, asymptomatic patients without neck pain or distracting injury, with a normal neurological examination and complete range of motion, radiographic evaluation is not recommended and only clinical clearance is necessary.[10] Those with neck tenderness and pain require multidetector CT (MDCT) which has a sensitivity of 97% to 100%.[1,10] Radiographs, flexion-distraction or neutral, have limited utility in the acute setting because of their high false-negative and false-positive rates.[10] Patients with presumed SCI should undergo MRI to determine the location and severity of the injury and to identify the cause of the spinal cord compression (eg, disk protrusion, hematoma development, vascular injury, osseous fragment or associated ligamentous injury).[11] While, there is no specific guideline for the timing of the MRI study, edema increases with time reducing the ability to properly evaluate spinal cord lesions.[11] Furthermore, ligamentous injury of cervical spine may not be clearly identifiable from MDCT images, but MRI images can reliably identify ligamentous injuries.[12] Therefore, it is recommended that patients presenting with a Glasgow Coma Scale of less than 15, midline tenderness with neurological symptoms, should be evaluated with MRI for possible ligamentous injury.[13]

Surgical Timing

Persistent compression of the spinal cord after the primary injury represents a reversible form of secondary injury which, if relieved quickly, can lead to reduced neural tissue damage and improved outcomes. Therefore, the time to decompression can be critical in the management of spinal trauma. Early surgical management of cervical SCI patients (<24 hours from injury) have shown to be associated with better motor function and neurological outcomes.[14] For cervical SCI, the Surgical Timing in Acute Spinal Cord Injury Study (STASCIS) trial demonstrated improved American Spinal Injury Association (ASIA) Impairment Scale (AIS) in patients who underwent decompression surgery within 24 hours of injury. Early decompression is also shown to be more cost effective for patients with motor complete and incomplete SCI.[15] Furthermore, at 12-month follow up, patients who were treated within 24-hour window had a 2.8 times greater odds of improvement AIS compared with those treated after the 24 hours window.[16] Recently, the benefits of surgical decompression with in first 8 hours of injury have been investigated. A study evaluating 70 patients with cervical SCI (35 patients each in early [<8 hours of injury] and late groups) showed that patients in the early group had better AIS grades, higher AIS conversation, and higher Spinal Cord Independence Measures at one year of follow-up.[17] Therefore, for those with cervical SCI, prompt decompressive surgery should be considered.

The benefits of early surgery in TL trauma are not fully clear. The Congress of Neurological Surgeons found that there is insufficient and conflicting evidence regarding the effect of timing of surgical intervention on neurological outcomes in patients with TL trauma.[18] The Congress recommends that early surgery (8 to 72 hours) should be considered as an option for TL trauma.[18] Benefits of early stabilization for TL trauma include improved neurological recovery, faster pulmonary recovery, improved pain control, shorter ICU stay, and shorter hospital stays.[19]

Surgical Management

The Thoracolumbar Injury Classification and Severity (TLICS) score[20] and the Subaxial Cervical Spine Injury Classification and Severity (SLIC) score[21] serve as clinical decision-making tools to assist in management of patients with thoracic and cervical spine injuries, respectively. TLICS and SLIC integrate the same three categories of injury characterization: injury morphology, integrity of the posterior ligamentous complex (PLC) for TLICS or discoligamentous complex (DLC) for SLIC, and neurological status (**Table 1**). Patients with a score of 3 or less should be managed nonsurgically, and a score of 5 or more warrants surgical intervention. A score of 4 can be managed surgically or nonsurgically based on surgeon's decision. However, a recent study showed that patients with a score of 4 that underwent surgery reported less pain.[22]

Ultimately, the objective of surgical intervention is to provide mechanical stability and prevent neurological deterioration. For patients with incomplete neurological injuries and undisrupted PLC, an anterior procedure is recommended.[1] If PLC and DLC are disrupted and there is evidence of nerve root injury, surgeons should consider posterior surgical approach if neurologically intact. If there is neurological injury, a combined AP approach should be adopted. In the case of complete neurological injury, aggressive decompression should be done promptly to prevent potential further neurological damage.[1]

Trauma

Trauma

Table 1

Comparison Between TLICS and SLIC

TLICS Characteristic	TLICS Score	SLIC Characteristic	SLIC Score
Injury morphology		**Injury morphology**	
No abnormality	0	No abnormality	0
Compression	1	Compression	1
Burst component	2	Burst component	2
Translation/rotation	3	Translation/rotation	3
Distraction	4	Distraction	4
Posterior ligamentous complex		**Disco ligamentous complex**	
Intact	0	Intact	0
Indeterminate	2	Indeterminate	1
Disrupted	3	Disrupted	2
Neurological status		**Neurological status**	
Intact	0	Intact	0
Nerve root injury	2	Nerve root injury	1
Complete cord injury	2	Complete cord injury	2
Incomplete cord injury	3	Incomplete cord injury	3
Cauda equina injury	3		

A total score of ≤3, nonsurgical management; 4, surgical or nonsurgical management; ≥5, surgical management

Comparison of Thoracolumbar Injury Classification and Severity (TLICS) score and Subaxial Cervical Spine Injury Classification and Severity (SLIC) score.
Adapted from Lee JY, Vaccaro AR, Lim MR, et al: Thoracolumbar injury classification and severity score: a new paradigm for the treatment of thoracolumbar spine trauma. *J Orthop Sci* 10[6]:671-675. Copyright 2005, with permission from Elsevier. with data from, Vaccaro AR, Koerner JD, Radcliff KE, et al: AOSpine subaxial cervical spine injury classification system. *Eur Spine* 2016;25(7):2173-2184.

Surgical Techniques

Minimally invasive spine surgery (MISS) techniques are valuable treatment modalities for the management of spine trauma. MISS techniques are based on the preservation of soft tissue, while maintaining the principles of spine decompression, stabilization, and deformity correction. Minimizing the physiologic burden associated with open procedures is one of the fundamental benefits of MISS. MISS approach has decreased blood loss and shorter surgical times and length of stay, when compared with traditional open procedures.[23] In spine trauma, MISS has largely been limited to the thoracic and lumbar spine. Minimally invasive techniques in the subaxial cervical spine are usually focused on surgical fixation utilizing anterior fixation techniques, thereby avoiding posterior dissection of paraspinal musculature. Minimally invasive lumbopelvic fixation (LPF) techniques have been shown to provide adequate biomechanical stability and appropriate fracture reduction for the management of patients with unstable sacral fractures.[24]

One controversy is the need for arthrodesis in the treatment of spine fractures. Nonfusion methods are effective in achieving stability and sagittal alignment, even after removal of implants. No difference is shown between fusion and nonfusion groups in terms of instrumentation failure, radiological parameters, and pain scores.[25]

Postoperative Management

Improved vigilance is essential for postsurgical spine trauma patients. Surgical intervention was found to be an independent predictor of adverse events, such as pneumonia and delirium. A study analyzing 390 patients with thoracolumbar trauma reported that adverse events were 6.2 times more likely to occur in patients who underwent surgery. Additionally, 75% of patients who presented with a neurologic deficit after spine trauma developed an adverse event compared with 25% of patients with similar injuries without neurological involvement.[26] Neurological status, implant failures, and surgical site infections are they key outcome metrics.[27] Depending on the level and severity of SCI, ICU stay may be required for patients postoperatively. Physical therapy and early mobilization play a critical role in recovery from the surgery as well as SCI. Plain radiographs at the time of discharge are recommended to assess spine stability in follow-up visits.

Complications

The complications after surgical intervention can determine the long-term outcome from spine trauma. In a study evaluating long-term (2.6 years) postoperative complications in patients with subaxial cervical spine fractures, 11% of patients had neck stiffness, 5% had severe neck pain, 6% reported hoarseness, and 9% had dysphagia. Of note, 98% of the patients had a successful fusion based on evaluation of CT scan.[28] More than 50% of patients with SCI experience at least one complication during their initial hospitalization. Age, extent of neurologic injury, mechanism of injury, and comorbidities increase the rate of complications.[29] Bowel and bladder incontinence can be observed depending on injury severity. Furthermore, for those immobilized due to their injury, pressure sores, adequate nutrition, and muscle atrophy can also present challenges.

Cervical Injuries

In the cervical spine, ligaments and facet joint capsules are critical in providing stability. Comparatively, in the thoracic and lumbar spine, bony articulations are responsible for stability. As a result, ligamentous distraction injury at the craniocervical junction and subaxial cervical spine can be unstable and associated with significant morbidity if missed.[12] Urgent decompression is generally recommended for cervical spine injury with evidence of SCI.

Occipitocervical Dissociation

Occipitocervical dissociation is reported in ~1% of patients that present with cervical spinal trauma. The true incidence of this injury may be higher, as improved hemodynamic and respiratory instability management as well as the widespread use of cervical stabilization allows for a greater proportion of patients with this injury to survive through prehospital transport.[30] Injuries to upper cervical spine are very difficult to detect with plain radiographs due to parallax effect at the occipitocervical junction and obscuration by the mastoid air cells. As a result, CT is recommended for identifying these injuries.[10,12]

Occipitocervical dissociation can be classified into three distinct morphologies. As part of the classification, the occipital condyles can be displaced anteriorly or posteriorly or remain in line but at a distance from the atlantoid facets[30]. Analysis of cervical radiographs have helped determine measures of instability such as Powers' ratio, condyle to C1 interval, basion-dens interval (BDI), and basion-axial interval (BAI).[30] A BDI of 10 mm in adults and 12 mm in pediatric patients is considered abnormal. BAI is abnormal if the anterior displacement is greater than 12 mm or posterior displacement is greater than 4 mm between the basion and posterior C2 line. Power's ratio compares measurements relating the skull base to C1 and is typically <0.9. When Power's ratio exceeds 1, occipitocervical dissociation should be suspected.[30]

Traction is sometimes used to realign type I and type III injuries; however, its use is controversial, as there can be neurological complication in 10% of traction cases. Craniocervical fixation by posterior occipitocervical fusion is the treatment of choice in most cases of traumatic occipitocervical dissociation.[30] If unable to perform surgery, patient should be stabilized using a rigid cervical collar or halo immobilization.

Atlas Fractures

Atlas fractures account for 2% to 13% of injuries of the cervical spine and 1% to 2% of all spinal injuries. In atlas fractures, isolated fractures involving the ring are highly unlikely, but a ring disruption is common.[31] Given that this fracture generally increases area for the spinal cord, neurologic injury is rare. Atlas fractures are classified into three types. Type I: isolated arch fractures, type II: fracture of the posterior and anterior arch, including bilateral anterior and posterior arch fractures also known as Jefferson burst fracture (**Figure 1**), and type III: unilateral lateral mass fractures.[32] The stability of C1 fractures depends on the integrity of the transverse atlantal ligament (TAL) which can be assessed with MRI.[32] Type I TAL injuries are those in which the TAL was injured without atlas fractures, and type II TAL injuries include avulsion fractures of atlas at the insertion of TAL.[32] Type I injuries should get early surgical fixation because of inherent instability; external immobilization is recommended for type II injuries.[32]

For atlas fractures, conservative management is generally recommended in the absence of gross spinal

Trauma

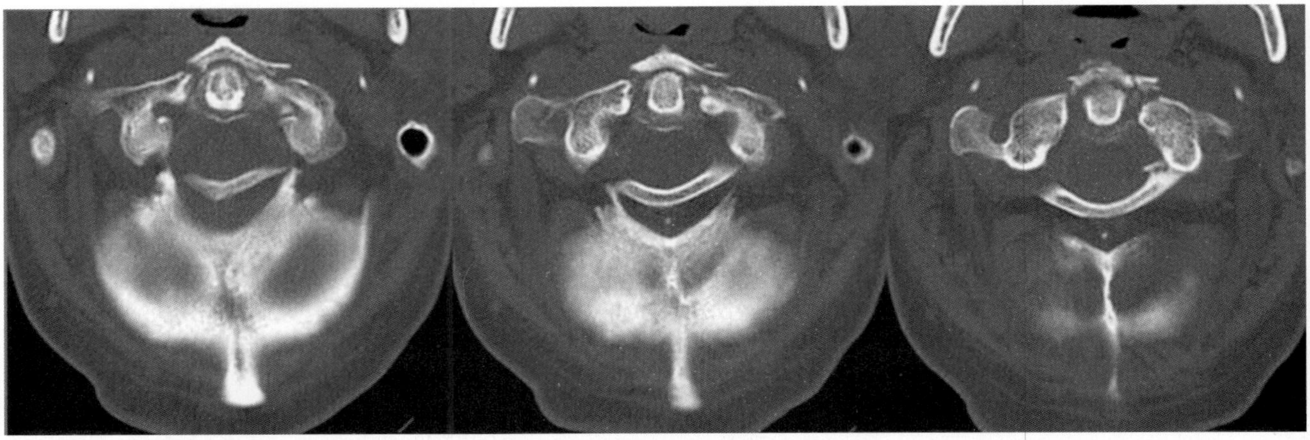

Figure 1 Axial C-Spine CT scan, Type II Atlas fractures, also known as Jefferson burst fracture, involving fractures of anterior and posterior arch.

instability. Nondisplaced isolated anterior or posterior arch fracture and lateral mass fracture (type I and III) are treated with external immobilization[32] The treatment plan for type II fracture is based on integrity of the TAL. Type II fractures with intact TAL are managed nonsurgically whereas those with ligamentous disruption can be treated with rigid immobilization or surgical stabilization and fusion.[32]

Odontoid Fractures

Odontoid fractures make up 9% to 15% of cervical spine fractures in adults. These injuries occur in a bimodal distribution and can be associated with severe morbidity and mortality. High-energy trauma episode in the younger population and trivial falls in elderly can cause odontoid fractures.[33] Odontoid fractures are classified into three subtypes. Type 1: fracture at the tip of dens, type II: fracture at the base of the dense that does not extend into the vertebral body or the C1-C2 articulation, and type III: fracture through the body of C2.[34]

Young patients without any risk factors for nonunion, minimal to no displacement, and no neurologic findings can be treated conservatively. High rates of stable union are common with conservative treatment at the expense of increased complications.[34] There is no significant difference in outcomes and need for revision surgery when comparing cervical orthosis (24%) to halo brace (17%).[35] For patients older than 65 years, there is an increased rate of nonunion, morbidity, and mortality when compared with a younger population.[34] Additionally, the halo vest is associated with significant morbidity in this population, especially increasing the risk of pulmonary complications.[36] For elderly, treatment for type I and type III fractures include a hard cervical orthosis. In cases where type III fracture is displaced greater than 5 mm, surgical stabilization is recommended to control vertical instability.[36] The treatment algorithm for type II fractures, however, is controversial and varies based on the patient. In isolated type II fractures, factors which promote nonunion include greater than 5 mm of displacement, 11° of angulation, or ≥2 mm of fracture gap. Surgery is warranted when these factors are present or if there is neurological involvement.[36] Octogenarians were shown to have adequate C1-C2 fusion with acceptably low mortality rate after surgical management of type II odontoid fractures.[37]

Surgical options for odontoid fractures options include a posterior C1-C2 fusion or direct anterior approach for osteosynthesis. The direct anterior approach may be more beneficial in younger patients because it conserves the range of motion at the atlantoaxial joint and reduces the risk of fracture displacement that occurs when placing the patient prone for the posterior approach. Because of the technical difficulty of the anterior procedure, a posterior approach is warranted in patients who display a barrel chest, have reverse obliquity, or have comminuted fractures.[38]

Traumatic Spondylolisthesis of Axis Vertebra (Hangman Fracture)

Traumatic spondylolisthesis of axis vertebra, also known as a hangman fracture, results from a high-energy traumatic episode and accounts for 5% of all cervical spine injuries.[39] Most hangman fractures can be treated nonsurgically, except for the higher grade injuries or injuries which fail conservative treatment after 3 months. Type I fractures are normally stable and can be treated with hard collar immobilization.[39] Most type II injuries can be managed with closed reduction and

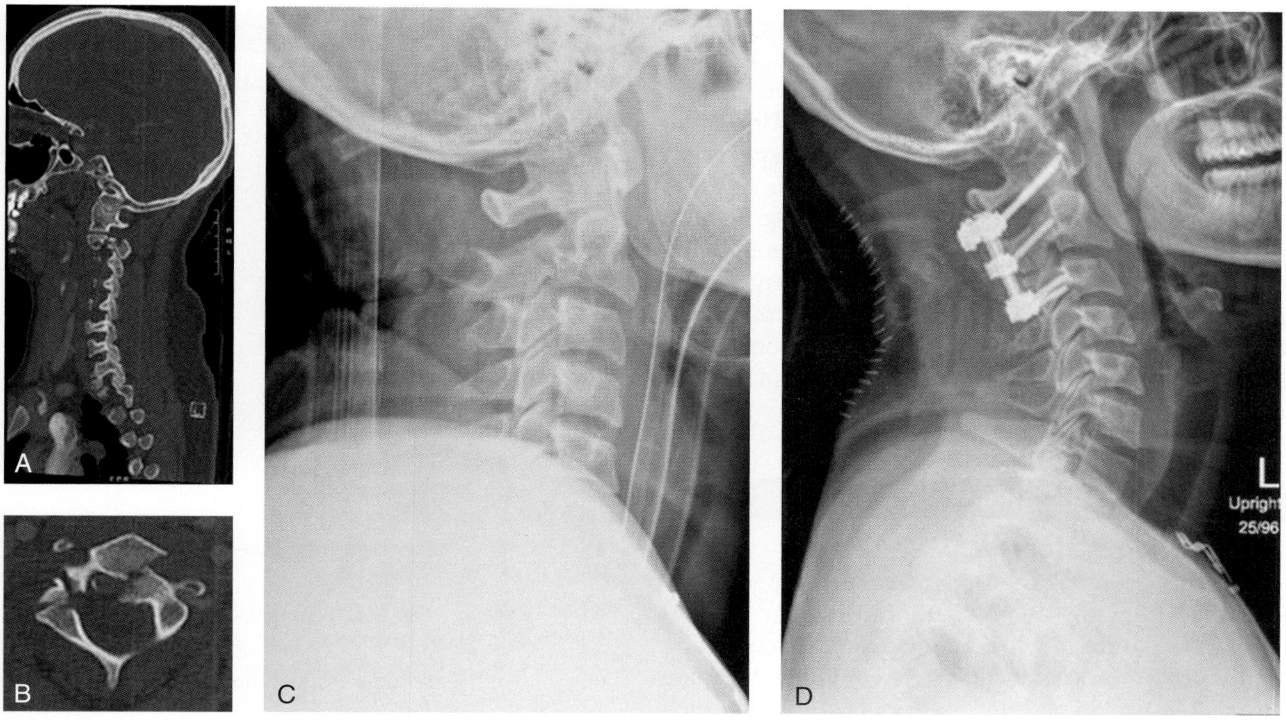

Figure 2 **A**, Sagittal CT; **B**, axial CT; **C**, preoperative lateral cervical radiograph; **D**, postoperative lateral cervical radiograph of axis hangman fracture.

a halo thoracic brace, except when there is substantial angulation, involvement of C2-C3 disk, or difficulty maintaining reduction. In these patients, if a C2 pedicle screw placement is possible, an isolated C2-C3 fusion should be performed. If pedicle screw placement is not practical, alternative options include a C2-C3 anterior cervical diskectomy and fusion (ACDF) or a C1-C3 posterior fusion. All type III fractures (**Figure 2**) require surgery and patients should be treated with a C1-C3 or C2-C3 fusion.[40]

Subaxial Cervical Spine Injuries

Subaxial injuries consist of cervical spine trauma from C3 to C7 with more than 50% of the cervical spine injuries located between C5 to C7.[41] The AOSpine subaxial spine classification system accounts for morphological features of the fracture, facet involvement, neurologic status, and case-specific modifiers.[42] It divides cervical injuries into four types: type A, compression; type B, tension band; type C, translation; and type F, facet[42] (**Figure 3**).

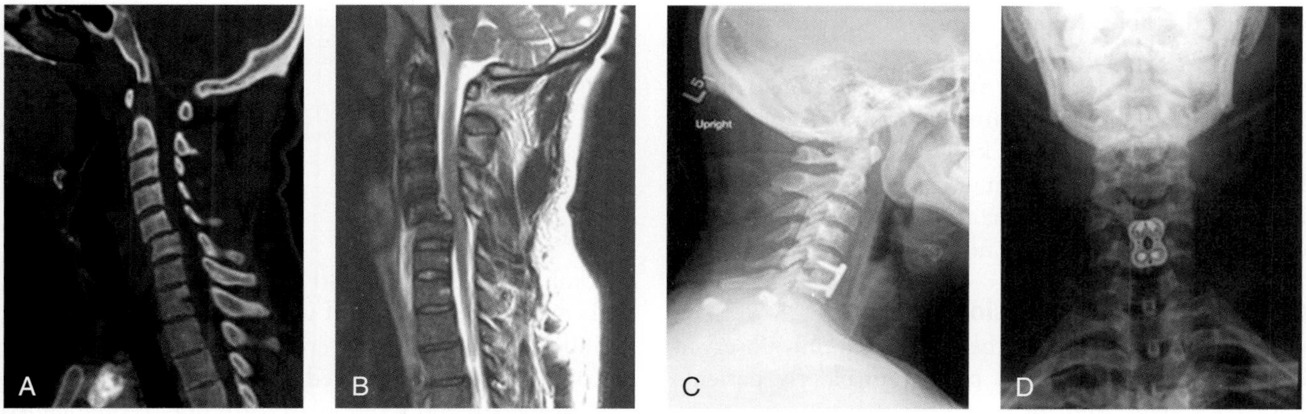

Figure 3 **A**, Sagittal CT; **B**, sagittal MRI; **C**, postoperative lateral cervical radiograph; **D**, postoperative AP radiograph of C5-C6 fracture-dislocation.

For subaxial spine injuries, urgent decompression is recommended if there is a concomitant SCI. In some cases, the decompression can be performed closed, delaying the need for surgical intervention. Under the AOSpine subaxial classification system, all type B and type C injuries require surgical intervention, whereas more severe and unstable type A injuries also require surgery.[42] Patients who have coexisting stiffening bone disease with a cervical fracture should undergo additional advanced imaging to find occult fractures and MRI to rule out epidural hematomas. Most commonly, these patients have an unstable fracture and require surgery.[41]

Thoracolumbar Injuries

Classification System

The TLICS score was proposed to develop a treatment algorithm for common thoracolumbar injuries and has been utilized when making clinical decisions.[20] Another common classification system is the AOSpine Thoracolumbar Spine Injury score (TL AOSIS) which focuses on describing the fracture characteristics.[43] The classification is based on three parameters: morphologic classification of the fracture, neurological status, and clinical modifiers. Three morphologic types are identified: type A, compression fractures, type B, tension band failure, and type C, dislocation or displacement[43] (**Table 2**). Based on the points, injuries with a TL AOSIS of <3 are managed nonsurgically and those with a score of >5 undergo surgical intervention. Injuries with a TL AOSIS of 4 or 5 can be managed surgically or nonsurgically.[43]

Compression Fractures

Compression fractures typically comprise of one vertebral level, do not have neurologic involvement, and are considered stable. Management options include early ambulation without bracing treatment, or orthosis, which may be beneficial in avoiding flexion load at the fracture site.[44] Surgical treatment should be considered when there is progressive kyphosis greater than 30°, loss of vertebral body height greater than 50%, increase in fracture angle greater than 10°, or presence of burdensome back pain despite nonsurgical management.[45]

Osteoporotic Compression Fractures

Compression fractures are the most commonly observed osteoporotic fractures and present in elderly patients with back pain after an insignificant traumatic event. Nonsurgical treatment should be employed in patients, encompassing bracing treatment, oral pain medication, and early mobilization.[44] If warranted, surgical options include kyphoplasty and vertebroplasty. However, due to complications, and mixed evidence on their efficacy, vertebroplasty and kyphoplasty are not recommended as an initial treatment modality.[45]

Table 2

AOSpine Thoracolumbar Spine Injury Classification System

Classification	Description	Points
Morphology		
Type-A	*Compression fractures*	
A0	No injury/process fracture	0
A1	Wedge/impaction	1
A2	Split/pincer type	2
A3	Incomplete burst	3
A4	Complete burst	5
Type B	*Tension band injuries*	
B1	Posterior transosseous disruption	5
B2	Posterior ligamentous disruption	6
B3	Anterior ligamentous disruption	7
Type C	*Translation injuries*	
C	Translation/displacement injuries	8
Neurological status		
N0	Intact	0
N1	Transient deficit	1
N2	Signs of radiculopathy	2
N3	Incomplete spinal cord injury	4
N4	Complete spinal cord injury	4
NX	Cannot be examined	3
Case-specific modifiers		
M1	Indeterminate injury to tension band	1
M2	Patient-specific comorbidity	0

The Thoracolumbar AOSpine Injury score (TL AOSIS) and classification system.

Data from Vaccaro AR, Oner C, Kepler CK, Dvorak M, et al: AOSpine thoracolumbar spine injury classification system: fracture description, neurological status, and key modifiers. *Spine* 2013;38(23):2028-2037.

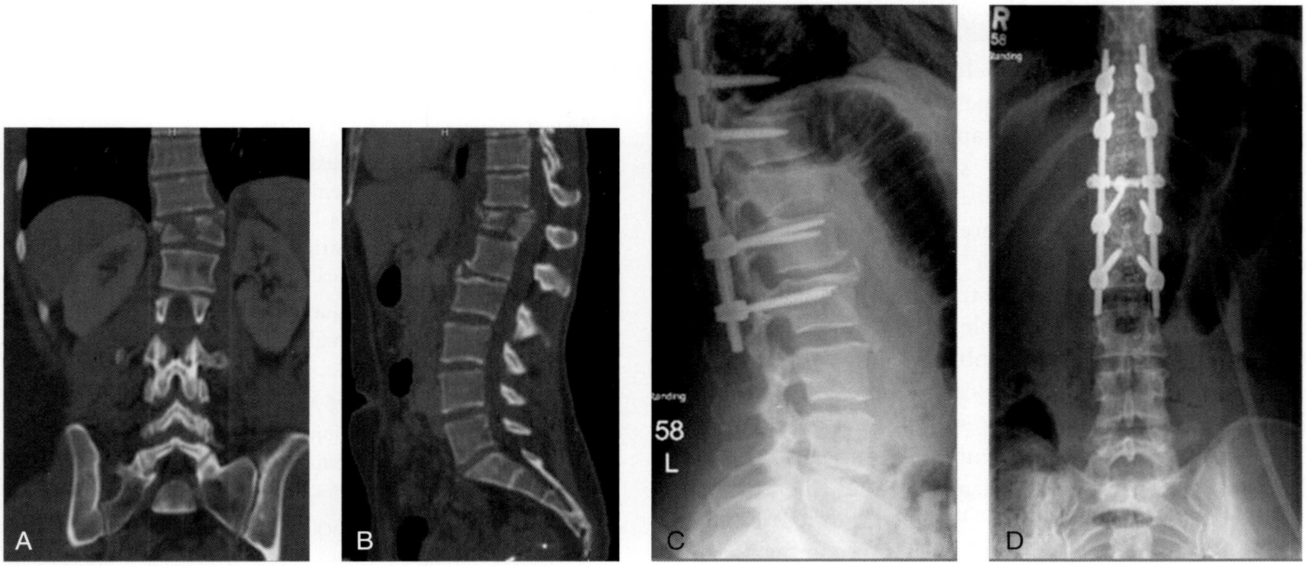

Figure 4 **A**, Coronal CT; **B**, sagittal CT; **C**, postoperative lateral thoracolumbar radiograph; **D**, postoperative AP thoracolumbar radiograph of a T12 burst fracture.

Burst Fractures Without Neurologic Injury

Options for burst fractures (**Figure 4**) without neurological injury include bed rest, immobilization with bracing treatment, and surgery with or without decompression. For burst fractures with less than 35° of kyphosis and without PLC involvement, early ambulation provides superior pain relief and improved functional outcomes at one-year follow-up. Conversely, burst fractures with PLC involvement are unstable and require surgical management. PLC compromise should be suspected in patients with vertebral compression >50%, angulation >25°, neurologic deficits, and positive MRI findings.[46]

Flexion-Distraction Injuries

Flexion-distraction injuries, also known as chance fractures, occur when the middle and posterior columns fail under tension, the anterior column fails under compression, and the PLC is disrupted. Isolated bony chance fracture can be treated nonsurgically with a hyperextension cast or orthosis for 3 months. However, comparative studies report worsening kyphosis, pain, and functional outcomes compared with surgery. Neurologically intact patients, polytrauma, or patients who are unable to tolerate external immobilization are candidates for MISS without fusion.[47]

Fractures With Incomplete Neurologic Injuries

The presence of incomplete neurological deficit in the context of trauma warrants surgical intervention; however, optimal surgical management is still controversial. Studies display the need for anterior column support in cases of extensive damage, kyphosis >30°, or fracture displacement of ≥2 mm.[45] Consideration should be given to the load-sharing system when deciding on the implementation of anterior support in addition to posterior fixation. Load-sharing score greater than 6 requires posterior fixation or combined anterior and posterior approach. Comparatively, a load-sharing score of less than 6 can be treated with short segment posterior fixation only.[48]

Fracture-Dislocations

Fracture-dislocations occur through a high-energy mechanism and can present with incomplete SCI. Patients with incomplete SCI benefit from early decompression, fracture reduction, and fusion with instrumentation. A posterior only approach is an effective option in absence of severe vertebral body comminution, extension of fragments into the spinal canal, or ventral cord compression. However, in these scenarios, additional direct anterior decompression with anterior column support may be required.[45]

Fractures of the Ankylosed Spine

Spinal fractures are four times as common in patients with ankylosing spondylitis. In ankylosed spine, progressively worsening ossification of the disks and ligaments of the spine reduce segmental mobility, increasing the risk of fractures. In these diseases, the fractures often involve all three columns and act in a similar manner to long bone fractures.[49]

Sacral Fractures

Sacral fractures are relatively rare and most (45%) occur with a concomitant pelvic ring injury. For suspected sacral fractures, inlet and outlet pelvic ring views are recommended, but CT scan is required because radiographs miss up to 50% of sacral fracture.[50] For management of sacral fracture, there is lack of rigorous clinical evidence; as a result, treatment is determined on a case-by-case basis. The treatment should take into account (1) associated stable or unstable pelvic ring fracture, (2) associated lumbosacral facet injury, (3) associated lumbosacral dislocation, and (4) neurologic injury and cauda equina or spinal cord compression. The potential benefits of neural decompression, stabilization, and patient mobilization should be carefully weighed against the risks.[50] For sacral fracture stabilization, minimally invasive LPF is a recommended to decrease blood loss. It is shown to maintain adequate reduction in follow-up radiographs.[24]

Summary

Traumatic spine injuries are common and can result in irreversible sensory, motor, or autonomic dysfunction. These injuries can have a devastating impact on the functional abilities of patients. SCI comprises compression, distraction, and shearing forces exerted directly on the spinal cord. Evaluation and management of these injuries includes a thorough physical examination, radiographs, and advanced imaging. Surgical or nonsurgical stabilization from early stage plays an important role in the long-term outcomes of these injuries. Fracture-specific classification systems such as the thoracolumbar injury classification and severity score are valuable for clinical decision making and are shown to have prognostic value.

Key Study Points

- Spinal cord injuries of the cervical and thoracolumbar region are associated with significant morbidity and mortality.
- Stabilization and treatment of these injuries in the acute setting are important and impact the long-term functional outcome of patient.
- Classification systems for fracture of the cervical and thoracolumbar region are important in determining the optimal management of patients with traumatic injuries.
- Both surgical and nonsurgical treatments play an important role in the stabilization and optimization of traumatic spine fractures.

Annotated References

1. Yue JK, Winkler EA, Rick JW, et al: Update on critical care for acute spinal cord injury in the setting of polytrauma. *Neurosurg Focus* 2017;43(5):E19.

   This study is a comprehensive review of the latest guidelines for the management of spinal cordy injury in patients with poly trauma. They discuss key management decisions such as stabilization, imaging, and surgical decisions. Level of evidence: V.

2. National Spinal Cord Injury Statistical Center: *Facts and Figures at a Glance*. Birmingham, AL, University of Alabama at Birmingham, 2018.

   Database from University of Alabama provides the most up-to-date figures on spinal cord injury. This is a valuable resource for the latest statistics on spinal cord injury and includes information on cost and outcomes. Level of evidence: III.

3. Kumar R, Lim J, Mekary RA, et al: Traumatic spinal injury: Global epidemiology and worldwide volume. *World Neurosurg* 2018;113:e345-e363.

   This is an excellent meta-analysis that assess the epidemiology, patient characteristics, and fracture types of traumatic spinal fractures across all World Health Organization regions and income groups. Level of evidence: III.

4. Katsuura Y, Osborn JM, Cason GW: The epidemiology of thoracolumbar trauma: A meta-analysis. *J Orthop* 2016;13(4):383-388.

   This is a meta-analysis discussing the rate of thoracolumbar fractures after blunt trauma. Provides an epidmiological description of thoracolumbar trauma. Level of evidence: III.

5. Savic G, DeVivo MJ, Frankel HL, et al: Long-term survival after traumatic spinal cord injury: A 70-year British study. *Spinal Cord* 2017;55(7):651-658.

   The longitudinal study spans 70 years and evaluates long-term survival in patients suffering from spinal cord injury. The study also identifies risk factors associated with mortality and estimates current life expectancy based on injury severity. Level of evidence: III.

6. Ahuja CS, Nori S, Tetreault L, et al: Traumatic spinal cord injury—repair and regeneration. *Neurosurgery* 2017;80(3S):S9-S22.

   This is a review paper that discusses the management of spinal cord injury while stressing the importance of early care. Medical as well as surgical therapies are discussed. Level of evidence: V.

7. Badhiwala JH, Ahuja CS, Fehlings MG: Time is spine: A review of translational advances in spinal cord injury. *J Neurosurg Spine* 2018;30(1):1-18.

   This review discuss new developments in the management of spinal cord injury including surgical decompression, neuroprotective agents, and clinical management. New translational therapies such as riluzole, minocycline, Neuro-Spinal Scaffold, and fibroblast growth factors are also discussed. Level of evidence: V.

8. Rogers WK, Todd M: Acute spinal cord injury. *Best Pract Res Clin Anaesthesiol* 2016;30(1):27-39.

This comprehensive review is critical to understanding the initial management of the spinal cord injuries in the trauma bay. They discuss surgical and nonsurgical interventions for all levels of spinal cord injuries. Level of evidence: V.

9. Wilson JR, Forgione N, Fehlings MG: Emerging therapies for acute traumatic spinal cord injury. *CMAJ (Can Med Assoc J)* 2013;185(6):485-492.
10. Shah LM, Ross JS: Imaging of spine trauma. *Neurosurgery* 2016;79(5):626-642.

Imaging is critical to effective management of spinal trauma. This review discusses the latest guidelines on imaging based on region of spinal trauma (cervical, thoracic, or lumbosacral). It also highlights the differences between imaging modalities.

11. Kumar Y, Hayashi D: Role of magnetic resonance imaging in acute spinal trauma: A pictorial review. *BMC Musculoskelet Disord* 2016;17:310.

Understanding and evaluating MRI is an important part of evaluation of spinal trauma. This study provides a guide for utilizing MRI in spinal trauma and uses images to help the reader better understand and analyze images. Level of evidence: V.

12. Chilvers G, Janjua U, Choudhary S: Blunt cervical spine injury in adult polytrauma: Incidence, injury patterns and predictors of significant ligament injury on CT. *Clin Radiol* 2017;72(11):907-914.

This retrospective study evaluates cervical spine trauma and determines the ideal imaging modalities for identify bony and ligamentous injury in the cervical spine. Level of evidence: III.

13. Duane TM, Young AJ, Vanguri P, et al: Defining the cervical spine clearance algorithm: A single-institution prospective study of more than 9,000 patients. *J Trauma Acute Care Surg* 2016;81(3):541-547.

The study developed an evidence-based algorithm for management of cervical spine trauma in the trauma setting with a focus on appropriate cervical spine clearance, optimal use of imaging, and appropriate spine consultations. Level of evidence: III.

14. Fehlings MG, Tetreault LA, Wilson JR, et al: A clinical practice guideline for the management of patients with acute spinal cord injury and central cord syndrome: Recommendations on the timing (</=24 hours versus >24 hours) of decompressive surgery. *Global Spine J* 2017;7(3 suppl):195S-202S.

Comprehensive review and expert opinion was used to establish these clinical guidelines for the management of spinal cord injury. These guidelines identify the key management questions for patients with spinal cord injuries and present clear and definitive recommendations. Level of evidence: V.

15. Furlan JC, Craven BC, Massicotte EM, Fehlings MG: Early versus delayed surgical decompression of spinal cord after traumatic cervical spinal cord injury: A cost-utility analysis. *World Neurosurg* 2016;88:166-174.

This study utilized the same population as the STASCIS trial to determine if earlier cervical spine surgery was more cost effective than later surgery. They showed that early decompression was more cost effective than delayed surgical decompression. Level of evidence: II.

16. Wilson JR, Tetreault LA, Kwon BK, et al: Timing of decompression in patients with acute spinal cord injury: A systematic review. *Global Spine J* 2017;7(3 Suppl):95S-115S.

The systematic review synthesizes the studies published to date regarding the timing of decompression surgery in patients with cervical spinal cord injury. This review is an important contribution to the discussion of early surgical intervention. Level of evidence: II.

17. Grassner L, Wutte C, Klein B, et al: Early decompression (< 8 h) after traumatic cervical spinal cord injury improves functional outcome as assessed by spinal cord independence measure after one year. *J Neurotrauma* 2016;33(18):1658-1666.

This retrospective review of 70 patients evaluates one-year outcomes of patients who underwent early (< 8 hours of injury) and late decompression after a spinal cord injury. Both the AIS and SCIM scales were used to determine outcome at one year. Level of evidence: III.

18. Eichholz KM, Rabb CH, Anderson PA, et al: Congress of neurological surgeons systematic review and evidence-based guidelines on the evaluation and treatment of patients with thoracolumbar spine trauma: Timing of surgical intervention. *Neurosurgery* 2019;84(1):E53-E55.

This study combines literature review with expert opinion to look at the available evidence for surgical timing of thoracolumbar trauma. They point out that the evidence for surgical timing for TL trauma is mixed with a broad range of definitions of "early" surgery (8 to 72 hours). Level of evidence: V.

19. O'Boynick CP, Kurd MF, Darden BV, Vaccaro AR, Fehlings MG: Timing of surgery in thoracolumbar trauma: Is early intervention safe?. *Neurosurg Focus* 2014;37(1):E7.
20. Lee JY, Vaccaro AR, Lim MR, et al: Thoracolumbar injury classification and severity score: A new paradigm for the treatment of thoracolumbar spine trauma. *J Orthop Sci* 2005;10(6):671-675.
21. Vaccaro AR, Hulbert RJ, Patel AA, et al: The subaxial cervical spine injury classification system: A novel approach to recognize the importance of morphology, neurology, and integrity of the disco-ligamentous complex. *Spine* 2007;32(21):2365-2374.
22. Mohamadi A, Googanian A, Ahmadi A, Kamali A: Comparison of surgical or nonsurgical treatment outcomes in patients with thoracolumbar fracture with score 4 of TLICS: A randomized, single-blind, and single-central clinical trial. *Medicine (Baltim)* 2018;97(6):e9842.

This randomized, single-blind, clinical trial aimed to compare the surgical and nonsurgical treatment of patients with TLICS score of 4. Outcomes measures assessed in the study included quality of life metrics. Level of evidence: I.

23. Tian F, Tu L-Y, Gu W-F, et al: Percutaneous versus open pedicle screw instrumentation in treatment of thoracic and lumbar spine fractures: A systematic review and meta-analysis. *Medicine* 2018;97(41):e12535.

The systematic review evaluates all available evidence for both percutaneous and open pedicle screw fixation in TL trauma. They find that percutaneous approach can replace open surgery and has decreased complications. Level of evidence: III.

24. Jazini E, Weir T, Nwodim E, et al: Outcomes of lumbopelvic fixation in the treatment of complex sacral fractures using minimally invasive surgical techniques. *Spine J* 2017;17(9):1238-1246.

The retrospective cohort study from a level 1 trauma center evaluated the use of minimally invasive lumbopelvic fixation for complex sacral fracture. They find adequate reduction, stabilization, and maintenance of correction using the minimally invasive LPF technique. Level of evidence: III.

25. Diniz JM, Botelho RV: Is fusion necessary for thoracolumbar burst fracture treated with spinal fixation? A systematic review and meta-analysis. *J Neurosurg: Spine SPI* 2017;27(5):584-592.

The systematic review evaluated the available evidence to determine that arthrodesis is not significant to maintain radiographic correction in TL trauma patients. Arthrodesis was associated with increased surgical time and higher intraoperative bleeding with no improvement in radiological parameters. Level of evidence: II.

26. Glennie RA, Ailon T, Yang K, et al: Incidence, impact, and risk factors of adverse events in thoracic and lumbar spine fractures: An ambispective cohort analysis of 390 patients. *Spine J* 2015;15(4):629-637.

27. Sadiqi S, Verlaan J-J, Mechteld Lehr A, et al: Universal disease-specific outcome instruments for spine trauma: A global perspective on relevant parameters to evaluate clinical and functional outcomes of thoracic and lumbar spine trauma patients. *Eur Spine J* 2017;26(5):1541-1549.

The study surveyed spine surgeons across the world to identify key metrics that they evaluate postoperatively in trauma patients. These metrics are thought to be important to the clinical and functional outcomes of patients. Level of evidence: V.

28. Fredo HL, Rizvi SA, Rezai M, et al: Complications and long-term outcomes after open surgery for traumatic subaxial cervical spine fractures: A consecutive series of 303 patients. *BMC Surg* 2016;16(1):56.

Long-term outcomes (2.6 years) of patients who underwent surgery for subaxial cervical spine trauma were evaluated in this study. The study population is interesting because 43% had spinal cord injury. The study also discussed outcomes with respect to AIS scale. Level of evidence: III.

29. Stricsek G, Ghobrial G, Wilson J, Theofanis T, Harrop JS: Complications in the management of patients with spine trauma. *Neurosurg Clin N Am* 2017;28(1):147-155.

This is a comprehensive study that reviews the complications commonly observed in patients with spinal cord injury. The review breaks down the complications into surgical and medical. They review different types of medical complications. Level of evidence: V.

30. Kasliwal MK, Fontes RB, Traynelis VC: Occipitocervical dissociation-incidence, evaluation, and treatment. *Curr Rev Musculoskelet Med* 2016;9(3):247-254.

This review article on occipitocervical dissociation discusses the epidemiology, clinical evaluation, initial stabilization, and management of patients. The article is comprehensive in its discussion of the management of occipitocervical injuries. Level of evidence: V.

31. Mead LB II, Millhouse PW, Krystal J, Vaccaro AR: C1 fractures: A review of diagnoses, management options, and outcomes. *Curr Rev Musculoskelet Med* 2016;9(3):255-262.

This review articles discusses the incidence, clinical evaluation, and management of patients with C1 fractures. Both surgical and nonsurgical management options are discussed in the article. Level of evidence: V.

32. Smith RM, Bhandutia AK, Jauregui JJ, Shasti M, Ludwig SC: Atlas fractures: Diagnosis, current treatment recommendations, and implications for elderly patients. *Clin Spine Surg* 2018;31(7):278-284.

This review discusses the management of atlas fractures with an emphasis on the elderly population. The management for the general population is also discussed. Level of evidence: V.

33. Sime D, Pitt V, Pattuwage L, Tee J, Liew S, Gruen R: Nonsurgical interventions for the management of type 2 dens fractures: A systematic review. *ANZ J Surg* 2013;84(5):320-325.

34. Hsu WK, Anderson PA: Odontoid fractures: Update on management. *J Am Acad Orthop Surg* 2010;18(7):383-394.

35. Waqar M, Van-Popta D, Barone DG, Sarsam Z: External immobilization of odontoid fractures: A systematic review to compare the halo and hard collar. *World Neurosurgery* 2017;97:513-517.

This systematic review evaluates the optimal management of odontoid fracture. The authors focus on the outcomes with halo and hard collar and evaluate the two techniques based on their respective failure and malunion rates. Level of evidence: IV.

36. Wagner SC, Schroeder GD, Kepler CK, et al: Controversies in the management of geriatric odontoid fractures. *J Orthop Trauma* 2017;31(suppl 4):S44-S48.

The study reviews literature to evaluate the optimal management of type II odontoid fractures in the elderly population. It discusses the factors to consider for surgical management and highlights surgical techniques to consider. Level of evidence: V.

37. Clark S, Nash A, Shasti M, et al: Mortality rates after posterior C1-2 fusion for displaced type II odontoid fractures in octogenarians. *Spine* 2018;43(18):E1077-E1081.

Octogenarians with type II odontoid fractures underwent surgical management and were shown to have acceptably low 30-day and 1-year mortality rates. Interestingly, this study showed that dysphagia was an independent risk factor for one-year mortality. Level of evidence: III.

38. Joaquim AF, Patel AA: Surgical treatment of type II odontoid fractures: Anterior odontoid screw fixation or posterior cervical instrumented fusion?. *Neurosurg Focus* 2015;38(4):E11.

39. Schleicher P, Scholz M, Pingel A, Kandziora F: Traumatic spondylolisthesis of the Axis vertebra in adults. *Global Spine J* 2015;5(4):346-358.

40. Al-Mahfoudh R, Beagrie C, Woolley E, et al: Management of typical and atypical hangman's fractures. *Glob Spine J* 2016;6(3):248-256.

This retrospective study of prospectively maintained database evaluates the outcomes with traumatic spondylolisthesis of the axis vertebrae. This study evaluated outcomes with rigid collar and halo immobilization. Level of evidence: III.

41. Joaquim AF, Patel AA: Subaxial cervical spine trauma: Evaluation and surgical decision-making. *Global Spine J* 2014;4(1):63-70.

42. Vaccaro AR, Koerner JD, Radcliff KE, et al: AOSpine subaxial cervical spine injury classification system. *Eur Spine J* 2016;25(7):2173-2184.

Expert consensus was used to help establish the classification system for subaxial cervical spine injury. The classification system is recommended to be used for surgical decisions as well as to establish uniformity across research on these injuries. Level of evidence: IV.

43. Vaccaro AR, Schroeder GD, Kepler CK, et al: The surgical algorithm for the AOSpine thoracolumbar spine injury classification system. *Eur Spine J* 2016;25(4):1087-1094.

This consensus paper establishes the optimal treatment pathway for patients with thoracolumbar spine trauma. The thoracolumbar AOSpine spine injury score (TL AOSIS) is proposed as a method for clinical decision making. Level of evidence: V.

44. Aebi M: Classification of thoracolumbar fractures and dislocations. *Eur Spine J* 2010;19(suppl 1):S2-S7.

45. Kim BG, Dan JM, Shin DE: Treatment of thoracolumbar fracture. *Asian Spine J* 2015;9(1):133-146.

46. Aras EL, Bunger C, Hansen ES, Søgaard R: Cost-effectiveness of surgical versus conservative treatment for thoracolumbar burst fractures. *Spine* 2016;41(4):337-343.

This study evaluates the total cost of managing TL burst fracture through either conservative or surgical methods. They study the cost of 85 patients over a 2-year span and find that, compared to conservative management, surgical management is not cost effective. Level of evidence: III.

47. Chu JK, Rindler RS, Pradilla G, Rodts GE, Ahmad FU: Percutaneous instrumentation without arthrodesis for thoracolumbar flexion-distraction injuries: A review of the literature. *Neurosurgery* 2017;80(2):171-179.

The role of percutaneous instrumentation without fusion in flexion distraction injuries is examined in this systematic review. They find that percutaneous instrumentation without fusion is a viable option without any increase in complications or loss of correction. Level of evidence: V.

48. Avanzi O, Landim E, Meves R, et al: Thoracolumbar burst fracture: Load sharing classification and posterior instrumentation failure. *Rev Bras Ortop* 2010;45(3):236-240.

49. Leone A, Marino M, Dell'Atti C, et al: Spinal fractures in patients with ankylosing spondylitis. *Rheumatol Int* 2016;36(10):1335-1346.

This comprehensive review of ankylosing spondylitis discusses the pathology, management, and complications of ankylosing spondylitis. They review recent changes with regard to management of spinal fractures in ankylosing spondylitis. Level of evidence: V.

50. Rodrigues-Pinto R, Kurd MF, Schroeder GD, et al: Sacral fractures and associated injuries. *Global Spine J* 2017;7(7):609-616.

This review of sacral fractures examines the clinical presentation, diagnosis, and management. They also discuss associated injuries including pelvis and soft-tissue injuries. Level of evidence: V.

Section 4
Shoulder

EDITOR

Grant E. Garrigues, MD

Chapter 23

Shoulder Anatomy and Biomechanics, Clinical Evaluation, Imaging

Robert J. Gillespie, MD • Michael T. Freehill, MD, FAOA

ABSTRACT

The shoulder possesses the most motion of any joint in the human body. Its function is highly dependent on its unique anatomy and biomechanical properties. Secondary to the complex musculoskeletal interactions of the shoulder, the physical examination and radiologic workup are detailed and require a thorough understanding. This chapter presents a thorough introduction and description of the shoulder and provides a basis for evaluation of many of the pathologies discussed in the chapters to follow.

Keywords: biomechanics; glenohumeral joint; MRI; rotator cuff; shoulder anatomy

Anatomy

Introduction

The shoulder is composed of a complex arrangement of unique osseous anatomy, multiple joints, and dynamic and static soft-tissue structures. The structural architecture of the multiple diarthrodial joints allows for the greatest range of motion (ROM) of any joint. Unfortunately, increased reliance upon ligamentous and muscular structures comes at the expense of biomechanical stability.

Dr. Gillespie or an immediate family member serves as a paid consultant to or is an employee of DJ Orthopaedics and Shoulder Innovations and is a member of a speakers' bureau or has made paid presentations on behalf of DJ Orthopaedics. Dr. Freehill or an immediate family member serves as a paid consultant to or is an employee of Integra; has received research or institutional support from Regeneration Technologies, Inc. and Smith & Nephew; and serves as a board member, owner, officer, or committee member of the American Academy of Orthopaedic Surgeons, the American Orthopaedic Society for Sports Medicine, the American Shoulder and Elbow Surgeons, the Arthroscopy Association of North America, and the International Society of Arthroscopy, Knee Surgery, and Orthopaedic Sports Medicine.

Osseous Anatomy

Scapula

The scapular plane generally is 30° anterior compared with the coronal plane. The scapula consists of a thin body serving as a critical site for muscular attachments and numerous bony processes, including the coracoid, glenoid, acromion, and scapular spine. Seventeen muscles originate or attach to the scapula (**Table 1**). The scapular spine separates two fossae (infraspinatus and supraspinatus) which house the infraspinatus and supraspinatus rotator cuff muscles. Two notches, the suprascapular and spinoglenoid, are present medial to the glenoid and are traversed by the transverse scapular ligament and occasionally an inferior transverse scapular ligament, respectively. These notches and ligaments are clinically relevant as they are implicated in compression and potential deficits of the suprascapular nerve.

The acromion is made up of three ossification centers: the pre- (tip), meso- (middle), and the meta-acromion (base) (**Figure 1**). Failure of fusion at these sites, generally by the age of 18 years, is termed "os acromiale" with the most common location being the junction between the meso- and meta-acromion.[1] The clinical relevance of this anatomic variant is that the mobile os acromiale can not only cause a painful articulation with the rest of the scapula, but can also predispose to full-thickness rotator cuff tears by impinging on the subacromial space. The normal space between the highest point in the humerus and the underside of the acromion, known as the acromiohumeral interval, can range from 7 to 14 mm, with spaces less than 7 mm being highly suggestive of a massive rotator cuff tear.[2]

The coracoacromial ligament connects the lateral coracoid to the anterior acromion and completes the coracoacromial arch. Ossification of the acromial attachment produces an enthesiophyte, colloquially known as a "bone spur," which is correlated with age and the presence of a rotator cuff tear. Changes in acromial morphology are classically described as one of three types: I, flat undersurface; II, curved undersurface; III, hooked undersurface. Type III has the highest propensity for subacromial pathology and external impingement.[3]

Table 1

Muscles Attaching to the Scapula

Muscle	Origin	Insertion	Innervation	Function
Trapezius[a]	Occipital bone to T12	Scapular spine, acromion, clavicle	Cranial nerve XI (Accessory)	Scapular elevation Scapular retraction (middle fibers)
Levator scapulae[a]	Transverse process of C1-C4	Medial border of scapula	Dorsal scapular	Scapular elevation
Rhomboid minor[a]	C7-T1	Medial border of scapula	Dorsal scapular	Scapular retraction
Rhomboid major[a]	T2-T5	Medial border of scapula	Dorsal scapular	Scapular retraction
Serratus anterior[a]	Ribs 1-9	Anterior surface medial border of scapula	Long thoracic	Scapular stability, protraction
Latissimus dorsi	T7-L5, ribs 10-12, iliac crest	Medial intertubercular groove of humerus	Thoracodorsal	Extension, adduction, internal rotation
Pectoralis minor	Ribs 3-5	Medial coracoid	Medial pectoral	Scapular protraction
Coracobrachialis	Coracoid tip	Anteromedial humerus	Musculocutaneous	Adduction, flexion
Biceps short head	Coracoid tip	Radial tuberosity	Musculocutaneous	Flexion of elbow, supination of forearm
Biceps long head[a]	Supraglenoid tubercle	Radial tuberosity	Musculocutaneous	Flexion of elbow, supination of forearm
Triceps long head	Infraglenoid tubercle	Olecranon of ulna	Radial and axillary	Extension of elbow
Deltoid	Lateral third clavicle, acromion, scapular spine	Deltoid tuberosity of humerus	Axillary	Abduction, flexion, extension
Subscapularis[a]	Subscapular fossa	Lesser tuberosity	Upper/lower subscapular	Humerus stabilization, internal rotation, adduction
Supraspinatus[a]	Suprascapular fossa	Greater tuberosity	Suprascapular	Humerus stabilization, abduction
Infraspinatus[a]	Infrascapular fossa	Greater tuberosity	Suprascapular	Humerus stabilization, external rotation
Teres minor[a]	Lateral border scapula	Greater tuberosity	Axillary	Humerus stabilization, external rotation
Teres major	Posterior inferior angle scapula	Medial to intertubercular groove of humerus	Lower subscapular	Adduction, internal rotation, extension

[a]Dynamic stabilizer of the glenohumeral joint.

The coracoid process, by virtue of its location in the deltopectoral interval, is considered the "lighthouse" of the deltopectoral approach to the shoulder. The coracoid comes off the upper base of the glenoid neck and moves generally in a more lateral direction. The coracoacromial and coracohumeral ligaments insert on the lateral side, the pectoralis minor tendon medially, and the coracoclavicular ligaments (conoid and trapezoid) into the base. The coracobrachialis and short head of the biceps originate from the tip of the process.

"Glenoid" is Latin for "pear shaped"—an apt description. The glenoid has a relatively flat subchondral surface with much of the depth of the glenoid made up by articular cartilage and the circumferential labrum. The average superior tilt is 5° and the mean retroversion is 6°, though the version to the axis of the scapular body can vary from 5° of anteversion to 10° of retroversion.[4]

Clavicle: The clavicle is the first bone to ossify (fifth week of gestation), and its medial epiphysis is the last ossification center to fuse between 20 and 25 years of

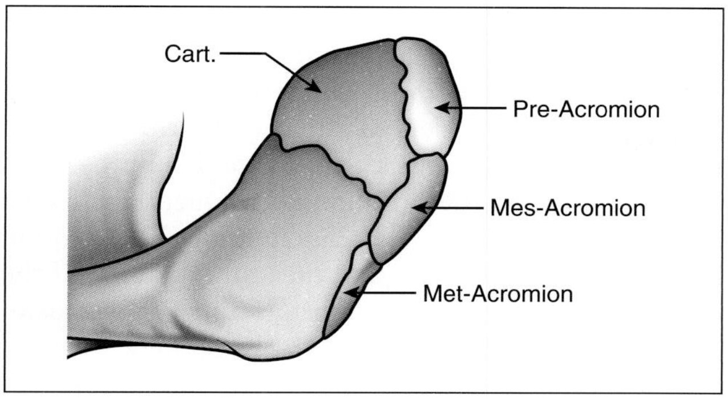

Figure 1 Illustration showing the ossification centers of the acromion. (Reproduced with permission from Sammarco VJ: Os acromiale: Frequency, anatomy, and clinical implications. *J Bone Joint Surg Am* 2000;82[3]:394-400.)

age making the clavicle the last bone to complete the ossification process. When viewed from anterior, the clavicle is relatively straight; however, in the transverse plane, it resembles more of an "S" shape.[5] The medial portion of the clavicle is convex anterior, and the lateral side is convex posterior. The primary blood supply is periosteal.

Proximal Humerus

The humeral head is spheroidal in shape in most individuals with an average diameter of 45 mm.[6] The bony architecture inferior to the articular surface is made up of the lesser (anterior) and greater (lateral) tuberosities. The greater tuberosity on average is 8 mm below the humeral articular surface.[6] These protuberances of bone serve as the attachment sites for the rotator cuff. The subscapularis attaches to the lesser tuberosity and the supraspinatus, infraspinatus, and teres minor attach to the greater tuberosity. The humeral head has an average retroversion of 25°, but there exists an SD of about 10°.[7] The head-shaft angle is roughly 135°.[6] The blood supply to the humeral head is made up of the ascending branch of the anterior humeral circumflex and arcuate arteries, but the posterior humeral circumflex is the main contribution.[8]

Joints

Glenohumeral

The glenohumeral (GH) joint relies upon complex musculoskeletal interactions between both static and dynamic soft-tissue structures to achieve stability. The joint is often thought of as a golf ball on a tee. The large ROM is achieved through rotation of the humeral head on the glenoid with minimal translation occurring.

Static Stabilizers

The static stabilizers are composed of the capsular glenohumeral ligaments, the coracohumeral ligament, the glenoid labrum, and articular congruity. These structures stabilize by anatomic architecture and position. The glenohumeral ligaments are made up of superior, middle, and inferior ligaments (**Figure 2**).

The superior glenohumeral ligament (SGHL) travels from the anterosuperior glenoid labrum to the humerus forming a pulley/sling medial to the bicipital groove. This helps to prevent medial or anterior-inferior translation of the long head of the biceps (LHB) tendon from the groove. Its principal function, however, is the primary static restraint to inferior translation at 0° of shoulder abduction.[9]

The middle glenohumeral ligament (MGHL) serves as the primary constraint against anterior and posterior translation with the shoulder in 45° to 60° of abduction.[10] The ligament inserts on the lesser tuberosity after originating from the anterior glenoid labrum. It is important during arthroscopic surgery to distinguish the MGHL running obliquely from the more horizontal (perpendicular to the glenoid) orientation of the subscapularis tendon (**Figure 3**). The ligament

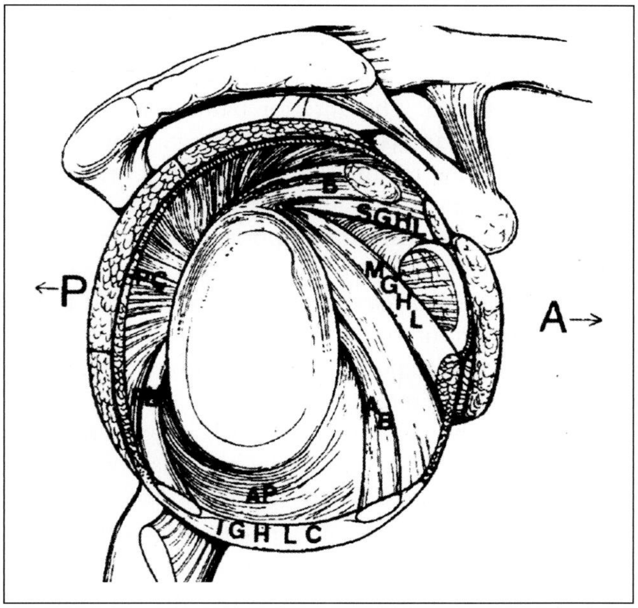

Figure 2 Illustration showing the ligaments of the glenohumeral joint. A = anterior, AP = axillary pouch, B= biceps, IGHL = inferior glenohumeral ligament, MGHL = middle glenohumeral ligament, P = posterior, SGHL = superior glenohumeral ligament. (Reproduced from O'Brien SJ, Neves MC, Arnoczky SP, et al: The anatomy and histology of the inferior glenohumeral ligament complex of the shoulder. *Am J Sports Med* 1990;18(5):449-456. [Figure 4])

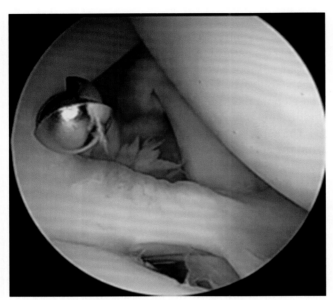

Figure 3 Arthroscopic view of anterior glenohumeral joint rotator interval in the lateral decubitus position. The middle glenohumeral ligament is running oblique (more horizontal) and the subscapularis running horizontal (vertical in this image) perpendicular to the glenoid. (courtesy Michael T. Freehill.)

can present with different sizes and characteristics discussed in more detail in the section on the glenoid labrum.

The inferior glenohumeral ligament (IGHL) is made up of anterior and posterior bands with an axillary pouch in between. The anterior band arises from the humerus to the anterior glenoid labrum. It acts as the primary restraint to anterior and inferior translation with the arm in 90° of abduction and external rotation.[11] This is the position of apprehension and is positive when a Bankart lesion involving this region present. The posterior band rises from the humerus and inserts into the posteroinferior glenoid labrum. It acts as the primary restraint to posterior and inferior translation at 90° of flexion and internal rotation.

The coracohumeral ligament (CHL) travels from the lateral coracoid, posterior to the coracoacromial ligament, to the humerus where it crosses both tuberosities bridging the bicipital groove and inserting into the rotator cable. Thus, it is a stabilizer to the LHB tendon. Its primary function, however, is a restraint to inferior translation in 0° of abduction and external rotation. The fibers of the CHL are arranged in a fashion to unwind with external rotation.[12]

The glenoid labrum is a circumferential fibrocartilage structure functioning to provide an increased depth to the glenoid cavity up to 50%, as well as increase the surface area for contact with the humeral head[13]. This helps to provide a concavity-compression of the joint. Smaller branches of three larger vessels provide the blood supply to the glenoid labrum with the anterosuperior aspect having the poorest blood supply. Areas of insertion into the labrum are frequently affected by pathologic lesions. These include the LHB tendon into the superior labrum and the anterior band of the IGHL leading to superior labrum anterior to posterior (SLAP) and Bankart lesions respectively. Normal anatomic variants in the anterosuperior labrum are frequent and should not be mistaken for pathology. These include a sublabral foramen, a sublabral foramen with a cord-like MGHL, and an absent anterosuperior labrum with a cord-like MGHL (the Buford complex).[14] Up to 14% of the population possess these variants, and surgical repair could lead to loss of motion notably in external rotation.

Two other anatomic areas are considered under the umbrella of static stabilizers. The first is the posterior capsule. Secondary to not possessing glenohumeral ligaments or "thickenings" akin to its anterior counterpart, the posterior capsule is much thinner at <1 mm.[15] Additionally, the cross-sectional area increases with posterior instability, a finding not present with anterior instability.[16] The posterior capsule can become thicker and contracted in overhead athletes leading to GH internal rotation deficit (GIRD). This is important as it changes the biomechanics of the shoulder in the late-cocking phase of throwing.[17] The humerus moves in a more posterosuperior direction and can lead to internal impingement—superior labral tearing or undersurface rotator cuff tearing of the anterior infraspinatus. Secondly, the triangular-shaped rotator interval is bordered by the anterior edge of the supraspinatus superiorly, the upper subscapularis inferiorly, and the lateral coracoid medially. It contains the SGHL, CHL, capsule, and the intra-articular portion of the LHB tendon. It can become contracted in adhesive capsulitis and become lax, demonstrating a sulcus sign, with inferior laxity.

Dynamic Stabilizers

While there are many muscles of the shoulder girdle, select ones act as dynamic stabilizers (**Table 1**). These include the rotator cuff (RC) musculature, the LHB tendon, and the scapulothoracic muscles. These muscles stabilize the glenohumeral joint via compression. The deltoid, innervated by the axillary nerve, is the largest and strongest shoulder girdle muscle and would provide an unopposed superior migration of the humerus without the counteraction of the aforementioned muscles. The deltoid, however, is not considered a dynamic stabilizer of the GH joint, as its primary function is shoulder abduction.

The RC is made up of the subscapularis, supraspinatus, infraspinatus, and the teres minor. The principal function of the RC is providing the dynamic stabilization for the GH joint. Whereas the static stabilizers act at the extremes of motion, the dynamic stabilizers act at the midrange of motion.

The scapulothoracic (ST) muscles play a critical role in the stability of the GH joint. The glenoid, as part of the scapula, can become malaligned with the humeral head with shoulder motion in the setting of ST dyskinesis. Along the medial border of the scapula, the levator scapulae and rhomboids minor and major attach. The largest of the ST muscles is the trapezius which serves as a scapular retractor with the upper fibers elevating the lateral angle of the scapula.[18] The serratus anterior has the highest percentage of maximal muscle activity with unresisted activities.[19] Dysfunction of the trapezius or the serratus anterior causes winging, lateral or medial respectively, of the scapula.

The LHB tendon remains controversial, but is considered by some a depressor of the humeral head. In vivo biomechanical studies show superior humeral head translation with LHB rupture[20] and depression with LHB activation.[21] Cadaveric models have reported decreased anterior, superior, and inferior translation at 55N,[22] but no significant changes at 11N,[23] leaving questions of the physiologic load required for this effect.

Acromioclavicular

The acromioclavicular (AC) joint is a small incongruent diarthrodial joint with a fibrocartilaginous intra-articular disk between the bony segments. Horizontal translatory stability of the joint is primarily provided by the superior (strongest) and posterior AC ligaments.[24] The coracoclavicular ligaments (conoid and trapezoid) are the primary stabilizers of vertical translation. The trapezoid ligament inserts 3 cm and the conoid ligament 4.5 cm from the distal end of the clavicle with the conoid being the more important stabilizer of the two. Although the clavicle can rotate up to 50° posteriorly with shoulder elevation, only 8° of rotation occurs through the AC joint itself.

Sternoclavicular

The sternoclavicular (SC) joint is a diarthrodial incongruous saddle joint with fibrocartilage surfaces and an intra-articular disk. It is the only articulation between the axial and upper appendicular skeleton. The posterior SC capsular ligaments are the strongest stabilizer to both anterior and posterior translation and inferior depression of the lateral end of the clavicle.[25] The anterior SC capsular ligament is the primary stabilizer to superior displacement. As previously mentioned, the medial clavicular physis may not ossify until 25 years of age; therefore it is important to distinguish SC dislocation from physeal fractures.[26] Motion of the SC joint of up to 30° occurs with 90° of elevation of the arm.[27]

Scapulothoracic

The scapulothoracic (ST) joint allows for motion of the scapula against the rib cage. This is not a diarthrodial joint, but can be considered a large articulation, lubricated by multiple bursae, between the scapula and the thorax. Sliding occurs between the medial border of the scapula and ribs 2 through 7. The primary motion is elevation and depression. Protraction and retraction are secondary motions important for clearance of the humeral head with overhead activities. Of note, the ratio of glenohumeral (GH) joint motion to ST motion is 2:1. Therefore, with full shoulder abduction, 120° of motion is contributed by the GH joint and 60° by the ST joint.

Clinical Evaluation

Patient History

Age and Sex

Most diseases of the shoulder occur during specific age ranges with the exception of autoinflammatory diseases or trauma. Osteoarthritis tends to affect older patients (>60 years of age),[28-30] while shoulder instability and labral pathology tend to occur in middle aged patients (40-60 years of age)[31-34] and young athletes.[31,35] Rotator cuff disease is divided between younger patients that experience acute injuries and older patients with chronic disease often due to repetitive microtrauma or degeneration.[36] Shoulder disease generally does not affect one sex more than the other. However, the following three conditions have significantly higher prevalence in women: multidirectional shoulder instability,[31] adhesive capsulitis,[37,38] and rotator cuff tear arthropathy.[39]

Pain

Shoulder pain is one of the most common reasons to see a physician and is reported to be responsible for as many as 30% of all primary care referrals to orthopaedic

Shoulder

surgeons.[39-42] The assessment of shoulder pain should start with a standard pain history: onset, location, duration, quality, and radiation. The patient's handedness, occupational history and leisurely activities, including repetitive overhead activities, heavy lifting, and sports should be discussed. Most shoulder conditions have distinguishing presenting features that can help narrow the differential diagnosis (**Table 2**).

Rotator cuff disease is a common cause of shoulder pain—including partial- and full-thickness rotator cuff tears.[43] Rotator cuff pain can have an acute onset following an injury or develop gradually over time.[44,45] In both acute and chronic cases, the patient usually describes a dull and aching pain in the lateral shoulder, frequently radiating into the deltoid insertion, worsening as the day progresses, and is exacerbated by shoulder movement, especially overhead.[44,45] Night pain and shoulder weakness are also frequent complaints.[43-45]

External shoulder "impingement" encompasses a variety of pathologies causing inflammation in the subacromial space—including subacromial bursitis, rotator cuff tendinitis, and LHB tenosynovitis which all may present similarly.[43,46,47] The typical presentation is subacute lateral shoulder pain that is exacerbated by shoulder movement, especially with overhead motion. In contrast is internal impingement, a diagnosis specific to

Table 2

Summary of Common Shoulder Presentations

Pathology	Common Presentation
Glenohumeral osteoarthritis	• Pain worse with activity and motion in all directions • Usually no pain at rest • Loss of range of motion, especially with external rotation (move to physical examination section) • Pain at night
Subacromial impingement	• Pain that is gradual, often with no apparent cause • Exacerbated by overhead motion and lifting objects outward • Pain at night
Adhesive capsulitis	• Diffuse pain • Stiffness with motion in all directions
Labral tear	• Vague pain that is felt deep in the shoulder • Worsens with activities • Popping and clicking sensation • Weakness • Decreased performance in athletes
Acromioclavicular joint injury	• Pain over the AC joint region • Occasional referred pain to the trapezius
Biceps tendinopathy	• Pain in the anterior region • Can radiate down the biceps • Similar presentation to rotator cuff tendinopathy
Rotator cuff tear	• Gradual onset of pain in the deltoid region • Exacerbated by overhead activities • Night pain • Acute weakness and pain with traumatic tear • Loss of active range of motion
Rotator cuff arthropathy	• Anterolateral pain • Pain exacerbated by overhead activities • Night pain • Stiffness

overhead athletes who repetitively place the shoulder in extreme positions of external rotation, extension, and abduction. This position causes contact between, and potential damage to, the undersurface of the rotator cuff and posterosuperior labrum.[48-50]

LHB tendinopathy usually occurs in combination with other shoulder pathology, coexisting with full-thickness rotator cuff tears 36% of the time in some studies,[51-53] and causes anteromedial shoulder pain that often radiates down the biceps into the arm.[54-56] Patients with a full-thickness tear of the LHB will often present with a Popeye deformity on examination. Recent studies have shown that up to 93% of these patients will have concomitant rotator cuff pathology.[51-53] Isolated biceps tendinopathy usually presents in younger athletes that participate in overhead sports such as baseball, softball, and volleyball.[57] Patients who develop biceps instability, frequently accompanying a superior border tear of the subscapularis which damages the medial portion of the biceps sling, will report that their symptoms began with an acute event that resulted in clicking or popping in the anterior shoulder and may even experience an audible snap when throwing.[57,58] Rotator cuff arthropathy (RCA) typically affects patients who are elderly and presents with progressively worsening shoulder pain that is accompanied by shoulder stiffness and decreased ROM.[59,60] The history may include an acute traumatic event or their condition could be the result of progressive degenerative disease of the rotator cuff and glenohumeral joint.[39,60,61] Patients often complain of night pain and can also have shoulder weakness.[39,61]

Lesions of the biceps-superior labrum complex which extend anterior to posterior (SLAP) are a frequently asymptomatic, nearly ubiquitous finding in older patients, but may be a source of disability in younger patients, especially overhead athletes.[62] Common mechanisms of injury include traction and compression of the shoulder, heavy lifting, and repetitive overhead motion in athletics.[62,63] Patients also often present with no obvious mechanism of injury.[63] Presentation consists of vague, deep shoulder pain that often is accompanied by clicking, popping, or snapping.[62,63] Pain is exacerbated by heavy lifting, pushing, and overhead motions and often radiates to the anterior or posterior aspects of the shoulder.[63]

Adhesive capsulitis, glenohumeral arthritis, and acromioclavicular (AC) joint disease all present with progressive diffuse pain that can limit mobility.[44] Adhesive capsulitis typically presents in middle-aged and elderly patients.[37] Patients are most frequently female and may have an endocrine imbalance (including diabetes mellitus, perimenopausal hormonal fluctuations, hyper- or hypothyroidism) or recent history of minor or major shoulder injury. Patients complain of diffuse, aching shoulder pain that initially is constant and accompanied by stiffness.[64] The sine qua non is anterior shoulder pain with passive external rotation to stretch the rotator interval with the arm at the side. The pain is exacerbated with movement in any direction, often wakes patients up at night, and interferes with daily activities—especially those behind the back.[44,65,66] If left untreated, the pain will subside somewhat, but the stiffness will progress to a point of limiting glenohumeral motion in all directions.[37,64] The complaints of glenohumeral arthritis are similar to those of adhesive capsulitis (as both involve synovitic processes) with the exception that the former also includes complaints of crepitus and follows a course of progressive deterioration in pain and ROM.[67] Plain radiographs are helpful in distinguishing these two diagnoses. Patients with AC joint disease present with pain specifically located above the AC joint, often radiating into the trapezius, that is worse with reaching across the body.[44]

Shoulder instability is commonly caused by macrotrauma, but often can be the result of repetitive microtrauma, including secondary to sports (swimming, gymnastics).[68] Patients with chronic instability will frequently have a sensations of apprehension—the uncomfortable feeling that shoulder is about to subluxate or dislocate.[69] Shoulder instability that results from acute trauma will also be accompanied by shoulder pain, especially with movement.[68]

Physical Examination

Inspection

The shoulder examination begins with inspection of the skin and superficial contour of the shoulder region. Both shoulders must be exposed for comparison. The acromioclavicular (AC) and sternoclavicular joints should be visualized for deformity. Muscle bulk should be assessed from both an anterior and posterior view. The anterior head of the deltoid can be visualized easily for atrophy, but the middle and posterior heads require active motion to make an accurate assessment. Skin lesions are usually secondary to underlying shoulder pathology. Ecchymoses can be observed in patients with traumatic injuries such as fractures, dislocations, or tendon ruptures. Erythema is often seen as a result of inflammation in the shoulder region that could be due to infection or a systemic inflammatory condition.

The resting position of the scapula can be observed but requires observation during motion to assess and confirm any abnormalities. Medial scapular winging caused by long thoracic nerve palsy can be observed, including a laterally prominent inferior scapula tip. Lateral scapular winging caused by spinal accessory nerve palsy can be identified by observing either excessive lateral rotation of the scapula or increased distance between the medial borders of each scapula.

Scapular dyskinesis can also be observed, often presenting with the affected scapula lower than normal and protracted. These patients often have painful crepitus with elevation and/or abduction of the arm that is relieved by the examiner stabilizing the scapula.[70] In addition, patients are often tender to palpation at scapular trigger points, areas of adhesion and inflammation caused by overworked and tightened muscles.[71] When scapular dyskinesis is suspected, it is recommended that dynamic scapular dyskinesis tests (SDT) be used.[72] The examiner observes the patient's medial and inferior scapular borders for winging, asymmetric, uncoordinated scapular elevation during elevation of the arm, and rapid downward rotation of the arm when lowing it from full flexion.[73]

Palpation

All of the joints in the shoulder region should be palpated for tenderness, deformity, or asymmetry. The sternoclavicular joint should be fixed in relation to the manubrium and nontender when palpated. Moving laterally down the clavicle, the acromioclavicular (AC) joint can be palpated and should be nontender and immobile in relation to the acromion. Lateral to the AC joint the acromion can be palpated. Finding the most lateral edge of the acromion can assist with palpating the greater tuberosity of the humerus.

The bicipital groove is palpated by having the patient rotate their forearm into the neutral position. In this position, the bicipital groove lies just distal to the readily palpable anterolateral corner of the acromion. To locate the groove, the examiner should rotate the arm internally and externally to palpate the grooves of the greater and lesser tuberosities. Tenderness in this region can be found in several pathologies such as rotator cuff tears and subacromial bursitis.

Pain with palpation of the greater tuberosity at the rotator cuff insertion, just distal to the lateral acromion, can indicate rotator cuff tear. Pain with palpation of the rotator interval, just lateral to the coracoid, may indicate a synovitic process including adhesive capsulitis or glenohumeral arthritis. Palpation of crepitus during rotation is indicative of glenohumeral arthritis when the arm is at the side and may be a sign of a full thickness rotator cuff tear as the "bare" tuberosity contacts the underside of the acromion if rotation is performed in 90° of scaption.

Table 3

Normal Maximum Range of Motion for the shoulder

Type of Motion	Normal Range of Motion
Flexion	170
Abduction	160
External rotation	80
Internal rotation	–70

Range of Motion

Range of motion (ROM) is assessed passively and actively for both shoulders. The three planes to assess ROM are elevation in the scapular plane, external rotation with the elbow near the side, and internal rotation using spinal segments as a reference point. The examiner begins with the normal shoulder to establish a normal ROM for evaluating the affected shoulder[74,75] (**Table 3**), and then will evaluate the affected shoulder for limitations in ROM to help narrow the differential diagnosis (**Table 4**). Examination of shoulder ROM

Table 4

Summary of Range of Motion in Common Shoulder Conditions

Pathology	Range of Motion (ROM)
Glenohumeral osteoarthritis	• ↓ passive ROM • ↓ active ROM • ↓ external rotation • ↓ forward flexion • ↓ internal rotation
Adhesive capsulitis	• ↓ passive ROM • ↓ active ROM • ↓ external rotation
Posterior shoulder dislocation	• shoulder locked in internal rotation
Rotator cuff disease	• Full passive ROM • ↓ active ROM

with the scapula fixed (supine) and free is imperative as scapulothoracic motion can contribute 20% to 30% of the overall motion of the shoulder.[74,75]

Neurovascular Examination

Shoulder pathology, especially trauma, can compromise the neurological and/or vascular status of a patient's upper extremity. Conversely, neurologic conditions, commonly cervical spine pathology, can mimic shoulder pathology. Therefore, clinical evaluation of patients with shoulder complaints should include neurovascular assessment of both upper extremities for comparison. The brachial, radial, and ulnar pulses can be palpated to test for adequate vascular perfusion. The integrity of the patient's peripheral nerves can be assessed by testing the strength and sensation of the upper extremity. The following motions should be assessed against resistance from the examiner: shoulder elevation and abduction and flexion and extension of the shoulder, elbow, wrist, and finger joints. The sensory distributions of the following nerves should be tested to ensure their sensory component is intact: axillary, musculocutaneous, medal brachial cutaneous, medial antebrachial cutaneous, median, radial, and ulnar nerves.

Special Tests

At the conclusion of any physical examination of the shoulder, specialty tests focused on specific pathology of the shoulder can be used to guide treatment and narrow the differential diagnosis. A summary of these physical examination findings can be found in **Tables 5-10.**

Imaging

Plain Radiograph and CT

Initially, all patients are usually asked to have AP and lateral plain radiographs of the shoulder related to their chief report. These images are often the only required studies needed for assessing acute shoulder trauma, including fractures or dislocations. Additionally, arthritis, calcific tendinitis, and osteolysis of the distal clavicle can be observed on plain radiograph.[76] CT imaging is frequently used to evaluate fractures of the shoulder, to assess for bony lesions in recurrent instability cases, or for preoperative templating for shoulder arthritis.[77]

MRI

MRI is the modality of choice for evaluating the rotator cuff, biceps, and subacromial/subdeltoid bursa.[78,79] T1-weighted MRI can reveal Hill-Sachs lesions and is often used with magnetic resonance (MR) arthrograms to provide a more detailed picture of the joint surfaces.[80] T2-weighted MRI provides better visualization of full thickness rotator cuff tears.[81]

Arthrography

Arthrography involves injection of contrast agent in conjunction with either an MRI or CT scan, enhancing imaging of the joint to enable better identification of normal structures and pathology involving the joint surfaces.[82] MR arthrography is considered the benchmark for evaluation for labral tears and rarely is indicated for evaluation of rotator cuff pathology.[79,82,83] When MRI or MR arthrography is contraindicated (eg, pacemaker, vascular clips), CT arthrography is indicated.

Ultrasonography

Ultrasonography is a low-cost alternative to MRI and arthrography for evaluating both skeletal and soft-tissue structures of the shoulder. It can provide

Table 5

Special Tests for the Acromioclavicular Joint

Test	Purpose	Description	Positive
AC shear	Test for AC path	• Patient sitting while examiner cups hands over the deltoid muscle with one hand on the clavicle and the other on the spine of the scapula • Examiner then squeezes the heels of hand together	• Abnormal movement
Horizontal adduction test	Test for AC joint damage or subacromial impingement	• Examiner stands behind the patient and places one hand on the posterior aspect of the shoulder to stabilize the joint • Using the other hand, the examiner grasps the patient's elbow and passively moves the shoulder into maximum horizontal adduction with the elbow in 90° of flexion	• Reproduces pain above the AC joint

Shoulder

Table 6

Special Tests for Shoulder Impingement Syndrome

Test	Purpose	Description	Positive
Hawkins test	Test for supraspinatus tendon impingement	• Shoulder is flexed to 90° with the elbow flexed to 90° as well • Examiner internally rotates the arm	• Pain felt during internal rotation
Neer impingement sign	Test for subacromial impingement	• Patient lies supine • Examiner brings the patient's arm into full elevation • Internal rotational torque is applied by the examiner to the patient's arm in this position	• Reproduces pain
Neer impingement test	Test for subacromial impingement	• Performed if the patient has a positive Neer sign • One percent lidocaine is injected into the subacromial space • Neer impingement maneuver is performed again	• Dramatic reduction in pain during the maneuver
Jobe-Yocum test	Testing for supraspinatus tendinitis	• Patient maintains their arm in 90° of elevation in the plane of the scapula • Arm is internally rotated with the thumb pointing down • Examiner applies a downward force to the patient's wrist	• Reproduces pain • Weak resistance from the patient secondary to pain
Internal rotation resistance test	Differentiate between intra-articular and subacromial impingement	• Patient stands with their arm in 90° of abduction and 80° external rotation • Examiner stands behind the patient and stabilizes the patient's elbow with one hand • Using the other the examiner grasps the patient's wrist to test both external and internal rotation strength	• If internal rotation is weaker than external rotation, that suggests internal impingement • If external rotation is weaker than internal rotation, that suggests subacromial impingement
Modified relocation test	Testing for internal impingement	• Patient lies supine with their arm hanging off the examination table • Arm is put into a position of maximal external rotation and is tested in three separate positions: 90°, 110°, and 120° of abduction • In each position, the examiner first applies an anterior load followed by a posterior load onto the shoulder	• Pain caused by an anterior force that is relieved by a posterior force
Painful arc testing	Rotator cuff impingement	• Patient elevates their arm in the scapular plane while maintaining a straight elbow • Patient can also fully elevate their arm and then slowly bring it down to their side	• Pain felt between 60° and 100° of abduction

immediate, real-time visualization of the rotator cuff, biceps tendon, and calcific deposits.[79,84-89] It can also be used to measure the subacromial space[90] and detect atrophy of rotator cuff muscles.[85,91] Additionally, as a result of providing images in real-time, ultrasonography can evaluate impingement in various positions and motions.[79,85,89] Ultrasonography is highly operator dependent and is not as useful for evaluating labral tears or rotator cuff tears that are very small or larger than 3 cm.[79,85]

Table 7

Special Tests for the Rotator Cuff

Test	Purpose	Description	Positive
Drop arm	Test for rotator cuff tear	• Patient abducts arm to 90° with the examiner's support • At 90°, the examiner removes their support and the patient slowly lowers their arm	• Patient is unable to slowly lower their arm and it "drops"
Empty can (Jobe sign)	Test for supraspinatus tendon tear	• Patient elevates their arm to 90° and extends it outward with full internal rotation of the shoulder • Forearm is pronated with the thumb turned downward toward the ground • Examiner stabilizes the shoulder while simultaneously pressing downward on the arm against resistance from the patient	• Reproduces pain
Belly Press	Tests for subscapularis tendon tear	• Patient places their hand on their abdomen area with the wrist extended • Patient presses their hand into their abdomen while maintain wrist extension	• Patient is unable to maintain wrist extension during maneuver • Reproduces pain
Bear hug	Tests for subscapularis tendon tear	• Patient brings hand across their body and places it onto the contralateral shoulder • Examiner holds the patient's elbow to prevent it from flexing during the maneuver • In this position, the patient pushes their hand down against the contralateral shoulder or against the examiner's hand	• Experiences pain during maneuver • Unable to push down
Lag sign	Test for infraspinatus and teres minor	• Patient holds arms by their side with their elbows flexed to 90° • Examiner externally rotates the patient's arm as far as it will go passively • Examiner releases the arm and patient holds their arm in that position	• Patient's arm internally rotates from where the examiner externally rotated it • Positive Lag sign is documented in degrees
Lift-off test	Tests for subscapularis tendon tear	• Patient places the dorsal aspect of their hand onto their lower back • Patient raises their hand off of their lower back against resistance from the examiner • If patient is unable to push against resistance, the examiner can pull the patient's hand off of the back and ask the patient to hold that position	• Reproduces pain • Unable to hold position if examiner pulls hand off of their back
Hornblower's	Test strength of teres minor	• Examiner elevates the patient's arm to 90° in the scapular plane • Patient flexes the elbow to 90° and laterally rotates their shoulder	• Reproduces pain • Patient shows weakness
Infraspinatus test	Test for infraspinatus strain	• Patient lets their arm hang at their side and flexes elbow to 90° • Examiner then applies a medial rotational force to the humerus against resistance from the patient	• Reproduces pain and/or the patient is unable to resist

Table 8

Special Tests for Shoulder Instability

Test	Purpose	Description	Positive
Sulcus sign		• Patient allows arm to hang relaxed and straight down • Examiner grasps the patient's elbow and applies traction inferiorly	• Depression in the skin (sulcus) occurs just below the acromion with inferior traction
Apprehension test		• Patient lies supine with both arms abducted to in 90° • Examiner externally rotates arm to 90°	• Patient is apprehensive during external rotation • If the patient reports pain, but no apprehension, then the test may be indicating rotator cuff tear
Relocation		• Often done after a positive apprehension test • Patient positioned supine with the arm abducted to 90° and the elbow flexed to 90° • Examiner applies a posterior force against the proximal arm forcing the humeral head from an anteriorly subluxated position to a centered position in the glenoid	• Patient no longer has apprehension • Patients with posterosuperior labral tears or internal impingement will have pain because the humeral head is forced against the torn labrum
Load and shift test	Test for capsular laxity	• Patient has arm slightly abducted with elbow supported (eg, by a pillow) and flexed to 90° • Examiner stabilizes the scapula with one hand • Using the other hand examiner grasps the approximates the humeral head into the glenoid fossa • Examiner applies an anterior and posterior force	• Excessive movement indicates laxity of the capsule
Posterior apprehension test	Tests for dislocation or posterior instability of the humerus	• Patient should be supine or sitting • Examiner elevates the patient's shoulder in the plane of the scapula to 90° while using the other hand to stabilize the scapula • Examiner applies a force onto the posterior aspect of the patient's elbow while horizontally adducting and internally rotating the arm	• Patient shows apprehension during the examination

Table 9

Special Tests for Biceps Tendon Pathology

Test	Purpose	Description	Positive
Speed test	Test for pathology of the biceps muscle or tendon	• Patient's arm is fully supinated and flexes forward to 90° against resistance from the examiner • Test is repeated with the forearm in full pronation	• Increased tenderness in the bicipital groove, especially with the arm supinated
Yergason test	Check the integrity of the transverse ligament across the bicipital groove of the humerus	• Patient sits while the examiner stands in front of them • Patient's elbow is flexed to 90° and the forearm is pronated while maintaining the proximal arm at their side • Patient actively supinates their arm while the examiner simultaneously provides resistance	• Localized pain at the bicipital groove
Ludington test	Tests for pathology of the long head of biceps tendon	• Patient's arm at their side with the elbow flexed to 90° and forearm in full pronation • Examiner grasps the patient's hand • Patient supinates their hand against resistance from the examiner	• Reproducing pain in the anterior shoulder or bicipital groove

Table 10

Special Tests for Labral Pathology

Test	Purpose	Description	Positive
Jerk test	Test for posterior instability/ torn posterior inferior labrum	• Examiner places their hand over the posterior aspect of the scapula and grasps the elbow with their other hand • Elevates the patient's arm to a position of 90° adduction and internal rotation • Examiner exerts an axial compression force to the humerus through the elbow while maintaining the horizontally abducted position • Compressive force is maintained as the examiner moves the arm into horizontal adduction.	• sharp pain in the shoulder with or without a clicking sound
Biceps load test I	Assess integrity of superior labrum	• Patient is in the supine position • Shoulder abducted to 90° and externally rotated with a supinated forearm • Examiner will begin by externally rotating the shoulder until the patient becomes apprehensive • In that position, the patient flexes the elbow against resistance from the examiner • if the patient's apprehension decreases with biceps contraction the test is negative	• Patient's pain remains the same or worsens with active biceps contraction against resistance
Biceps load test II	Test for SLAP lesion	• Patient is in the supine position • Shoulder elevated to 120° with their arm in full external rotation and forearm fully supinated • Elbow is bent to 90° and patient flexes elbow against resistance from the examiner	• Pain during elbow flexion
O'Brien test	Test for SLAP lesion	• Examiner stands behind the patient to perform test • Shoulder is flexed to 90° and adducted 15° toward the midline • Test is first performed with the patient's arm internally rotated with their thumb pointed toward the floor • Examiner will grab the patient's wrist and provide resistance against active adduction and flexion of the shoulder • Test is repeated with the patient's arm externally rotated and full forearm supination	• Pain or popping when the arm is internally rotated, and relief when the maneuver is performed with the arm externally rotated and forearm supination • Pain reproduced over the superior aspect of the shoulder or AC joint indicates AC joint pathology
SLAP-rehension test	Test for SLAP lesion and AC joint pathology	• Modified O'Brien's test where patient's arm is adducted to 45° instead of 15° • Examiner will grab the patient's wrist and provide resistance against active adduction and flexion of the shoulder (same as O'Brien's test)	• Pain or popping when the arm is internally rotated, and relief when the maneuver is performed with the arm externally rotated and forearm supination • Pain reproduced over the superior aspect of the shoulder or AC joint indicates AC joint pathology
Biceps tension test	Test for SLAP lesion	• Patient's elbow is positioned with full extension and forearm in supination • Patient flexes elbow forward to 90° against resistance from the examiner	• Reproduces pain

(continued)

Shoulder

Table 10

Special Tests for Labral Pathology (continued)

Test	Purpose	Description	Positive
Anterior slide test	Test for SLAP lesion	• Patient stands with both hands on their hips and thumbs along the posterior iliac crest • Examiner stands behind patient and *places one hand over the top of the acromion with the tips of the examiner's fingers just off the anterior edge of the acromion* • Examiner places other hand on the patient's elbow and pushes the arm forward against resistance from the patient	• Pain or click over the anterior shoulder
Crank test	Test for SLAP lesion	• Patient is in either sitting or supine position • Shoulder is flexed to 160° • Examiner applies axial loading through the humeral shaft onto the glenohumeral joint • In this position of axial loading, the arm is internally and externally rotated	• Reproduction of pain, catching, or a click
Pain provocation test		• Patient sits up and examiner stands behind them • Shoulder is placed in 90° of abduction and full external rotation • Patient's hand is first placed in full supination and then in full pronation • Patient is asked if supination or pronation induces more pain	• More pain felt when forearm is in pronation

SLAP = superior labrum anterior to posterior

Summary

The unique anatomy and complex biomechanical musculoskeletal interactions of the shoulder necessitate a complete knowledge and understanding of the physical examination and radiologic workup for both normal and pathologic shoulders. This chapter provides a detailed reference of the anatomy and biomechanical properties of the shoulder, allowing for a detailed discussion of the physical examination and radiologic evaluation of the shoulder.

Key Study Points

- Stability of the glenohumeral joint is achieved through a balance of dynamic and static stabilizers.
- The clavicle is the first bone to ossify (fifth week of gestation).
- The humeral head average retroversion is 25° (10° SD).
- The history and physical examination can narrow the diagnosis and allow for appropriate utilization of additional specialty tests of the shoulder.
- MRI is the modality of choice for evaluating the rotator cuff.

Annotated References

1. Sammarco VJ: Os acromiale: Frequency, anatomy, and clinical implications. *J Bone Joint Surg Am* 2000;82(3):394-400.
2. Petersson CJ, Redlund-Johnell I: The subacromial space in normal shoulder radiographs. *Acta Orthop Scand* 1984;55(1):57-58.
3. Bigliani LU, Morrison DS, April EW: The subacromial space in normal shoulder radiographs. *Orthop Trans* 1986;10:228.
4. Saha AK: Dynamic stability of the glenohumeral joint. *Acta Orthop Scand* 1971;42(6):491-505.
5. DePalma AF. *Surgery of the shoulder*, 3 ed. Philadelphia, Lippincott, 1983.
6. Iannotti JP, Gabriel JP, Schneck SL, Evans BG, Misra S: The normal glenohumeral relationships. An anatomical study of one hundred and forty shoulders. *J Bone Joint Surg Am* 1992;74(4):491-500.
7. Pearl ML, Volk AG: Retroversion of the proximal humerus in relationship to prosthetic replacement arthroplasty. *J Shoulder Elbow Surg* 1995;4(4):286-289.
8. Hettrich CM, Boraiah S, Dyke JP, Neviaser A, Helfet DL, Lorich DG: Quantitative assessment of the vascularity of the proximal part of the humerus. *J Bone Joint Surg Am* 2010;92(4):943-948.

9. Warner JJ, Deng XH, Warren RF, Torzilli PA: Static capsuloligamentous restraints to superior-inferior translation of the glenohumeral joint. *Am J Sports Med* 1992;20(6):675-685.
10. Burkart AC, Debski RE: Anatomy and function of the glenohumeral ligaments in anterior shoulder instability. *Clin Orthop Relat Res* 2002;(400):32-39.
11. O'Brien SJ, Neves MC, Arnoczky SP, et al: The anatomy and histology of the inferior glenohumeral ligament complex of the shoulder. *Am J Sports Med* 1990;18(5):449-456.
12. Rockwood CA: *The Shoulder*. 3 ed. Philadelphia, Elsevier, 2004.
13. Bigliani LU, Kelkar R, Flatow EL, Pollock RG, Mow VC: Glenohumeral stability. Biomechanical properties of passive and active stabilizers. *Clin Orthop Relat Res* 1996;(330):13-30.
14. Rao AG, Kim TK, Chronopoulos E, McFarland EG: Anatomical variants in the anterosuperior aspect of the glenoid labrum: A statistical analysis of seventy-three cases. *J Bone Joint Surg Am* 2003;85-A(4):653-659.
15. Bey MJ, Hunter SA, Kilambi N, Butler DL, Lindenfeld TN: Structural and mechanical properties of the glenohumeral joint posterior capsule. *J Shoulder Elbow Surg* 2005;14(2):201-206.
16. Dewing CB, McCormick F, Bell SJ, et al: An analysis of capsular area in patients with anterior, posterior, and multidirectional shoulder instability. *Am J Sports Med* 2008;36(3):515-522.
17. Grossman MG, Tibone JE, McGarry MH, Schneider DJ, Veneziani S, Lee TQ: A cadaveric model of the throwing shoulder: A possible etiology of superior labrum anterior-to-posterior lesions. *J Bone Joint Surg Am* 2005;87(4):824-831.
18. Wiedenbauer MM, Mortensen OA: An electromyographic study of the trapezius muscle. *Am J Phys Med* 1952;31(5):363-372.
19. Nuber GW, Jobe FW, Perry J, Moynes DR, Antonelli D: Fine wire electromyography analysis of muscles of the shoulder during swimming. *Am J Sports Med* 1986;14(1):7-11.
20. Warner JJ, McMahon PJ: The role of the long head of the biceps brachii in superior stability of the glenohumeral joint. *J Bone Joint Surg Am* 1995;77(3):366-372.
21. Pradhan RL, Itoi E, Kido T, Hatakeyama Y, Urayama M, Sato K: Effects of biceps loading and arm rotation on the superior labrum in the cadaveric shoulder. *Tohoku J Exp Med* 2000;190(4):261-269.
22. Pagnani MJ, Deng XH, Warren RF, Torzilli PA, O'Brien SJ: Role of the long head of the biceps brachii in glenohumeral stability: A biomechanical study in cadavera. *J Shoulder Elbow Surg* 1996;5(4):255-262.
23. Youm T, ElAttrache NS, Tibone JE, McGarry MH, Lee TQ: The effect of the long head of the biceps on glenohumeral kinematics. *J Shoulder Elbow Surg* 2009;18(1):122-129.
24. Renfree KJ, Wright TW: Anatomy and biomechanics of the acromioclavicular and sternoclavicular joints. *Clin Sports Med* 2003;22(2):219-237.
25. Bearn JG: Direct observations on the function of the capsule of the sternoclavicular joint in clavicular support. *J Anat* 1967;101:159-170.
26. Rockwood CA Jr: Fractures in adults, in: Rockwood CA, Green DP, eds: *Subluxations and Dislocations About the Shoulder*. Philadelphia, Lippincott, 1984, pp 722-947.
27. Inman VT, Saunders JB, Abbott LC: Observations of the function of the shoulder joint. 1944. *Clin Orthop Relat Res* 1996;(330):3-12.
28. Chillemi C, Franceschini V: Shoulder osteoarthritis. *Arthritis* 2013;2013:370231.
29. Kerr R, Resnick D, Pineda C, Haghighi P: Osteoarthritis of the glenohumeral joint: A radiologic-pathologic study. *AJR Am J Roentgenol* 1985;144(5):967-972.
30. Petersson CJ: Degeneration of the gleno-humeral joint. An anatomical study. *Acta Orthop Scand* 1983;54(2):277-283.
31. de Beer J, Bhatia DN: Shoulder instability in the middle-aged and elderly patients: Pathology and surgical implications. *Int J Shoulder Surg* 2010;4(4):87.
32. Onyekwelu I, Khatib O, Zuckerman JD, Rokito AS, Kwon YW: The rising incidence of arthroscopic superior labrum anterior and posterior (SLAP) repairs. *J Shoulder Elbow Surg* 2012;21(6):728-731.
33. Vogel LA, Moen TC, Macaulay AA, et al: Superior labrum anterior-to-posterior repair incidence: A longitudinal investigation of community and academic databases. *J Shoulder Elbow Surg* 2014;23(6):e119-26.
34. Weber SC, Martin DF, Seiler JG III, Harrast JJ: Superior labrum anterior and posterior lesions of the shoulder: Incidence rates, complications, and outcomes as reported by American board of orthopedic surgery. Part II candidates. *Am J Sports Med* 2012;40(7):1538-1543.
35. Wilk KE, Macrina LC, Cain EL, Dugas JR, Andrews JR: The recognition and treatment of superior labral (slap) lesions in the overhead athlete. *Int J Sports Phys Ther* 2013;8(5):579-600.
36. Green A: Chronic massive rotator cuff tears: Evaluation and management. *J Am Acad Orthop Surg* 2003;11(5):321-331.
37. Dias R, Cutts S, Massoud S: Frozen shoulder. *BMJ* 2005;331(7530):1453-1456.
38. Loyd JA, Loyd HM: Adhesive capsulitis of the shoulder: Arthrographic diagnosis and treatment. *South Med J* 1983;76(7):879-883.
39. Feeley BT, Gallo RA, Craig EV: Cuff tear arthropathy: Current trends in diagnosis and surgical management. *J Shoulder Elbow Surg* 2009;18(3):484-494.
40. Armed Forces Health Surveillance C: Arm and shoulder conditions, active component, U.S. Armed Forces, 2003-2012. *MSMR* 2013;20(6):18-22.
41. Bruls VE, Bastiaenen CH, de Bie RA: Non-traumatic arm, neck and shoulder complaints: Prevalence, course and prognosis in a Dutch university population. *BMC Musculoskelet Disord* 2013;14:8.
42. Greving K, Dorrestijn O, Winters JC, et al: Incidence, prevalence, and consultation rates of shoulder complaints in general practice. *Scand J Rheumatol* 2012;41(2):150-155.
43. Greenberg DL: Evaluation and treatment of shoulder pain. *Med Clin N Am* 2014;98(3):487-504.

44. Armstrong A: Evaluation and management of adult shoulder pain: A focus on rotator cuff disorders, acromioclavicular joint arthritis, and glenohumeral arthritis. *Med Clin N Am* 2014;98(4):755-775, xii.
45. Bishay V, Gallo RA: The evaluation and treatment of rotator cuff pathology. *Prim Care* 2013;40(4):889-910, viii.
46. Arce G, Bak K, Bain G, et al: Management of disorders of the rotator cuff: Proceedings of the ISAKOS upper extremity committee consensus meeting. *Arthroscopy* 2013;29(11):1840-1850.
47. Neer CS II: Anterior acromioplasty for the chronic impingement syndrome in the shoulder: A preliminary report. *J Bone Joint Surg Am* 1972;54(1):41-50.
48. Drakos MC, Rudzki JR, Allen AA, Potter HG, Altchek DW: Internal impingement of the shoulder in the overhead athlete. *J Bone Joint Surg Am* 2009;91(11):2719-2728.
49. Heyworth BE, Williams RJ III: Internal impingement of the shoulder. *Am J Sports Med* 2009;37(5):1024-1037.
50. Wright RW, Paletta GA Jr: Prevalence of the Bennett lesion of the shoulder in major league pitchers. *Am J Sports Med* 2004;32(1):121-124.
51. Desai SS, Mata HK: Long head of biceps tendon pathology and results of tenotomy in full-thickness reparable rotator cuff tear. *Arthroscopy* 2017;33(11):1971-1976.
52. Kowalczuk M, Kohut K, Sabzevari S, Naendrup JH, Lin A: Proximal long head biceps rupture: A predictor of rotator cuff pathology. *Arthroscopy* 2018;34(4):1166-1170.
53. Vestermark GL, Van Doren BA, Connor PM, Fleischli JE, Piasecki DP, Hamid N: The prevalence of rotator cuff pathology in the setting of acute proximal biceps tendon rupture. *J Shoulder Elbow Surg* 2018;27(7):1258-1262.
54. Ahrens PM, Boileau P: The long head of biceps and associated tendinopathy. *J Bone Joint Surg Br* 2007;89(8):1001-1009.
55. Nho SJ, Strauss EJ, Lenart BA, et al: Long head of the biceps tendinopathy: Diagnosis and management. *J Am Acad Orthop Surg* 2010;18(11):645-656.
56. Post M, Benca P: Primary tendinitis of the long head of the biceps. *Clin Orthop Relat Res* 1989(246):117-125.
57. Patton WC, McCluskey GM III: Biceps tendinitis and subluxation. *Clin Sports Med* 2001;20(3):505-529.
58. Curtis AS, Snyder SJ: Evaluation and treatment of biceps tendon pathology. *Orthop Clin N Am* 1993;24(1):33-43.
59. Jensen KL, Williams GR Jr, Russell IJ, Rockwood CA Jr: Rotator cuff tear arthropathy. *J Bone Joint Surg Am* 1999;81(9):1312-1324.
60. Nam D, Maak TG, Raphael BS, Kepler CK, Cross MB, Warren RF: Rotator cuff tear arthropathy: Evaluation, diagnosis, and treatment: AAOS exhibit selection. *J Bone Joint Surg Am* 2012;94(6):e34.
61. Ecklund KJ, Lee TQ, Tibone J, Gupta R: Rotator cuff tear arthropathy. *J Am Acad Orthop Surg* 2007;15(6):340-349.
62. Dodson CC, Altchek DW: SLAP lesions: An update on recognition and treatment. *J Orthop Sports Phys Ther* 2009;39(2):71-80.
63. Keener JD, Brophy RH: Superior labral tears of the shoulder: Pathogenesis, evaluation, and treatment. *J Am Acad Orthop Surg* 2009;17(10):627-637.
64. Guyver PM, Bruce DJ, Rees JL: Frozen shoulder – a stiff problem that requires a flexible approach. *Maturitas* 2014;78(1):11-16.
65. Neviaser RJ, Neviaser TJ: The frozen shoulder. Diagnosis and management. *Clin Orthop Relat Res* 1987;(223):59-64.
66. Nicholson GP: Arthroscopic capsular release for stiff shoulders: Effect of etiology on outcomes. *Arthroscopy* 2003;19(1):40-49.
67. Izquierdo R, Voloshin I, Edwards S, et al: Treatment of glenohumeral osteoarthritis. *J Am Acad Orthop Surg* 2010;18(6):375-382.
68. Rouleau DM, Hebert-Davies J, Robinson CM: Acute traumatic posterior shoulder dislocation. *J Am Acad Orthop Surg* 2014;22(3):145-152.
69. Goga IE: Chronic shoulder dislocations. *J Shoulder Elbow Surg* 2003;12(5):446-450.
70. Frank RM, Ramirez J, Chalmers PN, McCormick FM, Romeo AA: Scapulothoracic anatomy and snapping scapula syndrome. *Anat Res Int* 2013;2013:635628.
71. Roche SJ, Funk L, Sciascia A, Kibler WB: Scapular dyskinesis: The surgeon's perspective. *Shoulder Elb* 2015;7(4):289-297.
72. Kibler WB, Ludewig PM, McClure P, Uhl TL, Sciascia A: Scapular Summit 2009: Introduction. July 16, 2009, Lexington, Kentucky. *J Orthop Sports Phys Ther* 2009;39(11):A1-A13.
73. Kibler WB, Ludewig PM, McClure PW, Michener LA, Bak K, Sciascia AD: Clinical implications of scapular dyskinesis in shoulder injury: The 2013 consensus statement from the "scapular summit". *Br J Sports Med* 2013;47(14):877-885.
74. Mallon WJ, Herring CL, Sallay PI, Moorman CT, Crim JR: Use of vertebral levels to measure presumed internal rotation at the shoulder: A radiographic analysis. *J Shoulder Elbow Surg* 1996;5(4):299-306.
75. Matsen FA III, Lauder A, Rector K, Keeling P, Cherones AL: Measurement of active shoulder motion using the Kinect, a commercially available infrared position detection system. *J Shoulder Elbow Surg* 2016;25(2):216-223.
76. Willick SE, Sanders RK: Radiologic evaluation of the shoulder girdle. *Phys Med Rehabil Clin N Am* 2004;15(2):373-406.
77. Haapamaki VV, Kiuru MJ, Koskinen SK: Multidetector CT in shoulder fractures. *Emerg Radiol* 2004;11(2):89-94.
78. Opsha O, Malik A, Baltazar R, et al: MRI of the rotator cuff and internal derangement. *Eur J Radiol* 2008;68(1):36-56.
79. Singh JP: Shoulder ultrasound: What you need to know. *Indian J Radiol Imaging* 2012;22(4):284-292.
80. Sheridan K, Kreulen C, Kim S, Mak W, Lewis K, Marder R: Accuracy of magnetic resonance imaging to diagnose superior labrum anterior-posterior tears. *Knee Surg Sports Traumatol Arthrosc* 2015;23(9):2645-2650.
81. Morag Y, Jacobson JA, Miller B, De Maeseneer M, Girish G, Jamadar D: MR imaging of rotator cuff injury: What the clinician needs to know. *RadioGraphics* 2006;26(4):1045-1065.

82. Rhee RB, Chan KK, Lieu JG, Kim BS, Steinbach LS: MR and CT arthrography of the shoulder. *Semin Musculoskelet Radiol* 2012;16(1):3-14.

83. Roy EA, Cheyne I, Andrews GT, Forster BB: Beyond the cuff: MR imaging of labroligamentous injuries in the athletic shoulder. *Radiology* 2016;278(2):316-332.

84. Alasaarela E, Leppilahti J, Hakala M: Ultrasound and operative evaluation of arthritic shoulder joints. *Ann Rheum Dis* 1998;57(6):357-360.

85. Beggs I: Shoulder ultrasound. *Semin Ultrasound CT MR* 2011;32(2):101-113.

86. Farin PU, Jaroma H: Sonographic findings of rotator cuff calcifications. *J Ultrasound Med* 1995;14(1):7-14.

87. Kayser R, Hampf S, Pankow M, Seeber E, Heyde CE: Validity of ultrasound examinations of disorders of the shoulder joint. *Ultraschall der Med* 2005;26(4):291-298.

88. Nazarian LN, Jacobson JA, Benson CB, et al: Imaging algorithms for evaluating suspected rotator cuff disease: Society of Radiologists in Ultrasound consensus conference statement. *Radiology* 2013;267(2):589-595.

89. Read JW, Perko M: Shoulder ultrasound: Diagnostic accuracy for impingement syndrome, rotator cuff tear, and biceps tendon pathology. *J Shoulder Elbow Surg* 1998;7(3):264-271.

90. Azzoni R, Cabitza P, Parrini M: Sonographic evaluation of subacromial space. *Ultrasonics* 2004;42(1-9):683-687.

91. Sofka CM, Haddad ZK, Adler RS: Detection of muscle atrophy on routine sonography of the shoulder. *J Ultrasound Med* 2004;23(8):1031-1034.

Shoulder Instability, Rotator Cuff Disorders, Muscular Ruptures, Adhesive Capsulitis, Calcific Tendinitis

Jonathan C. Riboh, MD • Anshuman Singh, MD

ABSTRACT

The most common pathologic conditions of the shoulder involve the soft tissues. Rotator cuff disease, including calcific tendinitis and partial- and full-thickness tears, is a common source of weakness and pain. Traumatic and nontraumatic abnormalities of the glenohumeral capsule and ligaments lead to shoulder instability and dysfunction. It is important to review the diagnosis, decision making, treatment, and outcomes of rotator cuff disease, shoulder instability, and associated lesions.

Keywords: adhesive capsulitis; calcific tendinitis; multidirectional instability; rotator cuff tear; shoulder instability

Calcific Tendinitis

Pathophysiology

The prevalence of calcific tendinitis in a working population is 2.7%, with 35% of these shoulders being symptomatic. Calcific tendinitis typically affects patients aged 30 to 60 years and women more commonly than men. Those with endocrine disorders develop symptoms of calcific tendinitis at a younger age, experience symptoms for a longer duration, and have a higher rate of surgery.[1] The supraspinatus tendon is most often involved.

The precise pathogenesis of calcific tendinitis remains unclear, but an active, cell-mediated process is widely accepted.[2] Three main stages of calcification: precalcific, calcific, and postcalcific, are described. The precalcific stage consists of predominantly fibrocartilaginous metaplasia presumably within less vascular areas of the tendon. In the formative phase of the calcific stage, matrix vesicles unite to form calcium hydroxyapatite deposits that are separated by fibrocollagenous tissue. This phase can continue asymptomatically or cause pain secondary to subacromial bursitis or a mass effect of the calcific lesion. Without a clear trigger, the exquisitely painful resorption phase involves an inflammatory response.

Calcific tendinitis is generally self-limited, with most cases resolving spontaneously. The duration of each phase is highly variable. Pain is variable during the proliferative phase and is correlated with the macrophage activity during the resorptive phase (**Figures 1 and 2**).

Dr. Riboh or an immediate family member serves as a paid consultant to or is an employee of Stryker and has received research or institutional support from Sparta Biopharma. Neither Dr. Singh nor any immediate family member has received anything of value from or has stock or stock options held in a commercial company or institution related directly or indirectly to the subject of this chapter.

Evaluation

Given the possibility of asymptomatic calcific foci, it is important to exclude other sources of pain. Standard radiographic workup with oblique views will show the

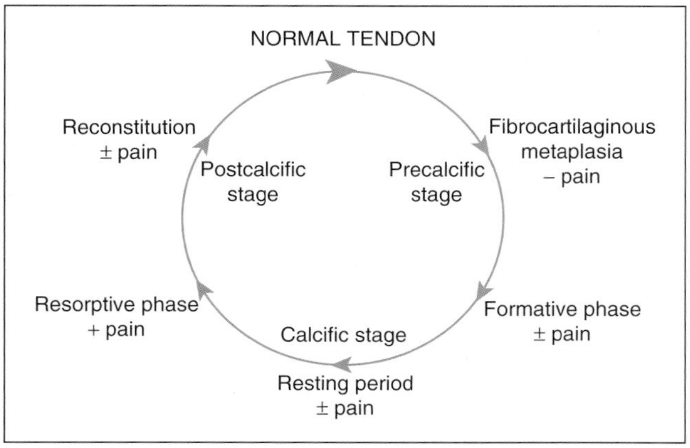

Figure 1 A schematic illustration showing the stages of calcific tendinitis. Note that the disease is generally self-limited, and pain is highly variable, but most prevalent in the resorptive phase. (Reproduced with permission from Uhthoff HK, Loehr JW: Calcific tendinopathy of the rotator cuff: pathogenesis, diagnosis, and management. *J Am Acad Orthop Surg* 1997;5(4):183-191.)

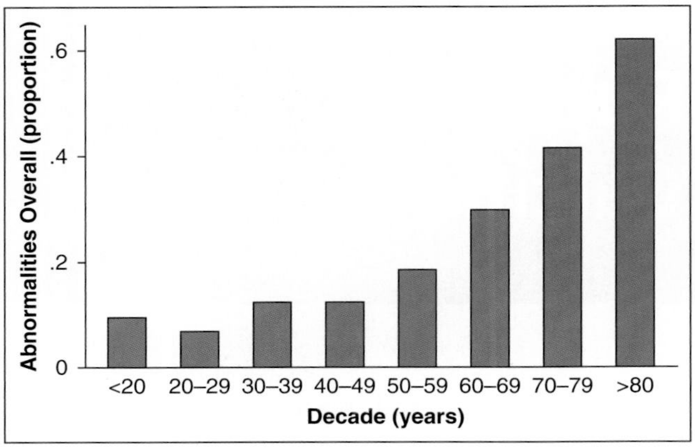

Figure 2 A graphic representation showing the prevalence of rotator cuff tears by decade. There is a sixfold increase in rotator cuff abnormalities between the fifth and ninth decades of life attributable to age-related degenerative changes coupled with decreased host healing potential. (Reprinted from Teunis TT, Lubberts B, Reilly BT, et al: A systematic review and pooled analysis of the prevalence of rotator cuff disease with increasing age. *J Shoulder Elbow Surg* 2014;23[12]:1913-1921, Copyright 2014, with permission from Elsevier.)

location of the deposit, typically 1.5 to 2 cm from the insertion. The calcification may be differentiated from dystrophic calcification, which occurs at the tendon insertion. MRI is not mandatory for workup of calcific tendinitis, but may identify concomitant pathology. Calcific deposits have low signal intensity on MRI sequences but can demonstrate surrounding edema on fluid-sensitive sequences.

On ultrasonography, calcific deposits are hyperechoic. In patients with symptomatic calcific tendinitis, ultrasonography reveals large fragmented deposits, positive power Doppler signal, and widening of the subacromial bursal space. Arc-shaped calcified deposits correspond to a dense homogeneous and generally less syptomatic deposit, whereas non–arc-shaped deposits (fragmented, nodular, and cystic) tend to be more painful, but have a higher rate of spontaneous resorption.

Treatment

Nonsurgical therapy with NSAIDs, physical therapy, and corticosteroid injections comprise first-line treatment. Prognostic factors were examined in 488 shoulders in which initial nonsurgical therapy failed. The failure rate at 6 months was 27%, and the probability of failure increased with bilateral disease, large calcifications, deposits underlying the anterior third of the acromion, and extension of the calcific deposits medial to the acromion.[2]

High-energy extracorporeal shockwave therapy (ESWT) leads to improvement in pain and outcome scores, but there is little consensus on the number of impulses and treatments performed for "low" and "high" energy ESWT. In one study 144 shoulders with calcific tendinitis were randomized into three groups: high-energy (0.32 mJ/mm^2) ESWT, low-energy (0.08 MJ/mm^2) ESWT, and placebo. At 6 months, both the high- and low-energy groups had statistically significant improvements compared with the placebo group, with the high-energy group substantially outperforming the low-energy group in terms of Constant score and visual analog scale (VAS).[3] High-energy ESWT may cause painful local reactions that require analgesia. Long-term data are lacking, but about 20% of patients will require arthroscopy 4 years after ESWT.[4]

Ultrasound-guided needle lavage involves localization of the calcific focus under local anesthesia and introducing a needle adjacent to or directly into the calcific deposit. Some authors describe the use of a single needle for aspiration and lavage, whereas others use two needles to maintain a route of egress. A mixture of anesthetic and saline is injected into the calcification, and calcific material is aspirated. An adjunct subacromial corticosteroid may be performed. Sometimes multiple sites are punctured in an effort to stimulate the resorptive inflammatory process. A recent randomized controlled trial comparing needle lavage and subacromial injection with subacromial injection alone found that, although both groups demonstrated improvement at 6 months, the needle lavage group had higher Constant scores and smaller residual calcifications and chose to undergo surgery at a lower rate.[5]

Arthroscopic localization and evacuation of the calcific focus is the treatment of choice for calcific tendinitis for which nonsurgical management has failed. In a study of 54 patients, 92% of patients had excellent results at a 2-year follow-up.[6] The role of acromioplasty has been debated, but it is clear that routine acromioplasty is not mandatory for a good outcome. In a study evaluating 99 shoulders at an average of 3 years after arthroscopic evacuation without acromioplasty or rotator cuff repair, 91% good to excellent results were reported.[7] The calcific focus should be débrided, but complete removal of the focus is not needed for a good outcome. Finally, concomitant rotator cuff tear (RCT) requiring repair is rare, with most studies demonstrating below a 10% rate of repair. Rotator cuffs that are repaired in the milieu of an inflammatory lesion such as calcific tendinitis may be more prone to stiffness and slow return of function (**Figure 3**).

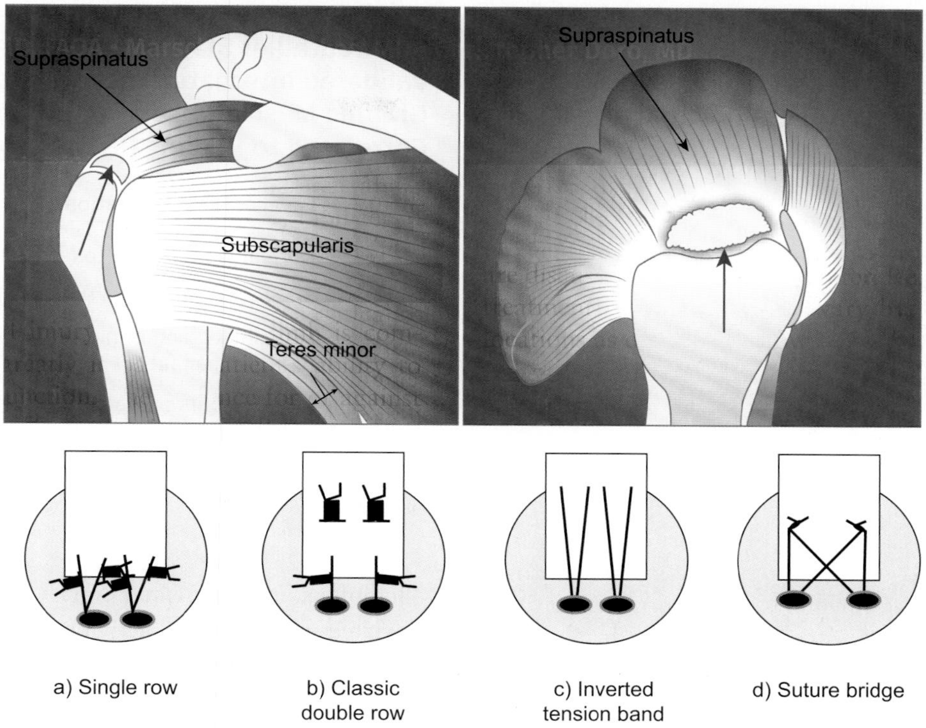

Figure 3 Illustration showing common rotator cuff repair configurations. There are multiple acceptable suture configurations for rotator cuff repair. The ideal construct is debated. Double row techniques are biomechanically superior, but likely do not yield better results in small and medium-sized tears. (Reproduced with permission from Rotator Cuff Tears: Surgical Treatment Options - OrthoInfo - AAOS. https://www.orthoinfo.org/en/treatment/rotator-cuff-tears-surgical-treatment-options/. Accessed October 11, 2019 and Andres BM, Lam PH, Murrell GAC. Tension, abduction, and surgical technique affect footprint compression after rotator cuff repair in an ovine model. *J Shoulder Elbow Surg* 2010;19(7):1018-1027, with permission of Elsevier. doi:10.1016/j.jse.2010.04.005.)

Rotator Cuff Tears

Pathophysiology

Atraumatic RCTs have a multifactorial pathophysiology. Intrinsic factors weaken the quantity, quality, and/or healing ability of the tendon. Age-related tendon changes include degeneration of the deep tendon layers, impaired vascularity, tendon swelling, and decreased regenerative capacity (**Figure 2**). Smoking negatively affects tendon vascularity in a dose-dependent manner. Hyperlipidemia increases the risk for RCT and recurrent tear, but this effect can be mitigated by control of serum hyperlipidemia with statins. Genetic factors contribute to an individual's risk of rotator cuff disease, with initial studies in twins demonstrating clustering of disease. Newer evidence implicates particular genetic loci in cuff disease[8] although the precise biological pathways are areas of ongoing study (**Table 1**).

Extrinsic factors contribute to rotator cuff tendinitis and tearing. These include high critical shoulder angle[9] and subcoracoid impingement, or dynamic factors such as poor scapular mobility and internal impingement. In young throwing athletes, internal impingement is caused by repetitive microtrauma during the late cocking and early acceleration phases of the throwing cycle between the underside of the rotator cuff at the junction of supraspinatus and infraspinatus tendons and the posterior-superior labrum. In older patients with some rotator cuff degeneration, the cuff may be overpowered by the deltoid and impinge into the coracoacromial arch creating a coracoacromial ligament enthesiophyte—a so-called "bone spur" and exacerbating the cuff disease.

Natural History

There is little agreement on what causes pain from an RCT. In a recent study, there was no correlation between pain, the size of RCT, age, and chronicity at the time of presentation.[10]

Longitudinal ultrasonographic studies have yielded significant data on the progression of RCTs. Individuals with asymptomatic tears were followed up for 5 years after they presented with symptoms on the contralateral side. Fifty-one percent of the cohort began having pain at

Table 1

Estimated Relative Risk for Development of Full-Thickness Rotator Cuff Tear (RCT). Note That These Factors Generally Impact Host Regenerative Capacity

Risk Factor for Rotator Cuff Tear	Estimated Relative Risk
Sibling with symptomatic rotator cuff tear	2.5
Age 70 vs age 50	2.5
Diabetes mellitus	2.1
Body mass index: morbid obesity	2.0
Hyperlipidemia	4.3
Well-treated hyperlipidemia w statins	1.8
Hypertension	2.1
Smoking	Over 2.0
Perioperative NSAIDs	–
Female sex	–
Quinolones	–
Oxidative stress	–

Table 2

The Goutallier Staging System is the Validated International Standard for Grading Muscle Degeneration and is Directly Correlated to Healing Probability

Stage	Level of Fatty Infiltration
0	Normal muscle with no fatty streak
1	Some fatty streaks in the muscle
2	Fatty infiltration is important, but more muscle exists than fat
3	Equal amounts of fat and muscle
4	More fat than muscle

Reprinted from Goutallier D, Postel JM, Gleyze P, et al: Influence of cuff muscle fatty degeneration on anatomic and functional outcomes after simple suture of full-thickness tears. *J Shoulder Elbow Surg* 12[6]:550-554, Copyright 2003, with permission of Elsevier.

an average of 2.8 years.[11] In a prospective study of small full-thickness tears in patients younger than 60 years, 49% of tears increased in size at 29 months.[12] Age older than 60 years, full-thickness tears, fatty infiltration, and symptoms are correlated with progression, but it is not clear which particular individuals will experience tear progression.

The progression of rotator cuff disease from tendinitis to degenerated full-thickness tear is a failure of biology. Animal and human studies of early stage disease demonstrate a biologically active and resilient musculotendinous unit that undergoes a productive inflammatory cycle in response to injury that leads to recovery of integrity and function. In some chronic tears, however, the tissue is unable to respond productively to the insult, resulting in deposition of disorganized connective, fatty, and fibrous tissue that is evident on CT and MRI, and classified most commonly by the Goutallier staging system (**Table 2**; **Figure 4**).

Evaluation

History and Physical Examination

A patient may present with a clear history of trauma resulting in acute pain and weakness, strongly suggesting acute RCT and warranting expeditious workup. In cases of chronic rotator cuff disease, patients often describe an insidious onset of lateral and/or anterior shoulder pain associated with overhead activities. Night pain is a common presenting symptom. A family or personal history of rotator cuff disease makes the diagnosis more likely.

Physical examination is critical in the workup of RCT. Basic examination consists of assessment of range of motion in the adducted and abducted positions, assessment of strength, and examination of associated structures such as the biceps and acromioclavicular joint. The empty can test has a sensitivity of 71.7% and a specificity of 64.6% for full-thickness supraspinatus tears. The lift-off and belly-press tests have high specificity but low sensitivity for full-thickness subscapularis tears. Patients with an external rotation lag sign at the side likely have a large posterosuperior tear involving the infraspinatus (**Table 3**). A positive hornblower sign suggests a massive posterosuperior cuff tear that prohibits the active positioning of the hand in space.

Diagnostic Studies

The goal of diagnostic imaging is threefold: determine the presence, size, orientation of the RCT; evaluate the healing capacity of the tendon; and assess associated pathology such as long head biceps tendinitis, acromioclavicular joint pathology, and arthrosis. This allows for risk stratification and optimizes treatment choice.

For full-thickness RCT, ultrasonography approaches the sensitivity and specificity of MRI for detecting the presence of a tear with an experienced practitioner. Ultrasonography is relatively inexpensive, allowing for dynamic testing, guided injections, and immediate feedback. MRI accurately assesses muscle, bone, and cartilage, which has advantages for surgical planning. MRI

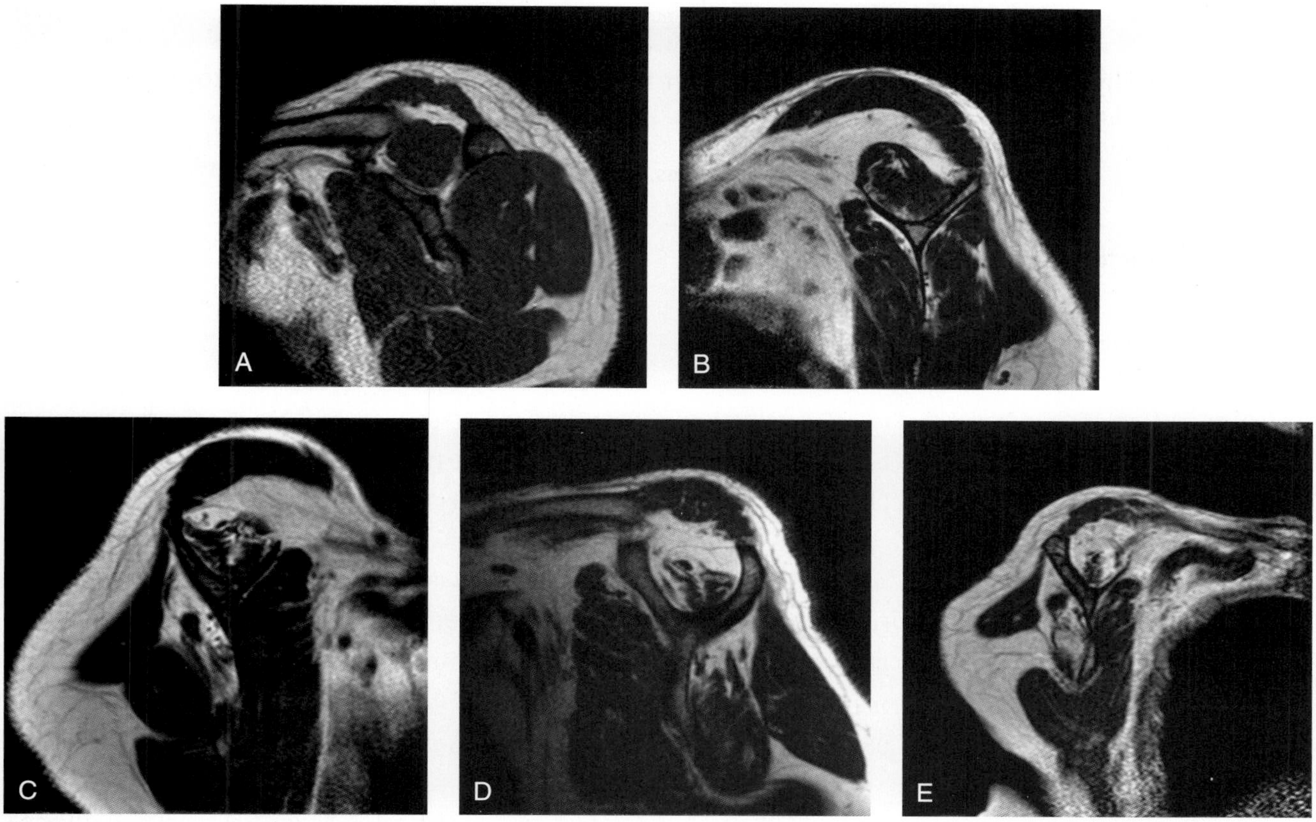

Figure 4 MRI cross sections of rotator cuff disease. The original Goutallier staging was described with CT imaging, but has been validated on MRI. (Reprinted from Schiefer M, Mendonca R, Magnanini MM, et al: Intraobserver and interobserver agreement of Goutallier classification applied to magnetic resonance images. *J Shoulder Elbow Surg* 2015;24[8]:1314-1321, Copyright 2015, with permission of Elsevier.)

continues to be the imaging modality of choice for most providers, with ultrasonography becoming common in certain centers.

Management of Partial-Thickness Rotator Cuff Tears

Nonsurgical Management

The literature available regarding the natural history, evaluation, and treatment of partial-thickness rotator cuff tear (PTRCT) is not as well developed as that for full-thickness RCT. The incidence of PTRCT ranges from 15% to 30% in asymptomatic individuals. The incidence of PTRCT is age dependent, with 6% of individuals younger than 40 years having an asymptomatic PTRCT, increasing to 26% of those older than 60 years.[13]

There are three main variants of PTRCT. The most common are partial articular supraspinatus tendon avulsion (PASTA) tears. These start lateral to the capsule on the less vascular articular side of the tendon. The second tear pattern is the bursal tear at the insertion of the superior cuff in the subacromial space, generally under the coracoacromial ligament. These may have a higher rate of progression than PASTA tears. Finally, there are PTRCTs secondary to internal impingement in athletes on the articular side of the supraspinatus and infraspinatus border, just adjacent to the posterosuperior labrum.

In terms of progression of tear size, the literature is highly variable for PTRCT. This is due to inconsistent inclusion criteria, follow-up, and imaging modalities between studies. In a 2017 study, MRI was used to follow up 122 individuals with partial- and full-thickness RCT for an average of 2 years. At final follow-up, 28/34 of symptomatic full-thickness RCTs (82.4%) and 23/88 of symptomatic partial-thickness tears (26.1%) increased in size.[14] PTRCT progression is likely slower than that for full-thickness RCT, which allows for more time for nonsurgical management without the risk of terminal degeneration.

Nonsurgical treatment of PTRCT includes oral and/or subacromial anti-inflammatory medications, physical therapy, pain medications, and biologic modalities such as platelet-rich plasma injections. Patients with smaller tears have a good outcome with nonsurgical management of PTRCT.

Table 3

Accuracy of Physical Examination Maneuvers for Rotator Cuff Disease or Full Rotator Cuff Tears From Quality Level 1-2 Studies

Finding	Rotator Cuff Condition	Studies, No.	% (95% CI)		LR (95% CI)	
			Sensitivity	Specificity	Positive	Negative
Pain Provocation Tests						
Painful arc[45]	Disease	1	71 (60-83)	81 (68-93)	3.7 (1.9-7.0)	0.36 (0.23-0.54)
Cross-body adduction[45]	Disease	1	75 (64-85)	61 (46-76)	1.9 (1.3-2.9)	0.42 (0.26-0.68)
Hawkins[44,45,48]	Disease	3[a]	76 (56-89)	48 (23-74)	1.5 (1.1-2.0)[b]	0.51 (0.39-0.66)[c]
Neer[45,48]	Disease	2[d]	64-68	30-61	0.98-1.6	0.60-1.1
Yocum[48]	Disease	1	79 (61-97)	40 (10-70)	1.3 (0.75-2.3)	0.53 (0.17-1.7)
Passive abduction[48]	Disease	1	74 (54-93)	10 (0-29)	0.82 (0.58-1.1)	2.6(0.35-20)
Strength Tests						
External rotation lag[47]	Full tear	1	47 (21-71)	94 (85-100)	7.2(1.7-31)	0.57 (0.35-0.92)
Internal rotation lag[47]	Full tear	1	97 (88-100)	83 (70-96)	5.6 (2.6-12)	0.04 (0.0-0.58)
Drop arm[45]	Disease	1	24 (13-34)	93 (85-100)	3.3 (1.0-11)	0.82 (0.70-0.97)
Dropping sign[47]	Full tear	1	73 (51-95)	77 (62-92)	3.2 (1.6-6.5)	0.35 (0.15-0.83)
Gerber (lift-off test)[44,48]	Disease	2[d]	34-68	50-77	1.4-1.5	0.63-0.85
Composite Test for Pain or Weakness						
External rotation resistance[44,e]	Disease	1	63 (49-77)	75 (69-82)	2.6 (1.8-3.6)	0.49 (0.33-0.72)
Full can[45]	Disease	1	75 (64-85)	68 (54-83)	2.4(1.5-3.8)	0.37 (0.23-0.60)
Patte[48]	Disease	1	58 (36-80)	60 (30-90)	1.4 (0.62-3.4)	0.70 (0.34-1.5)
Empty can (Jobe)[44,45,48]	Disease	3[a]	71 (49-86)	49 (42-56)	1.3 (0.97-1.6)[b]	0.64 (0.33-1.3)[f]
Resisted abduction[48]	Disease	1	58 (36-80)	20 (0-45)	0.72 (0.55-8.1)	2.1 (0.55-8.1)
Combinations of Findings						
Hawkins and Neer (both positive)[46]	Disease	1	78 (66-90)	50 (22-78)	16 (0.87-2.8)	0.43 (0.20-0.96)

CI, confidence interval; LR, likelihood ratio.

[a]Random-effects univariate estimates used because there were only three studies.

[b]I^2 = 45%, P = 0.16.

[c]I^2 = 0%, P = 0.75.

[d]Range because the test was only evaluated in two sets of data.

[e]Described as Patte test in Salaffi et al,[44] executed as external rotation resistance test.[25]

[f]I^2 = 70%, P = 0.04.

Reproduced with permission from Hermans J, Luime JJ, Meuffels DE, Reijman M, Simel DL, Bierma-Zeinstra SMA: Does this patient with shoulder pain have rotator cuff disease?: The rational clinical examination systematic review. *JAMA* 2013;310(8):837-847. doi:10.1001/jama.2013.276187. Copyright ©2013 American Medical Association. All rights reserved. (*Superscript numbers refer to references cited in Hermans et al.*)

Surgeons often use 50% of footprint tear as an indication for surgery for PTRCT. This recommendation began with a classic 1999 article discussing 65 patients with tear size of 50% or more who were treated with either arthroscopic acromioplasty alone or combined with mini-open rotator cuff repair.[15] Although significant for the size of the cohort and follow-up, patients were not randomized to acromioplasty versus repair, and there was no control group without repair. Thus although the "50% rule" is commonly used to determine when RCT should be repaired, the cutoff for a critical lesion is not well defined.

It is sensible to consider tear size as a continuum, to be considered with patient risk factors (**Table 1**), clinical presentation, desired activities, and response to conservative modalities, before indicating surgical intervention. Considering the high percentage of asymptomatic PTRCT with age, nonsurgical treatment is, not surprisingly, often highly effective. The ideal surgical candidate is young, active, medically uncomplicated, with a larger PTRCT of traumatic onset that has failed a trail of nonsurgical treatment.

Treatment of PTRCT

Surgical Management

In terms of surgical management, there are three primary options: débridement/acromioplasty only, in situ repair, or completion of the tear and repair with techniques similar to that used for full-thickness RCT.

Isolated acromioplasty and débridement of the PTRCT has 90% good results at 52 months.[16] Failure is associated with bursal-sided tear and larger tear size. Long-term studies suggest that favorable short-term results tend to regress with longer term follow-up. Fifty percent to 60% of athletes return to their previous level of competition.[17] Another compelling reason to consider alternatives is that isolated débridement does little to prevent the possibility of tear progression, with a risk of 34.5% (9 of 26 shoulders) at 8.4 years on follow-up ultrasonography.[18] Débridement is best reserved for small articular-sided PTRCT in elderly patients with low risk for progression.

In terms of arthroscopic repair, a main decision point is whether to complete the tear and use techniques similar to that for full-thickness RCT or to use an in situ technique, leaving the intact portion of the tendon. Biomechanical studies demonstrate superior properties of the in situ technique in cyclic loading and load to failure. Clinical outcomes between the two techniques, however, are similar and generally excellent. Multiple authors have reported that at midterm follow-up, 80% to 95% of tendons are healed,[19] and patient-reported outcomes and patient satisfaction are significantly better whether the tendon has healed or not. One study directly compared the completion technique with transtendon repair, reporting on 74 patients randomly assigned to treatment groups and followed up for a minimum of 2 years.[20] Both groups had similar improvements in Constant scores and VAS; however, the full-thickness conversion group had significantly greater improvement in postoperative strength. The literature does not clearly demonstrate the superiority of one technique over the other.

Management of Full-Thickness RCTs

Surgical Approach

There has been a transition from open, mini-open, arthroscopic-assisted open, and finally to fully arthroscopic repair techniques. Open cuff repair with transosseous sutures was regarded as the benchmark for decades. The mini-open technique avoids deltoid detachment and thus eliminates the risk of deltoid dehiscence. A randomized trial demonstrated superior results of mini-open technique at 3 months, but at 2 years there was no difference between mini- or full-open approaches.[21]

Although it is clear that arthroscopy allows for better diagnostic evaluation and the ability to address associated pathology, the ability of the surgeon to achieve the goal of a biomechanically robust repair with healing of tendon to bone is equivalent between groups. A systematic review demonstrated equivalent outcomes between groups, with the mini-open technique having a higher rate of complications including revision surgery and arthrofibrosis.[22]

Beach chair and lateral positioning are both acceptable for shoulder arthroscopy. The beach chair position does risk decreased cerebral perfusion. A few considerations will minimize this risk. First, recognized that cerebral autoregulation maintains perfusion in most scenarios, but may be compromised in an individual with significant baseline hypertension and/or with autonomic dysregulation that may result from certain medical conditions or medications. Second, noninvasive (cuff) blood pressure measurement in the arm, 20 cm below the level of the brain, means that cerebral pressure is about 15 mm Hg lower (correction: 1 mm Hg for each 1.25 cm) than the measured pressure. Finally, the surgeon and anesthesiologist should allow for mean arterial pressures of at least 60 mm Hg in healthy patients at the level of the brain, and in higher risk individuals mean arterial pressures of 80 mm Hg will allow some margin of error for periods of hypotension.

Role of Acromioplasty

Randomized trials of rotator cuff repair with and without acromioplasty demonstrate no benefit of routinely adding acromioplasty to arthroscopic rotator cuff repair. Pooled evidence from a systematic review of four randomized trials with a total of 354 patients followed up 2 years postoperatively did not support the routine use of partial acromioplasty with rotator cuff repair.[23] The available evidence points away from performing routine acromioplasty.

Shoulder

Results of Treatment

The benchmark for favorable long-term clinical outcome of full-thickness RCT is a healed rotator cuff tendon. This depends on both biology and the mechanics of the repair construct.

In terms of repair construct, double-row techniques are biomechanically superior to single-row techniques, but are more costly and time-consuming. For tears smaller than 3 cm, multiple randomized trials and systematic reviews demonstrate no clinical difference at short-term follow-up between patients treated with single-versus double-row rotator cuff repair technique.[24] There is evidence that suggests for tears larger than 3 cm, double row repair may result in better rates of healing and possibly better outcomes.[6,25]

Results of full-thickness rotator cuff repair are consistently good to excellent in the literature with predictable improvement in patient-reported outcomes, pain, strength, and return to work. Interestingly, postoperative rotator cuff integrity is not correlated with patient-reported outcomes or pain. Postoperative strength, however, is better in shoulders with healed rotator cuffs, but this difference is generally not reflected in patient satisfaction or scores. For example, in a study of arthroscopic repair for massive RCT, 94% had a retear by ultrasonography at final follow-up, but 72% of the cohort had an ASES score over 90 points.[26] Ten-year follow-up studies generally demonstrate durable clinical results and patient satisfaction.[27] Long-term data on rotator cuff integrity are lacking, but a reasonable estimate is that 70% to 90% of small to medium tears heal, whereas at least 50% of massive tears will retear.

Complications of Rotator Cuff Repair

Complications after rotator cuff repair include recurrent RCT, stiffness, slow return of function, and in less than 0.5% of cases, implant loosening, neurovascular injury, thromboembolic event, or deep infection. Stiffness presents in about 10% of cases, but about 3% do not improve with conservative measures, requiring capsular release.[28] About 30% of patients will not have recovered by 6 months.[29] Age, tear size, and preoperative motion are risk factors for delayed return of function.

The most common issue postoperatively is recurrent tear of the repaired rotator cuff. There is abundant evidence that the biologic capacity to heal is most affected by the individual's age. An ultrasonography study of 1,600 consecutive repairs at 6 months postoperatively demonstrated that retear is rare in those younger than 50 years and increases by 5% per decade with a sharp increase after age 70 years and beyond with a 34% rate after age 80 years.[30] Another study found that 86% of repaired supraspinatus tendons healed in patients younger than 65 years, whereas only 43% of the tendons healed in patients older than 65 years.[31] If the tendon heals at 1 year after surgery, there is a greater than 90% chance that it will remain healed at 2 years.[32]

Treatment of Massive RCTs

Débridement and Decompression

In select patients who are medically complicated, cannot rehabilitate, have goals limited to pain relief and light daily activities but with intact posterior rotator cuff and deltoid function, arthroscopic débridement of the shoulder with a limited acromioplasty and biceps tenotomy is an option. The coracoacromial arch must be preserved to prevent anterosuperior escape. The goal is pain relief, as strength will not improve, and the results will deteriorate over time. In a study of 31 patients with mean age of 70.6 years treated with débridement and biceps tenotomy for irreparable RCT, ASES scores improved from 24 to 70 and VAS pain scores decreased from 7.8 to 2.9 at 47 months.[33] The injured shoulder was not as functional as the contralateral side and showed radiographic progression of degenerative joint disease.

Partial Repair and Margin Convergence

Margin convergence involves placing sutures between the tendinous segments of a "U" or "L" shaped RCT to decrease the strain on the repair between the tendon edge and the tuberosity, theoretically reducing failure. Cadaver models of irreparable supraspinatus tear demonstrate that margin convergence progressively decreased strain on the subscapularis and infraspinatus repair. A partial repair should be attempted if the posterior force couple can be restored despite an irreparable supraspinatus. High-quality clinical evidence comparing partial repair to other techniques is lacking.

Tendon Transfer

Tendon transfer is used to augment weakened force couples resulting from irreparable RCT. Individuals with static subluxation, true pseudoparesis, or pain and stiffness attributable to degenerative joint disease are not candidates for tendon transfer.

The latissimus dorsi transfer has the most supporting data of tendon transfers for treatment of irreparable posterior-superior RCT. In a review of 58 shoulders 10 years after latissimus transfer for massive posterior-superior tear, the authors noted significantly improved Constant scores, pain, flexion, abduction, and strength.[34] An intact anterior force couple (subscapularis) is important to balance the transferred tendon and maximize outcome. Other factors that improve outcome are a functional deltoid, lack of preceding open shoulder surgery, male sex, and better preoperative strength. The latissimus transfer improves 1 to 2 kg of force in abduction.

Pectoralis major transfer is an option for irreparable anterosuperior RCT. Although there are several variants, the two predominant techniques involve transfer of the pectoralis major tendon over the conjoint tendon, or splitting the tendon and routing the sternal head under the conjoint tendon. The latter procedure is technically more challenging and puts the musculocutaneous nerve at risk, but has the biomechanical advantage of more closely matching the vector of the subscapularis than the more posterior to anterior vector of the pectoralis major over the conjoint tendon. The clinical results between the two techniques are not strong enough to recommend one over another. In a retrospective review of 28 patients treated with transfer over the conjoint tendon, Constant scores improved from 47% to 70% at 32 months.[35] Those with intact or repairable supraspinatus and infraspinatus muscles had superior outcomes to those without a functional infraspinatus.

An emerging technique is transfer of the latissimus and teres major to the lesser tuberosity for chronic subscapularis tears. This technique is safe, has a better vector than the pectoralis major in terms of a more anterior to posterior moment arm, is feasible with an arthroscopic-assisted technique, and is in phase as the involved tendons are all internal rotators of the shoulder.[36]

The lower trapezius tendon transfer is an emerging technique to address irreparable posterior-superior RCT. The advantages of this method include the most direct vector to the infraspinatus of the described donor options, and the redundancy of the large trapezius muscle minimizing the morbidity of harvest. The main downside is the need for allograft. In a review of open lower trapezius tendon transfer in 33 patients with a mean age of 53 years, there was a significant improvement in pain; shoulder subjective value; Disabilities of the Arm, Shoulder and Hand score; and range of motion (forward flexion, abduction, and external rotation) at a mean follow-up of 47 months.[37]

Reverse Total Shoulder Arthroplasty

As implants, techniques, and understanding of reverse total shoulder arthroplasty have improved, indications have expanded to include end-stage rotator cuff degeneration without degenerative joint disease. The outcomes of this procedure in physiologically older, low-demand individuals are well documented.[38] In a review of 60 individuals with isolated RCT treated with reverse total shoulder arthroplasty, flexion improved from 53° to 134°, external rotation from 33° to 51°, and ASES scores improved from 33 to 75 points at 52 months postoperatively. In a report of 10-year survivorship of reverse total shoulder arthroplasty for RCT with and without arthropathy, 10-year survivorship was 89% with revision as an end point, and 72% with Constant score less than 30 defined as failure.[39] Reverse total shoulder arthroplasty is a reliable option for irreparable RCT in low-demand individuals.

Emerging Techniques: Superior Capsular Reconstruction and Orthospace Balloon

Given the increasing elderly population, there is strong demand for better options for treatment of massive RCTs. Over the past 5 years, superior capsular reconstruction and the Orthospace balloon have been introduced to the market. The biodegradable subacromial spacer is designed is restore glenohumeral mechanics by reversing proximal humeral migration and restoring the fulcrum for elevation. Placement of the device is relatively quick and does not require extensive rehabilitation postoperatively. In addition, the implant does not prohibit future procedures. The subacromial balloon spacer is in widespread use in Europe and is currently being evaluated by the US FDA. One review of 39 patients at 32 months postoperatively found improvements in elevation, abduction, external rotation, and Constant score (45 to 76).[40] There are significant limitations in the outcome data, most significantly the lack of control groups to draw meaningful conclusions.

Superior capsular reconstruction is another option designed to avoid superior migration of a rotator cuff-deficient humeral head by reconstructing the capsular layer that connects the superior glenoid to the supraspinatus footprint. Preclinical data support that the dermal graft heals with tendon-like properties in animals, and that a reconstructed superior capsule depresses the humeral head and improves mechanics. The clinical literature is nascent, and limited by inconsistent graft size, variations in graft choice (fascia lata autograft vs dermal allograft), techniques, low power, and lack of control groups. At 1-year follow-up of 59 patients, pain, ASES, Subjective Shoulder Values, and motion significantly improved.[41] Although indications and prognostic factors remain an area of debate, concomitant partial repair of any repairable rotator cuff, thicker grafts, side-to-side repair with the posterior cuff, and patient selection of males with Hamada 1 or 2 arthropathy likely leads to optimal results.

When is a Rotator Cuff Not Repairable?

Patient satisfaction at midterm follow-up is not related to tendon integrity in low-demand individuals, but in younger and higher demand patients, integration of the motor unit to the tuberosity will lead to the best long-term outcomes. The three broad determinants of repair integrity are biology, repair construct, and postoperative management.

Patient factors such as age, smoking, lipid levels, genetics, prior surgery, and workers' compensation status negatively affect tendon healing to bone. Increased collagen content and fibrosis of the muscle-tendon unit make repair more technically difficult, and even if tendon healing is achieved, make the muscle less biologically responsive. This can be assessed by tear size, chronicity, atrophy, and Goutallier stage. These factors are all strongly correlated with failure, as small, acute tears of Goutallier stage 0 or 1 have a very high healing rate, whereas chronic two-tendon tears of Goutallier stage of 2 or more have a healing rate of only 20% to 30%.

Tendon rerupture is most likely to occur during the first 4 months postoperatively, when the tendon-to-bone integration is incomplete. Delaying active motion by 6 weeks or more may result in more pain, longer return of motion, but with less stress at the repair site. Earlier motion may be easier for the patient to tolerate but risks rerupture. Furthermore, early stiffness may lead to better long-term healing, as those with stiffness at 6 weeks had a higher rate of healing (30% tear) than those with better motion (64% retear).[42]

Role of the Biceps Tendon

The long head of the biceps tendon (LHBT) has been implicated in intra-articular shoulder pathology since Codman's writings nearly a century ago. Painful LHBT tendinitis may ensue from tears about the rotator interval or with any chronic inflammatory pathology of the glenohumeral joint. Clinical tests including the O'Brien, Yergason, Speed, and direct palpation tests have limited specificity, but along with a history of radiating anterior shoulder pain may inform the examiner of pain generation from the LHBT.

Other tools to evaluate biceps pathology include MRI, ultrasonography, and arthroscopic examination of the LHBT and its pulley. Of note, arthroscopic examination is limited to the intra-articular LHBT as well as the proximal groove, missing less common distal biceps groove lesions.

Treatment of LHBT pathology depends on concomitant injuries, patient factors, and surgeon preference. Isolated traumatic tears are generally treated nonsurgically with the potential rare exception of tenodesis for the dominant arm of a laborer or an individual who cannot tolerate deformity. In less physically demanding individuals who may tolerate deformity, arthroscopic tenotomy is acceptable. Outcomes are generally good to excellent, but tenotomy results in cosmetic deformity (Popeye) about 30% of the time, and vigorous activity may result in cramping pain of the biceps muscle belly.

For a patient who needs full supination strength and endurance, arthroscopic suprapectoral tenodesis may be performed for SLAP tears or in conjunction with rotator cuff repair. Finally, open or arthroscopic-assisted subpectoral tenodesis are options if biceps groove pathology is a concern. Sutures through bone tunnels have more cyclic displacement than anchors, keyhole, screw, or button techniques,[43] but there is no evidence that substantiates one approach or fixation method over another.

Shoulder Instability

Introduction

Shoulder instability is a common condition, especially in the young and athletic population. The estimated incidence is between 20 and 40 events per 100,000 people. The multicenter MOON Shoulder Instability group provided valuable insight into the epidemiology of patients undergoing surgical treatment of shoulder instability.[44] These patients are expectedly young (mean age 24 years) and frequently male (82% of the MOON cohort). Anterior instability represents approximately 80% of cases, whereas posterior and multidirectional instability account for 10% of cases each. Regardless of direction, most events (85%) are subluxations, with a small proportion (15%) being frank dislocations.

Anatomy

The shoulder is a minimally constrained ball-and-socket joint and, as a result, has the greatest mobility of any joint in the body. This comes at the expense of a relative propensity for instability. Glenohumeral stability is conferred by static and dynamic stabilizers.[45] Bony static stability is determined by the articular conformity between the humeral head and the glenoid, glenoid version and the coracoacromial arch. Soft-tissue static stabilizers include the glenoid labrum, the capsuloligamentous complex, and the rotator interval (**Figure 5**). Dynamic stability, the main mechanism in the shoulder, is provided primarily by the concavity compression of the rotator cuff pulling the humeral head into the

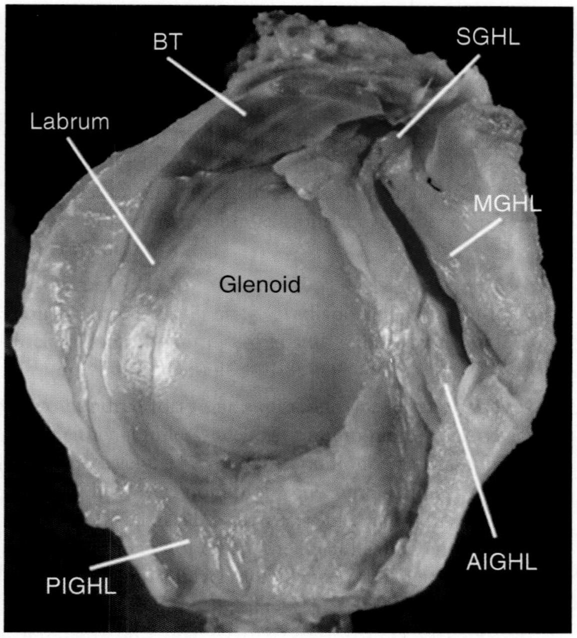

Anatomic Structure	Primary Function
SGHL	Restraint to inferior translation in adduction
MGHL	Restraint to anterior translation in abduction and external rotation
AIGHL	Most important restraint to anterior translation in abduction and external rotation
PIGHL	Most important restraint to posterior translation

Figure 5 The anatomy of the glenohumeral capsule and its thickenings, called glenohumeral ligaments, are demonstrated. AIGHL = anterior band of the inferior glenohumeral ligament; BT = biceps tendon; MGHL = middle glenohumeral ligament; PIGHL = posterior band of the inferior glenohumeral ligament; SGHL = superior glenohumeral ligament. (Left panel, Reprinted by permission from Springer Nature, Itoigawa Y, Itoi E: Anatomy of capsulolabral complex and rotator interval related to glenohumeral instability. *Knee Surg Sports Traumatol Arthrosc* 24[2]:343-349, Copyright 2016. doi:10.1007/s00167-015-3892-1.)

glenoid fossa, and also by the periscapular musculature moving the glenoid fossa to provide a stable base for the upper limb.

Anterior Instability

Natural History

Much of the understanding of the natural history of anterior shoulder instability can be credited to a landmark cohort of patients enrolled in the late 1970s and followed up for over 25 years.[46] Seventy percent of patients younger than 22 years had recurrent instability, with 50% requiring surgical stabilization. Regardless of age, glenohumeral posttraumatic arthritis developed in two-thirds of patients by the end of the 25-year period. A recent review of 26 studies summarized the natural history of anterior shoulder instability,[47] confirming high rates of recurrent instability across the board, with young age, male sex, and hyperlaxity being clear risk factors for failure of conservative treatment.

Decision Making and Nonsurgical Treatment

Perhaps the greatest challenge in treating patients with anterior shoulder instability is the decision-making process. An informed treatment decision should be guided by a thorough history and physical, careful examination of radiographs and MRI, and a discussion of the patient's activity goals including, potentially, the timing of athletic seasons.

For many patients after a first-time anterior shoulder instability event, nonsurgical treatment will be the optimal choice. Nonsurgical management is considered in preadolescents, older patients (older than 30 years), and/or in those with low activity demands, as well as in-season athletes. The definition of adequate nonsurgical treatment is subject to debate, but it typically involves a brief period of sling immobilization (3 to 7 days), followed by a course of structured rehabilitation focusing on cryotherapy, restoration of full range of motion, periscapular and rotator cuff strengthening to improve dynamic stabilizers, and finally stabilization and sport-specific drills.

Although the principles of nonsurgical management described above are helpful after a first-time dislocation, there is growing evidence that nonsurgical management in the face of recurrent instability has repercussions on the short- and long-term health of the shoulder. Multiple episodes of instability have been linked to increased attritional glenoid bone loss,[48] increased procedural complexity such as remplissage or coracoid transfer,[49] increased severity of glenoid chondral defects,[50] compromised outcomes at the time of surgical shoulder stabilization,[51] and higher rates of glenohumeral osteoarthritis.[52] In light of these data, there is growing enthusiasm for pursuing surgical stabilization after a first-time dislocation in the at-risk (eg, young and athletic) population.

Surgical Treatment

Once the decision has been made to pursue surgical intervention, a variety of surgical options are available.

Soft-Tissue Stabilization

In North America, arthroscopic anterior capsulolabral repair has become the most common surgical technique, accounting for more than 90% of surgical cases for anterior shoulder instability. An isolated arthroscopic soft-tissue stabilization is best suited for patients with little to no glenoid bone loss, minimal humeral bone loss, and good capsular and labral tissue quality. Although the overall reported outcomes of arthroscopic Bankart repair are excellent, there are growing data that this operation performs better for first-time rather than recurrent dislocators. A large 2017 cohort study showed subjective instability in 62% and revision surgery in 32% of patients undergoing arthroscopic Bankart repair after multiple episodes of instability—rates that were fourfold higher than in first-time dislocators.[53] This may be due to attritional bone loss, progressive capsular stretching, and labral degeneration with multiple dislocations.

The open Bankart procedure remains an excellent alternative to arthroscopic repair in patients without critical glenoid, humeral, or bipolar bone loss. An open Bankart repair typically involves a pants-over-vest capsular shift in addition to labral repair, and as such, the arthroscopic and open Bankart procedures are not biomechanically equivalent. Additionally, modern techniques allow an open Bankart procedure to be performed through a subscapularis split, minimizing the morbidity of subscapularis tenotomy. Numerous studies over the past 20 years have compared open and arthroscopic anterior stabilization, and these 22 studies were recently compiled in an excellent meta-analysis.[54] The authors found no difference in rates of recurrent instability or patient-reported outcomes between open and arthroscopic techniques. However, if the definition of recurrent instability is extended beyond frank dislocations to include apprehension and subluxations, open repairs outperform arthroscopic repairs.[55] Of particular interest are the results of open Bankart repair in contact athletes. Although only nonrandomized data are available, failure rates in all available studies are lower with open repairs in this population.[55] A unique scenario is a humeral avulsion of the glenohumeral ligaments, which should be identified preoperatively on MRI, and typically warrants an open repair with anchors back to the humeral neck.

Glenoid Bone Loss

Since the landmark description of glenoid bone loss, the "inverted-pear" glenoid, and their association with increased failure of soft-tissue shoulder stabilizations,[56] extensive research has confirmed the critical importance of glenoid bone stock in driving decision making and outcomes in shoulder instability. Although there is consensus on the importance of assessing glenoid bone loss, there is considerable heterogeneity in actually achieving this. The benchmark is to measure glenoid bone loss on a CT-based, 3D reconstruction of the glenoid, using a perfect circle to approximate the inferior two-thirds of the intact contralateral glenoid, and measuring the difference between this "perfect circle" and the injured glenoid contour (**Figure 6**). However, measures of glenoid bone loss are significantly affected by scapular positioning during measurement, the exact location of the best-fit circle, and the use of linear versus surface area measurements. Three-dimensional MRI quantification of glenoid bone has recently been validated as equivalent to CT-based measurements, provided specific bone-sensitive sequences are used.

Historically, 20% to 25% glenoid bone loss was the "critical amount," above which bony augmentation of the glenoid was recommended. However, in a 2015 paper, this definition of critical bone loss was brought into question.[57] In a well-designed cohort study, the authors demonstrated that patients with greater than 13.5% glenoid bone loss managed with arthroscopic Bankart repair had significantly decreased Western Ontario Shoulder Instability Index scores compatible with unacceptable outcomes, even in the absence of frank re-dislocation. Based on these findings, the category of patients with 13.5% to 20% glenoid bone loss may be better candidates for an open Bankart repair than an arthroscopic stabilization.

In cases with >20% glenoid bone loss, bony augmentation of the glenoid is the treatment of choice. This can be achieved by multiple techniques including the Bristow procedure (coracoid tip transfer), the Latarjet procedure (whole coracoid transfer), transfer of autograft bone (distal clavicle or iliac crest),

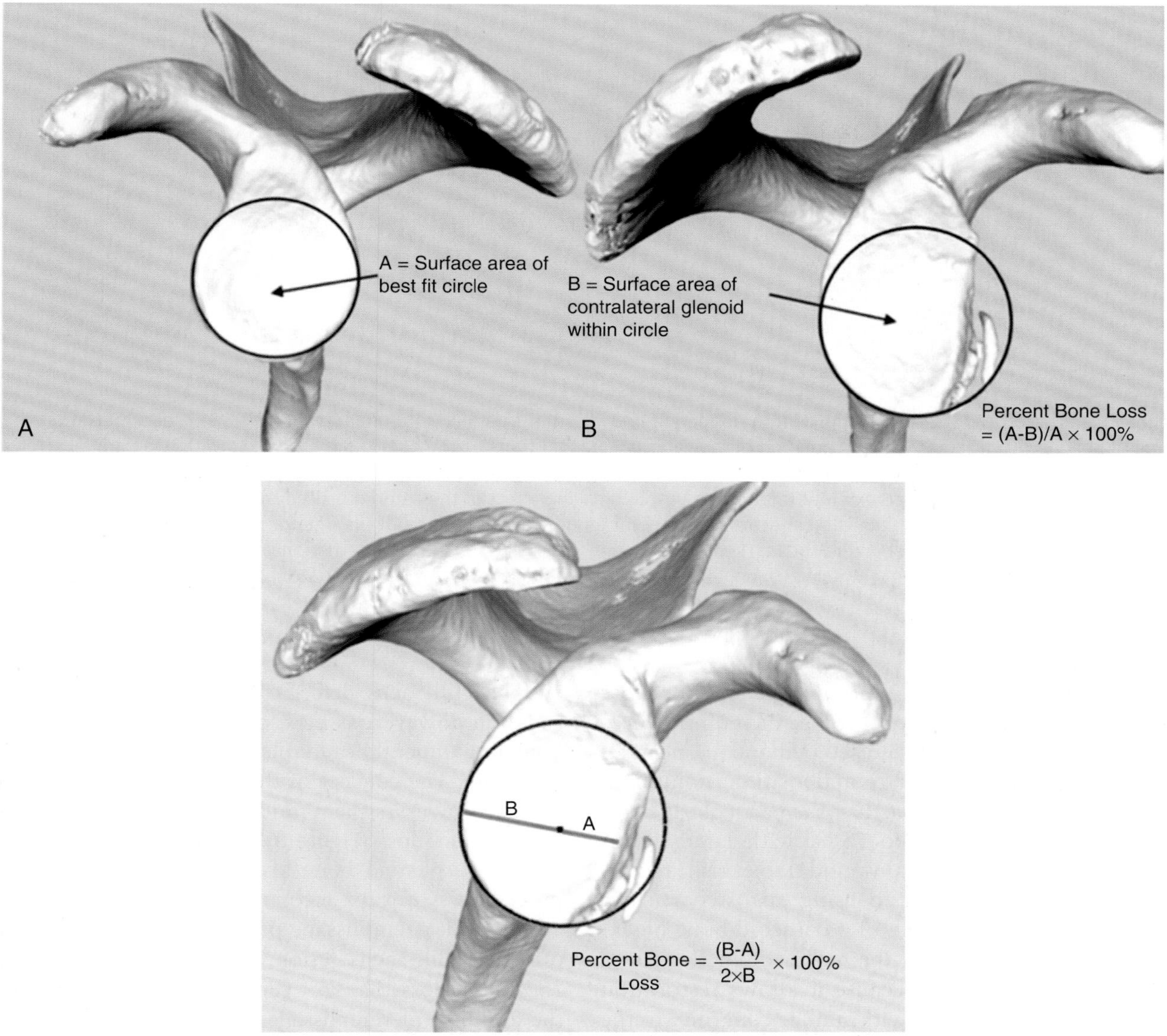

Figure 6 The percentage of glenoid bone loss can be calculated using two general techniques. The benchmark is to obtain bilateral three-dimensional CT images. A perfect circle that best fits the inferior two-thirds of the uninjured glenoid is created, and its surface area measured (A). This circle is then projected onto the injured glenoid. The surface area of injured glenoid contained within this circle (B) is measured, and the percentage of glenoid bone loss is calculated as (A − B)/(A) x 100%. If a CT scan of only the injured shoulder is available, a perfect circle estimating the inferior two-thirds of the native glenoid is created, with radius B. The distance from the center of this circle to the true glenoid edge anteriorly (A) is then measured. Percentage bone loss is calculated as (B − A)/(2 x B) x 100%. (Reprinted with permission from Bakshi NK, Cibulas GA, Sekiya JK, Bedi A: A clinical comparison of linear- and surface area–based methods of measuring glenoid bone loss. *Am J Sports Med* 2018;46[10]:2472-2477. doi:10.1177/0363546518783724.)

or transfer of an osteoarticular distal tibial allograft. The Latarjet procedure is considered the benchmark approach, because it increases shoulder stability by the "triple blocking effect (**Figure 7**)." Specifically, it (1) creates a dynamic sling of the conjoint tendon on the subscapularis in abduction and external rotation, (2) increases the bony dimensions of the glenoid, and (3) allows for reconstruction of the anterior capsule using the coracoacromial ligament. The Latarjet procedure can be performed open or arthroscopically, with similarly low recurrence (<5%) and complication rates with both.[58] However, the arthroscopic Latarjet is technically demanding, with longer surgical times and a longer learning curve. Regardless of surgical

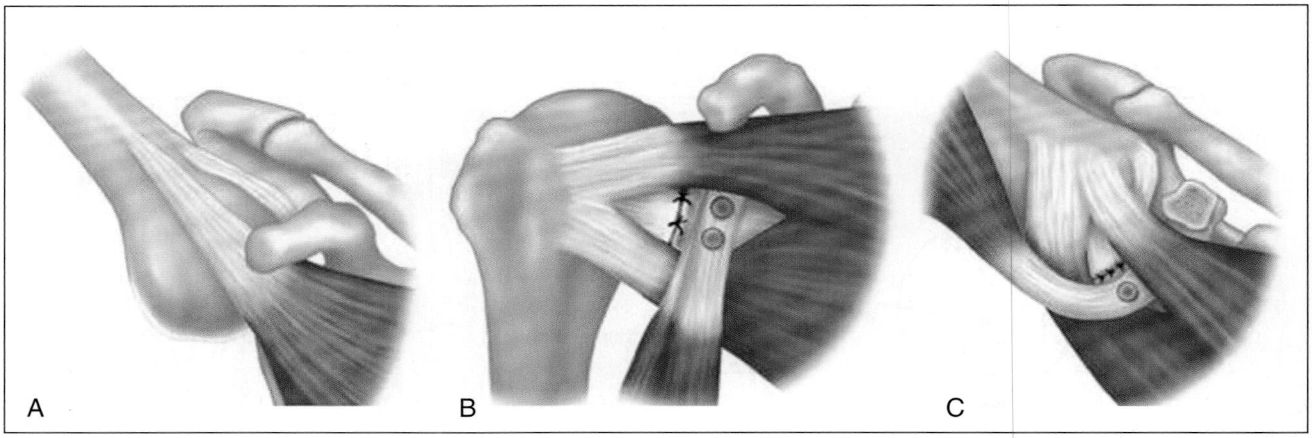

Figure 7 Latarjet procedure. **A,** With the arm in abduction and external rotation, anteroinferior displacement or subluxation of the humeral head is visualized. **B,** After completion of the Latarjet coracoid transfer, the coracoid graft is fixed with two parallel screws to the anterior glenoid neck through a split in the subscapularis. Repair of the capsule to the corarocaromial ligament stump is visualized. **C,** With the arm in abduction and external rotation, the triple blocking effect of the Latarjet procedure is visualized, with reconstruction of the glenoid surface area, the sling effect of the conjoint tendon, and tenodesis of the inferior portion of the subscapularis all contributing to restraint of the humeral head. (Republished with permission of Nancy International Ltd Subsidiary AME Publishing Company, from Mattern O, Young A, Walch G: Open latarjet: Tried, tested and true. *Ann Joint* 2017;2:65. doi:10.21037/aoj.2017.10.01.)

approach, bone block procedures for glenoid bone loss have a unique complication profile, including neurologic injury (axillary and musculocutaneous nerves), graft lysis, graft or hardware malposition, nonunion, and osteoarthritis.[59] Osteoarthritis is particularly common, estimated at 20% to 25%, with lateral graft positioning being the main modifiable risk factor. There is growing interest in using an osteoarticular distal tibial allograft in lieu of a coracoid bone block, in part because it reduces the technical challenges of the procedure, but also because it allows restoration of a true articular surface with similar congruity to the native glenoid and viable articular cartilage. The first large comparative series of distal tibial allograft (n = 50) and Latarjet procedures (n = 50) was recently published, showing equivalent patient-reported outcomes, failure, and complication rates at minimum 2-year follow-up.[60]

Humeral and Bipolar Bone Loss

Bone loss also commonly occurs on the humeral head (>90%), in the form of a Hill-Sachs deformity of the posterior-superior head. Hill-Sachs lesions can be described in terms of their depth, the amount of articular surface involved, their position with respect to the rotator cuff attachment, and their angle with respect to the long axis of the humerus. All of these factors will influence the likelihood that the Hill-Sachs lesion will "engage" with the anterior glenoid and contribute to shoulder instability.

The Hill-Sachs defect can rarely be considered in isolation however, as most cases will involve both glenoid and humeral head bone loss, referred to as bipolar bone loss. The concept of the glenoid track has helped standardize assessment and decision-making around bipolar bone loss (**Figure 8**).[61] For lesions with greater than 25% glenoid bone loss, a glenoid bone grafting procedure is always recommended, possibly with the addition of a remplissage procedure if there is also an off-track Hill-Sachs lesion. For cases with less than 25% bone loss, Bankart repair is recommended, with the addition of remplissage in the presence of an off-track humeral defect.

The remplissage procedure involves a capsulotenodesis of the infraspinatus into the humeral head defect, thereby preventing engagement of the Hill-Sachs by effectively making the lesion extra-articular in addition to providing a posterior restraint to anterior translation. The outcomes of this procedure are typically excellent with low complication rates.[62,63] However, although the available data on this topic are mixed, there is some concern about loss of shoulder rotation in overhead athletes, with ensuing difficulty returning to throwing sports, and remplissage should be considered cautiously in this population.[64] In cases of Hill-Sachs lesions extending beyond 40% of the articular surface, structural augmentation of the defect is required, either with an osteochondral allograft, focal metallic implants, or hemiarthroplasty.

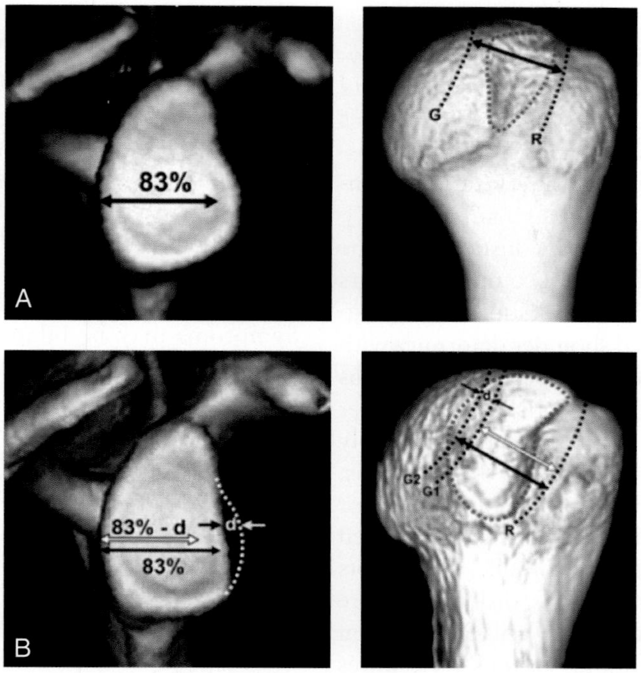

Figure 8 Technique for measuring the glenoid track on a three-dimensional CT scan. The length of the glenoid track is 83% of the maximum anterior-to-posterior diameter of the glenoid (**A**). The glenoid track length is then projected onto the humeral head extending medial from the rotator cuff attachment (R), creating the glenoid track line (G) on the humerus. This is then compared with the position of the Hill-Sachs defect (red dotted line, **B**). A defect that extends medial to G is considered off-track. When glenoid bone loss is present, the width of the defect (d) must be subtracted from the glenoid track. Thus, the original glenoid track line on the humerus (G2) must me brought laterally by the same distance (d) to create a more accurate line (G1) accounting for the bipolar bone loss. (Reprinted from Arthroscopy: The Journal of Arthroscopic & Related Surgery. Di Giacomo G, Eiji I, Burkhart SS. Evolving concept of bipolar bone loss and the hill-sachs lesion: From "engaging/non-engaging" lesion to "on-track/off-track" lesion. 30[1]:90-98, Copyright 2014, with permission from Elsevier. doi:10.1016/j.arthro.2013.10.004.)

Revision Anterior Instability Surgery

Addressing recurrent shoulder instability after prior surgical fixation is a uniquely challenging problem. Careful attention should be paid to the original surgical technique, plausible reasons for failure, and patient-specific risk factors—including bone loss (typically requiring 3D CT or 3D MRI), age, high-demand sports participation, and hyperlaxity. Although a revision arthroscopic Bankart repair is possible, high recurrent instability rates have been reported in the literature, between 30% and 45%.[65] The indications for an isolated arthroscopic Bankart revision are extremely narrow and are limited to patients with an inadequate primary repair (eg, 1-anchor repair), with no bone loss and well-preserved capsular quality. In settings with little to no glenoid bone loss, an open Bankart with capsular shift provides a reliable revision strategy. If more than 13.5% glenoid bone loss is present, or if an off-track Hill-Sachs is found, a Latarjet is likely the preferred option, though other graft options are certainly reasonable. It is important to note that remplissage has been recently shown to have high failure rates in the revision setting, as high as 35%.[66]

Posterior Instability

Clinical Presentation and Evaluation

The presentation of posterior instability is typically more subtle than anterior instability, and it is far less common, with an incidence rate of 4 per 1,000 person-years.[67] In most cases, no acute traumatic event occurs, and patients complain primarily of vague posterior shoulder pain. A focused history and physical examination, including the jerk, Kim, and posterior load shift tests, and a high index of suspicion can reveal the diagnosis. MRI is typically used to understand the anatomic injury pattern, which can include tears of the posterior labrum, posterior capsule, and variants such as the reverse humeral avulsion of the glenohumeral ligaments. In cases of recurrent instability, or if posterior glenoid bone loss is seen on plain radiographs, a CT scan may be required.

Decision Making and Nonsurgical Treatment

Nonsurgical treatment including physical therapy, activity modification, and anti-inflammatory agents should be considered for patients with minimal symptoms. This would also be the treatment of choice for voluntary posterior dislocators, in whom surgical intervention is contraindicated because of an extremely high failure rate.

A unique presentation of posterior instability is the locked posterior dislocation. This most commonly occurs with violent trauma or a seizure. This should be recognized promptly based on a fixed shoulder deformity with loss of shoulder rotation, and appropriate radiographs including an axillary view, CT, or MRI. The shoulder should be reduced by closed or open means in a timely fashion to reduce the risk of humeral head osteonecrosis. In addition, anterior capsular contracture and posterior capsular laxity develops within a few weeks of a missed dislocation which can dramatically complicate attempts at achieving stability. Fixed posterior dislocations are often associated with a large reverse Hill-Sachs lesion that requires surgical intervention. Various procedures have been described for this problem including the modified McLaughlin procedure (transfer of the lesser tuberosity and subscapularis into the humeral head defect), bone grafting and internal fixation of the humeral head, osteochondral allograft transfer to the defect, and hemiarthroplasty in severe cases.

Surgical Treatment

When nonsurgical treatment of posterior instability is unsuccessful, the benchmark treatment is an anchor-based arthroscopic capsulolabral repair. The outcomes of posterior stabilization are generally good, in a 2015 systematic review.[67] Recurrent instability rates are low (8%), and 90% return to sport. However, it should be noted that in throwers, only 58% were able to return to sport at the same level. Revision surgery is only required in 6% of patients with posterior instability, and the outcomes are far inferior to those of index surgery, with only 15% returning to sport at their preoperative level.

Posterior glenoid bone loss is less common than anterior loss, but can present significant challenge in the face of recurrent posterior instability. Although there is no consensus on the critical amount of posterior bone loss, recent biomechanical data suggest that beyond 20% posterior bone loss an isolated labral repair cannot restore adequate shoulder stability.[68] Large acute bony fragments can be included into a capsulolabral repair, yet chronic attritional bony injuries require grafting. This has been described using the iliac crest, distal tibia, or scapular spine, with either open or arthroscopic techniques.

Multidirectional Instability

Multidirectional shoulder instability (MDI) is a complex condition defined as symptomatic instability in at least two directions. Unlike unidirectional instability, the presentation is typically atraumatic and includes complaints of vague shoulder pain, decreased athletic performance with the arm, secondary shoulder girdle muscle spasm, and even distal neurologic symptoms from repetitive stretch to the brachial plexus. Symptoms may be bilateral, but in overhead athletes tend to be in the dominant arm. MDI is often, though not necessarily, associated with generalized joint laxity, whether from a congenital connective tissue disorder (Ehlers-Danlos, Marfan, etc) or from benign joint hypermobility. In patients with joint hypermobility, it is critical to differentiate shoulder laxity (increased translation on examination) from shoulder instability, as many lax shoulders are asymptomatic. It is recommended that all patients evaluated for shoulder instability be screened for joint hypermobility using the Beighton criteria.

In the absence of labral or capsular tears on MRI, nonsurgical treatment with physical therapy aimed at improving the dynamic stabilizers is considered the benchmark for MDI. If patients remain symptomatic in spite of 3 to 6 months of physical therapy, surgical shoulder stabilization may be required. In the absence of a congenital connective tissue disorder or severe joint hypermobility, an anchor-based pancapsular plication with labral repair as needed is considered an effective treatment.[69] However, it should be noted that the outcomes are more guarded than with unidirectional instability, with only 75% returning to sport and 25% to 40% experiencing postsurgical subluxations. Female sex, high Beighton score, and atraumatic onset of symptoms are strong negative predictors of outcome after pancapsular plication. In the presence of a high Beighton score or a known congenital connective tissue disorder, most experts recommend a formal open inferior capsular shift with or without augmentation of deficient collagen with allograft of xenograft patches.[70]

Muscular Ruptures

Muscular or musculotendinous ruptures of the shoulder (excluding rotator cuff injuries) are quite rare. These typically involve the long head of the biceps, the pectoralis major, the deltoid, or the latissimus dorsi. Biceps long head spontaneous rupture is seen in the elderly (often male) population, usually as the result of an eccentric contraction of the biceps during a fall. Treatment typically consists of observation, as the functional impact of a long head rupture is minimal. Patients should be counseled about the cosmetic "Popeye deformity" they can expect in their biceps.

In contrast, pectoralis major tears are most commonly seen in young, athletic males, typically during bench press. There is also an association with the use of anabolic steroids. Patients usually present after hearing a "pop" at the end of the eccentric phase of the bench press, when the bar is on the chest, with associated ecchymosis of the anterior shoulder and visible chest deformity. Isolated tears of the sternal head are most frequent, but full-thickness tears of both sternal and clavicular heads can occur. Although intramuscular and musculotendinous junction tears are typically irreparable, more distal injuries to the tendon should be treated with acute repair. Chronic or neglected tears often retract medially and may require interposition allograft reconstruction.

Avulsion injuries of the latissimus dorsi are extremely rare and are seen in competitive overhead athletes as the latissimus is a powerful decelerator of the arm during the follow-through phase. There is some controversy regarding the management of these injuries, with some authors showing a high rate of return to play, but others noting more guarded results with nonsurgical treatment and promising results have been described with primary repair of the latissimus to the humerus.

Finally, deltoid muscular ruptures can be seen rarely, usually as a result of iatrogenic injury after open rotator cuff surgery. Deltoid rupture can be a devastating complication, resulting in severe shoulder weakness and dysfunction, and when identified, should prompt acute surgical repair through trans-acromial drill holes as the rapid retraction and poor-suture holding qualities of the proximal deltoid tendon make repair challenging.

Summary

Labral and rotator cuff pathology are the most common sources of shoulder pain and dysfunction in adults. The treating provider must be familiar with common presenting symptoms, physical examination signs, and diagnostic imaging modalities to partner with the patient to choose the treatment with the highest chance of success with a reasonable risk profile. The options are highly variable and may require referral to a specialist, ranging from conservative management to tendon transfer and arthroplasty.

Key Study Points

- Anterior instability is the most common form of shoulder instability and is most common in young males active in contact sports.
- Decision making about treatment in anterior instability is complex, and assessment of glenoid and humeral bone loss, including calculation of the glenoid track, is of critical importance.
- Posterior and multidirectional instability represent about 10% each of shoulder instability. When nonsurgical treatment fails, arthroscopic stabilization, including capsular plication as necessary, is effective at treating these conditions.
- Steroid injection with physical therapy, extracorporeal shockwave therapy, ultrasound-guided needle lavage, and arthroscopic débridement are all valid options for treatment of rotator cuff calcific tendinitis.
- Patient-reported outcomes and pain are not correlated with rotator cuff healing on ultrasonography or MRI. Postoperative strength is better in individuals with healed rotator cuffs versus those with defects after repair.

Shoulder

Annotated References

1. Uhthoff HK, Loehr JW: Calcific tendinopathy of the rotator cuff: Pathogenesis, diagnosis, and management. *J Am Acad Orthop Surg* 1997;5:183-191.
2. Ogon P, Suedkamp N, Jaeger M, Izadpanah K, Koestler W, Maier D: Prognostic factors in nonoperative therapy for chronic symptomatic calcific tendinitis of the shoulder. *Arthritis Rheum* 2009;60:2978-2984.
3. Gerdesmeyer L, Wagenpfeil S, Haake M, et al: Extracorporeal shock wave therapy for the treatment of chronic calcifying tendonitis of the rotator cuff: A randomized controlled trial. *JAMA* 2003;290:2573-2580.
4. Daecke W, Kusnierczak D, Loew M: Long-term effects of extracorporeal shockwave therapy in chronic calcific tendinitis of the shoulder. *J Shoulder Elbow Surg* 2002;11:476-480.
5. de Witte PB, Selten JW, Navas A, et al: Calcific tendinitis of the rotator cuff: A randomized controlled trial of ultrasound-guided needling and lavage versus subacromial corticosteroids. *Am J Sports Med* 2013;41:1665-1673.
6. Pennington WT, Gibbons DJ, Bartz BA, et al: Comparative analysis of single-row versus double-row repair of rotator cuff tears. *Arthroscopy* 2010;26:1419-1426.

7. Maier D, Jaeger M, Izadpanah K, Bornebusch L, Suedkamp NP, Ogon P: Rotator cuff preservation in arthroscopic treatment of calcific tendinitis. *Arthrosc J Arthrosc Relat Surg* 2013;29:824-831.

8. Tashjian RZ, Granger EK, Farnham JM, Cannon-Albright LA, Teerlink CC: Genome-wide association study for rotator cuff tears identifies two significant single-nucleotide polymorphisms. *J Shoulder Elbow Surg* 2016;25:174-179.

The authors compared the genomes of 311 individuals with full-thickness RCT with a database of control subjects to search for nucleotide polymorphisms associated with the disease. They found two correlated single nucleotide polymorphisms associated with full-thickness RCT, lending evidence to hypothesis that there is a genetic component to rotator cuff disease.

9. Moor BK, Wieser K, Slankamenac K, Gerber C, Bouaicha S: Relationship of individual scapular anatomy and degenerative rotator cuff tears. *J Shoulder Elbow Surg* 2014;23:536-541.

This study retrospectively analyzed the scapular anatomy of shoulders with a simple radiographic measurement, the "critical shoulder angle." They found statistically significant differences in the angle between 92 asymptomatic individuals, 102 with osteoarthritis, and 102 patients with full-thickness RCT. These data support that there is a mechanical difference between those with arthritis and RC disease.

10. Dunn WR, Kuhn JE, Sanders R, et al: Symptoms of pain do not correlate with rotator cuff tear severity: A cross-sectional study of 393 patients with a symptomatic atraumatic full-thickness rotator cuff tear. *J Bone Joint Surg Am* 2014;96:793.

11. Yamaguchi K, Tetro AM, Blam O, Evanoff BA, Teefey SA, Middleton WD: Natural history of asymptomatic rotator cuff tears: A longitudinal analysis of asymptomatic tears detected sonographically. *J Shoulder Elbow Surg* 2001;10:199-203.

12. Safran O, Schroeder J, Bloom R, Weil Y, Milgrom C: Natural history of nonoperatively treated symptomatic rotator cuff tears in patients 60 years old or younger. *Am J Sports Med* 2011;39:710-714.

13. Sher JS, Uribe JW, Posada A, Murphy BJ, Zlatkin MB: Abnormal findings on magnetic resonance images of asymptomatic shoulders. *JBJS* 1995;77:10-15.

14. Kim Y-S, Kim S-E, Bae S-H, Lee H-J, Jee W-H, Park CK: Tear progression of symptomatic full-thickness and partial-thickness rotator cuff tears as measured by repeated MRI. *Knee Surg Sports Traumatol Arthrosc* 2017;25: 2073-2080.

The authors obtained MRI on 122 patients with full or partial RCT at presentation and at minimum 6 months later. The cohort was retrospectively analyzed for risk factors for progression. 53% increased tear size. Progression correlated with presenting tear size.

15. Weber SC: Arthroscopic debridement and acromioplasty versus mini-open repair in the treatment of significant partial-thickness rotator cuff tears. *Arthroscopy* 1999;15: 126-131.

16. Cordasco FA, Backer M, Craig EV, Klein D, Warren RF: The partial-thickness rotator cuff tear: Is acromioplasty without repair sufficient? *Am J Sports Med* 2002;30:257-260.

17. Reynolds SB, Dugas JR, Cain EL, McMichael CS, Andrews JR: Debridement of small partial-thickness rotator cuff tears in elite overhead throwers. *Clin Orthop Relat Res* 2008;466:614-621.

18. Kartus J, Kartus C, Rostgård-Christensen L, Sernert N, Read J, Perko M: Long-term clinical and ultrasound evaluation after arthroscopic acromioplasty in patients with partial rotator cuff tears. *Arthroscopy* 2006;22:44-49.

19. Kamath G, Galatz LM, Keener JD, Teefey S, Middleton W, Yamaguchi K: Tendon integrity and functional outcome after arthroscopic repair of high-grade partial-thickness supraspinatus tears. *JBJS* 2009;91:1055-1062.

20. Castagna A, Borroni M, Garofalo R, et al: Deep partial rotator cuff tear: Transtendon repair or tear completion and repair? A randomized clinical trial. *Knee Surg Sports Traumatol Arthrosc* 2015;23:460-463.

At a minimum of 2-year follow-up, there was no difference between treatment groups, in a randomized control trial of 74 patients with PASTA tears treated with transtendon repair or completion and repair.

21. Mohtadi NG, Hollinshead RM, Sasyniuk TM, Fletcher JA, Chan DS, Li FX: A randomized clinical trial comparing open to arthroscopic acromioplasty with mini-open rotator cuff repair for full-thickness rotator cuff tears: Disease-specific quality of life outcome at an average 2-year follow-up. *Am J Sports Med* 2008;36:1043-1051.

22. Nho SJ, Shindle MK, Sherman SL, Freedman KB, Lyman S, MacGillivray JD: Systematic review of arthroscopic rotator cuff repair and mini-open rotator cuff repair. *JBJS* 2007;89: 127-136.

23. Familiari F, Gonzalez-Zapata A, Ianno B, Galasso O, Gasparini G, McFarland EG: Is acromioplasty necessary in the setting of full-thickness rotator cuff tears? A systematic review. *J Orthop Traumatol* 2015;16:167-174.

A systematic review of four level I and II studies did not find support for routine acromioplasty in the setting of rotator cuff disease.

24. Burks RT, Crim J, Brown N, Fink B, Greis PE: A prospective randomized clinical trial comparing arthroscopic single-and double-row rotator cuff repair: Magnetic resonance imaging and early clinical evaluation. *Am J Sports Med* 2009;37:674-682.

25. Park J-Y, Lhee S-H, Choi J-H, Park H-K, Yu J-W, Seo J-B. Comparison of the clinical outcomes of single-and double-row repairs in rotator cuff tears. *Am J Sports Med* 2008;36: 1310-1316.

26. Galatz LM, Ball CM, Teefey SA, Middleton WD, Yamaguchi K: The outcome and repair integrity of completely arthroscopically repaired large and massive rotator cuff tears. *JBJS* 2004;86:219-224.

27. Wilson F, Hinov V, Adams G: Arthroscopic repair of full-thickness tears of the rotator cuff: 2-to 14-year follow-up. *Arthroscopy* 2002;18:136-144.

28. Randelli P, Spennacchio P, Ragone V, Arrigoni P, Casella A, Cabitza P: Complications associated with arthroscopic rotator cuff repair: A literature review. *Musculoskelet Surg* 2012;96:9-16.

29. Manaka T, Ito Y, Matsumoto I, Takaoka K, Nakamura H: Functional recovery period after arthroscopic rotator cuff repair: Is it predictable before surgery? *Clin Orthop Relat Res* 2011;469:1660-1666.

30. Diebold G, Lam P, Walton J, Murrell GA: Relationship between age and rotator cuff retear: A study of 1,600 consecutive rotator cuff repairs. *JBJS* 2017;99:1198-1205.

The authors evaluated retear by ultrasonography at 6 months post repair in 1,600 cases. They found that retear increases substantially by decade, with a retear rate of 5% in those younger than 50 years and culminating at 34% in those older than 80 years.

31. Boileau P, Brassart N, Watkinson DJ, Carles M, Hatzidakis AM, Krishnan SG: Arthroscopic repair of full-thickness tears of the supraspinatus: Does the tendon really heal? *JBJS* 2005;87:1229-1240.

32. Nho SJ, Adler RS, Tomlinson DP, et al: Arthroscopic rotator cuff repair: Prospective evaluation with sequential ultrasonography. *Am J Sports Med* 2009;37:1938-1945.

33. Liem D, Lengers N, Dedy N, Poetzl W, Steinbeck J, Marquardt B: Arthroscopic debridement of massive irreparable rotator cuff tears. *Arthroscopy* 2008;24:743-748.

34. Gerber C, Rahm SA, Catanzaro S, Farshad M, Moor BK: Latissimus dorsi tendon transfer for treatment of irreparable posterosuperior rotator cuff tears: Long-term results at a minimum follow-up of ten years. *JBJS* 2013;95:1920-1926.

35. Jost B, Puskas GJ, Lustenberger A, Gerber C: Outcome of pectoralis major transfer for the treatment of irreparable subscapularis tears. *JBJS* 2003;85:1944-1951.

36. Elhassan B, Christensen TJ, Wagner ER: Feasibility of latissimus and teres major transfer to reconstruct irreparable subscapularis tendon tear: An anatomic study. *J Shoulder Elbow Surg* 2014;23:492-499.

37. Elhassan BT, Wagner ER, Werthel J-D. Outcome of lower trapezius transfer to reconstruct massive irreparable posterior-superior rotator cuff tear. *J Shoulder Elbow Surg* 2016;25:1346-1353.

The authors retrospectively reviewed 33 patients at an average of nearly 4 years after lower trapezius transfer for massive superior rotator cuff tear. All but one patient improved functionally and on patient-reported outcomes. Greater than 60° of active preoperative flexion was associated with more functional gains.

38. Mulieri P, Dunning P, Klein S, Pupello D, Frankle M: Reverse shoulder arthroplasty for the treatment of irreparable rotator cuff tear without glenohumeral arthritis. *JBJS* 2010;92:2544-2556.

39. Favard L, Levigne C, Nerot C, Gerber C, De Wilde L, Mole D: Reverse prostheses in arthropathies with cuff tear: Are survivorship and function maintained over time? *Clin Orthop Relat Res* 2011;469:2469-2475.

40. Deranlot J, Herisson O, Nourissat G, et al: Arthroscopic subacromial spacer implantation in patients with massive irreparable rotator cuff tears: Clinical and radiographic results of 39 retrospective cases. *Arthrosc J Arthrosc Relat Surg* 2017;33:1639-1644.

39 consecutive shoulders treated with arthroscopic subacromial balloon implantation for symptomatic massive rotator cuff tears were followed up for a mean of 32 months. Pain decreased, range of motion improved, and there was narrowing of the acromiohumeral interval.

41. Denard PJ, Brady PC, Adams CR, Tokish JM, Burkhart SS: Preliminary results of arthroscopic superior capsule reconstruction with dermal allograft. *Arthrosc J Arthrosc Relat Surg* 2018;34:93-99.

A multicenter study retrospectively reviewed 59 patients at minimum 1 year after superior capsular reconstruction for massive irreparable cuff tear. 19% required an additional procedure in the study period and 45% of the grafts healed completely on MRI. Good results in terms of motion, ASES score, and pain were associated with 3 mm dermal grafts and Hamada 1 or 2 disease states.

42. Parsons BO, Gruson KI, Chen DD, Harrison AK, Gladstone J, Flatow EL: Does slower rehabilitation after arthroscopic rotator cuff repair lead to long-term stiffness? *J Shoulder Elbow Surg* 2010;19:1034-1039.

43. Mazzocca AD, Bicos J, Santangelo S, Romeo AA, Arciero RA: The biomechanical evaluation of four fixation techniques for proximal biceps tenodesis. *Arthrosc J Arthrosc Relat Surg* 2005;21:1296-1306.

44. Kraeutler MJ, McCarty EC, Belk JW, et al: Descriptive epidemiology of the MOON shoulder instability cohort. *Am J Sports Med* 2018;46:1064-1069.

45. Murray IR, Goudie EB, Petrigliano FA, Robinson CM: Functional anatomy and biomechanics of shoulder stability in the athlete. *Clin Sports Med* 2013;32:607-624.

46. Hovelius L, Rahme H: Primary anterior dislocation of the shoulder: Long-term prognosis at the age of 40 years or younger. *Knee Surg Sports Traumatol Arthrosc* 2016;24:330-342.

47. Galvin JW, Ernat JJ, Waterman BR, Stadecker MJ, Parada SA: The epidemiology and natural history of anterior shoulder instability. *Curr Rev Musculoskelet Med* 2017;10:411-424.

48. Nakagawa S, Ozaki R, Take Y, Mizuno N, Mae T: Enlargement of glenoid defects in traumatic anterior shoulder instability: Influence of the number of recurrences and type of sport. *Orthop J Sports Med* 2014;2:2325967114529920.

49. Denard PJ, Dai X, Burkhart SS: Increasing preoperative dislocations and total time of dislocation affect surgical management of anterior shoulder instability. *Int J Shoulder Surg* 2015;9:1.

50. Krych AJ, Sousa PL, King AH, Morgan JA, May JH, Dahm DL: The effect of cartilage injury after arthroscopic stabilization for shoulder instability. *Orthopedics* 2015;38:e965-e969.

51. Marshall T, Vega J, Siqueira M, Cagle R, Gelber JD, Saluan P: Outcomes after arthroscopic Bankart repair: Patients with first-time versus recurrent dislocations. *Am J Sports Med* 2017;45:1776-1782.

52. Buscayret F, Edwards TB, Szabo I, Adeleine P, Coudane H, Walch G: Glenohumeral arthrosis in anterior instability before and after surgical treatment: Incidence and contributing factors. *Am J Sports Med* 2004;32:1165-1172.

53. Hohmann E, Tetsworth K, Glatt V: Open versus arthroscopic surgical treatment for anterior shoulder dislocation: A comparative systematic review and meta-analysis over the past 20 years. *J Shoulder Elbow Surg* 2017;26: 1873-1880.

54. Miura K, Tsuda E, Tohyama H, et al: Can arthroscopic Bankart repairs using suture anchors restore equivalent stability to open repairs in the management of traumatic anterior shoulder dislocation? A meta-analysis. *J Orthop Sci* 2018;23(6):935-941.

55. Sanborn L, Arciero RA, Yang JS: Don't forget the open Bankart—Look at the evidence. *Annals of Joint* 2017;2.

56. Burkhart SS, De Beer JF: Traumatic glenohumeral bone defects and their relationship to failure of arthroscopic Bankart repairs: Significance of the inverted-pear glenoid and the humeral engaging hill-sachs lesion. *Arthrosc J Arthrosc Relat Surg* 2000;16:677-694.

57. Shaha JS, Cook JB, Song DJ, et al: Redefining "critical" bone loss in shoulder instability: Functional outcomes worsen with "subcritical" bone loss. *Am J Sports Med* 2015;43:1719-1725.

58. Horner NS, Moroz PA, Bhullar R, et al: Open versus arthroscopic latarjet procedures for the treatment of shoulder instability: A systematic review of comparative studies. *BMC Musculoskelet Disord* 2018;19:255.

59. Domos P, Lunini E, Walch G: Contraindications and complications of the Latarjet procedure. *Shoulder Elbow* 2018;10:15-24.

60. Frank RM, Romeo AA, Richardson C, et al: Outcomes of latarjet versus distal tibia allograft for anterior shoulder instability repair: A matched cohort analysis. *Am J Sports Med* 2018;46:1030-1038.

61. Di Giacomo G, Itoi E, Burkhart SS: Evolving concept of bipolar bone loss and the Hill-Sachs lesion: From "engaging/non-engaging" lesion to "on-track/off-track" lesion. *Arthrosc J Arthrosc Relat Surg* 2014;30:90-98.

62. Buza JA III, Iyengar JJ, Anakwenze OA, Ahmad CS, Levine WN: Arthroscopic Hill-Sachs remplissage: A systematic review. *JBJS* 2014;96:549-555.

63. Garcia GH, Wu H-H, Liu JN, Huffman GR, Kelly JD IV: Outcomes of the remplissage procedure and its effects on return to sports: Average 5-year follow-up. *Am J Sports Med* 2016;44:1124-1130.

64. Su F, Kowalczuk M, Ikpe S, Lee H, Sabzevari S, Lin A: Risk factors for failure of arthroscopic revision anterior shoulder stabilization. *JBJS* 2018;100:1319-1325.

65. Yang JS, Mazzocca AD, Arciero RA: Remplissage versus modified latarjet for off-track hill-sachs lesions with subcritical glenoid bone loss. *Orthop J Sports Med* 2017;5:2325967117S2325900274.

66. Lanzi JT, Chandler PJ, Cameron KL, Bader JM, Owens BD: Epidemiology of posterior glenohumeral instability in a young athletic population. *Am J Sports Med* 2017;45:3315-3321.

67. DeLong JM, Jiang K, Bradley JP: Posterior instability of the shoulder: A systematic review and meta-analysis of clinical outcomes. *Am J Sports Med* 2015;43:1805-1817.

68. Nacca C, Gil JA, Badida R, Crisco JJ, Owens BD: Critical glenoid bone loss in posterior shoulder instability. *Am J Sports Med* 2018;46:1058-1063.

69. Raynor MB, Horan MP, Greenspoon JA, Katthagen JC, Millett PJ: Outcomes after arthroscopic pancapsular capsulorrhaphy with suture anchors for the treatment of multidirectional glenohumeral instability in athletes. *Am J Sports Med* 2016;44:3188-3197.

70. Vavken P, Tepolt FA, Kocher MS: Open inferior capsular shift for multidirectional shoulder instability in adolescents with generalized ligamentous hyperlaxity or Ehlers-Danlos syndrome. *J Shoulder Elbow Surg* 2016;25:907-912.

Chapter 25

Shoulder Arthritis and Arthroplasty

Vahid Entezari, MD, MMSc • Eric T. Ricchetti, MD

ABSTRACT

The shoulder encompasses two diarthrodial joints—the glenohumeral (GH) joint and the acromioclavicular joint (AC)—and either can develop arthritis. Arthritic changes in the AC joint are common in patients older than 60 years with a low correlation between imaging and patient symptoms. Cortisone injection is effective in alleviating pain, and in patients who do not have lasting relief, distal clavicle excision (DCE) is an effective surgical treatment for symptomatic AC arthritis. One-third of patients older than 60 years with shoulder pain have GH arthritis. Primary GH osteoarthritis (OA) is common in elderly females and younger patients with manual labor and heavy weight-lifting habits. In addition to primary GH OA, secondary forms of GH arthritis include posttraumatic arthritis after proximal humerus or glenoid fracture, inflammatory arthritis (including rheumatoid arthritis, psoriatic arthritis, gout, and others), instability arthropathy and capsulorrhaphy arthropathy, osteonecrosis of the humeral head, cuff tear arthropathy in patients with long-standing rotator cuff failure, Charcot arthropathy, and arthropathy of hemophilia. In addition to a history and physical examination, evaluation of GH arthritis starts with plain radiographs. Advanced imaging such as CT and/or MRI may be ordered to assess glenoid and humeral morphology, rotator cuff integrity, and for preoperative planning. The modified Walch classification uses axial CT imaging to categorize primary GH OA based on glenoid erosion and humeral head subluxation. When arthritic changes are mild in young and active patients, arthroscopic débridement can be effective in delaying reconstructive surgery. Hemiarthroplasty is associated with high rate of glenoid erosion and revision, and its use should be limited to young patients with severe GH arthritis and high level of activity or patients with unipolar arthritic disease (eg, osteonecrosis of the humeral head with collapse but without significant glenoid chondral involvement). Anatomic total shoulder arthroplasty (ATSA) is the benchmark for surgical treatment of GH arthritis with an intact cuff with excellent mid- to long-term outcomes. There is a growing trend in performing ATSA with short stem and stemless humeral components and using augmented glenoid components to address glenoid bony deficiency. Reverse total shoulder arthroplasty (RTSA) has gained popularity in recent years for surgical treatment of rotator cuff arthropathy, comminuted proximal humerus fractures, irreparable rotator cuff tears without arthritis, and revision arthroplasty. Overall complications rate of anatomic and RTSA are reported as 10% and 16%, respectively. Glenoid component loosening, instability, and rotator cuff failure are the most common complications after ATSA, and instability, periprosthetic fracture, and infection are the most common complications after RTSA.

Dr. Entezari or an immediate family member serves as a paid consultant to or is an employee of DJ Orthopaedics and has received research or institutional support from OREF. Dr. Ricchetti or an immediate family member has received royalties from DJ Orthopaedics; is a member of a speakers' bureau or has made paid presentations on behalf of DJ Orthopaedics; serves as a paid consultant to or is an employee of DJ Orthopaedics; and serves as a board member, owner, officer, or committee member of the American Academy of Orthopaedic Surgeons, the American Board of Orthopaedic Surgery, Inc., and the American Shoulder and Elbow Surgeons.

Keywords: Acromioclavicular arthritis; hemiarthroplasty; reverse shoulder arthroplasty; shoulder arthritis; shoulder arthroplasty

Introduction

Shoulder arthritis is a degenerative process resulting in a loss of cartilage, synovitis, and capsular thickening, which frequently reduces joint mobility. With an aging population and a trend toward a more active lifestyle, the prevalence of symptomatic shoulder arthritis is rising. This chapter reviews and presents the current literature on presentation, evaluation, and treatment of acromioclavicular (AC) and glenohumeral (GH) arthritis.

Acromioclavicular Arthritis

The AC joint is a diarthrodial joint between the distal clavicle and acromial process. This joint is subjected to motion with hinging and translation during arm abduction and rotation around the long axis of the clavicle with forward elevation. The AC joint contains an intra-articular fibrocartilage disk which shows signs of degeneration starting in the second decade of life.[1] Radiographic AC joint narrowing is commonly seen in patients older than 60 years. Arthritis is the most common cause of pain in the AC joint and can be caused by degenerative, posttraumatic (prior AC dislocation, distal clavicle fracture or heavy lifting), septic, or inflammatory etiologies. Distal clavicle osteolysis is a distinct presentation of AC arthritis in young adults who frequently engage in overhead sports or repetitive heavy lifting.[2]

Presentation/Evaluation

Patients with AC arthritis generally present with pain localized to the AC joint, with occasional referred pain radiating into the trapezius, which is worse at night and aggravated by overhead and cross-body adduction activities. On examination, tenderness over the AC joint and positive provocative tests such as cross-body adduction (maximum adduction with the arm in 90° of forward flexion) or O'Brien compression test (resisted forward elevation causing pain only in internal rotation with arm in 90° of forward elevation and 10° of adduction) are highly suggestive of AC joint pathology.[3] Radiographic evaluation should include a Zanca view (AP view with 10° cephalad tilt), which avoids overlapping of the clavicle and the acromion. Common radiographic findings are joint space narrowing, osteophyte formation, and possibly joint malalignment in those patients with a history of AC dislocation. While radiographic findings are frequently asymptomatic, significant bone edema on MRI has a better correlation with symptomatic AC arthritis.[4] Despite this, the false-positive rate of MRI for true AC arthritis is reported to be as high as 82%.[5] Therefore, clinical correlation of any imaging findings is critical.

Treatment

The first-line of treatment for AC arthritis is nonsurgical, including rest, activity modification (avoiding repetitive overhead activities and heavy lifting), anti-inflammatory medications, cortisone injections, and physical therapy. Cortisone injections are highly effective in improving patients' pain and function in the short-term and although they commonly need to be repeated, studies show benefit for up to 5 years.[6] When nonsurgical interventions fail, open or arthroscopic DCE can be performed. There has been a trend toward arthroscopic DCE in recent years due to presumed lower complication rate, better cosmesis, and ability to evaluate other shoulder pathologies which are present in 98% of patients with symptomatic AC arthritis.[7] A biomechanical study demonstrated that DCE of more than 5 mm is sufficient to avoid any bony contact and resection of more than 15 mm risks causing coracoclavicular ligament incompetency.[8] A randomized clinical trial showed adding DCE to an arthroscopic rotator cuff repair in patients with symptomatic AC arthritis did not change patient reported outcomes at minimum 2-year follow-up.[9] This emphasizes the importance of having sound indications to perform DCE. Complications of DCE, although uncommon, include persistent pain, over resection causing instability, infection, heterotopic ossification, suprascapular nerve injury, and failure to completely address the pathology—most commonly with underresection of the posterosuperior distal clavicle.

Glenohumeral Arthritis

The glenohumeral (GH) joint is a diarthrodial, ball and socket type joint with the largest mobility of any joint in the body. GH arthritis is defined by degradation of articular cartilage and adaptations in the bone, labrum, and capsule that lead to increased joint friction and progressive loss of motion. Prevalence of GH arthritis in the general population is far less common than lower extremity weight-bearing joints. However, radiographic findings of GH arthritis are present in up to one-third of patients older than 60 years who have shoulder pain.[10] Risk factors for GH arthritis include genetic predisposition, age older than 70 years, female sex, occupation (eg, repetitive, heavy manual labor), inflammatory disease, prior shoulder dislocation, fracture, osteonecrosis, infection, rotator cuff tear, certain medical conditions (eg, hemophilia), and prior surgical procedure. A classification of GH arthritis and its common etiologies are presented in **Table 1**. We will briefly review the common etiologies of secondary GH arthritis.

Post-traumatic

A history of major or repetitive injury to the shoulder joint has been recognized as one of the leading causes

Table 1

Classification of Glenohumeral (GH) Arthritis Etiology

Type	Etiology
Primary	Idiopathic
Secondary	
Posttraumatic	Proximal humerus fracture
	Dislocation/recurrent instability
	Microtrauma (manual labor, heavy lifting)
Inflammatory	Crystal induced
	Rheumatoid arthritis (RA)
	Systemic lupus erythematous (SLE)
	Seronegative osteoarthropathies
Postsurgical	Capsulorrhaphy
	Rotator cuff repair
	Intra-articular hardware
Osteonecrosis	Corticosteroids
	Alcohol
	Chemo/radiation
	Sickle cell disease
	Metabolic disease (eg, Gaucher disease)
	Malignancy (eg, multiple myeloma)
	Trauma/dislocation
Septic	Acute purulent infection
	Chronic indolent infection
Cuff arthropathy	Massive rotator cuff tear
Neuropathic arthropathy	Syringomyelia
	Diabetes mellitus
Other	Arthropathy of hemophilia
	Chondrolysis from intra-articular pain pump

of GH arthritis. Repetitive injury may occur from heavy manual labor or excessive weight-lifting, while major injury most commonly occurs from intra-articular fracture (proximal humerus or glenoid) with joint incongruity that ultimately leads to GH arthritis. The incidence of posttraumatic arthritis is not well defined, possible due to a lack of specific features to distinguish it from primary GH OA if malunion is not present and slow progression of the disease. In addition to potential joint incongruity after healing, proximal humerus or intra-articular glenoid fractures may be associated with full-thickness cartilage loss that contributes to the development of long-term arthritic changes.

Inflammatory Arthritis

Rheumatoid arthritis (RA) is the most common inflammatory arthritis of the shoulder joint. RA affects 1% to 3% of the general population and is characterized by progressive joint destruction. The common features of RA and other inflammatory arthropathies (psoriatic arthritis, ankylosing spondylitis, etc.) include osteopenia, absence of typical osteoarthritic osteophytes, bipolar cystic changes, and joint space narrowing with joint line medialization from glenoid erosion in advanced phases of the disease.[11] The inflammatory changes can also lead to rotator cuff tendon attenuation and muscle atrophy. Widespread use of disease modifying agents have revolutionized the medical treatment of RA and other inflammatory arthropathies, helping patients to live with lower disease burden. Crystal induced arthropathies also fall under the category of inflammatory arthritis and are commonly reported in middle to advanced-age patients and are associated with poor kidney function or use of medications that affect production or excretion of uric acid in the body. Deposition of calcium hydroxyapatite (Milwaukee shoulder), calcium pyrophosphates (pseudogout), or monosodium urate monohydrate (goat) crystals into the joint results in an intense inflammatory reaction that can cause destructive GH arthritis. Milwaukee shoulder affects elderly women and has features of a rapidly progressive cuff tear arthropathy.[12]

Instability Arthropathy and Capsulorrhaphy Arthropathy

Neer identified shoulder dislocation as a cause of shoulder arthritis originally in 1982,[13] and later the term "dislocation arthropathy" was coined and linked to chronic recurrent instability. Marx et al reported a 10-fold increase in the risk of developing GH arthritis requiring shoulder arthroplasty in patients who had a history of prior shoulder dislocation.[14] Hovelius and Saeboe followed 223 patients with anterior dislocation for 25 years and reported age more than 25 years at the time of dislocation, high-energy sport, and alcohol use were linked to development of GH arthritis.[15] Besides dislocation itself, surgical treatment of instability can also lead to arthritic changes. Rapid loss of cartilage has been observed after arthroscopy and is referred to as postarthroscopic glenohumeral chondrolysis (PAGCL).[16] Overtightening of the anterior capsule

Shoulder

and possible excessive compression on the cartilage have been implicated in development of this complication. More commonly over the long term, overtightening of the anterior capsule can lead to contracture and abnormal GH mechanics that cause capsulorrhaphy arthropathy. The degenerative changes of capsulorrhaphy arthropathy are characterized by GH arthritis with eccentric posterior glenoid wear and posterior subluxation of the humeral head if the anterior capsule was overtightened. Prominent intra-articular hardware from surgical treatment (screws or anchors) can also cause cartilage destruction that leads to GH arthritis.[17]

Osteonecrosis of the Humeral Head

The humeral head is the second most common site for developing osteonecrosis in the body after the femoral head, but it is a relatively uncommon cause of GH arthritis. Osteonecrosis has a multifactorial etiology that leads to loss of blood supply to the humeral head and ultimately necrosis and articular collapse. Atraumatic osteonecrosis can be idiopathic or secondary to sickle cell disease, systemic lupus erythematosus, corticosteroid use, chemotherapy, alcohol use, and Caisson disease.[18] Traumatic osteonecrosis most commonly occurs following proximal humerus fractures but can also happen after shoulder dislocation or surgical fixation. Osteonecrosis is reported after zero to 34% of three- and four-part proximal humerus fractures and with a higher rate after surgical fixation of these fractures.[19] Hertel et al identified anatomic neck involvement, posteromedial metaphyseal extension of greater than 8 mm, and a disrupted medial hinge as prognostic factors for ischemia in proximal humerus fractures treated with open reduction and internal fixation.[20] Treatment of osteonecrosis depends on the disease stage and extent of humeral head collapse and involves nonsurgical management or arthroscopic débridement with core decompression for early stages without humeral head collapse, versus shoulder arthroplasty for more advanced stages of the disease with humeral head collapse. A resurfacing or standard hemiarthroplasty can be performed when collapse is present based on the extent of necrosis, with the goal of removing all of the necrotic bone with the implant. If arthritic changes also develop on the glenoid, TSA should be performed.

Rotator Cuff Tear Arthropathy

Rotator cuff tear arthropathy is defined as a constellation of soft tissue (eg, rotator cuff muscle atrophy and fatty infiltration) and bony (eg, femoralization of the humeral head and acetabulization of the acromial arch) adaptations that develop in response to a long-standing rotator cuff tear.[21] When the rotator cuff no longer provides dynamic stabilization of the humeral head in a large or massive rotator cuff tear and the GH joint cannot function as a stable fulcrum, the humeral head migrates upward, contacting the undersurface of the acromion and ultimately leading to the above-mentioned bony changes. The term cuff tear arthropathy was coined by Neer in 1983, and it was used to describe the end result of a chronic massive rotator cuff tear.[22]

Other Forms of Secondary Glenohumeral Arthritis

Neuropathic (Charcot) arthropathy can results in unexplained and severe joint destruction which is thought to be due to loss of protective and proprioceptive sensation of the GH joint. These patients should undergo evaluation for underlying diabetes mellitus or a syringomyelia of the cervicothoracic spine. Hemophilia is a rare inherited bleeding disorder that results in spontaneous bleeding into the joints and commonly affects the knee, ankle, elbow, and shoulder.[23] Recurrent intra-articular bleeding results in hemophilic arthropathy which involves synovial hyperplasia, fibrosis, and precipitation of iron product within the synovium in the first two decades of life. The use of continuous intra-articular pain pumps was found to be associated with a rapidly progressive GH arthritis that had features of PAGCL and was linked to the cytotoxic effect of bupivacaine analgesic on chondrocytes.[24] Since this discovery, the use of pain pumps has been abandoned, and evidence has shown that even a single injection of bupivacaine can result in reduction of chondrocyte cell population.

Presentation/Evaluation

Primary GH osteoarthritis commonly presents with activity-related joint pain which can radiate posteriorly with associated crepitus and a catching sensation with certain movements. With disease progression, patients usually report morning pain and stiffness and difficulty sleeping on the affected side. Surgeons should obtain information about the nature and pattern of pain, its location and relation to movement and sleep, timing of symptoms, comorbidities, and prior treatment including medications, cortisone injection, physical therapy, or surgeries.

On physical examination, the shoulder is inspected for any asymmetry, muscle atrophy (deltoid and posterior rotator cuff muscles), swelling or joint effusion, and the location of scars from prior surgeries should be noted. The examiner should palpate the AC joint, bicipital groove, and the anterior and posterior GH joint line for signs of tenderness. Active and passive range of motion (ROM) are tested to assess stiffness in all planes and should be compared with the contralateral side, which may also not be normal. Patients with cuff tear arthropathy can develop loss of the stable fulcrum of the GH joint with superior migration of the humeral head and loss of containment of the humeral head within the coracoacromial arch, leading to the examination findings of "anterosuperior escape," in which the humeral head becomes prominent anterosuperiorly with attempted active shoulder elevation, and "pseudoparalysis," in which active shoulder elevation is limited despite full passive shoulder ROM and intact neuromuscular function. Neurovascular status of the extremity including normal distal pulses and motor and sensory function of the axillary (by firing of all three heads of the deltoid muscle), median, ulnar, radial and, musculocutaneous nerves should be documented.

Imaging

Radiography

Initial imaging studies for GH arthritis should at minimum include true AP (Grashey view) and axillary views. Plain radiographs provide information about the type and severity of GH arthritis based on the degree of joint space narrowing, size and location of osteophytes, morphology of the glenoid, humeral head subluxation in any plane, and presence of calcifications, loose bodies, or implant/hardware from prior surgeries. Primary osteoarthritis typically demonstrates prominent osteophyte formation in advanced cases (**Figure 1**A). Surgeons should also take note of the overall bone quality, size of the intramedullary canal, and presence of an os acromiale or acromial erosion/stress fracture as they will have implications for surgical planning. Cuff tear arthropathy usually presents with GH arthritis and superior humeral head migration that in severe and long-standing arthritic cases results in AC arch erosion with concave deformity of the acromial undersurface known as "acetabulization" and rounding off of the greater tuberosity or "femoralization" of the proximal humerus (**Figure 1**B). Inflammatory arthritis can present in advanced cases with osteopenia, lack of osteophyte formation, cystic changes, central glenoid erosion, and joint line medialization (**Figure 1**C). The quality of plain radiographs is subjected to wide variation based on technique, patients' body habitus, and positioning of the shoulder relative to the radiograph beam. Measurements done on plain radiograph show 10% to 50% variation with only a 20° change in the angle of the radiograph beam.[25] Several studies have documented limitations of two-dimensional radiograph imaging in assessment of glenoid version, morphology, and quantifying the degree of glenoid bone loss.[26]

CT Scan

CT is a commonly utilized advanced imaging tool for evaluation of GH arthritis. CT allows for better assessment of glenoid version, inclination, morphology, and bone loss than plain radiographs and is commonly used for planning prior to shoulder arthroplasty. To achieve the best accuracy, CT images should be reconstructed in the scapular plane.[27]

Walch et al[28] used CT to classify glenoid morphology in primary GH osteoarthritis based on the pattern of glenoid wear and the subluxation of the humeral head relative to the scapular axis on the axial cuts (**Figure 2**A). Type A (59%) shows a well-centered humeral head with no subluxation and symmetric central glenoid wear, type B (32%) presents with posterior humeral head subluxation and posterior glenoid wear, and type C (9%) is a dysplastic glenoid with more than 25° of retroversion. Type A and B were further categorized as A1 and B1 if bony erosion was mild and A2 and B2 (biconcave) if bony erosion was advanced. Studies showed only fair interobserver reliability of the original Walch classification.[29] The classification was updated in 2016 by adding a type B3 glenoid with a monoconcave and posteriorly worn glenoid and a type D glenoid with anterior humeral head subluxation or glenoid anteversion (**Figure 2**B).[30] They demonstrated that both inter- and intraobserver reliability improved with the modified classification. Further modification of the Walch classification has included the addition of a C2 glenoid, in which a dysplastic C glenoid develops biconcavity from posterior glenoid wear.[31] It has been shown that the Walch classification has value in predicting natural history of GH osteoarthritis with A1 glenoids rarely developing posterior glenoid wear.[32] Also, surgical reconstruction of a glenoid with significant posterior glenoid bone loss can be technically challenging and ATSA without augmented glenoid components in these patients may have a less reliable outcome.[33]

Goutallier et al used CT to classify fatty infiltration of the rotator cuff muscles based on axial cuts as a surrogate for rotator cuff integrity and function.[34] Although the role of rotator cuff fatty infiltration in shoulder arthroplasty is not well understood, there are data to suggest that fatty infiltration negatively impacts patients' postoperative ROM and functional outcome.[35]

Shoulder

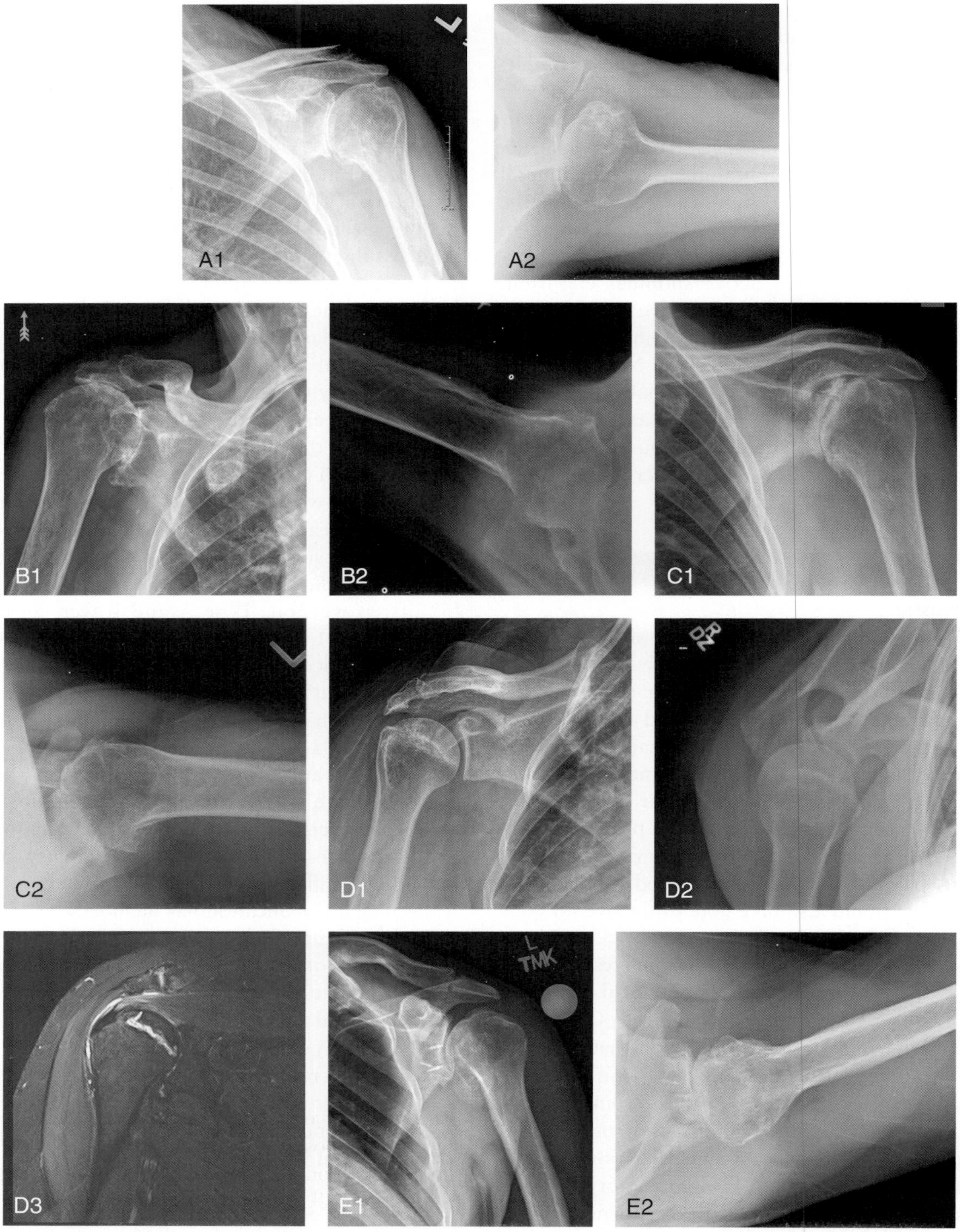

Figure 1 Radiographic appearance of glenohumeral (GH) arthritis. **A**, AP and axillary radiographs of primary GH arthritis with joint space narrowing and large osteophyte formation. In this particular case, the glenoid has B2 (biconcave) morphology with posterior glenoid wear. **B**, AP and axillary radiographs of cuff tear arthropathy with superior humeral head migration, anterosuperior glenoid wear, acetabularization of the acromion, and femoralization of the greater tuberosity. **C**, AP and axillary radiographs of inflammatory arthritis with joint space narrowing, minimal osteophyte formation, central glenoid erosion, and joint line medialization. **D**, AP and axillary radiographs and MRI of a steroid induced osteonecrosis of the humeral head with no collapse of the subchondral plate. **E**, AP and axillary radiographs of GH arthritis in a patient with a prior history of instability who underwent both arthroscopic and open anterior capsulorrhaphy. The axillary radiograph shows eccentric posterior glenoid wear and posterior subluxation of the humeral head that develops as a consequence of the anterior capsule being overtightened.

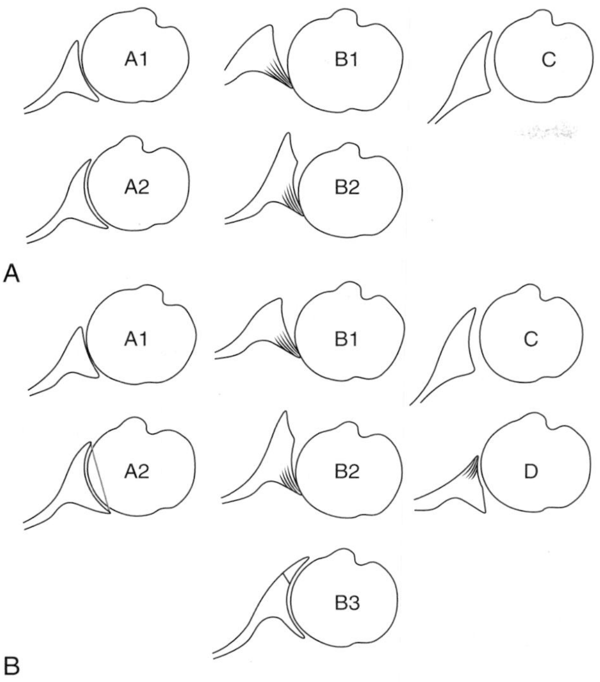

Figure 2 Illustrations of original (**A**) and modified (**B**) Walch classification of glenoid morphology in primary glenohumeral (GH) osteoarthritis. Type A shows a well-centered humeral head with no subluxation and symmetric glenoid wear. A1 has minimal central wear, while A2 has significant central wear with joint line medialization. Type B shows posterior humeral head subluxation and posterior glenoid wear. B1 has minimal posterior wear, while B2 has significant posterior wear and a distinct biconcave glenoid with native (paleoglenoid) and eroded (neoglenoid) facets. B3 type has severe posterior wear as the humeral head has progressively increased the size of the neoglenoid until a single concavity results. Type C is a dysplastic glenoid with more than 25° of retroversion, and type D is a glenoid with an anterior glenoid wear pattern. (Reprinted from Walch G, Badet R, Boulahia A, Khoury A: Morphologic study of the glenoid in primary glenohumeral osteoarthritis. *J Arthroplasty* 1999;14:756-760 Copyright 1999, with permission from Elsevier and Bercik MJ, Kruse K II, Yalizis M, Gauci MO, Chaoui J, Walch G: A modification to the Walch classification of the glenoid in primary glenohumeral osteoarthritis using three-dimensional imaging. *J Shoulder Elbow Surg* 2016;25:1601-1606, Copyright 2016, with permission from Elsevier.)

MRI

Another advanced imaging modality is MRI which has the ability to assess the bone, cartilage, and rotator cuff with high resolution without subjecting patients to radiation. Studies have shown that MRI can be used to assess glenoid version and morphology.[36] Similar to CT, MRI can be used to assess rotator cuff muscle atrophy and fatty infiltration, while also demonstrating the presence of significant partial-thickness or full-thickness rotator cuff tears.

Treatment

Nonsurgical Treatment

There is currently no therapeutic intervention to halt the natural history of primary GH arthritis. Nonsurgical treatment aims to minimize patients' symptoms, improve strength, and maintain mobility. The first line of treatment includes rest, activity modification, gentle physical therapy, anti-inflammatory, and analgesic medications. Long-term benefit of NSAID medications should be weighed against the risk of gastrointestinal irritation, cardiovascular disease, bleeding, and kidney damage. When NSAIDs are no longer effective, intra-articular cortisone injections can relieve pain but commonly need to be repeated and can lose effectiveness with serial injections over time. A systematic review found that despite their wide use, there is limited evidence on efficacy of cortisone injections for GH arthritis.[37] Cortisone injections in short succession (less than 3 months apart and more than 3 to 4 injections per year) are discouraged due to the potential effect on the bone and soft tissue around the shoulder. Although direct risk of infection from intra-articular cortisone injection is estimated to be 1 in 3,000 to 100,000, there is evidence to suggest that if a cortisone injection is given within 3 months of shoulder arthroplasty, it slightly, but statistically significantly, increases the risk of periprosthetic infection.[38] Although viscosupplementation with hyaluronic acid (HA) has only been FDA approved for use in knee arthritis, it has shown promising results for GH arthritis in several randomized trials. The largest clinical trial of 660 patients with GH osteoarthritis reported a threefold decrease in pain after HA injection compared with placebo at 26 weeks and a consensus panel recommended intra-articular HA injection in mild to moderate GH osteoarthritis.[39] Platelet-rich plasma (PRP) is an autologous derivative of whole blood and contains a variety of growth factors that can potentially modulate healing with a low risk of side effects. While several prospective studies have been conducted on the effect of PRP on knee OA, there is no dedicated study on PRP use in GH OA. The evidence in knee OA is mostly equivocal, with the most recent meta-analysis suggesting a possible small short-term effect on patient-reported outcomes.[40] Similarly, there are no studies on use of stem cell injections in GH OA. Due to their cost and limited evidence, these orthobiologics are considered experimental at this point for GH arthritis.

Surgical Treatment

Surgical options should be considered for patients who continue to have pain and disability despite nonsurgical management. Joint preservation procedures are considered in relatively young patients (<55 years) with mild to moderate GH arthritis and include arthroscopic débridement, capsular release, biceps tenodesis, and microfracture. If arthritic changes become severe in a young and active patient, the results of the armamentarium of options are mixed, including hemiarthroplasty, with or without the "ream and run" procedure or glenoid biologic resurfacing, and ATSA. Surgical options for an older patient with severe GH arthritis are more clearly defined, with both ATSA and RTSA showing excellent results. The choice between the two implant types is frequently dictated by the patient's rotator cuff status and degree of glenoid bone loss. The ATSA is commonly offered to a patient with an intact rotator cuff and mild to moderate glenoid bone loss, while RTSA is used for cuff tear arthropathy or GH arthritis cases with large full-thickness rotator cuff tears or severe glenoid bone loss.

Arthroscopic Débridement

Initial reports of arthroscopic treatment for GH arthritis showed favorable outcomes with 80% good to excellent outcomes and 83% improved shoulder ROM, but these were mostly short-term results and most deteriorated over time.[41] Other groups reported failure up to 60% after arthroscopic débridement and capsular release on average 10 months after surgery.[42] Millett et al[43] reported their results of comprehensive arthroscopic management (CAM) in 107 shoulders with average follow-up of 3.9 years and found 15.8% had to undergo TSA in less than 2 years. These patients underwent extensive chondroplasty, capsular release, osteophyte excision, axillary nerve neurolysis, subacromial decompression, loose body removal, and microfracture when indicated. Early failure in this cohort was associated with lower preoperative joint space, higher grade of arthritis, age older than 50 years, and Walch B2 and C type glenoids. In a relatively young and active patient with mild to moderate GH arthritis and minimal glenoid deformity who wants to avoid joint replacement, arthroscopic débridement is a viable option and may be a good temporizing measure until the patient is ready for shoulder arthroplasty. These procedures seem to work best in patients with mild arthritis, with a centered humeral head, where stiffness is severe and the main report.[44]

Hemiarthroplasty ± Biologic Resurfacing/Ream and Run

Hemiarthroplasty with or without glenoid reaming aims to relive pain and restore ROM by reconstructing proximal humeral anatomy and avoiding glenoid component placement, which historically has been the weak link in TSA. Hemiarthroplasty can be performed with resurfacing, short stemmed or stemless implant options to preserve humeral bone stock. Hemiarthroplasty for GH arthritis, however, has been associated with progressive glenoid erosion and high revision rates, particularly in the younger patient. One study reported glenoid erosion in 72% of patients younger than 50 years at 20 years and cited painful glenoid arthrosis as the main reason for revision after hemiarthroplasty.[45] The addition of biologic resurfacing of the glenoid using meniscus, anterior capsule, Achilles tendon, or acellular dermal allograft to hemiarthroplasty has also demonstrated high complication and revision surgery rates.[46] The "ream and run" procedure involves both a humeral hemiarthroplasty and concentric reaming of the glenoid with the aim of creating a concentric, centered bearing surface with the potential for biologic resurfacing with fibrous tissue covering the reamed glenoid surface. The rate of revision surgery for the ream and run procedure in some series has been reported to be 14% to 25% at minimum 2 years follow-up, while patients older than 60 years with no history of prior surgery and better preoperative function had more favorable outcomes.[47] While glenoid loosening remains the most common reason for revision of ATSA, attempts to avoid placement of a polyethylene glenoid component have had mixed success.[48]

Anatomic Total Shoulder Arthroplasty

In the patient with an intact rotator cuff and ample glenoid bone stock, ATSA has shown excellent results for improving ROM and decreasing pain in GH arthritis patients. ATSA is considered the benchmark for surgical treatment of primary GH arthritis, showing 93% implant survival at 10 years and 87% at 15 years (**Figure 3**A).[49] There is substantial evidence that ATSA provides better pain relief, ROM, and patient-reported outcomes than hemiarthroplasty. A multicenter study of 700 arthroplasties for GH arthritis showed better Constant score (96% versus 86%), forward elevation (145° versus 130°), and external rotation (42° versus 36°) for ATSA compared with hemiarthroplasty at minimum 2-year follow-up.[50] Similar results have been reported in patients younger than 50 years with 10 and 20 year implant survival rates of 97% and 84% for ATSA and 82% and 75% for hemiarthroplasty.[51]

Glenoid component loosening is the most common complication after ATSA. A systematic review between 2006 and 2012 found that after primary ATSA, radiolucent lines occur at a rate of 7.3% per year while only 1.2% become symptomatic with a revision rate of 0.8% per year.[52] A variety of patient factors (sex, glenoid morphology, rotator cuff status, and infection), surgical factors (cementing technique and implant seating), and implant factors (design and conformity) have been implicated in the risk of glenoid component loosening.[53] Currently,

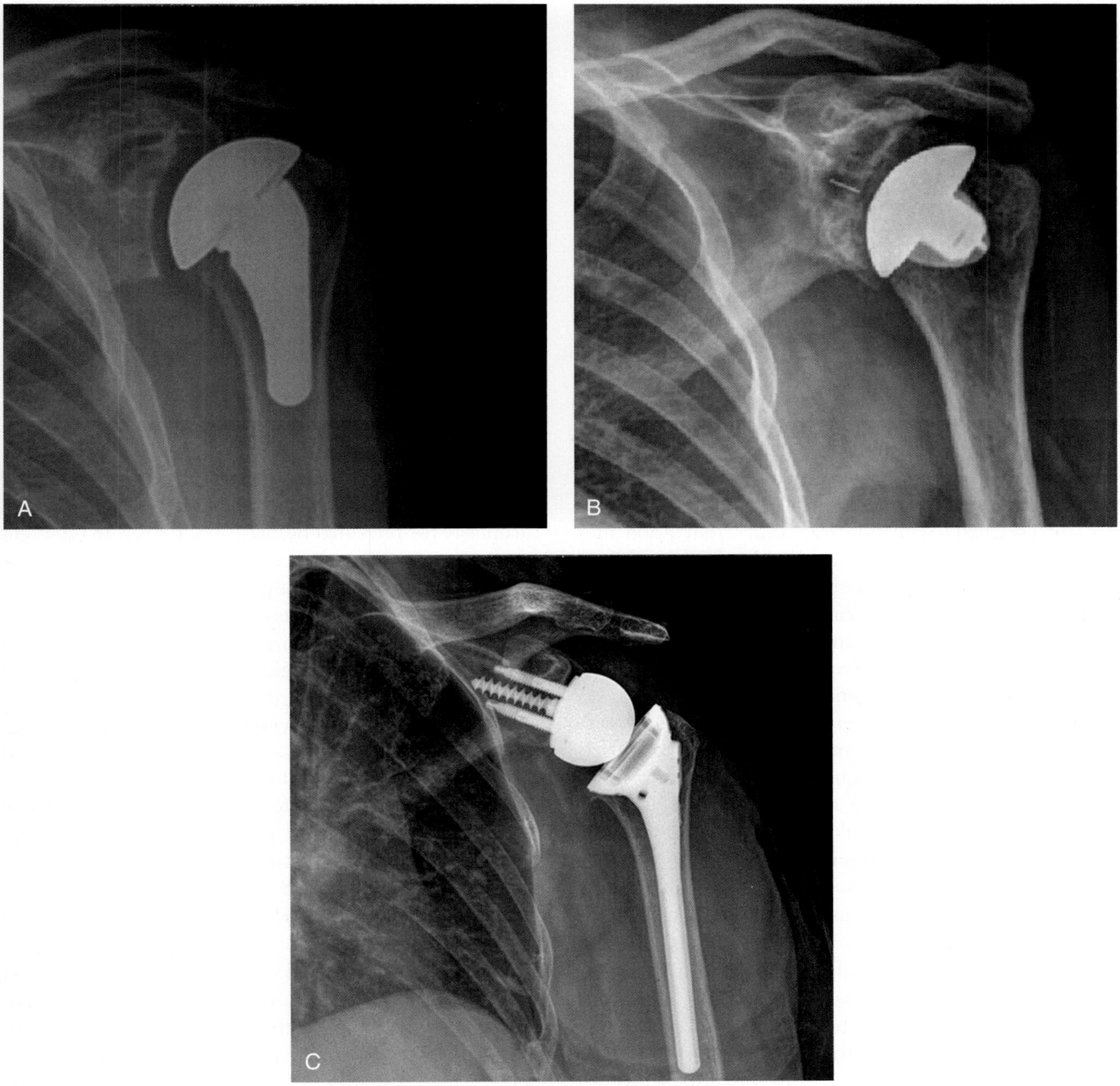

Figure 3 Radiographic appearance of total shoulder arthroplasty. **A**, Anatomic total shoulder arthroplasty using short stem humeral and polyethylene glenoid components. **B**, Anatomic total shoulder arthroplasty using stemless humeral and polyethylene glenoid components. **C**, Reverse total shoulder arthroplasty with lateralized glenosphere distalized and inferiorly tilted relative to the glenoid face.

all-polyethylene pegged glenoid components have better implant survivorship than keeled and metal-back glenoid designs.[54] Other determinants of the outcome after ATSA include Walch B2 glenoid, subscapularis function, and fatty infiltration of the rotator cuff. Approaches to address abnormal glenoid morphology with ATSA include in situ implantation, eccentric reaming, bone grafting, or use of augmented glenoid components.

The rate of implant failure on the humeral side remains very low and the desire to preserve proximal humeral bone stock has led to the evolution from long-stem to short-stem and stemless components. Short-stem implants have shown good clinical outcome with no sign of loosening in short- to midterm follow-up.[55] Stemless humeral components preclude the need for canal reaming and can be advantageous with shorter surgical time, less bleeding, and ease of revision (**Figure 3**B). Unlike resurfacing components, stemless components require a complete humeral head cut and thus allow easier access to the glenoid. A prospective multicenter trial of 149 patients with primary GH arthritis using a stemless humeral component showed significant improvement in Constant score (56% to 104%), forward elevation (103° to 147°) and external rotation (31° to 56°) at 2-year follow-up with no sign of radiographic humeral loosening, migration, or subsidence.[56]

Reverse Total Shoulder Arthroplasty

ATSA relies on the rotator cuff for stability and function. In the setting of a significant rotator cuff tear or fatty infiltration, the results of ATSA have been less predictable. While data show that small rotator cuff tears with no humeral head subluxation can be repaired at the time of ATSA with minimal impact on arm strength and patient-reported outcome, repair of moderate and large rotator cuff tears with humeral head subluxation may lead to poor functional outcome with ATSA, and these patients are better candidates for RTSA.[35,57] The goal of ATSA is to replicate normal joint biomechanics, but in patients with larger rotator cuff tears, dynamic stabilization of the joint is lost, resulting in edge loading of the glenoid component and implant loosening due to the rocking-horse phenomenon. The RTSA design with a "constrained" joint concept was introduced to address this problem, but early designs had a high failure rate due to high shear and stress at the bone-implant interface. The first RTSA implant developed with reliable outcomes was introduced by Grammont et al in 1987 with a large hemispheric glenosphere, medialized center of rotation, and a 155° humerosocket inclination angle to increase the length and tension of the deltoid muscle and improve stability.[58] Grammont specifically based his design on four biomechanical principals: (1) a fixed fulcrum of rotation, (2) the inherent stability of the constrained joint design, (3) medialization of the center of rotation, and (4) distalization of the humerus.[59] While initially reserved for cuff tear arthroplasty, RTSA is now also frequently used for irreparable rotator cuff tears without arthritis, comminuted proximal humerus fractures, revision shoulder arthroplasty, GH OA with significant glenoid bone loss, inflammatory arthritis where the rotator cuff may be at risk, chronic dislocations, tumors, and a variety of other indications. In recent years, lateralized baseplate designs have gained popularity and place the joint center of rotation in a more anatomic location, particularly in combination with decreased humerosocket inclination (135°), thus avoiding notching of the polyethylene humeral liner against the glenoid neck (**Figure 3**C).

The annual number of primary shoulder arthroplasties in the United States has been growing steadily since 2003 with FDA approval of RTSA, which in 2014 surpassed utilization of ATSA.[60] Early outcomes of RTSA were associated with high complication rates of up to 33%, but with improvement in implant design, surgical technique, and patient selection, complication rates have been in decline. The outcome of RTSA is dictated by the primary indication for use, with cuff tear arthropathy resulting in the best outcomes. Favard et al[61] retrospectively reviewed 527 cases of Grammont style RTSAs for cuff tear arthropathy and reported 89% implant survival at 10 years. Cuff et al reported similar minimum 10-year results in 96 cases of a lateralized RTSA design for irreparable rotator cuff tears with 90% implant survival.[62] However, ROM gains may be inferior in patients with rotator cuff arthropathy and younger age appears to be a negative prognostic factor for postoperative functional improvement.[63] The advantage of RTSA over hemiarthroplasty for proximal humerus fractures is that patient outcome appears to be less dependent on tuberosity healing.[64] Another emerging RTSA indication is treatment of GH OA with severe bone loss and intact rotator cuff. Mizuno et al reported the outcome of RTSA in patients with a biconcave glenoid and intact rotator cuff at an average 54 months.[65] Bone loss was addressed with bone grafting in 37% of patients and eccentric reaming for the remainder, with excellent clinical outcome and improvement in ROM and Constant scores.

One of the main differences between ATSA and RTSA is improvement in postoperative internal rotation. Cox et al compared postoperative patient-reported outcomes and ROM in 19 patients who had an ATSA in one shoulder and an RTSA in the other shoulder. All patients showed significant improvement in their ASES score and ROM compared with preoperative values, but patients with RTSA achieved lower internal rotation compared with the contralateral ATSA. Despite significant improvement in the outcome of RTSA in recent years, patients should be counseled regarding a higher complication rate and less reliable internal rotation compared with an ATSA. In addition, while RTSA can allow for abduction and forward elevation in a patient with preoperative pseudoparalysis, weakness or lag signs in external rotation at 0° and 90° abduction may not be corrected without a concomitant tendon transfer.[66]

Complications of Shoulder Arthroplasty

The rate of complications after shoulder arthroplasty has declined compared with a decade earlier. Bohsali et al[53] did a systematic review and reported the incidence of common complications following ATSA and RTSA

(**Tables 2 and 3**). They found that the 1-year mortality rate following shoulder arthroplasty is approximately 1% and the overall rate of complications is 10% for ATSA and 16% for RTSA.

There is no consistent definition for periprosthetic joint infection (PJI) of the shoulder in the literature.[67] The rate of infection after shoulder arthroplasty is reported as 1.2% to 3.0%, while the rate is 0.5% to 3.9% for ATSA and 5.1% to 10.0% for RTSA.[53] Shoulder PJI commonly presents as a painful arthroplasty with minimal clinical and laboratory findings typical for infection. This is mostly due to the predominance of indolent organisms, such as *Cutibacterium acnes* (formerly known as *Propionibacterium acnes*) (39% to 66%) and coagulates negative staph species (24% to 28%), in shoulder PJI.[68] Two-stage revision including aggressive débridement and antibiotic spacer placement, followed by prolonged IV antibiotics and second-stage reimplantation, was adopted from treatment of hip and knee PJI and showed 63% to 100% success in eradicating infection in short- to midterm follow-up.[69] However, one-stage revision has recently been advocated for the indolent infections common in shoulder PJI, with similar rates of eradication as two-stage revision. A systematic review found that average Constant score was 51 after one-stage revision and 41 after two-stage revision, presumably due to the decreased ROM secondary to the increased scarring of a two-stage procedure.[70] Hsu et al[71] compared patients who underwent one-stage revision for presumed *C acnes* infection with ≥2 positive cultures with patients with one or no positive cultures and showed that the patient-reported outcomes and need for revision was not different between the two groups.

The incidence of periprosthetic humeral fractures is reported as high as 4.6% after shoulder arthroplasty and is commonly associated with revision, osteoporosis, RA, prolonged steroid use, and history of frequent falls. According to the Swedish registry, intraoperative fractures are three times more common than postoperative fractures.[72] If the humeral implant is well-fixed, open reduction and internal fixation using a locking plate and screws or strut graft with cerclage wires is the preferred

Table 2

Complications of RSAs in Studies Published from 2006 to 2015*

Complication	No. of Shoulders	Percentage of All Complications	Percentage of All Shoulders
Instability	208	31.3	5.0
Periprosthetic fracture	138	20.8	3.3
Intraoperative	94	14.2	2.3
Postoperative	44	6.6	1.1
Infection	118	17.8	2.9
Component loosening	75	11.3	1.8
Glenoid	48	7.2	1.2
Humerus	27	4.1	0.7
Neural injury	50	7.5	1.2
Acromial and/or scapular spine fracture	40	6.0	1.0
Hematoma	21	3.2	0.51
Deltoid injury	6	0.9	0.15
Rotator cuff tear	4	0.6	0.10
VTE events	4	0.6	0.10
Deep venous thrombosis	2	0.3	0.05
Pulmonary embolus	2	0.3	0.05

*The 78 studies included a total of 4,124 shoulders (studies with mixed types of arthroplasties were excluded).

RSA = reverse shoulder arthroplasty; VTE = venous thromboembolism

Reprinted with permission from Bohsali KI, Bois AJ, Wirth MA. Complications of Shoulder Arthroplasty. *J Bone Joint Surg Am*. 2017;99:256-269. doi:10.2106/JBJS.16.00935.

Shoulder

Table 3

Complications of Anatomic TSAs in Studies Published from 2006 to 2015*

Complication	No. of Shoulders	Percentage of All Complications	Percentage of All Shoulders
Component loosening	135	39.1	4.0
Glenoid	130	37.7	3.9
Humerus	5	1.4	0.1
Glenoid wear	78	22.6	2.3
Instability	35	10.1	1.0
Rotator cuff tear	31	9.0	0.9
Periprosthetic fracture	23	6.7	0.69
Intraoperative	19	5.5	0.57
Postoperative	4	1.2	0.12
Neural injury	21	6.1	0.63
Infection	17	4.9	0.51
Hematoma	3	0.9	0.09
Deltoid injury	1	0.3	0.03
Deep venous thrombosis	1	0.3	0.03

*The 33 studies included a total of 3,360 shoulders (studies with mixed types of arthroplasty were excluded).

TSA = total shoulder arthroplasty

Reprinted with permission from Bohsali KI, Bois AJ, Wirth MA. Complications of Shoulder Arthroplasty. *J Bone Joint Surg Am* 2017;99:256-269. doi:10.2106/JBJS.16.00935.

surgical treatment. Loose implants should be revised with a longer humeral stem augmented with a locking plate or strut graft with bicortical screws distally and unicortical screws proximally reinforced by cerclage wires. In cases of severe proximal humeral bone loss that preclude rotational stability, using a proximal humeral allograft or tumor prosthesis should be considered.

Rotator cuff tears are uncommon in the setting of primary GH arthritis. Repair of partial and small full-thickness supraspinatus tears at the time of ATSA did not affect short-term clinical outcomes.[35] Nonetheless, attritional rotator cuff tear is a cause of possible late failure and revision of ATSA. Young et al conducted a multicenter study of secondary rotator cuff failure after ATSA with more than 5 years follow-up and showed 16.8% of patients develop moderate to severe superior subluxation of the humeral head on AP radiographs, which was associated with poor clinical and radiographic outcome.[73] Subscapularis failure after ATSA, which comprises 50% of rotator cuff failures in some series, may not be well tolerated and if associated with implant instability and poor function will lead to revision surgery.[74]

The Nordic shoulder arthroplasty registry recently reported 10-year survivorship data for RTSA and showed a 5% overall revision rate with infection as the most common cause of early revision and male sex as a significant predictor of failure.[75] RTSA is associated with a set of unique complications, particularly scapular notching, instability, and scapular stress fractures. Scapular notching is reported in 68% of Grammont style RTSAs and results from impingement of the polyethylene humeral liner with the scapular neck in adduction and external rotation. Although the clinical significance of mild to moderate notching is not well established, progressive forms of notching result in glenoid bone loss that can be associated with implant loosening. Scapular notching appears to be related to implant design and is less common in implants with a lateralized glenosphere and a more varus humerosocket inclination angle, where the polyethylene liner has less chance of coming into contact with the neck of the scapula. Instability is reported in 5% of patients following RTSA and commonly occurs in the anterosuperior direction during arm adduction, extension, and internal rotation when a patient is pushing up with the hand behind the back. Inadequate soft-tissue tension from implant malpositioning, deltoid dysfunction or proximal humeral bone loss, and mechanical impingement are common causes of instability. Closed reduction shoulder be attempted after a first-time dislocation,

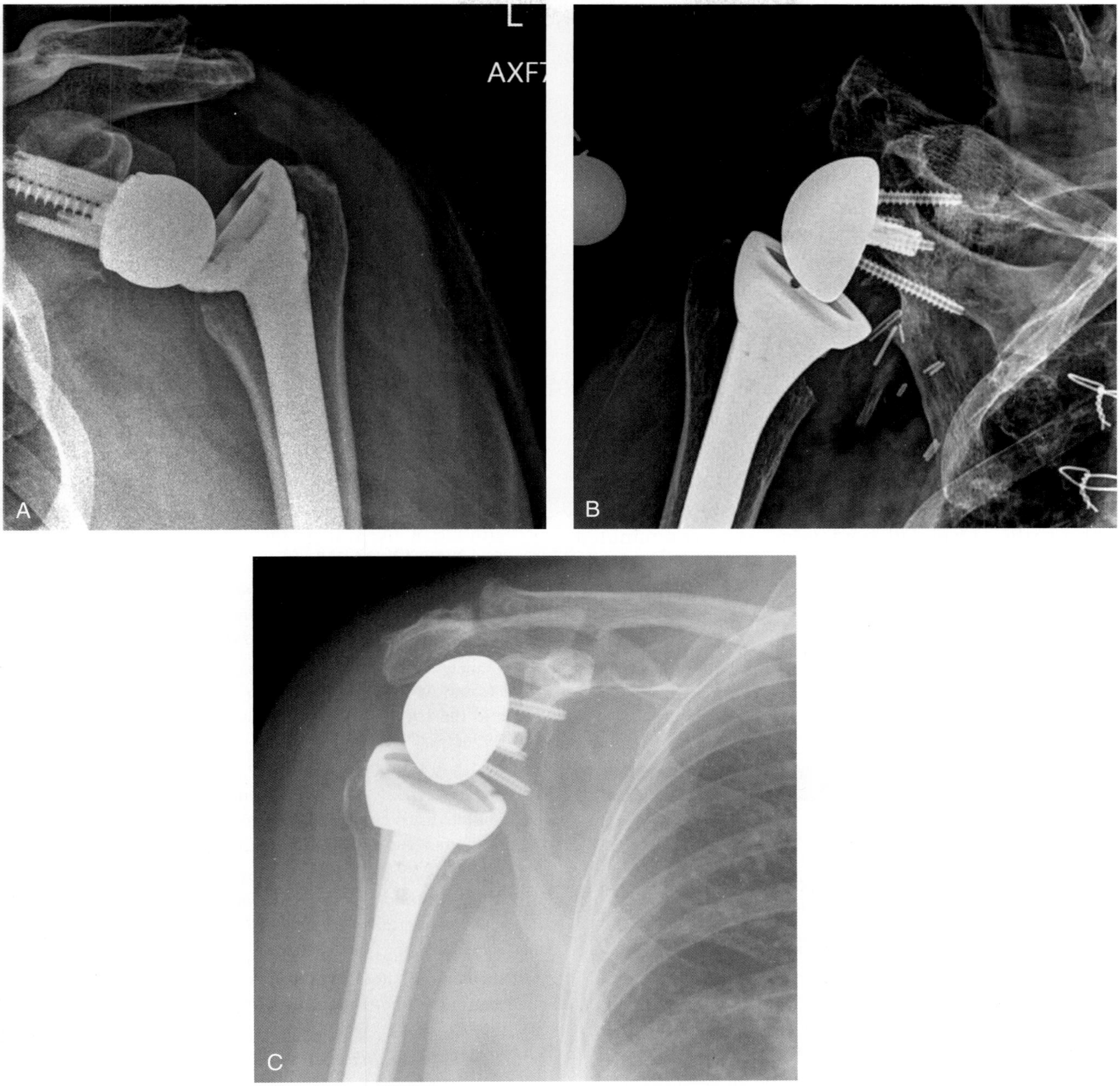

Figure 4 Radiographic appearance of common complications of reverse shoulder arthroplasty. **A**, Shoulder dislocation of a reverse total shoulder arthroplasty (TSA). **B**, Scapular notching in a reverse TSA with medialized center of rotation and valgus neck-shaft angle. **C**, Scapular fracture with extension to the spine of scapula and proximity to posterosuperior baseplate screw.

and the surgeon should be ready for revision surgery. Acromial stress fractures are reported in 1% to 5% of patients following RTSA and usually present with sudden onset of pain in the posterior aspect of the shoulder. They are thought to be related to tensioning of the deltoid in a patient with osteopenic or osteoporotic bone. Treatment is rest with an abduction pillow, as surgical fixation has been associated with a high complication and nonunion rate (**Figure 4**).

Summary

Arthritic changes in the AC joint are a common source of pain and commonly associated with advanced age, history of trauma, and repetitive heavy lifting. When rest, activity modification, and cortisone injections fail, DCE is an effective treatment option. Primary GH arthritis is common in elderly female and young patients with heavy lifting demands. Secondary GH arthritis includes posttraumatic arthritis after proximal humerus or glenoid fracture, inflammatory arthritis (including rheumatoid arthritis, psoriatic arthritis, gout, and others), instability arthropathy and capsulorrhaphy arthropathy, osteonecrosis of the humeral head, cuff tear arthropathy in patients with long-standing rotator cuff failure, Charcot arthropathy, and arthropathy of hemophilia. If activity modification, physical therapy, oral anti-inflammatory medications, and serial cortisone injection fail, surgical options include arthroscopic débridement, hemiarthroplasty, ATSA, and RTSA. Arthroscopic débridement can be effective in mild to moderate GH arthritis, but durability of results is unpredictable. Hemiarthroplasty is an option for young and active patients with severe GH arthritis, but glenoid erosion and need for early revision have been challenges in this patient population. ATSA is the benchmark for primary GH arthritis with an intact rotator cuff. In advanced cases of cuff tear arthropathy, severe glenoid bone loss, comminuted proximal humerus fractures and revision arthroplasty, RTSA has been a successful intervention. The outcome of shoulder arthroplasty has improved significantly in the past decade with better surgical technique, patient selection, and improved implant design, but RTSA continues to have a higher rate of complications compared with ATSA.

Key Study Points

- Arthroscopic débridement is an option for a young patient with mild to moderate GH arthritis, but durability of results is unpredictable. The best prognosis is in mild OA with a centered humeral head and stiffness as the chief report.
- Hemiarthroplasty is associated with a high rate of glenoid erosion and revision, and its use should be limited to a young patient with severe GH arthritis and a high level of heavy activity.
- ATSA is the benchmark for surgical treatment of primary GH arthritis with intact rotator cuff and ample glenoid bone stock.
- RTSA can address multiple issues including poor rotator cuff function, instability, and poor glenoid bone stock and is the treatment of choice in severe cuff tear arthropathy, and revision arthroplasty in elderly patients.
- The complication rate of RTSA is higher than ATSA and patients commonly achieve less internal rotation postoperatively.

Annotated References

1. Petersson CJ: Degeneration of the acromioclavicular joint. A morphological study. *Acta Orthop Scand* 1983;54:434-438.
2. Scavenius M, Iversen BF: Nontraumatic clavicular osteolysis in weight lifters. *Am J Sports Med* 1992;20:463-467.
3. Chronopoulos E, Kim TK, Park HB, Ashenbrenner D, McFarland EG: Diagnostic value of physical tests for isolated chronic acromioclavicular lesions. *Am J Sports Med* 2004;32:655-661.
4. Shubin Stein BE, Ahmad CS, Pfaff CH, Bigliani LU, Levine WN: A comparison of magnetic resonance imaging findings of the acromioclavicular joint in symptomatic versus asymptomatic patients. *J Shoulder Elbow Surg* 2006;15:56-59.
5. Stein BE, Wiater JM, Pfaff HC, Bigliani LU, Levine WN: Detection of acromioclavicular joint pathology in asymptomatic shoulders with magnetic resonance imaging. *J Shoulder Elbow Surg* 2001;10:204-208.
6. Hossain S, Jacobs LG, Hashmi R: The long-term effectiveness of steroid injections in primary acromioclavicular joint arthritis: A five-year prospective study. *J Shoulder Elbow Surg* 2008;17:535-538.
7. Brown JN, Roberts SN, Hayes MG, Sales AD: Shoulder pathology associated with symptomatic acromioclavicular joint degeneration. *J Shoulder Elbow Surg* 2000;9:173-176.
8. Branch TP, Burdette HL, Shahriari AS, Carter FM 2nd, Hutton WC: The role of the acromioclavicular ligaments and the effect of distal clavicle resection. *Am J Sports Med* 1996;24:293-297.
9. Park YB, Koh KH, Shon MS, Park YE, Yoo JC: Arthroscopic distal clavicle resection in symptomatic acromioclavicular joint arthritis combined with rotator cuff tear: A prospective randomized trial. *Am J Sports Med* 2015;43:985-990.
10. Nakagawa Y, Hyakuna K, Otani S, Hashitani M, Nakamura T: Epidemiologic study of glenohumeral osteoarthritis with plain radiography. *J Shoulder Elbow Surg* 1999;8:580-584.
11. Thomas T, Noel E, Goupille P, Duquesnoy B, Combe B: The rheumatoid shoulder: Current consensus on diagnosis and treatment. *Joint Bone Spine* 2006;73:139-143.
12. Nadarajah CV, Weichert I: Milwaukee shoulder syndrome. *Case Rep Rheumatol* 2014;2014:458708.
13. Neer CS 2nd, Watson KC, Stanton FJ: Recent experience in total shoulder replacement. *J Bone Joint Surg Am* 1982;64:319-337.
14. Marx RG, McCarty EC, Montemurno TD, Altchek DW, Craig EV, Warren RF: Development of arthrosis following dislocation of the shoulder: A case-control study. *J Shoulder Elbow Surg* 2002;11:1-5.
15. Hovelius L, Saeboe M: Neer Award 2008: Arthropathy after primary anterior shoulder dislocation–223 shoulders prospectively followed up for twenty-five years. *J Shoulder Elbow Surg* 2009;18:339-347.

16. Hansen BP, Beck CL, Beck EP, Townsley RW: Postarthroscopic glenohumeral chondrolysis. *Am J Sports Med* 2007;35:1628-1634.

17. Zuckerman JD, Matsen FA 3rd: Complications about the glenohumeral joint related to the use of screws and staples. *J Bone Joint Surg Am* 1984;66:175-180.

18. Harreld KL, Marker DR, Wiesler ER, Shafiq B, Mont MA: Osteonecrosis of the humeral head. *J Am Acad Orthop Surg* 2009;17:345-355.

19. Hettrich CM, Boraiah S, Dyke JP, Neviaser A, Helfet DL, Lorich DG: Quantitative assessment of the vascularity of the proximal part of the humerus. *J Bone Joint Surg Am* 2010;92:943-948.

20. Hertel R, Hempfing A, Stiehler M, Leunig M: Predictors of humeral head ischemia after intracapsular fracture of the proximal humerus. *J Shoulder Elbow Surg* 2004;13:427-433.

21. Ecklund KJ, Lee TQ, Tibone J, Gupta R: Rotator cuff tear arthropathy. *J Am Acad Orthop Surg* 2007;15:340-349.

22. Neer CS 2nd, Craig EV, Fukuda H: Cuff-tear arthropathy. *J Bone Joint Surg Am* 1983;65:1232-1244.

23. Sankaye P, Ostlere S: Arthritis at the shoulder joint. *Semin Musculoskelet Radiol* 2015;19:307-318.

24. Petty DH, Jazrawi LM, Estrada LS, Andrews JR: Glenohumeral chondrolysis after shoulder arthroscopy: Case reports and review of the literature. *Am J Sports Med* 2004;32:509-515.

25. Rozing PM, Obermann WR: Osteometry of the glenohumeral joint. *J Shoulder Elbow Surg* 1999;8:438-442.

26. Nyffeler RW, Jost B, Pfirrmann CW, Gerber C: Measurement of glenoid version: Conventional radiographs versus computed tomography scans. *J Shoulder Elbow Surg* 2003;12:493-496.

27. Bokor DJ, O'Sullivan MD, Hazan GJ: Variability of measurement of glenoid version on computed tomography scan. *J Shoulder Elbow Surg* 1999;8:595-598.

28. Walch G, Badet R, Boulahia A, Khoury A: Morphologic study of the glenoid in primary glenohumeral osteoarthritis. *J Arthroplasty* 1999;14:756-760.

29. Scalise JJ, Codsi MJ, Brems JJ, Iannotti JP: Inter-rater reliability of an arthritic glenoid morphology classification system. *J Shoulder Elbow Surg* 2008;17:575-577.

30. Bercik MJ, Kruse K II, Yalizis M, Gauci MO, Chaoui J, Walch G: A modification to the Walch classification of the glenoid in primary glenohumeral osteoarthritis using three-dimensional imaging. *J Shoulder Elbow Surg* 2016;25:1601-1606.

    This article presents modifications to the original Walch classification by addition of the B3 and D glenoids and a more precise definition of the A2 glenoid which results in better inter and intraobserver reliability. Level of evidence: Basic Science Study, Development or Validation of Classification System.

31. Iannotti JP, Jun BJ, Patterson TE, Ricchetti ET: Quantitative measurement of osseous pathology in advanced glenohumeral osteoarthritis. *J Bone Joint Surg Am* 2017;99:1460-1468.

    This article presents quantitative measurements of premorbid and pathologic glenoid anatomy using 3D gleboid vault and proposes addition of the B3 and C2 glenoid. Level of evidence: IV (Descriptive imaging study).

32. Walker KE, Simcock XC, Jun BJ, Iannotti JP, Ricchetti ET: Progression of glenoid morphology in glenohumeral osteoarthritis. *J Bone Joint Surg Am* 2018;100:49-56.

    This article shows asymmetric bone loss rarely develops in A1 glenoids, whereas initial posterior translation of the humeral head (B1 glenoids) may be associated with subsequent development and progression of posterior glenoid bone loss over time. Level of evidence: III (Prognostic).

33. Denard PJ, Walch G: Current concepts in the surgical management of primary glenohumeral arthritis with a biconcave glenoid. *J Shoulder Elbow Surg* 2013;22:1589-1598.

34. Goutallier D, Postel JM, Bernageau J, Lavau L, Voisin MC: Fatty muscle degeneration in cuff ruptures. Pre- and postoperative evaluation by CT scan. *Clin Orthop Relat Res* 1994:78-83.

35. Edwards TB, Boulahia A, Kempf JF, Boileau P, Nemoz C, Walch G: The influence of rotator cuff disease on the results of shoulder arthroplasty for primary osteoarthritis: Results of a multicenter study. *J Bone Joint Surg Am* 2002;84-A:2240-2248.

36. Lowe JT, Testa EJ, Li X, Miller S, DeAngelis JP, Jawa A: Magnetic resonance imaging is comparable to computed tomography for determination of glenoid version but does not accurately distinguish between Walch B2 and C classifications. *J Shoulder Elbow Surg* 2017;26:669-673.

    The authors compared the accuracy of MRI to CT for assessment of glenoid version and Walch classification and showed these are largely comparable modalities but MRI is less accurate at distinguishing between the B2 and C type glenoids. Level of evidence: III (Diagnostic Study).

37. Colen S, Geervliet P, Haverkamp D, Van Den Bekerom MP: Intra-articular infiltration therapy for patients with glenohumeral osteoarthritis: A systematic review of the literature. *Int J Shoulder Surg* 2014;8:114-121.

38. Werner BC, Cancienne JM, Burrus MT, Griffin JW, Gwathmey FW, Brockmeier SF: The timing of elective shoulder surgery after shoulder injection affects postoperative infection risk in Medicare patients. *J Shoulder Elbow Surg* 2016;25:390-397.

    This article demonstrates significant increase in postoperative infection in Medicare patients who underwent cortisone injection within 3 months before shoulder arthroscopy and arthroplasty. Level of evidence: III (Retrospective Case-Control Design Using Large Database Treatment Study).

39. Henrotin Y, Raman R, Richette P, et al: Consensus statement on viscosupplementation with hyaluronic acid for the management of osteoarthritis. *Semin Arthritis Rheum* 2015;45:140-149.

40. Shen L, Yuan T, Chen S, Xie X, Zhang C: The temporal effect of platelet-rich plasma on pain and physical function in the treatment of knee osteoarthritis: Systematic review and meta-analysis of randomized controlled trials. *J Orthop Surg Res* 2017;12:16.

This metanalysis shows that Intra-articular PRP injections probably are more efficacious in the treatment of knee OA in terms of pain relief and self-reported function improvement at 3, 6 and 12 months follow-up, compared with other injections, including saline placebo, HA, ozone, and corticosteroids. Level of evidence: I (Metanalysis of RCTs)

41. Weinstein DM, Bucchieri JS, Pollock RG, Flatow EL, Bigliani LU: Arthroscopic debridement of the shoulder for osteoarthritis. *Arthroscopy* 2000;16:471-476.
42. Skelley NW, Namdari S, Chamberlain AM, Keener JD, Galatz LM, Yamaguchi K: Arthroscopic debridement and capsular release for the treatment of shoulder osteoarthritis. *Arthroscopy* 2015;31:494-500.
43. Mitchell JJ, Warner BT, Horan MP, et al: Comprehensive arthroscopic management of glenohumeral osteoarthritis: Preoperative factors predictive of treatment failure. *Am J Sports Med* 2017;45:794-802.

    The authors present their average 2-year outcome of comprehensive arthroscopic management of GH arthritis and show that patients with less joint space and posterior glenoid bone loss were more likely to progress to early failure. Level of evidence: III (Case-Control Study).
44. Tao MA, Karas V, Riboh JC, Laver L, Garrigues GE: Management of the stiff shoulder with arthroscopic circumferential capsulotomy and axillary nerve release. *Arthrosc Tech* 2017;6:e319-e324.

    This study describes authors' preferred method for arthroscopic capsular release for management of severe, chronic glenohumeral joint contractures when conservative treatment fails. Level of evidence: V (Technique Paper).
45. Schoch B, Schleck C, Cofield RH, Sperling JW: Shoulder arthroplasty in patients younger than 50 years: Minimum 20-year follow-up. *J Shoulder Elbow Surg* 2015;24:705-710.
46. Namdari S, Alosh H, Baldwin K, Glaser D, Kelly JD: Biological glenoid resurfacing for glenohumeral osteoarthritis: A systematic review. *J Shoulder Elbow Surg* 2011;20:1184-1190.
47. Gilmer BB, Comstock BA, Jette JL, Warme WJ, Jackins SE, Matsen FA: The prognosis for improvement in comfort and function after the ream-and-run arthroplasty for glenohumeral arthritis: An analysis of 176 consecutive cases. *J Bone Joint Surg Am* 2012;94:e102.
48. Gartsman GM, Roddey TS, Hammerman SM: Shoulder arthroplasty with or without resurfacing of the glenoid in patients who have osteoarthritis. *J Bone Joint Surg Am* 2000;82:26-34.
49. Torchia ME, Cofield RH, Settergren CR: Total shoulder arthroplasty with the Neer prosthesis: Long-term results. *J Shoulder Elbow Surg* 1997;6:495-505.
50. Edwards TB, Kadakia NR, Boulahia A, et al: A comparison of hemiarthroplasty and total shoulder arthroplasty in the treatment of primary glenohumeral osteoarthritis: Results of a multicenter study. *J Shoulder Elbow Surg* 2003;12:207-213.
51. Sperling JW, Cofield RH, Rowland CM: Minimum fifteen-year follow-up of Neer hemiarthroplasty and total shoulder arthroplasty in patients aged fifty years or younger. *J Shoulder Elbow Surg* 2004;13:604-613.
52. Papadonikolakis A, Neradilek MB, Matsen FA 3rd: Failure of the glenoid component in anatomic total shoulder arthroplasty: A systematic review of the English-language literature between 2006 and 2012. *J Bone Joint Surg Am* 2013;95:2205-2212.
53. Bohsali KI, Bois AJ, Wirth MA: Complications of shoulder arthroplasty. *J Bone Joint Surg Am* 2017;99:256-269.

    This systematic review article presents rate and subtypes of the most common complications after anatomic and reverse TSA between 2006 and 2015. Level of evidence: III (Systematic review of clinical data).
54. Gartsman GM, Elkousy HA, Warnock KM, Edwards TB, O'Connor DP: Radiographic comparison of pegged and keeled glenoid components. *J Shoulder Elbow Surg* 2005;14:252-257.
55. Schnetzke M, Rick S, Raiss P, Walch G, Loew M: Mid-term results of anatomical total shoulder arthroplasty for primary osteoarthritis using a short-stemmed cementless humeral component. *Bone Joint J* 2018;100-B:603-609.

    This study reports the mid-term outcome of total shoulder arthroplasty using a short-stem humeral component resulted and shows that good clinical outcomes with no evidence of loosening can be achieved. Level of evidence: IV (Therapeutic case series).
56. Churchill RS, Chuinard C, Wiater JM, et al: Clinical and radiographic outcomes of the Simpliciti canal-sparing shoulder arthroplasty system: A prospective two-year multicenter study. *J Bone Joint Surg Am* 2016;98:552-560.

    This article reports results of a multicenter 2-year clinical outcome study on primary anatomic TSA for GH arthritis using the Simpliciti canal-sparing humeral implant. Level of evidence: IV (Therapeutic).
57. Simone JP, Streubel PH, Sperling JW, Schleck CD, Cofield RH, Athwal GS: Anatomical total shoulder replacement with rotator cuff repair for osteoarthritis of the shoulder. *Bone Joint J* 2014;96-B:224-228.
58. Boileau P, Watkinson DJ, Hatzidakis AM, Balg F: Grammont reverse prosthesis: Design, rationale, and biomechanics. *J Shoulder Elbow Surg* 2005;14:147S-161S.
59. Berliner JL, Regalado-Magdos A, Ma CB, Feeley BT: Biomechanics of reverse total shoulder arthroplasty. *J Shoulder Elbow Surg* 2015;24:150-160.
60. Palsis JA, Simpson KN, Matthews JH, Traven S, Eichinger JK, Friedman RJ: Current trends in the use of shoulder arthroplasty in the United States. *Orthopedics* 2018;41:e416-e423.

    The authors reports the current trends in the use of shoulder arthroplasty in the US including a growing number of reverse TSAs and declining number of hemiarthroplasties in the past decade. Level of evidence: IV (Therapeutic case series).
61. Favard L, Levigne C, Nerot C, Gerber C, De Wilde L, Mole D: Reverse prostheses in arthropathies with cuff tear: Are survivorship and function maintained over time? *Clin Orthop Relat Res* 2011;469:2469-2475.
62. Cuff DJ, Pupello DR, Santoni BG, Clark RE, Frankle MA: Reverse shoulder arthroplasty for the treatment of rotator cuff deficiency: A concise follow-up, at a minimum of 10 years, of previous reports. *J Bone Joint Surg Am* 2017;99:1895-1899.

This is a follow up study on a previously evaluated 94 patients (96 shoulders) who underwent reverse shoulder arthroplasty using a central compressive screw with 5.0-mm peripheral locking screws for end-stage rotator cuff deficiency and showed 90.7% implant survivorship at minimum 10 years. Level of evidence: IV (Therapeutic).

63. Hartzler RU, Steen BM, Hussey MM, et al: Reverse shoulder arthroplasty for massive rotator cuff tear: Risk factors for poor functional improvement. *J Shoulder Elbow Surg* 2015;24:1698-1706.

64. Boyle MJ, Youn SM, Frampton CM, Ball CM: Functional outcomes of reverse shoulder arthroplasty compared with hemiarthroplasty for acute proximal humeral fractures. *J Shoulder Elbow Surg* 2013;22:32-37.

65. Mizuno N, Denard PJ, Raiss P, Walch G: Reverse total shoulder arthroplasty for primary glenohumeral osteoarthritis in patients with a biconcave glenoid. *J Bone Joint Surg Am* 2013;95:1297-1304.

66. Boileau P, Chuinard C, Roussanne Y, Neyton L, Trojani C: Modified latissimus dorsi and teres major transfer through a single delto-pectoral approach for external rotation deficit of the shoulder: As an isolated procedure or with a reverse arthroplasty. *J Shoulder Elbow Surg* 2007;16:671-682.

67. Hsu JE, Somerson JS, Vo KV, Matsen FA III: What is a "periprosthetic shoulder infection"? A systematic review of two decades of publications. *Int Orthop* 2017;41:813-822.

This review article shows a great inconsistency in the literature regarding the definition of peroprosthetic shoulder infection. level of evidence: III (Systematic review of clinical data).

68. Pottinger P, Butler-Wu S, Neradilek MB, et al: Prognostic factors for bacterial cultures positive for *Propionibacterium acnes* and other organisms in a large series of revision shoulder arthroplasties performed for stiffness, pain, or loosening. *J Bone Joint Surg Am* 2012;94:2075-2083.

69. Strickland JP, Sperling JW, Cofield RH: The results of two-stage re-implantation for infected shoulder replacement. *J Bone Joint Surg Br* 2008;90:460-465.

70. George DA, Volpin A, Scarponi S, Haddad FS, Romano CL: Does exchange arthroplasty of an infected shoulder prosthesis provide better eradication rate and better functional outcome, compared to a permanent spacer or resection arthroplasty? A systematic review. *BMC Musculoskelet Disord* 2016;17:52.

This systematic review does not find a difference in infection eradication and functional improvement between established modalities for treatment of periprosthetic shoulder infection. Systematic Review of Reports of All Levels.

71. Hsu JE, Gorbaty JD, Whitney IJ, Matsen FA III: Single-stage revision is effective for failed shoulder arthroplasty with positive cultures for Propionibacterium. *J Bone Joint Surg Am* 2016;98:2047-2051.

The authors report that clinical outcomes after single-stage revision for *Propionibacterium* culture-positive shoulder were at least as good as the outcomes in revision procedures for control shoulders and two-stage revision might not be necessary in these patients. Systematic Review of Reports of All Levels.

72. Singh JA, Sperling JW, Schleck C, Harmsen WS, Cofield RH: Periprosthetic infections after total shoulder arthroplasty: A 33-year perspective. *J Shoulder Elbow Surg* 2012;21:1534-1541.

73. Young AA, Walch G, Pape G, Gohlke F, Favard L: Secondary rotator cuff dysfunction following total shoulder arthroplasty for primary glenohumeral osteoarthritis: Results of a multicenter study with more than five years of follow-up. *J Bone Joint Surg Am* 2012;94:685-693.

74. Elhassan B, Ozbaydar M, Massimini D, Diller D, Higgins L, Warner JJ: Transfer of pectoralis major for the treatment of irreparable tears of subscapularis: Does it work? *J Bone Joint Surg Br* 2008;90:1059-1065.

75. Lehtimaki K, Rasmussen JV, Mokka J, et al: Risk and risk factors for revision after primary reverse shoulder arthroplasty for cuff tear arthropathy and osteoarthritis: A Nordic Arthroplasty Register Association study. *J Shoulder Elbow Surg* 2018;27:1596-1601.

This article reports the midterm risk of revision after anatomic and reverse TSA from Nordic Arthroplasty Registry. Level of evidence: III (Retrospective Cohort Design Using Large Database, Treatment Study).

Section 5
Elbow

EDITOR

Surena Namdari, MD, MSc

Chapter 26

Anatomy, Biomechanics, Physical Examination, and Imaging of the Elbow

Mark E. Morrey, MD, MSc

ABSTRACT

The evaluation of the elbow requires an understanding of the anatomy, biomechanics, and diagnostic tests for this complex joint. This chapter will review the pertinent anatomy, functional biomechanics, physical examination, and imaging studies useful to the orthopaedic surgeons in the evaluation of the elbow joint. In particular, the bony architecture and an understanding of the ligaments and tendons necessary for stability and function in both normal and abnormal states are reviewed. Particular attention is paid to the functional biomechanics necessary when treating complex pathology. Key pearls in diagnostic tests including a comparison of different imaging studies and physical examination maneuvers necessary to diagnose various pathologies are discussed.

Keywords: elbow anatomy; elbow biomechanics; elbow evaluation; elbow imaging studies; elbow physical examination

Anatomy

Bony Anatomy

As a trocho-ginglymoid joint, the bony anatomy of the elbow is complex. It consists of medial and lateral articulations which afford bony stability to the elbow (**Figure 1, A**). On the medial side, the trochlea articulates with the ulna within the greater sigmoid notch to create the ulnohumeral, hinged or trochoid, portion of the elbow joint. There is highly congruent anatomy through almost 180° of articular contact with the exception of the bare area of the greater sigmoid notch of the ulna which is devoid of cartilage[1] (**Figure 1, C**).

The coronoid has a medial and lateral facet which buttresses the trochlea anteriorly. Just distal and medial to the coronoid is the sublime tubercle which provides the attachment site of the anterior bundle of the medial ulnar collateral ligament (MUCL) (**Figure 2, A**). The medial epicondyle forms the attachment site for the origins of the flexor pronator mass and is larger and more posteriorly oriented than the lateral epicondyle.

Laterally, the capitellum and radial head form the radiocapitellar joint. The radius is held in close approximation to the ulna at the proximal radioulnar joint (PRUJ) by the annular ligament (**Figure 1, C**). The area of the ulna which articulates with the margin of the radial head at the PRUJ is also known as the lesser sigmoid notch. The radial head is a concave elliptical structure, covered with articular cartilage along the radiocapitellar joint and approximately 270° of the articular margin; this articulates with both the capitellum and the lesser sigmoid notch. The less prominent lateral epicondyle is the origin of the lateral extensor musculature and just distal to it at the geometric center of the radiocapitellar articulation is the origin of the lateral ulnar collateral ligamentous (LUCL) complex (**Figure 2, B**).

The distal humeral articulation is angled 30° from the longitudinal axis, and the anterior humeral line should pass through the center of the axis of rotation (**Figure 3, C**). This is a critical landmark to understand during reconstructive efforts to avoid loss of flexion or extension. The axis of rotation is 5° to 7° angulated in the coronal plane to the epicondylar axis with the medial side more distal than the lateral side (**Figure 3, A** and **B**). The angulation accounts for the change in a valgus carrying angle to a more varus position as the elbow is flexed. There is a wide range of sizes of the radius and capitellum, but in the same individual, there is a high correlation between sides which is useful for surgical planning in cases where the capitellum or radius has been destroyed.[2]

Posteriorly, the olecranon allows for a broad attachment site of the triceps. The ulna medially bends approximately 8° at 8 cm from the tip of the olecranon. There is a slight anterior bow to the proximal ulna, and the articulation to the tip of the coronoid is approximately 30° from the long axis of the ulna in the sagittal plane (**Figure 3, D**) which can be useful when classifying fractures of the coronoid.

Dr. Morrey or an immediate family member has stock or stock options held in Tenex- stock.

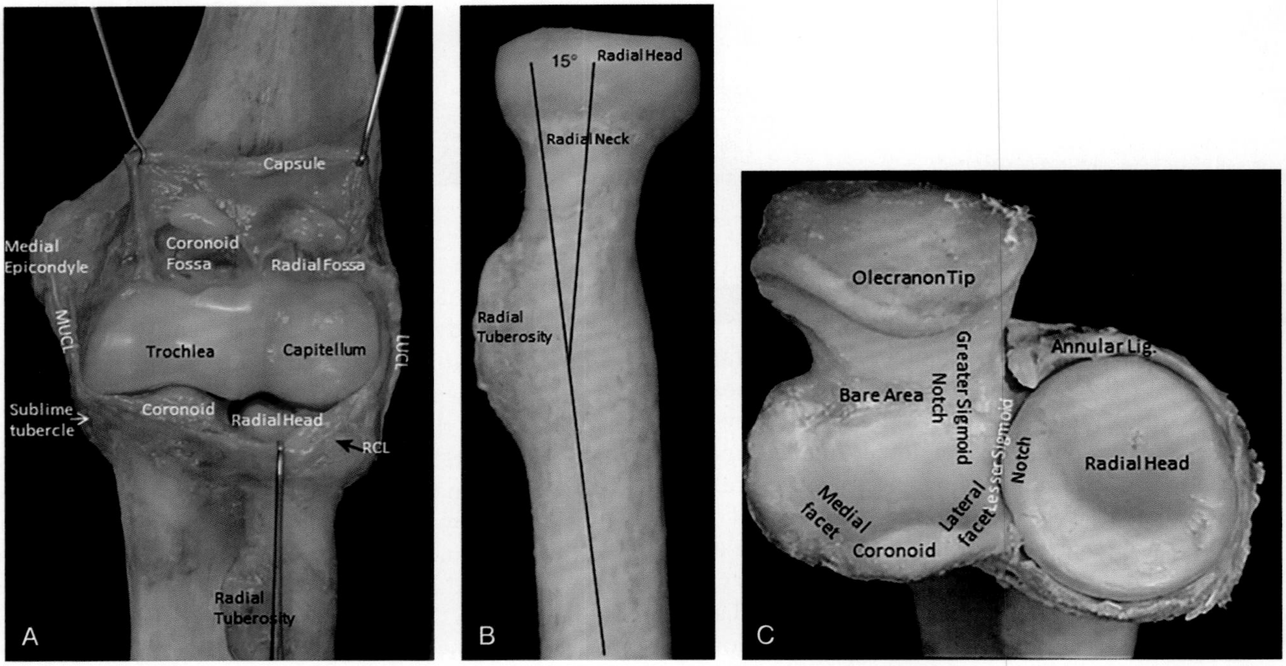

Figure 1 Photographs of elbow joint articulation as exposed through the capsule in (**A**) with the relevant bony landmarks and ligamentous attachment sites identified. **B**, shows the 15° of angular tilt from the long axis of the radius at the level of the radial tuberosity through the radial head and neck; (**C**) shows the ellipsoid radial head and annular ligament articulating with the lesser sigmoid notch within the proximal radial ulnar joint. The greater sigmoid notch and bare area are also identified in relationship to the olecranon tip and coronoid processes medial and lateral facets. LUCL = lateral ulnar collateral ligament; MUCL = medial ulnar collateral ligament; RCL = radial collateral ligament.

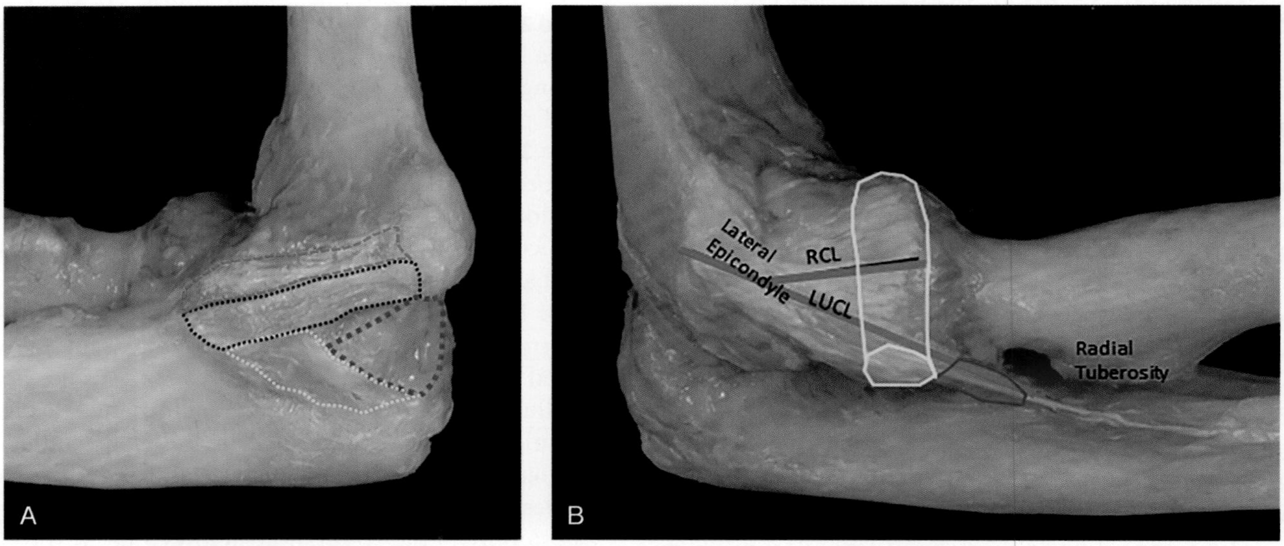

Figure 2 **A**, Photograph demonstrating that the medial ulnar collateral ligaments (MUCLs) are areas of capsular thickening which provide stability to the medial side of the elbow joint—The red dashed line is the anterior band of the anterior bundle; the dotted black line is the posterior band of the anterior bundle; the blue dotted line is the posterior bundle; and the yellow dotted line is the transverse bundle. **B**, Photograph of the lateral ulnar collateral ligament (LUCL) complex. The lines represent the approximate orientations of the radial collateral ligament (RCL) and lateral ulnar collateral ligament on the lateral side of the elbow. The yellow outline is the location of the annular ligament attachment proximal and deep to the ligamentous complex but intimately associated with it. The blue outline represents the ligamentous attachment site on the ulna of the LUCL proper.

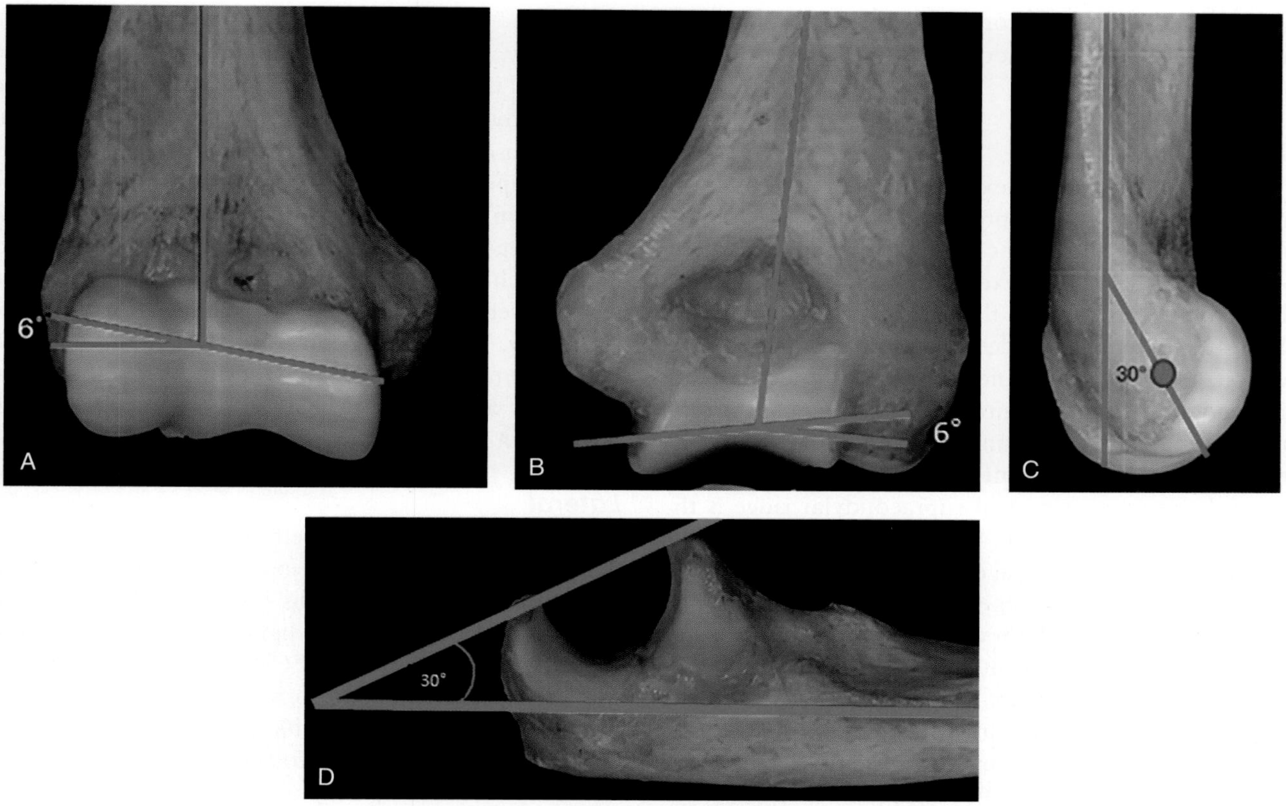

Figure 3 Cadaveric dissection photographs showing distal humeral articular angulation in anterior (**A**) and posterior (**B**) views in the coronal plane and sagittal plane in (**C**) and proximal ulnar articular angulation in the sagittal plan in (**D**).

Ligamentous Anatomy

The MUCL is the fan-shaped ligament and contains an anterior bundle, a posterior bundle, and a transverse band. It originates on the midportion of the medial epicondyle and inserts broadly and longitudinally to the sublime tubercle and medial margin of the olecranon[3,4] (**Figure 2, A**). Many fibers extend distally to fuse with the periosteum along the medial ulna, and recent studies have shown the benefit of this sleeve of tissue in force distribution along the ligament which is contiguous with septal tissue with contributions from the pronator teres and the flexor digitorum superficialis.[4,5]

The LUCL complex originates just distal to the lateral epicondyle at the geometric center of rotation of the capitellum and is composed of the radial collateral ligament (RCL) and LUCL (**Figure 2, B**). It fuses with the RCL and annular ligament (AL) and continues distally to insert on the supinator crest just distal to the AL insertion at the supinator crest of the ulna.[6]

Tendinous Anatomy

Multiple tendons cross the elbow joint to provide for both flexion, extension, pronation, and supination at the elbow and wrist. Broadly, there are two types of entheses, or tendinous attachments, to bone.[5,7,8] Fibrous attachments are more fleshy, broad, and indirect and typically arise from the metaphysis or diaphysis of the long bones and are grossly composed of very short tendinous or even muscular-appearing attachments. Muscles with these types of fibrous entheses around the elbow include the origin of the pronator teres (PT) on the medial side, extensor carpi radialis longus (ECRL) and brachioradialis (BR) and supinator on the lateral aspect, and origin of the brachialis and the deep head triceps from the metadiaphysis of the humerus anteriorly and posteriorly, respectively. The second type of attachment is the fibrocartilaginous enthesis which is associated with a direct attachment and a grossly recognizable tendon unit which typically attaches to the epiphysis or apophysis. Muscles with a fibrocartilaginous enthesis include the common flexor and extensor tendons, distal biceps and triceps tendons, and the insertion of the brachialis tendon.

Medial

On the medial side, the flexor tendons originate off the medial epicondyle from proximal to distal and superficial to deep including the flexor carpi radialis (FCR), palmaris longus (PL), flexor carpi ulnaris (FCU), and the humeral head of the flexor digitorum superficialis (FDS). These tendons coalesce to form a common flexor tendon group which is not easily separated because the tendon fibers interdigitate at their origins from the medial epicondyle. Just anterior and proximal to the insertion of the flexors off the medial epicondyle and along the anterior aspect of supracondylar ridge is the humeral origin of the PT. The deep ulnar head of the PT along with the humeral origin of the PT muscle form a tunnel through which the median nerve and brachial artery travel below the level of the lacertus fibrosus, a broad fascial attachment from the biceps brachii to the flexor pronator group, on the medial aspect of the elbow. These two structures pierce a fibrous septum between the FDS and ulnar head of the PT. This nerve can become compressed at this level causing pronator syndrome. The brachial artery divides and becomes the radial artery above and the ulnar artery below the ulnar head of PT muscle in the proximal forearm just distal to the articulation.

Anterior

Anteriorly, from the medial intermuscular septum to the lateral intermuscular septum and medial and lateral supracondylar ridges of the humerus originates the brachialis muscle which travels across the elbow to insert broadly upon the distal aspect of the coronoid on the proximal ulna anteriorly. Superficial to the brachialis is the biceps brachii. It is composed of a long and short head which fuse to form a common distal biceps tendon which inserts as a crescentic attachment to the radial tuberosity. This tendon spirals 90° with the long head inserting more proximal and posterior on the radial tuberosity and the short head more anterior and distal (**Figure 4, A** through **C**).

Lateral

On the lateral aspect of the elbow at the lateral epicondyle originates the common extensor tendon composed of the extensor carpi radialis brevis (ECRB), extensor digitorum (ED), extensor digiti minimi (EDM), and the extensor carpi ulnaris (ECU). Like the medial side, these tendons coalesce to form a common tendon that is not easily separated at its origin from the lateral epicondyle. Just proximal to the ECRB along the lateral column and intermuscular septum originates the ECRL muscle. Proximal to this origin is the origin of the BR in the distal third of the humerus. Both of these tendons arise from the humerus and intermuscular septum.

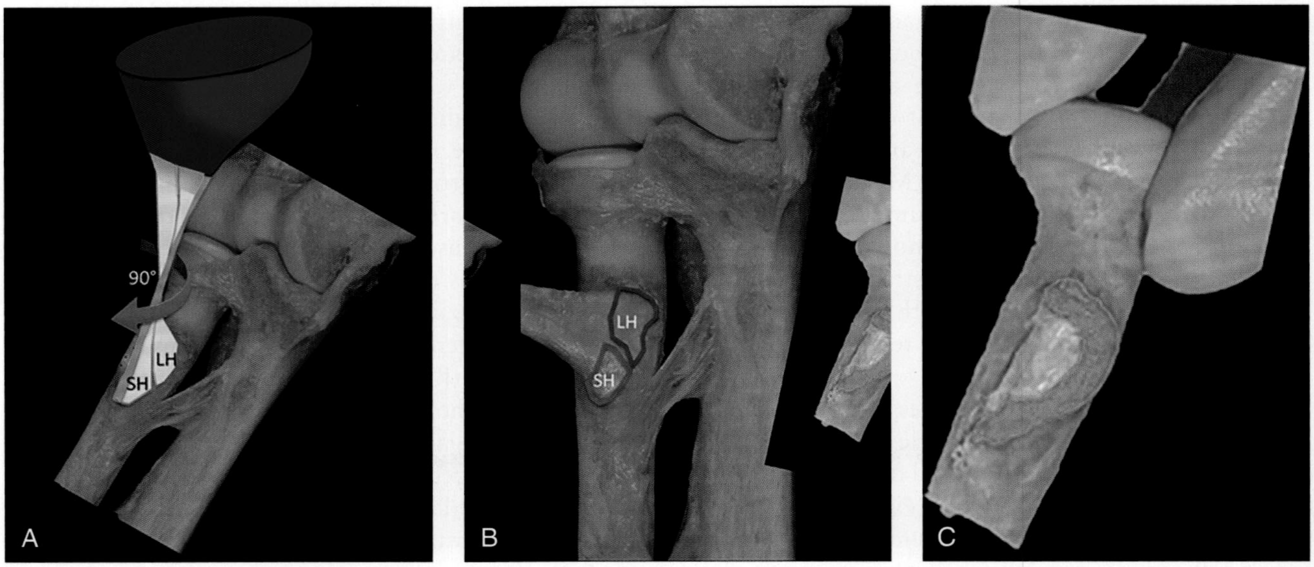

Figure 4 Cadaveric photograph with superimposed biceps tendon anatomy is illustrated. Biceps tendon anatomy is illustrated. **A**, shows how the short head (SH) spirals around the long head (LH) to attach more distally and anteriorly while the long head inserts more posteriorly and proximally in (**B**). The crescentic attachment site of the distal biceps tendon in (**C**).

Posterior

On the posterolateral aspect of the elbow is the origin of the anconeus from the posterior part of the humerus just proximal to the capitellum and posterior joint capsule. It inserts broadly along the posterior aspect of the ulna and is the first muscle palpable off the radial side of the ulna. The triceps tendon itself inserts onto the olecranon process with discrete heads and separate from the capsule. The medial head of the triceps inserts deep to and separately from the lateral and long heads on the olecranon[9] (**Figure 5, A** and **B**).

Biomechanics

Flexion-Extension

The normal arc of flexion-extension, although variable, ranges from 0° or slight hyperextension to 140 ° plus or minus 10°.[10-12] A functional arc of motion required for activities of daily living is about 30° to 130°.[13] While flexion and extension is one obvious role of the elbow joint, studies of passive motion at the elbow reveal that the elbow follows a more helical or vertical course of motion as measured from the intersection of the instantaneous axis within the sagittal plane.[14] This pattern has been attributed to the obliquity of the trochlear groove along which the ulna moves.[15] The amount of potential varus-valgus and axial laxity that occurs during elbow flexion averages about 3° to 4°.[15]

Center of Rotation

The axis of motion in flexion and extension has been the subject of many investigations. Fischer (1911), using Reuleaux technique, found the so-called *locus of the instant center of rotation* to be an area 2 to 3 mm in diameter at the center of the trochlea.[16] Fischer's observations were confirmed by use of the biplanar radiograph and CT scan in subsequent studies.[14] The axis of rotation passes through the center of the arcs formed by the trochlear sulcus and capitellum and can be identified from external landmarks. In the sagittal plane, the axis lies anterior to the midline of the humerus on a line that is collinear with the anterior cortex of the distal end of the humerus. The coronal orientation is defined by a line from the center of the projected center of the capitellum and from the anterior-inferior aspect of the medial epicondyle that corresponds to the projected center of the trochlea (**Figure 3, C**). In the coronal plane, a line perpendicular to the axis of rotation forms an angle of approximately 4° to 8° with the long axis of the humerus[15] (**Figure 3, A**). In the axial plane, this axis has been shown to be a mean of 14° externally rotated with respect to the plane formed by the posterior humerus and conversely internally rotated 3° to 8° relative to the plane of the epicondyles.[15,17] The reported variation in the elbow flexion axis is rather minimal. In fact, alterations of the axis by as much as 5 mm proximally, distally, anteriorly, or posteriorly have been shown to

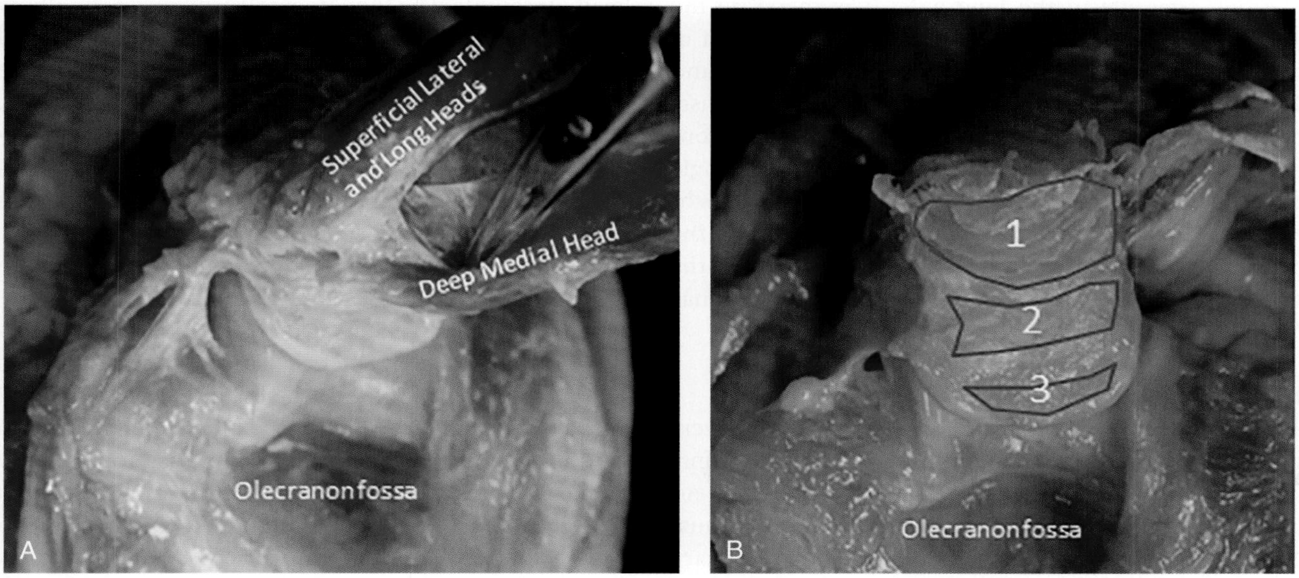

Figure 5 Triceps tendon anatomy is illustrated. **A**, shows the distinct insertions of the deep medial and superficial lateral and long tendinous heads. In **B**, the tendons have been removed, and 1 marks the superficial and long head insertion; 2, the deep medial head insertion; and 3, the capsular insertion on the posterior olecranon.

have only a slight effect on elbow kinematics. These data have helped to guide prosthetic development of less constrained but coupled elbow joint replacements designed to replicate the normal orientation and laxity of the elbow to prevent force transmission to the implant-cement and cement-bone interfaces.[15]

Forearm Rotation

The radius rotates around the ulna while centered on the capitellum, allowing forearm rotation or supination-pronation. Acceptable norms of pronation and supination are 75° and 85°, respectively. Fifty degrees in each direction is considered a functional arc of supination and pronation. Although variation exists, the rotational axis of the forearm is independent of elbow flexion and extension and considered to pass through the convex head of the radius in the proximal radioulnar joint.[18] Clinically and experimentally, greater than 10% angulation of either the radius or the ulna can cause functionally significant loss of forearm rotation.[15] Finally, the radius has been shown to migrate 1 to 2 mm proximally with pronation through a screw-home mechanism. This observation of physiologic radial laxity is relevant in instances of radial head replacement and examination maneuvers used to elicit pain on the lateral side of the elbow.

Carrying Angle

From an anatomic point of view, the carrying angle is based on the angles formed by the long axis of the humerus and ulna and the relative "tilt" of the articulations referable to the long axis. It is therefore the angle formed between the humerus and the forearm in the coronal plane and averages 10° to 15° for men and 13° to 18° for women, although much variation exists between age, race, sex, and body weight.[19-22] Some confusion has occurred regarding the change in this angle during flexion because of different measurement techniques. The specific varus/valgus relationship of the forearm to the humerus during flexion depends on the relative angular relationship of the humeral and ulnar articulations.

Elbow Stability

The elbow has both bony and soft tissue stabilizers that act statically and dynamically. Static constraints include the articulation and the capsular and ligamentous attachments. Dynamic stabilizers include the muscles which cross the elbow joint. The three primary stabilizers are the ulnohumeral articulation, the MUCL, and the LUCL complex (**Figure 2, A** and **B**). The secondary stabilizers are the radiocapitellar articulation, the common flexor tendon, the common extensor tendon, and the joint capsule. The primary ligamentous stabilizer of the elbow to valgus stress is the MUCL on the medial side.[15]

The LUCL is the primary stabilizer to posterior lateral rotatory instability on the lateral side. The coronoid process medial and lateral facet is the most important stabilizer of the elbow and provides a buttress to anterior dislocation and medial and lateral instability. In particular, the medial coronoid provides significant resistance to varus posterior medial rotatory instability (VPMRI).[23,24] Serial resection of the coronoid leads to significant instability and <50% loss of coronoid height. Recent computational studies show that with loss >2.5 mm of the medial buttress isolated repair of the LUCL is not capable of restoring rotation or angulation.[25]

Posteriorly the olecranon prevents anterior and varus and valgus instability. The articulation is unlocked from the olecranon fossa at approximately 30° of flexion, and at this point, forces are transmitted directly to the ligamentous stabilizers. Resection of normal bone of the posterior medial olecranon, as in valgus extension overload syndrome can lead to significantly increased forces across the MUCL.[26]

Clinical Examination

Physical examination of the elbow is essential to correct diagnosis and should focus on functional anatomy. The elbow is functionally critical because it places the hand in space and allows the hand to be brought to the torso, head, or mouth. The fundamental elements of the elbow examination are characteristic of other musculoskeletal examinations and include inspection, palpation, range of motion (ROM), strength, stability, and special tests. It is important to recognize that these examination elements are dynamic, and adequate assessment oftentimes combines examination maneuvers to fully elucidate the elbow pathology.

A comprehensive physical examination aids in the diagnosis of specific pathologies related to the functional anatomic elements which include nerves, muscles and tendons, ligaments, articular elements, and bone. On a practical basis, the examination is focused based on the history which is the most valuable tool to guide the clinical examination. The location, quality or type, context, duration, and severity of elbow pain are all important to understanding patients' pathology and focus the physical examination. Prior treatments including surgical interventions and injections can also help in making the correct diagnosis. When considering intervention, it is extremely helpful to determine the symptom trajectory, that is, if the pain is getting better, worse, or remaining constant over a period of time. Finally, a working knowledge of the pathologic conditions affecting different locations around the elbow is paramount to making a correct diagnosis. Specific pathologic conditions as they relate to elements of the history and the physical examination maneuvers which aid in identifying the pathology are listed in **Table 1**.

Inspection

Many alterations in the skeletal anatomy are often detectable by simple observation as much of the elbow joint is subcutaneous. As with other joints, it is often helpful to compare the elbow of interest to the normal contralateral side. For example, soft-tissue swelling and muscle atrophy or derangement is easily observed with comparison to the contralateral side (**Figure 6**). Scars or prior incisions should be observed and documented.

Table 1

Conditions Affecting the Elbow by Anatomic Compartment

Lateral	Characteristic Elements of the History	PE Manuevers to Elicit	Imaging Studies to Evaluate
Cutaneous neuritis (PACN, LABCN)	Burning or radiating pain; "I want to cut my arm off"	Direct palpation or percussion ie, Tinel test	Ultrasonography-guided diagnostic injection
Radial tunnel syndrome (PIN entrapment)	Extensor musculature "forearm aching" (PIN)	Wrist flexion and forearm pronation Rule of nines test Weakness and pain with resisted long finger extension	Ultrasonography-guided diagnostic injection EMG
Lateral elbow tendinopathy, ie, "tennis elbow"	Pain lifting things from a bag with a pronated hand, turning doorknobs, taking milk from the fridge, shaking hands, taking a laptop out of a bag, bumping lateral elbow.	Direct palpation ECRB origin Tennis elbow shear test Pain along with resisted wrist or long finger extension Laptop test	MRI if LUCL is suspected as part of pathology Ultrasonography
Posterolateral rotatory instability	Do not trust the elbow Feeling of giving way, or instability when pushing out of a chair with arms	PLR drawer PLR pivot shift Supinated push-up test	MRI
Plica	Pop with associated pain and then "feels better"	Direct palpation "click" with flexion and pronation (anterior) Direct palpation "click" with extension and supination (posterior)	MRI Dynamic ultrasonography
Trauma (RH, LE, Cap)	History of acute traumatic event and then pain	Direct palpation Pain with pronosupination or flexion and extension	Plain radiograph CT with 3D reconstruction
Radiocapitellar arthrosis (post trauma)	Distant trauma or surgery	RC load test (pain with pronation and resisted extension)	CT with 3D reconstruction
OCD or osteonecrosis	Gradual loss of motion +/− pain Catching and locking if loose bodies present	RC load test (pain with pronation and resisted extension)	CT with 3D reconstruction MRI

(continued)

Elbow

Table 1

Conditions Affecting the Elbow by Anatomic Compartment (continued)

Lateral	Characteristic Elements of the History	PE Manuevers to Elicit	Imaging Studies to Evaluate
Partial biceps tendon tear (occasional)	Pain in the lateral arm with resisted supination	Direct palpation of radial tuberosity with arm in pronation elicits crepitus and pain	MRI or ultrasonography
Medial			
Medial elbow tendiopathy or tendon tear	Pain washing the face or carrying objects with arm in a supinated position	Direct palpation flexor > pronator tendon origin Face press examination Server tray examination Resisted flexion TEST Moving valgus TEST (pain between 30° and 60° flexion)	MRI or ultrasonography
Snapping triceps	Pain with flexion with a pop or snap and often tingling into the fingers (if ulnar nerve involved)	Palpation with flexion	Ultrasonography
Ulnar neuritis or neuropathy	Ring and small finger go to sleep when elbow is flexed, ie, while reading in bed or wakes them up at night	Direct palpation/Tinel test	Ultrasonography or MRI
MUCL strain tear or instability	Decreased control and velocity while pitching (athlete) History of trauma and dislocation	Milking manuever Moving valgus stress test	MRI
Valgus extension overload	Decreased ROM and pain with deceleration and follow through	Valgus extension overload examination Arm bar examination	CT with 3D reconstruction MRI
Varus posteromedial rotatory instability	Decreased ROM after traumatic dislocation with continued varus deformity and pain with activities with the arm away from the body	Gravity assisted varus grind test	CT with 3D reconstruction
Ulnohumeral arthritis	History of inflammatory conditions or trauma	Painful ROM through the midarc with or without a load	Radiograph or CT with 3D reconstruction
Trauma (medial epicondyle or condyle fracture)	History of trauma	Direct palpation valgus stress, moving valgus stress test	Radiograph or CT with 3D reconstruction
MABCN neuroma or neuritis	Localized pain or burning with an area of hypersensitivity over an area of injury or prior surgery	Palpation or tinel test	Ultrasonography-guided injection
Median nerve compression	Vague forearm pain that may radiate from hand to forearm	Palpation or tinel test	Ultrasonography EMG
Posterior			
Posterior impingement primary OA with osteophyte formation	Pain when extending the arm and at the end of the day	Posterior arm bar or extension test	CT with 3D reconstruction

The radial collateral ligament resists varus stress throughout the arc of elbow flexion with varying contributions of the anterior capsule and articular surface in extension. The LUCL complex consists of the RCL and the LUCL. They have a common origin, and the RCL maintains consistent patterns of tension as it inserts and interdigitates with the annular ligament throughout the arc of flexion.[39] To properly assess collateral ligament integrity, the elbow should be flexed to about 15° to 30°. This relaxes the anterior capsule and removes the olecranon from the fossa. Varus stress is best applied with the humerus in full internal rotation and forearm supination. Valgus instability is best measured with the arm in 10° of flexion and full pronation.

Valgus Instability

The milking maneuver test for medial instability is performed by grabbing the thumb of the affected side's thumb with the elbow in about 90° of flexion as if the patient is throwing a ball. This may reproduce pain along the MUCL in cases of insufficiency. However, it is a static examination, and diagnostic accuracy may be improved by performing the moving valgus stress test (**Figure 7, A**).[40] This test is performed similar to the milking maneuver but is dynamic. It begins with the patient in a fully flexed throwers position, and the examiner applies a constant valgus torque while the patient extends the elbow. It is considered positive if the pain is reproduced between 120° and 70° of flexion and most commonly at 90° of flexion (**Figure 7, A**). Valgus extension overload represents a chronic attrition of the MUCL, and physical examination findings include reproduction of pain with an arm bar test. In this test, the patient's shoulder is placed at 90° of forward flexion, full internal rotation, and the patient's hand is placed on the examiner's shoulder. The examiner creates a forced extension by pulling down on the olecranon.

Rotatory Instability

Insufficiency of the LUCL is responsible for posterolateral instability of the elbow, which can be demonstrated in several ways.[30] Two tests are the lateral pivot shift and the posterior lateral rotatory drawer. Both are best performed with the patient supine and arm in forward flexion overhead. The patient's forearm is fully supinated, and the examiner grasps the wrist or forearm and slowly moves the elbow from extension to flexion while applying valgus and supination movements and an axial compressive force. This produces a rotatory subluxation of the ulnohumeral joint at about 40° of flexion. The rotation dislocates the radiohumeral joint posterolaterally by a coupled motion. As the elbow approaches extension, a posterior prominence (the dislocated radiohumeral joint) is noted with an obvious dimple in the skin proximal to the radial head (**Figure 7, B** and **C**). As the arm is gently flexed, the radial head reduces with a clunk. Unfortunately, pain or apprehension may render this maneuver difficult to execute unless performed under anaesthesia. The posterolateral rotatory drawer test is a gentler examination that can be reliably reproduced. This is performed when the elbow is slightly flexed and a valgus load is places while the forearm is grasped and gently lifted while being supinated. The radial dimple will be seen to disappear with this maneuver as the ulna rolls off the humerus and is then considered positive. Two other very simple tests for apprehension are the push-up and the chair push-up tests in which the patient attempts to perform a standard push-up or lift themselves from an arm chair by pushing down on the armrest with a supinated forearm, respectively. Apprehension or inability to perform the tests alerts the examiner that instability is likely.

VPMRI can best be assessed with the gravity-assisted varus grind test in which the arm is abducted away from the body to provide a varus stress with the weight of the arm against gravity in which the arm is then flexed and extended (**Figure 7, D**). Crepitus is considered positive, and anteromedial facet pathology, LUCL, and posterior bundle of the MUCL disruption should be suspected. Stability testing can also routinely be performed with fluoroscopy and ultrasonography, which can significantly aid in making the diagnosis with objective measurements.

Imaging

Proper selection of imaging studies can be crucial to the diagnosis and to guide treatment in pathologic conditions of the elbow. **Table 2** lists the uses of each of the imaging modalities and the advantages and disadvantages of each.

Plain Radiographs

Plain radiographs are by far the most useful screening tool for elbow pathology. Standard radiographs include the AP view and lateral views. Oblique views may be useful in cases of lateral or medial pathology. A true lateral view superimposes the medial and lateral trochlear ridges with that of the capitellar articulation. The anterior and posterior fat pads can be useful clues in instances of elbow effusion due to trauma.

CT Scan

The CT scan is increasingly recognized as an invaluable modality for evaluation and treatment of bony pathologies of the elbow. The use of 3D reconstruction

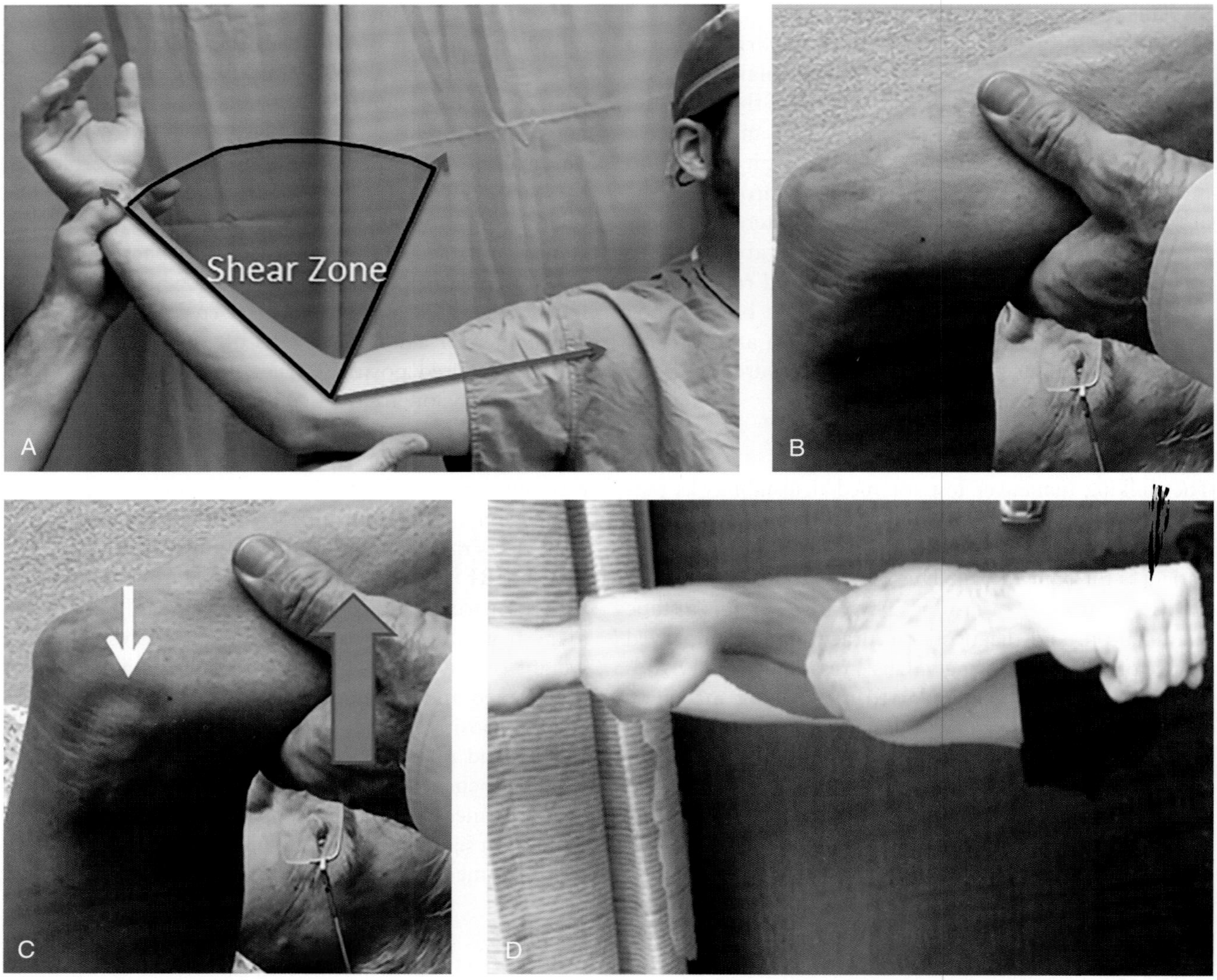

Figure 7 Photographs of physical examination and maneuvers for instability. (**A**) The moving valgus stress test is done with the patient in a fully flexed throwers position. The examiner applies a constant valgus torque while the patient fully extends the elbow. It is considered positive if the pain is reproduced between the shear zone of 120° and 70° of flexion and most commonly at 90° of flexion. **B** and **C**, demonstrates a posterior lateral rotatory drawer test. The forearm is slightly flexed, and an upward force is applied to the forearm in full supination. Note the dimple that is formed as the radial head subluxates in a patient with signs of posterior lateral rotatory instability. **D**, shows the gravity-assisted varus posterior medial rotatory grind test. With the arm fully abducted, it is gently brought through flexion and extension. Grinding and pain or an obvious subluxation are signs of varus posterior medial rotatory instability (VPMRI).

is extremely helpful for surgical planning for complex fracture patterns, but also cases involving reshaping of the distal articulation such as osteocapsular arthroplasty in the setting of primary osteoarthritis or posttraumatic conditions with associated elbow stiffness due to heterotopic ossification or significant osteophyte formation. CT can be invaluable in demarcating the paths of nerves and their relationship to bony prominences or ectopic bone prior to surgical intervention.[41]

Image quality with high-spatial and high-contrast resolution is paramount in CT for accurate diagnosis. Unfortunately, artifact from metal or motion can reduce the image quality immensely and can limit accurate evaluation in precisely the instance it is most needed—fracture healing. In the elbow, indwelling metal is a common hindrance, but there now exist modern-generation CT scanners which can effectively reduce metallic artifact, allowing clear visualization of the underlying bone in most cases.[42] Specifically, dual-energy CT (DECT) postprocessing has been extremely effective in reducing metal artifact when compared with conventional CT.[43] In fact, this technology is so specific it can be used to

Table 2

Uses, Advantages, and Disadvantages of Different Imaging Modalities for the Elbow

Imaging Modality	Uses	Advantages	Disadvantages
Radiograph	Excellent screen for fracture, can be used for dynamic assessment with examination under fluoroscopy, complementary with MRI for suspected osteomyelitis, screening or follow-up evaluation of prosthetic devices	Low cost, low radiation dose, excellent cortical bone detail	Lower resolution to other imaging modalities, poor for soft tissues
CT	Articular and complex fractures, osteochondritis dissecans (OCD) lesions, boney tumors (osteoid osteoma), heterotopic ossification and synostoses, crystalline arthropathy, nonunion, infection, implant component malposition	Superior bone detail, fast acquisition times, can distinguish inflammatory crystalline disease from infection (dual-energy CT), cost	Ionizing radiation, need the appropriate technology for high resolution
MRI	Soft-tissue conditions including tendon tears and tendinopathies, chronic and acute ligament injuries, nondisplaced articular lesions, osteonecrosis prior to collapse, early inflammatory arthropathy, soft-tissue tumors, infection	Excellent soft-tissue detail and identification of edema, no ionizing radiation, cost	Length of scan, prone positioning for scans is not well tolerated by many patients, can "overcall" nonpathologic conditions
Ultrasonography	Tendinopathies and tendon rupture (first line), ligamentous injury, nerve entrapment syndromes, puncture wounds with suspected foreign body	Dynamic real-time assessment, portable, flow velocity of blood supply, ability to inject for diagnostic purposes under direct visualization, no ionizing radiation or long scan times associated with MRI	Technical expertise of the user, poor for deep bone or articular lesions

differentiate the inflammatory urate crystals present in gout from calcium pyrophosphate and hydroxyapatite deposition diseases.[44] These modalities can also be used to determine implant malposition as in the case of total elbow arthroplasty (**Figure 8, A** through **E**). One potential downside to CT is the amount of radiation exposure typically needed for a high-resolution image. While this is certainly a concern, recent innovations are allowing for dose modulation without degrading image quality.

Magnetic Resonance Imaging

MRI is useful for the diagnosis of most soft-tissue pathologies about the elbow. It can additionally be used to identify occult fracture. The patient is positioned prone in the scanner with the arm above the head in the so-called superman position. One downside is this position can be uncomfortable, depending on the length of the scan. As with CT, MRI imaging is typically performed in three planes: axial, coronal, and sagittal. Coronal images are particularly useful to visualize the tendon and ligamentous attachments. The plane of imaging can also be changed to align with the anatomic structure in question, such as the biceps tendon with the use of a flexion, abduction, and supination (FABS) view.

The selection of imaging sequences used to evaluate the elbow differs among institutions and typically includes a combination of T1, T2, proton density (PD), and short tau inversion recovery sequences. Intravenous gadolinium-based contrast material is indicated in cases of suspected neoplasm, infection, or inflammatory process. MRI following intra-articular injection of dilute gadolinium-based contrast material (MR arthrogram) can be used if there is suspicion of a ligament tear, loose body, or osteochondritis dissecans with articular flap tears. Nerve entrapment syndromes can also be evaluated by MRI. Often, there is surrounding edema or areas of calibre change within the nerves on fluid-sensitive sequences.

Fat saturation is often used on T2 and proton density sequences and improves visualization of bone marrow or soft-tissue edema as in cases of infection or

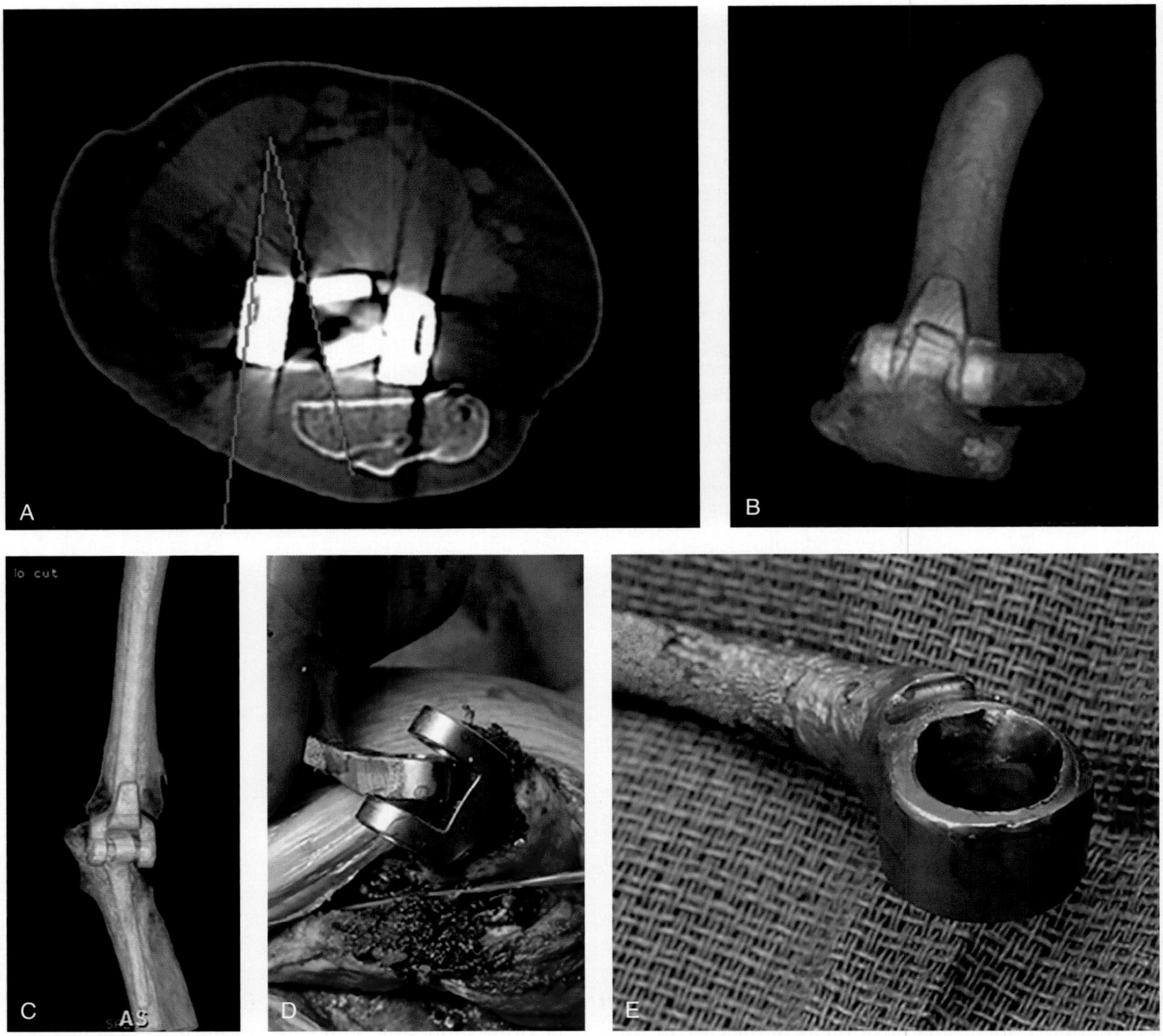

Figure 8 Dual-energy CT (DECT) with metal suppression to evaluate component malposition in TEA. **A**, is 2-D axial image showing significant rotational malalignment between humeral and ulnar components. **B** and **C**, show 3-D image with "ghosting" which shows the orientation of the implant within the bone. (**D** and **E**) Photographs show the in situ malposition and the metal wear trough (*) from the medial side of the component.

tumor. MRI at higher field strengths (1.5-3 T) is preferable because of the superior signal-to-noise ratio (SNR) which improves spatial resolution and decreases scan times.[45] Unfortunately, imaging artifacts such as chemical shift, metallic susceptibility, and pulsation artifact are accentuated at higher field strengths (particularly 3 T). Therefore, if metallic hardware is in the region of interest, scans are performed at lower field strengths. Finally, the amount of energy transferred to the patient increases with the square of the field strength, which can produce heat.[45]

Ultrasonography

Ultrasonography is being used increasingly for the evaluation of ligaments, tendons, and nerves. The elbow is suited to ultrasonography given its relatively subcutaneous location and the ability to perform a dynamic evaluation of the elbow, including provocative maneuvers, ultrasonic palpation, and a resolution not afforded by either CT or MRI when hardware is in place. Furthermore, not only diagnoses, but treatment can be performed utilizing ultrasonography-guided injections and procedures. Finally, a recent European

Society of Musculoskeletal Radiology Delphi-based consensus paper concluded that ultrasonography may be the first-line imaging technique for the assessment of tendinopathies, synovitis, septic arthritis, joint effusions, and nerve compression syndromes.[46] Because of the nature of how ultrasonography works, a drawback is that it is not as expedient for evaluating bony structures as radiographs and CT. Additionally, ultrasonography is also dependent on the skill of the ultrasonographer and may not be of equal quality in all practice environments.

As with the physical examination, the elbow is divided into four compartments for routine ultrasonography diagnostic practice: anterior, lateral, posterior, and medial. Specific structures in each of the quadrants are orthogonally examined in short and long axis views. The anatomic structures are then sonographically characterized according to four visual criteria: echogenicity, echotexture, vascularity, and anisotropy.[47] Structures that appear white or bright are described as being echogenic or hyperechoic, and represent regions with ultrasonic impedance such as a normal tendon or ligament and bone. Regions that are relatively darker are described as being hypoechoic (or of decreased echogenicity), representing structures with less acoustic impedances including normal muscle and degenerative tendon. Anechoic is a term describing a uniformly black region, such as fluid within bursae, that is devoid of internal reflections. Echotexture is a term used to describe the pattern of acoustic shadows within an individual structure such as fibrillated ligament and tendon patterns. When indicated, dynamic imaging can be performed to assess for nerve instability or tendon or collateral ligament injury. Detailed scanning reference guidelines are available on the European Society of Musculoskeletal Radiology (ESSR) website.[48]

Summary and Conclusions

The evaluation of the elbow requires an intimate understanding of the anatomy, biomechanics, and diagnostic tests for this complex joint. The relevant anatomy provides a foundation to understanding the functional biomechanics, physical examination maneuvers, and imaging studies useful in its evaluation. In particular, stability is conferred to the elbow by the bony articular anatomy, which is highly congruent, and the ligamentous structures on the medial and lateral sides. These structures should be the focus of the examiners' physical examination and choice of diagnostic studies to uncover underlying pathologic conditions.

Key Study Points

- The anatomy of the elbow is complex and a thorough understanding helps the clinician to a) understand the biomechanics b) perform the physical exam maneuvers and c) order appropriate imaging studies to diagnose elbow pathology and direct treatment.
- The normal elbow has a range of motion from 0° to 140° from extension to flexion and 75° and 85° in pronation and supination respectively. Pathological entities frequently affect the arc of motion and a functional arc in each plane is 100° for flexion and extension and forearm rotation.
- Elbow stability is determined by primary and secondary stabilizers. Injury to these structures causes elbow instability. The three primary stabilizers are the ulnohumeral articulation, the MUCL, and the LUCL complex on the medial and lateral sides respectively. Secondary stabilizers are the radiocapitellar articulation, the common flexor tendon, the common extensor tendon, and the joint capsule.
- The physical exam is directed by history and location of the patients pain in the anterior, posterior, medial or lateral aspect of the elbow. Pathologic entities associated with these discreet compartments aide the examiner in detecting pathologic conditions.
- Proper selection of imaging studies can be aide the diagnosis and guide treatment and each of the imaging modalities have advantages and disadvantages. Plain radiographs remain the hallmark and the best screening test.

Annotated References

1. Karbach LE, Elfar J: Elbow instability: Anatomy, biomechanics, diagnostic maneuvers, and testing. *J Hand Surg Am* 2017;42(2):118-126.

   This article reviews the elbow's complex bony and ligamentous anatomy and the biomechanical characteristics important to understanding the maneuvers and testing used to diagnose elbow instability patterns.

2. Vanhees M, Shukla DR, Fitzsimmons JS, et al: Anthropometric study of the radiocapitellar joint. *J Hand Surg Am* 2018; 43(9):867.e1-867.e6.

   This study examined relationship between the size of the radial head and the size of the capitellum and whether there were differences between the right and left elbows. Investigators found a high correlation between the long outer diameter of the radial head and the vertical height of the capitellum as well its anterior width and between the left and the right elbow.

Elbow

3. Kholinne E, Zulkarnain RF, Lee HJ, et al: Functional classification of the medial ulnar collateral ligament: An in vivo kinematic study with computer-aided design. *Orthop J Sports Med* 2018;6(3):2325967118762750.

This study analyzed ligament functional properties and kinematics at the level of the MUCL fibers. This study provides MUCL group coverage area and kinematic function for each degree of motion arc, allowing selective reconstruction of the MUCL according to mechanism of injury and dominant fibers affected.

4. Labott JR, Aibinder WR, Dines JS, Camp CL: Understanding the medial ulnar collateral ligament of the elbow: Review of native ligament anatomy and function. *World J Orthop* 2018;9(6):78-84.

The MUCL of the elbow, is comprised of the anterior bundle, posterior, and transverse ligament, is commonly injured in overhead throwing athletes. The anterior bundle is the strongest component of the ligamentous complex and the primary restraint to valgus stress and is further subdivided into anterior and posterior bands which provide reciprocal function with the anterior band tight in extension, and the posterior band tight in flexion. This review consolidates existing literature regarding the native anatomy, biomechanical, and clinical significance of the entire medial ulnar collateral ligament complex.

5. Hoshika S, Nimura A, Yamaguchi R, et al: Medial elbow anatomy: A paradigm shift for UCL injury prevention and management. *Clin Anat* 2019;32:379-389.

The aim of this study was to anatomically clarify the medial side of the elbow joint in terms of the tendinous structures and joint capsule. A descriptive anatomical study of 23 embalmed cadaveric elbows was conducted.

6. Camp CL, Fu M, Jahandar H, et al: The lateral collateral ligament complex of the elbow: Quantitative anatomic analysis of the lateral ulnar collateral, radial collateral, and annular ligaments. *J Shoulder Elbow Surg* 2019;28(4):665-670.

Examination of the LUCLs, radial collateral ligaments, and annular ligaments in 10 cadaveric elbows were measured for surface areas, origin and insertion footprint areas, distances between perceived footprint centers and geometric footprint centroids, distances to key landmarks, and ligament isometry were measured. The LUCL origin center was 10.7 mm from the lateral epicondyle and insertion was 3.3 mm from the apex of the supinator crest helping guide surgeons for reconstruction.

7. Killian ML, Cavinatto L, Galatz LM, et al: The role of mechanobiology in tendon healing. *J Shoulder Elbow Surg* 2012;21(2):228-237.

8. Zelzer E, Blitz E, Killian ML, Thomopoulos S: Tendon-to-bone attachment: From development to maturity. *Birth Defects Res Part C Embryo Today - Rev* 2014;102(1):101-112.

9. Barco R, Sánchez P, Morrey ME, et al: The distal triceps tendon insertional anatomy—implications for surgery. *JSES Open Access* 2017;1(2):98-103.

Muscle insertions of the triceps have 3 distinct insertional areas to the olecranon corresponding to the posterior capsular insertion, the deep muscular portion, and the superficial tendinous portion of the triceps. The deep muscular head corresponds to the medial head of the triceps and the tendinous portion corresponded to the long and lateral heads and the triceps and the width at insertion was 2.6 cm and was 1.1 cm from the tip of the olecranon.

10. *Joint Motion: Method of measuring and recording*. Chicago, American Academy of Orthopedic Surgeons, 1965.

11. Boone DC, Azen SP: Normal range of motion of joints in male subjects. *J Bone Joint Surg Am* 1979;61(5):756-759.

12. Wagner C: Determination of the Rotary flexibility of the elbow joint. *Phys Ther Rev* 1977;39:47.

13. Askew LJ, An K-N, Morrey BF, et al: Functional evaluation of the elbow: Normal motion requirements and strength determination. *Orthop Trans* 1981;5:304.

14. Adikrishna A, Kekatpure AL, Tan J, et al: Vortical flow in human elbow joints: A three-dimensional computed tomography modeling study. *J Anat* 2014;225(4):390-394.

15. Morrey ME, Sanchez-Sotelo J, Morrey BF, eds: *Morrey's The Elbow and Its Disorders*, ed 5. Philadelphia, PA, Elsevier, 2018, p 1144.

16. Fick R: Handbuch der anatomie und mechanik der gelenke, unter berucksichtigung der bewegenden muskeln. *Jena* 1904;2(299).

17. Sabo MT, Athwal GS, King GJ: Landmarks for rotational alignment of the humeral component during elbow arthroplasty. *J Bone Joint Surg Am* 2012;94(19):1794-1800.

18. Fraysse F, Thewlis D: Comparison of anatomical, functional and regression methods for estimating the rotation axes of the forearm. *J Biomech* 2014;47(14):3488-3493.

19. Atkinson WB, Elfman H: The caring angle of the human arm as a secondary symptom character. *Anatomy Rec* 1945;91:49.

20. Beals RK: The normal carrying angle of the elbow. *Clin Orthop* 1976;119:194.

21. Keats TE, Teeslink R, Diamond AE, Williams JH: Normal axial relationships of the major joints. *Radiology* 1966;87:904.

22. Lanz T, Wachsmuth W. *Praktishe Anatomie*. Berlin, Springer-Verlag, 1959.

23. Pollock JW, Brownhill J, Ferreira L, et al: The effect of anteromedial facet fractures of the coronoid and lateral collateral ligament injury on elbow stability and kinematics. *J Bone Joint Surg Am* 2009;91(6):1448-1458.

24. Hartzler RU, Llusa-Perez M, Steinmann SP, et al: Transverse coronoid fracture: When does it have to be fixed? *Clin Orthop Relat Res* 2014;472(7):2068-2074.

25. Karademir G, Bachman DR, Stylianou AP, Cil A: Posteromedial rotatory incongruity of the elbow: A computational kinematics study. *J Shoulder Elbow Surg* 2018;28(2):371-380.

The effect of different anteromedial coronoid fracture patterns with different combinations of ligamentous repairs was examined to determine if smaller fractures could be treated with ligamentous repair alone versus larger fragments needing a combination of ligament, bony repair or reconstruction. The study concluded that LUCL repair alone is sufficient to restore kinematics for small fractures as long as deep flexion is avoided and with a posteriormedial bundle repair kinematics were restored to normal and larger fractures need bone and ligament repairs.

26. Kamineni S, ElAttrache NS, O'Driscoll SW, et al: Medial collateral ligament strain with partial posteromedial olecranon resection. A biomechanical study. *J Bone Joint Surg Am* 2004;86(11):2424-2430.
27. Morrey BF, Chao EY: Passive motion of the elbow joint: a biomechanical study. *J Bone Joint Surg Am* 1979;61A:63.
28. Childress HM: Recurrent over nerve dislocation at the elbow. *Clin Orthop* 1975;108:168.
29. O'Driscoll SW, Goncalves LB, Dietz P: The hook test for distal biceps tendon avulsion. *Am J Sports Med* 2007;35(11):1865-1869.
30. O'Driscoll SW, Morrey BF, An KN: Intra-articular pressuring capacity of the elbow. *Arthroscopy* 1990;6:100.
31. Loh YC, Lam W, Stanley J, Soames R: A new clinical test for radial tunnel syndrome–the rule-of-nine test: A cadaveric study. *J Orthop Surg* 2004;12(1):83-86.
32. Youm Y, Dryer RF, Thambyrajah K, et al: Biomechanical analysis of forearm pronation – supination and elbow flexion-extension. *J Biomech* 1979;12:245.
33. Docherty MA, Schwab RA, Ma OJ: Can elbow extension be used as a test of clinically significant injury?. *South Med J* 2002;95(5):539-541.
34. O'Neill OR, Morrey BF, Tanaka S, An KN: Compensatory motion in the upper extremity after elbow arthrodesis. *Clin Orthop Relat Res* 1992(281):89-96.
35. Elkins EC, Ursula ML, Khalil GW: Objective recording of the strength of normal muscles. *Arch Phys Med* 1951;33:639.
36. Provins KA, Salter N: Maximum torque exerted about the elbow joint. *J Appl Physiol* 1955;7:393.
37. Rasch PJ: Effect of position of forearm on strength of the elbow flexion. *Res Q* 1955;27:393.
38. Williams M, Stutzman L: Strength variations through the range of motion. *Phys Ther Rev* 1959;39:145.
39. Regan WD, Korinek SL, Morrey BF, An KN: Biomechanical study of ligaments about the elbow joint. *Clin Orthop* 1991;271:170.
40. O'Driscoll SW, Lawton RL, Smith AM: The "moving valgus stress test" for medial collateral ligament tears of the elbow. *Am J Sports Med* 2005;33(2):231-239.
41. Bachman DR, Kamaci S, Thaveepunsan S, et al: Preoperative nerve imaging using computed tomography in patients with heterotopic ossification of the elbow. *J Shoulder Elbow Surg* 2015;24(7):1149-1155.
42. Roth TD, Buckwalter KA, Choplin RH: Musculoskeletal computed tomography: Current technology and clinical applications. *Semin Roentgenol* 2013;48(2):126-139.
43. Zhou C, Zhao YE, Luo S, et al: Monoenergetic imaging of dual-energy CT reduces artifacts from implanted metal orthopedic devices in patients with factures. *Acad Radiol* 2011;18(10):1252-1257.
44. Desai MA, Peterson JJ, Garner HW, Kransdorf MJ: Clinical utility of dual-energy CT for evaluation of tophaceous gout. *RadioGraphics* 2011;31(5):1365-1375; discussion 1376-7.
45. Ramnath RR: 3T MR imaging of the musculoskeletal system (Part I): Considerations, coils, and challenges. *Magn Reson Imaging Clin N Am* 2006;14(1):27-40.
46. Klauser AS, Tagliafico A, Allen GM, et al: Clinical indications for musculoskeletal ultrasound: A delphi-based consensus paper of the European Society of Musculoskeletal Radiology. *Eur Radiol* 2012;22(5):1140-1148.
47. Smith J, Finnoff JT: Diagnostic and interventional musculoskeletal ultrasound: Part 1. Fundamentals. *PM R* 2009;1(1):64-75.
48. Radiology, ESoM: *Musculoskeletal ultrasound technical guidelines. II.* Elbow, 2015; Available at: http://www.essr.org/html/img/pool/elbow.pdf2015.

Chapter 27

Elbow Degenerative Conditions and Nerve Disorders

Matthew L. Ramsey, MD • Jason S. Klein, MD

ABSTRACT

The elbow is a complex joint that is prone to pain and dysfunction. There are several pathologies that result in arthritis and stiffness with a wide variety of nonsurgical and surgical treatment options. There also are several important neurovascular structures that cross the elbow en route to supplying the forearm and hand. Two nerve disorders where the pathology originates around the elbow include cubital tunnel and radial tunnel syndromes. This chapter will address the etiologies, treatments, and outcomes for elbow arthritis, stiffness, and nerve compression disorders.

Keywords: Cubital and radial tunnel syndrome; elbow arthritis

Introduction

The elbow is a complex synovial hinge joint made up of three articulations (the ulnohumeral, radiocapitellar, and radioulnar) as well as the surrounding ligaments, capsule, and muscles. The delicate interplay of these structures as well as elbow's unique geometry places the elbow at unique risk for dysfunction. Patients with arthritis may complain of pain and stiffness, which is particularly debilitating when one loses the motion required for most activities of daily living. Functional range of motion has been defined as a 100° flexion/extension arc (30° to 130° of flexion) and 100° pronation/supination arc (50° of supination and 50° of pronation).[1] Historically, inflammatory arthritides such as rheumatoid arthritis were a common cause of elbow joint arthritis. However, with the introduction of disease modifying antirheumatic drugs (DMARDs), patients have been better able to slow the progression of inflammatory conditions. Nonetheless, rheumatoid arthritis continues to be a challenging cause of elbow arthritis and stiffness. Other causes not covered in this chapter include septic arthritis, crystalline arthropathy, and hemophilia.

Dr. Ramsey or an immediate family member has received royalties from Integra (Ascension) and Zimmer; has stock or stock options held in Aevumed and Trice Medical; is a member of a speakers' bureau or has made paid presentations on behalf of Integra (Ascension) and Zimmer; serves as a paid consultant to or is an employee of Integra (Ascension) and Zimmer; has received research or institutional support from Integra (Ascension) and Zimmer; and serves as a board member, owner, officer, or committee member of the Rothman Institute. Neither Dr. Klein nor any immediate family member has received anything of value from or has stock or stock options held in a commercial company or institution related directly or indirectly to the subject of this chapter.

Etiologies

Primary osteoarthritis most commonly affects middle-aged males (~50 years old), manual laborers, throwing athletes, and heavy weight lifters. The prevalence is estimated to be less than 2% of the population. The primary pathology of elbow osteoarthritis is loss of articular cartilage with resulting osteophyte formation on the olecranon process, coronoid process, and their respective fossae (**Figure 1**). Secondary resultant changes involve osteophyte formation along the margin of the radial head as well as formation of loose bodies that may result in mechanical block or crepitance. Most patients initially complain of pain at terminal limits of motion as a result of capsular stretch and osteophyte impingement at the extremes of motion, with or without mechanical symptoms. Later in the disease process, pain through the mid arc of motion develops as the extent of cartilage loss progresses.

Rheumatoid arthritis (RA) is the most common inflammatory arthritis of the elbow. Unlike primary osteoarthritis, RA frequently involves the elbow joint, can be bilateral, and often involves other joints. Affecting ~1% to 2% of the population, it involves the

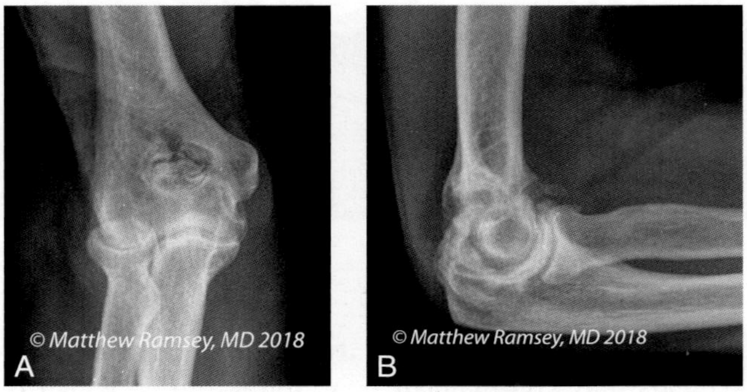

Figure 1 (**A**) AP and (**B**) lateral radiographs of an elbow with advanced osteoarthritis. Notice the periarticular osteophytes.

elbow joint in 20% to 50% of patients.[2,3] Rheumatoid arthritis causes an intense inflammatory synovitis that leads to progressive joint destruction. In the elbow, this involves the ulnohumeral joint early in the disease process, becoming pan articular as the disease progresses. Pockets of inflamed synovium can invade surrounding soft tissues, sometimes leading to radial and ulnar nerve compression and neuropathy. End-stage disease may result in ligamentous attenuation and instability.

Unlike RA and primary osteoarthritis, posttraumatic arthritis of the elbow can affect any age or sex. Posttraumatic arthritis is a common complication following traumatic soft-tissue injury, fracture, or surgery.[4] Fractures involving the articular surface may lead to advanced cartilage loss, particularly if the joint surface is not anatomically aligned following treatment. Ligamentous insufficiency may also lead to articular wear and progressive posttraumatic arthritis. Therefore, understanding the cause of posttraumatic arthritis is extremely important when considering management options.

Evaluation

A thorough history and physical examination are invaluable to understanding the type of disease process and the degree that the condition affects the patient. Understanding whether the patient has pain throughout the arc of motion or only at terminal limits as well as any associated mechanical symptoms or instability is of paramount importance. Associated conditions such as cubital tunnel syndrome must be considered and evaluated to provide optimal recommendations on management. From an imaging perspective, plain radiographs should be obtained during the initial workup to evaluate the articular surface and bony anatomy. CT scans with 3D reconstructions may be useful for evaluating the extent and location of disease and for surgical planning. MRI may be useful to evaluate the status of the soft tissues including the medial and lateral collateral ligamentous complexes. Electromyography and nerve conduction studies (EMG/NCS) may be useful to evaluate the degree of nerve compression and contribution to the elbow pain and/or dysfunction. Evaluating all of these findings in the context of the patient's age, activity level, expectations, handedness, and more will guide patient-physician shared decision for a given elbow condition.

Nonsurgical Treatment

Nonsurgical management is appropriate for early stages of elbow arthritis, particularly when the patient reports mild pain and a functional arc of motion. Treatment options include rest, activity modification, nonsteroidal anti-inflammatory medications (NSAIDs), corticosteroid injections, bracing treatment, and physical therapy. Although NSAIDs are an effective treatment modality, patients must be appropriately counseled about and followed up for possible development of gastrointestinal ulcers, kidney damage, or uncontrolled increases in blood pressure. Physical therapy (PT) can be beneficial, particularly when focused on pain control, anti-inflammatory modalities, maintaining strength, and preserving range of motion. However, PT should be done cautiously as aggressive passive stretch or strengthening of an arthritic, stiff elbow can worsen inflammation and increase pain. Steroid injections are a maintenance therapy that can provide pain relief but does not improve structural impediments to function. They should be limited to no more than three to four injections per year. Hyaluronic acid (HA) injections have gained support in the treatment of arthritis affecting other joints, particularly the knee. However, there is currently no evidence that HA injections improve conditions like posttraumatic osteoarthritis of the elbow.[5] Additionally, these medications are not FDA approved for use in the elbow and therefore have limited use in the treatment of elbow arthritis. Splinting (both dynamic and static) may be beneficial in cases of soft-tissue contracture. However, when the ulnohumeral articulation is involved, success may be limited, and similar to PT, splinting can actually exacerbate inflammation resulting in increased pain.

Nonsurgical medical management has become the mainstay of treatment for rheumatoid elbows thanks to the introduction of new disease modifying antirheumatic drugs (DMARDs) in the last 20 to 30 years. In addition to methotrexate, sulfasalazine, and leflunomide, new biologic agents such as TNF-α inhibitors, IL-6 inhibitors, B-cell inhibitors, and T-cell costimulator inhibitors have further improved the ability to reduce systemic inflammation and joint synovitis thereby slowing joint destruction and disease progression. Some studies have even found complete resolution of elbow arthritis signs and symptoms in patients taking DMARDs for rheumatoid arthritis.[6] Although these drugs have been revolutionary for the treatment of rheumatoid arthritis and other inflammatory conditions, they can alter a patient's ability to mount an immune response to infection. Therefore, concerns persist regarding increased infection and malignancy risks. When considering surgery, most experts recommend discontinuing the use of these biologic agents for 4 to 5 half-lives before a planned procedure to enhance surgical healing while limiting the risk of autoimmune flare.[7,8]

Surgical Management

If pain and functional limitation persist despite some or all of the nonsurgical measures discussed above, then surgical options may be considered. The appropriate surgical treatment must factor in the patients age, activity level, expectations, degree of pathologic changes, patient health, and surgeon experience. Although total elbow arthroplasty (TEA) is an option to treat elbow arthritis, implant durability and weight-bearing restrictions limit its widespread application to older, sedentary patients. Other options include open versus arthroscopic capsular release/débridement, interposition arthroplasty, arthrodesis, and resection arthroplasty. The following is a brief description of when each type of procedure may be used to treat certain elbow conditions.

Débridement, Synovectomy, Capsular Release, and Loose Body Removal

Open and arthroscopic débridement, synovectomy, capsular release, and loose body removal are effective treatment options for rheumatoid arthritis and early posttraumatic and osteoarthritis before the joint space and cartilage are completely lost (**Figure 2**). Synovectomy may delay disease progression and reduce the incidence of painful synovitis associated with inflammatory arthropathies. Both open and arthroscopic procedures can be performed to remove loose bodies and encroaching osteophytes on the humerus and the ulna to eliminate impingement and increase end range motion.

Open Versus Arthroscopic Débridement

Over the last 20 to 30 years, the literature supports both open and arthroscopic approaches as methods to obtain similar pain relief, patient satisfaction, and functional improvements even up to 10 years postoperatively.[9-12] The advantages of arthroscopic surgery are improved visualization, decreased morbidity, shorter rehabilitation, and less soft-tissue trauma. Arthroscopic elbow débridement should be carefully considered in patients who have undergone previous elbow surgery or who have had trauma resulting in distorted anatomy due to concerns of nerve injury with portal placement. Previous ulnar nerve transposition is a relative contraindication to arthroscopy and may require identification of the nerve before establishing medial portals. Additionally, an arthroscopic procedure is contraindicated in a patient with an ankylosed elbow that may prevent safe cannula entry or joint distension.

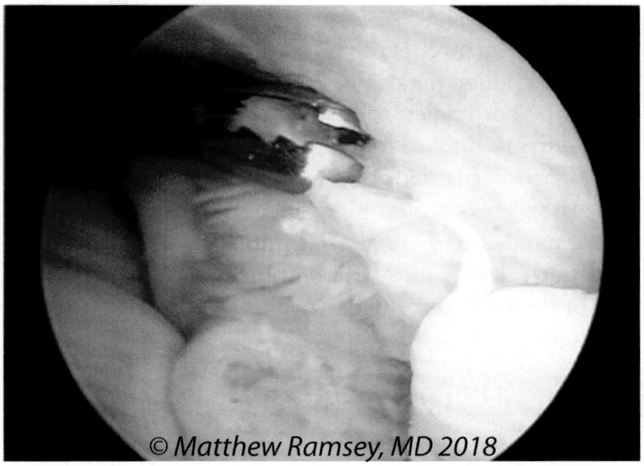

Figure 2 Arthroscopy photograph of a patient with rheumatoid arthritis with an active synovitis and loose body in the anterior compartment of the elbow.

A retrospective review by Galle et al[12] showed significant improvement in range of motion, pain, and outcomes for mild to moderate OA following arthroscopic débridement in 31 patients at a mean follow-up of 3.4 years. While concern exists about injury to neurovascular structures with arthroscopic elbow surgery, several studies have shown that it is safe when performed by trained surgeons.[11,13,14] In an effort to maximize motion gains, capsulectomy may be performed but increase the risk of iatrogenic injury to surrounding neurovascular structures. Greater improvement in the arc of range of motion was noted within the first few months when a capsulectomy was performed with the débridement, but no statistically significant difference in final range of motion were noted when compared with a cohort of patients who underwent débridement alone.[15] Therefore, routine capsulectomy may not be worth the risk in all cases.

Elbow

When ulnar nerve symptoms are present preoperatively or if preoperative elbow flexion is less than 90°, open ulnar nerve decompression or transposition should be performed followed by arthroscopic or open débridement and capsular release. Neither the open nor arthroscopic débridement should be considered in patients with complete loss of joint spaced, ankylosed joints, painful mid arc range of motion, or elbow instability seen in advanced RA because of the limited success of the procedure with advanced disease.

Interposition Arthroplasty

Interposition arthroplasty is an option to consider for patients who are seeking pain relief but would like to avoid restrictions associated with elbow arthroplasty (**Figure 3**). A variety of tissues have been proposed for use in interposition arthroplasty, including allograft and autograft dermis, Achilles tendon, fascia lata, and synthetic grafts. Interposition arthroplasty can be performed with or without a hinged external fixator. A study with midterm follow-up of 6 years noted poor or fair results and/or the need for revision surgery in 32 of 45 cases (71%).[16] In a more recent retrospective review, 18 consecutive cases of interposition arthroplasty were reviewed. At least one revision procedure was required in 15/18 patients (83%), including four that were converted to a total elbow replacement, two converted to an arthrodesis, and one that went on to revision interposition arthroplasty.[17] Factors that have been found to be predictive of a successful outcome include preserved elbow stability, relatively well preserved bony anatomy, intraoperative adequacy of joint release, stable resurfacing, and careful wound closure and management.[18] Patients should be counseled about the high risk of complications and revision with interposition arthroplasty before proceeding with surgery.

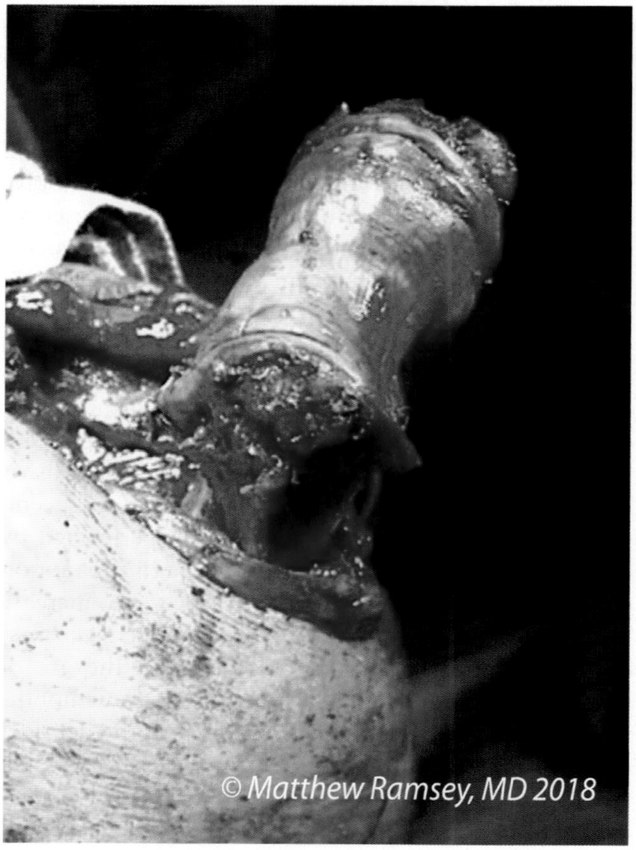

Figure 3 Intraoperative photograph of an interposition arthroplasty performed with a dermal allograft.

Elbow Arthroplasty

In more advanced disease or in the setting of unreconstructable distal humeral fractures, distal humeral hemiarthroplasty (DHH) or TEA may be considered (**Figure 4**). DHH is reserved for higher demand patients who wish to remain active and have preserved humeral and ulnar bone stock. Unfortunately, anatomic humeral implants, which are required for DHH, are not FDA approved for use in the United States and are no longer commercially available even though they have been successfully used in this application off label. Because of the unlinked nature of the construct, however, the patients should be counseled about a different set of risks and complications associated with DHH including wear on the native ulna and radial head leading to pain and possibly instability in the future. In the setting of unreconstructable distal humerus fracture, if the condyles and the integrity of the attached collateral ligaments cannot be reconstructed to achieve elbow stability, a linked TEA may be necessary. The authors of a series of 121 cases of DHH for unreconstructable distal humerus fractures with a mean 37.5 months follow-up reported 61% excellent, 25% good, 8% fair, and 6% poor functional outcomes based on the MEPS (Mayo Elbow Performance Score) scoring system.[19] These results were comparable to the results that have been reported for TEA for fracture. Risk factors for poorer outcomes included those who had an olecranon osteotomy at the time of surgery and younger patients. Five of the 121 required conversion to a TEA. Although the rate of aseptic loosening was low, the rates of ulnar and radial head wear were significant and progressive with time.[19] A recent study demonstrated that regardless of implant size, the elbow joint kinematics were altered after DHH, resulting in changes in joint tracking, which may cause abnormal articular contact, loading, pain, and progressive cartilage wear.[20]

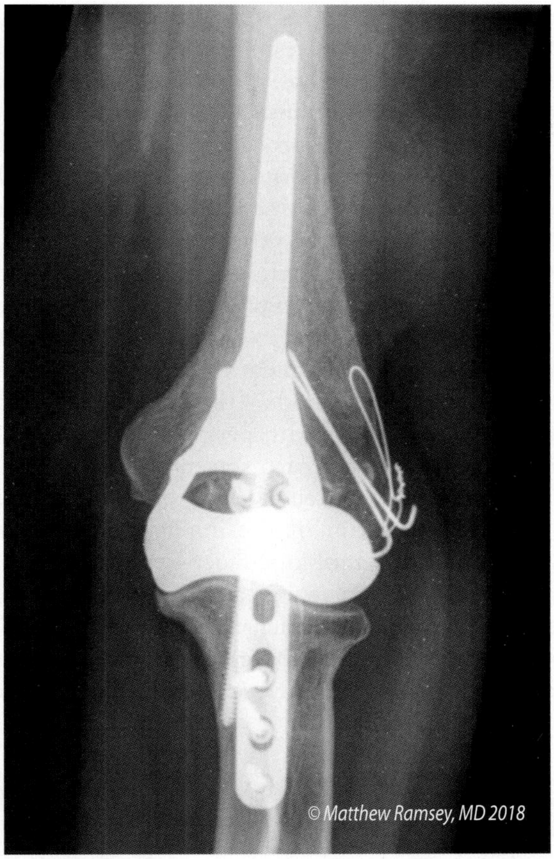

Figure 4 AP radiograph of a distal humeral hemiarthroplasty (DHH) for fracture of the distal humerus performed through an olecranon osteotomy. Notice fixation of the medial condyle component of the fracture to reestablish integrity of the medial collateral ligament.

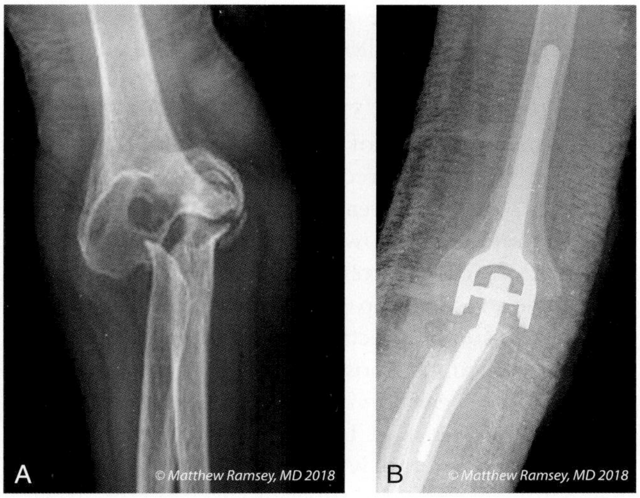

Figure 5 **A**, Preoperative AP radiograph of a patient with advance rheumatoid arthritis of the elbow. **B**, Postoperative AP radiograph following linked total elbow arthroplasty.

TEA is considered in lower demand, elderly patients who have failed conservative and other surgical alternatives who can comply with the activity limitations postoperatively (**Figure 5**). Historically, TEA was reserved for rheumatoid arthritis patients. However, with improved implant design and increasing surgeon experience, there has been a broader application of TEA for patients suffering from posttraumatic arthritis, distal humerus fractures, and primary OA. Contraindications for TEA include persistent infection and loss of motor function of the elbow flexors. The status of the humeral condyles and ligamentous stability play a significant role in deciding whether to use an unlinked or linked prosthesis. In the absence of ligamentous or bony support, a linked device is mandatory. Early reporting focused on pain relief, range of motion, and survival rates for linked and unlinked designs. However, with expanding indications for TEA, it is more insightful to analyze TEA outcomes by the underlying pathology. For rheumatoid arthritis, Sanchez-Sotelo et al reported on the long-term outcomes of linked semiconstrained elbow arthroplasty. At final follow-up, the authors had an 11% revision rate or removal of prosthesis (20% for infection, 80% for mechanical failure) and a 23% incidence of bushing wear. The overall survival rate at 10, 15, and 20 years was 92%, 83%, and 68%, respectively. Risk factors for implant revision included male sex, history of concomitant traumatic pathology, and implantation of the ulnar component with a PMMA surface finish[21] (**Figure 6**). When evaluating results based on the etiology for TEA, trauma (57%) and inflammatory arthritis (27%) were the two most common causes for implant failure and revision in one case series.[22] Pham et al reported on the long-term outcomes of 54 patients with an average 7-year follow-up (range 2 to 16 years) who underwent a linked TEA, noting a 24% complication and a 97%

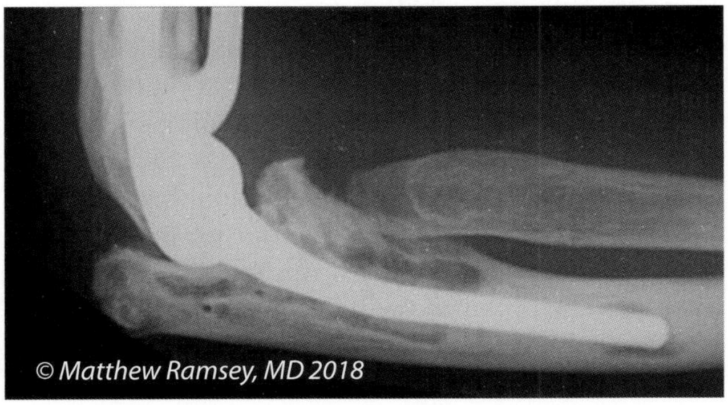

Figure 6 Lateral radiograph of a patient with a PMMA precoated ulnar component with progressive osteolysis about the distal tip and proximal aspect of the implant.

and 85% survival rate at 5 and 10 years follow-up, respectively. At final follow-up, patients had an average MEPS of 91 (range, 55 to 100), QuickDASH score of 34 points (range, 0 to 75), and a statistically significant improvement in range of motion ($P < 0.0001$).[23] In the setting of fracture, Barco et al reported on long-term outcomes of patients treated with TEA for fracture. At 10-year minimum follow-up, the mean VAS was 0.6, flexion 123°, loss of extension 24°, MEPS 90.5. Eleven percent developed deep infections and 18% required implant revision or resection for various reasons including infection, ulnar loosening, and ulnar component fractures. The mean survival rates for elbows with rheumatoid arthritis before fracture were 85% at 5 years and 76% at 10 years, whereas those without baseline rheumatoid arthritis had superior survival rates at 92% at both 5 and 10 years follow-up.[24]

Regardless of the indication, TEA is best reserved for older, less active patients given the 5 to 10 lb weight-lifting restriction following surgery. In a study on the outcomes of TEA in patients less than 50 years old (mean age, 37 years; range 22 to 47 years), Schoch et al documented an 82% complication rate among the 11 linked TEAs completed over a 5-year period. Six elbows sustained mechanical failures predominantly on the ulnar side. Despite the high complication rate, patients' pain improved on average from 8.0 to 4.9, mean DASH at final follow-up (average 3.2 years, range 1.8 to 5.5 years) was 42.9, and MEPS for surviving implants were rated as excellent (2), good (1), and fair (2). Therefore, surgeons should remain cautious about the use of TEA in young patients because of the increased risk of complications such as mechanical failure and need for revision.[25]

In the setting of primary osteoarthritis, TEA may be a reasonable option to provide pain relief. In one case series with an average follow-up of 8.9 years, 20 patients with primary OA underwent TEA between 1984 and 2011. Complications included mechanical failure (three patients), infection requiring I&D (one patient), bony ankylosis (one patient), radial head component failure (one patient), and humeral loosening or component fracture (two patients). In those without failure, pain improved but the range of motion was relatively unchanged compared with preoperative examination.[26]

In the setting of revision arthroplasty, similar outcomes can be obtained to the primary setting but with a higher complication rate. In a review of 19 revision TEAs at an average of 57 months follow-up, the MEPS and VAS were both significantly improved compared with preoperatively with combined good to excellent results in 53% of the patients and average range of motion of 123°. All elbows were stable, but three cases (19%) showed nonprogressive osteolysis around the prosthesis. Despite 58% of the patients suffering from postoperative complications, 87% were satisfied with the results of the revision procedure. Therefore, revision TEA can lead to satisfactory results, less pain, and better elbow function but with a higher complication rate as compared with primary procedures.[27]

One of the most devastating complications of elbow arthroplasty is infection (**Figure 7**). Treatment options include a one- or two-stage exchange arthroplasty with implant removal and treatment with intravenous antibiotics. Streubel et al reported on their experience treating 23 consecutive patients with periprosthetic joint infection (PJI) of the elbow with a staged protocol.

This protocol consisted of a first-stage irrigation and débridement, retention of the implants, manufacture and application of antibiotic-laden cement beads, and organism-specific intravenous antibiotics followed by a repeat irrigation and débridement with re-linkage of the implant and long-term suppressive antibiotic therapy. At a mean follow-up of 7.1 years, they did find good

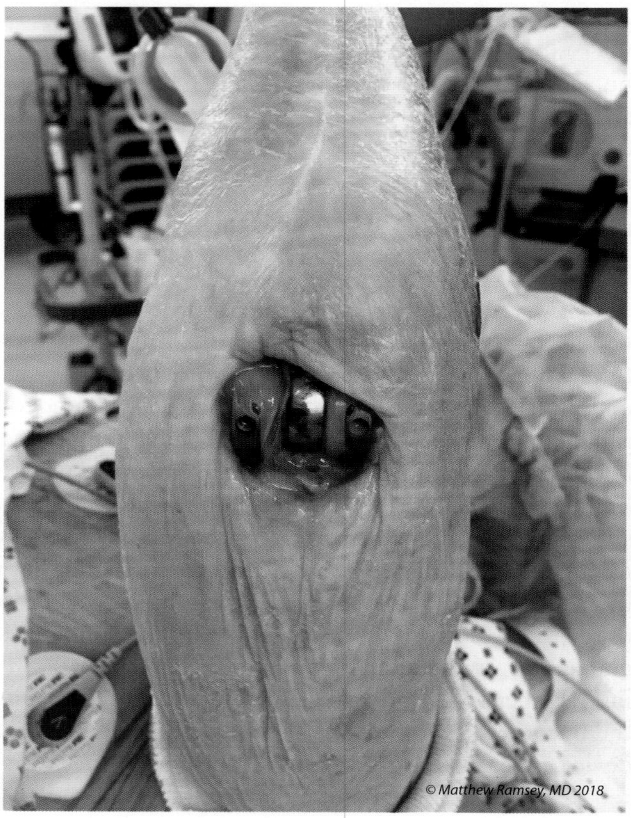

Figure 7 Intraoperative photograph of a patient with an infected total elbow arthroplasty with compromise of the soft-tissue envelope.

or excellent outcomes in 15/23 patients. However, the function was unfavorable as compared with an uncomplicated TEA. Additionally, seven patients required further débridement including one that underwent implant removal for persistent infection.[28] Ultimately, irrigation and débridement may be successful in acute infections, particularly with microorganisms that are sensitive to antibiotic therapy. Two-stage reimplantation is most commonly considered for chronic and resistant infections. When infection cannot be eradicated, when frail patients cannot tolerate multiple procedures, or when painless range of motion and function cannot be restored, resection arthroplasty can be performed.[29]

In some instances, the radiocapitellar compartment may develop advanced OA with preservation of the ulnohumeral joint. This may develop as a result of trauma, osteonecrosis or osteochondral lesion of the capitellum, primary degenerative arthritis, or previous radial head arthroplasty.[30,31] If nonsurgical or surgical treatment does not provide symptomatic relief, radiocapitellar arthroplasty may be considered. Several case series have been published over the last 5 to 10 years with encouraging results.[32-34] Early results demonstrated moderate functional recovery, reduction in pain, improved range of motion postoperatively, and high implant survival at final follow-up.[32] Others have reported similar results, but highlighted potential complications including asymptomatic loosening of the radial component, heterotopic bone requiring excision,[35] or progressive ulnohumeral arthritis.[34]

Elbow arthrodesis should be reserved for patients who are not candidates for joint arthroplasty or as a salvage procedure following unsuccessful elbow arthroplasty (**Figure 8**). In these cases, elbow arthrodesis is a consideration with goals of achieving stability and pain relief, while avoiding amputation. The procedure is not routinely performed because the remaining upper extremity joints cannot completely compensate for the loss of elbow motion following arthrodesis. Additionally, there is no ideal position of elbow fusion for all activities of daily living. Therefore, before a planned elective elbow arthrodesis, casting the elbow in various degrees of flexion can simulate the final arthrodesis and may help the patient and surgeon decide on the position that best serves their needs. In a study of patients with elbow arthrodesis performed for acute trauma or posttraumatic arthritis, the authors found that 10 of 12 patients required an additional procedure (42% of the elbows had nonunion or delayed union, and infection developed in 33% of the elbows). The poor results led the authors to conclude that "this is a procedure of last resort and should be performed when no other options exist."[36]

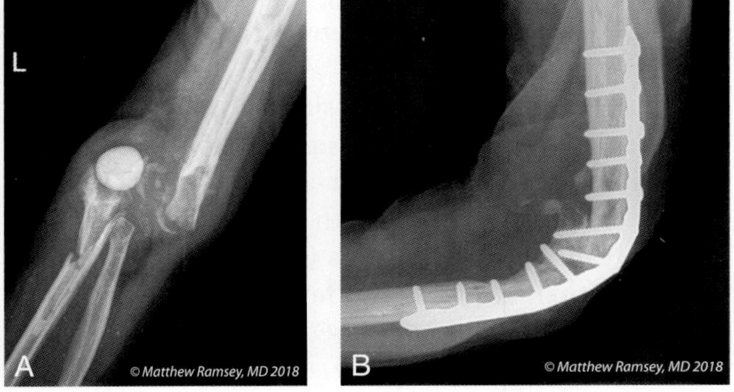

Figure 8 **A**, Preoperative AP radiograph of a patient following resection of a recurrently infected total elbow arthroplasty. **B**, Lateral radiograph following successful arthrodesis.

Nerve Disorders

Several nerves innervate the upper extremity and some are more susceptible to entrapment and compression than others. There are many etiologies for nerve compression including, but not limited to, previous trauma, surgery, and nearby hardware. Nerve disorders can occur in isolation or in conjunction with any of the arthritides affecting the elbow. When considering surgical management of arthritis, careful evaluation of associated nerve disorders must be undertaken and treated with the underlying arthritis. The two most common nerve disorders about the elbow are cubital tunnel (ulnar nerve) and radial tunnel (radial nerve) syndromes.

Cubital Tunnel Syndrome

Cubital tunnel syndrome is the second most common peripheral nerve entrapment disorder of the upper extremity after carpal tunnel syndrome. Although compression of the ulnar nerve may occur anywhere along its course through the arm, the most common site of entrapment is about the elbow. The ulnar nerve's posterior location and superficial course make it particularly susceptible to irritation, compression, and traction particularly with elbow motion. A cadaver study using three-dimensional modeling found that elbow flexion diminished the volume of the cubital tunnel and elongated the nerve; this finding suggested that both compression and nerve tension can contribute to cubital tunnel syndrome.[37] Ulnar nerve compression may also stem from space occupying lesions, compression proximally at the ligament of Struthers (medial intermuscular septum), and fascial bands distally between the ulnar and humeral heads of the flexor carpi ulnaris, or about the roof of the cubital tunnel in patients with an anconeus epitrochlearis.

The diagnosis of cubital tunnel syndrome again starts with the history of numbness and tingling in the ulnar one and one-half digits of the affected upper extremity and at times pain and numbness along the ulnar forearm and elbow. Later in the disease process, patients may complain of grip weakness and hand atrophy. The clinical manifestations of cubital tunnel syndrome include dysesthesias in the small finger and ulnar side of the ring finger exacerbated by prolonged elbow flexion (elbow flexion testing). More advanced findings include intrinsic muscle weakness of the hand, hypothenar wasting, and resulting functional impairment. EMG/NCS may be ordered to confirm the extent of compression as well as sites (including identifying additional sites of compression such as above the elbow in the cervical spine).

First-line treatment includes NSAIDs, night splints to avoid elbow flexion, elbow pads, and behavioral modification. If a patient fails to respond, surgical decompression may be achieved arthroscopically or by open means.

In a recent meta-analysis, both in situ decompression and decompression with transposition showed clinical improvement with no significant differences in electrodiagnostic or clinical outcomes.[38] Although both procedures decrease the overall strain on the nerve, anterior transposition still demonstrates increased regional strain when the arm is in extension, whereas in situ decompression shows increased strain value in flexion. This suggests that both procedures still lead to positional increase in strain in the nerve that influences the method of treatment of ulnar neuropathy.[39]

Predictors of surgical outcome after in situ ulnar nerve decompression have been extensively studied. Recently, one study evaluated 235 patients who underwent cubital tunnel decompression between 2010 and 2014 and found that 88.5% had satisfactory outcomes. The patients with longer and more severe preoperative symptoms were more likely to report unsatisfactory outcomes.[40] However, patients may improve with ulnar nerve decompression even in the setting of muscular atrophy. In another study, 42 consecutive cases of cubital tunnel syndrome with muscular atrophy were treated with in situ decompression (67%) or submuscular transposition (33%). At 6-month follow-up, 45% of patients noted improvement in sensory deficits and 57% showed improvement in motor deficits. At mean final follow-up of 39.8 months, 76% of patients had improvement in their atrophy and nearly 80% were satisfied with the postoperative result. Again, patients with a longer duration of atrophy and/or pseudoneuroma identified at the time of surgery were less likely to experience improvement in their atrophy.[41]

Another surgical option to treat cubital tunnel is medial epicondylectomy. Although most patients improve following this procedure, younger age, associated workers' compensation claims, lesser disease severity, and preoperative opioid use were all associated with the need for revision surgery.[42] Care must be taken when performing this procedure not to compromise the integrity of the ulnar collateral ligament.

Arthroscopic ulnar nerve decompression at the time of arthroscopic débridement and contracture release has been reported with encouraging results, particularly in patients without muscular wasting on presentation.[43] However, delayed-onset ulnar neuropathy (DOUN) has been described in this patient population. Significant risk factors for DOUN include preoperative diagnosis of heterotopic ossification, preoperative neurological symptoms, and limited preoperative arc of motion.[44] When evaluating the method of managing the ulnar nerve at the time of arthroscopic débridement and contracture release, it was found that DOUN could be avoided with a limited open ulnar nerve decompression or transposition. Therefore, if the ulnar nerve needs to be managed at the time surgery, the current recommendation is open management of the nerve regardless of whether the débridement and contracture release is performed open or arthroscopically.[45]

For the surgical treatment of recurrent cubital tunnel, some authors advocate for revision neurolysis with amniotic membrane wrapping. Of 18 patients who underwent this procedure following at least two previous failed decompressions, the authors noted significant improvements in VAS and DASH outcome measures as well as pinch strength and elbow motion. They conclude that ulnar neurolysis with amniotic membrane allograft wrapping is a safe and effective treatment for patients with debilitating recurrent cubital tunnel syndrome.[46]

Finally, an ulnar nerve lesion following TEA is a troubling complication with significant consequences. In a study of 82 elbows that underwent TEA, 78 of the patients were treated with in situ decompression alone. Of those 78, 4 patients (5%) experienced postoperative ulnar nerve symptoms of which 2 resolved with observation and 2 required subsequent neurolysis and transposition. Conversely, two of the four patients (50%) who had an ulnar nerve transposition at the time of TEA without preoperative symptoms developed ulnar nerve symptoms postoperatively. Unless the nerve is maltracking or has significant preoperative dysfunction, the authors recommend avoiding transposition to decrease nerve handling and possible nerve lesions.[47]

Radial Tunnel Syndrome

Radial tunnel syndrome is a painful syndrome of the elbow and forearm caused by compression of the motor branch of the radial nerve known as the posterior interosseous nerve (PIN) at the level of the proximal forearm. The symptoms include forearm pain but usually do not result in any weakness or functional deficits. The pain can be made worse by repetitive pronosupination of the forearm, supination against resistance, and resisted third finger extension against resistance with the elbow in extension. The most frequent sites of nerve compression include around the fibrous bands overlying the radiocapitellar joint, along the medial edge of the extensor carpi radialis brevis, along the distal superficial edge of the supinator, along the proximal aponeurotic edge of the supinator known as the "arcade of Frohse," near a recurrent leash of vessels just proximal to the lateral epicondyle that swells with repetitive use. The diagnosis is largely clinical as confirmatory EMG studies are negative given that there is no involvement of the nerve conduction capacity of the nerve. Local anesthetic injection about the nerve can relieve symptoms and can help confirm the diagnosis and differentiate it from the other diagnoses, which include lateral epicondylitis, PIN syndrome, and cervical radiculopathy.

First-line treatment is activity modification, temporary splinting, and nonsteroidal anti-inflammatory medications. Occasionally, a corticosteroid injection can be diagnostic and therapeutic. When resistant or recurrent, surgical release via a number of open approaches may be entertained with expected improvement in pain in upwards of 67% to 92% of patients in some studies over the course of the first year postoperatively, particularly when combined with a release of the superficial branch of the radial nerve.[48-50]

Summary

The elbow is prone to several different pathologies including arthritis, stiffness, and nerve compression disorders. There is a wide spectrum of treatment options that should be tailored to the patient's complaints in the context of his or her life. The data highlighted in this chapter will help guide nonsurgical and surgical treatment for these conditions.

Key Study Points

- Disease modifying antirheumatic drugs (DMARDs) are effectively managing patients with rheumatoid arthritis of the elbow, limiting disease progression and the need for surgical intervention such as total elbow arthroplasty.
- There are several etiologies of elbow arthritis. When conservative management fails, the appropriate surgical treatment must factor in the patient's age, activity level, expectations, degree of pathologic changes, patient health, and surgeon experience.
- Open or arthroscopic débridement may be effective in the treatment of early arthritis, whereas interposition arthroplasty or total elbow arthroplasty is best reserved for more advanced cases.
- Total elbow arthroplasty outcomes differ based on etiology and indication for surgery. TEA is best reserved for low demand, elderly patients who will be able to comply with the 5-lb weightlifting restriction imposed postoperatively to protect the implants from bearing wear, hardware loosening, or failure.
- The two most common nerve entrapment disorders about the elbow are cubital tunnel and radial tunnel, both of which should be initially managed conservatively before considering surgical intervention.

Annotated References

1. Nandi S, Maschke S, Evans PJ, Lawton JN: The stiff elbow. *Hand* 2009;4:368-379.
2. Stenstrom CH, Nisell R: Assessment of disease consequences in rheumatoid arthritis: A survey of methods classified according to the International Classification of Impairments, Disabilities, and Handicaps. *Arthritis Care Res* 1997;10:135-150.
3. Soojian MG, Kwon YW: Elbow arthritis. *Bull NYU Hosp Jt Dis* 2007;65:61-71.
4. Myden C, Hildebrand K: Elbow joint contracture after traumatic injury. *J Shoulder Elbow Surg* 2011;20:39-44.
5. Brakel RW, Eygendaal D: Intra-articular injection of hyaluronic acid is not effective for the treatment of post-traumatic osteoarthritis of the elbow. *Arthroscopy* 2006;22(11):1199-1203.
6. Brasington R: TNF-α antagonists and other recombinant proteins for the treatment of rheumatoid arthritis. *J Hand Surg Am* 2009;34(2):349-350.
7. Scott DL: Biologics-based therapy for the treatment of rheumatoid arthritis. *Clin Pharmacol Ther* 2012;91(1):30-43.

8. Saleh KJ, Kurdi AJ, El-Othmani MM, et al: Perioperative treatment of patients with rheumatoid arthritis. *J Am Acad Orthop Surg* 2015;23:e38-e48.
9. Wada T, Isogai S, Ishii S, Yamashita T: Debridement arthroplasty for primary osteoarthritis of the elbow. *J Bone Joint Surg Am* 2004;86(2):233-241.
10. Morrey BF: Primary degenerative arthritis of the elbow: Treatment by ulnohumeral arthroplasty. *J Bone Joint Surg Br* 1992;74:409-413.
11. Savoie FH III, Nunley PD, Field LD: Arthroscopic management of the arthritic elbow: Indications, technique, and results. *J Shoulder Elbow Surg* 1999;8(3):214-219.
12. Galle SE, Beck JD, Burchette RJ, Harness NG: Outcomes of elbow arthroscopic osteocapsular arthroplasty. *J Hand Surg* 2016;41:184-191.

    Case series highlighting arthroscopic osteocapsular arthroplasty as a safe and effective treatment for early to moderate primary elbow OA. Level of evidence: IV (Therapeutic).
13. Krishnan SG, Harkins DC, Pennington SD, Harrison DK, Burkhead WZ: Arthroscopic ulnohumeral arthroplasty for degenerative arthritis of the elbow in patients under fifty years. *J Shoulder Elbow Surg* 2007;16(4):443-448.
14. Adams JE, Wolff LH III, Merten SM, Steinmann SP: Osteoarthritis of the elbow: Results of arthroscopic osteophyte resection and capsulectomy. *J Shoulder Elbow Surg* 2008;17(1):126-131.
15. Isa AD, Athwal GS, King GJW, MacDermid JC, Faber KJ: Arthroscopic debridement for primary elbow osteoarthritis with and without capsulectomy: A comparative cohort study. *Shoulder Elbow* 2017;10(3):223-231.

    Comparative study demonstrating no difference in final ROM or complications when arthroscopic elbow débridement with or without capsulectomy is performed. Level of evidence: III (Therapeutic, Retrospective cohort study).
16. Larson AN, Morrey BF: Interposition arthroplasty with an Achilles tendon allograft as a salvage procedure for the elbow. *J Bone Joint Surg Am* 2008;90(12):2714-2723.
17. Laubscher M, Vochteloo A, Smit AA, Vrettos BC, Roche JL: A retrospective review of a series of interposition arthroplasties of the elbow. *Shoulder Elbow* 2014;6:129-133.
18. Chen DD, Forsh DA, Hausman MR: Elbow interposition arthroplasty. *Hand Clin* 2011;27(2):187-197.
19. Phadnis J, Watts AC, Bain GI: Elbow hemiarthroplasty for the management of distal humeral fractures: Current technique, indications and results. *Shoulder Elbow* 2016;8(3): 171-183.

    Review of the literature, indications, contraindications, and results on their series of hemiarthroplasty for distal humeral fracture in the elderly as an alternative treatment to total elbow arthroplasty. Level of evidence: IV.
20. Desai SJ, Athwal GS, Ferreira LM, Lalone EA, Johnson JA, King G: Hemiarthroplasty of the elbow: The effect of implant size on kinematics and stability. *J Shoulder Elbow Surg* 2014;23:946-954.
21. Sanchez-Sotelo J, Baghdadi Y, Morrey BF: Primary linked semiconstrained total elbow arthroplasty for rheumatoid arthritis: A single institute experience with 461 elbows over three decades. *J Bone Joint Surg Am* 2016;98(20):1741-1748.

    Case series report on the long-term outcomes of linked semiconstrained elbow arthroplasty in the setting of rheumatoid arthritis. Level of evidence: IV (Therapeutic).
22. Perretta D, Leeuwen W, Dyer G, Ring D, Chen N: Risk factors for reoperation after total elbow arthroplasty. *J Shoulder Elbow Surg* 2017;26:824-829.

    Case series on TEA to evaluate for rates of revision surgery (41%) as well as risk factors for revision surgery. TEA completed for trauma was the greatest risk factor associated with revision at 51% followed by inflammatory arthritis at 27% and osteoarthritis at 11%. Level of evidence: IV.
23. Pham TT, Delclaux S, Huguet S, Wargny M, Bonnevialle N, Mansat P: Coonrad-Morrey total elbow arthroplasty for patients with rheumatoid arthritis: 54 prostheses reviewed at 7 years' average follow-up (maximum, 16 years). *J Should Elbow Surg* 2018;27:398-403.

    Fifty-four patients implanted with a Coonrad-Morrey TEA were followed up for an average of 7 years (range 2 to 16) to evaluate complication rates and postoperative functional outcomes for patients with rheumatoid arthritis. At final follow-up, they noted satisfactory outcomes despite a high complication rate. Level of evidence: IV (Therapeutic).
24. Barco R, Streubel PN, Morrey BF, Sanchez-Sotelo J: Total elbow arthroplasty for distal humeral fractures: A ten-year-minimum follow-up study. *J Bone Joint Surg Am* 2017;99(18):1525-1531.

    Review of 44 patients who underwent TEA for fracture to evaluate survival rates, complication rates, and outcomes scores at a minimum of 10 years follow-up. Level of evidence: IV (Therapeutic).
25. Schoch B, Wong J, Abboud J, Lazarus M, Getz C, Ramsey M: Results of total elbow arthroplasty in patients less than 50 years old. *J Hand Surg Am* 2017;42:797-802.

    Review of TEA results in patients younger than 50 years. Compared with an older population, these higher demand patients are at increased risk for complications such as mechanical failure. Level of evidence: V (Therapeutic).
26. Schoch BS, Werthel JD, Sanchez-Sotelo J, Morrey BF, Morrey M: Total elbow arthroplasty for primary osteoarthritis. *J Shoulder Elbow Surg* 2017;26(8):1355-1359.

    Case series detailing complication rates, survival rates, and outcomes of TEA for patients with a history of primary OA of the elbow. Although the complication rate was high, mechanical failure rates were relatively low, leading the authors to conclude that TEA is a reliable surgical option for patients with primary elbow OA. Level of evidence: IV (Case series; Treatment study).
27. Viveen J, Prkic A, Koenraadt K, Kodde IF, The B, Eydendaal D: Clinical and radiographic outcome of revision surgery of total elbow prosthesis: Midterm results in 19 cases. *J Shoulder Elbow Surg* 2017;26:716-722.

Report on the midterm clinical and radiographic results of 19 patients who underwent revision TEA, noting a high complication rate but satisfactory results with improved pain and elbow function. Level of evidence: IV (Case series; Treatment study).

28. Streubel PN, Simone JP, Morrey BF, Sanchez-Sotelo J, Morrey ME: Infection in total elbow arthroplasty with stable components: Outcomes of a staged surgical protocol with retention of the components. *Bone Joint J* 2016;98-B:976-983.

    Report on the encouraging outcomes of 23 patients with infected TEA treated with an unlinking of the implant, irrigation and débridement, antibiotic beads, retention of components, and then staged I&D and relinkage with average follow-up of 7.1 years. Level of evidence: IV (Therapeutic).

29. Sanchez-Sotelo J, Zarkadas P, Throckmorton T, Morrey B: Elbow resection for deep infection after total elbow arthroplasty: Surgical technique. *JBJS Essent Surg Tech* 2012;2(1):e5.

30. Murata H, Ikuta Y, Murakami T: An anatomic investigation of the elbow joint, with special reference to aging of the articular cartilage. *J Shoulder Elbow Surg* 1993;2:175-181.

31. Aherns PM, Redfern DRM, Forester AJ: Patterns of articular wear in the cadaveric elbow joint. *J Shoulder Elbow Surg* 2001;10:52-56.

32. Giannicola G, Angeloni R, Mantovani A, et al: Open debridement and radiocapitellar replacement in primary and post-traumatic arthritis of the elbow: A multicenter study. *J Shoulder Elbow Surg* 2012;4:456-463.

33. Heijink A, Morrey BF, Eygendaal D: Radiocapitellar prosthetic arthroplasty: A report of 6 case and review of the literature. *J Shoulder Elbow Surg* 2014;23(6):843-849.

34. Kachooei AR, Heesakkers N, Heijink A, The B, Eygendaal D: Radiocapitellar prosthetic arthroplasty: Short-term to midterm results of 19 elbows. *J Shoulder Elbow Surg* 2018;27:726-732.

    Report on the midterm functional and radiographic results of elbows following radiocapitellar prosthetic arthroplasty. Level of evidence: IV (Case series; Treatment study).

35. Bigazzi P, Biondi M, Ceruso M: Radiocapitellar prosthetic arthroplasty in traumatic and post-traumatic complex lesions of the elbow. *Eur J Orthop Surg Traumatol* 2016;26:851-858.

    Case series evaluating the success of radiocapitellar prosthetic arthroplasty in the setting of acute traumatic as well as posttraumatic conditions. Level of evidence: IV (Case series; Treatment study).

36. Reichel LM, Wiater BP, Friedrich J, Hanel DP: Arthrodesis of the elbow. *Hand Clin* 2011;27(2):179-186.

37. James J, Sutton LG, Werner FW, Basu N, Allison MA, Palmer AK: Morphology of the cubital tunnel: An anatomical and biomechanical study with implications for treatment of ulnar nerve compression. *J Hand Surg Am* 2011;36(12):1988-1995.

38. Chen HW, Ou S, Liu GD, et al: Clinical efficacy of simple decompression versus anterior transposition of the ulnar nerve for the treatment of cubital tunnel syndrome: A meta-analysis. *Clin Neurol Neurosurg* 2014;126:150-155.

    There was no substantial difference in clinical outcomes between patients with a simple decompression and patients with an anterior transposition of the ulnar nerve for cubital tunnel syndrome. The complication rate was substantially higher in those who underwent anterior transposition.

39. Foran I, Vaz K, Sikora-Klak J, Ward SR, Hertzen ER, Shah SB: Regional ulnar nerve strain following decompression and anterior subcutaneous transposition in patients with cubital tunnel syndrome. *J Hand Surg Am* 2016;41:e343-e350.

    Evaluation of regional ulnar nerve stress following in situ decompression versus decompression and anterior transposition. Anterior transposition increases strain in extension and decreases strain in flexion in comparison to in situ decompression alone. Level of evidence: III.

40. Kong L, Bai J, Yu K, Zhang B, Zhang J, Tian D: Predictors of surgical outcome after in situ ulnar nerve decompression for cubital tunnel syndrome. *Ther Clin Risk Manag* 2018;14:69-74.

    Review of 235 patients who underwent CuTR with an 85% satisfaction rate. Patients with more severe preoperative symptoms are more at risk for poor postoperative outcomes. Level of evidence: IV.

41. Bruder M, Dutzmann S, Rekkab N, Quick J, Seifer V, Marquardt G: Muscular atrophy in severe cases of cubital tunnel syndrome: Prognostic factors and outcome after surgical treatment. *Acta Neurochir* 2017;159:537-542.

    Ulnar nerve release can be effective in improving manifestations of cubital tunnel syndrome, even in the setting of muscular atrophy. Level of evidence: IV.

42. Gaspar MP, Jacoby SM, Osterman AL, Kane PM: Risk factors predicting revision surgery after medial epicondylectomy for primary cubital tunnel syndrome. *J Shoulder Elbow Surg* 2016;25:681-687.

    Medial epicondylectomy is a reasonable treatment option to address cubital tunnel syndrome. However, younger patients, workers' compensation cases, patients with less severe disease, and patients on preoperative opioids tended to experience poorer outcomes and require revision surgery. Level of evidence: IV.

43. Kovachecvich R, Steinmann P: Arthroscopic ulnar nerve decompression in the setting of elbow osteoarthritis. *J Hand Surg* 2012;37A:663-668. Level of evidence: IV.

44. Blonna D, Huffman GR, O'Driscoll SW: Delayed-onset ulnar neuritis after release of elbow contractures: Clinical presentation, pathological findings, and treatment. *Am J Sports Med* 2014;42(9):2113-2121.

45. Blonna D, O'Driscoll SW : Delayed-onset ulnar neuritis after release of elbow contractures: Preventative strategies derived from a study of 563 cases. *Arthroscopy* 2014;30(8):947-956.

46. Gaspar MP, Abdelfattah HM, Welch IW, Vosbikian MM, Kane PM, Rekant MS: Recurrent cubital tunnel syndrome treated with revision neurolysis and amniotic membrane nerve wrapping. *J Shoulder Elbow Surg* 2016;25:2057-2065.

    Recurrent cubital tunnel syndrome may be effectively treated with repeat neurolysis and amniotic membrane wrapping to improve postoperative outcomes, pinch strength, and elbow range of motion. Level of evidence: IV.

47. Dachs RP, Vrettos BC, Chivers DA, Du Plessis JD, Roche SJ: Outcomes after ulnar nerve in situ release during total elbow arthroplasty. *J Hand Surg Am* 2015;40:1832-1837.

48. Lawrence T, Mobbs P, Fortems Y, Stanley JK: Radial tunnel syndrome: A retrospective review of 30 decompressions of the radial nerve. *J Hand Surg Br* 1995;20(4):454-459.

49. Jebson PJ, Engber WD: Radial tunnel syndrome: Long-term results of surgical decompression. *J Hand Surg Am* 1997;22(5):889-896.

50. Sotereanos DG, Varitimidis SE, Giannakopoulos PN, Westkaemper JG: Results of surgical treatment for radial tunnel syndrome. *J Hand Surg Am* 1999;24(3):566-570.

Chapter 28

Tendinopathy, Elbow Ligament Reconstruction, and Throwing Injuries

Christopher S. Ahmad, MD • James N. Irvine, Jr, MD

ABSTRACT

Elbow disorders come in a variety of both acute injuries and chronic conditions from overuse. Tendinopathy of the elbow is incredibly common, yet treatment strategies tend to vary based on surgical training with recent graduates gravitating away from surgical intervention while also performing more cases arthroscopically. Acute ligamentous injuries, notably those to the ulnar collateral ligament, have seen a recent spike in the rate of surgeries being performed, particularly in younger patients. Tendon disruptions around the elbow to include the triceps and biceps are problems generally resulting from eccentric loads and commonly managed surgically.

Keywords: collateral ligaments of the elbow; distal biceps injury; distal triceps injury; elbow tendinopathy

Introduction

Pathologies and injuries around the elbow can commonly occur from chronic overuse of the joint in manual laborers and overhead athletes or following trauma. The laborer and athlete typically experience injuries due to repetitive use of dynamic and static stabilizers of the elbow joint. Traumatic injuries are often the result of excessive eccentric loads or distracting forces that are biomechanically distinct from throwing injuries. Tendinopathies about the elbow are prevalent disorders with lateral epicondylosis, also known as "tennis elbow," representing the most commonly diagnosed elbow condition.[1] Medial epicondylosis occurs much less frequently and is associated with chronic overuse of the flexor-pronator tendon complex and excessive valgus stress.[2] Injury to the biceps and triceps including strains and complete ruptures are less frequent, but the muscle groups play an important role during the acceleration and deceleration phases of throwing.[3] For elbow disorders in the overhead athlete, this chapter will focus on throwing motion as it has been well documented that the valgus stress created (exceeding 60 N m) during late cocking and early acceleration phases can exceed the failure strength (22 N m) of the medial ulnar collateral ligament (UCL) and result in attenuation or rupture.[4]

Dr. Ahmad or an immediate family member has received royalties from Arthrex, Inc.; serves as a paid consultant to or is an employee of Arthrex, Inc.; has stock or stock options held in At Peak; and has received research or institutional support from Arthrex, Inc., Major League Baseball, and Stryker. Neither Dr. Irvine nor any immediate family member has received anything of value from or has stock or stock options held in a commercial company or institution related directly or indirectly to the subject of this chapter.

Tendinopathy

Medial Epicondylosis

Medial epicondylar tendinopathy of the elbow is a pathology of the flexor-pronator muscle group at its origin overlying the medial epicondyle. The etiology of the disease has been associated with overuse of the flexor-pronator muscle group and has a predilection for certain occupations as well as sports such as golf, baseball, and racquet sports. Patients typically present in the fourth or fifth decades of life. Most of the literature on this process has described this clinical entity as an "epicondylitis" as it was believed to be an inflammatory process. Histological analysis of the disease process revealed a very brief inflammatory period followed by microtearing, collagen architectural disruption and an incomplete vascular response, and, finally, an angiofibroblastic degeneration. The explanation of this "tendinosis" process is actually based on lateral epicondylosis which is 7 to 10 times more common, but the same pathophysiological process is thought to be from an imbalance between persistent microtrauma and a vascular healing response.[5]

A patient's history is critical to differentiating this disease process from other pathologies on the medial side of the elbow such as valgus extension overload, ulnar neuritis, UCL injury, or even cervical radiculopathy. The pain associated with medial epicondylosis is typically insidious in nature and is made worse with specific activities or upper extremity motions for throwing and swinging. In the overhead throwing athlete, if pain occurs during the acceleration phase over the medial elbow, it may indicate medial epicondylosis. A history of fluoroquinolone use is also a vital piece of information as it has been associated with increased rates of tendinopathy and rupture. Focused examination of the medial elbow generally yields pain to palpation over the medial epicondyle, but pain with resisted forearm pronation has been described as the most sensitive examination finding. Patients should be evaluated for ulnar neuritis in this setting as 60% of patients requiring surgery for their medial epicondylosis have concomitant ulnar neuritis.[2]

Plain radiographs of the elbow should always be performed as part of the workup for the etiology of medial-sided elbow pain. Given the older age of presentation of most cases of medial epicondylosis, it is helpful to rule out arthritis as a possible source of pain. A proper diagnosis does not necessarily require advanced imaging but ultrasonography and MRI have the added ability to evaluate the surrounding soft tissues as well as demonstrate objective findings consistent with medial epicondylosis. Ultrasonography has a sensitivity of 95% and specificity of 92% with focal hypoechoic areas and intratendinous calcifications representing the typical findings during evaluation.[6] MRI has been described as the standard of care for radiographic diagnostic purposes and is extremely helpful if trying to rule out or identify concomitant pathology (**Figure 1**). When reviewing MRI scans for medial epicondylosis a positive finding on the T2-weighted sequence will likely demonstrate intermediate to high signal intensity within the proximal flexor-pronator mass.[2]

Though the data are limited, nonsurgical treatment of this condition is successful in 85% to 90% of cases.[2] The first step in treatment is rest from the offending repetitive motions and activities that are pain generators. Counterforce bracing treatment, physical therapy as well as sports-specific evaluation to modify technique have been described as providing relief and minimizing symptoms. Medical management with systemic and topical NSAIDs, localized injection with corticosteroids, as well as biologics such as platelet-rich plasma (PRP) have also been studied. In a prospective study comparing corticosteroid with saline injections, the treatment group only saw benefit at the 6-week time point but no added benefit by 3 months following injection.[7] A recent review of a national database determined that age younger than 65 years and obesity (body mass index [BMI] >30 kg/m^2) were risk factors for failing therapeutic injections.[8] Another approach, which has previously been attempted, involves dry needling of the tendon to generate a bleeding and vascularized response coupled with an injection of autologous blood, provided a decrease in visual analog scale scores in 17 of 20 patients at 10 months after the intervention.[9]

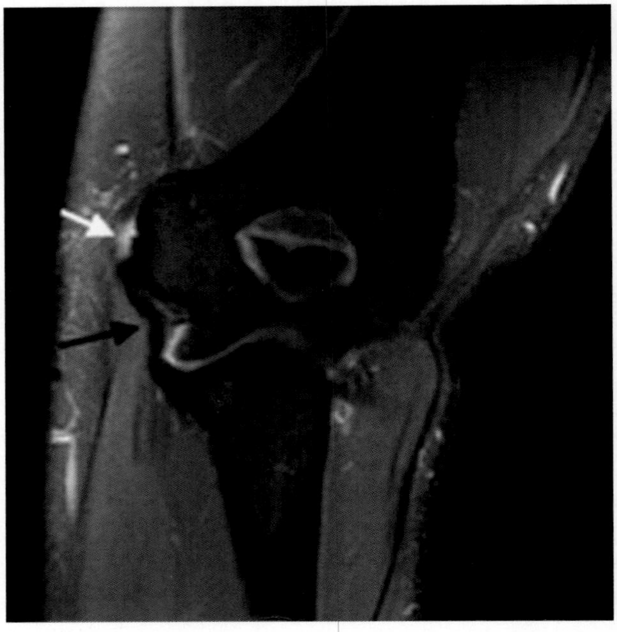

Figure 1 Coronal T2 magnetic resonance image of the ulnohumeral joint demonstrates medial epicondylosis (white arrow) of the flexor-pronator muscle group. This finding occurs following a brief inflammatory period followed by microtearing, collagen architectural disruption and an incomplete vascular response, and finally angiofibroblastic degeneration. An intact ulnar collateral ligament (black arrow) is seen just distal to the diseased tendon origin.

After failure of nonsurgical treatment for 4 to 6 months, surgical options may be explored. In isolated cases of medial epicondylosis without evidence of ulnar neuritis, localized epicondylar débridement is the treatment of choice. Also, patients who either lacked concomitant ulnar neuritis or had only mild ulnar neuropathy had good to excellent results in 96% of cases, but when moderate to severe ulnar neuropathy was present, this number dropped to 40%.[10] The presence of ulnar nerve symptoms appears to be the most important factor when evaluating outcomes following surgical débridement, but the management of the nerve (simple decompression vs transposition) has not been studied to date.

Lateral Epicondylosis

Lateral epicondylosis affects 1% to 3% of the population and is the most commonly diagnosed painful elbow problem.[11] It is also commonly referred to as "tennis elbow"; this term was first used 1883 by H.P. Major who noted an increased prevalence of the disorder among people playing tennis.[12] This condition tends to affect athletes and workers requiring repetitive wrist extension during their mid-30s to 50s and commonly involves the dominant arm.

Similar to its counterpart on the medial side of the elbow, this pathological condition is caused by repetitive contraction of the forearm extensor muscles leading to microtrauma and tearing of the common extensor tendon. The most commonly involved tendon is the origin of the extensor carpi radialis brevis. Over time, the body attempts to heal the repetitive trauma through revascularization while fibroblasts migrate to the area and attempt to lay down new collagen material. Unfortunately, a disorganized collagen matrix is produced as well as a vascular hyperplasia resulting in an entity known as angiofibroblastic tendinosis according to histopathological analysis. One anatomical theory that has been proposed to initiate this cascade of events is extensor carpi radialis brevis impingement upon the lateral edge of the capitellum based on a cadaver study.[13]

Patients presenting with tennis elbow will complain of pain directly over the origin of the common forearm extensor tendon and may report a radiating pain down the arm. Rarely is there history of a trauma, but they may report a recent increase in strenuous activity involving the elbow due from a combination of wrist and elbow extension while having a clenched fist. They often complain of a weakened grip or pain while shaking hands, and typically the pain is only present during activation of the extensor muscles of the forearm and less frequently is present during a resting state. When examining the patient, pain and symptoms are commonly reproduced when having them keep their elbow extended and perform resisted wrist extension. Clinical examination is usually sufficient for making the diagnosis of lateral epicondylosis but it is important to consider additional diagnoses such as a hypertrophic plica, osteoarthritis, rheumatoid arthritis, radial tunnel syndrome as well as referred pain from the neck in patients with cervical radiculopathy.

AP and lateral radiographs of the elbow are the first study of choice and are often normal. Both ultrasonography and MRI have been reported as useful adjuncts to aid in diagnosis and are usually obtained following a period of failed conservative management. According to a 2013 MRI study, there was a very high rate of concomitant pathology involving the lateral ulnar collateral ligament (LUCL) (91.67%, 22 of 24) in patients who had been symptomatic anywhere from 1 week to 15 years.[14] There was also a strong correlation between the extent of injury to the common extensor tendon and involvement of the LUCL. The authors of the MRI study recommend preoperative MRI evaluation for anyone undergoing surgery for lateral epicondylosis given the correlation with LUCL injury and possible need to address this pathology to avoid destabilization of the elbow with the potential for posterolateral rotatory instability in the setting of an incompetent LUCL.

Nonsurgical management of tennis elbow consists of a myriad of treatment options with most patients never requiring surgical treatment. According to a recent systematic review of nonsurgical treatment of lateral epicondylosis, there was no conclusive evidence of an optimal treatment approach.[15] As with other tendinopathies, treatment begins with rest and avoidance of activities which re-create the pain. For cases involving novice tennis players, review and adjustment in their backhand technique may be beneficial, as they more commonly have a flexed wrist at the time of impact of their backhand shots which creates greater eccentric contractions of the extensor muscles leading to microtears in the tendon. High-level players tend to have a more extended wrist position just before impact, which reduces the eccentric forces transmitted across the origin of the common extensor tendon. Physical therapy to include basic stretching exercises as well as multimodality approaches with iontophoresis, electrical stimulation, and friction massages have been described with evidence that eccentric extensor strengthening exercises coupled with a multimodal treatment have clinical benefits.[16] Some may elect to try an orthosis at the wrist or elbow to provide pain relief.

A separate approach to this problem entails use of oral, topical, and injectable anti-inflammatory and biologic agents. Although the underlying pathophysiology of lateral epicondylosis is not purely an inflammatory condition, use of NSAIDs are commonly prescribed as part of the initial treatment. Use of topical NSAIDs has demonstrated some benefits over placebo with associated risk notable for skin rash. A Cochrane review failed to find enough evidence to recommend oral NSAIDs given mixed results as well as documented gastrointestinal side effects.[17] Corticosteroids have historically been used in an attempt to treat tennis elbow, whereas in more recent years PRP has been used in an attempt to deliver a more biologic approach for treating the condition. A recent review of studies comparing the effectiveness of PRP with corticosteroids revealed that PRP seems to have a longer lasting effect, while corticosteroids appear to have a more rapid onset in providing pain relief but are shorter lived.[18] Treatment failure after 6 to 12 months of nonsurgical approaches may warrant surgical intervention. According to a review of nonsurgical treatment failure in the management of patients with tennis elbow, the following risk factors were identified:

workers' compensation claim, previous elbow injection, presence of radial tunnel syndrome, history of previous orthopaedic surgery, and symptoms for greater than 1 year.[11]

Several approaches have been described to include percutaneous release of the extensor tendon, open resection of the diseased tendon as well as arthroscopic resection (**Figure 2**). In a recent review of the American Board of Orthopaedic Surgery database of cases submitted for Part II examination, surgeons with fellowship training in shoulder and elbow or sports medicine were more likely to perform arthroscopic surgery for tennis elbow compared with hand surgeons, and there were no self-reported differences in the complications rates between open (4.4%) and arthroscopic (5.5%) procedures. The breakdown of approaches was as follows: percutaneous tenotomy (6.4%), débridement only (46.3%) and débridement with tendon repair (47.3%).[19] Surgical management of tennis elbow can be highly successful with return to activities and sport around 90%.

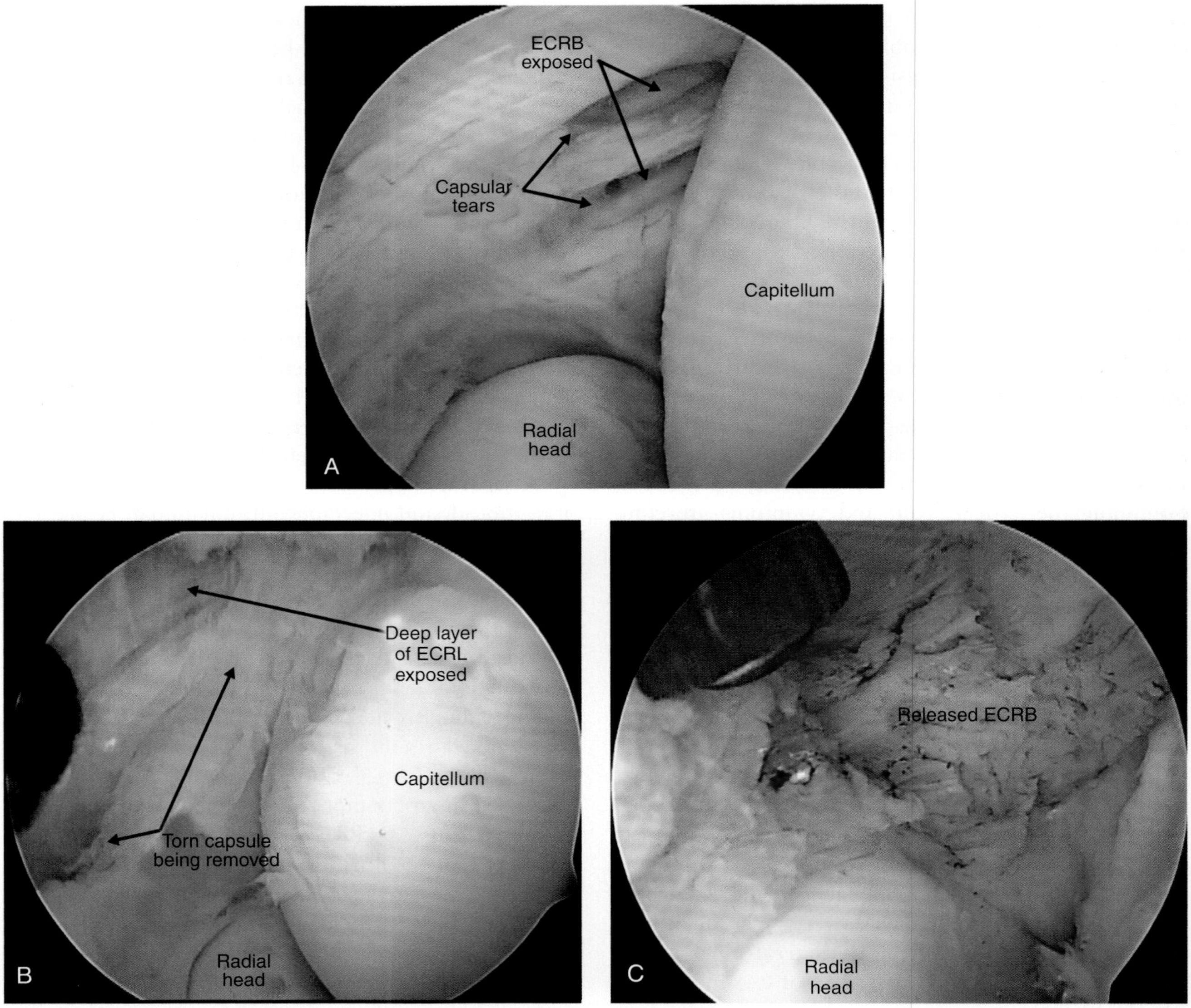

Figure 2 Arthroscopic images of lateral epicondylitis via the proximal anteromedial portal. **A**, The capitellum, radial head, and capsular tears are visualized. **B**, After capsular débridement, the deep extensor carpi radialis longus (ECRL) is exposed. **C**, The diseased extensor carpi radialis brevis (ECRB) origin is resected off its origin using a radiofrequency probe. (Reproduced from Baker CL Jr: Arthroscopic release for lateral epicondylitis, in Yamaguchi K, King GJW, McKee MD, O'Driscoll SWM, eds: *Advanced Reconstruction: Elbow*. Rosemont, IL, American Academy of Orthopaedic Surgeons, 2007, pp 25-30.)

Distal Biceps Injury

Distal biceps tendon ruptures typically occur in the dominant arm of males during the fifth to sixth decade of life and at a rate of 1.2 per 100,000 persons per year.[20] They are associated with a traumatic event which causes a sudden, eccentric load to a flexed and supinated forearm. Common risk factors include anabolic steroid use, body building, and smoking.[20]

The patient may recall an audible pop over the anterior elbow and may have difficulty contracting the biceps muscle. Inspection of the soft tissues tends to demonstrate swelling of the soft tissues in the antecubital fossa.[21] The hook test is a valuable diagnostic tool where an examiner has the patient's elbow in 90° of flexion and full supination then hooks a finger around the lateral edge of the distal biceps tendon as it spans the antecubital fossa and has proven 100% sensitivity and specificity for making a prompt diagnosis.[21] Additional clinical findings to support the diagnosis include retraction of the muscle belly with a visible bulge (reverse Popeye deformity), weakness in flexion and supination, as well as bruising. Missed injuries have been attributed to the examiner actually palpating an intact brachialis tendon, which is an intramuscular tendon at the level of the antecubital fossa and cannot be hooked away from an underlying muscle belly as in the case of an intact distal biceps tendon.[21] Furthermore, the hook test allows for the distinction between complete avulsion which results in an abnormal hook test versus a partial avulsion which yields a painful hook test. Advanced imaging with MRI or ultrasonography is helpful in cases of partial avulsions as it can assess the biceps insertion. Obtaining an MRI view of the elbow during flexion, abduction, and supination can be done by having the patient's elbow flexed to 90°, shoulder fully abducted, and forearm supinated to allow for optimal evaluation of the tendon along its long axis and minimizes error by reducing volume averaging.[22]

Nonsurgical management of acute, complete distal biceps tendon avulsions has been suggested in patients who are poor hosts with multiple medical comorbidities and historically has demonstrated a 40% loss of supination strength and 30% loss in flexion strength.[23] Another study reported similar loss in supination strength but return of flexion strength that is 93% of the contralateral uninjured side.[24] Substantial debate still surrounds the management of partial injuries but greater than 50% tendon involvement may benefit from surgical intervention. In general, successful nonsurgical treatment of partial distal biceps ruptures is uncommon.[25]

Surgical management of complete injuries in active patients and athletes are ideally performed within 4 weeks of injury or else they are classified as chronic ruptures which have been associated with muscle atrophy, tendon shortening due to scar formation, and ultimately may require a tendon graft for reconstruction.[26] Single- and two-incision techniques have been described in the literature and were compared in a prospective randomized controlled trial.[27] No differences in outcomes were reported between the two techniques American Shoulder and Elbow Surgeons score, Disabilities of the Arm, Shoulder and Hand score, or the Patient-Rated Elbow Evaluation score. Notable differences included the two-incision group had greater isometric flexion strength at 1 year (104% vs 94%) but also had a lower complication rate of lateral antebrachial cutaneous nerve palsies compared with the single-incision approach (3/43 vs 19/47). Lateral antebrachial cutaneous nerve palsies have been attributed to aggressive retraction and are known to represent the most common complication of distal biceps tendon repair. Other associated complications include PIN palsy, radial sensory nerve injury, heterotopic ossification, infection, and rerupture. A review of the MEDLINE, Cochrane, and Embase databases reported complication rates of 26.4% for suture anchors, 20.4% for bone tunnels, 44.8% for intraosseous screws, and 0% for cortical button fixation when analyzing outcomes of distal biceps tendon repair.[28]

Distal Triceps Injuries

Distal triceps injuries are the least common of all tendon injuries, commonly involve young men, and are the result of a forceful eccentric load during active triceps contraction. Activities and sports such as weight lifting and football, which often require elbow extension against heavy loads, are risk factors for these injuries. Football players are at a higher risk for these injuries than the general population, and positions that involve blocking are at greatest risk.[29]

When patients present with a distal triceps rupture, they may recall an audible pop following a fall onto an outstretched hand, direct blow to the triceps, or a sudden forced flexion of the elbow. They will often report pain over the olecranon with a possible palpable defect as well as pain to palpation and pain at terminal extension of the elbow. They may also lack full active motion or be unable to extend against gravity. Plain radiographs to include AP, lateral, and oblique views of the elbow are standard imaging, and the lateral view can help identify an avulsion fracture of the olecranon process (fleck sign) which is pathognomonic for a rupture of the triceps[30] (**Figure 3**). Advanced imaging with MRI or ultrasonography can be

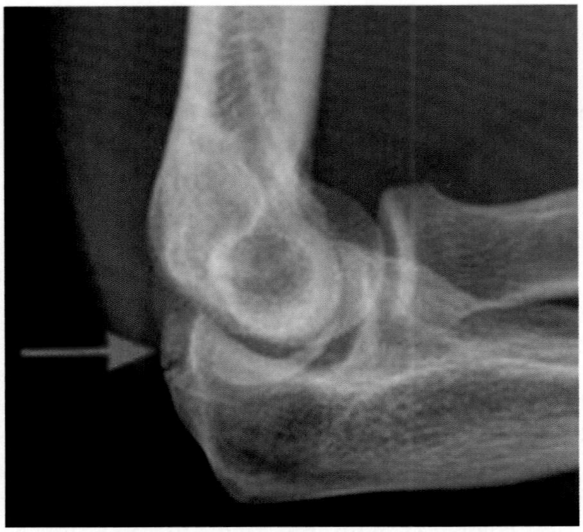

Figure 3 Lateral radiograph of the elbow demonstrates a minimally displaced fleck sign (red arrow), which indicates an injury to the triceps tendon insertion. MRI is warranted to fully appreciate the extent of the injury.

used to distinguish partial from complete injuries, with MRI having the ability to identify rupture location as well as other soft-tissue disruptions.

Nonsurgical management has been described for partial tears of the distal triceps with disruption within the muscle or musculotendinous junction having good healing potential. Conservative treatment includes a 3- to 4-week period of immobilization at 30° flexion, followed by gradual increases in flexion and motion as tolerated beyond 4 weeks. Partial tears in athletes may require surgical intervention. In a study of 10 professional football players with partial triceps tendon injuries, 6 of 10 players were able to return to play following conservative management, whereas 3 required surgery due to continued pain and weakness and 1 player attempted to practice while wearing an elbow brace and subsequently suffered a complete rupture of the triceps.[31] Timing of surgical repair or reconstruction is also an important consideration as delayed treatment of partial tears may require upward of a year postoperatively to achieve full recovery compared with 3 to 4 months in those repaired in the acute setting.[32]

Surgical management is considered for most complete triceps tendon injuries with poor surgical hosts representing the rare exception. Both suture anchors and transosseous bone tunnels have been described as surgical techniques for primary repair. Ideally, surgical repair should occur within 2 weeks of injury, and it has been associated with greater mean range of motion and peak strength when compared with patients undergoing triceps tendon reconstruction. Instances such as delayed presentation or failure of conservative management of a partial tear may necessitate tendon reconstruction due to scar tissue formation and retraction. For cases necessitating reconstruction, an anconeus rotation flap technique has been described if the tissue is viable and a large tendon defect does not exist.[33] An Achilles tendon allograft has also been described, but there are limited data to support this technique.

Timing of return to sport following surgical repair has been described, but there are limited data. Most would agree that 4 to 6 months of recovery time is necessary before returning to the field or work, as there are reports of rerupture in patients who return sooner.[32] Associated complications following triceps tendon repair include wound healing issues, ulnar nerve neurapraxia and rerupture.[34]

UCL Injuries

The UCL is subject to injury in overhead athletes (most commonly baseball pitchers) due to repetitive valgus forces that are imposed on the throwing elbow. Reconstruction of the UCL, also referred to as "Tommy John surgery", has gained a lot of attention in the media, likely due to the prolonged rehabilitation period and the more than 10% of Major League Baseball (MLB) pitchers who have undergone the surgery.[35] Recent 10-year epidemiologic data from New York State revealed a 193% increase in UCL reconstructions between 2002 and 2011.[36] One growing concern is the age in which the surgery is being performed as one study revealed that 56.8% of UCL reconstructions were in adolescents between 15 and 19 years of age with a nearly 10% annual growth rate between 2007 and 2011.[37] Risk factors, which some attribute to this recent rise, include high-velocity pitches, high pitch counts, curveballs, sliders, lifting weights during the season, increased weight, showcase events, and pitchers in warm-weather climates who ultimately play in more games, leading to increased number of annual pitches.[38]

The UCL is the main restraint to valgus stress and is composed of the anterior, posterior, and oblique bundle, which is also known as the transverse ligament. The anterior bundle consists of anterior and posterior bands with the anterior band playing the most important role against valgus stress in the throwing athlete. The anterior band provides valgus constraint at 30°, 60°, and 90° of flexion and coconstraint with the posterior band at 120° of flexion. In comparison, the posterior band provides primary coconstraint at the higher flexion angle and secondary constraint at 30° and 90°. Dynamic support and stability is provided by the flexor carpi ulnaris and flexor digitorum superficialis.

The throwing athlete imparts extreme tensile forces on the UCL during late cocking and acceleration phases that surpass the maximal tensile strength of the ligament during high-velocity pitches.[39] Patients with these injuries may report a "pop" or pain at the time of injury whereas others may be more insidious in nature and noticed due to considerable loss of accuracy and maximal pitch speed. Patients may also present with the subjective report of apprehension or instability at a flexion arc of 70° to 120°. Evaluation by the team physician oftentimes reveals pain to palpation directly over the ligament and a positive moving valgus stress test which is performed with valgus stress applied to the elbow while moving the arm from flexion to extension (**Figure 4**).

Valgus stress radiographs can also aid in diagnosis of UCL tears. In a recent study, stress radiographs on elbows with confirmed UCL tear by MRI opened an average of 0.6 mm for full-thickness tears compared with 0.1 mm for partial tears.[39] These numbers differ from the 3 mm of opening that has been previously quoted in the literature as being diagnostic of a UCL injury and may be attributed to the Telos stress device (SE 2000; Telos, Weiterstadt, Germany), which provided 15 daN of valgus stress in the more recent study compared with a manual stress test in the comparative study.[40] Conventional MRI is capable of detecting full-thickness tears but the more subtle partial tears are more difficult to recognize and diagnose. The use of magnetic resonance arthrography has a reported sensitivity of 86% for partial-thickness tears and specificity of 100% and is the study of choice[41] (**Figure 5**). A recent MRI-based classification system has been published in hopes of improving communication of UCL injuries as well as guiding treatment options and is composed of four types: I, low-grade partial tear with edema in UCL; II, high-grade partial tear; III, complete tear in one location; IV, complete tear in more than one location.[42] The clinical use of dynamic ultrasonography has been gaining traction as it has the ability to dynamically assess ligamentous competence as opposed to the static modalities previously listed. Dynamic ultrasonography is a good alternative because it can readily yield reproducible results when used in the training room, office, has associated lower costs, and is a noninvasive approach.[43]

Nonsurgical management begins with rest from throwing for a period of at least 3 months or other motions and activities that would exacerbate the injury by applying a valgus force across the elbow joint. Rehabilitation of the shoulder and elbow includes flexor-pronator strengthening, analysis and possible correction of weaknesses within the kinetic chain, fine tuning of throwing mechanics, stretching exercises if glenohumeral internal rotation deficits are present, and a progressive throwing program beginning at 3 months if symptoms have resolved. Nonsurgical treatment was effective in one study for 13 of 31 (42%) overhead throwing athletes with UCL injuries with an average return to sport of 24.5 weeks.[44] Biologic augmentation has also been

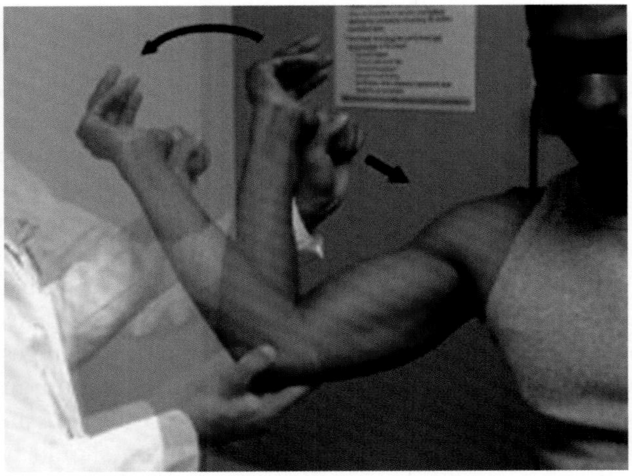

Figure 4 Clinical photograph showing examination of the ulnar collateral ligament using the moving valgus stress test. The test is performed by applying a valgus stress to the elbow while moving the arm from flexion to extension as shown in the photograph.

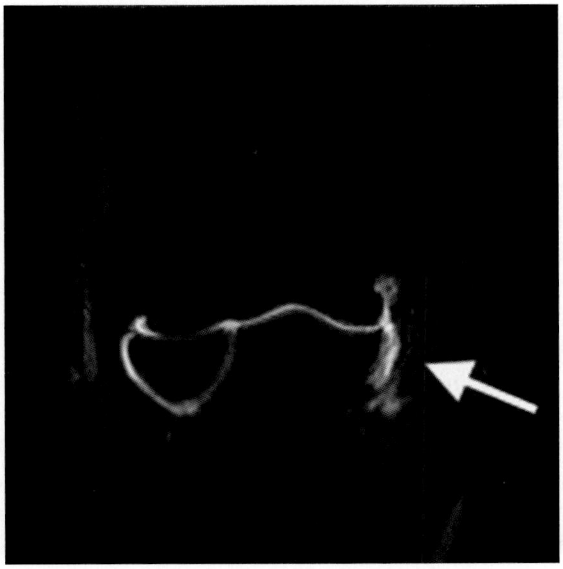

Figure 5 Coronal T2 MRI with intra-articular (magnetic resonance arthrography) contrast demonstrates a complete tear of the ulnar collateral ligament (white arrow) off of its insertion onto the sublime tubercle.

explored in the setting of partial UCL tears treated with a PRP injection which allowed 88% of players to return to sport after 12 weeks of rest and rehabilitation.[45] Larger prospective studies are needed to understand optimal PRP composition for enhancing the biologic healing response of partial ligament and tendon injuries.

Indications for surgery on UCL tears include (1) failure of nonsurgical management in symptomatic nonthrowing athletes, (2) partial tears in athletes in whom a comprehensive rehabilitation program has failed, and (3) complete tear of the anterior bundle of the UCL in throwing athletes who wish to return to sport. Surgical treatment may entail either direct repair or ligament reconstruction. Direct repair is less often a viable option as it generally requires a younger host who presents with an avulsion type injury. In recent years, a considerable amount of research has been dedicated to determining optimal surgical techniques which maximize the chance of return to sport while also minimizing the risk of a surgical complication. One of the early modifications of Jobe's successful technique was described in a 1996 study, which was a muscle-splitting approach through the anterior fibers of the flexor carpi ulnaris as opposed to taking down the flexor-pronator musculature coupled with submuscular transposition of the ulnar nerve.[46] This was an important modification as the complication rate first described by Jobe et al in 1986 was an astounding 32%, many of which were postoperative ulnar neuropathies.[47] The muscle-splitting approach has increased the rate of excellent results by nearly 20% (87% vs 70%), significantly reduced the complication rate (7% vs 23%), and greatly cut back on the rate of postoperative neuropathy (6% vs 20%) compared with patients who had the flexor-pronator mass taken down and ulnar nerve transposed.[48] Over time, management of the ulnar nerve transitioned from a submuscular to subcutaneous technique in an effort to reduce the complication rate until finally there was an abandonment of obligatory ulnar nerve transpositions. Cases in which ulnar nerve transposition was abandoned had a higher rate of excellent results (89% vs 75%), less complications (6% vs 14%), and less than half of the ulnar neuropathies.[48]

A few years following transition to a muscle-splitting approach, a modification of the Jobe technique, known as the docking technique, was described in a 2002 study, and it ultimately led to easier graft passage, tensioning, and fixation.[49] The ulnar tunnels are prepared in a similar fashion near the sublime tubercle as originally described by Jobe. There is a single humeral tunnel and the limbs of the graft are brought through the tunnel and exit out two separate drill holes and are tied over a bone bridge.

Complications of the surgery include injury to the ulnar nerve, medial antebrachial cutaneous nerve, fracture of the ulna or humeral epicondyle, stiffness, and heterotopic ossification.[50,51] In a 2015 study, the rate of return to play was 86.2% with those who underwent reconstruction using a docking technique having the highest return to play at 97%.[52] In a recent report, pitchers in Major League Baseball who underwent Tommy John surgery were found to have decreases in their presurgical fastball velocity with the greatest drop in speed noted for players aged 35 years and older (91.7 vs 88.8 mph, $P = 0.0048$).[50]

Lateral Collateral Ligament of the Elbow

The lateral collateral ligament complex is composed of four components: (1) the radial collateral ligament, (2) the LUCL, (3) the annular ligament, and (4) the accessory collateral ligament and the LUCL. Injuries to this complex and specifically the LUCL are commonly associated with simple elbow dislocations. The elbow is second only to the shoulder as the most commonly dislocated joint in the human body and nearly half occur during sporting events. The most common underlying mechanism involves direct contact with another person (46.9%) followed closely by contact with the ground (46%).[53]

In 1991, the sequence of events was described that take place during an elbow dislocation and termed posterolateral rotatory instability (PLRI).[54] In the acute setting, there is usually an obvious deformity of the elbow, and the patient may present with neurological changes involving the ulnar, median, or radial nerve. Depending on the presentation of the injury, some have argued for sideline reduction if an elbow dislocation is suspected while others recommend obtaining plain radiographs to evaluate for possible fracture prior to reduction.[55] AP and lateral radiographs are typically sufficient to identify an elbow dislocation as well as any additional bony injuries. Elbow instability has been suggested if there is radiographic evidence of a positive "drop sign" which is when there is an ulnohumeral distance of at least 4 mm[56] (**Figure 6**). These patients should be followed closely because they may require a surgical stabilization procedure.

Closed reduction of the elbow should be performed as soon as radiographs confirm dislocation and absence of any fractures or concomitant neurological changes. A combination of sedation and muscle relaxation are commonly utilized to ease the process of successful closed reduction. Repeat clinical evaluation should be performed and documented following closed reduction. Treatment of simple elbow dislocations that are stable throughout an arc of motion following reduction has been shown to benefit from 2 days of immobilization

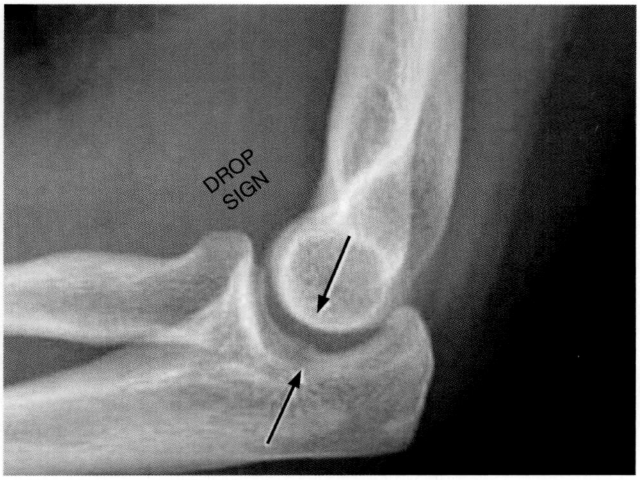

Figure 6 Lateral radiograph of the ulnohumeral joint demonstrates the drop sign, which indicates a noncongruent reduction. This finding usually occurs because of periarticular muscle pain–related atony and hemarthrosis. If only axial distraction (no medial or lateral translation of the joint) exists, the elbow can be treated with isometric exercises and overhead rehabilitation can be considered. The patient should be followed with weekly radiographs to ensure improvement. (Reproduced with permission from Pipicelli JG, Chinchalkar SJ, Grewal R, King GJ: Therapeutic implications of the radiographic "drop sign" following elbow dislocation. *J Hand Ther* 2012;25[3]:346-353, quiz 354, Copyright 2012, with permission from Elsevier. doi:10.1016/j.jht.2012.03.003.)

and then early motion to avoid stiffness according to a recent randomized trial.[57] In instability cases, the elbow is braced with an extension block just before the point of dislocation and should be maintained for 3 to 4 weeks. Following discontinuation of the brace a stretching program should begin immediately to avoid long-term stiffness.

Persistent instability following a trial of bracing treatment may require LUCL repair or reconstruction because it has been identified as the essential lesion in PLRI. At the time of injury, the LUCL usually avulses from the lateral epicondyle and has the potential for direct repair in the acute setting (<4 to 6 weeks after trauma) but more often requires reconstruction in cases presenting beyond this time point. Patients tend to do well following LUCL repair or reconstruction. In one study, 94% of patients were satisfied with their outcomes at a mean follow-up of 44 months; and among this same group of patients, 83% were able to return to their preinjury level of activity. One patient in the study required revision for treatment of a failed graft.[58] In a separate study looking at both direct repairs and reconstructions, 86% (38 of 44) were satisfied at their final follow-up (mean 6 years). Aside from persistent instability (five patients, two had revision surgery), one had surgery for heterotopic ossification and three others had posttraumatic arthritis necessitating interposition arthroplasty of the elbow.[33]

Return to sport following simple elbow dislocation varies depending on the extent of the injury and presence of instability following reduction. These athletes should be treated on a case-by-case basis and should not return to sport until they have a painless and normal range of elbow motion. Focused clinical examination maneuvers including the valgus and PLRI tests should not reproduce the pain. In cases that are able to be managed nonsurgically, time away from sport is typically 2 to 4 weeks but can range anywhere from 3 months to a year following surgical repair or reconstruction.

Summary

Injuries involving the elbow are oftentimes associated with repetitive overuse. Disorders that involve chronic tendinopathy respond well to nonsurgical management. In recalcitrant cases, successful results can be achieved with surgical intervention. Partial and complete tears of the UCL in high-level throwers typically necessitate surgical repair or reconstruction. As for injuries involving the distal biceps, distal triceps, and LUCL, they are typically acute in nature whether from an excessive eccentric contraction or elbow dislocation and warrant surgery in most instances.

Key Study Points

- Recent 10-year epidemiological data out of New York State revealed a 193% increase in UCL reconstructions between 2002 and 2011.
- In a recent review of the American Board of Orthopaedic Surgery database of cases submitted for Part II examination, surgeons with fellowship training in shoulder and elbow or sports medicine were more likely to perform arthroscopic surgery for tennis elbow compared with hand surgeons, and there were no self-reported differences in the complications rates between open (4.4%) and arthroscopic (5.5%) procedures. The breakdown of approaches was as follows: percutaneous tenotomy (6.4%), débridement only (46.3%), and débridement with tendon repair (47.3%).
- Treatment of simple elbow dislocations that are stable throughout an arc of motion following reduction has been shown to benefit from 2 days of immobilization and then early motion to avoid stiffness according to a recent randomized trial.

Annotated References

1. Cohen MS, Romeo AA, Hennigan SP, Gordon M: Lateral epicondylitis: Anatomic relationships of the extensor tendon origins and implications for arthroscopic treatment. *J Shoulder Elbow Surg* 2008;17(6):954-960.
2. Amin NH, Kumar NS, Schickendantz MS: Medial epicondylitis: Evaluation and management. *J Am Acad Orthop Surg* 2015;23(6):348-355.
3. Stucken C, Ciccotti MG: Distal biceps and triceps injuries in athletes. *Sports Med Arthrosc Rev* 2014;22(3):153-163.
4. Fleisig GS, Andrews JR, Dillman CJ, Escamilla RF: Kinetics of baseball pitching with implications about injury mechanisms. *Am J Sports Med* 1995;23(2):233-239.
5. Regan W, Wold LE, Coonrad R, Morrey BF: Microscopic histopathology of chronic refractory lateral epicondylitis. *Am J Sports Med* 1992;20(6):746-749.
6. Park GY, Lee SM, Lee MY: Diagnostic value of ultrasonography for clinical medial epicondylitis. *Arch Phys Med Rehabil* 2008;89(4):738-742.
7. Stahl S, Kaufman T: The efficacy of an injection of steroids for medial epicondylitis. A prospective study of sixty elbows. *J Bone Joint Surg Am* 1997;79(11):1648-1652.
8. Degen RM, Cancienne JM, Camp CL, Altchek DW, Dines JS, Werner BC: Patient-related risk factors for requiring surgical intervention following a failed injection for the treatment of medial and lateral epicondylitis. *Phys Sportsmed* 2017;45(4):433-437.

   The authors determined that risk factors related to failure of a therapeutic injection for the treatment of medial epicondylitis were obesity and age younger than 65 years, and age younger than 65 years, diabetes mellitus, smoking history, and peripheral vascular disease for lateral epicondylitis. Patients with these risk factors were more likely to undergo subsequent surgical treatment. Level of evidence: III.
9. Suresh SP, Ali KE, Jones H, et al: Medial epicondylitis: Is ultrasound guided autologous blood injection an effective treatment? *Br J Sports Med* 2006;40(11):935-939; discussion 939.
10. Gabel GT, Morrey BF: Operative treatment of medical epicondylitis. Influence of concomitant ulnar neuropathy at the elbow. *J Bone Joint Surg Am* 1995;77(7):1065-1069.
11. Knutsen EJ, Calfee RP, Chen RE, et al: Factors associated with failure of nonoperative treatment in lateral epicondylitis. *Am J Sports Med* 2015;43(9):2133-2137.
12. Major H: Lawn-tennis elbow. *BMJ* 1883.
13. Bunata RE, Brown DS, Capelo R: Anatomic factors related to the cause of tennis elbow. *J Bone Joint Surg Am* 2007;89(9):1955-1963.
14. Qi L, Zhu Z-F, Li F, Wang R-F: MR imaging of patients with lateral epicondylitis of the elbow: Is the common extensor tendon an isolated lesion?. *PLoS One* 2013;8(11):e79498.
15. Lian J, Mohamadi A, Chan JJ, et al: Comparative efficacy and safety of nonsurgical treatment options for enthesopathy of the extensor carpi radialis brevis: A systematic review and meta-analysis of randomized placebo-controlled trials. *Am J Sports Med* 2019;47(12):3019-3029.

    The authors compared efficacy and safety of nonsurgical treatment of enthesopathy of the extensor carpi radialis brevis and determined that all treatments provided only limited relief of pain.
16. Cullinane FL, Boocock MG, Trevelyan FC: Is eccentric exercise an effective treatment for lateral epicondylitis? A systematic review. *Clin Rehabil* 2014;28(1):3-19.
17. Pattanittum P, Turner T, Green S, Buchbinder R: Non-steroidal anti-inflammatory drugs (NSAIDs) for treating lateral elbow pain in adults. *Cochrane Database Syst Rev* 2013(5):CD003686.
18. Ben-Nafa W, Munro W: The effect of corticosteroid versus platelet-rich plasma injection therapies for the management of lateral epicondylitis: A systematic review. *SICOT J* 2018;4:11.

    The authors found that corticosteroid injections provided short-term rapid improvement of symptoms in the management of lateral epicondylitis. Platelet-rich plasma had a slower but longer-term effect. Level of evidence: II.
19. Wang D, Degen RM, Camp CL, McGraw MH, Altchek DW, Dines JS: Trends in surgical practices for lateral epicondylitis among newly trained orthopaedic surgeons. *Orthop J Sports Med* 2017;5(10):2325967117730570.

    The authors review current practice trends for surgical management of lateral epicondylitis among new US orthopaedic surgeons using the American Board of Orthopaedic Surgeons database. Level of evidence: III.
20. Safran MR, Graham SM: Distal biceps tendon ruptures: Incidence, demographics, and the effect of smoking. *Clin Orthop Relat Res* 2002;(404):275-283.
21. O'Driscoll SW, Goncalves LB, Dietz P: The hook test for distal biceps tendon avulsion. *Am J Sports Med* 2007;35(11):1865-1869.
22. Giuffre BM, Moss MJ: Optimal positioning for MRI of the distal biceps brachii tendon: Flexed abducted supinated view. *AJR Am J Roentgenol* 2004;182(4):944-946.
23. Schmidt CC, Brown BT, Sawardeker PJ, et al: Factors affecting supination strength after a distal biceps rupture. *J Shoulder Elbow Surg* 2014;23(1):68-75.
24. Freeman CR, McCormick KR, Mahoney D, et al: Nonoperative treatment of distal biceps tendon ruptures compared with a historical control group. *J Bone Joint Surg Am* 2009;91(10):2329-2334.
25. Behun MA, Geeslin AG, O'Hagan EC, King JC: Partial tears of the distal biceps brachii tendon: A systematic review of surgical outcomes. *J Hand Surg Am* 2016;41(7):e175-e189.
26. Darlis NA, Sotereanos DG: Distal biceps tendon reconstruction in chronic ruptures. *J Shoulder Elbow Surg* 2006;15(5):614-619.

27. Grewal R, Athwal GS, McDermid JC, et al: Single versus double-incision technique for the repair of acute distal biceps tendon ruptures: a randomized clinical trial. *J Bone Joint Surg Am* 2012;94(13):1166-1174.

28. Watson JN, Moretti VM, Schwindel L, Hutchinson MR: Repair techniques for acute distal biceps tendon ruptures: A systematic review. *J Bone Joint Surg Am* 2014;96(24):2086-2090.

29. Finstein JL, Cohen SB, Dodson CC, et al: Triceps tendon ruptures requiring surgical repair in national football League players. *Orthop J Sports Med* 2015;3(8):2325967115601021.

30. Keener JD, Sethi PM: Distal triceps tendon injuries. *Hand Clin* 2015;31(4):641-650.

31. Mair SD, Isbell WM, Gill TJ, et al: Triceps tendon ruptures in professional football players. *Am J Sports Med* 2004;32(2):431-434.

32. van Riet RP, Morrey BF, Ho E, et al: Surgical treatment of distal triceps ruptures. *J Bone Joint Surg Am* 2003;85-A(10):1961-1967.

33. Sanchez-Sotelo J, Morrey BF: Surgical techniques for reconstruction of chronic insufficiency of the triceps. Rotation flap using anconeus and tendo achillis allograft. *J Bone Joint Surg Br* 2002;84(8):1116-1120.

34. Thomas JR, Lawton JN: Biceps and triceps ruptures in athletes. *Hand Clin* 2017;33(1):35-46.

Rupture of the biceps is more common than triceps rupture. Surgical management is most effective; nonsurgical management is used for partial ruptures.

35. Cain EL Jr, Andrews JR, Dugas JR, et al: Outcome of ulnar collateral ligament reconstruction of the elbow in 1281 athletes: Results in 743 athletes with minimum 2-year follow-up. *Am J Sports Med* 2010;38(12):2426-2434.

36. Hodgins JL, Vitale M, Arons RR, Ahmad CS: Epidemiology of medial ulnar collateral ligament reconstruction: A 10-year study in New York state. *Am J Sports Med* 2016;44(3):729-734.

The frequency of UCL reconstruction is steadily increasing in New York State. It is important to emphasis public education on the risks associated with overuse throwing injuries and prevention strategies.

37. Erickson BJ, Nwachukwu BU, Rosas S, et al: Trends in medial ulnar collateral ligament reconstruction in the United States: A retrospective review of a large private-payer database from 2007 to 2011. *Am J Sports Med* 2015;43(7):1770-1774.

38. Lyman S, Fleisig GS, Andrews JR, et al: Effect of pitch type, pitch count, and pitching mechanics on risk of elbow and shoulder pain in youth baseball pitchers. *Am J Sports Med* 2002;30(4):463-468.

39. Bruce JR, Hess R, Joyner P, et al: How much valgus instability can be expected with ulnar collateral ligament (UCL) injuries? A review of 273 baseball players with UCL injuries. *J Shoulder Elbow Surg* 2014;23(10):1521-1526.

40. Thompson WH, Jobe FW, Yocum LA, et al: Ulnar collateral ligament reconstruction in athletes: Muscle-splitting approach without transposition of the ulnar nerve. *J Shoulder Elbow Surg* 2001;10(2):152-157.

41. Schwartz ML, al-Zahrani S, Morwessel RM, et al: Ulnar collateral ligament injury in the throwing athlete: Evaluation with saline-enhanced MR arthrography. *Radiology* 1995;197(1):297-299.

42. Joyner PW, Bruce J, Hess R, Mates A, Mills FB IVth, Andrews JR: Magnetic resonance imaging-based classification for ulnar collateral ligament injuries of the elbow. *J Shoulder Elbow Surg* 2016;25(10):1710-1716.

The authors proposed a new classification system for UCL injuries based on MRI findings regarding severity and location of the injury to better guide management options.

43. Shanley E, Smith M, Mayer BK, et al: Using stress ultrasonography to understand the risk of UCL injury among professional baseball pitchers based on ligament morphology and dynamic abnormalities. *Orthop J Sports Med* 2018;6(8):2325967118788847.

The authors suggest that ultrasonographic evaluation of UCL morphology may indicate risk of UCL injury in pitchers and may improve player assessment. Level of evidence: II.

44. Rettig AC, Sherrill C, Snead DS, et al: Nonoperative treatment of ulnar collateral ligament injuries in throwing athletes. *Am J Sports Med* 2001;29(1):15-17.

45. Podesta L, Crow SA, Volkmer D, et al: Treatment of partial ulnar collateral ligament tears in the elbow with platelet-rich plasma. *Am J Sports Med* 2013;41(7):1689-1694.

46. Smith GR, Altchek DW, Pagnani MJ, et al: A muscle-splitting approach to the ulnar collateral ligament of the elbow. Neuroanatomy and operative technique. *Am J Sports Med* 1996;24(5):575-580.

47. Jobe FW, Stark H, Lombardo SJ: Reconstruction of the ulnar collateral ligament in athletes. *J Bone Joint Surg Am* 1986;68(8):1158-1163.

48. Vitale MA, Ahmad CS: The outcome of elbow ulnar collateral ligament reconstruction in overhead athletes: A systematic review. *Am J Sports Med* 2008;36(6):1193-1205.

49. Rohrbough JT, Altchek DW, Hyman J, et al: Medial collateral ligament reconstruction of the elbow using the docking technique. *Am J Sports Med* 2002;30(4):541-548.

50. Lansdown DA, Feeley BT: The effect of ulnar collateral ligament reconstruction on pitch velocity in major League baseball pitchers. *Orthop J Sports Med* 2014;2(2):2325967114522592.

51. Andrachuk JS, Scillia AJ, Aune KT, et al: Symptomatic heterotopic ossification after ulnar collateral ligament reconstruction: Clinical significance and treatment outcome. *Am J Sports Med* 2016;44(5):1324-1328.

52. Erickson BJ, Chalmers PN, Bush-Joseph CA, et al: Ulnar collateral ligament reconstruction of the elbow: A systematic review of the literature. *Orthop J Sports Med* 2015;3(12):2325967115618914.

53. Dizdarevic I, Low S, Currie DW, et al: Epidemiology of elbow dislocations in high school athletes. *Am J Sports Med* 2016;44(1):202-208.

54. O'Driscoll SW, Bell DF, Morrey BF: Posterolateral rotatory instability of the elbow. *J Bone Joint Surg Am* 1991;73(3):440-446.

55. McGuire DT, Bain GI: Management of dislocations of the elbow in the athlete. *Sports Med Arthrosc Rev* 2014;22(3):188-193.

56. Coonrad RW, Roush TF, Major NM, Basamania CJ: The drop sign, a radiographic warning sign of elbow instability. *J Shoulder Elbow Surg* 2005;14(3):312-317.

57. Iordens GI, Van Lieshout EMM, Schep NWL, et al: Early mobilisation versus plaster immobilisation of simple elbow dislocations: Results of the FuncSiE multicentre randomised clinical trial. *Br J Sports Med* 2017;51(6):531-538.

The authors compared outcome of early mobilization and plaster immobilization in patients with a simple elbow dislocation and hypothesized that early mobilization is safe and effective and would lead to earlier functional recovery.

58. Olsen BS, Sojbjerg JO: The treatment of recurrent posterolateral instability of the elbow. *J Bone Joint Surg Br* 2003;85(3):342-346.

Elbow

Section 6
Hand and Wrist

EDITOR

Alexander Y. Shin, MD

Chapter 29

Anatomy, Evaluation, Clinical Examination, and Imaging

Nina Suh, MD, FRCSC • David M. Brogan, MD, MSc • Kimberly K. Amrami, MD

ABSTRACT

Accurate evaluation of hand and wrist injuries is imperative to assist the clinician making treatment management decisions. To assist the reader, this chapter will discuss hand and wrist anatomy, clinical examination techniques and tests, and relevant imaging modalities.

Keywords: CT; hand anatomy; metal suppression; MRI; physical examination; wrist anatomy

Introduction

Hand and wrist injuries are among the most common injuries of the upper extremity. Prior to the discussion of the management and treatment options for both acute and chronic pathologies, the clinician must initially perform a thorough history and physical examination. This chapter will address the fundamental concepts of hand and wrist anatomy, clinical examination, and imaging upon which the clinician may build their clinical acumen to pursue greater understanding of the clinical problem at hand.

Dr. Suh or an immediate family member serves as a paid consultant to or is an employee of Shire. Dr. Brogan or an immediate family member is a member of a speakers' bureau or has made paid presentations on behalf of Arthrex, Inc. and Trimed; has received research or institutional support from Axogen; and serves as a board member, owner, officer, or committee member of the American Society for Surgery of the Hand and the Member of Board of Governors for Missouri State Orthopaedic Association. Neither Dr. Amrami nor any immediate family member has received anything of value from or has stock or stock options held in a commercial company or institution related directly or indirectly to the subject of this chapter.

Anatomy: Refinement in the Understanding of Wrist/Hand Anatomy

Osseous Anatomy

The wrist is composed of the distal portion of the radius that articulates with the ulnar head through the sigmoid notch as well as the eight carpal bones that articulate with the distal radius through the concave scaphoid and lunate facets. The wrist serves as a link between the hand and forearm unit and allows for wrist flexion, extension, ulnar deviation, radial deviation, and dart-throw motion by coordinated movement through the radiocarpal, ulnocarpal, and midcarpal joints.

Classically, the distal radial volar tilt is reported to be approximately 11° (range: 5° to 20°); however, nonuniform volar tilt has been reported with the greatest tilt found at the radial edge of the scaphoid fossa and the least tilt at the center of the lunate fossa (15.2° + 4.9° and 9.2° + 2.4°, respectively).[1,2] Furthermore, radial inclination and ulnar variance averages 23° and 1 mm negative, respectively, although significant variability is present.[3]

The distal radioulnar joint (DRUJ) in conjunction with the proximal radioulnar joint (PRUJ) permits supination and pronation through rotation of the radius around the stationary ulna.[4] However, the DRUJ is intrinsically unstable due to the radius of curvature of the sigmoid notch being nearly twice that of the articulating ulnar head as well as the sigmoid notch being dorsally open wedge-shaped (10°) with the dorsal length on average being greater than the volar length (10 versus 6 mm).[5] In fact, further characterization of DRUJ shape has been explored with flat face, ski slope, "C" type, and "S" type being described in the literature for axial plane assessments and coronal plane descriptions including vertical (38%), oblique (50%), and reverse obliquity (12%).[6] As a result, dorsopalmar and proximal-distal translation of the ulnar head occurs with forearm rotation.

Meanwhile, the carpus is arranged into two rows with the scaphoid, lunate, triquetrum, and pisiform in the proximal row and the trapezium, trapezoid, capitate, and hamate in the distal row. The pisiform is the only carpal bone that is noncontributory to wrist motion while the scaphoid is the only carpal bone that serves as a linkage between the proximal and distal rows. Further distally, the hand is composed of four fingers each with a singular metacarpal and three phalanges (proximal, middle, and distal) as well as a thumb with a singular metacarpal and two phalanges (proximal and distal). Each metacarpal is composed of a head, neck, shaft, and base while each phalanx is composed of a head, shaft, and base.

Ligamentous Anatomy

The ligaments of the wrist are divided into extrinsic and intrinsic ligaments with further subdivision into radiocarpal or ulnocarpal ligaments and volar or dorsal ligaments. The major volar radiocarpal ligaments include the radioscaphoid, radioscaphocapitate, long radiolunate, and short radiolunate ligaments while the major volar ulnocarpal ligaments include the ulnocapitate, ulnolunate, and ulnotriquetral ligaments.[7] The volar ligaments form an inverted V-configuration to prevent dorsovolar subluxation of the carpus; however, an intraligamentous sulcus between the radioscaphocapitate and long radiolunate ligaments exists, known as the space of Poirier, that is a well-described area of capsular weakness frequently affected in perilunate injuries.[7]

Conversely, only dorsal radiocarpal ligaments exist as no defined ligaments are found between the ulna and carpus dorsally. The main dorsal radiocarpal ligaments include the dorsal radial triquetrum (aka dorsal radiocarpal) and dorsal intercarpal ligament that traverses between the triquetrum, trapezoid, capitate, lunate, and scaphoid.[8] The dorsal ligaments contribute to carpal stability and alignment, and the importance of the dorsal ligamentous structures for scaphoid stability, in particular, has been explored through anatomical studies of the dorsal capsule-scapholunate septum that attaches the dorsal aspect of the scapholunate interosseous ligament to the dorsal intercarpal ligament.[9]

The intrinsic wrist ligaments connect adjacent carpal bones with the principal intrinsic ligaments being the scapholunate and lunotriquetral ligaments. The scapholunate ligament is composed of the dorsal (strongest), proximal (membranous), and volar segments, and disruption leads to dorsal intercalated segmental instability.[8] Similarly, the lunotriquetral ligament is composed of the dorsal, proximal (membranous), and volar (strongest) segments, and disruption leads to volar intercalated segmental instability.[8]

The DRUJ is principally stabilized statically by the triangular fibrocartilage complex (TFCC) and the interosseous membrane.[4] Meanwhile, the extensor carpi ulnaris (ECU) and deep head of the pronator quadratus act as dynamic stabilizers. The primary soft-tissue restraint, the TFCC, is composed of the ulnocarpal ligaments (ulnolunate, ulnocapitate, and ulnotriquetral ligaments), ECU tendon subsheath, volar and dorsal radioulnar ligaments, proper articular disk, and the meniscus homologue. The primary ligamentous stabilizers of the DRUJ are the volar and dorsal radioulnar ligaments that originate from the sigmoid notch and traverse ulnarly to divide into superficial and deep limbs with the former attaching at the base and midportion of the ulnar styloid while the latter attaches to the ulnar fovea. It is the foveal attachments that are the most important for conferring stability to the DRUJ.[10]

The metacarpophalangeal joint of the finger is reinforced by the capsule, volar plate, and laterally by the deep transverse metacarpal ligament. Similarly, the proximal interphalangeal joint (PIP) is stabilized by proper and volar accessory collateral ligaments as well as the volar plate that thickens proximally to form strong checkrein ligaments. Meanwhile, the distal interphalangeal joint is analogous to the PIP joint ligamentous structure but is further stabilized by the direct attachments of the extensor and flexor tendons.

Special consideration should be given to the thumb carpometacarpal joint ligamentous structures that include the volar oblique (aka palmar beak), intermetacarpal, dorsoradial, and dorsal oblique ligaments. The volar oblique is thought to the primary restraint to dorsal subluxation/dislocation and is often reconstructed after trapeziectomy for thumb arthritis.[11]

Muscular Anatomy

The volar musculature of the wrist assists with wrist, finger, and thumb flexion and forearm pronation. It includes the flexor carpi radialis, palmaris longus, flexor carpi ulnaris, pronator teres, flexor digitorum superficialis, flexor digitorum profundus, flexor pollicis longus, and pronator quadratus.

Contrarily, the dorsal musculature assists with wrist, finger, and thumb extension as well as forearm supination. The superficial dorsal compartment includes the brachioradialis, extensor carpi radialis longus, extensor carpi radialis brevis, extensor carpi ulnaris, and anconeus. The first three previously mentioned tendons are also known as the mobile wad. The intermediate dorsal compartment consists of the extensor digitorum communis and extensor digiti minimi tendons while the deep compartment consists of the abductor pollicis longus, extensor pollicis longus, extensor pollicis brevis, extensor indicis proprius, and the supinator.

The muscles of the hand include the thenar muscles (abductor pollicis brevis, flexor pollicis brevis, and opponens pollicis), hypothenar muscles (abductor digiti minimi, flexor digiti minimi, and opponens digiti minimi), interossei muscles (four dorsal and three palmar), lumbricals, and adductor pollicis muscle which in concert allow movement of the hand and fingers.

Neurovascular Anatomy

The principal motor and sensory neurologic structures of the hand and wrist include the median, radial, and ulnar nerves.[12] The median nerve supplies the volar forearm flexor pronator muscles, thenar muscles, and the first and second lumbricals. Its terminal branches include the anterior interosseous nerve, palmar cutaneous nerve, recurrent motor branch, and digital sensory nerves to the radial 3.5 digits. The radial nerve via the posterior interosseous nerve branch supplies the dorsal forearm extensor supinator muscles while distally its radial sensory nerve branch divides into distal sensory branches supplying the dorsal thumb, first web space, and dorsal aspect of the index and long fingers. Lastly, the ulnar nerve supplies the flexor carpi ulnaris, flexor digitorum profundus of the ring and small finger, adductor pollicis, deep head of the flexor pollicis brevis, interossei, third and fourth lumbricals, and hypothenar muscles. Its sensory component includes the dorsal sensory branch of the ulnar nerve.

The vascular supply of the wrist and hand is comprised of the radial and ulnar arteries that combine to form the superficial and deep palmar arch.[13] The former is formed by the anastomosis of the ulnar artery and superficial palmar branch of the radial artery while the latter is formed by the anastomosis of the radial artery and deep palmar branch of the ulnar artery. The deep palmar arch branches into the palmar metacarpal branches to supply the fingers while the princeps pollicis artery arises off of the radial artery. Meanwhile, the superficial palmar arch branches into the common palmar digital branches.

Evaluation and Clinical Examination: Current Concepts

Clinical evaluation of the injured or dysfunctional hand and wrist can be a daunting task. Painless and full hand function requires seamless integration of joints, muscles, and nerves to complete even the most basic task. Patients often have difficulty accurately describing their symptoms and may incorrectly attribute pathology to a perceived deficit, whether real or imagined. The task of the astute clinician is to combine the patient history with a careful physical examination to pinpoint or at least narrow the scope of possible pathologic processes. Diagnostic tests such as imaging and serum laboratory studies are useful in this determination but can be expensive, time consuming, and often nonspecific. Therefore, a careful physical examination is essential to direct care and future testing if indicated.

With so many structures in such a small space, a systematic method to approaching the physical examination is essential. Some clinicians may prefer to organize their examination by anatomic location or region of the hand, while others may choose to proceed by organ system or pathology. This section will review recent literature in the systematic approach to evaluation of the wrist and hand.

Fractures

While open fractures and obvious deformities may not pose a diagnostic dilemma, more subtle presentations of minimally displaced fractures may prove challenging to detect. Observation and palpation of an injured hand often leads to the identification of occult fractures that may be a source of pain. Careful palpation of each of the metacarpal and carpal bones is essential, and observation of the patient's ability to make a tight composite fist yields information about the status of the phalanges. Any perceived pain should be explored with palpation of the affected area to identify step-offs or possible fractures to better direct imaging. This is particularly true in the diagnosis of scaphoid fractures. Negative plain films may be unreliable in diagnosing nondisplaced scaphoid fractures, making the physical examination critical for timely diagnosis.[14] In a recent meta-analysis, the presence of snuffbox tenderness was found to have a 96% sensitivity in diagnosis of a scaphoid fracture, although the specificity was only 39%.[15]

In addition to tenderness, the clinician should inspect for evidence of edema and deformity. Fractures of the distal radius may result in radial deviation or volar/dorsal angulation of the wrist with significant swelling. Metacarpal and phalangeal fractures may also present with clinical deviation or malrotation. Some digital overlap (<50% of nail plate) is common in uninjured fingers,[16] but obvious malrotation that interferes with grip should be identified and is a relative indication for surgical treatment (**Figure 1**). Results of this can be quite good. The authors of a 2017 study[17] retrospectively assessed 28 patients who underwent open reduction and internal fixation of metacarpal and phalangeal fractures to correct rotational malalignment. The average angulation corrected during surgery was 11.9°, with an average of 254° total active motion. No patient had recurrent scissoring.

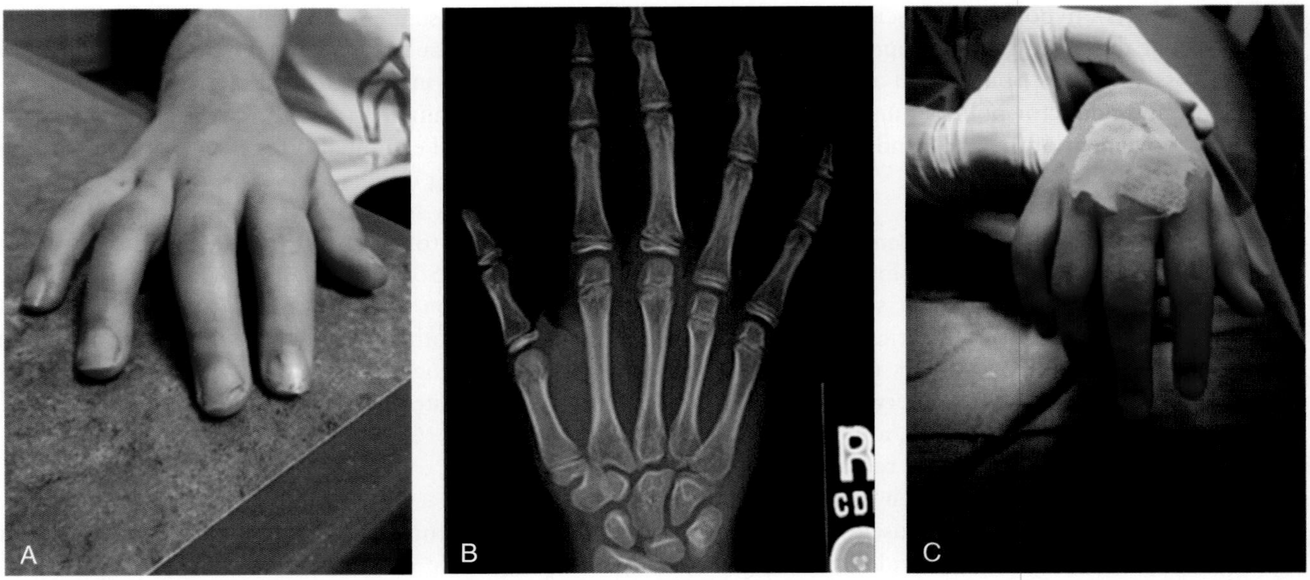

Figure 1 Clinical photograph of an 8-year-old with a long finger proximal phalanx fracture and obvious clinical malrotation (**A**), despite minimal fracture displacement on radiographs (**B**). After closed reduction and percutaneous pinning, the deformity is corrected (**C**).

Ligamentous Injury and Instability

Ligamentous injuries in the hand often manifest as pain with loading of the joint. Scapholunate ligament injury is a common complaint encountered by hand surgeons and manifests as dorsal wrist pain over the scapholunate ligament. The scaphoid shift test has been described as a method of assessing for a globally unstable scaphoid; a similar dynamic test that attempts to shift the scaphoid posteriorly has also been described.[18] However, laxity on physical examination alone can be misleading, as generalized ligamentous laxity can lead to false-positives. This was demonstrated in a recent case report that described dynamic scapholunate instability that began spontaneously at 6 weeks postpartum and subsequently resolved 4 months after cessation of nursing.[19] Therefore, isolated ligamentous laxity should be interpreted with caution in patients who lack a history of trauma.

Diagnosis of injury to the ulnar collateral ligament (UCL) of the metacarpophalangeal joint of the thumb can also be quite difficult, particularly when attempting to differentiate between a partial and complete tear. Classically, a complete tear of the ligament presents with more than 35° of laxity in full extension or greater than 15° compared with the contralateral side or lack of a fixed end point.[20] However, given the difficulty in assessing instability, MRI and ultrasound remain popular tools for the diagnosis of this injury. A prospective cohort study investigated the utility of physical examination in this diagnosis by assessing the accuracy of a resident physician's examination in the emergency room compared with MRI—considered the gold standard.[21] Thirty patients were determined to have a UCL tear by MRI, and 73% of these had clear physical examination findings consistent with this, while another 27% had an inconclusive examination—highlighting the difficulty of determining the diagnosis in the acute setting.

Another source of instability in the wrist can occur due to disruption of the ligaments of the DRUJ. Ballotment of the DRUJ is one of the physical examination maneuvers utilized to assess for instability—this is performed by grasping the distal radius with one hand and the distal ulna with the other and providing a relative translational force between the two. A recent biomechanical study assessed the intra- and inter-rater reliability of this technique and found that its accuracy in detecting instability was improved by holding the carpal bones fixed to the radius during assessment.[22]

Evaluation of Tendinopathy

Tendinopathy is a common pathology seen by hand surgeons, but rarely presents a significant diagnostic dilemma. Flexor tenosynovitis manifests as locking and catching of the digit, with pain over the A1 pulley of the flexor tendon sheath. Similarly, DeQuervain tenosynovitis is readily diagnosed by its localization to the first dorsal compartment on the radial aspect of the wrist. However, ulnar-sided wrist pain can have multiple etiologies, but recent attention has focused on the potential pathophysiology of structures on the peripheral aspect of the TFCC. The ECU synergy test has been previously described as a maneuver to differentiate between intra-articular and extra-articular ulnar wrist pathology.[23] The forearm is held in supination, and the physician stabilizes the thumb and long finger, asking the patient to radially abduct the thumb while the ECU tendon is palpated. Dorsal ulnar wrist pain during this maneuver is thought to be consistent with ECU pathology. The sensitivity of this test was more recently explored utilizing ultrasound as a reference standard in a prospective study of 40 wrists.[24] The authors found a sensitivity of 73.7% and a specificity of 85.7%, suggesting it is a useful tool in evaluating the complex nuances of ulnar-sided wrist pain.

Evaluation of Neuropathy

Disorders of the peripheral nervous system routinely manifest in the upper extremity as hand numbness and tingling, with more severe cases leading to intrinsic atrophy and objective weakness. However, subtle presentations may prove to be a diagnostic challenge, as multiple site of compression may contribute to a constellation of symptoms. The scratch collapse test has gained notoriety in recent years as an adjunct diagnostic tool in evaluation of compressive neuropathy, particularly as a technique to identify the precise location of compression. First described in 2008, the test evaluates the patient's ability to perform resisted bilateral shoulder external rotation. Light scratching of the area of nerve compression results in transient weakness in shoulder external rotation (**Figure 2**), resulting in a positive test.[25] The original series of 278 subjects described a sensitivity of 64% and 69% for carpal and cubital tunnel, respectively, with a specificity of 99% for both syndromes.[25] Accuracy was determined to be 82% for carpal tunnel syndrome and 89% for cubital tunnel syndrome. However, more recent evaluation of the accuracy of the test to diagnose carpal tunnel syndrome with blinded examiners reported a sensitivity of 24%, a specificity of 60%, and an accuracy of 31% compared with electrodiagnostic studies.[26] This was a series of 40 patients referred to a physiatrist for nerve conduction studies and examined by physicians instructed in the test, but unfamiliar with the significance of each test result. These recent results are more in line with those reported by authors of previous studies examining its role in diagnosis of carpal tunnel syndrome: one study reported a sensitivity of 31% but a specificity of 61%.[27] While this examination maneuver may contribute to the clinical diagnosis of peripheral entrapment neuropathy, caution should be exercised in its interpretation.[27]

Response to operative treatment of carpal tunnel syndrome can also be difficult to predict, as some patients will have complete resolution of symptoms, while others demonstrate persistent symptoms. Jansen

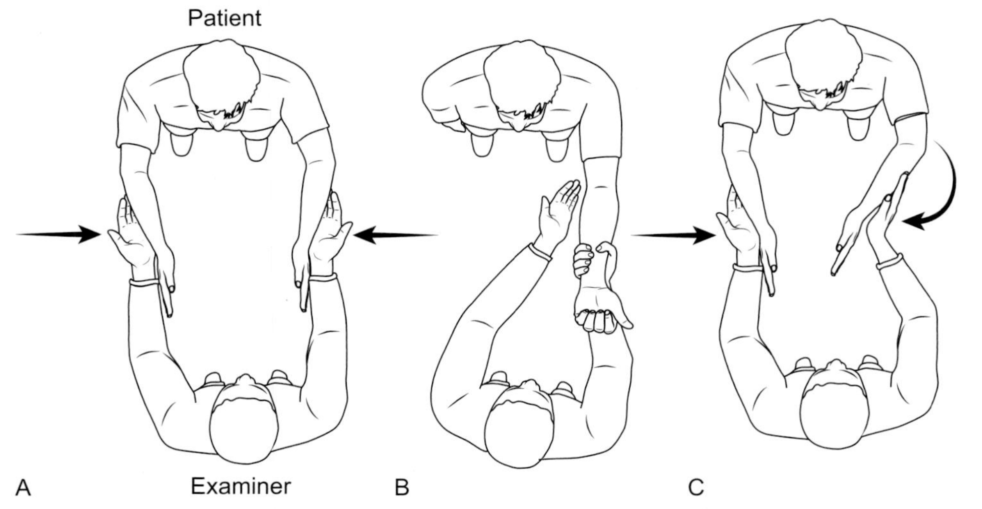

Figure 2 Illustration of the scratch-collapse test. **A**, Examiner resists external rotation of the patient's shoulders. **B**, The examiner scratches the area of possible nerve compression. **C**, A positive test results in weakness in the patient's ability to externally rotate the shoulder against resistance. (Reproduced with permission from Cheng CJ, Mackinnon-Patterson B, Beck JL, Mackinnon SE: Scratch collapse test for evaluation of carpal and cubital tunnel syndrome. *J Hand Surg* 2008;33[9]:1518-1524, Copyright 2008, with permission from Elsevier.)

et al. evaluated 1,049 patients undergoing carpal tunnel release at 11 centers in the Netherlands and found that low preoperative Boston Carpal Tunnel Questionnaire (BCTQ) scores helped predict a smaller improvement in symptoms postoperatively.[28] Similarly, presence of other comorbid hand conditions such as trigger finger, ulnar neuropathy, and basilar thumb arthritis also predicted less improvement postoperatively. However, when the Quick Disabilities of the Arm, Shoulder and Hand (Quick-DASH) was utilized as an outcomes measure, severity of disease did not correlate to postoperative improvement at 2 weeks and 3 months, in a separate study of 199 patients. All patients showed improvement at 2 weeks regardless of preoperative severity.[29]

Imaging: Advances in Imaging of the Hand and Upper Extremity

In the last several years, there have been technological advances in all modalities which have great promise for enhancing imaging of the hand and wrist. The hand and wrist places unique demands in imaging compared with other, larger joints and body parts. The highest spatial resolution, the smallest fields of view (often 8 cm or less), and best tissue contrast are required to obtain the most accurate information in support of clinical care. Close collaboration between surgeons and radiologists is essential to optimize tailoring imaging to specific indications and needs.

Radiography

Since Roentgen's famous radiograph of his wife's hand, radiography has been a mainstay of diagnosis for the hand and wrist. Two-dimensional (2D) film screen radiography originally relied on taking exposures in multiple planes and then exposing individual films to create a permanent x-ray image on film. Since the 1990s, there has been rapid transition away from analog acquisitions toward digital options for both image acquisition and storage. The current standard, fully digital radiography has some advantages and disadvantages for imaging of the hand and wrist. The obvious advantage is the availability of images for viewing across digital platforms rather than requiring a physical copy of the radiograph. This leads to lower costs for handling and storage (although equipment costs are substantially higher than conventional radiograph machines).

Conventional tomography, developed in the 1930s as a way to diminish overlap in radiographic images, was largely replaced by computed tomography (CT) by the 1990s. There has been a revival of x-ray tomography in the last several years using digital acquisition techniques. This has been specifically applied to areas such as the wrist, lung, and breast. For the wrist, it has been proposed as an alternative to CT for clinical problems such as fracture healing, but its application is limited, and it is not widely available.

Computed Tomography

CT has long been the preferred technique for diagnosis and surgical planning for fractures of the wrist. Images can be acquired at a resolution of 0.1 mm or less in acquisition times under 5 minutes. The images can then be reconstructed in multiple planes and three-dimensional (3D) models created. CT is also a useful technique for following fracture healing due to its ability to image trabecular and cortical bridging with high confidence. CT can be combined with arthrography of the wrist, but this is rarely indicated unless MRI cannot be performed for safety or other reasons.

There have been two developments in CT imaging that have had a significant impact on hand and wrist imaging. Both rely on established technology which has now become commercially available.

Conventional CT uses a single energy source to acquire images, typically in the range of 140 kVp, which generates the familiar image—dense (white) bone and less dense (gray) soft tissues. When a second, lower energy acquisition is performed (usually in the range of 80 kVp), it is possible to further discriminate tissue properties by comparing their Hounsfield densities at the different energies. This technique has been used to distinguish monosodium urate from calcium oxalate stones in the kidney; in the hand and wrist, it is used to assess for the presence of gout by identifying urate deposits. This has become a standard technique for rheumatologic imaging to distinguish gout from osteoarthritis or other types of inflammatory arthritis.[30] The radiation dose is the same as conventional CT and both standard and "urate" images are generated, with the urate deposits typically being color coded and superimposed on the conventional images (**Figure 3**, **A** and **B**). Both 2D and 3D images are generated using this technology. The latest musculoskeletal application of dual-energy CT is termed "calcium subtraction," whereby the calcium in an image is subtracted, which in the case of orthopedic imaging highlights the presence of bone marrow edema for improved detection of nondisplaced fractures or fractures in very osteopenic patients without the use of MRI. While most useful for imaging of the hip, it has been applied to the wrist (**Figure 4**, **A** through **C**).[31]

Cone beam CT is an exciting "new" technology, first developed in 1996 and in common use for dental applications, that is important because it does not require the kind of installation and cost related to a conventional CT scanner but can provide images approaching CT

5. Omokawa S, Iida A, Kawamura K, et al: A biomechanical perspective on distal radioulnar joint instability. *J Wrist Surg* 2017;6:88-96.

The authors explore the anatomy and kinematics of the DRUJ with a further discussion of the clinical implications of DRUJ instability. Level of evidence: III.

6. Tolat AR, Stanley JK, Trail IA: A cadaveric study of the anatomy and stability of the distal radioulnar joint in the coronal and transverse planes. *J Hand Surg [Br]* 1996;21:587-559.

7. Berger RA, Landsmeer JM: The palmar radiocarpal ligaments: A study of adult and fetal human wrist joints. *J Hand Surg Am* 1990;15(6):847-854.

8. Berger RA: The ligaments of the wrist. A current overview of anatomy with considerations of their potential functions. *Hand Clin* 1997;13(1):63-82.

9. Tommasini Carrara de Sambuy M, Burgess RM, Cambon-Binder A, Mathoulin CL: The anatomy of the dorsal capsule-scapholunate septum: A cadaveric study. *J Wrist Surg* 2017;6(3):244-247.

The DCSS was identified and characterized using cadaver specimens. Level of evidence: IV.

10. Haugstvedt J-R, Berger RA, Nakamura T, Neale P, Berglund L, An K-N: Relative contributions of the ulnar attachments of the triangular fibrocartilage complex to the dynamic stability of the distal radioulnar joint. *J Hand Surg Am* 2006;31(3):445-451.

11. Bakri K, Moran SL: Thumb carpometacarpal arthritis. *Plast Reconstr Surg* 2015;135(2):508-520.

12. Seiler JG, Daruwalla JH, Payne SH, Faucher GK: Normal palmar anatomy and variations that impact median nerve decompression. *J Am Acad Orthop Surg* 2017;25:e194-e203.

Review article describing normal palmar anatomy. Level of evidence: V.

13. Zarzecki MP, Popieluszko P, Zayachkowski A, Pekala PA, Henry BM, Tomaszewski KA: The surgical anatomy of the superficial and deep palmar arches: A meta-analysis. *J Plast Reconstr Aesthet Surg* 2018;71(11):1577-1592.

A meta-analysis of 4841 palmar arches in 36 studies whose aim was to identify the pooled prevalence estimate of palmar vasculature in the hand. Level of evidence: II.

14. Sobel AD, Shah KN, Katarincic JA: The imperative nature of physical exam in identifying pediatric scaphoid fractures. *J Pediatr* 2016;177:323-323.e1.

The authors use a representative case description to illustrate the importance of physical examination on diagnosis of scaphoid fractures—recommendations for management of such fractures are outlined. Level of evidence: V.

15. Gemme S, Tubbs R: What physical examination findings and diagnostic imaging modalities are most useful in the diagnosis of scaphoid fractures? *Ann Emerg Med* 2015;65(3):308-309.

16. Tan V, Kinchelow T, Beredjiklian PK: Variation in digital rotation and alignment in normal subjects. *J Hand Surg Am* 2008;33(6):873-878.

17. Lee S, Lee S, Lee J-K, Sim Y, Choi D-S, Han S-H: Surgical treatment of metacarpal and phalangeal fracture with rotational malalignment. *J Korean Soc Surg Hand* 2017;22(3):189-195.

The authors present a retrospective review of a series of 28 cases of metacarpal or phalangeal malrotation requiring operative treatment. Average motion, correction of angulation, and strength are reported with an average follow-up greater than 1 year. Level of evidence: IV.

18. Lane LB: The scaphoid shift test. *J Hand Surg Am* 1993;18(2):366-368.

19. Miller EK, Tanaka MJ, LaPorte DM, Humbyrd CJ: Pregnancy-related ligamentous laxity mimicking dynamic scapholunate instability: A case report. *JBJS Case Connect* 2017;7(3):e54.

This is a case report of spontaneous postpartum ligamentous wrist laxity as well as a discussion of the effects of various hormones on ligamentous laxity. Level of evidence: IV.

20. Mayer SW, Ruch DS, Leversedge FJ: The influence of thumb metacarpophalangeal joint rotation on the evaluation of ulnar collateral ligament injuries: A biomechanical study in a cadaver model. *J Hand Surg Am* 2014;39(3):474-479.

21. Mahajan M, Tolman C, Würth B, Rhemrev SJ: Clinical evaluation vs magnetic resonance imaging of the skier's thumb: A prospective cohort of 30 patients. *Eur J Radiol* 2016;85(10):1750-1756.

The article reports a single institution, prospective cohort series of patients suspected to have acute ulnar collateral ligament insufficiency and compares diagnostic sensitivity of physical examination with MRI. Level of evidence: I.

22. Onishi T, Omokawa S, Iida A, et al: Biomechanical study of distal radioulnar joint ballottement test. *J Orthop Res* 2017;35(5):1123-1127.

This is a cadaveric biomechanical study of 5 specimens assessing the sensitivity of the DRUJ ballotement test in detecting DRUJ injury, with and without immobilization of the carpus during the test. Level of evidence: I.

23. Ruland RT, Hogan CJ: The ECU synergy test: An aid to diagnose ECU tendonitis. *J Hand Surg Am* 2008;33(10):1777-1782.

24. Sato J, Ishii Y, Noguchi H: Diagnostic performance of the extensor carpi ulnaris (ECU) synergy test to detect sonographic ECU abnormalities in chronic dorsal ulnar-sided wrist pain. *J Ultrasound Med* 2016;35(1):7-14.

The authors report a clinical series comparing the sensitivity and specificity of the ECU synergy test with ultrasound for the diagnosis of ECU abnormalities. Level of evidence: II.

25. Cheng CJ, Mackinnon-Patterson B, Beck JL, Mackinnon SE: Scratch collapse test for evaluation of carpal and cubital tunnel syndrome. *J Hand Surg Am* 2008;33(9):1518-1524.

26. Simon J, Lutsky K, Maltenfort M, Beredjiklian PK: The accuracy of the scratch collapse test performed by blinded examiners on patients with suspected carpal tunnel syndrome assessed by electrodiagnostic studies. *J Hand Surg Am* 2017;42(5):386.e1-386.e5.

Forty patients were examined by blinded examiners to assess the accuracy of the scratch collapse test to determine carpal tunnel syndrome with electrodiagnostic testing as the reference standard. Level of evidence: II.

Hand and Wrist

27. Makanji HS, Becker S, Mudgal CS, Jupiter JB, Ring D: Evaluation of the scratch collapse test for the diagnosis of carpal tunnel syndrome. *J Hand Surg Eur Vol* 2014;39(2):181-186.

28. Jansen M, Evers S, Slijper H, et al: Predicting clinical outcome after surgical treatment in patients with carpal tunnel syndrome. *J Hand Surg Am* 2018;43(12):1098-1106.

This is a large study of more than 1,000 patients treated with carpal tunnel release and followed for 6 months after surgery. The authors identify a number of factors predictive of poor outcome after carpal tunnel release. Level of evidence: II.

29. Rivlin M, Kachooei AR, Wang ML, Ilyas AM: Electrodiagnostic grade and carpal tunnel release outcomes: A prospective analysis. *J Hand Surg Am* 2018;43(5):425-431.

The authors report a prospective study evaluating factors influencing patient response to open carpal tunnel release. Level of evidence: II.

30. Bongartz T, Glazebrook KN, Kavros SJ, et al: Dual-energy CT for the diagnosis of gout: An accuracy and diagnostic yield study. *Ann Rheum Dis* 2015;74(6):1072-1077.

31. Ali IT, Wong WD, Liang T, et al: Clinical utility of dual-energy CT analysis of bone marrow edema in acute wrist fractures. *AJR Am J Roentgenol* 2018;210(4):842-847.

Dual-energy CT with calcium subtraction is an emerging method for assessing for the presence of bone marrow edema and occult fractures on noncontrast CT. For patients unable to undergo MRI, this is a viable alternative for diagnosing radiographically occult scaphoid and other hand and wrist fractures. Level of evidence: III.

32. De Cock J, Mermuys K, Goubau J, et al: Cone-beam computed tomography: A new low dose, high resolution imaging technique of the wrist, presentation of three cases with technique. *Skeletal Radiol* 2012;41(1):93-96.

33. Koenig H, Lucas D, Meissner R, The wrist: a preliminary report on high-resolution MR imaging. *Radiology* 1986;160(2):463-467.

34. Yin ZG, Zhang JB, Kan SL, et al: Diagnostic accuracy of imaging modalities for suspected scaphoid fractures: Meta-analysis combined with latent class analysis. *J Bone Joint Surg Br* 2012;94(8):1077-1085.

35. Burke CJ, Alizai H, Beltral LS, Regatte RR: MRI of synovitis and joint fluid. *J Magn Reson Imaging* 2019 [Epub ahead of print].

Contrast-enhanced MRI has become the standard for diagnosing and following rheumatologic disease in the hand and wrist. This paper evaluates MRI for erosions and other bone changes in addition to assessing synovitis. MRI can be used for both qualitative and quantitative assessments. Level of evidence: III.

36. Jungmann PM, Agten CA, Pfirrmann CW, et al: Advances in MRI around metal. *J Magn Reson Imaging*, 2017;46(4):972-991.

This paper reviews technical advances in MRI in the presence of metal which improve visualization of structures in the postoperative hand and wrist. Level of evidence: IV.

Chapter 30

Bone and Soft-Tissue Infections of the Hand and Wrist

Nicholas Pulos, MD • Scott M. Tintle, MD

ABSTRACT

In the past decade the literature on bone and soft-tissue infections of the hand and wrist has been dominated by three main themes: preventing surgical site infection, the rising incidence of more virulent infections, and case reports of unusual pathogens in both immunocompetent and immunocompromised patients. This chapter not only covers these topics but also presents a review of the latest evidence for diagnosing and treating specific bone and soft-tissue infections of the hand and wrist.

Keywords: Atypical infection; flexor tenosynovitis; hand abscess; osteomyelitis; surgical site infection

Introduction

Infections of the hand and wrist make up a significant number of emergency department visits and surgical hand surgery procedures. In the past decade, literature on this topic has been dominated by three main themes: preventing surgical site infection, the rising incidence of more virulent infections, and case reports of unusual pathogens in both immunocompetent and immunocompromised patients. The routine use of preoperative antibiotics in clean hand surgery cases is being scrutinized. In patients presenting with hand infections requiring surgical intervention, more than half are now due to methicillin-resistant *Staphylococcus aureus* (MRSA). Delays in the proper diagnosis and treatment of these and other infections caused by atypical organisms can be threatening to both limb and life.

Dr. Pulos or an immediate family member is a member of a speakers' bureau or has made paid presentations on behalf of Trimed. Dr. Tintle or an immediate family member serves as a board member, owner, officer, or committee member of Society of Military Orthopaedic Surgeons.

Soft-Tissue Infections

Surgical Site Infection

Concomitant with a rise in WALANT and a transition toward increased office-based procedures, the need for surgical antimicrobial prophylaxis has been called into question. Across several recent studies the infection rate following carpal tunnel release and similar procedures is consistently less than 1% regardless of the whether antibiotics are provided. In 454,987 Medicare patients undergoing carpal tunnel release, Werner et al reported a 0.32% infection rate.[1] A multistate, commercial insurance database study of 516,986 patients used propensity-score matching to find no difference in the risk for surgical site infection between patients who received antibiotic prophylaxis and those who did not.[2] These database studies have been corroborated by a large clinical study, which reported a 0.35% infection rate for clean, elective, hand surgeries performed at an outpatient surgical center. Again, no difference was found between patients who received antibiotics and those who did not.[3] Some minor hand procedures may be safely performed in the emergency department or office with a similarly low infection rate.[4] Finally, a randomized, double-blind study of 1,340 patients undergoing hand surgery found no decrease in infection rates with the administration of preoperative antibiotics. This led the authors to conclude that there is little evidence to support the routine use of preoperative antibiotics in hand surgery.[5]

Reported factors associated with the development of a surgical site infection include younger age, male sex, obesity, tobacco use, alcohol use, diabetes, and other medical comorbidities.[1,3] More important than the diagnosis of diabetes itself, however, may be the patient's HbA1c level. Patients with a preoperative HbA1c greater than 8 are at a significantly increased risk for surgical site infection.[6] Other relevant risks for infection include prolonged surgical time[7] and delayed treatment for open hand fractures.[8]

A prospective study comparing surgical site preparation techniques found that prep-stick application led to more unprepared areas of skin compared with immersed, sterile gauze sponges. The areas most at risk were distal to the PIP joint such as the hyponychium and finger pulp.[9] A prospective randomized trial comparing preparation solutions found that the use of DuraPrep and Betadine was associated with significantly fewer positive cultures than ChloraPrep. However, the authors note that the majority of positive cultures identified were *Bacillus* species, a rare cause of postoperative infection.[10]

Whether to bury Kirschner wires and their effect on surgical site infection have been debated across multiple studies including two randomized controlled trials. A recently published retrospective series indicated that 7% of percutaneously placed K-wires were complicated by infection requiring intervention, but other groups have reported infection rates approaching 20%.[11] Among 695 patients treated with K-wires for fractures in the hand and wrist, exposed K-wires were more likely to be treated for pin-site infection (17.6%) than K-wires placed beneath the skin (8.7%).[12]

Hand Cellulitis and Abscesses

Hand involvement is an independent risk factor for hospital admission for patients presenting to the emergency department with cellulitis.[13] Community-acquired MRSA (CA-MRSA) hand infections increased rapidly in prevalence over the past two decades, but may be decreasing as polymicrobial infections become more frequent.[14] Anywhere from 30% to 70% of surgical hand infections are MRSA related. Prolonged hospitalization, chronic illness, IV drug abuse, and prior hand infection are known risk factors. The results of a systematic review recommend empiric coverage for CA-MRSA should be provided if local prevalence rates exceed 10% to 15%.[15] Furthermore, a prospective randomized trial of patients presenting to a county emergency department diagnosed with MRSA hand infections demonstrated increased cost and mean hospital stay for patients treated with cefazolin compared with vancomycin. The trial was cut short when the incidence of MRSA infection in their study was found to be 72%.[16] Alarmingly, multidrug-resistant strains of MRSA are being increasingly reported with a higher incidence of resistance to clindamycin and levofloxacin. Risk factors for such pathogens at an urban center included young age, intravenous drug use, and nosocomial infection.[14,17] This should be considered when selecting empiric antibiotic therapy.

For patients with fluctuance concerning for abscess, ultrasonography may be of value as a diagnostic test. Ultrasonography was shown to have a 78.4% positive predictive value of identifying an abscess and a negative predictive value of 90% to rule out an abscess in a series of 179 patients.[18] Early antibiotic administration should be provided and has not been shown to greatly reduce bacterial culture growth from hand abscess so long as decompression is performed within 24 hours.[19] After surgical decompression, débridement, and irrigation of the abscess, packing is often used, at least initially, to allow for continued drainage. No difference has been shown between different soaks and daily dressing changes in clearing the infection postoperatively.

Patients with immunosuppression are being increasingly encountered because of malignancies, transplants, or autoimmune disorders. In a matched cohort study, the most frequent immunosuppressive medication among patients with upper extremity infections was glucocorticoids. Infections in immunosuppressed patients were more likely to involve deeper structures such as joints, bone, tendons, and muscle.[20] Additionally, these patients are at a higher risk for atypical infections. They should be treated rapidly and aggressively as their potential for increased morbidity is high.

Flexor Tenosynovitis

The clinical diagnosis of flexor tenosynovitis is classically made with the use of Kanavel signs. However, only slightly more than half of patients will exhibit all four signs and thus how best to apply these signs to patients suspected of having an infection is debated. Pang et al[21] found that fusiform swelling was the most common sign (97% of patients) and that pain with passive extension of the digit was most specific (**Figure 1**). This is in contrast to a similar study by Kennedy et al which reported pain with passive extension to be the most sensitive sign and tenderness along the tendon sheath to be the most specific. Additionally, they identified three independent predictors of flexor tenosynovitis: tenderness along the sheath, pain with passive extension, and duration of symptoms less than 5 days. Patients with all three findings had an 87.9% likelihood of having the diagnosis compared with zero in patients with none of these signs or symptoms.[22] It should also be noted that Kanavel signs are not uniformly present in children and adolescents.[23] Furthermore, inflammatory markers such as white blood cell count (WBC), erythrocyte sedimentation rate (ESR), and C-reactive protein (CRP) are not sensitive enough to be used as a screening tool for ruling out flexor tenosynovitis in concerning patients. However, an elevation in any of these markers increases the likelihood of infection. The presence of a subcutaneous abscess on initial presentation is associated with poorer outcomes.[24]

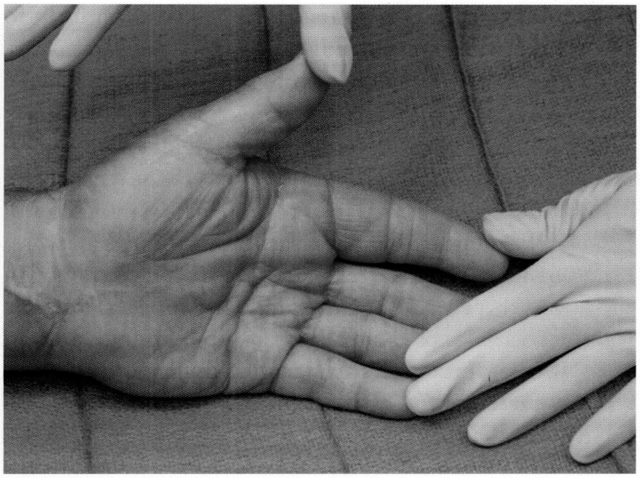

Figure 1 Photograph showing fusiform swelling of an index finger. (Used with permission of Mayo Foundation for Medical Education and Research. All rights reserved.)

Patients who present with symptoms for less than 24 hours may undergo a trial of nonsurgical therapy with intravenous antibiotics. Ketonis et al[25] demonstrated in a cadaver study that *S aureus* readily forms thick biofilms on flexor tendons, suggesting the well-known role for surgical treatment. A variety of surgical approaches have been described. A recent systematic review reported excellent range of motion in 74% of patients treated with limited exposure of the sheath and closed catheter irrigation compared with 26% of patients treated with open surgical drainage.[26] The most common pathogens identified are *S aureus* and beta-hemolytic *Streptococcus*.[27] At a pediatric center, MRSA was the most commonly identified pathogen.[23] Infection with beta-hemolytic *Streptococcus* is associated with the need for more operations to eradicate infection and prolonged hospital stays. Rare pathogens in flexor tenosynovitis cultures recently reported include *Shewanella algae*,[28] *Nocardia nova*,[29] and *Mycobacterium* species.[30] Antibiotics are an important component of any surgical treatment. However, the ideal route of administration and duration has not been determined.[26] The use of catheter irrigation postoperatively has not been shown to improve outcomes in clinical studies.

Unfortunately, 14.2% patients will require at least one additional surgical intervention according to a recent retrospective, single-center study.[24] Worse outcomes are associated with older age, a delay in receiving antibiotics, and certain comorbidities.[21,31] In one series, 5 of 20 diabetic patients and all 3 patients on renal dialysis required an amputation because of complications from flexor tenosynovitis.[27]

Septic Arthritis

As few as 5% of patients presenting to the emergency department with an inflamed, atraumatic wrist joint will have a diagnosis of septic arthritis. In a review of 104 such patients at an academic medical center, a successful joint aspiration was able to be obtained in fewer than half.[32] This emphasizes the importance of using the history and physical examination to determine the need for surgical intervention.

In a separate, retrospective comparison, patients with nonseptic arthritis were more likely to have chronic kidney disease, preexisting gout, or both compared with patients with confirmed septic arthritis. All infected patients had normal serum uric acid levels and two or more raised inflammatory markers with a mean CRP significantly higher compared with nonseptic group.[33] This finding is not consistent across studies and the possibility of a septic, gouty wrist does exist. However, diabetic and immunosuppressed patients may be more prone to develop septic arthritis.

Surgical treatments for septic arthritis include aspiration, arthroscopic débridement, or open arthrotomy with irrigation and débridement. A retrospective review of 36 patients reported increased repeat procedures required in patients initially treated with open versus arthroscopic irrigation and débridement.[34] After surgical drainage, a short course of intravenous antibiotics (less than 1 week) followed by oral antibiotics for 2 to 3 weeks successfully treated most cases of septic arthritis in the hand and wrist. *S aureus* is the most commonly isolated organism.

Necrotizing Fasciitis

Approximately 600 to 1,200 cases of necrotizing fasciitis are reported each year in the United States.[35] When the infection is monomicrobial, it is most often caused by beta-hemolytic *Streptococcus* or *Vibrio* species. Polymicrobial infections are common and often involve aerobic and anaerobic organisms.

The initial diagnosis of necrotizing fasciitis is made on clinical examination in addition to available imaging studies and a constellation of laboratory results, such as the laboratory risk indicator for necrotizing fasciitis (LRINEC) score[36] (**Table 1**). Using a cutoff of 6 points, the positive predictive value of a patient having necrotizing fasciitis is 92%. The negative predictive value is 96%.[36] The utility of the LRINEC score for *Vibrio*-related skin infections, however, has been called into question.[37] In *Vibrio vulnificus*–infected patients, a LRINEC score ≥2 and hemorrhagic bullous or blistering skin lesions were significant predictors of NSTI.[37] In a systematic

Table 1

Laboratory Risk Indicator for Necrotizing Fasciitis (LRINEC) Score

Variable	Score
C-reactive protein (mg/dL)	
<15	0
≥15	4
WBC (1/mm³)	
<15,000	0
15,000-25,000	1
>25,000	2
Hemoglobin (g/dL)	
>13.5	0
11.0-13.5	1
<11.0	2
Na (mmol/L)	
≥135	0
<135	2
Creatinine (mg/dL)	
≤1.6	0
>1.6	2
Glucose (mg/dL)	
≤180	0
>180	1

Reprinted from Wong CH, Khin LW, Heng KS, Tan KC, Low CO: The LRINEC (Laboratory Risk Indicator for Necrotizing Fasciitis) score: a tool for distinguishing necrotizing fasciitis from other soft tissue infections. *Crit Care Med* 2004;32(7):1535-1541. doi:10.1097/01.CCM.0000129486.35458.7D.

review, the most common risk factors for developing necrotizing fasciitis included IV drug abuse, smoking, trauma, and diabetes.[38]

Although advanced imaging is not necessary for confirmation, a CT scan scoring system based on presence of fascial air, muscle/fascial edema, fluid tracking, lymphadenopathy, and subcutaneous edema has been described.[39] Findings on MRI include abnormal signal intensity on fat-suppressed T2-weighted images at least 3 mm in thickness. However, many of the same MRI findings are seen in nonnecrotizing soft-tissue infections. Definitive diagnosis and treatment of necrotizing fasciitis is made in the operating room with fascial biopsy and thorough surgical débridement.

Administration of broad-spectrum antibiotics and treatment of shock are equally important. Given the high incidence of polymicrobial and *Vibrio*-related necrotizing soft-tissue infections, maintaining broad-spectrum antibiotic coverage until definitive culture results are available is advised.[35]

Most series report patients requiring an average of three débridements. Amputation and mortality rates range from 20% to 25%.[36,38] Severe hypoalbuminemia, thrombocytopenia, and increased neutrophil bands are significant risk factors for mortality in patients infected with *Vibrio* species. Improvements in early diagnosis, wound care, and critical care delivery have decreased the mortality rate over the past decade.[40]

Bite Wounds

The hand is the most common site for bite injuries and although many bites are self-treated, an estimated 50% of people will suffer such an injury in their lifetime. Fight bites are sustained when a clenched fist strikes a human tooth resulting in a traumatic soft-tissue injury. Among a series of 147 patients, 100% of those with fight bite injuries over the PIP joint and 95% with MCP injuries were found to have sustained a traumatic arthrotomy. In most patients, initial culture results were negative. When identified, *viridans* group streptococci and enterococci were the most common pathogens. The authors note that while *Eikenella corrodens* is the classically described pathogen associated with human bite injuries, it is difficult to culture in vitro and many patients in their series received antibiotics before obtaining cultures.[41] Regardless, broad-spectrum antibiotics are the first-line treatment and a low threshold to explore the wound for traumatic arthropathy is prudent. All patients following MCP joint injuries achieved satisfactory or good outcomes, compared with no good outcomes in patients with PIP involvement.[41] Late presentation increases the risk for amputation.

Dog bites account for 80% to 90% of all domestic animal bites and are often sustained while separating two fighting animals. Nygaard et al reported on a series of 81 patients who presented with dog bite injuries. Fifty-one patients required surgery with *S aureus*, *Pasteurella multocida*, and *Haemophilus influenza* being the most common pathogens. Dog bites present with large traumatic wounds due to tearing of soft tissue, whereas cat bites frequently appear small and innocuous. However, the zone of injury often extends deep into the soft tissues. In a series of 193 patients treated for cat bite injuries by Babovic et al, 30% of patients required hospitalization. Twenty percent of patients required at least one irrigation and débridement. There was an increased risk for hospitalization in patients who smoke, were immunocompromised, presented with erythema and swelling, or if the bite was over joint or tendon. *P multicoda* was the most common pathogen identified.[42] Domestic bird bites are similar to cat bites in that their beaks are able to penetrate deep into the soft tissue. In addition to irrigation and débridement, broad-spectrum antibiotics should be administered to cover both gram-positive and gram-negative organisms typically found in oral and respiratory flora of psittacine birds including *Staphylococcus* species, *Pasteurella*, *Escherichia coli*, *Salmonella*, and *Proteus*.

Most hand infections attributable to wild animal bites and stings are polymicrobial. Hand surgeons should approach these injuries with a high degree of suspicion. A recent systematic review of such injuries highlights that the existing evidence in the treatment of wild animal bites is largely based on level IV and V studies.[43]

Bone Infections

Osteomyelitis of the hand is uncommon, presenting in up to 6% of all hand infections and just 10% of all cases of osteomyelitis[44] (**Figure 2**). In the hand, the distal phalanx is most commonly involved, followed

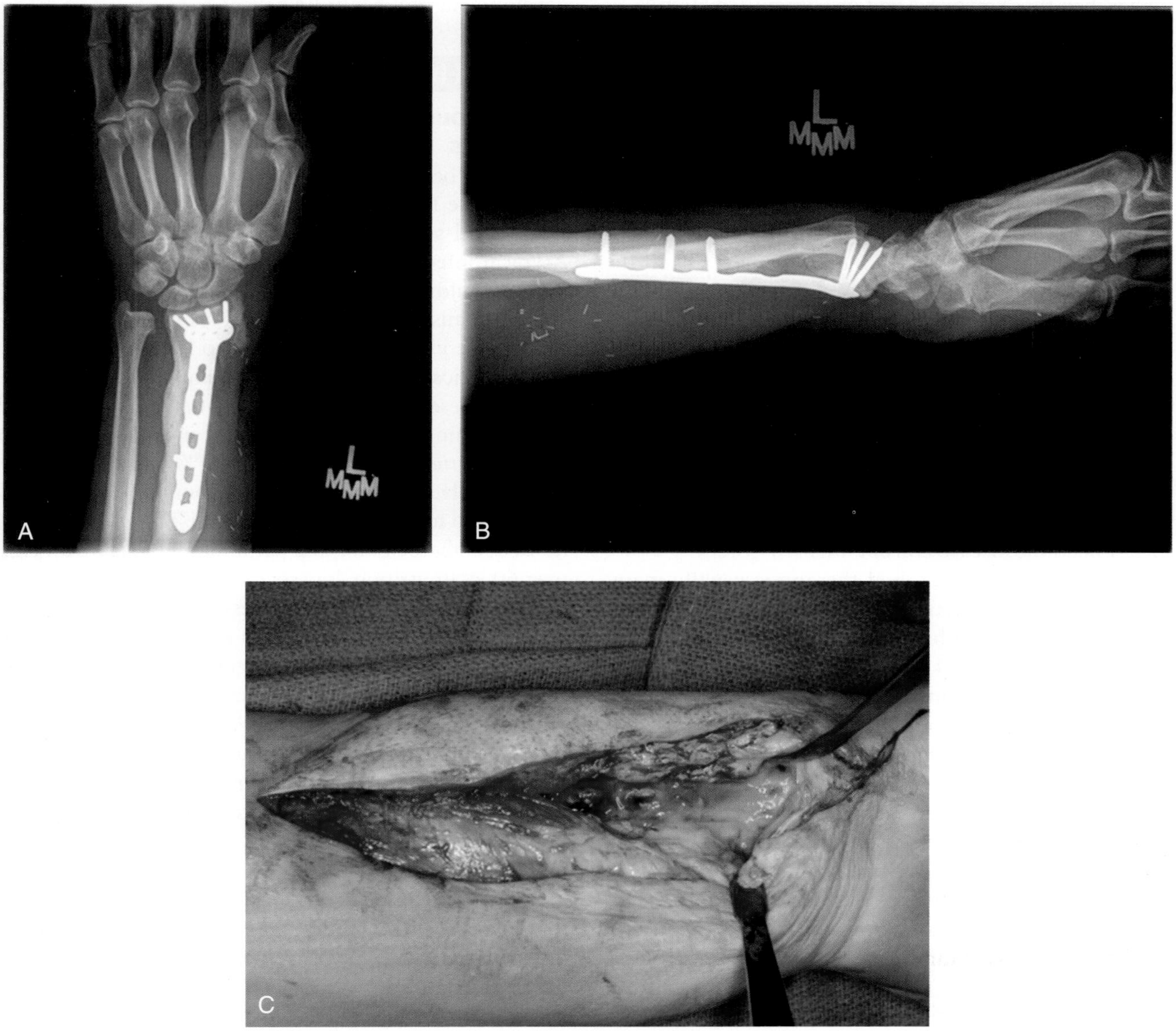

Figure 2 **A, B**, AP and lateral radiographs status-post volar plating of a Gustilo-Anderson type IIIC injury concerning for osteomyelitis. **C**, Intraoperative photograph with significant purulent tissue involving the distal radius. (Used with permission of Mayo Foundation for Medical Education and Research. All rights reserved.)

by the proximal phalanx and metacarpal.[45] In 70% of cases, a single bone is affected.[45] This is consistent with penetrating trauma being the most common cause of osteomyelitis in the hand. However, crush injuries, open fractures, surgical fracture treatment, contiguous spread from adjacent soft-tissue infections and joints, and hematogenous seeding are all possible etiologies.

Immunocompromised patients and children are particularly at risk for hematogenous osteomyelitis. One institution reported a 2.8-fold increase in the annualized per capita incidence of osteomyelitis in children over a 20-year period coinciding with a rise in the incidence of MRSA infections.[46] There appears to be a racial disparity with hospitalization rates among African American children higher than those among Asian or Hispanic children.[47]

In a prospective cohort of hand and forearm infections, diabetic patients were more likely than nondiabetic patients to present with osteomyelitis. Furthermore, the infection was more likely to be polymicrobial or fungal, located more proximal in the upper extremity, and the result of an idiopathic or unknown mechanism. Among diabetic patients, poor glycemic control is associated with the need for repeat débridements.[20]

MRI, CT, and 3-phase bone scans may add to the radiographic diagnosis made on plain radiographs, but all have poor sensitivity and specificity. Deep tissue cultures are the most accurate method of diagnosis. *S aureus* and *S epidermidis* are the most common infecting organism, but regional variation exists in the epidemiology of osteomyelitis. The presence of an indolent course suggests a fungal or mycobacterial cause. The empiric antibiotic choice is generally driven by the local prevalence of CA-MRSA and the recommendations of local infectious disease consultants.

Intravenous antimicrobial therapy is usually maintained until an appropriate clinical and laboratory response has been observed. In acute osteomyelitis, early transition to oral therapy has not been shown to increase the risk of treatment failure and avoids the risk of prolonged intravenous therapy.[48] In children, there is evidence to suggest that oral antibiotics alone, either as the primary treatment or as postoperative therapy, are effective for the treatment of hand osteomyelitis.[49] Despite decades of research on the treatment of osteomyelitis, the best antibiotic agents, route, and duration of therapy have yet to be conclusively determined.

Débridement to remove all infected bone is the mainstay of surgical treatment of osteomyelitis. In case of failure to eradicate the infection following surgical débridement, amputation is the definitive treatment. Masquelet described the induced membrane technique for bone defects in the hand. In this two-stage procedure, a bony defect created following surgical débridement is first replaced with antibiotic-impregnated cement. After clearance of the infection based on clinical and laboratory findings, a biological pseudomembrane allows for placement of cancellous bone graft to reconstitute the bone. For cases involving metacarpophalangeal and interphalangeal joints, Aime et al[50] described a single-stage procedure to replace the articulation with antibiotic-eluting methyl methacrylate spacer as definitive treatment.

In a classic study on osteomyelitis in the hand, the overall amputation rate was 39% despite aggressive surgical and medical management. Delayed diagnosis and treatment led to higher rates of amputation and development of a Marjolin's ulcer.[45]

Atypical Infections

Tuberculous and Nontuberculous Mycobacterial Infections

There has been an increased interest in atypical infections of the hand due to immigration, an aging population, and survival of immunocompromised patients. Atypical infections affecting the hand are often caused by tuberculous and nontuberculous *Mycobacteria* and fungi. Because there are often delays in proper diagnosis of these infections which lead to long-term sequelae and complications, a heightened awareness of their frequency, presentation, and treatment is prudent.

The main causative organism of tuberculosis (TB) is *Mycobacterium tuberculosis*. Only 2% of musculoskeletal TB involves the wrist. The most common presentation in the hand and wrist is tenosynovial TB with rice bodies frequently seen on gross pathology[51,52] (**Figure 3**). Age over 60, malnutrition, low socioeconomic status, alcohol abuse, diabetes, immunosuppression, exposure to TB, and local steroid injection are all identified risk factors.[52]

True to its monicker, "the great mimicker" several radiological patterns of tuberculous osteomyelitis in the hand have been described.[51] Unifocal tuberculous osteomyelitis of the hand is more common in children, whereas multifocal and disseminated tuberculosis is seen most commonly in adults and immunocompromised patients, respectively. Definitive diagnosis is made on biopsy.

Kotwal and Khan recommended 18 months of drug therapy for TB of the hand starting with four-drug regimen. Surgical treatment with open or arthroscopic débridement and incision and drainage of abscesses is reserved for cases that do not respond to medical treatment. Conservative treatment is successful in most cases.[53]

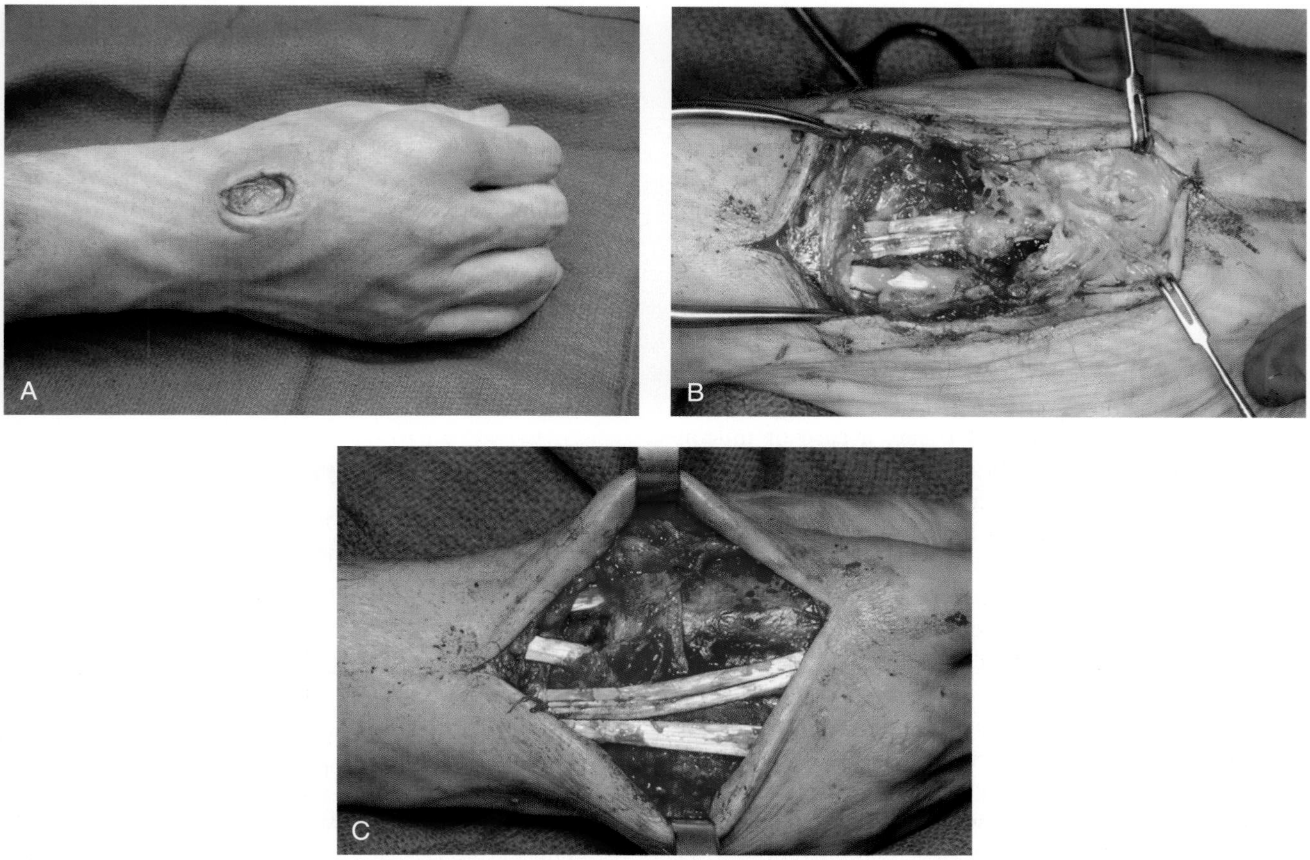

Figure 3 **A**, Photograph showing chronic dorsal hand wound infected with *Mycobacterium haemophilum* after an initial trauma to the index finger. **B**, Intraoperative photograph showing dorsal exposure demonstrating caseating yellow tissue with rice bodies involving the extensor tendons. **C**, Intraoperative photograph showing extensor tendons after débridement. (Used with permission of Mayo Foundation for Medical Education and Research. All rights reserved.)

Nontuberculous mycobacterial infections are often diagnosed late because of indolent presentation and lack of clinical suspicion. Atypical organisms such as *Mycobacterium marinum*, *Mycobacterium kansasii*, and *Mycobacterium xenopi* thrive in lower temperatures making the distal extremity susceptible to infection.[30] *M marinum* is most the commonly isolated pathogen.[54] Similar to tuberculosis, *M marinum* infections in the hand may involve the skin, tenosynovium, joints, or bone.

Cheung et al reviewed 166 cases of *M marinum* in the hand. Most patients were initially treated as autoimmune or idiopathic synovitis with an average delay in presentation of 4.9 months. Delayed antibiotic administration and inappropriate treatment with steroid injections were associated with unsatisfactory outcomes.[55] Lopez et al reported a mean 9-month symptomatic period before accurate diagnosis. Fifty-nine percent of patients were immunocompetent and most could not identify a cause of infection.[54] In another series, clinical presentation, diagnostic delay, and diagnostic testing results were similar between immunocompetent and immunocompromised patients. Although treatment differed between the two groups (more aggressive débridement and longer antibiotic course), outcomes were similar.[56] Cheung et al[55] stratified clinical presentations into benign and aggressive types, which guided both prognosis and therapeutic treatment plan. These studies highlight the need to keep *M marinum* in the differential diagnosis of patients with chronic finger swelling a stiffness following a puncture wound.

Although *M marinum* is associated with aquatic hand injuries, skin flora are the most common bacterial infections associated with aquatic hand injuries. Other pathogens unique to the aquatic environment include *Vibrio species, Aeromonas hydrophila, and Erysipelothrix rhusiopathiae.*

Fungal Infections

Fungal infections of the upper extremity are rare and largely affect immunocompromised patients. These may be cutaneous, subcutaneous, or deep fungal infections.

Deep fungal infections of the hand are frequently opportunistic and several pathogens have been implicated. In a series of 10 patients with fungal tenosynovitis, 8 were immunocompromised. Three separate pathogens were identified. The most common symptom was a subacute mild tenosynovitis. The median delay to diagnosis was 6 months. Despite extensive surgical débridement and antimicrobial therapy, O'Shaugnessy et al[57] reported a 30% recurrence rate.

Deep mucormycosis infections in immunocompetent patients have been reported as well, most commonly associated with grossly contaminated open wounds involving soil or agricultural facilities. Although largely isolated to the skin and soft tissue, a case of mucormycosis osteomyelitis in an intravenous drug user following an automobile accident was recently reported. Mucormycosis can be both life- and limb-threatening. Recognition of this uncommon diagnosis in high-risk patients with destructive lesions or indolent infections is necessary for successful outcomes. Treatment includes early, aggressive surgical débridement and antifungal therapy.

Blastomycosis is endemic to parts of the United States and should be suspected in chronic hand infections refractory to antibiotic therapy. Blastomycosis in immunocompetent patients with extensor tenosynovitis has been reported.[58] Blastomycotic osteomyelitis in the hand is similarly rare and often clinically unsuspected, leading to delays in diagnosis and treatment.

Based on the results of 100 patients undergoing surgical débridement of acute deep infections of the upper extremity, Kazmers et al recommended surgeons consider obtaining atypical cultures including fungal and acid-fast bacillus (AFB) despite the low incidence of positive findings. Owing to the potential benefit of accurately identifying the offending pathogen, intraoperative purulence at the time of surgical débridement should not deter the surgeon from obtaining atypical cultures.[59]

Summary

Over the past decade there has been mounting evidence to support not using prophylactic antibiotics in routine clean hand surgery cases. As we use our antibiotic armamentarium to combat infections, there has been a rise in antibiotic resistance relevant to the orthopaedic surgeon treating the hand and wrist. Both immunocompetent and immunocompromised patients may be infected with atypical organisms and an indolent course refractory to traditional antibiotics should raise clinical suspicion for such pathogens.

Key Study Points

- There is little evidence to support the use of prophylactic antibiotics in several outpatient hand surgery cases in most patients.
- Roughly half of all surgical hand infections may be due to drug-resistant organisms such as MRSA.
- Immunocompromised and immunocompetent patients are at risk for infection with atypical microbes.

Annotated References

1. Werner BC, Teran VA, Deal DN: Patient-related risk factors for infection following open carpal tunnel release: An analysis of over 450,000 Medicare patients. *J Hand Surg* 2018;43:214-219.

   The authors reported a 0.32% rate of postoperative infection for patients undergoing open CTR in a Medicare database. Level of evidence: II (Prognostic).

2. Li K, Sambare TD, Jiang SY, Shearer EJ, Douglass NP, Kamal RN: Effectiveness of preoperative antibiotics in preventing surgical site infection after common soft tissue procedures of the hand. *Clin Orthop Relat Res* 2018;476:664-673.

   Antibiotic prophylaxis for common soft-tissue procedures of the hand was not associated with a reduction in postoperative infection risk among 516,986 patients in a commercial insurance database. Level of evidence: III (Therapeutic).

3. Bykowski MR, Sivak WN, Cray J, Buterbaugh G, Imbriglia JE, Lee WP: Assessing the impact of antibiotic prophylaxis in outpatient elective hand surgery: A single-center, retrospective review of 8,850 cases. *J Hand Surg* 2011;36:1741-1747.

4. Jagodzinski NA, Ibish S, Furniss D: Surgical site infection after hand surgery outside the operating theatre: A systematic review. *J Hand Surg Eur Vol* 2017;42:289-294.

   A systematic review of hand procedures done outside the operating theater identified three studies which did not report a single infection and two studies which reported an identical infection rate of 0.4%. Level of evidence: IV.

5. Aydin N, Uraloğlu M, Yilmaz Burhanoğlu AD, Sensöz O: A prospective trial on the use of antibiotics in hand surgery. *Plast Reconstr Surg* 2010;126:1617-1623.

6. Werner BC, Teran VA, Cancienne J, Deal DN: The association of perioperative glycemic control with postoperative surgical site infection following open carpal tunnel release in patients with diabetes. *Hand* 2017;14(3):324-328.

   Among diabetic patients in a national private-payer database, increased HbA1c levels were associated with increased surgical site infection rates after CTR. The authors suggest a perioperative threshold between 7 and 8 poses an increased risk.

7. Hosseini P, Mundis GM Jr, Eastlack R, et al: Do longer surgical procedures result in greater contamination of surgeons' hands? *Clin Orthop Relat Res* 2016;474:1707-1713.

Twenty cases among three spine surgeons were analyzed and showed that duration of surgery correlates with hand recontamination. Recolonization became detectable after 5 hours of operating.

8. Ketonis C, Dwyer J, Ilyas AM: Timing of debridement and infection rates in open fractures of the hand: A systematic review. *Hand* 2017;12:119-126.

A systematic review of 1,669 open hand fractures demonstrated a 4.6% infection rate. Administration of antibiotics was correlated with the risk of infection, but not timing of débridement.

9. Seigerman DA, Rivlin M, Bianchini J, Liss FE, Beredjiklian PK: A comparison of two sterile solution application methods during surgical preparation of the hand. *J Hand Surg* 2016;41:698-702.

A comparison of hand surgical preparation techniques among healthy volunteers found a higher contamination rate when prep-stick applicators were used compared to immersed gauze sponges. The distal finger was most at risk.

10. Xu PZ, Fowler JR, Goitz RJ: Prospective randomized trial comparing the efficacy of surgical preparation solutions in hand surgery. *Hand* 2017;12:258-264.

In a randomized controlled trial of 240 patients undergoing clean, elective, soft-tissue hand surgery, DuraPrep and Betadine were found to be superior to ChloraPrep for skin decontamination.

11. van Leeuwen WF, van Hoorn BT, Chen N, Ring D: Kirschner wire pin site infection in hand and wrist fractures: Incidence rate and risk factors. *J Hand Surg Eur Vol* 2016;41:990-994.

In a retrospective review of 1,213 patients who underwent percutaneous K-wire fixation for hand and/or wrist fractures, 7% of patients required oral antibiotics, early pin removal, or revision surgery related to a pin site infection. Level of evidence: III.

12. Ridley TJ, Freking W, Erickson LO, Ward CM: Incidence of treatment for infection of buried versus exposed Kirschner wires in phalangeal, metacarpal, and distal radial fractures. *J Hand Surg* 2017;42:525-531.

Among 695 patients treated with K-wire fixation for hand and/or wrist fractures, the authors found an increased infection rate in the exposed K-wire group (16.4%) compared with buried K-wires (9.2%). Metacarpal fractures were most at risk. Level of evidence: IV (Therapeutic).

13. Volz KA, Canham L, Kaplan E, Sanchez LD, Shapiro NI, Grossman SA: Identifying patients with cellulitis who are likely to require inpatient admission after a stay in an ED observation unit. *Am J Emerg Med* 2013;31:360-364.

14. Kistler JM, Thoder JJ, Ilyas AM: MRSA incidence and antibiotic trends in urban hand infections: A 10-year longitudinal study. *Hand* 2019;14(4):449-454.

Over a 10-year period, the annual incidence of MRSA culture positive hand infections at an urban medical center decreased, concomitant with an increase in polymicrobial infections. MRSA resistance to clindamycin and levofloxacin increased during the study period as well.

15. Harrison B, Ben-Amotz O, Sammer DM: Methicillin-resistant *Staphylococcus aureus* infection in the hand. *Plast Reconstr Surg* 2015;135:826-830.

16. Janis JE, Hatef DA, Reece EM, Wong C: Does empiric antibiotic therapy change hand infection outcomes? Cost analysis of a randomized prospective trial in a county hospital. *Plast Reconstr Surg* 2014;133:511e-518e. [Erratum in *Plast Reconstr Surg* 2014;134:580.]

17. Tosti R, Trionfo A, Gaughan J, Ilyas AM: Risk factors associated with clindamycin-resistant, methicillin-resistant *Staphylococcus aureus* in hand abscesses. *J Hand Surg* 2015;40:673-676.

18. Halim A, Shih Y, Dodds SD: The utility of ultrasound for diagnosing purulent infections of the upper extremity. *Hand* 2015;10:701-706.

19. Trionfo A, Thoder JJ, Tosti R: The effects of early antibiotic administration on bacterial culture growth from hand abscesses. *Hand* 2016;11:216-220.

A retrospective review of 88 consecutive hand abscesses that received empiric antibiotics prior to incision and drainage reported an overall 90% positive culture growth rate. Furthermore, 96% of isolates were susceptible to the given antibiotic.

20. Sharma K, Pan D, Friedman J, Yu JL, Mull A, Moore AM: Quantifying the effect of diabetes on surgical hand and forearm infections. *J Hand Surg* 2018;43:105-114.

Using a prospective cohort of diabetic and nondiabetic patients, the authors conclude that diabetes exacerbates the surgical burden of upper extremity infections. Specifically, the infections seen were more proximal, deeper, with more antibiotic resistance, leading to poorer outcomes. Level of evidence: I (Prognostic).

21. Pang HN, Teoh LC, Yam AK, Lee JY, Puhaindran ME, Tan AB: Factors affecting the prognosis of pyogenic flexor tenosynovitis. *J Bone Joint Surg Am* 2007;89:1742-1748.

22. Kennedy CD, Lauder AS, Pribaz JR, Kennedy SA: Differentiation between pyogenic flexor tenosynovitis and other finger infections. *Hand* 2017;12:585-590.

Among adult patients undergoing surgical consultation for PFT, sensitivity of the Kanavel signs ranged from 91.4% to 97.1%. Independent predictors of infection were tenderness along the sheath, pain with passive extension, and duration of symptoms less than 5 days.

23. Brusalis CM, Thibaudeau S, Carrigan RB, Lin IC, Chang B, Shah AS: Clinical characteristics of pyogenic flexor tenosynovitis in pediatric patients. *J Hand Surg* 2017;42:388.e381-388.e385.

The authors found that the presence of Kanavel signs are a meaningful indicator of PFT, but are not uniformly present in children and adolescents. MRSA was the most commonly identified pathogen in this retrospective series of 32 pediatric patients. Level of evidence: IV (Therapeutic).

24. Muller CT, Uckay I, Erba P, Lipsky BA, Hoffmeyer P, Beaulieu JY: Septic tenosynovitis of the hand: Factors predicting need for subsequent debridement. *Plast Reconstr Surg* 2015;136:338e-343e.

25. Ketonis C, Hickcock NJ, Ilyas AM: Rethinking pyogenic flexor tenosynovitis: Biofilm formation treated in a cadaveric model. *J Hand Microsurg* 2017;9:131-138.

Fresh human cadaveric tendons were harvested and inoculated with *S aureus* for 48 hours. Using confocal laser scanning microscopy, investigators were able to identify bacterial attachment with dense biofilm formation, best treated with a combination of antibiotics (vancomycin) and corticosteroids.

26. Giladi AM, Malay S, Chung KC: A systematic review of the management of acute pyogenic flexor tenosynovitis. *J Hand Surg Eur Vol* 2015;40:720-728.

27. Karagergou E, Rao K, Harper RD: Parameters affecting the severity and outcome of pyogenic digital flexor tenosynovitis. *J Hand Surg Eur Vol* 2015;40:100-101.

28. Fluke EC, Carayannopoulos NL, Lindsey RW: Pyogenic flexor tenosynovitis caused by *Shewanella algae*. *J Hand Surg* 2016;41:e203-e206.

The authors report a case of complicated flexor tenosynovitis caused by *S algae*, which is rare, but virulent, and associated with traumatic water exposure.

29. Wilhelm A, Romeo N, Trevino R: A rare cause of pyogenic flexor tenosynovitis: Nocardia nova. *J Hand Surg* 2018;43:778.e771-778.e774.

A case of trigger thumb release complicated by *N nova* infection which manifested as pyogenic flexor tenosynovitis and acute carpal tunnel syndrome is presented.

30. Senda H, Muro H, Terada S: Flexor tenosynovitis caused by *Mycobacterium arupense*. *J Hand Surg Eur Vol* 2011;36:72-73.

31. Born TR, Wagner ER, Kakar S: Comparison of open drainage versus closed catheter irrigation for treatment of suppurative flexor tenosynovitis. *Hand* 2017;12:579-584.

Twenty-four patients treated for PFT with either open drainage through a single incision or closed catheter irrigation were identified. Similar pain scores, function, and need for revision surgery were reported between the two groups.

32. Skeete K, Hess EP, Clark T, Moran S, Kakar S, Rizzo M: Epidemiology of suspected wrist joint infection versus inflammation. *J Hand Surg* 2011;36:469-474.

33. Kang G, Leow MQH, Tay SC: Wrist inflammation: A retrospective comparison between septic and non-septic arthritis. *J Hand Surg Eur Vol* 2018;43:431-437.

Seventy-seven patients admitted for wrist inflammation were retrospectively reviewed. Nonseptic patients were more likely to have chronic kidney disease and/or preexiting gout. All infected patients had normal serum uric acid levels and two or more raised inflammatory markers. Level of evidence: IV.

34. Sammer DM, Shin AY: Comparison of arthroscopic and open treatment of septic arthritis of the wrist. *J Bone Joint Surg Am* 2009;91:1387-1393.

35. Koshy JC, Bell B: Hand infections. *J Hand Surg* 2019;44(1):46-54.

The authors provide a review of hand infections with a focus on identifying serious hand infections and maintaining a heightened awareness of pathogens whose course may result in delayed identification and management.

36. Wong CH, Khin LW, Heng KS, Tan KC, Low CO: The LRINEC (Laboratory Risk Indicator for Necrotizing Fasciitis) score: A tool for distinguishing necrotizing fasciitis from other soft tissue infections. *Crit Care Med* 2004;32:1535-1541.

37. Chao WN, Tsai SJ, Tsai CF, et al: The Laboratory Risk Indicator for Necrotizing Fasciitis score for discernment of necrotizing fasciitis originated from *Vibrio vulnificus* infections. *J Trauma Acute Care Surg* 2012;73:1576-1582.

38. Angoules AG, Kontakis G, Drakoulakis E, Vrentzos G, Granick MS, Giannoudis PV: Necrotising fasciitis of upper and lower limb: A systematic review. *Injury* 2007;38(suppl 5):S19-S26.

39. McGillicuddy EA, Lischuk AW, Schuster KM, et al: Development of a computed tomography-based scoring system for necrotizing soft-tissue infections. *J Trauma* 2011;70:894-899.

40. Psoinos CM, Flahive JM, Shaw JJ, et al: Contemporary trends in necrotizing soft-tissue infections in the United States. *Surgery* 2013;153:819-827.

41. Shewring DJ, Trickett RW, Subramanian KN, Hnyda R: The management of clenched fist 'fight bite' injuries of the hand. *J Hand Surg Eur Vol* 2015;40:819-824.

42. Babovic N, Cayci C, Carlsen BT: Cat bite infections of the hand: Assessment of morbidity and predictors of severe infection. *J Hand Surg* 2014;39:286-290.

43. Israel JS, McCarthy JE, Rose KR, Rao VK: Watch out for wild animals: A systematic review of upper extremity injuries caused by uncommon species. *Plast Reconstr Surg* 2017;140:1008-1022.

A systematic review identified 71 articles relevant to the treatment of wild animal bites, the vast majority of which were level IV and level V evidence. Their results suggest that the majority of such infections are polymicrobial.

44. Waldvogel FA, Medoff G, Swartz MN: Osteomyelitis: A review of clinical features, therapeutic considerations and unusual aspects. *N Engl J Med* 1970;282:198-206.

45. Reilly KE, Linz JC, Stern PJ, Giza E, Wyrick JD: Osteomyelitis of the tubular bones of the hand. *J Hand Surg* 1997;22:644-649.

46. Gafur OA, Copley LA, Hollmig ST, Browne RH, Thornton LA, Crawford SE: The impact of the current epidemiology of pediatric musculoskeletal infection on evaluation and treatment guidelines. *J Pediatr Orthop* 2008;28:777-785.

47. Okubo Y, Nochioka K, Testa M: Nationwide survey of pediatric acute osteomyelitis in the USA. *J Pediatr Orthop B* 2017;26:501-506.

Using the Kids Inpatient Database, the authors calculated the annual rates of hospitalization due to acute osteomyelitis at 1.34 to 1.66 per 100,000 children. Black children and those living in very low median household income regions were more likely to be hospitalized. Level of evidence: II.

48. Zaoutis T, Localio AR, Leckerman K, Saddlemire S, Bertoch D, Keren R: Prolonged intravenous therapy versus early transition to oral antimicrobial therapy for acute osteomyelitis in children. *Pediatrics* 2009;123:636-642.

49. Kargel JS, Sammer DM, Pezeshk RA, Cheng J: Oral antibiotics are effective for the treatment of hand osteomyelitis in children. *Hand (N Y)* 2018 Aug 3:1558944718788666. doi: 10.1177/1558944718788666. [Epub ahead of print].

In a retrospective review of 21 patients with acute osteomyelitis of the hand initially treated with oral antibiotics, only 3 patients required conversion to intravenous administration. All patients who underwent débridement were successfully treated with orals antibiotics only. Level of evidence: II.

50. Aime VL, Kidwell JT, Webb LH: Single-stage treatment of osteomyelitis for digital salvage by using an antibiotic-eluting, methylmethacrylate joint-spanning spacer. *J Hand Surg* 2017;42:480.e481-480.e487.

A series of 12 patients who underwent joint spanning, antibiotic-eluting, methyl methacrylate spacer placement as definitive treatment for digital tenosynovitis is presented with 77% successfully treated in a single stage.

51. Al-Qattan MM, Al-Namla A, Al-Thunayan A, Al-Omawi M: Tuberculosis of the hand. *J Hand Surg* 2011;36:1413-1421; quiz 1422.

52. Woon CY, Phoon ES, Lee JY, Puhaindran ME, Peng YP, Teoh LC: Rice bodies, millet seeds, and melon seeds in tuberculous tenosynovitis of the hand and wrist. *Ann Plast Surg* 2011;66:610-617.

53. Kotwal PP, Khan SA: Tuberculosis of the hand: Clinical presentation and functional outcome in 32 patients. *J Bone Joint Surg Br* 2009;91:1054-1057.

54. Lopez M, Croley J, Murphy KD: Atypical mycobacterial infections of the upper extremity: Becoming more atypical? *Hand* 2017;12:188-192.

The authors present a retrospective review of their patients with nontuberculous mycobacterial infections. *M marinum* made up the majority of infections, many of which were not associated with marine water. The mean symptomatic period prior to diagnosis was 9 months.

55. Cheung JP, Fung B, Ip WY, Chow SP: *Mycobacterium marinum* infection of the hand and wrist. *J Orthop Surg* 2012;20:214-218.

56. Sotello D, Garner HW, Heckman MG, Diehl NN, Murray PM, Alvarez S: Nontuberculous mycobacterial infections of the upper extremity: 15-Year experience at a tertiary care medical center. *J Hand Surg* 2018;43:387.e381-387.e388.

A retrospective review of 44 patients with nontuberculous mycobacterial infections was performed. Forty-five percent of patients were immunocompromised. Although treatment regimens differed, outcomes were similar between immunocompromised and immunosuppressed patients. Timely diagnosis had the greatest impact on patient outcome. Level of evidence: IV (Therapeutic).

57. O'Shaughnessy MA, Tande AJ, Vasoo S, Enzler MJ, Berbari EF, Shin AY: A rare diagnosis: Recognizing and managing fungal tenosynovitis of the hand and upper extremity. *J Hand Surg* 2017;42:e77-e89.

The authors review 10 patients with fungal tenosynovitis of the upper extremity. Eight patients were immunosuppressed. The average delay to diagnosis was 6 months. The majority of patients were successfully treated with débridement and antifungal therapy, but 30% of infections recurred. Level of evidence: V (Therapeutic).

58. Popa MA, Jebson PJL, Condit DP: Blastomycotic extensor tenosynovitis of the hand: A case report. *Hand* 2012;7:323-326.

59. Kazmers NH, Fryhofer GW, Gittings D, Bozentka DJ, Steinberg DR, Gray BL: Acute deep infections of the upper extremity: The utility of obtaining atypical cultures in the presence of purulence. *J Hand Surg* 2017;42:663.e661-663.e668.

The authors review 100 patients who underwent surgical débridement of a deep upper extremity infection. Atypical cultures were positive for 7% of patients and influenced treatment in only 4%. However, the presence of purulence was not predictive. Level of evidence: IV (Diagnostic).

Chapter 31

Neuropathies, Vascular Conditions: Buerger's, Raynaud's; Degenerative Conditions

Ryan D. Endress, MD • Robert J. Spinner, MD • Ashley Pistorio, MD • Philip Blazar, MD • Ross Puffer, MD

ABSTRACT

Nontraumatic pathologic conditions of the upper extremity, such as neuropathy, vascular disease, and degenerative arthritis can have a profound effect on function and quality of life. Most of these conditions are progressive in nature with a variable course and end point in individual patients. A thorough understanding of the risk factors and progression of each condition will aid in decision making for best practices in workup, longitudinal observations, and treatment options as well as management of complications.

Keywords: brachial plexopathy; Buerger disease; carpal tunnel syndrome; cubital tunnel syndrome; interphalangeal joint arthrodesis; interphalangeal joint arthroplasty; osteoarthritis; Parsonage-Turner syndrome; Raynaud disease; vaso-occlusive disease; vasospastic disease

Upper Extremity Neuropathies

Carpal Tunnel Syndrome

Carpal tunnel syndrome is the most common compression neuropathy of the upper extremity. The mean age at diagnosis is 50 years. It is more common in women than men by nearly four times, and by the age of 65 years, the prevalence is approximately 5.1% for women and 1.3% for men. Risk factors for carpal tunnel syndrome include obesity, pregnancy, hypothyroidism, diabetes mellitus, and menopause.[1] The proposed mechanisms for association of carpal tunnel syndrome with these conditions range from hormonal changes to edema, yet no consensus has been reached regarding the role that these risk factors play in the pathophysiology of carpal tunnel syndrome. The recent American Academy of Orthopaedic Surgeons (AAOS) guidelines list body mass index (BMI) and high hand repetition rate as factors with strong evidence of increased risk for development of carpal tunnel syndrome.[2]

The diagnosis is made by clinical history, physical examination, and supportive diagnostic testing with exclusion of other possible disorders. Classically, carpal tunnel syndrome presents with nocturnal paresthesias in a median nerve distribution that gradually worsen as nerve injury progresses, leading to sensory loss and thenar muscle atrophy late in the disease course. Many patients report pain in the hand and may even report symptoms that are not directly referable to the median nerve, yet a strong clinical history should direct the clinician to the diagnosis even when patient-reported symptoms are not classic. A positive Tinel sign at the wrist or development of symptoms after provocative Phalen maneuver can aid in the diagnosis; however, the reported specificity of these tests can vary from 55% to 100% for Tinel sign at the wrist and 54% to 98% for Phalen test, so these maneuvers are most reliable as adjuncts to other diagnostic tests.[2]

Nerve conduction studies remain a useful diagnostic tool in carpal tunnel syndrome, as focal demyelination can be assessed by delayed conduction velocities of the median nerve at the wrist. Needle electromyography is currently considered an optional adjunct to nerve conduction studies and is mostly used to differentiate carpal tunnel syndrome from other possible causes. Documenting muscle atrophy and fibrillations on needle EMG can assist with identifying severity of the disease and help with prognostication, but often thenar atrophy and abductor pollicis brevis weakness can be detected

Dr. Spinner or an immediate family member serves as a paid consultant to or is an employee of Mayo Medical Ventures. Dr. Pistorio or an immediate family member serves as a board member, owner, officer, or committee member of the American Society for Surgery of the Hand. None of the following authors or any immediate family member has received anything of value from or has stock or stock options held in a commercial company or institution related directly or indirectly to the subject of this chapter: Dr. Endress, Dr. Blazar, and Dr. Puffer.

on physical examination. Advances in ultrasonography technology have allowed rapid diagnosis of carpal tunnel syndrome by identification of enlarged, hypoechoic median nerve fascicles proximal to the carpal tunnel. Controversy remains as to whether ultrasonography evaluation could replace electrophysiology in the diagnosis of carpal tunnel syndrome. MRI and/or ultrasonography imaging should be considered in patients who have new, persistent, or recurrent symptoms after surgery to delineate the etiology of the symptoms, either due to incomplete ligament division, iatrogenic injury, or other cause.

Initial management depends on severity of the condition at presentation, but for mild and/or moderate symptoms, initial conservative management via hand therapy, activity modification with splinting and corticosteroid injection should be considered as there is strong evidence supporting their use as an initial management.[2,3] Surgical decompression of the transverse carpal ligament is the benchmark procedure for the treatment of carpal tunnel syndrome. Many techniques have been developed for division of the transverse carpal ligament, including standard open carpal tunnel release, endoscopic release, ultrasonography-guided release, and thread carpal tunnel release. Improving ultrasonography has allowed for better real-time visualization of the carpal tunnel and median nerve, allowing for new techniques such as hydrodissection and carpal tunnel release with a thread device or retractable blade.[4] These emerging techniques are still under evaluation, and long-term outcomes are not yet available. At this time, there has been no definitive difference in long-term functional outcome between open and endoscopic carpal tunnel release; however, patients undergoing endoscopic release often have a more abbreviated recovery with less incisional pain. This is contrasted with an increased cost of the procedure, and a slightly higher rate of iatrogenic transient neurapraxia. Postoperative complications include nerve, arterial, or tendon injury (0.5% incidence) and complex regional pain syndrome (2.1% to 5%). More recently, mini-open carpal tunnel release has been performed by many surgeons, with a limited, targeted incision (1.5 to 2 cm), with low complication rates and high rates of patient satisfaction.[5] No approach has yet demonstrated superiority over other techniques currently in use in large, randomized controlled surgical trials.

Recurrent symptoms after carpal tunnel release can occur and are thought to be due to scarring, tenosynovitis, and/or adhesive tethering. Rates of recurrent symptoms may be as high as 4.5%. Recurrent symptoms should be differentiated from persistent symptoms, which may be due to an incompletely divided ligament during the index procedure or incorrect diagnosis. Repeat open median nerve neurolysis is often performed when symptoms recur, either by itself or in conjunction with local tissue flaps or wraps; however, neither approach has demonstrated superiority for treatment of recurrent carpal tunnel symptoms.[6]

Cubital Tunnel Syndrome

Cubital tunnel syndrome is the second most common entrapment neuropathy of the upper extremity behind carpal tunnel syndrome. While pain is not a common symptom of cubital tunnel syndrome, an aching pain localized to the elbow or proximal forearm may be reported by patients. Typically patients present with worsening sensory numbness of the hand and digits in an ulnar distribution, with progression to involve motor weakness of the hypothenar musculature, and clawing of the hand due to loss of intrinsic musculature. The incidence is reported to be nearly 21 cases per 100,000 people per year.[7]

The diagnosis is made by clinical history and physical examination, with adjunct electrophysiology and imaging as needed. A detailed ulnar nerve examination should be performed with particular attention to the presence or absence of sensation in the distribution of the dorsal ulnar cutaneous nerve. This sensory branch innervates the ulnar aspect of the dorsum of the hand and arises from the ulnar nerve approximately 6 cm proximal to the wrist. If sensation is diminished in this territory, the localization is proximal to the dorsal ulnar cutaneous nerve and is likely within the cubital tunnel. With preserved dorsal sensation, the lesion may be localized to Guyon canal in the wrist. For this reason, electrophysiology is helpful to ensure proper diagnosis and targeted treatment. In some patients, subluxation or dislocation of the ulnar nerve during elbow flexion can be palpated and may be associated with increased symptoms. Ulnar nerve mobility may also be associated with dislocation of the medial head of the triceps; identification of the dislocating structures is important as it may affect surgical decision making. Increasingly, MRI and ultrasonography imaging techniques are being utilized to aid in the diagnosis of ulnar neuropathy at the elbow by demonstrating hypoechoic, enlarged nerve fascicles (ultrasonography sensitivity 46% to 100%, specificity 43% to 97%) and enlarged, T2-hyperintense nerve lesions proximal to a point of compression with distal muscle atrophy (MRI, as high as 95% sensitivity and 80% specificity).[8] These techniques can be helpful adjuncts in the preoperative setting, but also when evaluating recurrent or persistent symptoms.

After diagnosis of cubital tunnel syndrome has been made, conservative management via activity modification, anti-inflammatory medications, and therapy can be attempted, but many cases require surgical intervention. The most commonly utilized techniques for ulnar nerve surgery within the cubital tunnel include in situ decompression and anterior transposition. Techniques and extent of decompression vary; some surgeons simply unroof the cubital tunnel, while others do more of a circumferential neurolysis from the distal third of the arm (arcade of Struthers), through the cubital tunnel, to distal (Osborne fascia).[7] Anterior transposition of the nerve can be performed subcutaneously, intramuscularly, or in a submuscular fashion. Transposition involves more mobilization of the nerve and more extensive degrees of dissection of the soft tissues around the elbow. Along with the proximal medial intermuscular septum and the arcade of Struthers, particular attention must be paid to structures that may tether the nerve distally after transposition, including branches of the medial antebrachial cutaneous nerve, vascular branches from the ulnar artery, Osborne fascia, ulnar motor branches to the flexor carpi ulnaris, the distal intermuscular septum, the flexor-pronator muscle origin, and the investing fascia of the flexor digitorum superficialis overlying the ulnar nerve.[9]

A recent Cochrane review demonstrated no difference in symptom severity scores at follow-up (6 and 12 months) between in situ decompression and anterior transposition techniques; however, there was insufficient evidence to recommend a best treatment.[10] In situ decompression has a reported success rate of 65.3% to 94.1%, and subcutaneous transposition has a reported success rate of 77.7% to 94%; however, these cohorts are small and subject to significant publication bias. Complications from both approaches include ulnar instability, infection, and medial antebrachial cutaneous nerve injury, and rates are reported to be 3% for in situ decompression and higher (up to 14%) for transposition, likely due to a more extensive dissection required to complete the nerve transposition. Rates of secondary surgery were higher in patients undergoing anterior transposition (in situ release 2.5% vs anterior transposition 11.1%).[11] In view of these similar outcomes but higher complication and revision surgery rates, a recent trend has been for more surgeons to perform in situ decompression rather than ulnar nerve transposition. Endoscopic techniques are being increasingly utilized, and outcomes have been similar to in situ decompression for symptom relief and return to work, with higher scar satisfaction among patients.[12] While controversy over which technique is superior remains, anterior transposition should be considered in patients where ulnar nerve subluxation/dislocation is apparent and reproducible during elbow flexion on physical examination. In patients with ulnar neuropathy and no evidence of active subluxation, in situ decompression is feasible and cost-effective.

Recurrent or persistent symptoms after surgery can be difficult to treat; however, recent evidence suggests that in patients with recurrent symptoms, a significant proportion (77%) can experience either motor and/or sensory improvement, with 23% achieving complete recovery from symptoms at final follow-up after revision cubital tunnel decompression, although this may be due to pain relief even when neurologic findings do not improve.[13] Thus, revision surgery should be considered for these patients, with particular attention paid to the seven identified structures distal to the medial epicondyle that may cause persistent compression or deformation of the ulnar nerve post surgery.[9]

Radial Tunnel Syndrome

Radial tunnel syndrome is a highly controversial disorder. It has been described as compression of the posterior interosseous nerve (PIN) compression by the leading edge of the supinator muscle (arcade of Frohse), vascular structures (leash of Henry), or a fibrous edge of the extensor carpi radialis brevis. The syndrome is characterized by deep, aching pain in the proximal forearm without sensory disturbance or motor weakness and a normal EMG. There is significant overlap with other conditions, including lateral epicondylitis. It is often considered together with PIN syndrome; however, it is a distinct entity involving only pain without motor deficit, and radial tunnel syndrome does not progress to PIN palsy over time. It is a rare diagnosis, with a reported annual incidence of 0.03% in the general population, although incidence is also controversial, with some believing the diagnosis is much more common. Mean age at diagnosis is 30 to 50 years, occurring more commonly in women in some series, but with an even sex distribution in others.[14]

Symptoms include nocturnal pain that wakes the patient from sleep and is centered approximately 5 cm distal to the lateral epicondyle (and not directly over the lateral epicondyle). Physical examination is notable for preserved muscle strength in posterior interosseous-innervated muscles and intact sensation in the superficial radial nerve distribution. The "rule of nine" test involves drawing nine equal squares inside a larger square on the anterior forearm just distal to the elbow crease. Pain should be located within the lateral squares, which roughly approximates the anatomic

Hand and Wrist

course of the PIN. Provocative testing includes resisted supination of the arm and/or hyperextension of the wrist against resistance. Electrophysiological studies are nearly always normal, with no changes noted in nerve conduction velocities or on needle EMG of the posterior interosseous-innervated musculature. It has been reported that the PIN carries pain fibers that may be affected, yet not evaluated on electrophysiology. However, if the posterior interosseous is compressed to the point of nerve injury, electrophysiological findings should likely be demonstrated.[14] Imaging of the radial nerve and its branches in the elbow, either via ultrasonography or MRI, is important, as mass lesions compressing the PIN can mimic the controversial radial tunnel syndrome. It should be noted that flattening of the PIN on ultrasonography can be seen as it enters the supinator muscle even in normal patients, which can further complicate the diagnosis of radial tunnel syndrome.[15] Diagnostic blocks of the radial nerve more proximally in the elbow region can be performed to help isolate the radial nerve as a source of the pain syndrome. Radial tunnel syndrome should be a diagnosis of exclusion, and other potential causes of lateral elbow pain should be definitively ruled out, including lateral epicondylitis and supinator/common extensor overuse conditions.

Treatment begins conservatively, involving physical therapy, splinting, anti-inflammatory medications, and activity modification.[14] There has been some suggestion of improvement in pain after a single steroid injection of the PIN in the proximal forearm for treating radial tunnel syndrome, although further evaluation of steroid treatments are needed.[16] Surgical exploration and neurolysis may be considered in patients with symptoms that are refractory to nonsurgical measures. Surgical decompression via different surgical approaches (anterior, posterior, or muscle-splitting) should focus on complete neurolysis of the radial nerve at its bifurcation including its branches (deep radial/PIN and superficial radial nerve). Any constrictive vasculature should be cauterized and divided, and fibrous bands of regional musculature should be decompressed if there is evidence of nerve injury.[14] Outcomes after surgical decompression have varied substantially, with successful pain relief reported in 10% to 95% of cases, while others have suggested that no evidence has been found demonstrating effective surgical or nonsurgical treatment of radial tunnel syndrome. Recent literature suggests that routine release of the PIN in cases of lateral epicondylitis does not improve outcomes, so diagnosis of radial tunnel syndrome should be certain before planned PIN decompression.[17]

Radial tunnel syndrome remains controversial. It should be considered a diagnosis of exclusion, with surgical decompression of the PIN as a last resort for patients with persistent proximal forearm pain without another reasonable diagnosis after prolonged conservative management.

Idiopathic Brachial Plexitis (Parsonage-Turner Syndrome)

Idiopathic brachial plexitis is thought to be a rare neurologic condition with an incidence of approximately 2 to 3 cases per 100,000 people per year in the general population, nevertheless, it is becoming recognized increasingly by hand, shoulder, and peripheral nerve surgeons.[18] Originally described in a classic series in 1948 by Drs. Parsonage and Turner, both neurologists in the United Kingdom, the syndrome is often anteceded by significant pain in the region of the shoulder, followed by delayed weakness of muscles in the distribution of involved nerves. Typically, the pain is present for days to weeks, after which muscle weakness and visible atrophy may develop. Nerves typically affected include the axillary, suprascapular, dorsal scapular, long thoracic, as well as the anterior and posterior interosseous. Recovery is variable and occurs over the subsequent months. The underlying pathophysiology is thought to be an autoimmune reaction to nerve tissue, initiated by an external trigger, such as viral illness, flu shot, or a significant stressor, such as surgery or trauma.

The involvement of multiple, distinct nerves at varying locations can lead to a complex pattern of weakness that can mimic other disorders of nerve, including compression syndromes of the upper extremity or even brachial plexus trauma. Recent clinical studies have called into question certain mononeuropathies (AIN, PIN, long thoracic, suprascapular) previously thought to be due to isolated compression syndromes, but on detailed clinical and electrodiagnostic examinations, subtle findings are present in distinct, yet coexistent nerve territories, suggesting an underlying inflammatory etiology rather than isolated compression.[19-22] A careful history is important in achieving the correct diagnosis of idiopathic brachial plexitis, and attention should be paid to the initial onset of significant pain, followed by weakness several weeks later. Shoulder pain was present in 71% of patients in one series.[23] When the clinical history of pain, followed by multiple mononeuropathies, or uncommon brachial plexus involvement is demonstrated, idiopathic brachial plexitis should be included in the differential diagnosis. Electrophysiology and magnetic resonance (MR) imaging can be very helpful in making the ultimate diagnosis. EMG and nerve conduction studies can delineate a pattern of denervation that is likely caused by multiple, distinct areas of plexus or peripheral nerve involvement. MR imaging can identify T2 hyperintensities of the brachial plexus and/or peripheral nerves that do not appear to be due to extrinsic compression from local structures as well as denervation in a patchy pattern of muscles.

Targeted treatment strategies have not yet been elucidated, as the true underlying pathophysiologic mechanisms have not yet been fully described. Administration of steroids or immunoglobulins has been attempted, and one study demonstrated some improvement in pain and faster recovery in some patients who received steroids within 1 month of symptom onset; however, this study was retrospective in nature. A Cochrane review determined that currently there is no significant evidence to support the routine use of steroids in treatment of idiopathic brachial plexitis. Rates of recovery are variable, and initial recovery may not begin until 1 year after onset with maximal recovery occurring over a 2- to 3-year interval. Nearly 66% will recover M4 strength, and some can achieve M5 strength with continued, active physical therapy.[23] Some have advocated surgical exploration and interpositional grafting or nerve transfer as a treatment strategy, but this approach (particularly the timing of surgical reconstruction) remains controversial given the favorable outcomes in many (but not all) patients and the delayed onset of reinnervation seen in some. Secondary reconstruction should be considered for incomplete or poor recovery.

Nontraumatic Vascular Conditions of the Upper Extremity

Introduction and Vascular Anatomy

Nontraumatic upper extremity vascular disorders can be classified as vasospastic, occlusive, or a combination of vasospastic and occlusive. The natural history of hand and digital ischemia is challenging to define because of varying causes and treatments for each. In general, mild to moderate ischemia has a favorable prognosis, whereas severe ischemia with ulceration and the coexistence of a connective tissue disease show higher rates of ulcer recurrence and lead to more amputations. Acute ischemic conditions can usually be treated with good outcomes if early intervention is achieved and the inciting incident can be eliminated. Chronic ischemic conditions can prove more challenging, and treatments range from medical to surgical and are largely dictated by the natural history of the condition and severity of the ischemia.

The brachial artery bifurcates just distal to the antecubital crease. Three major sources provide collateral flow across the elbow and may serve as a means of continued perfusion to the limb despite injury to the brachial artery: the deep brachial artery, the superior ulnar collateral artery, and the inferior ulnar collateral artery. After the bifurcation, the radial artery courses deep to the brachioradialis and bicipital aponeurosis and superficial to the biceps tendon, pronator teres, flexor digitorum superficialis, and then flexor pollicis longus. At the wrist flexion crease, the radial artery lies between the brachioradialis and flexor carpi radialis tendons. After the ulnar artery branches from the brachial artery, it branches off the common interosseous artery and courses on the superficial surface of the flexor digitorum profundus, joins the ulnar nerve, and reaches the wrist flexion crease deep and radial to the flexor carpi ulnaris tendon. In the hand, there are three major vascular arches, one dorsal and two palmar, which all communicate at multiple levels. The superficial palmar arch supplies three to four common digital arteries and the deep palmar arch supplies three to four palmar metacarpal arteries. The dorsal arch supplies the dorsal metacarpal arteries (**Figure 1**).

Variable anatomy is more common in the radial artery than in the ulnar artery. A high origin of the radial artery is defined as being proximal to the antecubital fossa and can take off from the brachial or axillary arteries. While this is reported historically as occurring in up to 14%, a recent small cohort of ischemic limbs undergoing angiography reported a much higher incidence of 38%.[24] Other variations include absence or duplication of the radial artery. In the hand, the superficial palmar arch is complete in most patients and the deep arch is complete in nearly all patients.[25] The superficial arch is often made complete by communication between the superficial branch of the ulnar artery in Guyon canal and the superficial volar branch of the radial artery. One important anatomic variation is the embryological remnant of a persistent median artery, which can communicate with the superficial palmar arch, thus making it complete.[26]

Vasospastic Conditions

In Raynaud disease, paroxysmal pallor or cyanosis occurs in the digits of the hands or feet due to cold-induced vasoconstriction of the digital arteries, precapillary arterioles, and cutaneous arteriovenous shunts. The condition is due to an exaggerated central and local vasomotor response to emotion or cold. Raynaud disease is classified as primary or secondary, depending on whether it is an isolated condition or associated with

Hand and Wrist

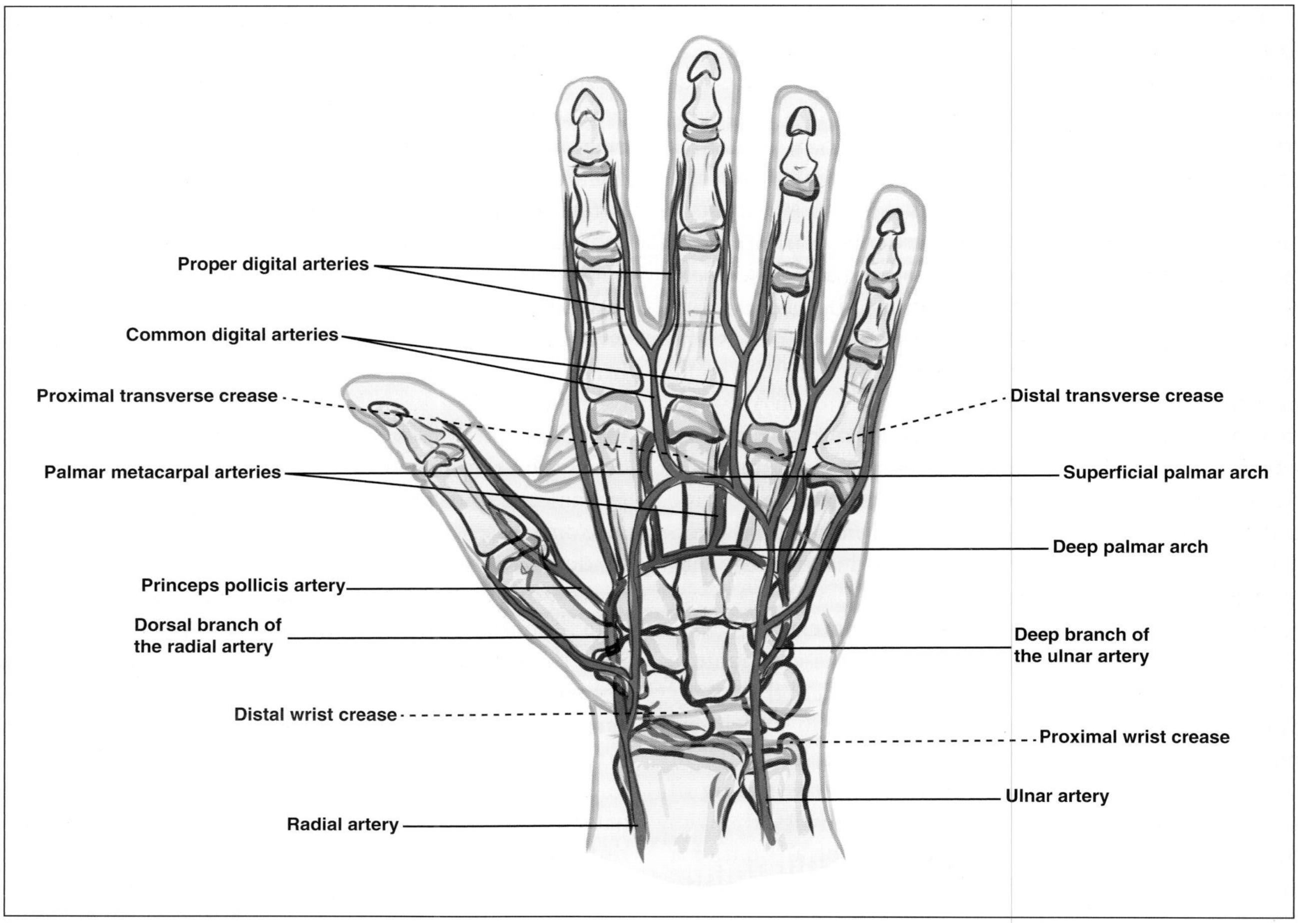

Figure 1 Illustration showing the arterial anatomy of the hand depicting bony and surface landmarks.

another condition, mainly connective tissue disease. Primary Raynaud disease typically presents in young women; symptoms are elicited by thermal or emotional stress, rarely results in necrosis, and responds to nonsurgical measures. Secondary Raynaud phenomenon may be complicated by occlusive events and may be further classified based on the presence or absence of adequate collateral circulation. Digital ulcers are extremely painful cutaneous necrotic lesions at the digital pulp or overlying bony prominences and occur in up to 50% of patients with scleroderma. Recurrent ischemic episodes, overall diminished blood flow, and repetitive microtrauma are all thought to contribute to the development of digital ulcers. Complications can include progressive ischemia leading to gangrene and infection, which can progress to osteomyelitis.

Vasospastic conditions can be statically and dynamically measured. As with any presentation of possible vascular insufficiency in the upper extremity, thorough history and physical examination is crucial and should include probing questions regarding systemic vascular disease, autoimmune disease, digit and nail inspection, and a bedside Allen test. Flow can be confirmed by handheld Doppler and/or ultrasonography. Dynamic studies include Doppler fluxometry, plethysmography, cold stress testing, and capillaroscopy. Nail fold videocapillaroscopy is the best noninvasive diagnostic technique for detecting morphofunctional changes in the microcirculation and is accepted in early diagnosis and monitoring of primary and secondary Raynaud disease.[27] Typical capillaroscopic features are 10 to 30 capillaries per 1 mm and hairpin-shaped loops arranged in parallel rows, while ischemic changes include morphologically changed capillaries, enlarged loops, diminished loop density, microhemorrhages, and, most importantly, avascular areas.[27] Formal angiography remains the benchmark; however, CT and MR angiography can be noninvasive alternatives.[28]

Raynaud phenomenon and digital ulcers are managed nonsurgically with pain medications, avoidance of stimulators of vasospasm, meticulous wound care, and antibiotics for infected ulcers. Pharmaceutical treatment options include calcium channel blockers, angiotensin-converting enzyme inhibitors, angiotensin receptor blockers, alpha-1 antagonists, antiplatelet and anticoagulant therapies, selective serotonin reuptake inhibitors, endothelin receptor antagonists, phosphodiesterase inhibitors, and statins.[29] In the case of failed pharmacologic treatment, the standard method of choice has sometimes been thoracoscopic upper thoracic sympathectomy, with reported short-term success despite a high symptom recurrence rate.[30] Indeed, surgical intervention may be required when medical treatments fail, and there is an increasing frequency or severity of vasospastic episodes, digital pain, or multiple recurrent digital ulcerations. Digital sympathectomy and arterial bypass are the two main treatment options. A bupivacaine block has been described as one method to predict the potential benefit of digital sympathectomy (**Figure 2**). Botulinum toxin can be utilized as a

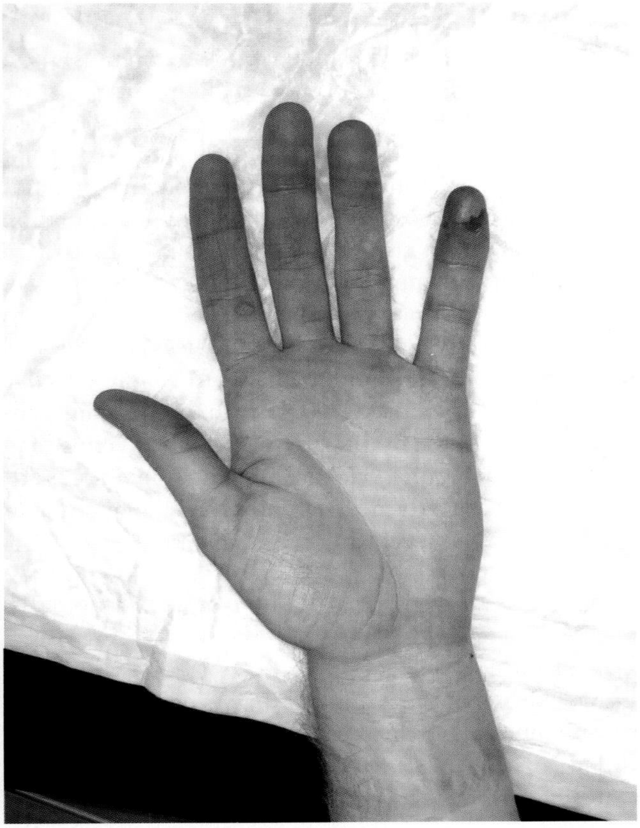

Figure 2 Photograph of patient with Raynaud phenomenon who had severe enough constriction on the ulnar digits to have ulceration. This picture is after the flow has been restored to the ulnar digits via ulnar nerve block at the wrist. Note the contrast to the radial side.

chemical sympathectomy to address vasospasm and has been shown to be highly effective at least in the short term.[31,32] Chronic digital ischemia in scleroderma is also due to fibrosis of the adventitia ,and periarterial sympathectomy involves adventitial stripping of the common digital arteries and the palmar arch as well as ulnar and radial arteries at the wrist. In cases where preoperative angiography shows occlusion, bypass should be performed in addition to periarterial sympathectomy, as initial healing was equivalent, but long-term recurrence of ulceration was improved when bypass was added.[11]

Occlusive Conditions

Occlusive disease of the hand includes thrombus formation with or without aneurysm; adventitial, medial, or intimal changes secondary to plaque or mural thrombus; and embolism with distant thrombosis. Ischemia results from inadequate flow secondary to lack of adequate collateral vessels or vasospasm of existing collaterals. Isolated vaso-occlusive disease includes acute or acute on chronic conditions such as embolism and aneurysm, peripheral vascular disease, vasculitis, and chronic posttraumatic thrombosis.

Arterial thrombosis can occur from local chronic trauma as well as thromboembolic events from underlying conditions such as atrial fibrillation atherosclerosis and vasculitis. While most thromboembolic events in the upper extremity are cardiac in origin, repetitive trauma such as the use of crutches and hypothenar hammer syndrome have been described. An acute event will usually have good outcome if intervention is undertaken promptly to include anticoagulation alone, catheter-directed thrombolysis, stenting, angioplasty, or thrombectomy depending on the size and location of the target vessel. Overall there is a high incidence of recurrence due to underlying conditions as well as poor patient compliance with medical therapies.[33]

Aneurysms of the upper extremity can result from repetitive blunt trauma and are of two basic types: (1) False (pseudo) aneurysms occur secondary to vessel wall penetration and subsequent hemorrhage in which the hematoma in the soft tissue organizes, fibroses, and recanalizes in continuity with the true vessel but is devoid of an endothelial lining. (2) True aneurysms occur usually after repetitive injury to the vessel and result in a gradual dilatation of the vessel. Both true and false aneurysms are characterized by slow progression that leads to thrombosis or embolism and may be diagnosed clinically by the presence of distal ischemia with an expanding mass. Distal ischemia typically occurs from embolization. Both Doppler ultrasonography and arterial duplex imaging are effective in identifying aneurysms, but arteriography can differentiate true aneurysms from malignancy, arteriovenous malformations, and neural tumors.

Various forms of vasculitis can affect the upper extremity including Wegener, giant cell, and Takayasu arteritis. Duplex arterial ultrasonography can be a useful tool in diagnosing arteritis and typically demonstrates the presence of dark hypoechoic circular vascular wall thickening around the artery lumen, occlusion, and thrombosis. CT/MR or formal angiography can show long segments of smooth arterial stenosis or smooth tapered occlusions of affected arteries alternating with areas of normal caliber, ectasia, and thrombosis.

Vasculitis should be treated expectantly. Systemic corticosteroids are usually first line, as well as other immunosuppressives. Critically occluded vessels of sufficient caliber have been stented in some cases, but this has not been universally feasible at the level of the mid-forearm and wrist. With irreversible hand ischemia, vascular reconstruction using grafts can be considered if the underlying condition is controlled medically, although any reconstruction effort could be compromised due to ongoing inflammation. Treatment of aneurysms depends on a number of factors, including whether a critical vessel is involved as well as the extent of collateral flow and vasomotor tone. Treatment options include ligation and resection, excision of the damaged wall with patch grafting, resection with end-to-end repair, and resection with an interpositional graft. Thrombolytic treatment is considered experimental in the treatment of upper extremity aneurysms although in the case of known thrombosis, catheter-directed thrombolytic therapy is a useful therapeutic option in the setting of severe acute hand and digital ischemia. Thrombolytic therapy performed for chronic thrombus appears to have much less benefit and is unlikely to be successful for thrombus that is present for more than 2 weeks.[34]

Combined Occlusive and Vasospastic Conditions

The ulnar artery at the wrist is the most common site of arterial aneurysms of the upper extremity due to being superficial and overlying the hook of the hamate. The dorsal branch of the artery tethers the main artery, preventing it from being displaced off the hook of hamate during traumatic episodes. Repetitive trauma damages the medial wall of the artery, leading to thrombosis, occlusion, distal embolization, and aneurysmal degeneration and expansion. Hypothenar hammer syndrome is a rare vascular disorder resulting from injury to the ulnar artery at the level of Guyon canal. Although most commonly associated with hand-intensive laborers such as mechanics and construction workers, it has also been diagnosed in athletes engaged in squash, golf, weight-lifting, martial arts, baseball, basketball, volleyball, tennis, football, and hockey.[35] Treatment of hypothenar hammer syndrome includes nonsurgical approaches such as cessation of the offending activity, calcium channel blockers, and antiplatelet/anticoagulant therapy, with surgical options and thrombolytic therapy reserved for those with severe or refractory symptoms.[36] Treatment options depend on the Doppler measured segmental arterial pressures (DBI) confirming adequate or inadequate collateral flow to provide nutrients to the tissues. For DBI >0.7, a Leriche sympathectomy is often performed. For inadequate collateral circulation (DBI <0.7) arterial reconstruction is required and can include end-to-end repair if the segment is short, resection and in line graft, bypass graft, or reversal of flow. Long-term patency rates of reconstructed vessels appear to be much higher when autologous arterial graft is used instead of vein.[37]

Buerger disease (thromboangiitis obliterans) is a nonatherosclerotic, segmental inflammatory disease that usually affects small- and medium-sized arteries, veins, and nerves in the extremities. The etiology is not completely understood but involves hereditary susceptibility, tobacco exposure, and immune and coagulation responses. Even in critical limb ischemia, there is often no possibility of improvement with revascularization, and the only option is pharmacological treatment. Moderate-quality evidence across studies has suggested that intravenous prostacyclin analogue is more effective than aspirin for eradicating rest pain and healing ischemic ulcers, but the oral form is not more effective than placebo. Low-quality evidence suggests there is no difference between prostacyclin and a prostaglandin analogue for healing ulcers and relieving pain.[38]

Degenerative Arthritis of the Digits

Epidemiology

Osteoarthritis of the hand and digits is one of the most common entities treated by a hand surgeon, especially in patients older than 65 years. While the underlying cause of arthritis remains under debate, it is generally accepted that genetic factors, mechanical stress, overuse, and inflammatory disorders all play important roles in the progressive loss of articular cartilage. Women are affected more commonly than men; the distal interphalangeal (DIP) joint is the most common location, followed by the thumb carpometacarpal (CMC) joint. Regardless of etiology, symptomatic arthritis in the digits can result in the inability to perform functions critical to the hand.

Evaluation

Patients most commonly present with pain, swelling, and loss of motion, with characteristic findings in each joint. Osteoarthritic changes are radiographically most common at the distal interphalangeal (DIP) joint, and least common at the metacarpophalangeal (MCP) joint. At the (MCP) joint the characteristic findings include joint swelling, volar subluxation, and a flexion contracture. Extensor tendon subluxation and ulnar drift may be present due to failure of the sagittal bands, although this is less common than in patients with rheumatoid arthritis. The proximal interphalangeal (PIP) joint frequently demonstrates flexion contractures along with characteristic swelling and osteophyte formation known as Bouchard nodes. Similar swelling at the DIP joint is known as Heberden nodes and may occur in association with a mucous cyst at this level. Radiographs including AP, lateral, and oblique views centered over the joint in question are typically sufficient for diagnosis. The Brewerton view, obtained with the hand supine and MCP flexed 45° to 60°, can help further characterize the MCP joint. Advanced imaging modalities such as CT and MRI are seldom necessary, but may be utilized to characterize early stages of cartilage loss or in posttraumatic deformities. Furthermore, symptoms do not always correlate with the severity of radiographic arthritis.

Distal Interphalangeal Joint Arthritis

DIP osteoarthritis is the most location of OA in the hand. Radiographs frequently do not match patients' symptoms, and often the only symptom may be a cosmetic deformity of the digit (Heberden node) or an overlying mucous cyst. Furthermore, the degree of deformity does not correlate with the degree of functional impairment. Treatment is based on patient symptoms and the degree of arthrosis. Nonsurgical treatment consists of splinting and either oral or topical anti-inflammatory medications as well as patient education. Steroid injections, while possible, are difficult and cumbersome to localize into the DIP joint. Surgical treatment is chosen for patients with pain, deformity, or functional impairment of the digit. For patients with lesser osteoarthritic changes and symptoms as well as cosmetic deformity, DIP joint débridement, osteophyte removal, and mucous cyst excision are often adequate. For patients with advanced arthritic changes, DIP fusion is the standard of care. A variety of fusion techniques have been described including interosseus wiring, axial compression screws, tension band constructs, and lag screw fixation. All techniques utilize the same principles of joint preparation to cancellous bone, preservation of bone stock, avoidance of nail plate injury, and fusion in 10° to 15° of flexion. Regardless of technique, fusion rates approach 90% to 100% in reported studies.

DIP arthroplasty remains an uncommon procedure with limited indications. The primary advantage is the preservation of range of motion; however, since only 15% of digital flexion occurs at the DIP joint, this benefit is limited to a select few patients. Sierakowski et al reviewed 131 DIP arthroplasties at midterm follow-up.[39] Mean postoperative motion was 40° with an average extension lag of 11° and pain improved from 8/10 to 1/10. Complications included three joints with cellulitis, one osteomyelitis, two joints with persistent instability, and one with persistent mallet deformity. The authors propose a lateral approach with preservation of the extensor tendon to reduce the risk of postoperative deformity. Given the risk of postoperative complications and current success rate of DIP fusion, DIP arthroplasty should remain a limited treatment option for only a select few patients.

Proximal Interphalangeal Joint Arthritis

Similar to the DIP joint, PIP joint osteoarthritis presents with pain, swelling, and functional impairment of the digit. Bouchard nodes are bony protuberances at the PIP joint pathognomonic for osteoarthritis (**Figure 3**). Radiographic findings include joint space narrowing, sclerosis, subchondral cysts, and osteophyte formation. PIP joint range of motion is often maintained until late stages of the disease process, but loss of motion at the PIP joint is more of a functional concern than at the DIP. Initial management consists of rest, splinting, NSAIDS, education, and steroid injections for symptomatic relief. For patients with recalcitrant symptoms, PIP joint fusion and PIP joint arthroplasty are the treatments of choice.

The decision between arthroplasty and arthrodesis is based on functional requirements, desire for range of motion, grip strength, and stability of the digit. In the index finger, requirements for lateral pinch stability and opposition against the thumb makes it a poor candidate for PIP arthroplasty. Vitale et al compared

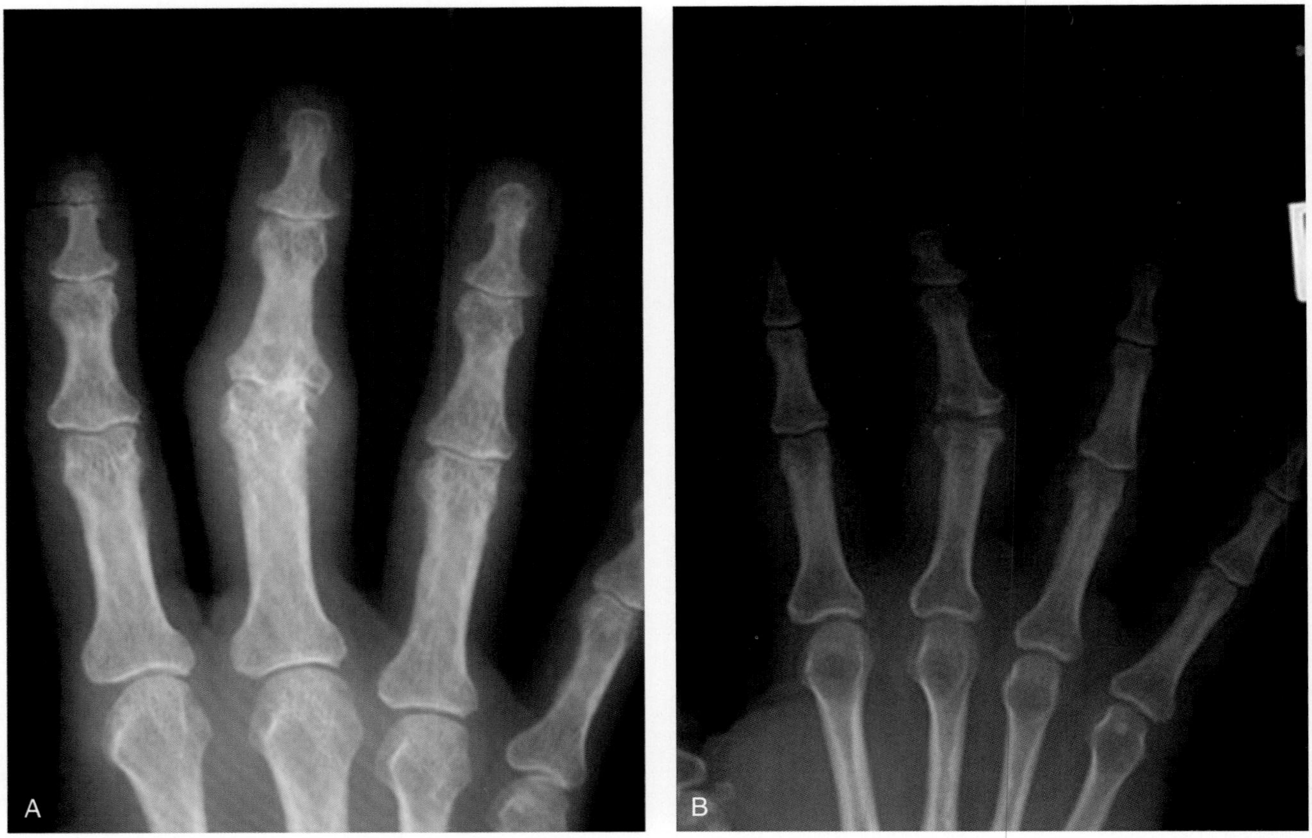

Figure 3 **A**, Radiograph showing proximal interphalangeal (PIP) joint osteoarthritis of the long finger with ulnar deviation deformity. **B**, Radiograph of post-op follow-up after replacement with silicone arthroplasty—note the coronal plane deformity in the digit.

outcomes of arthrodesis versus arthroplasty in the index finger PIP joint and found no difference in pain relief, satisfaction, or Michigan Hand Questionnaire outcome scores between the two. The arthroplasty group had a significantly higher number of mean complications postoperatively, and a 4.3 times higher risk of complication compared with arthrodesis.[40] In the ulnar digits, PIP arthroplasty can preserve motion that improves grip strength and function in the hand. The decision for arthroplasty or arthrodesis must be tailored to each patient's individual needs. PIP arthrodesis can be accomplished utilizing many of the same techniques for the DIP joint. The position of optimal fusion varies in each digit—but generally accepted values are 40°, 45°, 50°, and 55° for the index, long, ring and little finger, respectively.

Recent studies have focused on approaches, techniques, and outcomes for PIP arthroplasty. Trumble et al reviewed surface replacement arthroplasties performed on 21 patients with a volar approach.[41] Average postoperative range of motion was 87° with no evidence of implant subsidence at follow-up. Proubasta et al reviewed 36 PIP arthroplasties performed through a volar approach.[42] The arc of active motion of the PIP joint improved from 33° to 72°. Patient satisfaction averaged 4.8/5, and all patients stated they would repeat the surgery. Wolfe et al concluded that the volar approach offers the advantage of maintaining the integrity of the extensor mechanism while allowing early postoperative motion.[43] No randomized trial has been conducted yet comparing the dorsal and volar approaches.

Options for PIP arthroplasty include silicone replacement and surface replacement implants, including metal on polyethylene and pyrolytic carbon. Long-term results of silicone implants have generally shown good outcomes for pain relief, but high rates of implant fractures and small improvements in range of motion. Surface replacement arthroplasties have generally shown a trend toward better range of motion, but higher complication rates requiring revision surgery. Bales et al reviewed 10-year outcomes of silicone PIP joint arthroplasties and found a 90% 10-year implant survival rate, with predictable pain relief and maintenance of preoperative joint range of motion.[44]

Long-term outcomes following surface replacement arthroplasty have shown improved range of motion but higher complication rates compared with silicone arthroplasty or fusion. A prospective randomized trial comparing pyrolytic carbon, metal on polyethylene and silicone arthroplasties found a tendency toward greater range of motion but markedly higher postoperative complication rates in surface replacement arthroplasty.[45] Jennings et al reviewed 43 surface replacement arthroplasties with 10-year follow-up and noted good pain relief with an average of 55° arc of motion. However, over 25% of patients required revision arthroplasty, most commonly for early implant loosening.[46] Murray et al reported an implant failure rate of 11% at five years and 16% at 15 years for surface replacement arthroplasty.[47] Average postoperative motion was 40° with good VAS pain scores at long-term follow-up. Interestingly, a recent study found that patients undergoing multiple PIP joint arthroplasties actually had similar outcomes and improved revision-free survival rates compared with patients undergoing single digit PIP arthroplasties.[48] The authors suggest that replacement of multiple PIP joints does not increase the risk of postoperative complications or implant revision.

Recent studies have also investigated the outcomes following PIP hemiarthroplasty and revision PIP arthroplasties. Pettersson et al performed 42 hemiarthroplasties on PIP joints with mean follow-up of 4.6 years. Overall pain scores improved to 2/10 with postoperative arc of motion of 40°. Four implants were revised for failure to either arthrodesis or silicone arthroplasty.[49] Wagner et al reviewed 75 revision PIP arthroplasties at 10-year follow-up. Twenty-five percent of patients required a second revision surgery for infection, instability, flexion contracture, or heterotopic ossifications. Implant survival rate was 70% at 5 years but with a high risk of postoperative complications.[50]

In spite of the high-complication profile compared with arthrodesis, PIP arthroplasty continues to be an option for patients desiring range of motion and potentially improved grip strength. Harris et al surveyed patients with PIP joint OA and found the majority of patient's preferred surgical attributes characteristic of arthroplasty compared with those associated with arthrodesis.[51] Therefore, patient selection and expectation is critical in the decision between silicone arthroplasty, surface replacement arthroplasty, and arthrodesis.

Metacarpophalangeal Joint Arthritis

Arthritis of the MCP joint can be attributed to trauma, degenerative, inflammatory, or crystalline etiologies. Thumb MCP arthritis is more common than the digits, and the treatment of choice remains MCP fusion. The large degree of motion in the thumb CMC joint allows patients to tolerate arthrodesis of the MCP joint with little functional consequence. By contrast, MCP arthritis of the digits is commonly associated with rheumatoid arthritis, and joint arthroplasty is favored over arthrodesis to maintain digital motion. Options for MCP arthroplasty include silicone replacement and surface replacement arthroplasty.

Silicone MCP arthroplasty has generally shown improved functional outcomes, pain and good revision-free survival rates at long-term follow-up. While the rate of radiographic implant fracture is much higher than clinical failure, this does not correlate with functional outcomes of need for revision surgery (**Figure 5**). Studies examining risk factors for implant wear have shown that that ulnar deviation of the digit increases wear rate and chance of implant fracture.[52] Implant fractures typically occur at the hinge or distal junction of the hinge and the stem.[53] Boe et al reviewed 325 consecutive silicone arthroplasties—although there was a high incidence of radiographic implant fracture, the 15-year revision-free survival rate was 95%.[54] Patients reported significant improvement in pain and MCP range of motion. Morell et al studied 31 patients with silicone MCP arthroplasties and found a 97% revision-free survival rate at 15-year follow-up. A recent cost-effectiveness analysis of silicone arthroplasty in rheumatoid arthritis demonstrated improved patient outcomes at 5 years were achieved at costs ranging from $787 to $1,150 when measured by the Michigan Hand Outcomes Questionnaire. Taken together, these studies suggest that despite a higher rate of radiographic implant failure, silicone MCP arthroplasty provides good long-term functional outcomes and a low risk of revision surgery. Patients must be informed that recurrent ulnar drift after MCP arthroplasty is fairly common, although it is not always an indication for revision implant surgery.

Surface replacement arthroplasty is generally reserved for younger patients who place higher demands on the digit. The outcomes of surface replacement arthroplasty in the MCP joint have generally been more favorable than the PIP joint. Dickson et al reviewed 51 implants at 10-year follow-up.[55] Mean range of motion was 54° with a VAS pain score of 1. Overall revision-free survival was 88% at 10 years, and the degree of radiographic loosening or

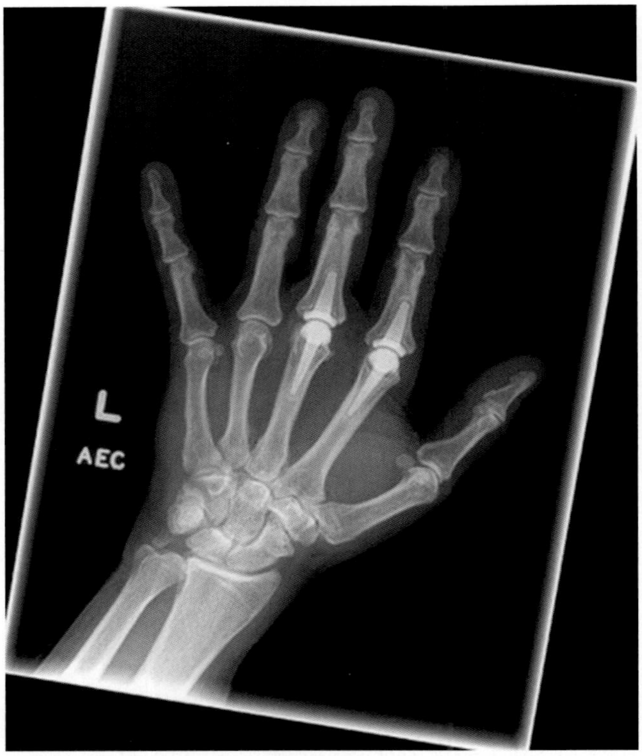

Figure 4 Example radiograph of metacarpophalangeal (MCP) pyrocarbon arthroplasty at long-term follow-up.

subsidence did not correlate with the need for revision. Chojnowski et al found similar results for 18 patients undergoing pyrocarbon arthroplasties.[56] At an average, 5-year follow-up arc of motion was 40° and DASH scores improved by 18 points. Pyrocarbon arthroplasty is also a viable solution for the treatment of traumatic injuries to the MCP joint. Houdek et al reviewed patients with MCP pyrocarbon arthroplasties performed within 24 hours of traumatic injury—there were no implant revisions, and mean range of motion was 56° (**Figure 4**).[57]

The most common complications following MCP arthroplasty include dislocation, stiffness, periprosthetic fracture, and implant loosening.[55] The risk of periprosthetic fractures is approximately 3% in both primary and revision surgery—this is increased by the use of pyrocarbon implants and noncemented fixation. Other studies examining MCP dislocations identified implant fracture, component loosening, and soft-tissue deficiency as the most common cause of MCP dislocations. All dislocations treated nonsurgically ultimately failed. Revision soft-tissue stabilization procedures have demonstrated only a 28% success rate, while revision arthroplasty for dislocation has shown a 71% success

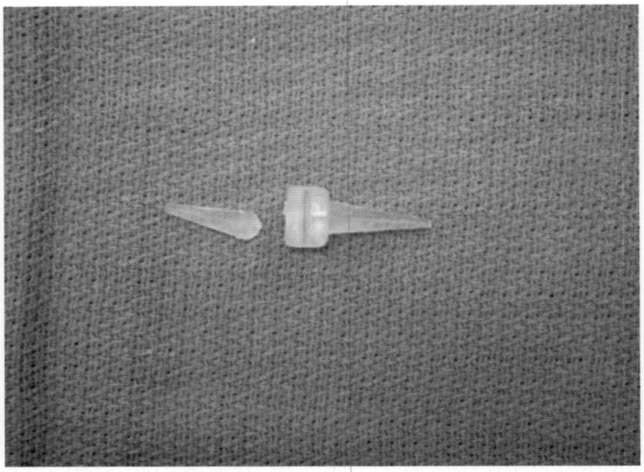

Figure 5 Photograph of implant fracture after silicone arthroplasty. Note fracture location at the junction of the hinge and stem.

rate. Silicone revisions have demonstrated significantly improved outcomes compared with surface replacement revisions.

Summary

Nontraumatic pathologic conditions of the upper extremity, such as neuropathy, vascular disease, and degenerative arthritis, can be sometimes difficult to diagnose, and it is crucial to recognize common clinical presentations of each condition with appropriate history and physical examination, followed by well-chosen diagnostic studies as needed to confirm the suspected diagnosis. Compression neuropathies with intermittent symptoms are generally treated first with physical therapy and splinting prior to proceeding to surgical decompression; however, constant symptoms or motor involvement are cues to proceed with surgical intervention to preserve remaining nerve function. Idiopathic brachial plexopathy, often preceded by shoulder pain, can progress to severe weakness in the distribution of effected nerves and patients generally have a slow and variable course of recovery despite interventions. Vascular conditions of the upper extremity can be occlusive or vasospastic in nature, and a thorough workup is imperative to determine the cause and formulate an appropriate treatment plan, ranging from lifestyle modification to pharmaceutical to surgical intervention. Degenerative osteoarthritis of the digits can have a profound effect on daily functions and lifestyle of patients, and treatment for pain is tailored to the individual's age and occupation to optimize outcome.

Study Facts/ Key Study Points

- Compression neuropathies occur at known anatomic locations in the upper extremity and are diagnosed by clinical history and examination which may be augmented by the addition of electrodiagnostic studies of sensory and motor function of the individual nerves.
- Idiopathic brachial plexitis has an insidious onset and can involve weakness in multiple but well-defined nerve distributions. There is no good evidence for steroid administration or surgical intervention, and most will have recovery with a variable functional end point over the course of multiple months to more than one year.
- Nontraumatic vascular conditions can cause a range of symptoms from intermittent discomfort to critical limb ischemia. It is of utmost importance to elucidate whether the presenting condition is occlusive versus vasospastic, as the management for each is vastly different and early intervention is often critical for tissue preservation.
- Degenerative arthritis in the finger joints can cause severe functional deficit, and the treatment algorithm is largely based on relief of pain symptoms which improves function, with the choice of nonsurgical management or surgical intervention (arthrodesis versus arthroplasty) based on patient lifestyle and usual level of physical activities.

Annotated References

1. Pourmemari MH, Shiri R: Diabetes as a risk factor for carpal tunnel syndrome: A systematic review and meta-analysis. *Diabet Med* 2016;33(1):10-16.

   This meta-analysis suggests that both type 1 and type 2 diabetes are risk factors for carpal tunnel syndrome. Level of evidence: I.

2. Graham B, Peljovich AE, Afra R, et al: The American Academy of Orthopaedic Surgeons evidence-based clinical practice guideline on: Management of carpal tunnel syndrome. *J Bone Joint Surg Am* 2016;98(20):1750-1754.

   This is a consensus clinical guideline for managing carpal tunnel syndrome. Level of evidence: I.

3. Padua L, Coraci D, Erra C, et al: Carpal tunnel syndrome: Clinical features, diagnosis, and management. *Lancet Neurol* 2016;15(12):1273-1284.

   This is a review of clinical symptoms, physical examination findings, and best approaches for assessment of carpal tunnel syndrome and to guide treatment decisions. Level of evidence: V.

4. Hebbard PD, Hebbard AIT, Tomka J, et al: Ultrasound-guided microinvasive carpal tunnel release using a novel retractable needle-mounted blade: A cadaveric study. *J Ultrasound Med* 2018;37(8):2075-2081.

   This is a cadaveric study of ultrasound (US)-guided microinvasive carpal tunnel release using a novel needle-based tool, the microi-Blade. Level of evidence: VI.

5. Zhang D, Blazar P, Earp BE: Rates of complications and secondary surgeries of mini-open carpal tunnel release. *Hand (N Y)* 2018: p 1558944718765226.

   The rates and types of complications and secondary surgeries after mini-open carpal tunnel release were examined and show the short-term complication and secondary surgery rates of mini-open carpal tunnel release are low. Patients with diabetes mellitus, chronic kidney disease, and cervical radiculopathy should be counseled regarding risks of complication and secondary surgery. Level of evidence: IV.

6. Pace GI, Zale CL, Gendelberg D, Taylor KF: Self-reported outcomes for patients undergoing revision carpal tunnel surgery with or without hypothenar fat pad transposition. *Hand (N Y)* 2018;13(3):292-295.

   To compare the outcomes of patients undergoing revision carpal tunnel decompression with and without hypothenar fat pad transposition, the authors perform a retrospective review of all patients undergoing revision carpal tunnel surgery at a single institution between reveal no difference in self-reported symptom severity and functional scores between patients undergoing revision carpal tunnel surgery with repeat decompression alone or decompression with fat pad transposition. Level of evidence: IV.

7. Carlton A, Khalid SI: Surgical approaches and their outcomes in the treatment of cubital tunnel syndrome. *Front Surg* 2018;5:48.

   This review provides an updated summary of the current literature on outcomes for various surgical treatments for cubital tunnel syndrome. None of the techniques in this review has demonstrated universal superiority above all others, but all appear to be effective in the treatment of cubital tunnel syndrome. The only consensus seems to be that transposition is preferred where the ulnar nerve tends to subluxate either on preoperative or intraoperative examination. Level of evidence: V.

8. Terayama Y, Uchiyama S, Ueda K, et al: Optimal measurement level and ulnar nerve cross-sectional area cutoff threshold for identifying ulnar neuropathy at the elbow by MRI and ultrasonography. *J Hand Surg Am* 2018;43(6):529-536.

   This establishes imaging criteria for diagnosing compressive ulnar neuropathy at the elbow (UNE) have recently been established as the maximum ulnar nerve cross-sectional area (UNCSA) upon MRI and/or ultrasonography (US) showing that by measuring UNCSA with MRI or US at 1 cm proximal to the ME, patients with and without UNE could be discriminated at a cut-off threshold of 11.0 mm^2 with high sensitivity, specificity, and reliability. Level of evidence: III.

9. Felder JM III, Mackinnon SE, Patterson MM: The 7 structures distal to the elbow that are critical to successful anterior transposition of the ulnar nerve. *Hand (N Y)* 2018:1558944718771390.

This is a cadaveric study defining anatomical structures distal to the medial epicondyle that should be recognized by all surgeons performing ulnar nerve transposition to prevent postoperative neuropathy. Level of evidence: VI.

10. Caliandro P, La Torre G, Padua R, et al: Treatment for ulnar neuropathy at the elbow. *Cochrane Database Syst Rev* 2016;11:CD006839.

This is a meta-analysis of nine randomized controlled trials evaluating the effectiveness and safety of conservative and surgical treatment in UNE. Only two studies of treatment of ulnar neuropathy used conservative treatment as the comparator. The available comparative treatment evidence is not sufficient to support a multiple treatment meta-analysis to identify the best treatment for idiopathic UNE on the basis of clinical, neurophysiological, and imaging characteristics. Level of evidence: I.

11. Zhang D, Earp BE, Blazar P: Rates of complications and secondary surgeries after in situ cubital tunnel release compared with ulnar nerve transposition: A retrospective review. *J Hand Surg Am* 2017;42(4):294 e1-294 e5.

In contrasting the rate and types of complications and secondary surgeries for in situ cubital tunnel release and ulnar nerve transposition, the short-term complication rates of cubital tunnel surgery are low (3.2%), but higher for patients with chronic kidney disease. The secondary surgery rate after cubital tunnel surgery was 5.7% overall, but higher for patients with prior elbow trauma and for patients undergoing ulnar nerve transposition. Level of evidence: IV.

12. Krejci T, Večeřa Z, Krejčí O, et al: Comparing endoscopic and open decompression of the ulnar nerve in cubital tunnel syndrome: A prospective randomized study. *Acta Neurochir* 2018;160(10):2011-2017.

This prospective randomized comparison of endoscopically assisted surgery with open surgical techniques in the treatment of cubital tunnel syndrome (CUTS) demonstrates equal satisfactory outcomes in the treatment of CUTS. Level of evidence: II.

13. Natroshvili T, et al: Results of reoperation for failed ulnar nerve surgery at the elbow: A systematic review and meta-analysis. *J Neurosurg* 2018:1-16.

This systematic review and meta-analysis of studies on persistent or recurrent ulnar nerve compression show that the majority of patients had relief from their complaints after reoperation for recurrent or persistent ulnar nerve compression at the elbow following a previous surgery. Level of evidence: I.

14. Moradi A, Ebrahimzadeh MH, Jupiter JB: Radial tunnel syndrome, diagnostic and treatment dilemma. *Arch Bone Jt Surg* 2015;3(3):156-162.

This review article highlights radial tunnel syndrome and helps to describe clinical presentation, workup, and treatment options. Level of evidence: V.

15. Raeburn K, Burns D, Hage R, et al: Cross-sectional sonographic assessment of the posterior interosseous nerve. *Surg Radiol Anat* 2015;37(10):1155-1160.

The PIN was identified with ultrasound and classified by measurements of the cross-sectional area (CSA), anteroposterior (AP) and lateral (L) distances were taken immediately proximal and distal to the arcade of Frohse in order to provide reference values for the PIN in healthy individuals at the arcade of Frohse. Level of evidence: VI.

16. Marchese J, Coyle K, Cote M, et al: Prospective evaluation of a single corticosteroid injection in radial tunnel syndrome. *Hand (N Y)* 2018:1558944718787282.

Background: The role of corticosteroid injections in the treatment of radial tunnel syndrome (RTS) has not been evaluated in depth. The purpose of this study was to evaluate the utility of a single corticosteroid injection as a therapeutic modality for RTS. Methods: We enrolled 40 patients with a clinical diagnosis of RTS. Our primary outcome was the quick Disabilities of the Arm, Shoulder and Hand (qDASH) score at 1 year. Each patient was then treated with a single corticosteroid injection in the proximal forearm at the PIN. Patient follow-up occurred at 2 weeks, 3 months, and 1 year. Results: The cohort had a mean age of 49 years, and 35 patients completed 1 year of follow-up. Outcomes based on qDASH and visual analog scale (VAS) showed significant improvement from baseline, with mean qDASH decreasing from 49.4 ± 7.0 points to 35.8 ± 7.5 points (P = 0.03) and 28.5 ± 7.3 points (P = 0.01) at 12 and 52 weeks, respectively, and VAS decreasing from 6.0 ± 0.8 points to 3.4 ± 0.9 points (P = 0.005) and 2.9 ± 0.8 points (P = 0.003) at 12 and 52 weeks, respectively. During the study period, 8 of 35 patients (23%) failed nonsurgical treatment and went on to surgical decompression of the PIN. A minimal clinically important difference in qDASH was achieved in 57% of subjects at 1-year follow-up. Conclusions: Nonsurgical management with corticosteroid injection can be used as a therapeutic measure with potential long-term benefits in the treatment of RTS.

17. Tsolias A, Detrembleur C, Druez V, et al: Effect of radial nerve release on lateral epicondylitis outcomes: A prospective, randomized, double-blinded trial. *J Hand Surg Am* 2018.

This is a prospective, randomized, double-blind single-center clinical trial in 54 patients treated surgically for lateral epicondylitis, without any EMG or imaging sign of compression of the PIN at the arcade of Frohse and demonstrates that radial nerve release, in association with surgical treatment for lateral epicondylitis, was not associated with greater improvement. Type of study/level of evidence: I.

18. van Alfen N: Clinical and pathophysiological concepts of neuralgic amyotrophy. *Nat Rev Neurol* 2011;7(6):315-322.

Neuralgic amyotrophy—also known as Parsonage-Turner syndrome or brachial plexus neuritis—is a distinct and painful peripheral neuropathy that causes episodes of multifocal paresis and sensory loss in a brachial plexus distribution with concomitant involvement of other PNS structures (such as the lumbosacral plexus or phrenic nerve) in a large number of patients. The phenotype can be limited or extensive and the amount of disability experienced also varies between patients, but many are left with residual disabilities that affect their ability to work and their everyday life. Both idiopathic and hereditary forms exist. The latter form is genetically heterogeneous, but in 55% of affected families, neuralgic amyotrophy is associated with a point mutation or duplication in the SEPT9 gene on chromosome 17q25. The disease is thought to result from an underlying genetic predisposition, a susceptibility to mechanical injury of the brachial plexus (possibly representing disturbance of the epineurial blood-nerve barrier), and an immune or autoimmune trigger for the attacks. The precise pathophysiological mechanisms are still unclear; treatment is empirical, and preventive measures are not yet available. This review provides an overview of the current clinical and pathophysiological concepts and research topics in neuralgic amyotrophy.

19. Maldonado AA, Amrami KK, Mauermann ML, Spinner RJ: Nontraumatic "isolated" posterior interosseous nerve palsy: Reinterpretation of electrodiagnostic studies and MRIs. *J Plast Reconstr Aesthet Surg* 2017;70(2):159-165.

    Introduction: Different hypotheses have been proposed for the pathophysiology of PIN palsy, namely compression, nerve inflammation, and fascicular constriction. We hypothesized that critical reinterpretation of electrodiagnostic (EDX) studies and MRIs of patients with a diagnosis of PIN palsy could provide insight into the pathophysiology and treatment. Materials and Methods: We retrospectively reviewed patients with a diagnosis of nontraumatic PIN palsy and an upper extremity EDX and MRI. The original EDX studies and MRIs were reinterpreted by a neuromuscular neurologist and musculoskeletal radiologist, respectively, both blinded to our hypothesis. Results: 15 patients met the inclusion criteria, ie, having an "isolated" PIN palsy. Four patients (27%) had a defined mass compressing the PIN. The remaining 11 patients (73%) presented with at least one finding incompatible with the compression hypothesis: physical examination revealed that weakness in muscles was not innervated by the PIN in four patients (36%); EDX abnormalities not related to the PIN were found in four patients (36%); and reinterpretation of the MRIs showed muscle atrophy or nerve enlargement beyond the territory of the PIN in nine patients (82%), without any evidence of compression of the PIN in the proximal forearm. Conclusion: The 11 patients in our series with presumed isolated and idiopathic PIN palsy had evidence of a more diffuse nerve-muscle involvement pattern, without any radiologic signs of nerve compression of the PIN itself. These data would favor an inflammatory pathophysiology when a structural lesion compressing the nerve is ruled out with imaging.

20. Maldonado AA, Amrami KK, Mauermann ML, Spinner RJ: Reinterpretation of electrodiagnostic studies and magnetic resonance imaging scans in patients with nontraumatic "isolated" anterior interosseous nerve palsy. *Plast Reconstr Surg* 2016;138(5):1033-1039.

    Background: Different hypotheses have been proposed for the pathophysiology of anterior interosseous nerve palsy: compression, fascicular constriction, or nerve inflammation (Parsonage-Turner syndrome). The authors hypothesized that critical reinterpretation of electrodiagnostic studies and magnetic resonance imaging scans of patients with a diagnosis of anterior interosseous nerve palsy could provide insight into the pathophysiology and treatment. Methods: A retrospective review was performed of all patients with a diagnosis of nontraumatic anterior interosseous nerve palsy and an upper extremity MRI scan. The original electrodiagnostic study and MRI scan reports were reinterpreted by a neuromuscular neurologist and musculoskeletal radiologist, respectively, both blinded to the authors' hypothesis. Results: 16 patients met the inclusion criteria as having "isolated" anterior interosseous nerve palsy. Physical examination revealed weakness in muscles not innervated by the anterior interosseous nerve in five cases (31%), and electrodiagnostic studies showed abnormalities not related to the anterior interosseous nerve in 9 of 15 cases (60%). In all cases, reinterpretation of the MRI scans demonstrated atrophy in at least one muscle not innervated by the anterior interosseous nerve and did not reveal any evidence of compression of the anterior interosseous nerve. Conclusions: All patients in the authors' series with presumed isolated anterior interosseous nerve palsy had MRI evidence of a more diffuse muscle involvement pattern, without any radiologic signs of nerve compression of the anterior interosseous nerve branch itself. These data strongly support an inflammatory pathophysiology.

21. Maldonado AA, Zuckerman SL, Howe BM, et al: "Isolated long thoracic nerve palsy": More than meets the eye. *J Plast Reconstr Aesthet Surg* 2017;70(9):1272-1279.

    Introduction: Two main hypotheses have been proposed for the pathophysiology of long thoracic nerve (LTN) palsy: nerve compression and nerve inflammation. We hypothesized that critical reinterpretation of EDX studies and MRIs of patients with a diagnosis of nontraumatic isolated LTN palsy could provide insight into the pathophysiology and, potentially, the treatment. Material and Methods: A retrospective review was performed of all patients with a diagnosis of nontraumatic isolated LTN palsy and an EDX and brachial plexus or shoulder MRI studies performed at our institution. The original EDX studies and MR examinations were reinterpreted by a neuromuscular neurologist and musculoskeletal radiologist, respectively, both blinded to our hypothesis. Results: Seven patients met the inclusion criteria as having a nontraumatic isolated LTN palsy. Upon reinterpretation, all of them were found to have findings not consistent with an isolated LTN. On physical examination, three of them (43%) presented with weakness in muscles not innervated by the LTN. Four of them (57%) had additional EDX abnormalities beyond the distribution of the LTN. Five of them (71%) had MRI evidence of enlargement of nerves or denervation atrophy of muscles outside the innervation of the LNT, without evidence of compression of the LTN in the middle scalene muscle. Conclusion: In our series, all seven patients, originally diagnosed as having an isolated LTN, on reinterpretation, were found to have a more diffuse muscle/nerve involvement pattern, without MR findings to suggest nerve compression. These data strongly support an inflammatory pathophysiology.

22. Le Hanneur M, et al: "Isolated" suprascapular neuropathy: Compression, traction, or inflammation? *Neurosurgery* 2018.

    Background: Several hypotheses have been proposed for the pathophysiology of suprascapular nerve (SSN) palsy, including compression, traction, and nerve inflammation. Objective: To provide insight into the pathophysiology of isolated nontraumatic SSN palsy by performing critical reinterpretations of EDX studies and MR images of patients with such diagnosis. METHODS: We retrospectively reviewed all patients referred to our institution for the past 20 years with a diagnosis of nontraumatic isolated suprascapular neuropathy who had an upper extremity EDX study and a shoulder or brachial plexus MR scan. Patient charts were reviewed to analyze their initial clinical examination, and their original EDX study and MR images were reinterpreted by an experienced neurologist and a musculoskeletal radiologist, respectively, both blinded from the authors' hypothesis and from each other's findings. RESULTS: Fifty-nine patients were included. Fifty of them (85%) presented with at least 1 finding that was inconsistent with an isolated SSN palsy. Forty patients (68%) had signs on physical examination beyond the SSN distribution. Thirty-one patients (53%) had abnormalities on their EDX studies not related to the SSN. Twenty-two patients (37%) had denervation atrophy in other muscles than the spinati, or neural hyperintensity in other nerves than the SSN on their MR scans, without any evidence of SSN extrinsic compression. Conclusion: The great majority of patients with presumed isolated SSN palsy had clinical, electrophysiological, and/or imaging evidence of a more diffuse pattern of neuromuscular involvement. These data strongly support an inflammatory pathophysiology in many cases of "isolated" SSN palsy.

23. Milner CS, Kannan K, Iyer VG, et al: Parsonage-turner syndrome: Clinical and epidemiological features from a hand surgeon's perspective. *Hand (N Y)* 2016;11(2):227-231.

    A retrospective evaluation of patients with Parsonage-Turner syndrome (PTS) characterizing clinical features of all PTS patients seen over a 9-year period and highlights both the rarity and atypical spectrum of clinical presentation of PTS, especially considering the more common involvement found for AIN and PIN. Level of evidence: VI.

24. Polfer EM, Sabino JM, Giladi AM, Higgins JP: Anatomical variation of the radial artery associated with clinically significant ischemia. *J Hand Surg Am* 2018.

    In this retrospective review, the authors investigate the incidence of radial artery anatomical variations in patients with clinically significant distal upper extremity (UE) ischemia and find that the incidence of high radial artery takeoff was found more frequently in patients with distal UE ischemia requiring angiogram than in reported population data. Level of evidence: IV.

25. van Leeuwen MAH, Hollander MR, van der Heijden DJ, et al: The ACRA anatomy study (assessment of disability after coronary procedures using radial access): A comprehensive anatomic and functional assessment of the vasculature of the hand and relation to outcome after transradial catheterization. *Circ Cardiovasc Interv* 2017;10(11).

    Although incompleteness of the superficial palmar arch is common, digital blood supply is always preserved by a complete deep palmar arch. Preprocedural patency tests have thus no added benefit to prevent ischemic complications of the hand. Incompleteness of the SPA is not associated with a loss of upper extremity function after transradial catheterization. Level of evidence: III.

26. Bijannejad D, Azandeh S, Javadnia F, et al: Persistent median artery in the carpal tunnel and anastomosis with superficial palmar arch. *Case Reports Plast Surg Hand Surg* 2016;3(1):25-27.

    Persistent median artery (PMA) originates from the brachial artery and anastomoses with the superficial palmar arch (SPA). As the PMA may be the cause of carpal tunnel syndrome and SPA is the main source of arterial supply, knowledge of which are important for the hand surgical interventions. Level of evidence: VI.

27. Berks M, Dinsdale G, Murray A, et al: Automated structure and flow measurement – a promising tool in nailfold capillaroscopy. *Microvasc Res* 2018;118:173-177.

    Patients with systemic sclerosis, primary Raynaud phenomenon, and healthy controls were imaged using a novel capillaroscopy system to evaluate structural and blood flow measurements and is able to distinguish patients with SSc from those with PRP/HC. Level of evidence: IV.

28. Nagpal P, Maller V, Garg G, et al: Upper extremity runoff: Pearls and pitfalls in computed tomography angiography and magnetic resonance angiography. *Curr Probl Diagn Radiol* 2017;46(2):115-129.

    This review article discusses relevant imaging anatomy of the upper extremity arteries, presents CT and MRI protocols, briefly describes the state-of-the-art CT and MRI of various pathologies affecting the upper extremity arteries, and summarizes the important pearls needed for busy practicing radiologist. Level of evidence: V.

29. Mouthon L, Carpentier PH, Lok C, et al: Controlling the digital ulcerative disease in systemic sclerosis is associated with improved hand function. *Semin Arthritis Rheum* 2017;46(6):759-766.

    This is a multicenter observational study investigating the impact of controlling the ulcerative disease on disability, pain, and quality of life in SSc patients receiving bosentan. Level of evidence: IV.

30. Karapolat S, Turkyilmaz A, Tekinbas C: Effects of endoscopic thoracic sympathectomy on Raynaud's disease. *J Laparoendosc Adv Surg Tech* 2018;28(6):726-729.

    The authors describe examples and outcomes of endoscopic thoracic sympathectomy (ETS) in the treatment of Raynaud disease that is treatment-resistant with severe symptoms and serious complications, disturbed social and daily lives, and impaired quality of life. Level of evidence: VI.

31. Motegi SI, Uehara A, Yamada K, et al: Efficacy of botulinum toxin B injection for Raynaud's phenomenon and digital ulcers in patients with systemic sclerosis. *Acta Derm Venereol* 2017;97(7):843-850.

This is a randomized double-blinded, controlled trial demonstrating that 1,000 and 2,000 U botulinum toxin-B injections significantly suppressed the activity of Raynaud phenomenon and digital ulcers in patients with SSc without serious adverse events. Level of evidence: II.

32. Bello RJ, Cooney CM, Melamed E, et al: The therapeutic efficacy of botulinum toxin in treating scleroderma-associated Raynaud's phenomenon: A randomized, double-blind, placebo-controlled clinical trial. *Arthritis Rheumatol* 2017;69(8):1661-1669.

This is a randomized, double-blind, placebo-controlled clinical trial using laboratory-based Doppler imaging flow data, physical examination, and patient-reported outcomes to assess the therapeutic efficacy of local injections of botulinum toxin type A (Btx-A) in improving blood flow to the hands of patients with Raynaud phenomenon (RP) secondary to scleroderma. Level of evidence: II.

33. Chisari A, Pistritto AM, Bellosta R, et al: Upper limb ischemia from arterial thromboembolism: A comprehensive review of incidence, etiology, clinical aspects, diagnostic tools, treatment options and prognosis. *Minerva Cardioangiol* 2016;64(6):625-634.

This is a review of upper limb thromboembolism with a purpose to providing cardiologists and critical care physicians with the essential tools to recognize and treat upper limb thromboembolism, identifying and correcting also its risk factors and causes. Level of evidence: V.

34. Wong VW, Major MR, Higgins JP: Nonoperative management of acute upper limb ischemia. *Hand (N Y)* 2016;11(2):131-143.

A guide for the nonsurgical treatment of acute upper limb ischemia includes anticoagulation therapy as the mainstay of both treatment and prevention of AULI. Because AULI patients often have underlying cardiac and/or systemic disease, a multidisciplinary approach is essential to minimize complications and prevent future occurrences. Level of evidence: V.

35. Swofford BP, Swofford DP: Management of hypothenar hammer syndrome a case report. *American Journal of Case Reports* 2018;19:150-152.

The authors present a case of hypothenar hammer syndrome and review the treatment of this condition. Level of evidence: VI.

36. Shukla H, Yaghdjian V, Koleilat I: A case of intra-arterial thrombolysis with alteplase in a patient with hypothenar hammer syndrome but without underlying aneurysm. *SAGE Open Med Case Rep* 2018;6:2050313X17748866.

This is a case report of acute unilateral arterial hand ischemia requiring catheter-directed thrombolysis with Alteplase therapy in a patient with acute occlusive arterial thrombosis of the left ulnar artery and review of this minimally invasive alternative to open surgical revascularization. Level of evidence: VI.

37. de Niet A, Van Uchelen JH: Hypothenar hammer syndrome: Long-term follow-up after ulnar artery reconstruction with the lateral circumflex femoral artery. *J Hand Surg Eur Vol* 2017;42(5):507-510.

The authors performed ulnar artery reconstructions with the descending branch of the lateral circumflex femoral artery and compared these with previously performed venous reconstructions. The patency rate of venous reconstructions in hypothenar hammer syndrome is significantly lower. Arterial grafting for hypothenar hammer syndrome has superior patency compared with venous grafting. Level of evidence: IV.

38. Cacione DG, Macedo CR, Baptista-Silva JC: Pharmacological treatment for Buerger's disease. *Cochrane Database Syst Rev* 2016;3:CD011033.

This is a meta-analysis of five randomized controlled trials (total 602 participants) compared prostacyclin analogue with placebo, aspirin, or a prostaglandin analogue, and folic acid with placebo. Moderate quality evidence suggests that intravenous iloprost (prostacyclin analogue) is more effective than aspirin for eradicating rest pain and healing ischaemic ulcers in Buerger disease, but oral iloprost is not more effective than placebo. Very-low- and low-quality evidence suggests there is no difference between prostacyclin (iloprost and clinprost) and the prostaglandin analogue alprostadil for healing ulcers and relieving pain respectively in severe Buerger disease. Very-low-quality evidence suggests there is no difference in pain scores and amputation rates between folic acid and placebo, in people with Buerger disease and hyperhomocysteinaemia. Level of evidence: I.

39. Sierakowski A, Zweifel C, Sirotakova M, et al: Joint replacement in 131 painful osteoarthritic and post-traumatic distal interphalangeal joints. *J Hand Surg Eur Vol* 2012;37(4):304-309.

This study reports the results of Swanson replacement of DIP joints for painful osteoarthritis and ongoing pain after injury. Level of evidence: IV.

40. Vitale MA, Fruth KM, Rizzo M, et al: Prosthetic arthroplasty versus arthrodesis for osteoarthritis and posttraumatic arthritis of the index finger proximal interphalangeal joint. *J Hand Surg Am* 2015;40(10):1937-1948.

Comparing outcomes of prosthetic arthroplasty versus arthrodesis to treat index finger PIP joint arthritis demonstrate that the decision for prosthetic arthroplasty versus arthrodesis in the index finger of patients with osteoarthritis or posttraumatic arthritis must be made with patient goals in mind and in light of greater risk of complications associated with arthroplasty. Level of evidence: IV.

41. Trumble TE, Heaton DJ: Outcomes of surface replacement proximal interphalangeal joint arthroplasty through a volar approach: A prospective study. *Hand (N Y)* 2017;12(3):290-296.

SR arthroplasty, when performed through a volar approach, allows for early range of motion and greater improvements in arc of motion, DASH score, and patient satisfaction. Level of evidence: IV.

42. Proubasta IR, Lamas CG, Natera L, Millan A: Silicone proximal interphalangeal joint arthroplasty for primary osteoarthritis using a volar approach. *J Hand Surg Am* 2014;39(6):1075-1081.

The authors retrospectively reviewed proximal PIP joints that were replaced with Avanta silicone implants and found that the volar approach to PIP joint silicone arthroplasty offers the advantages of maintaining the integrity of the extensor mechanism, providing pain relief, and improving postoperative range of motion with minimal complications. Level of evidence: IV.

43. Stoecklein HH, Garg R, Wolfe SW: Surface replacement arthroplasty of the proximal interphalangeal joint using a volar approach: Case series. *J Hand Surg Am* 2011;36(6):1015-1021.

Outcomes (range of motion, function, and pain relief) of the volar approach to PIP joint surface replacement arthroplasty (SRA) were examined in active, high-demand patients based on a single surgeon using the volar approach. Level of evidence: IV.

44. Bales JG, Wall LB, Stern PJ: Long-term results of Swanson silicone arthroplasty for proximal interphalangeal joint osteoarthritis. *J Hand Surg Am* 2014;39(3):455-461.

45. Daecke W, Kaszap B, Martini AK, et al: A prospective, randomized comparison of 3 types of proximal interphalangeal joint arthroplasty. *J Hand Surg Am* 2012;37(9):1770-1779 e1-3.

This is a prospective, randomized, multicenter trial that demonstrates surface replacement arthroplasty devices have a tendency for a temporarily superior maximum postoperative ROM, but markedly higher postoperative complication and explantation rates were observed compared with the silicone spacer implantation. Level of evidence: II.

46. Jennings CD, Livingstone DP: Surface replacement arthroplasty of the proximal interphalangeal joint using the SR PIP implant: Long-term results. *J Hand Surg Am* 2015;40(3):469-473.e6.

Long-term results of PIP joint surface replacement arthroplasty for arthritis using the SR PIP implant (Small Bone Innovations, New York, NY) are comparable with those reported using other implants. This and other studies suggest that this procedure is not appropriate for most rheumatoid joints. Level of evidence: IV.

47. Murray PM, Linscheid RL, Cooney WP, et al: Long-term outcomes of proximal interphalangeal joint surface replacement arthroplasty. *J Bone Joint Surg Am* 2012;94(12):1120-1128.

This retrospective study was performed to examine long-term outcomes of PIP joint prosthetic surface replacement with a proximal cobalt-chromium (CoCr) and distal ultra-high–molecular-weight polyethylene component over 30 years at a single institution. PIP surface replacement arthroplasty is a reliable treatment alternative for pain and deformity due to PIP joint osteoarthritis and rheumatoid arthritis. Level of evidence: IV.

48. Srnec JJ, Wagner ER, Rizzo M: Impact of multi- versus single finger proximal interphalangeal joint arthroplasty: Analysis of 249 fingers treated in 15 years. *J Hand Surg Eur Vol* 2018;43(5):524-529.

The authors retrospectively reviewed and compared the outcomes and complications associated with single and multiple digit PIP joint arthroplasties and showed similar, or even slightly improved, rates of complications, reoperation, and revision surgery, PIP joint arthroplasty performed on multidigits results in no worse outcomes compared with single digit PIP joint arthroplasty. Level of evidence: IV.

49. Pettersson K, Amilon A, Rizzo M: Pyrolytic carbon hemiarthroplasty in the management of proximal interphalangeal joint arthritis. *J Hand Surg Am* 2015;40(3):462-468.

50. Wagner ER, Luo TD, Houdek MT, et al: Revision proximal interphalangeal arthroplasty: An outcome analysis of 75 consecutive cases. *J Hand Surg Am* 2015;40(10):1949-1955.e1.

The authors retrospectively examined the outcomes and complications associated with revision PIP joint arthroplasty, finding that PIP joint arthroplasty in the revision setting represents a challenge for surgeons and was associated with a 70% 5-year survival but with a high incidence of complications. Instability was associated with worse outcomes. Level of evidence: IV.

51. Harris CA, Shauver MJ, Yuan F, et al: Understanding patient preferences in proximal interphalangeal joint surgery for osteoarthritis: A conjoint analysis. *J Hand Surg Am* 2018;43(7):615-624.e4.

In comparing preferences for arthroplasty versus arthrodesis among patients with PIP joint osteoarthritis (OA) by quantifying the patient-assigned utility of each operation's attributes, the authors identify relevant surgical attributes, including a literature review, surgeon survey, and pretest patient pilot test to build a set of discrete choice experiments. In aggregate, patients prefer surgical attributes characteristic of arthroplasty (ability to preserve joint motion and grip strength) relative to those associated with arthrodesis (decreased need for revision surgery, lower costs, and shorter revision surgery times). Level of evidence: III.

52. Drayton P, Morgan BW, Davies MC, et al: A biomechanical study of the effects of simulated ulnar deviation on silicone finger joint implant failure. *J Hand Surg Eur Vol* 2016;41(9):944-947.

Silicone finger arthroplasties are used widely, especially for MCP joint replacement in patients with inflammatory arthritis. Implant failure is well recognized. The rates of failure in vivo differ substantially from experience in vivo. One cause of failure is felt to be postoperative ulnar deviation. The aim of our study was to test the effect of ulnar deviation testing on silicone finger implants. We tested twelve implants in three groups of four implants. The implants were submerged in a bath of Ringer solution at 370°C throughout the experiment and tested in a rig held in 0°, 10°, and 20° deviation. The rig was cycled at 1.5 Hz from 0° to 90°. The implants were inspected every 500,000 cycles until a total of 4 million cycles. There was consistently increased wear and supination plastic deformity in going from 0° to 20° deviation. This study confirms the adverse effects of ulnar deviation on silicone finger implant wear. It is likely that this combines with lateral pinch forces and sharp bone edges to cause catastrophic silicone implant failure. Level of evidence: III.

53. Joyce TJ, Giddins G: Sites of fractures in explanted NeuFlex(R) silicone metacarpophalangeal joint prostheses. *J Hand Surg Eur Vol* 2018:1753193418774500.

Explanted NeuFlex(R) MCP joint prostheses were examined to identify the failure modes of these implants including location of fracture. Level of evidence: VI.

54. Boe C, Wagner E, Rizzo M: Long-term outcomes of silicone metacarpophalangeal arthroplasty: A longitudinal analysis of 325 cases. *J Hand Surg Eur Vol* 2018:1753193418778461.

This is an analysis of 325 consecutive MCP arthroplasties at a single institution, which show improvements in their postoperative pain levels and MCP arc of motion. Overall, pain relief and functional improvement are reliable, although silicone implants do not protect from progression of coronal plane deformity and have a high fracture rate. Level of evidence: IV.

55. Dickson DR, Badge R, Nuttall D, et al: Pyrocarbon metacarpophalangeal joint arthroplasty in noninflammatory arthritis: Minimum 5-year follow-up. *J Hand Surg Am* 2015;40(10):1956-1962.

Outcomes, complications, and survivorship of pyrocarbon MCP joint arthroplasty in noninflammatory arthropathy were evaluated by retrospective review and show good pain relief, a functional range of motion, and high satisfaction were seen in the majority of patients. All implant revisions were performed within 18 months of the index procedure. This may represent technical issues rather than problems with the implant. Level of evidence: IV.

56. Simpson-White RW, Chojnowski AJ: Pyrocarbon metacarpophalangeal joint replacement in primary osteoarthritis. *J Hand Surg Eur Vol* 2014;39(6):575-581.

The purpose of this retrospective cohort study was to evaluate the outcomes of primary pyrocarbon MCP joint replacements for primary osteoarthritis and showed good patient satisfaction with initial complication reporting. Level of evidence: IV.

57. Houdek MT, Wagner ER, Rizzo M, Moran SL: Metacarpophalangeal joint arthroplasty in the setting of trauma. *J Hand Surg Am* 2015;40(12):2416-2420.

In analyzing outcome of pyrocarbon MCP joint implants with traumatic nonreconstructible articular cartilage loss, MCP joint arthroplasty was performed safely in the setting of acute complex open MCP joint trauma. Patients had preservation of adequate MCP joint motion and experienced little pain. Level of evidence: IV.

Chapter 32

Tendon Injuries and Tendinopathies of the Hand and Wrist

Mark A. Vitale, MD, MPH • Andrew D. Sobel, MD • Ryan P. Calfee, MD, MSc • Kristofer S. Matullo, MD, MPH

ABSTRACT

Flexor and extensor tendon injuries to the hand and wrist challenge the surgeon, therapist, and patient. Substantial research has advanced our surgical treatment of both flexor and extensor tendon injuries, including novel surgical materials, repair or reconstruction techniques, and "wide-awake" analgesia. Rehabilitation strategies have evolved to promote earlier motion for both flexor and extensor tendon repairs and reconstructions. Imperfect outcomes remain common for flexor tendon injuries. Tendinopathies of the hand and wrist, including tenosynovitis of the first through sixth extensor tendon compartments and trigger finger, are common conditions that can be diagnosed by a thorough history and examination. Treatment is similar for most of these tendinopathies, and newer research has advanced both the nonsurgical and surgical management of these conditions.

Keywords: de Quervain tenosynovitis; extensor tendon laceration; flexor tendon laceration; hand therapy; trigger finger

Dr. Calfee or an immediate family member has received research or institutional support from Medartis and serves as a board member, owner, officer, or committee member of the American Society for Surgery of the Hand. Dr. Matullo or an immediate family member serves as a paid consultant to or is an employee of Synthes and serves as a board member, owner, officer, or committee member of the American Society for Surgery of the Hand. Neither of the following authors nor any immediate family member has received anything of value from or has stock or stock options held in a commercial company or institution related directly or indirectly to the subject of this chapter: Dr. Vitale and Dr. Sobel.

Introduction

Tendon disorders of the hand and wrist represent a broad range of conditions caused by sharp or blunt trauma, overuse, or underlying inflammatory pathology. Flexor or extensor tendon lacerations and avulsions about the hand and wrist pose distinct challenges when compared with tendinous injuries in other parts of the body, and these injuries generally require surgical treatment to regain function. In contrast, tendinopathies of the hand and wrist represent a common group of conditions that can often be successfully treated nonsurgically, but if conservative management fails, surgical management generally consists of release of the involved tendon compartments.

Flexor Tendon Injuries

Pathophysiology and Anatomy

Flexor tendon injuries most commonly occur following penetrating trauma, although flexor digitorum profundus (FDP) avulsions are common closed flexor tendon injuries. The four flexor digitorum superficialis (FDS), four FDP, and flexor pollicis longus (FPL) tendons take distinct origins proximally in the forearm and medial elbow and insert in the base of the middle phalanges of the fingers, the distal phalanges of the fingers, and distal phalanx of the thumb, respectively. Upon reaching the proximal phalanx, the FDS tendons divide at "Camper's chiasm" into radial- and ulnar-sided slips which allow for the emergence of the FDP tendons to more superficial positions.

The digital pulley system is a network of five annular (A_1 to A_5) and three cruciate (C_1 to C_3) pulleys with a palmar aponeurotic pulley (**Figure 1**). The thumb has classically been described as having an A_1, A_2, and oblique (A_o) pulley, although more recently, a pulley of variable orientation and morphology (A_v) has been defined between the A_1 and A_o pulleys.[1] The pulleys keep the flexor tendons tightly applied to the phalanges which optimizes the tendon's ability to flex the digit and provide a smooth gliding surface for the tendons.

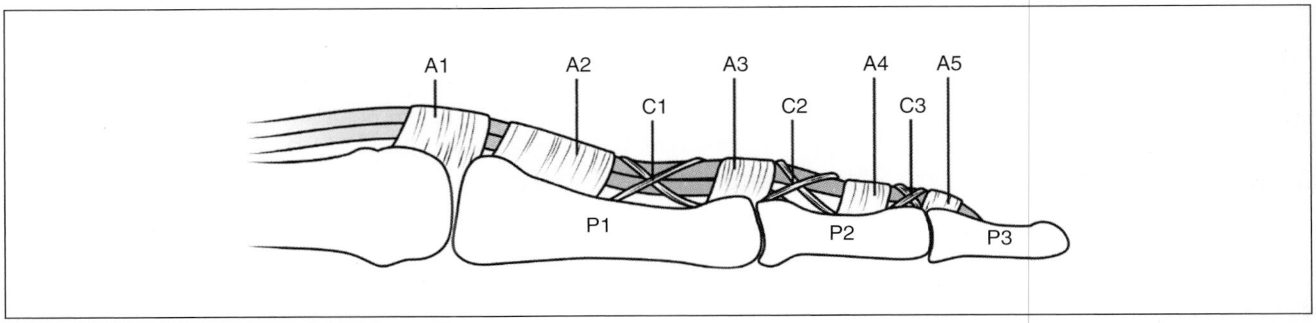

Figure 1 Illustration demonstrating the anatomy of the flexor tendon sheath and associated pulley system of the finger. (Reproduced with permission from Adams JE, Habbu R: Tendinopathies of the hand and wrist. *J Am Acad Orthop* 2015;23[12]:741-750. doi:10.5435/JAAOS-D-14-00216.)

The path of the flexor tendons from the forearm to the fingertips is divided into zones I-V,[2] and different aspects of treatment may be dictated according to the anatomic zone. Zone II, referred to as "no man's land," has received the most attention given the historically poor results of primary repair due to the need to preserve the tight flexor pulley system and the two tendons that must glide adhesion-free to restore function. The thumb has three distinct zones along the extent of the FPL tendon distal to the carpal tunnel.

Diagnostic Evaluation

Physical examination should identify the location of wounds realizing that even small penetrating injuries can completely lacerate tendons. Flexor tendon injury disrupts the normal digital cascade and alters the normal tenodesis effect (**Figure 2**). Palpation may elicit areas of bulk at the location of a retracted tendon stump. Neurologic examination should include assessment of two-point discrimination on the radial and ulnar borders of each digit to detect associated nerve injury. The vascular status of digits may be assessed by capillary refill or Doppler. An evaluation of active FDP and FDS tendon flexion should be done systematically for each digit. Zone I flexor tendon injuries should be evaluated with radiographs to assess for the presence and location of an avulsed fragment and/or fracture of the distal phalanx.

Tendon Repair

Ultimately, the overall goals of flexor tendon repair are to regain function and strength by maximizing the tendon's intrinsic healing potential, preventing gapping of the repair >3 mm, and countering increasing resistance to gliding in the initial postoperative period while minimizing adhesion formation. This requires a strong repair with well-coapted ends at an appropriate tension. Many factors play a role in the repair strength at surgery including the injury location, tissue quality, and repair method.

Technical Considerations for Repairs in Zone I

Though intratendinous injuries are possible within zone I, FDP avulsion (ie, jersey finger) is more common and the repair strategy requires repairing tendon to bone. The Leddy and Packer classification describes three avulsion injury patterns, although more recently a fourth pattern has been described in which the tendon dissociates from the bone fragment,[3] and a fifth pattern has been described in which there is concomitant fracture of the distal phalanx with tendon avulsion.[4] These repairs require stability but not gliding at the repair site, and the outcomes from avulsion repairs are good with return of functional distal interphalangeal (DIP) joint motion, minor interphalangeal joint contractures, and few infections.[5] The FDP tendon may be repaired to the distal phalanx with either "pull out" sutures tied over a button or the nail plate directly, via suture anchors placed into the distal phalanx, or via a hybrid technique of anchors and a button. Comparable clinical outcomes were found

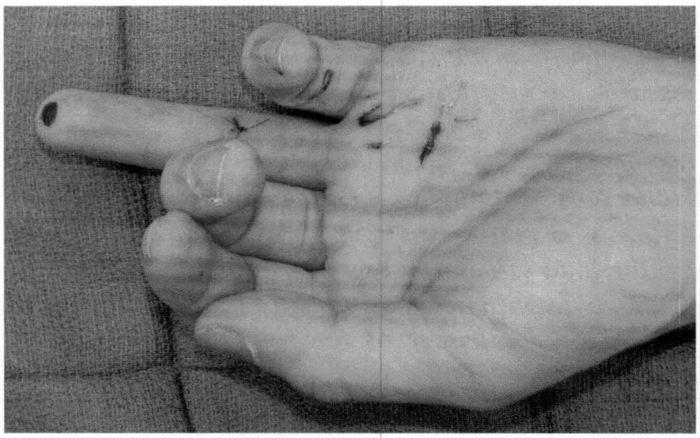

Figure 2 Photograph demonstrating obvious change in resting finger cascade with flexor digitorum superficialis (FDS) and flexor digitorum profundus (FDP) lacerated in ring finger. (Photo courtesy of Ryan S. Calfee, MD, MSc.)

between the two techniques in a clinical series of 26 patients with FDP avulsions, although a significantly quicker return to work was found in the group with suture anchor repair by about 2.5 weeks.[5] Recently hybrid suture anchor-button fixation was shown in a biomechanical study to have less gapping and result in a stronger repair compared with button or suture anchor repair only constructs.[6] If the patient presents in a delayed fashion, the tendon cannot be advanced, or the FDS tendon is also compromised, staged reconstruction may be considered. In the setting of preserved active proximal interphalangeal (PIP) flexion, the FDP injury is either ignored or the DIP may be fused for stable function. While reported surgical outcomes of repair and reconstruction are generally good to excellent, quadrigia (loss of adjacent digit flexion) is a possible complication with overadvancement of the repaired/reconstructed tendon.

Technical Considerations for Strengthening Flexor Repairs Zone II

Given the relative frequency and historically poorer outcomes of zone II tendon injuries in comparison to injuries within the other zones, the preponderance of recent research has focused on repairs in zone II. Strength of repair at time zero is improved by using larger caliber suture given increased tensile properties of the material,[7] although increasing the number of "core" sutures crossing the repair site may have a more important effect.[8] Considering the impact of suture-tendon interaction, using looped suture may increase the chance of suture pullout, core suture purchase of less than 0.7 cm compromises repair strength, and dorsally biased core suture may optimize repair stability.[9] When using looped suture, a cadaveric study demonstrated no demonstrable mechanical benefit to making a single knot versus cutting the suture and tying two knots to secure the repair.[10] The addition of a running epitendinous suture can improve strength and reduce bulk and irregularity at the repair site.

There have been numerous suturing techniques developed for tendon coaptation with variable numbers of core sutures, presence of locking loops, orientation of core sutures, and technical requirements. The modified Kessler repair is commonly utilized for its technical ease, although many have studied alternative techniques such as the cruciate, Savage, Winters-Gelberman, Tang, and Strickland which have greater numbers of core sutures and greater strength. No consensus technique exists although recent mechanical testing of porcine tendon repairs demonstrated greater strength of Tang type repairs over a modified Lim-Tsai technique with each incorporating six core strands.[11] In a similar porcine model, the asymmetric Pennington technique demonstrated superior fatigue strength and gap resistance over other conventional six strand techniques.[12] Regardless of technique, a minimum of four core suture strands crossing the repair site is considered necessary for early active motion rehabilitation.[13]

Technical Considerations for Improved Gliding of Zone II Repairs

Although there are advantages in increasing the number of core sutures and suture caliber, increased repair site bulk may also increase in gliding resistance during tendon motion potentially contributing to gap formation and rupture. To reduce bulk, some have advocated resecting a slip of the FDS tendon as it improves gliding and maintains strong PIP joint flexion.[14] The use of knotless, barbed suture has also been studied as a means to reduce bulk, and while nonclinical studies show promise to reduce bulk and result in equal or improved strength to knotted repairs,[15] these findings have not been replicated in all studies.[16,17] Others have focused on the pulley system as a modifiable component of tendon function. Expansion of the pulley system has been described, although this may result in peritendinous adhesions and tendon bowstringing.[18,19] Historical concerns of bowstringing, decreased tendon excursion and increased work of flexion pulley release have been questioned by more recent research showing that leaving an intact A_2 pulley increases the rate of rupture and gliding resistance[20] and decreases strength of tendon repair.[21] A recent clinical study of flexor tendon repair in zone II with complete A_2 pulley release (with other pulleys intact) showed no significant bowstringing.[22]

There is an increasing interest in performing tendon repairs with patients "wide-awake" without intravenous sedation or a tourniquet with the use of lidocaine with epinephrine as it gives the surgeon real-time feedback on repair gapping, gliding resistance, and triggering and allows for intraoperative instruction and patient feedback.[23] Use of the wide-awake approach for flexor tendon repair has demonstrated low rupture rates which has been attributed to intraoperative assessment of gapping.[24]

Biologic and Adjunctive Considerations

While many earlier studies have focused on the optimization of suture placement and orientation, recent studies have attempted to study biologic adjuncts to either reduce adhesion formation or hasten repair site strength. Lubricin has shown promise as a means to reduce gliding resistance; however, its use may decrease repair site strength.[25,26] Attempts at modulating repair site strength have been made with the use of adhesive-[27] and cross-linking agent-[28]coated sutures and early results have been promising. Mesenchymal stem cell and growth factor applications have been promising in vitro, though effective delivery of these agents remains unsolved.[29]

Tendon Reconstruction

In the setting of chronic, retracted tendons and tissue loss from trauma, advancement of the tendon for direct repair is unadvisable. The flexor pulley system is often unsuitable for tendon gliding and extraordinary approaches to advance the chronically injured tendon risks contracture or quadrigia. As such, tendon reconstruction in either one or two stages, with intra- or extrasynovial tendon grafts, is considered for the appropriate patient willing to undergo lengthy rehabilitation.

Single-Stage Reconstruction

Current indications for single-stage grafting are reserved to chronic injuries where a proximal tendon stump can be identified and the flexor sheath is not scarred or damaged. Improved understanding of differences in healing mechanisms of intrasynovial and extrasynovial tendons promoted clinical study into single-stage reconstruction with intrasynovial grafts which have yielded good results. In a recent canine model of 24 FDP tendon reconstructions, use of an intrasynovial allogeneic graft produced less adhesions and improved gliding but less tendon-bone healing compared with extrasynovial autologous grafts.[30]

Two-Stage Reconstruction

Two-stage reconstruction is the most common strategy and allows for assessment and treatment of concomitant injuries to the pulley system, bones, skin, and neurovascular structures. Many derivations of silicone rod placement and subsequent grafting through the developed pseudosheath have been developed, though all require delay until full range of motion. As a result, the second stage is typically delayed at least 2 months. Grafting is commonly completed with extrasynovial tendons such as palmaris longus, though utilization of a concomitantly lacerated FDS, part of which is intrasynovial, has been shown to yield good outcomes. Tenolysis may be required as a third stage.

Rehabilitation

The rehabilitation of flexor tendon repairs has undergone tremendous evolution resulting in improved motion and decreased rupture rates. It has been shown that flexor tendons tend to heal with increased strength, vascularity, and gliding and less motion restriction with early initiation of passive motion exercises.

One of the primary goals of repair is reestablishment of an active motion arc, and the total active motion (TAM) is significantly enhanced when patients complete early passive motion exercises. These exercises include passively flexing the digits at the metacarpophalangeal (MCP), PIP, and DIP joints, and depending on the protocol, often with changes in wrist position during the exercises. Passive motion protocols that have been developed that have been mainstays of rehabilitation for decades. Place-and-hold exercises have been shown to have improved TAM compared with passive exercises alone.[31] More recently, and especially with the utilization of wide-awake surgery in which the repair can be tested in real time, TAM protocols have been increasingly utilized. A recent survey of the American Society for Surgery of the Hand found that 20% of surgeons used some "wide-awake" surgery and surgeons were roughly evenly divided between active and passive motion rehabilitation.[32] Patients are able to actively flex and extend the digit with the repaired tendon within a few days of repair with TAM protocols. Though the results are promising, direct comparative studies with higher levels of evidence have not shown substantial difference of one rehabilitation protocol over another.[13]

Although advances in repair and reconstruction techniques and rehabilitation have improved outcomes, complications and subpar outcomes are common after flexor tendon repair. Among the potential complications generally related to surgery on the hand and digits, adhesion formation and tendon rupture predominate negative flexor tendon repair outcomes. Ultrasonography or MRI can be helpful in the setting of loss of active flexion and maintenance of passive motion to distinguish between adhesion and tendon rupture. Adhesion formation is especially prone to develop in zone II. Tenolysis may be performed to address adhesions after a minimum of three months after index surgery to ensure adequate healing of tendon repair and any associated fractures/injuries as well as an appropriate trial of therapy to regain passive digital motion.

Postoperative flexor tendon rupture may develop from noncompliance with restrictions, especially in the setting of an appropriate repair, although repair using inadequate techniques can contribute to gapping and failure. Revision of the repair may be considered after acute rupture if there are identifiable and correctable causes of rupture (eg, not enough core sutures, triggering or increased gliding resistance without pulley venting/release, etc.). Reconstruction is appropriate in the compliant patient with a subacute to chronic rupture.

Extensor Tendon Injuries

Pathophysiology and Anatomy

Extensor tendon injuries are less common than flexor tendon injuries within the upper extremity. The technical aspects of surgical treatment of extensor tendon injuries are generally more straightforward, and the surgical outcomes are generally better than those of flexor tendon injuries in the hand and wrist due to specific anatomical differences in the extensor and flexor tendon systems. Extensor tendon injuries most commonly occur following traumatic lacerations, attritional ruptures, forced flexion events (eg, mallet fingers), or resisted extension events (eg, sagittal band injuries after "flicking" the finger).

As the extensor tendons of the hand and wrist originate within the proximal to midforearm and extend to the distal phalanx, the structure of the extensor tendons transforms from a more cord-like structure into a flatter, broader tendon, eventually becoming contiguous with the extensor hood at the level of the MCP joint. As the tendon moves distally, the ultimate effect on distal joints also changes. The extensor tendons at midforearm are responsible for wrist and MCP joint extension, while the terminal tendon moves only the distal phalanx. With this knowledge, repairs at various levels require differing rehabilitation techniques which allow mobilization of some joints with protected or complete immobilization of others. This is significantly different from the flexor tendons, where the tendons are responsible for digital and wrist flexion regardless of location. Treatment of extensor tendon injuries depends not only on the amount of tendon that is lacerated, but also on the location zone of the tendon injury,[2] similar to flexor tendon injuries.

Diagnostic Evaluation

As in the case of flexor tendon lacerations, a thorough examination of wounds, resting stance of the digits, palpation, neurovascular examination, and evaluation of wrist and digital motion should be performed for each digit. In some cases, the diagnosis of extensor tendon injury may not be clear, and diagnostic imaging can be helpful in confirming diagnosis. Radiographs are useful in the assessment of mallet finger extensor injuries to determine the presence of bony involvement and/or DIP joint subluxation. Ultrasonography may also be a useful adjunct to diagnose extensor tendon injuries. To determine the accuracy of ultrasonography in diagnosing extensor tendon injuries, a recent cadaveric study evaluated 27 lacerations with underlying extensor tendon transections and 41 "sham" lacerations with intact extensor tendons.[33] Dynamic ultrasonography imaging had 100% sensitivity, 100% specificity, and a positive predictive value of 1.0 compared with static ultrasonography imaging which resulted in 85% sensitivity, 89% specificity, and 88% accuracy in determining extensor tendon lacerations from "sham" incisions.

Surgical Repair

Technical Considerations for Zone I Repairs

Closed extensor zone I injuries of the finger (ie, mallet finger) are successfully managed with extension splinting, but open zone I injuries require repair which can be challenging, and the development of a future extensor lag is a potential unwanted outcome. Typically, after tendon repair, immobilization of the DIP joint is accompanied with active motion and rehabilitation of the PIP and MCP joints. One recent retrospective study of 50 patients evaluated the outcomes of suture repair and splinting with or without the addition of supplemental transarticular DIP Kirschner wire (K-wire) fixation.[34] Surprisingly, additional use of the K-wire led to increased extensor lag with no other difference in ultimate range of motion.

Technical Considerations for Strengthening Extensor Tendon Repairs

The choice of suture technique is often debated and changes with location of injury and shape of the tendon. Repair strength of these various techniques is often demonstrated in cadaveric studies. A recent prospective study looking at in vivo repairs of zone V extensor tendon lacerations compared a roll stitch with a modified Kessler technique in 36 digits.[35] At final follow-up, flexion and total active motion were equal with improved extensor lag in the roll stitch technique.

Considerations in Partial Extensor Tendon Lacerations

Historically, injuries involving less than 50% of the tendon have been left to heal by secondary intention, and injuries involving 50% or more of the tendon have been repaired and rehabilitated depending on the zone of injury. This standard was called into question in a prospective study involving 45 tendons in 39 manual workers.[36] All of these patients had lacerations injuring between 50 and 90% of the extensor tendons in zones II, IV, and VI-XIII of the fingers or zones T-II, T-IV, and T-V of the thumb. Patients underwent nonresistive active mobilization for 4 weeks followed by resistive exercises and a return to work at 6 weeks after injury. At 8 to 9 months final follow-up, all patients had full motion and returned to work and no cases of rupture were reported.

Biologic and Adjunctive Considerations

Patients with complex finger injuries can often have significant soft-tissue injury and underlying loss of tendon and periosteum. With exposed bone and tendon grafting, adhesion and scar are risks of surgery that may limit postoperative range of motion. One study reported on six digits in four patients with complex finger injuries who underwent periosteal grafting with a slip of inverted extensor retinaculum autograft from the ipsilateral wrist sutured onto the phalanx with the tendon side dorsal.[37] The extensor tendons were then repaired. At an average follow-up of 1.5 years, all fingers had near normal strength and range of motion.

Surgical Reconstruction

In chronic extensor tendon injuries, injuries to the stabilizing sagittal bands or injuries to extensor tendons with compromised tissues, such as those with rheumatoid arthritis (RA), surgical reconstruction rather than repair may be considered, although extensor tendon anatomy does not have the same limitations that the flexor tendon system demands of maintaining a patent, gliding flexor tendon sheath. A recent study reported on the results of a technique to reconstruct either a traumatic or nontraumatic radial sagittal band rupture with resultant extensor tendon subluxation using the residual sagittal band.[38] In this technique, the radial paratenon is sutured to the undersurface of the radial sagittal band component and then further secured with the attachment of the radial sagittal band to the ulnar side of the extensor tendon. In their series of 13 patients, all recovered with full range of motion and no repeat subluxation at 14 months after surgery.

Reconstruction of the extensor tendon can at times be challenging owing to a lack of local grafting material. In a cadaveric study followed by one clinical patient, the flexor-tendon Paneva-Holevitch technique was adapted utilizing the extensor indicis proprius (EIP) tendon as a local graft choice.[39] In this staged technique, the EIP tendon is attached to the extensor digitorum communis (EDC) with eventual release and turn-down of the EDC from the forearm. This method allows sufficient tendon length to repair to the PIP joint.

Another report described a two-staged extensor tendon reconstruction of 6 patients and 19 tendons with extensor tendon loss in zone VI with or without zone VII involvement.[40] These patients underwent placement of silicone rods and soft-tissue coverage procedures with eventual palmaris longus grafting from the EDC tendons distally to a divided extensor carpi radialis tendon proximally. All patients developed complete or near complete MCP joint flexion; however, minor extensor lags developed in 15 of 19 fingers.

Rehabilitation

Recent research has attempted to elucidate the optimal postoperative rehabilitation protocols for extensor tendon injuries. In a recent literature review comparing two types of early active motion rehabilitation protocols after zone V and VI extensor tendon repairs, the authors concluded that relative motion extension splinting protocols allow an earlier return to function with no difference in complication rates compared with early active range of motion protocols.[41] Another review of 11 studies was performed evaluating therapy protocols from zone IV through zone VIII. While a high level of evidence was noted to be lacking, there was support for early active motion rehabilitation, but the optimal orthotic splint design could not be determined.[42]

The relative motion "yoke" splint has been evaluated as a protective orthotic for extensor tendon injuries allowing early active relative motion with slight modifications verified as successful for protecting repair and allowing rehabilitation of extensor tendon injuries from zone IV through zone VII. One study evaluated the use of a yoke splint to protect extensor tendon repairs of the fingers coupled with a wrist orthotic to decrease wrist motion.[43] A comparative 4- versus 6-week rehabilitation program was undertaken by 63 patients yielding no significant differences in outcomes as a function of rehabilitation program.

Tendinopathies of the Hand and Wrist

Tendinopathy is a nonspecific term used to describe a tendon disorder occurring anywhere along its course, and stenosing tenosynovitis refers to inflammation of a tendon and corresponding thickening of its enveloping sheath, although these terms are sometimes used interchangeably. Tendinopathies of the hand and wrist represent a common group of conditions which may affect any of the associated extensor or flexor tendons from the forearm to the digits resulting in swelling, pain, and/or limitations in motion. The underlying pathophysiology of these disorders may involve different etiologies. Many are believed to be caused by "overuse" resulting in swelling of an affected musculotendinous unit and/

or its associated sheath or fibro-osseous tunnel from repetitive motion, although the degree to which overuse or occupational exposure truly plays a role has not been definitively determined. Another etiology may be inflammatory pathology seen in patients with RA or crystalline disease (eg, gout) which may eventually lead to tenosynovitis or even tendon rupture. Additionally systemic disorders such as diabetes mellitus (DM) or thyroid disease may result in tendon adhesions or tendon/sheath thickening. Generally an absence of inflammatory cells is seen histologically in these conditions. This section will focus on the most common tendinopathies of the extensor and flexor compartments of the hand and wrist, including de Quervain tenosynovitis, intersection syndrome, extensor carpi ulnaris (ECU) tenosynovitis, and trigger finger, although tendinopathies including flexor carpi radialis (FCR) and third dorsal compartment, fourth dorsal compartment, and fifth dorsal compartment tenosynovitis are less common conditions.

Extensor Tendinopathies

de Quervain Tenosynovitis

de Quervain tenosynovitis or syndrome is the most commonly occurring tendinopathy of the extensor tendons of the wrist. The first dorsal compartment lies on the most radial aspect of the distal radius, and the fibro-osseous tunnel of the first compartment contains the abductor pollicis longus (APL) and extensor pollicis brevis (EPB) tendons (**Figure 3**). There is a variable anatomy of the first dorsal compartment with multiple tendon slips of the APL often present. Additionally, a septum that separates the various slips of the APL from a distinct subcompartment of the EPB has been noted in 34% to 47% of wrists.

The diagnosis can be made solely on history and physical examination. Patients present with radial-sided wrist pain exacerbated by thumb motion or radioulnar deviation of the wrist, swelling on the radial aspect of the wrist, and occasionally popping or triggering on the radial side of the wrist. Patients may report a history lifting a child or pet, cross-country skiing, or may have history of trauma to the radial side of the wrist. This condition affects women up to six times more often than men and is associated with the dominant hand during middle age. Additionally, de Quervain tenosynovitis is associated with pregnancy, the postpartum period, and lactation.

Examination may reveal swelling or warmth over the first dorsal compartment. Palpation reveals tenderness over the first dorsal compartment, and a small retinacular ganglion cyst may be present. Eichhoff described

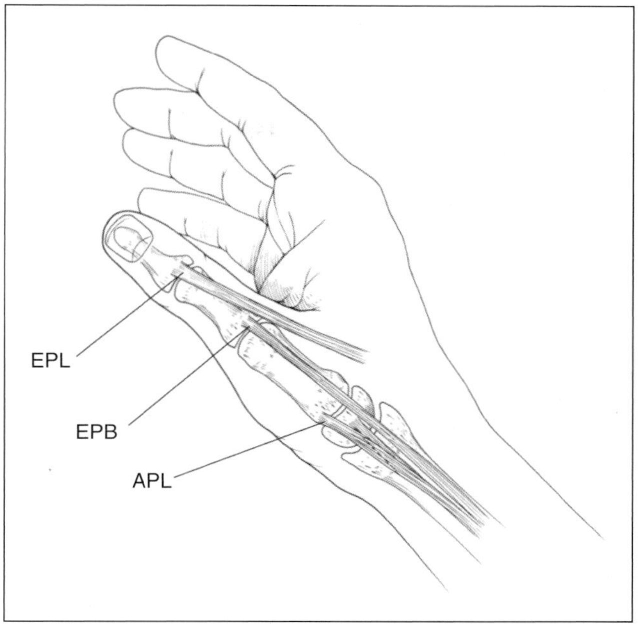

Figure 3 Illustration demonstrating the anatomy of the first dorsal compartment of the wrist, including the insertions of the abductor pollicis longus (APL) and extensor pollicis brevis (EPB) tendons. (Reproduced with permission from Ilyas AM, Ast M, Schaffer AA, Thoder J: de Quervain tenosynovitis of the wrist. *J Am Acad Orthop* 2007;15[12]:757-764.)

a physical examination maneuver often misinterpreted as the Finkelstein test,[44] in which the examiner asks the patient to grasp their thumb in the palm with the other digits while the examiner passively ulnarly deviates the wrist. The EPB entrapment test was described to assess for the presence of a separate subcompartment for the EPB.[45] The patient is asked to extend the thumb MCP joint against resistance and then to palmarly abduct the thumb against resistance. The test is considered positive for a separate compartment when the first maneuver is more painful than the second and has shown to be 81% sensitive, but only 50% specific for a separate EPB compartment. The Wrist Hyperflexion and Abduction of the Thumb (WHAT) test was described as a dynamic test to isolate the tendons within the first extensor compartment.[46] With the wrist maximally flexed, the patient is asked to abduct their thumb against the examiner's resistance, and a positive test reproduces pain. This test has been shown to have a greater sensitivity (0.99) and specificity (0.29) than the Eichhoff test alone (sensitivity 0.89, specificity 0.14).

Imaging is not necessary when patients have typical history and physical examination findings, but radiographs of the wrist can be helpful to rule out concomitant conditions such as carpometacarpal joint,

Hand and Wrist

scaphotrapeziotrapezoidal, or radioscaphoid arthritis. Ultrasonography may also be a useful test to verify thickness of the retinaculum overlying the APL and EPB.

Initial management options include oral nonsteroidal anti-inflammatory drugs (NSAIDs), thumb spica splinting, hand therapy, or corticosteroid injections. Thumb spica splinting alone has been shown to be successful in 14% to 18% of patients.[47,48] Physical therapy may include education on activity modification, modalities, tendon-gliding exercises, and custom forearm-based thumb spica splints. Iontophoresis, phonophoresis, and low-level laser therapy have been used to treat de Quervain tenosynovitis, but generally the evidence for efficacy is scant and limited to small series or anecdotal reports.[49]

Despite a lack of histological inflammatory changes seen in the first dorsal compartment,[50] corticosteroid injections in the first dorsal compartment have been shown to be highly effective.[51,52] The success rate has been shown to be poorer if an associated septum is present within the first dorsal compartment.[45] The incidence of soft-tissue complications has been reported to be as high as 31% for injections in de Quervain tenosynovitis.[53] Risks of corticosteroid injections include skin depigmentation and skin and subcutaneous tissue atrophy, transient elevation of blood glucose levels, and tendon rupture.

A recent cadaveric study reported on the accuracy of anatomic landmark-guided versus ultrasonography-guided injections in the first dorsal compartment using 43 cadaveric specimen receiving latex dye injections into the compartment with one of the two techniques.[54] If ultrasonography imaging identified a septated first dorsal compartment, the needle was redirected and a portion of the dye was injected around the EPB. Ultrasonography had a sensitivity of 75% and a specificity of 92% in detecting a septated compartment. Of specimen with a septated compartment, 75% (6 of 8) of specimen with ultrasonography-guidance versus 33% (2 of 6) of specimen with anatomic landmark-guidance demonstrated dye infiltration around the EPB, although there was not a statistically significant difference.

In cases of failed conservative management, surgical release of the first dorsal compartment is considered. After the sheath is released, the surgeon should inspect for the presence of a separate subcompartment for the two tendons, as failure to release a subcompartment is considered a common cause of residual symptoms or recurrence. Potential surgical complications include volar subluxation of the first dorsal compartment tendons, superficial radial nerve neuroma, or residual symptoms. A recent retrospective review of 200 patients diagnosed with de Quervain syndrome attempted to examine which patient- or disease-specific factors were associated with electing to undergo surgical management.[55] Surgically treated patients were more likely to have Medicaid insurance and a history of psychiatric illness, controlling for other factors, supporting the use of a biopsychosocial framework when treating this condition.

Intersection Syndrome

Second dorsal compartment tenosynovitis, also known as intersection syndrome, is much less common than de Quervain tenosynovitis. This is a tenosynovitis that occurs where the second extensor compartment tendons, the extensor carpi radialis longus (ECRL) and extensor carpi radialis brevis (ECRB), cross under the muscle bellies of the first compartment tendons, the APL and EPB, proximal and ulnar to the first dorsal compartment. The point of crossover, or intersection, is the point where tenosynovitis in this condition develops.[56]

The ECRL and ECRB insert on the second and third metacarpals, respectively. Similar to the first dorsal compartment, there is some variability in the anatomy of the second dorsal compartment. Three variants of the radial wrist extensors have been described with a 10% to 20% incidence: the extensor carpi radialis intermedius (ECRI), extensor carpi radialis accessorius (ECRA), and extensor carpi radialis tertius (ECRT).[57] It is unknown whether the presence of an additional radial wrist extensor might contribute to intersection syndrome.

Similar to de Quervain tenosynovitis, the diagnosis is usually made solely on a thorough history and examination. This disorder is more common in athletes such as rowers, weight-lifters, or other athletes who perform repetitive wrist extension. Patients may complain of pain and swelling on the dorsal aspect of their wrist. Patients may sometimes report palpable or audible crepitus at the intersection point with wrist motion. The location of pain is proximal and ulnar to the first dorsal compartment, approximately 6 cm proximal to the radial styloid (**Figure 4**). Pain is elicited with active wrist extension, and direct palpation of the point of intersection is painful.

Nonsurgical treatment consists of oral NSAIDs, activity modification, immobilization in a wrist splint in 15° to 30° of extension, and consideration of a corticosteroid injection. Therapy modalities including hydrocortisone phonophoresis over the point of maximal tenderness have been noted anecdotally to relieve pain, but there is a paucity of clinical evidence to support this modality.[58] A corticosteroid injection is performed at

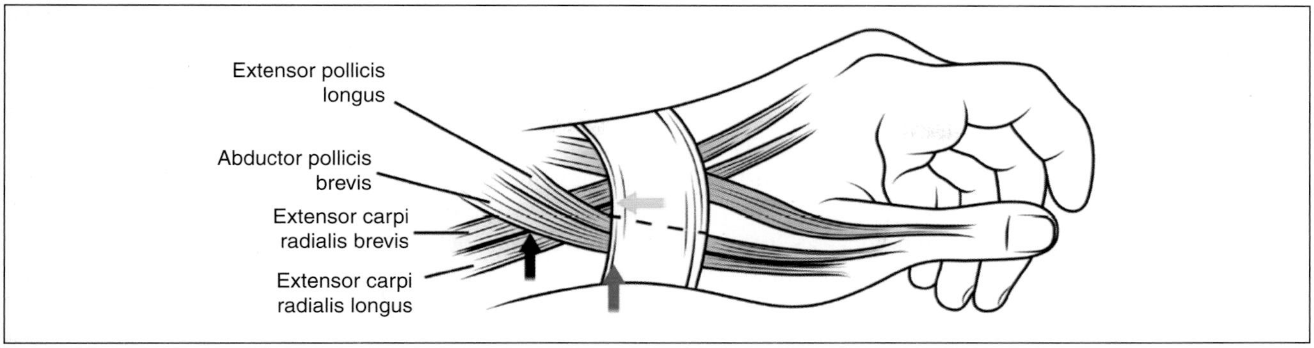

Figure 4 Illustration demonstrating the anatomy of the first (blue arrow) and second (yellow arrow) dorsal compartments, differentiating the locations of de Quervain syndrome (blue arrow) and intersection syndrome (black arrow). (Reproduced with permission from Adams JE, Habbu R: Tendinopathies of the hand and wrist. *J Am Acad Orthop* 2015;23[12]:741-750. doi:10.5435/JAAOS-D-14-00216.)

the point of intersection. In cases in which conservative treatment fails, surgical release is an option. Surgical treatment involves releasing the second dorsal compartment distal to the point of intersection, but there is scant published literature reporting clinical outcomes.[56]

Extensor Carpi Ulnaris Tenosynovitis

ECU tenosynovitis is a relatively common cause of ulnar-sided wrist pain. Similar to the first dorsal compartment, the sixth dorsal compartment of the wrist has a well-developed, separate fibro-osseous canal for the ECU tendon that is distinct from that of the second through fifth compartments of the wrist. ECU tenosynovitis can be difficult to differentiate from triangular fibrocartilage complex (TFCC) pathology as the source of ulnar-sided wrist pain because the ECU and its subsheath are in close proximity to each other. Additionally, it is important to differentiate between ECU tendinitis and ECU instability/subluxation, as these two conditions are treated differently.

Patient history can be helpful in this differentiation. ECU subluxation is often the result of a traumatic injury in which the ECU subsheath overlying the distal ulna ruptures whereas ECU tendinitis typically occurs following overuse, particularly athletes using a club or racquet, or may be idiopathic in nature. Patients will complain of pain and swelling on the ulnar side of the wrist that is exacerbated with gripping or wrist extension.

Physical examination typically reveals swelling of the ECU tendon and point tenderness over the tendon sheath at the level of the distal ulna. The ECU synergy test has been described to differentiate between ECU pathology and TFCC or other intra-articular pathology.[59] This involves grasping the patient's thumb and long fingers and asking the patient to radially deviate the thumb against resistance with the forearm supinated. The examiner's other hand palpates the ECU and the flexor carpi ulnaris. Pain with this maneuver suggests ECU pathology rather than TFCC pathology.

Imaging studies can be helpful in the workup of ECU tenosynovitis, as they are in general workup of ulnar-sided wrist pain. Radiographs as well as PA grip view may be helpful to evaluate positive ulnar variance that may be seen in ulnar impaction syndrome. In addition to ruling out other possible sources of ulnar-sided wrist pain, MRI may be helpful in the differentiation of isolated ECU tenosynovitis versus ECU subluxation in which rupture of the ECU subsheath and/or dislocation of the ECU tendon may be seen (**Figure 5**). Dynamic ultrasonography can be helpful to rule out ECU subluxation and has the benefit that examination of the contralateral wrist can be performed for comparison.

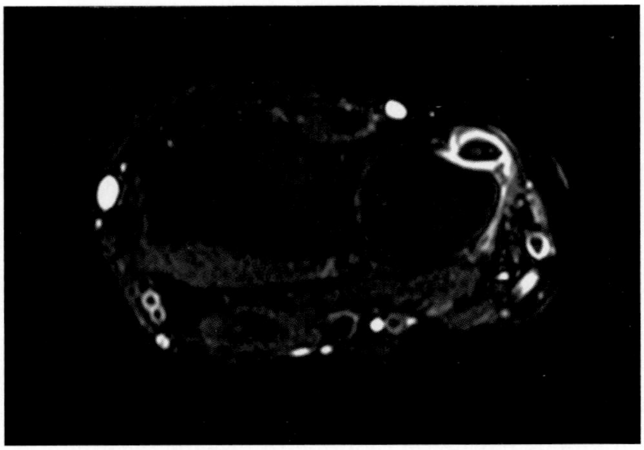

Figure 5 Axial T2-MRI demonstrates peritendinous fluid deep to the subsheath tracking below the overlying extensor retinaculum with extensor carpi ulnaris (ECU) tenosynovitis with surrounding subsheath disruption at the level of the osseous sulcus. (Reprinted from Ruchelsman DE, Vitale MA: Extensor carpi ulnaris subsheath reconstruction. *J Hand Surg Am* 2016;41[11]:e433-e439, Copyright 2016, with permission from Elsevier.)

Conservative treatment includes NSAIDs, activity modification, immobilization, and hand therapy. Corticosteroid injections can be useful both therapeutically and also diagnostically in the workup of other sources of ulnar-sided wrist pain, although ECU tendon rupture has been reported with local corticosteroid injections.

Surgical treatment is considered in cases of failed conservative management. This is accomplished via a dorsal approach over the sixth extensor compartment with release of the sixth compartment subsheath. While symptomatic ECU instability is a concern, studies have not reported tendon subluxation regardless of whether the sheath or retinaculum was repaired. In the setting of a subluxating ECU, the tendon may be stabilized by creating a pulley from the retinaculum after the ECU has been released from its sheath. A number of techniques have been described, but one recently described technique involves reconstructing the subsheath with a radially based extensor retinacular sling and planing the dorsoradial wall of the ulnar groove to prevent snapping of the ECU.[60]

Flexor Tendinopathies

Stenosing Flexor Tenosynovitis

Also known as trigger finger, stenosing flexor tenosynovitis of the A_1 pulley is the most common tendinopathy seen, with about a 2% to 3% prevalence. Various demographic factors may play a role. A higher incidence is in patients with DM, RA, and in women. In this condition, changes occur in the pulley system, including thickening of the A_1 pulley as well as the flexor tendons, most notably in the FDP (**Figure 1**). There is believed to be a multifactorial etiology, with genetic factors, systemic conditions such as renal insufficiency, thyroid disease, RA and DM, and occupational exposure.

Patients may present with pain at the level of the A_1 pulley, swelling, triggering, or locking of the affected digit. Patients often report worsening of locking of their affected digit at nighttime or early in the morning. Physical examination may show tenderness over the A_1 pulley, triggering provoked with digital compression of the A_1 pulley, and in chronic cases a PIP joint contracture.

Initial conservative management may include NSAIDs, splinting, hand therapy, and corticosteroid injections. Splints immobilizing either the MCP, PIP, or DIP joints have been reported to provide relief in 40% to 87% of cases.[61-63] Splinting may be cumbersome and prolonged use may cause digital stiffness. Supervised hand therapy often attempts to develop differential gliding between the FDS and FDP tendons, and one randomized controlled trial found that therapy had a 69% success rate at 3 months.[64]

Corticosteroid injections into the A_1 pulley region or flexor tendon sheath have been shown to be highly successful. Recurrence of symptoms is more common in the setting of DM, multiple affected digits, and other associated tendinopathies. Complications of corticosteroid injections may include fat atrophy, temporary elevation of blood glucose in diabetic patients, and rarely tendon or pulley rupture. The administration of trigger finger injections may cause substantial pain and anxiety as well. A prospective randomized controlled trial in 2017 evaluated the efficacy of administration of needle-free jet 2% lidocaine for pain reduction prior to corticosteroid injection compared with simultaneous 1% lidocaine injection with corticosteroid through a single syringe.[65] Patients treated with the needle-free jet lidocaine had significantly lower mean pain scores on a visual analog score compared with those in the control group (3.3 versus 4.6 visual analog scale). Patients also had a higher expected pain preinjection than they actually experienced postinjection.

The long-term efficacy of corticosteroid injections for trigger finger has been studied. One retrospective case series examined 366 first-time corticosteroid injections for trigger fingers with a minimum follow-up of 5 years.[66] The authors reported a 45% overall long-term success rate after a single injection at the time of latest follow-up. Eighty-four percent of treatment failures occurred in the first 2 years, suggesting that patients who continue to experience symptoms relief 2 years after injection are likely to maintain long-term success. Another more recent retrospective study investigated the long-term efficacy of repeat corticosteroid injections for trigger finger.[67] This series analyzed 292 cases of repeat corticosteroid injections for trigger fingers. Second injections provided long-term treatment success in 39% of trigger fingers. Of those receiving a third injection, 39% had long-term success. Median times-to-failure for second and third injections were 371 and 407 days, respectively. Advancing age and injection for trigger thumb were associated with success of second injections.

Surgical treatment is considered when conservative management fails. Open and percutaneous techniques have been used to release the A_1 pulley. Open release is the most well-established technique and is associated with a high proportion of excellent results. In 2017, a randomized controlled trial compared the results of ultrasonography-guided corticosteroid injection versus open surgical release in a group of 165 patients.[68] At 12 months, the study showed a 49% and 99% success rate after injection and surgical treatment, respectively, with a significantly higher pain score in the corticosteroid injection group at latest follow-up. There were, however, more severe complications after surgery, including 3 wound infections and 1 iatrogenic nerve injury following surgery compared with 11 steroid flare reactions and 2 instances of fat necrosis following injections.

A recent decision analysis compared the costs associated with immediate surgery versus attempted corticosteroid injection in diabetic patients given the high rate of failure of corticosteroid injections in diabetic patients.[69] The results showed that initial surgical release was the least costly treatment (overall cost $642), which resulted in a 32% and 39% cost reduction when compared with treatment with one or two corticosteroid injections, respectively.

The rising popularity of wide-awake analgesia specifically for A_1 pulley release offers the advantages allowing assessment of active finger motion after release to confirm the lack of triggering after release, in addition to avoiding the risks of anesthesia and being more cost effective.[23] If the finger still triggers after A_1 release, additional pathology such as an A_0 pulley—a stenosing portion of the superficial palmar fascia—or structural changes in the FDS or FDP should be investigated. Complications of open release include injury to the neurovascular bundles, wound complications, stiffness, and bowstringing if the A_2 pulley is complete divided.

Percutaneous release of the A_1 pulley may be done with various instruments including hypodermic needles, knife blades, or special percutaneous devices with or without ultrasonography guidance. Cadaveric studies have demonstrated that the A_1 pulley can be safely divided without injury to adjacent tendinous or neurovascular structures. For instance, a 2016 cadaveric study of 155 digits of unembalmed cadavers with restored perfusion investigated percutaneous A_1 release with an 18-gauge needle with and without ultrasonography guidance.[70] Seventy-four percent of A_1 pulleys were completely released, 24% were partially released, and 2% were not released. There were no complete tendon injuries, but 23% of specimens had scoring of the flexor tendon. There were no digital nerve lacerations, but there was one digital artery laceration (1%). There was no difference in successful pulley release rates or injury rates between ultrasonography-assisted and blind percutaneous release techniques.

Summary

The treatment of flexor and extensor tendon injuries to the hand has evolved over the years based on a large body of basic science and clinical investigation. Zone II flexor tendon injuries still represent the greatest technical and rehabilitation challenge. The treatment of extensor tendon injuries is generally technically easier and results in better clinical outcomes overall compared with flexor tendon injuries, although surgical techniques, materials, and rehabilitation protocols continue to evolve. Biologic modifications to accelerate healing and rehabilitation may be the next major advance to improve the care for flexor and extensor tendon injuries. Diagnosis and management of tendinopathies of the hand and wrist, including tenosynovitis of the first through sixth dorsal compartments and trigger finger, is relatively straightforward, but future research is needed to determine optimal management.

Key Study Points

- While zone II flexor tendon injuries challenge the surgeon, therapist, and patient, multistrand repair (≥4 core strands) and early motion protocols result in functional outcomes.
- In the setting of chronic flexor or extensor tendon injuries of the hand and wrist, one- or two-stage tendon reconstruction techniques should be used instead of tendon repair.
- Wide-awake analgesia has allowed for intraoperative assessment of flexor or extensor tendon repair/reconstruction as well as surgical treatment of tendinopathies of the hand and wrist and is a safe and cost-effective alternative to intravenous sedation or general anesthesia.
- Tendinopathies of the flexor and extensor tendons of the hand and wrist are common conditions that may be managed conservatively with immobilization, NSAIDs, therapy, and corticosteroid injections, and surgical treatment typically involves release of the associated tendon sheath.

Annotated References

1. Schubert MF, Shah VS, Craig CL, Zeller JL: Varied anatomy of the thumb pulley system: Implications for successful trigger thumb release. *J Hand Surg Am* 2012;37(11):2278-2285.

2. Kleinert HE, Verdan C: Report of the Committee on Tendon Injuries (International Federation of Societies for Surgery of the Hand). *J Hand Surg Am* 1983;8(5 pt 2):794-798.

3. Trumble TE, Vedder NB, Benirschke SK: Misleading fractures after profundus tendon avulsions: A report of six cases. *J Hand Surg Am* 1992;17(5):902-906.

Hand and Wrist

4. Al-Qattan MM: Type 5 avulsion of the insertion of the flexor digitorum profundus tendon. *J Hand Surg Am* 2001;26(5):427-431.

5. McCallister WV, Ambrose HC, Katolik LI, Trumble TE: Comparison of pullout button versus suture anchor for zone I flexor tendon repair. *J Hand Surg Am* 2006;31(2): 246-251.

6. Lee SK, Fajardo M, Kardashian G, Klein J, Tsai P, Christoforou D: Repair of flexor digitorum profundus to distal phalanx: A biomechanical evaluation of four techniques. *J Hand Surg Am* 2011;36(10):1604-1609.

7. Taras JS, Raphael JS, Marczyk SC, Bauerle WB: Evaluation of suture caliber in flexor tendon repair. *J Hand Surg Am* 2001;26(6):1100-1104.

8. Osei DA, Stepan JG, Calfee RP, et al: The effect of suture caliber and number of core suture strands on zone II flexor tendon repair: A study in human cadavers. *J Hand Surg Am* 2014;39(2):262-268.

9. Bernstein DT, Alexander JJ, Petersen NJ, Lambert BS, Noble PC, Netscher DT: The impact of suture caliber and looped configurations on the suture-tendon interface in zone II flexor tendon repair. *J Hand Surg Am* 2019;44(2):156.e1-156.e8

   A cadaveric study of 4-strand flexor tendon repairs determined that 3-0 caliper suture failed more frequently by suture pullout under progressive cyclic loading compared with a 4-0 caliper suture. Level of evidence: NA (cadaveric study).

10. Gil JA, Skjong C, Katarincic JA, Got C: Flexor tendon repair with looped suture: 1 versus 2 knots. *J Hand Surg Am* 2016;41(3):422-426.

    Cadaveric study of flexor tendon repairs determined that two knots did not increase repair strength compared to one knot. Level of evidence: NA (cadaveric study).

11. Kang GH, Wong YR, Lim RQ, Loke AM, Tay SC: Cyclic testing of the 6-strand Tang and modified Lim-Tsai flexor tendon repair techniques. *J Hand Surg Am* 2018;43(3):285. e1-285.e6.

    Porcine tendon study that identified that the Tang repair was stronger than the modified Lim-Tsai repair with cyclic loading. Level of evidence: NA (animal study).

12. Kozono N, Okada T, Takeuchi N, Shimoto T, Higaki H, Nakashima Y: A biomechanical comparison between asymmetric Pennington technique and conventional core suture techniques: 6-strand flexor tendon repair. *J Hand Surg Am* 2018;43(1):79.e1-79.e8.

    Tendon study comparing six-strand core repair strengths. The asymmetric Pennington technique resulted in increase repair strength and reduced gap formation. Level of evidence: NA (cadaveric study).

13. Prowse P, Nixon M, Constantinides J, Hunter J, Henry A, Feldberg L: Outcome of zone 2 flexor tendon injuries: Kleinert versus controlled active motion therapy regimens. *Hand Ther* 2011;16(4):102-106.

14. Zhao C, Amadio PC, Zobitz ME, An K-N: Gliding characteristics of tendon repair in canine flexor digitorum profundus tendons. *J Orthop Res* 2001;19(4):580-586.

15. Zhao C, Amadio PC, Zobitz ME, An K-N: Resection of the flexor digitorum superficialis reduces gliding resistance after zone II flexor digitorum profundus repair in vitro. *J Hand Surg Am* 2002;27(2):316-321.

16. Shin JY, Kim JS, Roh S-G, Lee N-H, Yang K-M: Biomechanical analysis of barbed suture in flexor tendon repair versus conventional method. *Plast Reconstr Surg* 2016;138(4):666e-674e.

    Systematic review and meta-analysis of flexor tendon literature was performed to examine barbed suture use. The authors concluded that barbed sutures were similar to conventional suture regarding ultimate strength and gap force. Level of evidence: V.

17. O'Brien FP, Parks BG, Tsai MA, Means KR: A knotless bidirectional-barbed tendon repair is inferior to conventional 4-strand repairs in cyclic loading. *J Hand Surg Eur* 2016;41(8):809-814.

    This tendon repair study performed zone II repairs and determined that barbed sutures were inferior to cruciate repairs with 4-0 suture. Level of evidence: NA (cadaveric study).

18. Bunata RE, Simmons S, Roso M, Kosmopoulos V: Gliding resistance and triggering after venting or A2 pulley enlargement: A study of intact and repaired flexor tendons in a cadaveric model. *J Hand Surg Am* 2011;36(8):1316-1322.

19. Paillard PJ, Amadio PC, Zhao C, Zobitz ME, An KN: Pulley plasty versus resection of one slip of the flexor digitorum superficialis after repair of both flexor tendons in zone II: A biomechanical study. *J Bone Joint Surg Am* 2002;84-A(11):2039-2045.

20. Tang JB, Xie RG, Cao Y, Ke ZS, Xu Y: A2 pulley incision or one slip of the superficialis improves flexor tendon repairs. *Clin Orthop Rel Res* 2007;456:121-127.

21. Cao Y, Tang JB: Strength of tendon repair decreases in the presence of an intact A2 pulley: Biomechanical study in a chicken model. *J Hand Surg Am* 2009;34(10):1763-1770.

22. Moriya K, Yoshizu T, Tsubokawa N, Narisawa H, Hara K, Maki Y: Clinical results of releasing the entire A2 pulley after flexor tendon repair in zone 2C. *J Hand Surg Eur* 2016;41(8):822-828.

    This case series reported overall positive results after flexor tendon repairs that required A2 pulley releases. Level of evidence: IV.

23. Lalonde D, Bell M, Benoit P, Sparkes G, Denkler K, Chang P: A multicenter prospective study of 3,110 consecutive cases of elective epinephrine use in the fingers and hand: The Dalhousie Project clinical phase. *J Hand Surg Am* 2005;30(5):1061-1067.

24. Higgins A, Lalonde DH, Bell M, McKee D, Lalonde JF: Avoiding flexor tendon repair rupture with intraoperative total active movement examination. *Plast Reconstr Surg* 2010;126(3):941-945.

25. Zhao C, Sun Y-L, Kirk RL, et al: Effects of a lubricin-containing compound on the results of flexor tendon repair in a canine model in vivo. *J Bone Joint Surg Am* 2010;92(6):1453-1461.

26. Zhao C, Ozasa Y, Reisdorf RL, et al: Engineering flexor tendon repair with lubricant, cells, and cytokines in a canine model. *Clin Orthop Rel Res* 2014;472(9): 2569-2578.

27. Linderman SW, Kormpakis I, Gelberman RH, et al: Shear lag sutures: Improved suture repair through the use of adhesives. *Acta Biomater* 2015;23:229-239.

28. Thoreson AR, Hiwatari R, An K-N, Amadio PC, Zhao C: The effect of 1-ethyl-3-(3-dimethylaminopropyl) carbodiimide suture coating on tendon repair strength and cell viability in a canine model. *J Hand Surg Am* 2015;40(10): 1986-1991.

29. Linderman SW, Gelberman RH, Thomopoulos S, Shen H: Cell and biologic-based treatment of flexor tendon injuries. *Oper Tech Orthop* 2016;26(3):206-215.

This review article discusses the use of biologic and cellular adjuncts to improve flexor tendon repairs in an effort to reduce complications. Level of evidence: NA (review article).

30. Wei Z, Reisdorf RL, Thoreson AR, et al: Comparison of autograft and allograft with surface modification for flexor tendon reconstruction: A canine in vivo model. *J Bone Joint Surg Am* 2018;100(7):e42.

This canine tendon study examined FDP reconstructions. They found that intrasynovial allografts with surface modification reduced adhesions but had impaired healing compared to use of an extrasynovial autograft. Level of evidence: NA (animal study).

31. Trumble TE, Vedder NB, Seiler JG, Hanel DP, Diao E, Pettrone S: Zone-II flexor tendon repair: A randomized prospective trial of active place-and-hold therapy compared with passive motion therapy. *J Bone Joint Surg Am* 2010;92(6):1381-1389.

32. Gibson PD, Sobol GL, Ahmed IH: Zone II flexor tendon repairs in the United States: Trends in current management. *J Hand Surg Am* 2017;42(2):e99-e108.

This study surveyed hand surgeons and determined that most reported using a four-strand repair with either 3-0 or 4-0 suture. Variability existed among surgeons for preferred rehabilitation. Level of evidence: NA (survey).

33. Dezfuli B, Taljanovic MS, Melville DM, Krupinski EA, Sheppard JE: Accuracy of high-resolution ultrasonography in the detection of extensor tendon lacerations. *Ann Plast Surg* 2016;76(2):187-192.

A cadaveric study evaluating the ability of static and dynamic ultrasound to differentiate between lacerated extensor tendons and nonlacerated controls. Sensitivities, specificities, and positive predictive values of 88%, 89%, and 0.88 for static imaging and 100%, 100%, and 1.0 for dynamic imaging, respectively, were obtained. Level of evidence: NA (cadaveric study).

34. Simonian M, Dan M, Graan D, Lumsdaine W, Meads B: Suture and splint compared with k-wire fixation for open zone 1 extensor tendon injuries. *Ann Plast Surg* 2018;81(2):176-177.

A retrospective cohort analysis between zone 1 extensor tendon injuries treated with suture repair and splinting with or without supplemental K-wire fixation was performed. Final outcomes did not differ with regard to range of motion or splint time, but the K-wire group had an increased flexor lag. Level of evidence: III.

35. Namazi H, Mozaffarian K, Golmakani MR: Comparison of roll stitch technique and core suture technique for extensor tendon repair at the metacarpophalangeal joint level. *Trauma Mon* 2016;21(1):e24563.

Patients with extensor tendon lacerations at the MCP joint repaired with either a roll stitch technique had superior outcomes to those treated with a modified Kessler technique. Level of evidence: III.

36. Al-Qattan MM: Conservative management of partial extensor tendon lacerations greater than half the width of the tendon in manual workers. *Ann Plast Surg* 2015;74(4):408-409.

37. Barr JS, Schneider L, Sharma S: Reconstruction of a functional gliding surface with extensor retinaculum in extensor tendon reconstruction in the digits. *Ann Plast Surg* 2014;72(2):155-158.

38. Lee JH, Baek JH, Lee JS: A reconstructive stabilization technique for nontraumatic or chronic traumatic extensor tendon subluxation. *J Hand Surg Am* 2017;42(1):e61-e65.

A surgical technique article utilizing a ruptured residual portion of the sagittal band for reconstruction of extensor tendon subluxation. Level of evidence: IV.

39. Pierrart J, Tordjman D, Otayek S, Douard R, Mahjoubi L, Masmejean E: Two-stage extensor tendon graft using the Paneva-Holevitch procedure: A new technique. *Hand Surg Rehabil* 2018;37(1):12-15.

A cadaveric feasibility study evaluating the Paneva-Holevitch technique for extensor tendon repairs. Level of evidence: NA (cadaveric study).

40. Al-Qattan MM: Two-staged extensor tendon reconstruction for zone 6 extensor tendon loss of the fingers: Indications, technique and results. *J Hand Surg Eur* 2015;40(3):276-280.

41. Collocott SJ, Kelly E, Ellis RF: Optimal early active mobilisation protocol after extensor tendon repairs in zones V and VI: A systematic review of literature. *Hand Ther* 2018;23(1):3-18.

A systematic review comparing the results of controlled active motion protocols compared with relative motion extension splinting protocols after extensor tendon repair in zones V and VI. End results were similar, but relative motion extension splinting protocols provided an earlier return to work. Level of evidence: NA (systematic review).

42. Wong AL, Wilson M, Girnary S, Nojoomi M, Acharya S, Paul SM: The optimal orthosis and motion protocol for extensor tendon injury in zones IV-VIII: A systematic review. *J Hand Ther* 2017;30(4):447-456.

A systematic review comparing extensor tendon rehabilitation protocols demonstrating early active motion to be the more favorable rehabilitation technique. Level of evidence: NA (systematic review).

43. Svens B, Ames E, Burford K, Caplash Y: Relative active motion programs following extensor tendon repair: A pilot study using a prospective cohort and evaluating outcomes following orthotic interventions. *J Hand Ther* 2015;28(1):11-18.

44. Elliot BG: Finkelstein's test: A descriptive error that can produce a false positive. *J Hand Surg Br* 1992;17(4):481-482.

45. Alexander RD, Catalano LW, Barron OA, Glickel SZ: The extensor pollicis brevis entrapment test in the treatment of de Quervain's disease. *J Hand Surg Am* 2002;27(5):813-816.

46. Goubau JF, Gobau L, Van Tongel A, Van Hoonacker P, Kerckhove D, Berghs B: The wrist hyperflexion and abduction of the thumb (WHAT) test: A more specific and sensitive test to diagnose de Quervain tenosynovitis than the Eichhoff's test. *J Hand Surg Eur* 2014;39(3):286-292.

47. Richie CA III, Briner WW Jr: Corticosteroid injection for treatment of de Quervain's tenosynovitis: A pooled quantitative literature evaluation. *J Am Board Fam Pract* 2003;16(2):102-106.

48. Earp BE, Han CH, Floyd E, Rozental TD, Blazar PE: de Quervain tendinopathy: Survivorship and prognostic indicators of recurrence following a single corticosteroid injection. *J Hand Surg Am* 2015;40(6):1161-1165.

49. Hartzell TL, Rubinstein R, Herman M: Therapeutic modalities – An updated review for the hand surgeon. *J Hand Surg Am* 2012;37(3):597-621.

50. Read HS, Hooper G, Davie R: Histological appearance in postpartum de Quervain's disease. *J Hand Surg Br* 2000;25(1):70-72.

51. Mardani-Kivi M, Mobarakeh MK, Bahrami F, Hashemi-Mortlagh K, Saheb-Ekhtiari K, Akhoondzadeh N: Corticosteroid injection with or without thumb spica cast for de Quervain tenosynovitis. *J Hand Surg Am* 2014;39(1):37-41.

52. Witzak JW, Masear VR, Meyer RD: Triggering of the thumb with de Quervain's stenosing tendovaginitis. *J Hand Surg Am* 1990;15(2):265-268.

53. Pace CS, Blanchet NP, Isaacs JE: Soft tissue atrophy related to corticosteroid injection: Review of the literature and implications for hand surgeons. *J Hand Surg Am* 2018;43(6):558-563.

An analysis of the incidence of soft-tissue complications from corticosteroid injections encountered by hand surgeons, with a discussion of the underlying pathophysiology of soft-tissue atrophy and treatment strategies. Level of evidence: V.

54. Kutsikovich J, Merrell G: Accuracy of injection into the first dorsal compartment: A cadaveric ultrasound study. *J Hand Surg Am* 2018;43(8):777.e1-777.e5.

A cadaveric investigation of the accuracy of ultrasonography- versus anatomic-guided injections into the first dorsal compartment in specimen with and without a septated first dorsal compartment. Ultrasonography did not increase the accuracy of injections overall, but there was a nonstatistically significant increase in the rate of successful injection into a septated compartment with use of ultrasound. Level of evidence: NA (cadaveric study).

55. Kazmers NH, Liu TC, Gordon JA, Bozentka DJ, Steinberg DR, Gray BL: Patient- and disease-specific factors associated with operative management of de Quervain tendinopathy. *J Hand Surg Am* 2017;42(11):931.e1-931.e7.

The patient- and disease-specific factors influencing the decision to seek surgical management of de Quervain syndrome was analyzed in a retrospective review of 200 patients. Regression analysis identified that those with Medicaid insurance and psychiatric illness were associated with surgical treatment, supporting the use of a biopsychosocial framework when treating patients. Level of evidence: IV.

56. Grundberg AB, Regan DS: Pathologic anatomy of the forearm: Intersection syndrome. *J Hand Surg Am* 1985;10(2):299-302.

57. Andring N, Kennedy SA, Iannuzzi NP: Anomalous forearm muscles and their clinical relevance. *J Hand Surg Am* 2018;43(5):455-463.

A review of the most common anomalous forearm muscles encountered and the implications of management of symptomatic anomalous muscles. Level of evidence: NA (review article).

58. Strickland JW, Idler RS, Creighton JC: de Quervain's stenosing tenosynovitis. *Indiana Med* 1990;83(5):340-341.

59. Ruland RT, Hogan CJ: The ECU synergy test: An aid to diagnose ECU tendonitis. *J Hand Surg Am* 2008;33(10):1777-1782.

60. Ruchelsman DE, Vitale MA: Extensor carpi ulnaris subsheath reconstruction. *J Hand Surg Am* 2016;41(11):e433-e439.

A review of ECU subsheath injury and a description of a novel ECU subsheath reconstruction technique for symptomatic ECU tendon instability. Level of evidence: V.

61. Valdes K: A retrospective review to determine the long-term efficacy of orthotic devices for trigger finger. *J Hand Ther* 2012;25(1):89-95.

62. Colbourn J, Heath N, Manary S, Pacifico D: Effectiveness of splinting for the treatment of trigger finger. *J Hand Ther* 2008;21(4):336-343.

63. Rodgers JA, McCarthy JA, Tiedeman JJ: Functional distal interphalangeal joint splinting for trigger finger in laborers: A review and cadaver investigation. *Orthopedics* 1998;21(3):305-309.

64. Salim N, Abdullah S, Sapuan J, Haflah NH: Outcome of corticosteroid injection versus physiotherapy in the treatment of mild trigger fingers. *J Hand Surg Eur* 2012;37(1):27-34.

65. Earp BE, Stanbury SJ, Mora AN, Blazar PE: Needle-free jet lidocaine administration for preinjection anesthesia in trigger finger injection: A randomized controlled trial. *J Hand Surg Am* 2017;42(8):618-622.

A prospective randomized trial of pain and anxiety of patients receiving trigger finger injections with or without a needle-free topical J-tip lidocaine application prior to injection showed that use of the J-tip demonstrated a lower mean pain. Both groups also anticipated more pain than they actually experienced. Level of evidence: I.

66. Wojahn RD, Foeger NC, Gelberman RH, Calfee RP: Long-term outcomes following a single corticosteroid injection for trigger finger. *J Bone Joint Surg Am* 2014;96(22):1849-1854.

67. Dardas AZ, Vandenberg J, Shen T, Gelberman RH, Calfee RP: Long-term effectiveness of repeat corticosteroid injections for trigger finger. *J Hand Surg Am* 2017;42(4):227-235.

A retrospective case series of 292 patients with repeat corticosteroid injections to determine the long-term success rate of repeat injections for trigger fingers and to identify predictors of success. Thirty-nine percent of second and third corticosteroid injections for trigger finger yielded long-term relief. Level of evidence: IV.

68. Hansen RL, Sondergaard M, Lange J: Open surgery versus ultrasound-guided corticosteroid injection for trigger finger: A randomized trial with 1-year follow-up. *J Hand Surg Am* 2017;42(5):359-366.

This randomized controlled trial analyzed 165 patients that received wither open surgery or ultrasonography-guided corticosteroid injection with 1-year follow-up. Open surgery was superior to ultrasound-guided corticosteroid injections, but complications with surgery were more severe. Level of evidence: I.

69. Luther GA, Murthy P, Blazar PE: Cost of immediate surgery versus non-operative treatment for trigger finger in diabetic patients. *J Hand Surg Am* 2016;41(11):1056-1063.

This cost analysis identified four treatment strategies: (1) one steroid injection followed by surgery, (2) two steroid injections followed by surgery, (3) immediate surgery in the operating room, and (4) immediate surgery in the clinic. The results showed that the least costly strategy was immediate surgery in the clinic, assuming a corticosteroid injection failure rate of at least 34%. Level of evidence: NA (economic analysis).

70. Hoang D, Lin AC, Essilfie A, et al: Evaluation of percutaneous first annular pulley release: Efficacy and complications in a perfused cadaveric study. *J Hand Surg Am* 2016;41(7):e165-e173.

A perfused cadaveric model of 155 digits was used to determine the efficacy and safety of percutaneous A_1 pulley release with an 18-gauge needle. There were 74% of A_1 pulleys completely released, and there were no significant digital artery or flexor tendon lacerations, but scoring of the flexor tendon was seen in 23% of cases, and 1% of digital arteries were lacerated. Level of evidence: NA (cadaveric study).

Chapter 33

Hand and Wrist Reconstruction: Microsurgery and Replantation

Peter C. Rhee, DO, MSc • Rudolph H. Houben, MD • Allen T. Bishop, MD

ABSTRACT

The mangled upper extremity consists of severe injuries to the bone, soft tissues, vessels, and/or nerves with associated contamination. Management of the mutilated hand and wrist starts with a thorough assessment of injured structures and should focus on radical initial wound débridement and excision of nonviable tissue. A goal-directed approach should be maintained to systematically reconstruct the upper extremity while preventing infectious complications, minimizing residual deformity, and restoring function. When amputations are present, adherence to the principles of replantation and revascularization can result in successful limb salvage.

Keywords: Amputation; damage control; débridement; limb salvage; mangled upper extremity; replantation; revascularization

Introduction

The mangled upper extremity can pose tremendous challenges in the acute and reconstructive stages. A mangled upper extremity is defined by trauma that results in severe injuries to three of four tissue types, such as bone, soft tissues, vessels, and nerves.[1] The trauma is typically a result of a high-energy injury with a crushing, tearing, and/or cutting mechanism that is often associated with marked contamination and segmental loss of the previously mentioned tissue types.[2] Successful reconstruction of the mangled upper extremity is largely based upon the outcomes of the initial surgical treatment that in turn is dependent on the adequacy of débridement. Once a stable bony framework and a clean, viable wound bed have been established, staged reconstruction can be performed toward the goal of achieving a functional upper extremity.

Reconstruction of the Traumatized Hand and Wrist: Principles of Treatment

Goals of Treatment

The primary goal in managing the patient with a mangled upper extremity is to preserve life. Often in the setting of the mangled upper extremity, patients may have sustained other life-threatening injuries, thus "life before limb" always remains the chief priority. In line with preservation of life, all sources of hemorrhage must be emergently controlled with pressure, tourniquets, or direct vessel ligation to prevent fatal exsanguination. In severe cases, a completion amputation should be considered in the hemodynamically unstable patient with a hemorrhagic, mangled upper extremity.[3] Otherwise, the guidelines set forth by the Advanced Trauma Life Support program should be followed.

An early assessment of the viability of the injured upper extremity will provide a clear indication between attempting limb salvage or proceeding with early complete amputation. Careful consideration should be performed to determine if the morbidity of multiple failed attempts at reconstruction or the limited function that can be expected with limb salvage outweigh the benefits of proceeding directly to a primary amputation.[3] However, unless the mutilated upper extremity is clearly beyond the indication for limb salvage, the initial management should be directed toward limb salvage.

Acute management of the mangled upper extremity must be goal-oriented which includes preventing infectious complications, minimizing residual disability, and restoring function. An important concept in limb salvage

Dr. Rhee or an immediate family member is a member of a speakers' bureau or has made paid presentations on behalf of Trimed and serves as a board member, owner, officer, or committee member of the American Association for Hand Surgery, the American Society for Surgery of the Hand, and the Clinical Orthopaedic Society. Neither of the following authors nor any immediate family member has received anything of value from or has stock or stock options held in a commercial company or institution related directly or indirectly to the subject of this chapter: Dr. Houben and Dr. Bishop.

requiring multiple staged procedures is that the surgeon who will be performing the limb reconstruction should be involved in surgical planning from the initial débridement. The reconstructive surgeon must visualize the end result and the pathway in which that can be achieved.[4] Thus, staged procedures, such as incisions, skeletal fixation, vascular repair, and soft tissue coverage, can be strategically planned in a sequential fashion toward the end goal without inadvertently eliminating a surgical option secondary to poor and disjointed planning.

Biomechanics of Hand Function

Understanding the functional role of each digit in the hand is necessary when initially managing the mutilated hand. The index and long fingers serve as stable posts upon which an opposable thumb can perform various forms of pinch. Ulnarly, the ring and small finger act as mobile units, afforded though the motion at the carpometacarpal joints, to perform several forms of grasp. Lastly, the hand rests upon the wrist that positions the hand in space and can optimize digit function and strength.

To perform basic tasks, the mutilated hand must be reconstructed with some structural principles. At a minimum, the hand requires a stable wrist with two opposing digits that are stable enough to withstand the force of pinch.[5] In addition, a cleft must be present between the two digits to accommodate prehensile movement and the digits must be pain-free and senate. Most importantly, a stable wrist is mandatory to preserve the forces generated by the extrinsic flexor and extensor tendons that are exerted onto the remaining digits. Although loss of the thumb can be restored with free toe-to-thumb transfer, the highest priority should be toward salvaging the thumb given the fact that its loss results in a 40% loss of function and 25% loss of total body function.[6]

Patient Assessment

Patient Characteristics

The patient's preinjury functional status, occupation, handedness, general medical status, psychology, and socioeconomic status are important factors that influence the results of reconstructing the mangled upper extremity.[7] Additionally, comorbidities such as diabetes or cardiopulmonary disease can affect the outcomes of limb salvage as well and should be considered in the overall assessment of the patient.[6,8] All of these factors, in concert, will determine the physiologic drive of the patient to heal their injuries and to participate in the rehabilitation after their definitive reconstructive procedures.

Injury Characteristics

The mechanism of injury is another important factor when determining the appropriate management of the mutilated hand and wrist. The zone of injury from a sharp penetrating mechanism will be considerably less than that of a blast injury. Similarly, a crush injury will typically not have the degree of contamination as an agricultural or industrial injury. These various mechanisms have implications on the management of associated skeletal, neurovascular, and soft-tissue injuries. Additionally, time from injury to presentation is also of importance since irreversible tissue necrosis can occur with prolonged ischemia. The recommended ischemia time prior to replantation or revascularization for the digits is 12 hours of warm and 24 hours of cold ischemia.[6] In more proximal levels of injury, 6 hours of warm and 12 hours of cold ischemia are the recommended limits for attempted limb salvage.[9]

Injury Severity Scores

Although predictive scores can be calculated to guide the decision for limb salvage versus primary amputation in the mangled lower limb, it may not be applicable to the upper extremity.[10] The Mangled Extremity Severity Score (MESS) takes into account the age of the patient, magnitude of shock based on the systolic blood pressure, limb ischemia, and the extent of bone and soft-tissue injuries to predict the success of limb salvage.[11] An injured limb with a MESS of seven points or higher is recommended to undergo amputation. However, the MESS was devised for the lower extremity that inherently has greater muscle mass and less collateral circulation than the upper extremity.

A hand specific injury severity score may be predictive of final outcome after limb salvage. The Hand Injury Severity Score (HISS) was developed to measure the extent of hand injuries and to permit comparisons of treatment results between institutions.[12] It takes into account the severity of injury to the skin, bone, tendon, and nerves of each finger with a score ranging from 0 (no injury) to 826 (maximum severity).[13] Matsuzaki et al noted that the HISS could be utilized to accurately predict the functional outcome and return to work status in patients who had sustained mutilating hand injuries.[13]

Initial Management

Damage control procedures in the acute stage include wound débridement, irrigation, bone stabilization, revascularization, fasciotomy, and temporizing soft-tissue coverage or placement of a negative-pressure wound therapy dressing. Upon initial evaluation, the patient should be administered intravenous antibiotics and tetanus toxoid. If the patient has not received a tetanus booster within the past 5 years, tetanus immunoglobulin is also administered.[14]

Wound Débridement

Although radical excision is the mainstay of initial wound débridement, marginal tissue should be preserved and excessive skin excision should be avoided in the initial débridement.[3] Color, consistency, contractility, and the capacity to bleed are the dogmatic tenets of assessing muscle viability; however, the surgeon's distinction of muscle viability in the mangled upper extremity is often incorrect. Sassoon et al[15] noted that in 35 muscle specimens that the surgeon declared as nonviable or necrotic, 21 (60%) specimens were identified as normal or mildly inflamed under histologic evaluation and were erroneously excised. Therefore, débridement should be aggressive; however, marginal tissue can be observed between serial débridement to allow for declaration of viability.

The principles of wound débridement are outlined in **Table 1**. Bone fragments with viable soft-tissue attachments and no significant contamination should be left in place to be utilized for later reconstruction.[3] In addition, intact longitudinal structures such as blood vessels, nerve, and tendons should be preserved to enhance final function in the hand.[3] In more proximal levels of injury where completion amputation may be necessary, the uninjured distal segment or the "spare part" can be utilized as a free tissue transfer to provide soft-tissue coverage to preserve residual limb length.[16] Similarly, vascularized skin flaps should not be excised as they can be utilized as fillet flaps to cover adjacent areas of soft-tissue loss (**Figure 1**).

If possible, wound débridement should be performed under tourniquet control to permit adequate visualization during wound exploration and to limit blood loss.[17] The bloodless field afforded through the use of a tourniquet allows for a thorough and expeditious exploration

Table 1

Principles of Initial Wound Management

1. Radical initial débridement
2. Restore tissue viability
3. Relieve the pressure of hematoma
4. Systematically inspect all structures
5. Preserve as much viable skin as possible
6. Preserve all surgical options

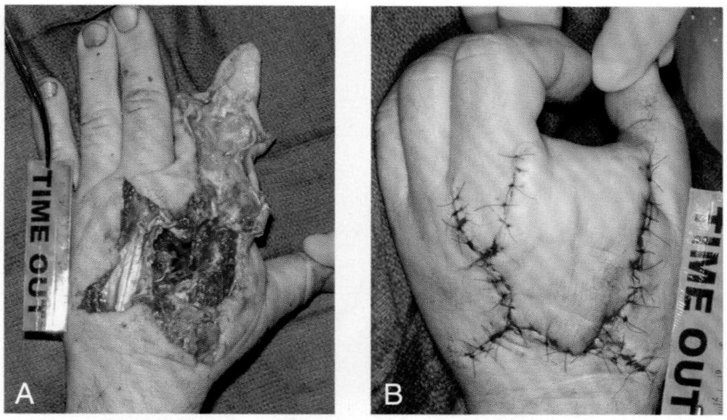

Figure 1 Photographs demonstrating the use of a vascularized skin as a fillet flap. Patient sustained traumatic loss of the second ray with preservation of the vascularized volar soft tissue (**A**). This skin flap was utilized to cover the area of soft-tissue loss on the dorsum of the hand (**B**).

of the wound to systematically evaluate and detect any injured structures.[2] Once all critical structures have been examined, release of the tourniquet and the resultant hyperemia will provide an assessment of tissue viability and declare those areas of nonviable tissue that should be radically excised.

High-pressure irrigation should not be performed in heavily contaminated wounds to prevent driving contaminants deeper into the tissues and causing pressure-related soft-tissue damage.[14] The addition of antibiotics or soap into the irrigation does not provide any supplementary benefit and may even lead to higher revision surgery rates.[18,19] It is recommended to irrigate the wound with copious amounts of sterile normal saline under a low-pressure system.

Skeletal Injuries

In the initial stage, fractures within the hand and wrist should be stabilized to achieve and maintain proper length, rotation, and alignment. Due to the magnitude of soft-tissue contamination and other associated injuries, anatomic reduction and internal fixation should not be performed.[20] In the hand and carpus, Kirschner-wires (K-wires) are typically utilized while in the wrist and forearm (**Figure 2**), external fixation is most effective in providing fracture stability. Wrist spanning plate fixation can be utilized in the acute and subacute setting for select cases and is dictated by the degree of contamination and soft issue injury.[21] In the presence of multilevel injuries in the upper extremity, stabilizing structures from a proximal to distal direction is recommended to restore a stable foundation upon which the reconstruction of more distal structures can be performed.

Hand and Wrist

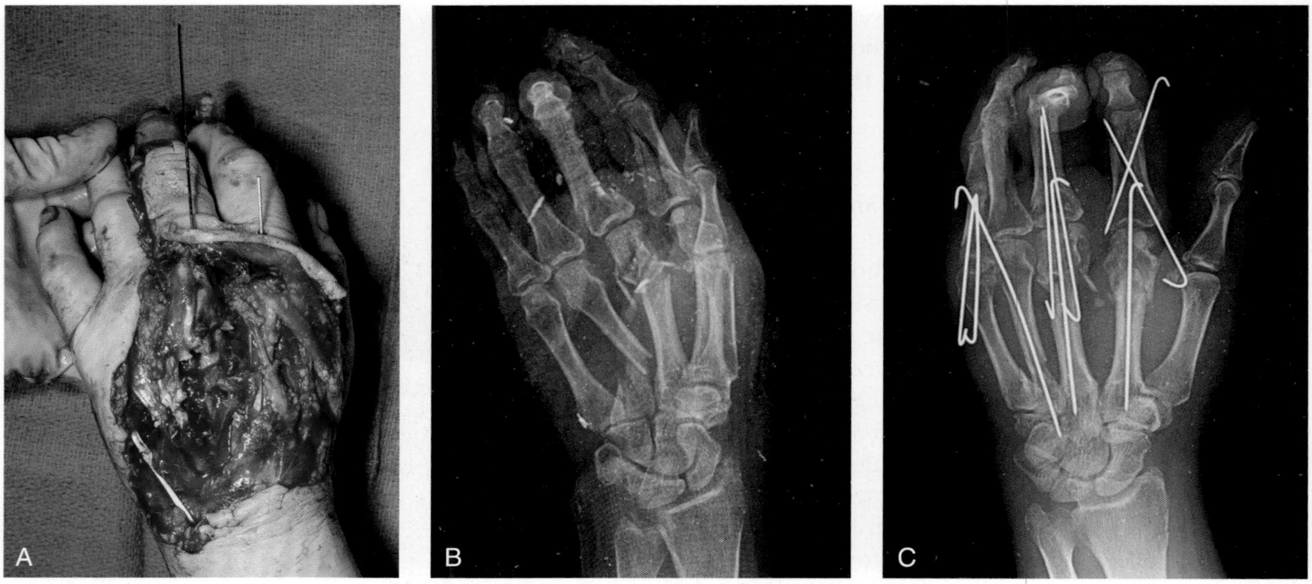

Figure 2 **Initial skeletal fixation in a mutilated hand with Kirschner-wires**. Photograph showing that the patient sustained multiple soft-tissue (**A**) and skeletal (**B**) injuries in a rollover motor vehicle accident. Injury (**B**) and postoperative (**C**) PA radiographs are shown.

Injuries to the hand can lead to soft-tissue and intrinsic joint contractures which can be extremely limiting. Injuries to the radial side of the hand can often lead to first web space contractures from crush or avulsion mechanisms and even from minor lacerations. Therefore, these contractures should be prevented with temporary K-wire transfixation or external fixation of the first ray in maximal palmar and radial abduction (**Figure 3**) for the first 4 to 6 weeks. Similarly, any trauma to the hand, carpus, or wrist can result in metacarpophalangeal (MCP) joint extension contractures secondary to a variety of reasons, mainly due to the sequelae of edema within the periarticular structures.[22] This can be prevented by positioning the MCP joints in a flexed position with either an orthosis or temporary MCP joint K-wire transfixation with early range of motion.

Skeletal defects can be initially managed with antibiotic-impregnated polymethyl-methacrylate (PMMA) cement spacers to provide local antibiotic delivery, obliterate the dead space, and stimulate the formation of an induce membrane.[23-25] Bishop et al[26] noted that vancomycin eluted from PMMA cement at an increasing volume of up to 8 days and continued to be observed in the effluent until 60 days. Aho et al[27] performed a histologic evaluation of an induced membrane that was consistent with a maturing, vascularized fibrous tissue with the highest membrane samples of osteogenic factors such as VEGF, IL-6, and Col-1, at 4 weeks of age. Based on these findings, a staged secondary procedure for cement spacer removal and bone grafting should be performed at approximately 4 to 6 weeks after initial cement spacer implantation.[25,27]

Vascular Injuries

Vascular injuries must be expediently addressed to reestablish blood flow when distal perfusion is absent. Arterial injury involving the brachial artery may still provide adequate perfusion distally through an intact profunda brachii artery and its collateral vessels that span the elbow.[28] Similarly, in the presence of an intact superficial and/or deep arch, perfusion to the hand can be present despite transection of either the radial or ulnar artery. As such, either artery can be ligated in the acute setting if the hand remains perfused. However, if critical ischemia is present, revascularization must be performed.

Vascular shunts can be inserted to temporarily establish blood flow prior to definitive revascularization when other life-preserving procedures are being performed, during patient transport to a facility that can provide higher level of care, or prior to performing skeletal stabilization techniques.[29] Shunts are intended to be temporary, up to 6 hours, until definitive vascular repair or reconstruction can be performed urgently. The use of routine systemic anticoagulation with vascular shunts is debatable; however, it is recommended in stable patients who do not have any other contraindications.[2,3,29] Nonetheless,

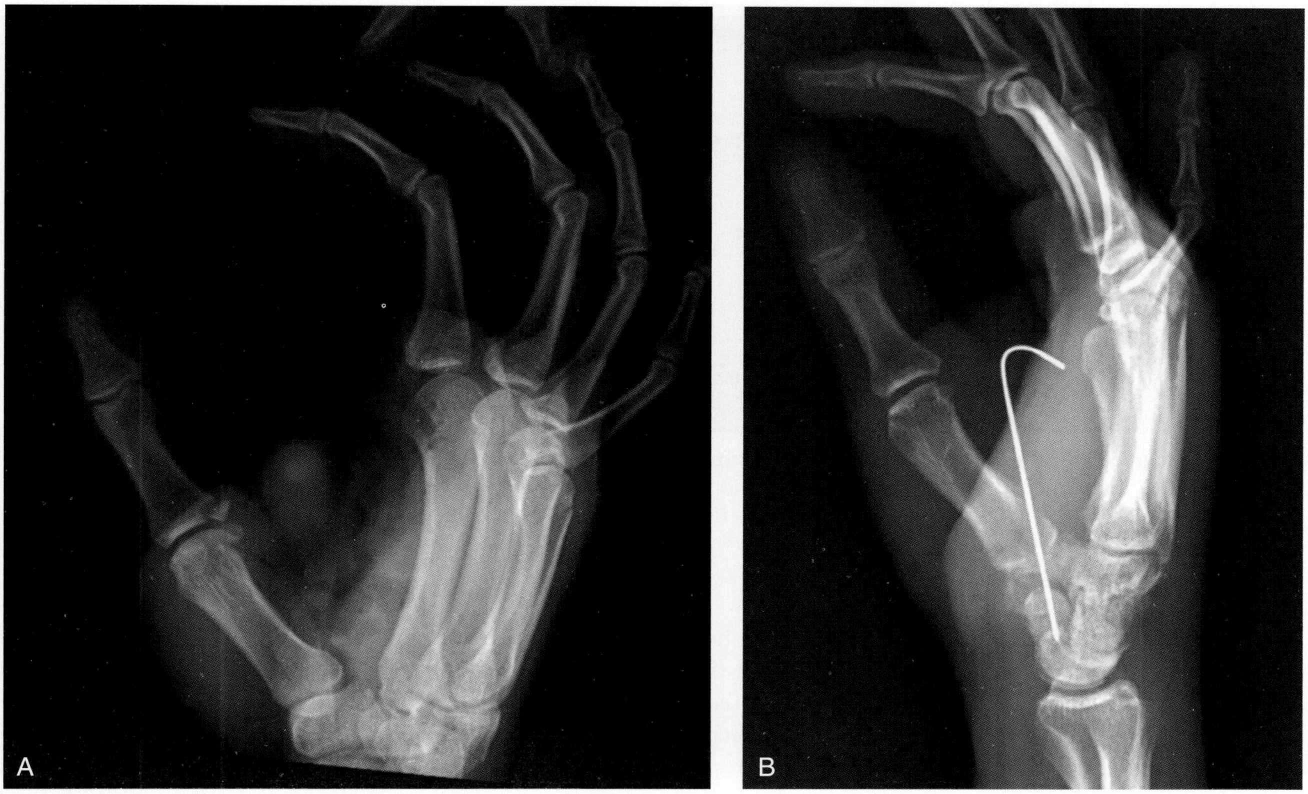

Figure 3 Radiographs demonstrating the prevention of first web space contracture. Patient sustained a blast injury to the first web space (**A**). At the time of initial management, the trapeziometacarpal joint was temporarily transfixed with a Kirschner wire to keep the joint reduced while maintaining the first ray in maximal palmar and radial abduction (**B**).

prolonged use of intraluminal shunts have been reported patency up to 52 hours without systemic anticoagulation.[30]

Revascularization in the mangled upper extremity often requires vein graft reconstruction due to the extensive zone injury and segmental vessel loss. Paramount to successful vessel reconstruction is a healthy and clean wound bed. This can be facilitated by performing a thorough débridement and obtaining adequate vein graft length that can be routed out of the zone of injury. Fox et al[31] noted that in eight mangled extremities that required amputation after vascular reconstruction, five were associated with contaminated wounds and infected grafts. It is of utmost importance to provide soft-tissue coverage over vein grafts and ligated arterial stumps which may otherwise desiccate and/or breakdown the anastomosis leading to complications such a thrombosis or hemorrhage.[32]

Nerve Injuries

Acute primary repair of traumatic nerve injuries in the mangled extremity is challenging due to the inability to macroscopically detect the zone of injury which may lead to a neuroma-in-continuity or failure of nerve regeneration if the coapted nerve ends undergo progressive fibrosis. Therefore, it is advocated to place a large, colored suture temporarily into the nerve stump that can also be sutured into the adjacent tissues to prevent retraction and aid in identifying the nerve during a staged secondary procedure (**Figure 4**).[3] In addition, segmental nerve loss is common in high-energy trauma to the upper extremity and tension-free primary repair is often not possible necessitating nerve graft or conduit reconstruction.[33] Thus, it is recommended to stage nerve reconstruction until the zone of neural injury has declared itself and the wound bed is clean, well-vascularized, with adequate soft-tissue coverage.[34]

Soft-Tissue Injuries

Primary closure should not be performed in the mangled upper extremity and wounds should be left open to allow for egress of contaminated fluid while minimizing soft-tissue tension on the wound periphery which otherwise could lead to progressive tissue necrosis and potentiate the risk of infection.[3,14] Emergency-free soft-tissue coverage has been advocated in the past to

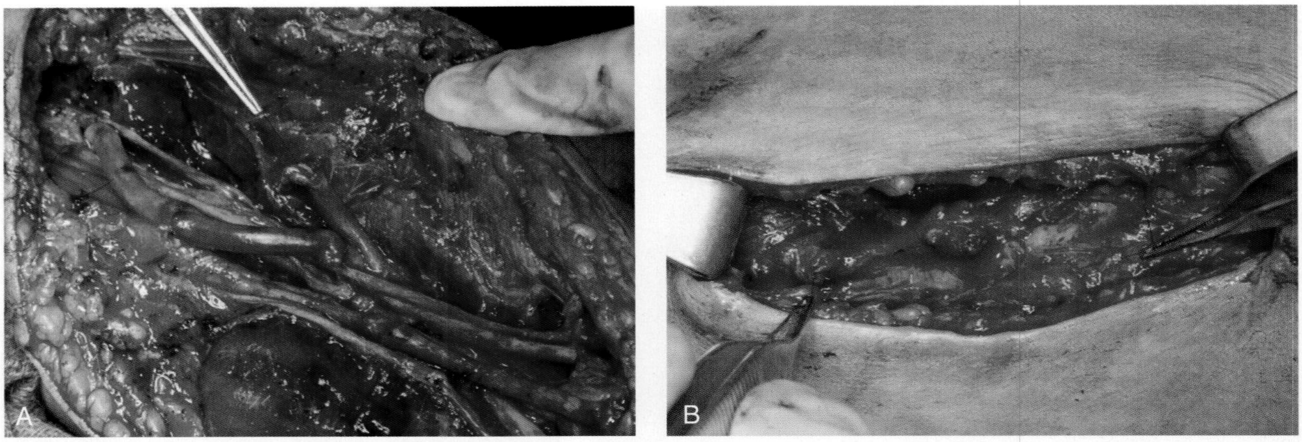

Figure 4 Photographs demonstrating the identification sutures placed into transected nerve stumps. This patient sustained a gunshot wound into the brachium that resulted in transection of the median nerve and the brachial artery that required vein graft reconstruction. The nerve ends were tagged with sutures (blue suture held by forceps) to prevent retraction and to facilitate later identification (**A**). At the time of staged nerve reconstruction, 4 weeks from injury, the tagging sutures (blue sutures held by forceps) were easily identified amidst the scar tissue to assist with nerve stump exposure (**B**).

minimize the development of severe infection; however, with the advent of negative-pressure wound therapy (NPWT) and dermal substitutes, emergent-free or pedicle soft-tissue transfer is not necessary.[35] In fact, in areas of contaminated soft-tissue loss, NPWT can promote granulation and angiogenesis, remove edema, and reduce wound surface area that can even obviate the need for free tissue transfer.[36] However, caution must be maintained when applying a NPWT dressing over exposed tendon, nerve, or vascular structures as secondary injuries can occur.

Tendon injuries can be repaired in the acute setting to minimize tendon retraction and to reestablish the agonist-antagonist relationship across the joints. However, in the mutilated upper extremity, tendon injuries are often not amenable to primary end-to-end repairs. The mechanism of injury can lead to a segmental defect in the tendons that can be reconstructed with tendon grafts. In more proximal lesions where the myotendinous junction or the muscle belly itself has been lost, acute tendon transfers can be performed. However, tendon reconstruction and transfers should only be performed in the acute setting if the wound bed is clean, well vascularized, and can be covered with viable soft tissue; the patient can participate in postoperative rehabilitation; and further surgical procedures are not planned through the zone of tendon reconstruction which can lead to progressive scarring.

Vigilance must be maintained to detect compartment syndrome in the mangled upper extremity and a low-threshold should exist to perform fasciotomies, particularly in the setting of crush or vascular injuries. The diagnosis of compartment syndrome can be aided by calculating a difference of 20 mm Hg or less between the diastolic blood pressure and the intracompartment pressure.[37] However, it may be difficult to accurately obtain intracompartment pressures in the mangled upper extremity, especially in the setting of multilevel skeletal injuries which can affect intracompartmental pressures.[37] Given the fact that compartment syndrome is a clinical diagnosis, forearm (3 compartments), hand (10 compartments), and even digital fasciotomies should be considered in the setting of tense compartments and/or after revascularization of a previously ischemic upper extremity that can lead to a reperfusion injury.

Replantation: Indications and Outcomes

The ability to replant severed body parts, now well standardized and routine in the practice of hand surgery, required a sequence of technical advances. The development of the operating microscope early in the 20th century led in the 1960s to its application for anastomosis of small vessels. During this period, rapid development of the necessary instruments and fine sutures with swedged atraumatic needles enabled routine successful replantation of amputated arms, hands, and ultimately individual digits. Subsequent experience has further improved microsurgical tools and techniques, and defined appropriate candidates for these complex procedures. Using current methods and appropriate patient selection, replantation has become a standard procedure with predictable outcomes.

It is important to recognize, however, that not all severed or dysvascular tissues should have attempted microvascular reconstruction. The morbidity and even potential mortality of these procedures, particularly in proximal levels is not insubstantial, and must be weighed with the likelihood of a successful outcome of a replantation procedure. In this regard, survival alone is not the only criterion. Restoration of both limb form and function is the goal. Adequate active motion and sensation in particular, sufficient to improve rather than hinder extremity use is the goal. Identification of patients and injuries most likely to have a satisfactory functional outcome has become the focus of recent investigations, together with analyses of cost-effectiveness and surgical efficiency.[38]

Regional Differences

In real-world practice, surgeons in different regions or different units of a given region or country execute these well documented principles differently and are strongly affected by patients' desires in deciding whether or how to replant.[39] A cultural desire to replant most amputations and surgeon's experience resulting from the need to treat frequent digit amputations account in part for reported differences in number and survival rate in different parts of the world.[39] The frequency of replantation surgery in adults has undergone a gradual reduction over time in the United States, England, and Europe. While in part attributable to improved safety standards in industry, it is also likely that many Western surgeons choose not to replant some amputations based on a variety of other factors.

Fortunately, we now have the benefit of 50 years of clinical experience, which provides necessary guidance in selecting appropriate candidates for replantation well as other reconstructive alternatives. All options must be kept in mind at the time of initial patient evaluation.

Replantation and Revascularization

Traumatic injury to the upper limb may result in a complete amputation or result in a distal segment without any blood supply, but with some remaining attachment of any tissue type. Reattachment of a completely severed body part is termed "replantation," while restoring viability to an incompletely amputated part with a remaining soft-tissue connection, no matter how minimal, is appropriately referred to as "revascularization."

Replantation Team

Certainly successful replantation is likely to have better outcomes when performed by a team experienced in microvascular surgery and equipped to add lengthy surgical procedures on short notice. A microsurgeon operating alone is less likely to maintain a high success rate than an organized team. Not surprisingly, in the United States, the majority of these operations take place in teaching facilities, large or urban hospitals.[40] Although the indications for replantation, discussed below, are generally agreed upon, a higher proportion of amputations are selected for replantation surgery at teaching hospitals than other clinical settings.[40] Hospital volume does directly affect outcomes for many high-risk surgical procedures, including reported success rates for digit replantation in one American study.[41] Interestingly, no increased risk of failure was found when replantations were performed by senior level trainees at a major German trauma center as compared with attending hand surgeons, due to extensive microsurgical experience and "appropriate supervision."[42]

Most authors recommend the use of two or more surgical teams in polydigit replantation, allowing simultaneous preparation of the proximal stumps and the amputated parts. The ability to have more than one skilled microsurgeon during neurorrhaphy and microvascular repair is also a distinct advantage during these demanding procedures.

Decision Making

The indications for replantation may be broadly divided as absolute or relative based upon age, mechanism and number of fingers in digit amputations, level of amputation, and mechanism of injury (**Table 2**). Similarly, contra-indications are also generally agreed upon, when factors such as severe avulsion or mangling injury, excessive ischemia time, or significant comorbidity and associated injuries make replantation inadvisable (**Table 3**).

Table 2

Indications for Replantation

Absolute indications

1. Any incomplete amputation (revascularization)
2. Any childhood amputation
3. Any thumb, of any mechanism
4. Multiple digits other than thumb
5. Transmetacarpal and wrist level amputations

Relative indications

1. Single digit distal to the flexor digitorum superficialis insertion
2. Ring avulsion injury
3. Major limb amputations (proximal to the wrist) with acceptable ischemic time

Table 3

Contraindications to Replantation

Absolute contraindications
1. Severely crushed or mangled parts
2. Significant comorbidity or associated injury
3. Severe vascular disease
4. Prolonged warm > cold ischemia in major limb replantations
Relative contraindications
1. Avulsion mechanism
2. Segmental amputation
3. Mentally unstable patients (self-inflicted amputations)
4. Prolonged normothermic ischemia in fingers

While the indications and contraindications for replantation provided in these tables provide general guidelines for preoperative decisions, they are at best generalizations. The ultimate best plan must be individualized for the patient and his or her clinical situation.

Culture and societal differences affect not only the incidence of amputation, but also the decision to proceed with amputation. Societal stigmatization of digit amputations in some cultures, particularly in Asia, makes replantation more likely, particularly at very distal (fingertip) level and in more complex injury, such as segmental injury.[39,43]

Indications for Replantation or Revascularization (Table 2)

Pediatric Amputations

Pediatric amputations commonly occur from saws or axes, motor vehicle accidents, or crush/avulsions in machinery, bicycle chains, or door slams.[44] Most if not all amputated parts in a child should undergo an attempt at replantation, not only to improve future function but also for psychosocial adaptation. It is unfortunate that in reality not all children are treated equally in America. Squitieri et al found that only 40% of cases are generally taken to the OR—a rate higher than adults, but lower than expected. Of these, white patients and those with private health insurance are more likely to undergo replantation than other children.[45]

The anticipated success of pediatric replantation is less than adult injury. Not only are structures smaller, but significant differences in anatomy (unossified structures, presence of growth plates) and physiology (including a higher tendency for vasospasm) account for higher failure rates. Nevertheless, functional results tend to be superior in young patients in both recovery of motion and sensation. Childhood amputation injuries at any level and by any mechanism thus remain absolute indications for attempted replantation.

Thumb Amputations

The thumb provides 40% to 50% of hand function. Because of its critical role in prehension, it has been demonstrated to be of use even when little motion distal to the carpometacarpal joint is present or sensation is absent. Because of its importance, any thumb amputation regardless of level or mechanism of injury should be considered an absolute indication for replantation (**Figure 5**).

Multiple-Digit Amputation

Although multiple digits are generally agreed to be appropriate indication, controversy still exists regarding selection and best position for polydigit replantation. The level of amputation, degree of injury of each stump, and amputated digit must be considered, if any reattached finger is to have reasonable function. Particularly in crush or avulsion mechanism injury, the amputated digit with the least damage should be placed onto the least injured stump as a heterotopic replantation. Priority should be given to thumb reconstruction, either with a heterotopic replant or later thumb reconstruction.

Single Digit Amputations

Single digits are generally agreed to be indicated for replantation only when the resulting function will not compromise hand function. Single finger amputations at or proximal to the proximal interphalangeal (PIP) joint should not generally be reattached. Active range of motion averaged 35° for replanted digits amputated proximal to the PIP joint.[38] Proximal level finger amputations are likely to be stiff, cold intolerant, and often the cause of diminished hand dexterity.

Specific indications for single digit replantation include amputations distal to the PIP joint with an intact flexor digitorum superficialis (FDS) insertion, fingertip (distal to distal interphalangeal [DIP] joint) level amputations without distal crush injury, and some ring avulsion injuries. In these specific circumstances, a reasonable chance for restoration of function exists.

Single Digit Amputations with Intact Flexor Digitorum Superficialis

Amputations distal to the FDS insertion generally permit satisfactory PIP joint motion and restore digit length. Function is superior to primary closure even if the distal joint motion is poor, and cosmesis is greatly enhanced.

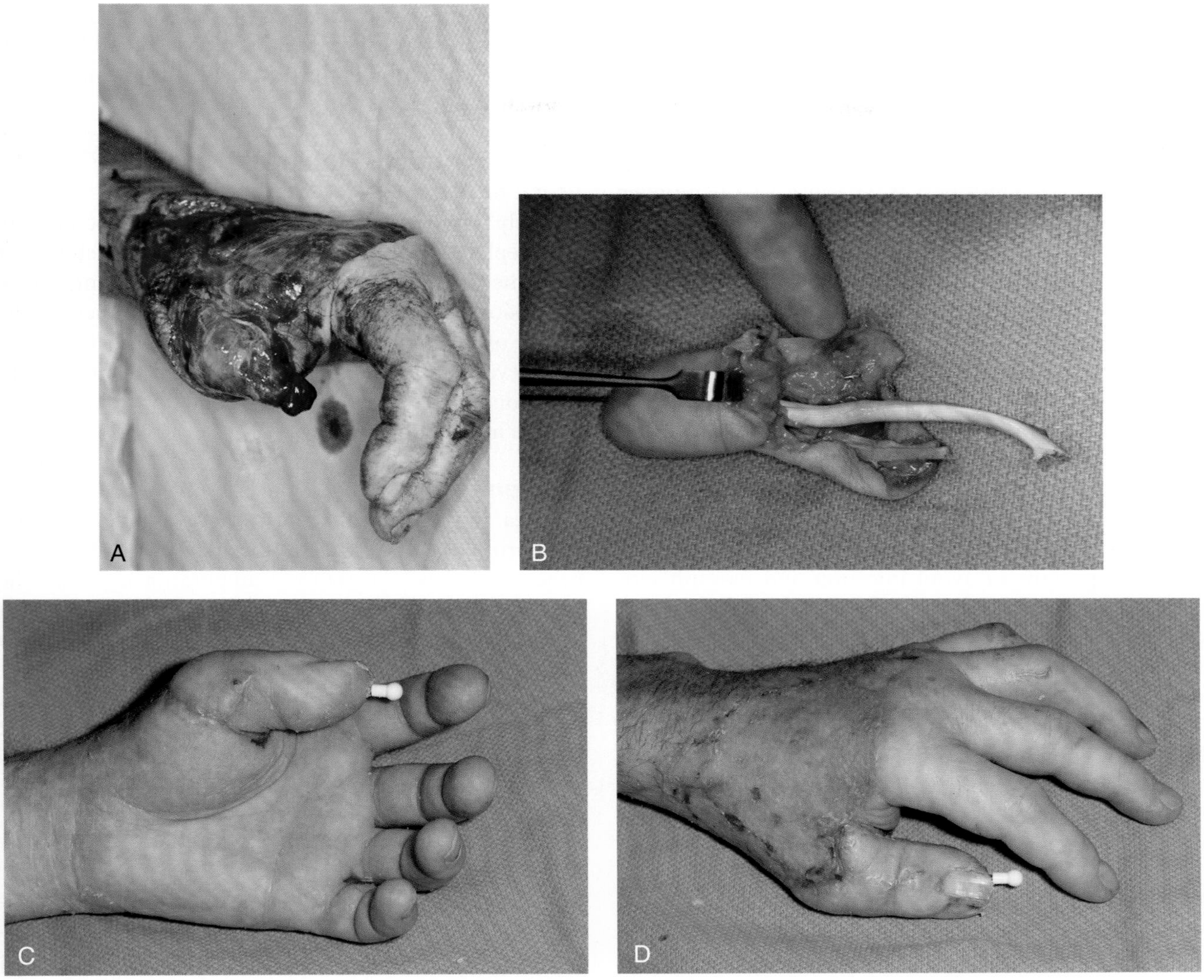

Figure 5 Photographs showing avulsion amputation of the thumb. Despite the mechanism, amputation of the thumb is an absolute indication for attempted replantation due to functional loss with shortening and closure, residual hand (**A**) and amputated part (**B**). Final clinical photographs after successful replantation and soft-tissue coverage, volar (**C**) and dorsal hand views (**D**).

Distal Level Single Digit Amputations

Recent improvements in supermicrosurgery, including better microscopes, now permit repair of small (0.3 to 0.8 mm) vessels and thus replantation of fingertip level amputations (distal to the DIP joint).[46] While these procedures are uncommon in the United States, evidence from Asian countries demonstrates their ability to provide cosmetic coverage and preservation of digital length with results better than stump revision and closure. Results are best with sharp mechanisms, and most functional in index and long rather than ring or small fingers as reflected by DASH (Disabilities of the Arm, Shoulder and Hand) scores.[47] A large Korean series of distal replantation included most cases, including those with severe soft-tissue injuries.[48] The overall survival rate was 78%, even though the most common type of vascular repair was revascularization of one artery only, most commonly with an interposed vein graft and no vein repair. Of these cases, interpositional vein grafts were used in 65%. In many such cases, no nerve repair is possible, but satisfactory sensation frequently results, as well as high levels of patient satisfaction with appearance and function.

Ring Avulsion Injuries

Although the conventional recommendation for treatment of Urbaniak class III ring avulsions (those with complete degloving and absent blood supply) has been revision amputation, more recent studies demonstrate the ability to successfully perform replantation. This is particularly true if the PIP joint and FDS tendon are intact.[49] A meta-analysis of 32 ring avulsion papers found the mean survival rate for avulsion replantation to be 66%, and the mean total active motion (TAM) of complete finger avulsions 174°, despite a large number of patients in the included studies having a DIP joint arthrodesis.[50] The mean 2-point discrimination (2PD) in patients after replantation was 10 mm (n = 32). These very satisfactory functional outcomes challenge the practice.

Transmetacarpal-Level Amputations

Amputation through the metacarpals results in severe loss of hand function, and attempted replantation is absolutely indicated at this level to restore grasp and result in useful restoration of digit length, motion, and sensibility. Débridement of muscle from the amputated part is important to avoid infection and may obviate intrinsic plus contracture. In a large series of 174 metacarpal ray amputations, only 14 were deemed unsalvageable.[51] The remainder had attempted replantation, with 86% survival, repairing from two to five arteries. At mean 9 years follow-up, results were judged excellent in 11, good in 11, fair in 10 and poor in 6 patients. Seventy-eight percent had measurable two-point discrimination averaging 14.7 mm (range 6 to 25 mm) and total active motion averaged 154° per injured digit.

Wrist Amputations

At this level, replantation is also desirable. Preservation of wrist motion will depend upon the particulars of the injury, and the potential need to shorten the skeletal elements to enable soft-tissue management. Reconstruction of median and ulnar nerves, extrinsic flexors, and extensors permits some function, but the prognosis for finger intrinsic recovery is poor.

Major Limb Replantation

Risk of significant morbidity and even mortality from bleeding, reperfusion injury (myoglobinemia in particular), wound issues, and infection may occur.

A significant amount of muscle in the amputated part requires expedited transport with immediate cooling of the limb. The patient must be brought immediately to the operating room to expedite revascularization. Examination in the operating room should evaluate for muscle rigor which if present, replantation is contraindicated. The use of a vascular shunt is advisable prior to bone stabilization, to allow immediate arterial flow. Free outflow of venous blood is allowed initially to flush myoglobin and other products of ischemia and reperfusion prior to establishing venous return. Blood loss may require resuscitation in the OR, as well as evaluation for associated injuries.

Contraindications (Table 3)

Crush or Avulsion Mechanism

Severely traumatized parts will be unlikely to be successfully replanted. Clinical judgement must be exercised at the time of initial inspection and débridement before a decision is reached. Considerations must include the degree of functional loss (greater with thumb and proximal level amputation) and the surgical team's ability to reconstruct multiple tissues (bone and joint, nerve, muscle and tendon, skin).

Mechanism of Injury

Injuries are broadly divided in the available literature as sharp, crush, or avulsion mechanisms. Prognosis is generally lowest for avulsion amputations, due to the extensive longitudinal injury to soft tissues. Crush injury carries a variable prognosis, depending upon location and extent. A recent meta-analysis found that an odds-ratio comparison of success rates for crush and avulsion to sharp amputation demonstrates that a digit is 5.17 times more likely to be replanted successfully after a clean amputation than after either crushing or avulsion injury.[52]

Age

Replantation is also less commonly performed in older individuals. Diminished range of motion and poorer recovery of sensation have been demonstrated, as well as higher rates of transfusion and increased need for support after discharge. However, successful replantation was reported in 91% of patients older than 60 years in a recent review.[53] Age older than 70 years remained a significant predictor of poorer outcome in this study, but not an absolute contraindication.

Ischemia Time

Muscle tolerates ischemia poorly. It is critical that ischemia time be minimized and muscle survival optimized during transport and initial care with cooling of the amputated part. Warm ischemia time greater than 6 hours is an absolute contraindication in parts containing muscle, as myonecrosis may cause renal damage and risk of sepsis. For digit-only replantation, successful replantation with cold ischemia time of up to 96 hours has been reported, although classic recommendations have been 12 hours of warm or 24 hours cold ischemia time.[46]

Comorbidities and Other Factors

Systemic factors will influence the likelihood of replanted digit survival. Recent reviews found heavy smoking (>20 cigarettes/d), age, and ischemia time >12 hours were risk factors for replant failure.[53,54] A preoperative history of smoking is not an absolute contraindication for surgery, although it is clear that postoperative continuation increases the risk of failure and complications. Poor overall health, polytrauma, and atherosclerosis are also frequently mentioned factors that enter into decision making prior to replantation.

Principles of Digit Replantation

Initial Management

Cold storage (4°C) may permit replantation of a major limb as late as 12 hours, and a digit for at least 24 hours. Wrap the amputated part in most gauze, place in a sealed plastic bag, and place on ice. Similarly, incompletely amputated parts should be wrapped and cooled in situ to improve likelihood of replantability and survival. Prior to transport and/or in the emergency department, antibiotic and tetanus prophylaxis should be administered, with fluid resuscitation and warming as needed.

When possible, the patient and family should be informed about treatment options, including replantation and shortening. The risks and benefits of replantation, the possibility of need for nerve, bone, skin or vein grafting, and the time course of surgery and anticipated hospital stay. The recovery time, possible need for secondary surgery, and expected outcome should be presented to enable their active participation in preoperative decision-making.

During initial patient evaluation, much time may be saved by bringing the amputated part(s) directly to the operating room in advance of the patient. This allows débridement and preparation of the amputated part before the patient arrives in the theatre. Major limb replant patients *must* be brought directly to surgery, to facilitate immediate restoration of circulation.

Delay in digit replantation is not to be generally recommended, given the proven association of ischemia time with survival and function. However, in digit replantation with short cold ischemia times, delay until the morning operating room schedule has been reported to not adversely affect outcome.[55]

Once in the operating room, a urinary catheter is positioned prior to surgery. A regional nerve block is frequently useful not only for pain management, but also for its sympatholytic effect (vasodilation). Maintaining patient core temperature is important in any microsurgical procedure for this same purpose, both during and following replantation. A warm operating room (>80°F or 27°C), use of a warming blanket, and core temperature monitoring during surgery should be routine.

Steps of Digit Replantation

Inspection of the Amputated Part

Irreparable damage to distal vessels may be evidenced by the presence of the *red line sign*, a hemorrhagic stripe seen in the skin along the midlateral aspect of the avulsed digit. A twisted, corkscrew-like appearance of the digital artery, the *ribbon sign*, provides evidence of intimal damage and a poor prognosis. Resection of this damaged portion of the vessel is mandated to improve chances for success. Photographs of the stump and amputated part should generally be made, primarily for a medicolegal record should replantation not be performed.[46]

Débridement

Adequate débridement is vital before replantation. The zone of injured soft tissues is greatest with avulsion injury and further affected by warm ischemia time.[39] Nonviable tissue must be débrided and vascular repairs performed on healthy vessels. To achieve this, shortening the bone of the amputated digit is the simplest primary way to facilitate débridement and soft-tissue repair.[39]

Structure Identification

Midlateral incisions are made in the stump and amputated part, folding dorsal skin distally to identify dorsal veins and extensor tendons. Similarly, the palmar structures are carefully exposed. The use of small hemoclips to tag dorsal veins, arteries, and nerves during this process will avoid the need for a later search for previously dissected structures in a bloody field. Grasping sutures may be preplaced in the flexor tendons and mattress sutures in the extensor tendons. Preparation for bone fixation with preplacement of interosseous wires or K-wires may also be performed on the amputated part at this time. With structures now identified, débrided, and tagged, replantation proceeds in a step-wise fashion.

Bone Fixation

Bone fixation should almost always include a shortening step. I prefer to shorten the bone of finger amputations approximately 1 cm in all but very sharp, "guillotine-like" amputations. This may be done either at the amputated part or stump. In many cases, skeletal shortening will solve issues caused by resection of damaged or contaminated vessels, skin, and other soft tissues and potentially avoid the need to use vein and/or nerve grafts. Joint damage requires fusion or arthroplasty with the same shortening goals.

Bone fixation should be expeditious and rigid. I prefer the use of interosseous wires, as they meet both requirements and generally do not require removal later. Many other methods have been reported, including plate and screw fixation. Rigid internal fixation permits early active movement, with potential improved functional outcome, although more dissection often leads to more scar tissue formation.[56]

Repair Extensor Tendons

Extensor tendons are repaired following bone fixation, using nonabsorbable mattress sutures in the conventional manner.

Repair Flexor Tendons

Similarly, flexor tendons are repaired with grasping sutures. Placement of core sutures individually in proximal and distal tendons permits a more rapid sequence of repairs, particularly in polydigit replantation when more than one team is working on the amputated digits.

Arterial Repair

Authors differ in preference in order of vein and arterial repair. Those who advocate repairing the artery first cite the ability to rapidly revascularize the part, demonstrate adequate inflow and properly select veins for outflow. The disadvantage is bleeding from the veins, particularly in polydigit replants, making subsequent steps more difficult and resulting in undesirable blood loss.

Direct repair may be possible in sharp mechanisms and in local crush injury with adequate bone shortening. Use of reversed veins, generally harvested from the forearm or dorsum of the foot, is necessary to bridge gaps. Synthetic grafts are not used in the hand, and arterial grafts seldom chosen although not unreasonable from an expendable source such as a thoracodorsal system branch, obtainable from the ipsilateral extremity. Transposition of an adjacent digital artery may also salvage flow to a single digit injury such as a ring avulsion.[57] During preparation and microsurgery, bathing the vessels with lidocaine or papaverine is desirable to minimize vasospasm.

Venous Repair

Veins previously identified and tagged are most easily repaired by careful dissection from the dorsal skin to maximize length. Ligation of one or more small branches may also be used to effectively elongate the vein as needed. A gap between proximal and distal vein may require an interposed vein graft, assuming adequate débridement and bone shortening had already been performed to minimize the effect of tissue loss. Transposition of an adjacent digital vein is another effective means to reconstruct a gap without need for graft. Inability to repair venous outflow will result in venous congestion. Outflow from the nail bed with removal of the nail plate with hourly rubbing with heparin-soaked pledgets or use of medicinal leeches may occasionally salvage such a digits.

Nerve Repair

Direct repair may be possible with adequate skeletal shortening in local crush and sharp injury. Traumatized stumps should be resected until healthy fascicular detail is observed. Repair must be tension-free. This may be facilitated by longitudinal dissection of the nerve stumps for a few centimeters proximal and/or distal. When insufficient, a nerve graft should be used. Small gaps in purely sensory digital nerves may be managed with decellularized allograft or use of autogenous graft sources such as the posterior interosseous, sural nerve, or an antebrachial cutaneous nerve. In fingertip-level replantation, inability to repair digital nerves is common, yet recovery of protective sensation generally occurs.

Obtain Skin Coverage

Loose skin closure is important to prevent vascular compression. The midlateral incisions may be loosely approximated or even left open if necessary to heal by secondary intention. Transverse wounds should be closed. Venous flow-through flaps may provide coverage in larger defects or when both skin and vein defects exist simultaneously. Negative pressure wound therapy for skin defects after replantation has been reported to be well tolerated, maintaining replant survival and allowing wound granulation.[58]

Thumb Replantation Technique

The thumb's unique position in the hand makes a direct palmar approach for vascular reconstruction difficult. Repair of the large proper ulnar digital artery is particularly challenging due to the pronated position of the thumb relative to the other digits.

In addition, obtaining adequate exposure and positioning of the thumb can be challenging under a surgical microscope. Proximal vessels may be injured well proximal to the bone level. Rather than dissect the proximal circulation of the thumb into thenar muscle, a simpler alternative will facilitate success and reduce surgical time. Instead, an interposition reversed venous graft may be placed with the hand positioned palm-down on the hand table, extending from the radial artery in the anatomic snuff box directly to the proper ulnar digital artery of the thumb (**Figure 6**).[59]

Once the initial bone fixation and tendon and nerve repairs are completed, a vein graft is harvested from the forearm. The hand is then positioned with the forearm pronated and palm-down on the hand table. This position permits easy access to the dorsal veins and proper ulnar digital artery. The majority of the remainder of the operation can be completed comfortably and quickly. The vein graft previously harvested is used to bridge radial artery in the anatomic snuffbox to the ulnar digital artery.

Multiple Digit Replantation Technique

Approach: Sequence

The use of two or more surgical teams is highly desirable to diminish operating time and improve outcomes. To reduce surgical time, digits are replanted using the structure-by-structure method, first obtaining bony fixation in all digits, followed by tendon repairs before any vascular repairs are performed.[60] This method will reduce surgical time and result in high levels of digit survival. In one recent study, mean surgical time was 313 minutes for four or five digits, with an 87.5% digit survival rate and 61% excellent or good functional outcomes using Chen criteria.[61]

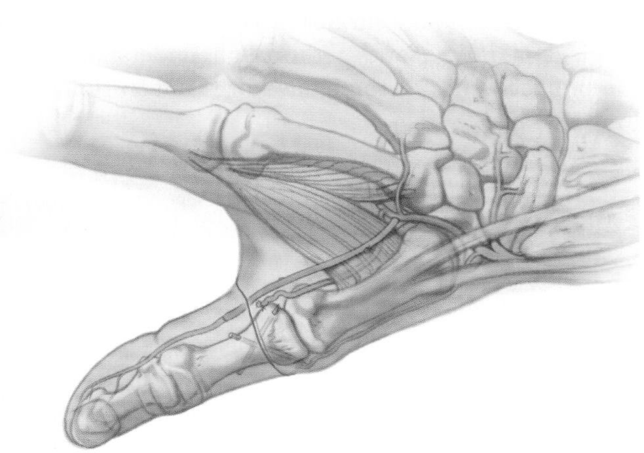

Figure 6 **Illustration demonstrating that replantation of the thumb is facilitated by arterial reconstruction with a bridging vein graft from a dorsal exposure.** Bone fixation, tendon repair, and nerve repairs are performed first, followed by vein graft harvest from the forearm. Arterial reconstruction is next performed from a dorsal exposure, grafting end-to-side to the radial artery in the snuff box and end-to-end to the proper ulnar digital artery. Venous repair from the same exposure then follows.

Selection and Location of Digits

As previously discussed, priority is given to the least damaged digits and stumps, frequently leading to placement of a digit in a heterotopic location. Priority is given to the thumb, then other digits. Portions of an otherwise unreplantable digit may also be used heterotopically as a source of spare parts for specific defects. For example, the use of a neurovascular fillet flap may facilitate soft-tissue cover, or a finger joint from placed within an otherwise less severely injured finger.[62]

Temporary ectopic replantation, allowing recovery of crushed recipient sites, and placement of digits on the forearm when wrist-level amputations cannot be replanted are other reported means to improve functional outcomes.[63,64]

Aftercare

Monitoring

Skin color, capillary refill, and tissue turgor are clinically visible measures that should be used in the postoperative assessment of digit perfusion. Venous congestion will be evident by cool skin temperatures, bluish discoloration, rapid capillary refill, and swelling. Arterial insufficiency results in pallor, loss of skin turgor, and loss of capillary refill. Use of a hypodermic needle to prick the pulp will provide useful information regarding congestion or insufficient inflow. Skin temperature has been used for decades, noting a drop in temperature of at least 1°C/h over 2 hours to correlate with arterial thrombosis. Transcutaneous oxygen sensors provide a continuous measurement that may be of value, and laser Doppler flowmetry has also been reported as useful. In one such study, replanted digit flow values were compared with that of an adjacent unaffected digit.[65] The resulting perfusion index (defined as the revascularized digit perfusion value divided by that of the normal digit) was found to have an ideal value of 0.397.

Anticoagulation

Topical lidocaine or papaverine is routinely used during surgery to minimize local vasospasm, and systemic heparin when intraoperative thrombosis occurs. There is otherwise little or no consensus on ideal postoperative anticoagulation. Heparin carries risk of thrombocytopenia and bleeding, which is reduced with low-molecular-weight heparin. Aspirin at a low dose blocks the cyclo-oxygenase pathway, and dextran provides both antiplatelet and heparin-like effects, with some risk of major adverse effects (anaphylaxis, renal failure, cardiac failure, bleeding). Of these, aspirin in the most commonly used agent, at a dose of 3 mg/kg. Reports vary in the utility of postoperative anticoagulation. For example: The survival rates of digits from patients who received dextran with those treated with low-molecular-weight heparin, dextran with prostaglandin E1, or no antithrombotic therapy were not significantly different. Antithrombotic therapies showed no significant benefit for digit replantation in patients receiving papaverine.[66]

Venous thrombosis and congestion is the usual finding in a failing replant. Removal of the nail plate and application of a heparin-soaked pledge to a small nail bed incision is one potential solution. Use of leeches to improve venous outflow may also provide immediate relief of the problem (**Figure 7**). Although the use of a leech will produce prolonged local anticoagulation, risk of infection with *Aeromonas hydrophila* or other organisms require antibiotic prophylaxis.[67] Sluggish inflow results from uncorrected congestion, at times resulting in subsequent arterial thrombosis. Venous congestion improves by 4 to 6 days postoperatively due to new outflow connections.

Temperature Control

Maintaining patient core temperature is important in any microsurgical procedure for this same purpose, both during and following replantation. A warm operating room (>80°F or 27°C), use of a warming blanket, and core temperature monitoring during surgery should be routine. Postoperatively, similar environmental controls should be used for a minimum of 24 hours.[46]

Caffeine

Avoidance of caffeine is generally recommended following microsurgery, to avoid peripheral vasoconstriction. A recent study has questioned this dictum, noting no change in digital blood flow following the ingestion of 100 mg of caffeine by healthy volunteers, as measured by laser Doppler flow monitoring.[68]

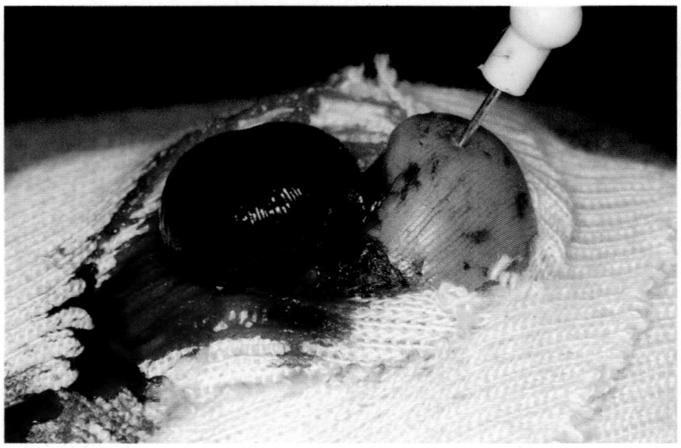

Figure 7 Photograph demonstrating that medicinal leeches may be used to diminish venous congestion.

Rehabilitation

Digit replantation results may be optimized with a graded rehabilitation program. Each case is unique, and decisions based upon factors such as fixation rigidity, quality of tendon repair, and wound status. Edema is controlled by elevation, and the dressing monitored to avoid excessive compression. Protective splintage is important, and early active and/or passive range of motion is helpful to obtain a functional outcome. Protocols similar to those of flexor tenorrhaphy are useful to avoid excessive initial force.

Values for replant survival vary considerably by global region, mechanism, and level of injury. While survival rates in the 80% to 90% range have been reported, most studies are less optimistic, particularly with avulsion mechanisms. Tendon adhesions, fracture nonunion, and joint stiffness are common, with need for subsequent surgery in up to 60% of replanted digits.

Summary

Severe trauma to the upper extremity can lead to mutilating hand and wrist injuries that may be associated with amputations. Although acute management of the mangled upper extremity can be daunting, understanding the goals of care and the principles of wound débridement can guide the surgeon in obtaining a healthy and stable limb upon which staged reconstruction can be carried out. In the presence of an amputation, meticulous surgical technique, methodical surgical planning, and a thorough understanding of the biomechanics of the hand can result in functional limb salvage.

Key Study Points

- The primary goal in managing the patient with a mangled upper extremity is to preserve life.
- The quality of wound débridement dictates the outcome of limb salvage.
- Thoughtful staged surgical planning is necessary to avoid limiting surgical options for reconstruction.
- Individual patient consideration is necessary to determine if replantation is indicated in distal amputations of the digits.
- Vein interposition graft from the digital artery to the radial artery within the anatomic snuff box can facilitate thumb replantation or revascularization.

Annotated References

1. Gregory RT, Gould RJ, Peclet M, et al: The mangled extremity syndrome (M.E.S.): A severity grading system for multisystem injury of the extremity. *J Trauma* 1985;25(12):1147-1150.
2. Bumbasirevic M, Stevanovic M, Lesic A, Atkinson HD: Current management of the mangled upper extremity. *Int Orthop* 2012;36(11):2189-2195.
3. Mathieu L, Bertani A, Gaillard C, et al: Surgical management of combat-related upper extremity injuries. *Chir Main* 2014;33(3):174-182.
4. Sabapathy SR, Bhardwaj P: Setting the goals in the management of mutilated injuries of the hand – Impressions based on the Ganga Hospital experience. *Hand Clin* 2016;32(4):435-441.

   The authors present a review article discussing the need for improved access for care in patients who have sustained mutilating hand injuries. They present clear goals that are utilized in the author's institution that treats an underserved population. Level of evidence: V.
5. Baltzer HL, Moran SL: The biomechanical impact of digital loss and fusion following trauma: Setting the patient up for success. *Hand Clin* 2016;32(4):443-463.

   In this review article, the authors discuss the biomechanics of the hand, in particular the function of the digits in performing various grip and pinch activities. Additionally, the authors present a function based treatment principle to optimize the results after digit amputation. Level of evidence: V.
6. Hegge T, Neumeister MW: Mutilated hand injuries. *Clin Plast Surg* 2011;38(4):543-550.
7. Bueno RA Jr, Neumeister MW: Outcomes after mutilating hand injuries: Review of the literature and recommendations for assessment. *Hand Clin* 2003;19(1):193-204.
8. Brown HC, Williams HB, Woolhouse FM: Principles of salvage in mutilating hand injuries. *J Trauma* 1968;8(3):319-332.
9. Wilhelmi BJ, Lee WP, Pagenstert GI, May JW Jr: Replantation in the mutilated hand. *Hand Clin* 2003;19(1):89-120.
10. Togawa S, Yamami N, Nakayama H, Mano Y, Ikegami K, Ozeki S: The validity of the mangled extremity severity score in the assessment of upper limb injuries. *J Bone Joint Surg Br* 2005;87(11):1516-1519.
11. Johansen K, Daines M, Howey T, Helfet D, Hansen ST Jr: Objective criteria accurately predict amputation following lower extremity trauma. *J Trauma* 1990;30(5):568-572; discussion 572-573.
12. Campbell DA, Kay SP: The Hand Injury Severity Scoring System. *J Hand Surg* 1996;21(3):295-298.
13. Matsuzaki H, Narisawa H, Miwa H, Toishi S: Predicting functional recovery and return to work after mutilating hand injuries: Usefulness of Campbell's Hand Injury Severity Score. *J Hand Surg* 2009;34(5):880-885.
14. Yaffe MA, Kaplan FT: Agricultural injuries to the hand and upper extremity. *J Am Acad Orthop Surg* 2014;22(10):605-613.
15. Sassoon A, Riehl J, Rich A, et al: Muscle viability revisited: Are we removing normal muscle? A critical evaluation of dogmatic debridement. *J Orthop Trauma* 2016;30(1):17-21.

    The authors obtained 36 muscle biopsies from trauma patients to compare surgeon's impression of tissue viability to histologic assessment of viability. They noted that in 60% of patients, the surgeon's distinction of nonviable tissue was incorrect on histologic exam. Level of evidence: II.
16. Russell RC, Neumeister MW, Ostric SA, Engineer NJ: Extremity reconstruction using nonreplantable tissue ("spare parts"). *Clin Plast Surg* 2007;34(2):211-222, viii.
17. Brown PW: War wounds of the hand revisited. *J Hand Surg* 1995;20(3 Pt 2):S61-S67.
18. Anglen JO: Wound irrigation in musculoskeletal injury. *J Am Acad Orthop Surg* 2001;9(4):219-226.
19. The FLOW Investigators, Bhandari M, Jeray KJ, et al: A trial of wound irrigation in the initial management of open fracture wounds. *N Engl J Med* 2015;373(27):2629-2641.
20. Possley DR, Burns TC, Stinner DJ, et al: Temporary external fixation is safe in a combat environment. *J Trauma* 2010;69(suppl 1):S135-S139.
21. Ruch DS, Ginn TA, Yang CC, Smith BP, Rushing J, Hanel DP: Use of a distraction plate for distal radial fractures with metaphyseal and diaphyseal comminution. *J Bone Joint Surg Am* 2005;87(5):945-954.
22. Bhardwaj P, Sankaran A, Sabapathy SR: Skeletal fixation in a mutilated hand. *Hand Clin* 2016;32(4):505-517.

    The authors present a review of the various methods to provide skeletal fixation in the mutilated hand such as Kirschner wires, plate and screw constructs, and external fixators. In addition, they recommend staged reconstruction in the setting of segmental bone loss. Level of evidence: V.
23. Masquelet AC: Induced membrane technique: Pearls and pitfalls. *J Orthop Trauma* 2017;31(suppl 5):S36-S38.

    In this review article, the author who had initially described the technique of induced membrane formation discusses the procedure in great detail with pearls for effectively performing the staged procedures. Level of evidence: V.
24. Herisson O, Masquelet AC, Doursounian L, Sautet A, Cambon-Binder A: Finger reconstruction using induced membrane technique and ulnar pedicled forearm flap: A case report. *Arch Orthop Trauma Surg* 2017;137(5):719-723.

    The authors present a case to illustrate the utility of an induce membrane in a contaminated, mutilated hand to reconstruct skeletal defects in the hand. In this case, the patient underwent staged procedures with functional limb. Level of evidence: IV.
25. Micev AJ, Kalainov DM, Soneru AP: Masquelet technique for treatment of segmental bone loss in the upper extremity. *J Hand Surg* 2015;40(3):593-598.
26. Bishop AR, Kim S, Squire MW, Rose WE, Ploeg HL: Vancomycin elution, activity and impact on mechanical properties when added to orthopedic bone cement. *J Mech Behav Biomed Mater* 2018;87:80-86.

The authors performed mechanical and elution testing of Palacos polymethyl-methacrylate bone cement mixed with vancomycin. They noted vancomycin can elute from the cement for up to 60 days. Level of evidence: II.

27. Aho OM, Lehenkari P, Ristiniemi J, Lehtonen S, Risteli J, Leskela HV: The mechanism of action of induced membranes in bone repair. *J Bone Joint Surg Am* 2013;95(7):597-604.
28. Weber MA, Fox CJ, Adams E, et al: Upper extremity arterial combat injury management. *Perspect Vasc Surg Endovasc Ther* 2006;18(2):141-145.
29. Starnes BW, Beekley AC, Sebesta JA, Andersen CA, Rush RM Jr: Extremity vascular injuries on the battlefield: Tips for surgeons deploying to war. *J Trauma* 2006;60(2):432-442.
30. Granchi T, Schmittling Z, Vasquez J, Schreiber M, Wall M: Prolonged use of intraluminal arterial shunts without systemic anticoagulation. *Am J Surg* 2000;180(6):493-496; discussion 496-497.
31. Fox CJ, Gillespie DL, O'Donnell SD, et al: Contemporary management of wartime vascular trauma. *J Vasc Surg* 2005;41(4):638-644.
32. Geer DA, Olson DW: Vascular graft coverage in peripheral vascular injuries. *Mil Med* 1986;151(4):224-226.
33. Panattoni JB, Ahmed MM, Busel GA: An ABC technical algorithm to treat the mangled upper extremity: Systematic surgical approach. *J Hand Surg* 2017;42(11):934.e1-934.e10.

    In this review article, the authors present an algorithm of evaluating and managing the mangled upper extremity. They recommend bony stabilizing, tendon and nerve repair or reconstruction, and soft-tissue coverage to salvage the limb. Level of evidence: V.

34. Wang E, Inaba K, Byerly S, et al: Optimal timing for repair of peripheral nerve injuries. *J Trauma Acute Care Surg* 2017;83(5):875-881.

    The authors present a retrospective study on the motor and sensory outcomes in traumatic peripheral nerve injuries. They noted that patient characteristics and injury level influenced final outcomes over surgical factors such as time from injury to nerve repair. Level of evidence: III.

35. Ng ZY, Askari M, Chim H: Approach to complex upper extremity injury: An algorithm. *Semin Plast Surg* 2015;29(1):5-9.
36. Morykwas MJ, Simpson J, Punger K, Argenta A, Kremers L, Argenta J: Vacuum-assisted closure: State of basic research and physiologic foundation. *Plast Reconstr Surg* 2006; 117(7 suppl):121S-126S.
37. Leversedge FJ, Moore TJ, Peterson BC, Seiler JG III: Compartment syndrome of the upper extremity. *J Hand Surg* 2011;36(3):544-559; quiz 560.
38. Prucz RB, Friedrich JB: Upper extremity replantation: Current concepts. *Plast Reconstr Surg* 2014;133(2):333-342.
39. Tang JB, Wang ZT, Chen J, Wong J: A global view of digital replantation and revascularization. *Clin Plast Surg* 2017;44(2):189-209.

    Survival rates of digital replantation range from 65% to 85% in most countries. A few extremely difficult digital replantations illustrate how surgeons have challenged themselves in pushing the limits of microsurgery in salvaging amputated digits. Level of evidence: V.

40. Friedrich JB, Poppler LH, Mack CD, Rivara FP, Levin LS, Klein MB: Epidemiology of upper extremity replantation surgery in the United States. *J Hand Surg* 2011;36(11):1835-1840.
41. Mahmoudi E, Chung KC: Effect of hospital volume on success of thumb replantation. *J Hand Surg* 2017;42(2):96-103.e105.

    Regionalization of digit replantation procedures to high volume centers can achieve the highest rate of successful revascularization. Patient-level logistics models were used to examine the association between a hospitals annual thumb replantation volume and the probability success. Level of evidence: II.

42. Kotsougiani D, Ringwald F, Hundepool CA, et al: Safety and suitability of finger replantations as a residency training procedure: A retrospective cohort study with analysis of the initial postoperative outcomes. *Ann Plast Surg* 2017;78(4):431-435.

    Finger replantations can be applied as a safe procedure in residency training under standardized conditions and do not negatively affect quality of care. Retrospective comparison study in which two patients cohorts were compared. Level of evidence: III.

43. Maroukis BL, Shauver MJ, Nishizuka T, Hirata H, Chung KC: Cross-cultural variation in preference for replantation or revision amputation: Societal and surgeon views. *Injury* 2016;47(4):818-823.

    US society and surgeon surveys were compared to Japanese society and surgeon surveys. Japanese society and surgeons had a stronger preference for replantation than American society and surgeons, possibly attributed to cultural differences. Level of evidence: II.

44. Abzug JM, Kozin SH: Pediatric replantation. *J Hand Surg* 2014;39(1):143-145.
45. Squitieri L, Reichert H, Kim HM, Steggerda J, Chung KC: Patterns of surgical care and health disparities of treating pediatric finger amputation injuries in the United States. *J Am Coll Surg* 2011;213(4):475-485.
46. Wolfe VM, Wang AA: Replantation of the upper extremity: Current concepts. *J Am Acad Orthop Surg* 2015;23(6):373-381.
47. Hattori Y, Doi K, Ikeda K, Estrella EP: A retrospective study of functional outcomes after successful replantation versus amputation closure for single fingertip amputations. *J Hand Surg* 2006;31(5):811-818.
48. Kim WK, Lim JH, Han SK: Fingertip replantations: Clinical evaluation of 135 digits. *Plast Reconstr Surg* 1996;98(3):470-476.
49. Adani R, Marcoccio I, Castagnetti C, Tarallo L: Long-term results of replantation for complete ring avulsion amputations. *Ann Plast Surg* 2003;51(6):564-568; discussion 569.

50. Sears ED, Chung KC: Replantation of finger avulsion injuries: A systematic review of survival and functional outcomes. *J Hand Surg* 2011;36(4):686-694.

51. Paavilainen P, Nietosvaara Y, Tikkinen KA, Salmi T, Paakkala T, Vilkki S: Long-term results of transmetacarpal replantation. *J Plast Reconstr Aesthet Surg* 2007;60(7):704-709.

52. Dec W: A meta-analysis of success rates for digit replantation. *Tech Hand Up Extrem Surg* 2006;10(3):124-129.

53. Kwon GD, Ahn BM, Lee JS, Park YG, Chang GW, Ha YC: The effect of patient age on the success rate of digital replantation. *Plast Reconstr Surg* 2017;139(2):420-426.

Analyses of all age groups older than 20 demonstrated a significant increase in failure rate in those aged 70 years and older. The authors demonstrated a high rate of digit replantation success in elderly patients. Level of evidence: III.

54. Zhu X, Zhu H, Zhang C, Zheng X: Pre-operative predictive factors for the survival of replanted digits. *Int Orthop* 2017;41(8):1623-1626.

Univariate and multivariate analyses were performed to evaluate the correlation between potential risk factors and failure rate. Heavy cigarette consumption, increased age, noncut injury and prolonged ischemia time were risk factors for replant failure. Level of evidence: III.

55. Woo SH, Cheon HJ, Kim YW, Kang DH, Nam HJ: Delayed and suspended replantation for complete amputation of digits and hands. *J Hand Surg* 2015;40(5):883-889.

56. Ross M, Bollman C, Couzens GB: Use of low-profile palmar internal fixation in digital replantation. *Tech Hand Up Extrem Surg* 2015;19(4):147-152.

57. Ozaksar K, Toros T, Sugun TS, Kayalar M, Kaplan I, Ada S: Finger replantations after ring avulsion amputations. *J Hand Surg Eur Vol* 2012;37(4):329-335.

58. Dadaci M, Isci ET, Ince B, et al: Negative pressure wound therapy in the early period after hand and forearm replantation, is it safe? *J Wound Care* 2016;25(6):350-355.

Negative pressure wound therapy (75 mm Hg) can be used in the intermittent mode in order to improve wound healing and shorten the period to start physical therapy in the early period after replantation and revascularization. Level of evidence: III.

59. Wagner ER, Bishop AT, Shin AY: Venous bridge arterial grafting for thumb replantation. *Hand* 2017;12(3):272-276.

The authors describe a novel technique to bridge the dorsal radial artery to the ulnar digital artery of the thumb. Eight patients were retrospectively followed and remained viable. This novel arterial reconstruction has shown promise in thumbs replantation. Level of evidence: III.

60. Camacho FJ, Wood MB: Polydigit replantation. *Hand Clin* 1992;8(3):409-412.

61. Kwon GD, Ahn BM, Lee JS, Park YG, Ha YC: Clinical outcomes of a simultaneous replantation technique for amputations of four or five digits. *Microsurgery* 2016;36(3):225-229.

The results of 43 cases have been reviewed and showed that simultaneous replantation technique of four or five digit amputations may provide and alternative method to shorten surgical time, reduce complication rates and enhance high survival rate. Level of evidence: III.

62. Kokkoli E, Spyropoulou GA, Shih HS, Feng GM, Jeng SF: Heterotopic procedures in mutilating hand injuries: A synopsis of essential reconstructive tools. *Plast Reconstr Surg* 2015;136(5):1015-1026.

63. Zhang GL, Chen KM, Zhang JH, Wang SY: Hand reconstruction using heterotopic replantation of amputated index and little fingers. *Chin J Traumatol* 2011;14(5):316-318.

64. Nazerani S, Motamedi MH: Ectopic single-finger transplantation, a novel technique for nonreplantable digits: Assessment of 24 cases-presenting the "piggyback" method. *Tech Hand Up Extrem Surg* 2009;13(2):65-74.

65. Chu YY, Yu DY, Chang CW, Fang F, Liao HT: Determination of a threshold compromise value for the perfusion index by laser Doppler imaging after digital revascularization. *J Hand Surg Eur Vol* 2017;42(6):633-639.

Assessment of laser Doppler imaging to monitor the microcirculation in replanted digits (103 cases). The authors believe that by establishing a threshold, laser Doppler imaging should provide a reliable and objective assessment for the development of perfusion compromise after replantation. Level of evidence: III.

66. Zhu H, Zhu X, Zheng X: Antithrombotic therapies in digit replantation with papaverine administration: A prospective, observational study. *Plast Reconstr Surg* 2017;140(4):743-746.

Survival rates of 477 digits of 319 patients after replantation were assessed for three different antithrombotic therapies. Different antithrombotic therapies showed no significant benefit for digit re-plantation in patients receiving papaverine. Level of evidence: II.

67. Levine SM, Frangos SG, Hanna B, Colen K, Levine JP: *Aeromonas* septicemia after medicinal leech use following replantation of severed digits. *Am J Crit Care* 2010;19(5):469-471.

68. Knight R, Pagkalos J, Timmons C, Jose R: Caffeine consumption does not have an effect on digital microvascular perfusion assessed by laser Doppler imaging on healthy volunteers: A pilot study. *J Hand Surg Eur Vol* 2015;40(4):412-415.

Section 7

Hip and Femur

EDITOR

Jeffrey A. Geller, MD

Chapter 34

Anatomy and Biomechanics, Evaluation, Clinical Examination, and Imaging of the Hip

Hany Bedair, MD • Maureen K. Dwyer, PhD, ATC

ABSTRACT

The hip is a complex joint which allows for motion in multiple planes and serves as the axis to propel the body forward into motion. Extensive knowledge of anatomy and normal function of the hip is critical to identifying pathologies and developing successful treatment strategies. The hip is an inherently stable joint, supported by its bony morphology, the strong capsuloligamentous complex surrounding it, and the multitude of muscles acting upon it. Any alteration to normal joint morphology can place the hip at risk for pathology, because of the effect on joint loading and function. A comprehensive clinical examination of the hip should include a thorough history, gait analysis, palpation, and special tests. Multiple imaging modalities are available to assess patients with hip pain; however, findings from imaging studies should be used in accordance with clinical examination findings to confirm a suspected diagnosis.

Keywords: biomechanics; hip anatomy; hip clinical examination; imaging

Introduction

The hip is a complex joint which allows for motion in multiple planes and serves as the axis to propel the body forward into motion. Extensive knowledge of anatomy and normal function of the hip is critical to identifying pathologies and developing successful treatment strategies. This chapter describes the basic anatomy and biomechanics of the hip and provides an overview of clinical examination principles and diagnostic imaging approaches.

Osseous and Ligamentous Anatomy

The hip is a multiaxial joint formed by the articulation between the pelvis and femur, which connects the axial skeleton and the lower extremity. The hemipelvis comprises three bones, the ilium, ischium, and pubis, which unite at the triradiate cartilage within the concave acetabulum. The shape and depth of the acetabulum is formed by the appearance of ossification centers around the end of the first decade of life, with complete fusion occurring around 18 to 19 years of age.[1] The ilium is a large flat bone that forms the majority of the coxal bone. Forming the ilium's superior margin, the iliac crest terminates anteriorly at the anterior superior iliac spine (ASIS) and posteriorly at the posterior superior iliac spine (PSIS). Inferior to the ASIS and PSIS are the anterior and posterior inferior iliac spines (AIIS and PIIS). These bony landmarks are clinically important areas of the physical examination and serve as attachment points for various muscles. Directly below the PIIS is the greater sciatic notch through which the large sciatic nerve travels to pass out of the pelvis, and into the thigh. The ischium, a small L-shaped bone, forms the posteroinferior margin of the pelvis. The thickened portion of its body, the ischial tuberosity, is easily palpable posteriorly and also serves as the large attachment site for multiple muscle groups. Anteriorly, the pubis bone consists of a body and two rami that connect superiorly to the ilium and inferiorly to the ischium to form the obturator foramen, an important anatomical landmark that serves as a conduit for arteries and nerves. The obturator foramen is covered by a strong membrane that provides surface area for muscle attachments. The hemipelvises unite anteriorly at the pubic symphyses and articulate posteriorly with the sacral ala to form the sacroiliac (SI) joint.

Dr. Bedair or an immediate family member serves as a paid consultant to or is an employee of Smith & Nephew; has stock or stock options held in DEF Medical and Osteon Holdings; and has received research support from Zimmer. Neither Dr. Dwyer nor any immediate family member has received anything of value from or has stock or stock options held in a commercial company or institution related directly or indirectly to the subject of this chapter.

The acetabulum comprises an articular crescent-moon–shaped lunate surface and a nonarticular central fossa that serves as the attachment point for the ligamentum teres. The acetabulum is incomplete inferiorly, forming a notch through which vital blood vessels and nerves pass to supply the joint. Attached to the rim of the acetabulum is the acetabular labrum, a fibrocartilaginous ring that extends the articulating surface area and increases femoral head coverage.[2] The labrum is triangular in cross section,[2-4] which contributes to its ability to create a pressurized seal of the central compartment of the hip during loading.[5,6] Only the external one-third of the labrum contains blood vessels, leaving the majority of the structure avascular,[7] limiting its healing ability following injury. The labrum is highly innervated, with the presence of both mechanoreceptors and nociceptors.[8] The labrum is absent in the area of the inferior acetabular notch, where the transverse acetabular ligament serves as the continuation of the labrum, connecting the anterior and posterior lunate surfaces of the acetabulum.[7,9]

The femoral head forms two-thirds of a sphere, with a small depression at its center from which the ligamentum teres extends to connect to the acetabular notch, blending with the transverse ligament. This connection provides a means by which the femoral head receives its blood supply via the acetabular branch of the obturator artery, named the artery of the ligamentum teres. The head is covered with articular cartilage and is connected to the shaft by the femoral neck, with the long axis of head and neck projecting superomedially at an angle to that of the obliquely oriented shaft. The neck-shaft angle averages 125°,[10] which allows for greater mobility as it places the head and neck more perpendicular to the acetabulum in a neutral position. Normal version, the head-neck angle in the frontal plane, averages 15 to 20°.[11] The angular projection of the femoral head and neck in relation to the obliquely placed acetabulum allows for the rotary movements at the hip and prevents impingement. At the junction of the neck and shaft are the greater and lesser trochanters, which are connected by the intertrochanteric line anteriorly and the intertrochanteric crest posteriorly. These bony prominences serve as important bony landmarks as well as attachment sites for thigh and pelvic muscles.

The hip is surrounded by a dense fibrous capsule extending from the periphery of the acetabulum to the intertrochanteric line of the femoral neck. The capsule enhances joint stability by preventing translation of the femoral head in the acetabulum.[12] Reinforcing the capsule are the three main ligaments that support the hip. Anteriorly, the Y-shaped iliofemoral ligament is the thickest and strongest of the three. The medial portion of the ligament connects the anterior inferior iliac spine to the anterior intertrochanteric line, while the lateral portion originates slightly superior to the medial arm and attaches to the anterior greater trochanter. The iliofemoral ligament functions to limit external rotation,[39-41] while, in isolation, the lateral arm limits extension of the joint.[39] Extending from the ischial margin of the acetabulum to the greater trochanter of the femur, the ischiofemoral ligament provides support posteriorly and restricts internal rotation motion.[39] Inferiorly, the pubofemoral ligament extends from the obturator crest of the pubic bone to the femoral neck and acts to limit abduction of the joint. Deep fibers from all three ligaments merge to form the zona orbicularis, which circumvents the femoral neck, adding vital stability to the anterosuperior portion of the joint capsule.[11] The zona orbicularis provides the greatest contribution to resisting dislocation forces.[13]

Muscular Anatomy

Multiple muscles cross the hip, providing motion in all three cardinal planes and enhancing joint stability. The muscles are organized into four compartments based on their location and function—the gluteal region, anterior compartment, medial compartment, and posterior compartment.

Anterior Compartment

The anterior compartment consists of the sartorius, iliopsoas, quadriceps, and pectineus muscles. The most superficial muscle, the sartorius is the longest muscle in the body, running obliquely from the ASIS to insert on the proximal medial tibia at the pes anserine. The sartorius acts to flex, abduct, and laterally rotate the femur at the hip and flexes the leg at the knee. The iliopsoas muscle is a composite of the iliacus, psoas major, and psoas minor muscles, whose fibers merge to form a conjoined tendon that attaches to the lesser trochanter of the femur. The iliacus muscle originates from the iliac crest, iliac fossa, and sacrum, whereas the psoas major originates from the transverse processes, bodies, and disks of the T12-L5 vertebrae. The psoas minor originates from the body and intervertebral disks of T12 and L1 vertebrae. The iliopsoas muscle is the prime flexor of the femur at the hip and contributes to lateral rotation, whereas the psoas major contributes to spinal stabilization. The quadriceps muscle group consists of four muscles—the vastus lateralis, vastus medialis, vastus intermedius, and rectus femoris muscles. The rectus femoris muscle originates on the ASIS, whereas the vasti muscles originate along the anterior proximal shaft of the femur. Together, they form a conjoined tendon that attaches directly to the base of the patella and indirectly to the tibial tuberosity via the patellar ligament. As a group, the quadriceps muscle flexes the leg at the knee. The rectus femoris is the only one of the four to contribute to hip motion, assisting with hip flexion. With the exception of the psoas major and psoas minor muscles, which are innervated by the anterior rami of lumbar nerves, all muscles in the anterior compartment are innervated by the femoral nerve.

Gluteal Region

The gluteal region is organized into two layers of muscles—superficial and deep. The largest and most superficial of the gluteal muscles, the gluteus maximus originates from the outer surface of the ilium, the sacrum, coccyx, and sacrotuberous ligament and inserts into the iliotibial tract and gluteal tuberosity. As the strongest extensor and lateral rotator of the hip, the gluteus maximus is most active against resistance and when rising from sitting. The gluteus medius originates from the external ilium between the superior and posterior gluteal lines and attaches to the greater trochanter, whereas the gluteus minimus extends from the external ilium between the anterior and inferior gluteal lines and attaches to the greater trochanter, anterior to the gluteus medius. The tensor of fascia lata extends from the ASIS to insert into the iliotibial tract. The tensor of fascia lata contributes to abduction and medial rotation of the thigh. The primary function of the gluteus medius and minimus is to stabilize the pelvis during single limb support.[14] With the exception of the gluteus maximus, which is innervated by the inferior gluteal nerve, the muscles of the superficial gluteal region are innervated by the superior gluteal nerve.

The deep layer of the gluteal region consists of a group of small, deep muscles which primarily serve to stabilize the head of the femur in the acetabulum. This group of muscles includes the piriformis, the superior and inferior gemelli muscles, the obturator internus, and the quadratus femoris muscles. Most of these muscles insert on the medial surface of the greater trochanter, whereas the quadratus femoris originates laterally on the ischial tuberosity and attaches to the quadrate tubercle of the femur. The obturator internus and superior gemelli muscles are innervated by the nerve to the obturator internus, whereas the inferior gemelli and quadratus femoris are innervated by the nerve to the quadratus femoris. The superior and inferior gemelli muscles, piriformis muscle, and obturator externus muscle also assist in external rotation of the femur. The obturator internus muscle assists in internal rotation of the femur at the hip.

Medial Compartment

The medial compartment consists of the adductor muscle group, gracilis, and obturator externus muscles. The adductor muscle group comprises three muscles—the adductor longus, adductor brevis, and adductor magnus. The adductor longus originates on the body of the pubis and attaches distally to the linea aspera of the femur. The shortest of the three, the adductor brevis originates at the body and inferior rami of the pubis and attaches to the pectineal line of the femur at the proximal linea aspera. The adductor magnus is a composite muscle, with the adductor portion originating at the ischial and pubic rami and inserting at the gluteal tuberosity and linea aspera, whereas the hamstring portion originates at the ischial tuberosity and inserts at the adductor tubercle of the femur. The gracilis muscle originates at the inferior ramus of the pubis and attaches to the medial upper tibia at the pes anserine. The obturator externus originates from the margins of the obturator foramen and the obturator membrane and attaches to the trochanteric fossa of the femur. All of the muscles in the medial compartment are innervated by the obturator nerve, with the exception of the hamstring portion of the adductor magnus, which is innervated by the tibial portion of the sciatic nerve. The adductor longus, adductor brevis, and gracilis muscles all contribute to active adduction of the femur at the hip, whereas the gracilis muscle also assists with flexion and medial rotation.

Posterior Compartment

The posterior compartment of the thigh consists of the hamstring muscles. The medial hamstring muscles, the semimembranosus and semitendonosus originate at the ischial tuberosity, with the former attaching to the posterior part of the medial tibial condyle and the latter to the superior medial tibia at the pes anserine. The long head of the biceps femoris originates at the ischial tuberosity and the short head originates at the linea aspera and lateral supracondylar line of the femur, with both attaching to the fibular head. The hamstrings are innervated by the sciatic nerve and function to extend the thigh at the hip and flex the leg at the knee. The medial hamstrings also contribute to medial rotation of the leg and the lateral hamstrings to lateral rotation.

Hip Biomechanics

The orientation and depth of the articulating surfaces of the hip result in an inherently stable joint; however, the acetabulum has a slightly smaller diameter than the femoral head, resulting in the hip being slightly incongruous.[15] This incongruity is important for optimizing load transmission[16,17] and permitting the arthrokinematic motions of gliding and rolling.[18] Rotary movements of the femoral head in the acetabulum orient it to properly allow the hip to move through large ranges of motion without impinging. Motion at the hip occurs in all three axes, resulting in flexion-extension, abduction-adduction, and internal-external rotation movements. The degree of active motion occurring at the hip in a single plane averages 120° of flexion, 20° of extension, 45° of abduction, 30° of adduction, and 30° to 35° of internal and external rotation.[19-21] However, during normal activities of daily life, the hip generally functions within a smaller range of motion. Normal gait requires 40° of sagittal plane hip motion, with limited frontal and transverse plane motion at the hip.[22] Sagittal plane motion requirements are greater for activities such as stair climbing, kneeling, and sitting cross-legged, with hip flexion averaging 90°.[23,24]

As stated previously, the incongruity of the hip is important in the distribution of loads applied to joint surfaces. Contact areas are limited to the anterior and posterior lunate surfaces during light loads; however, as loads increase, such as those experienced during the stance phase of gait, the entire acetabular surface will become weight bearing.[25] Contact stresses are highly variable between individuals and activity, with the highest stresses observed anteriorly during stair descent and superioposteriorly during stair ascent.[26,27] Alterations in joint morphology and orientation can result in significant increases in stresses incurred by the cartilaginous surfaces of the joint and may predispose these individuals to degenerative conditions. External forces acting upon the hip are also affected by joint morphology and vary greatly with the type of activity, ranging from 2 to 4 times body weight during gait[42] up to and exceeding 8 times body weight during unanticipated stumbling.[43] The resultant forces acting upon the hip are primarily dictated by the muscles that act upon it. Muscles are the primary contributor to hip contact forces, with contributions from gravitational and centrifugal forces totalling less than 5%.[44] During gait, the gluteus medius muscle provides the greatest contribution to the superior and medial forces, with lesser contribution from gluteus maximus.[44] Alteration to the force-producing capabilities of muscles disrupts normal joint mechanics, resulting in abnormal force distribution that places the hip at increased risk for pathology.[45,46]

Physical Examination

Given that the presentation of many hip disorders is nonspecific and can be referred to or from other regions, obtaining a thorough history and physical examination is important to ascertain the underlying cause of pain. Assessing the onset, duration, and location of symptoms, along with what factors exacerbate or alleviate pain, is important to determining its causes. For many patients with hip pain, there may not be a known precipitating event and the presentation of symptoms occurs gradually over months or years, versus acute pain secondary to trauma. In these instances, identifying changes to activity type or training regime can help differentiate between conditions.[47] Patients should also be asked to provide any previous history of the present condition or any previous treatments undertaken for the hip, whether operative or nonoperative. In addition, documenting any family history of hip conditions is important, as certain genetic conditions can affect the hip, such as Ehlers-Danlos syndrome.

The location of pain can be a strong indicator of the underlying pathology. Anterior groin pain is most associated with intra-articular pathologies which may include labral tears, degenerative changes, synovial pathologies, loose bodies, and osteonecrosis. Outside of intra-articular condition, anterior groin pain can also be the result of extra-articular conditions, such as hip flexor strains, iliopsoas snapping syndrome, or femoral stress fractures. Pain along the lateral thigh is often associated with greater trochanteric bursitis, iliotibial band syndrome, or abductor tendon tears or tendinitis. Pain in the posterior region of the hip and pelvis could be the result of muscle pathologies, such as piriformis syndrome and hamstring muscle tears; however, posterior pain can often be the result of referred pain from the sacroiliac joint or low back. A comprehensive evaluation should include examination of these structures as well.

Clinical Examination

A comprehensive clinical examination of the hip should be standardized and comprehensive, and the patient should be assessed while standing, supine, lateral, and prone. The standing examination should include gait analysis, anatomical alignment of the pelvis and spine, motion, and the Trendelenburg test. Analysis of gait should be performed in an area where the patient can take 6 to 8 consecutive strides. Observation of foot contact angle, pelvic obliquity, and limb length should be done both from the front and back. Antalgic gaits are characterized by a shortened stride length or shortened time in stance phase, limping, or abductor deficiency, resulting in a Trendelenburg gait.[28] Assessment of anatomical alignment is performed via palpation of important bony landmarks to ensure symmetry side to side and front to back, including the iliac crests, ASIS, and PSIS. The Trendelenburg test should be performed to assess stability and strength during single limb standing. Any increase in pelvic or trunk inclination would indicate a positive test.[29]

The clinical examination in supine should include measures of leg length and passive range of motion, palpation, and performance of provocative maneuvers to assess the presence of specific pathologies. The flexion, abduction, external rotation test (FABER) can help differentiate between pain derived from the hip, with reproduction of pain anteriorly, or from the sacroiliac joint, with reproduction of pain posteriorly. A modification of the FABER test can also be used to determine the presence of internal snapping hip syndrome. From the FABER position, the hip is actively extended and internally rotated, attempting to reproduce the catching of the iliopsoas tendon over the iliopectineal eminence. The flexion, adduction, and internal rotation test (FADDIR), or impingement test, assesses for the presence of intra-articular pathologies, and the Thomas test is used to evaluate for the presence of hip flexor contractures. The dynamic internal rotary (DIRIT) and external rotary (DEXRIT) impingement tests are useful to determine the presence of femoroacetabular impingement.[30] Additional tests that can be performed in the supine position would be the straight leg raise (SLR) to test for lumbar radiculopathy or the log roll to test for capsular insufficiency.

The lateral examination should include assessment of abductor muscle strength, palpation of the greater trochanter and iliotibial band, and two special tests. Tenderness at the tip of the greater trochanter may indicate abductor muscle tears or tendinitis, whereas tenderness distal to the greater trochanter is more indicative of hip trochanteric bursitis. Ober's test is performed with the patient in side-lying position, with a positive test indicating contracture of the iliotibial band. The piriformis test places the hip in flexion and internal rotation, which would cause compression of the sciatic nerve in the presence of piriformis syndrome. With the patient in the prone position, the Craig test can be performed to assess femoral anteversion, as well as Ely test to assess for rectus femoris contracture and irritation of the femoral nerve. Physical examination tests can be helpful in isolating out a cause of symptoms, but should be used in accordance with clinical examination findings.

Imaging

Multiple imaging technologies are available to assist with diagnosing the causes of hip pain in accordance with findings from the clinical examination. Plain radiographs are the first imaging studies obtained for patients presenting with hip pain and can determine the presence of fractures, degenerative changes, and abnormal joint morphology. The type of radiographic imaging performed is dependent upon the suspected pathology. Standard AP radiographs of the hip and pelvis are obtained to examine bony architecture, check for evidence of joint space narrowing or changes to bone quality, and quantify femoral head coverage. The Dunn view and frog leg view are appropriate to measure α angle to determine the presence of impingement.[31]

Magnetic Resonance Imaging

For patients suspected of soft tissue or intra-articular pathology, MRI is the modality of choice, given its superior sensitivity and specificity.[32] Conventional MRI is effective at identifying osteochondral injuries, musculotendinous pathologies, and inflammation. However, magnetic resonance arthrography (MRA) is more appropriate to determine injuries to the labrochondral structures and the ligamentum teres and identify the presence of loose bodies and synovial chondromatosis.[33] In the accurate detection and staging of articular cartilage lesions, the utility of MRA is reduced, with sensitivity reported to be less than 50% compared with arthroscopic findings.[34] Recent advances in MRI imaging techniques, such as delayed gadolinium-enhanced MR imaging and T2* mapping, allow for a more in-depth analysis of the structure of articular cartilage[35] and were effective at detecting early changes to the articular cartilage surfaces of patients with hip dysplasia and femoroacetabular impingement.[36]

Computed Tomography

CT scans are effective for examining cortical and cancellous bone and can be used to create three-dimensional reconstructions of the hip for use in surgical planning. Measurements of femoral head coverage and acetabular and femoral impingement can also be performed reliably using CT images.[37]

Ultrasonography

Although ultrasonography is a valuable tool to examine pediatric hip conditions, its utility in evaluating the adult hip is limited. Ultrasonography can be an effective modality to identify musculotendinous disruptions, effusions associated with intra-articular pathology, or inflammatory conditions, such as bursitis.[38] Ultrasonography is also being increasingly used for targeted injections into muscles, tendons, or intra-articularly around the hip, for use with corticosteroids or biologic treatments emerging as a more recognized modality.

Summary

The complexity of the hip and pelvic region can make accurate diagnosis of painful conditions difficult. A thorough understanding of normal anatomy and biomechanics is necessary to identify pathology and determine the appropriate course of treatment. Because many hip conditions present with similar symptoms, a comprehensive clinical examination is required to determine a differential diagnosis. Many imaging modalities are available to assist with identifying causes of hip pain; however, findings from imaging studies should complement clinical examination findings to provide the most accurate diagnosis.

Key Study Points

- The hip is a complex multiaxial joint capable of producing large forces and moving the thigh through large ranges of motion.
- Any alteration to joint morphology or function can place the hip at risk for pathology.
- A thorough history is essential to differentiating between common causes of hip pain. Clinical examination tests and imaging findings should be used to confirm a suspected clinical diagnosis.

Annotated References

1. Moore KL, Dalley AF, Agur AMR: *Clinically Oriented Anatomy*, ed 5. Philadelphia, Lippincott Williams & Wilkins, 2006.
2. Tan V, Seldes RM, Katz M, Freedhand AM, Klimkiewicz JJ, Fitzgerald RH: Contribution of acetabular labrum to articulating surface area and femoral head coverage in adult hip joints: An anatomic study in cadavera. *Am J Orthoped* 2001;30(11):809-812.
3. Lecouvet FE, Vande Berg BC, Malghem J, et al: MR imaging of acetabular labrum: Variations in 200 asymptomatic hips. *Am J Roentgenol* 1996;167:1025-1028.
4. Won Y-Y, Chung I, Chung N, Song K: Morphological study on the acetabular labrum. *Yonsei Med J* 2003;44(5):855-862.
5. Hlavacek M: The influence of the acetabular labrum seal, intact articular superficial zone and synovial fluid thixotropy on squeeze-film lubrication of a spherical synovial joint. *J Biomech* 2002;35:1325-1335.
6. Ferguson SJ, Bryant JT, Ganz R, Ito K: An in vitro investigation of the acetabular labral seal in hip joint mechanics. *J Biomech* 2003;36(2):171-178.
7. Peterson W, Peterson F, Tillman B: Structure and vascularization of the acetabular labrum with regard to the pathogenesis and healing of labral lesions. *Arch Orthop Trauma Surg* 2003;123:283-288.
8. Kim YT, Azuma H: The nerve endings of the acetabular labrum. *Clin Orthop Relat Res* 1995;320:176-181.
9. Lohe F, Eckstein F, Sauer T, Putz R: Structure, strain and function of the transverse acetabular ligament. *Acta Anat* 1996;157:315-323.
10. Boese CK, Dargel J, Oppermann J, et al: The femoral neck-shaft angle on plain radiographs: A systematic review. *Skeletal Radiol* 2016;45(1):19-28.

    The authors performed a systematic review to identify normative values for femoral neck-shaft angle on x-ray. The average angle was 129°. Level of evidence: I.
11. Torry MR, Schenker ML, Martin HD, Hogoboom D, Philippon M: Neuromuscular hip biomechanics and pathology in the athlete. *Clin Sports Med* 2006;25:179-197.
12. Smith MV, Costic RS, Allaire R, Schilling PL, Sekiya JK: A biomechanical analysis of the soft tissue and osseous constraints of the hip joint. *Knee Surg Sports Traumatol Arthrosc* 2014;22(4):946-952.
13. Ito H, Song Y, Lindsey DP, Safran MR, Giori NJ: The proximal hip joint capsule and the zona orbicularis contribute to hip joint stability in distraction. *J Orthop Res* 2009;27(8):989-995.
14. Gottschalk F, Kourosh S, Leveau B: The functional anatomy of tensor fasciae latae and gluteus medius and minimus. *J Anat* 1989;166:179-189.
15. Konrath GA, Hamel AJ, Olson SA, Bay B, Sharkey NA: The role of the acetabular labrum and the transverse acetabular ligament in load transmission in the hip. *J Bone Joint Surg Am* 1998;80-A(12):1781-1788.
16. Gu D, Hu F, Wei J, Dai K, Chen Y. Contributions of non-spherical hip joint cartilage surface to hip joint contact stress. Annual International Conference of the IEEE; August 30–September 3, 2011; Boston, MA.
17. von Eisenhart R, Adam C, Steinlechner M, Müller-Gerbl M, Eckstein F: Quantitative determination of joint incongruity and pressure distribution during simulated gait and cartilage thickness in the human hip joint. *J Orthop Res* 1999;17(4):532-539.
18. Menschik F: The hip joint as a conchoid shape. *J Biomech* 1997;30(9):971-973.
19. Magee D: *Orthopedic Physical Assessment*, ed 4. Pennsylvania, Saunders, 2002.
20. Roach KE, Miles TP: Normal hip and knee active range of motion: The relationship to age. *Phys Ther* 1991;71:656-665.
21. Moreside JM, McGill SM: Quantifying normal 3D hip ROM in healthy young adult males with clinical and laboratory tools: Hip mobility restrictions appear to be plane-specific. *Clin Biomech* 2011;26(8):824-829.
22. Perry J: *Gait analysis, in Normal and Pathological Function*. Thorofare, NJ, Slack, 1992.

23. Hemmerich A, Brown H, Smith S, Marthandam SS, Wyss UP: Hip, knee, and ankle kinematics of high range of motion activities of daily living. *J Orthop Res* 2006;24(4):770-781.
24. Lamontagne M, Beaulieu ML, Beaule PE: Comparison of joint mechanics of both lower limbs of THA patients with healthy participants during stair ascent and descent. *J Orthop Res* 2011;29(3):305-311.
25. Greenwald AS, Haynes DW: Weight-bearing areas in the human hip joint. *J Bone Joint Surg Br* 1972;54(1):157-163.
26. Harris MD, Anderson AE, Henak CR, Ellis BJ, Peters CL, Weiss JA: Finite element prediction of cartilage contact stresses in normal human hips. *J Orthop Res* 2012;30(7):1133-1139.
27. Anderson AE, Ellis BJ, Maas SA, Weiss JA: Effects of idealized joint geometry on finite element predictions of cartilage contact stresses in the hip. *J Biomech* 2010;43(7):1351-1357.
28. Kendall KD, Patel C, Wiley JP, Pohl MB, Emery CA, Ferber R: Steps toward the validation of the Trendelenburg test: The effect of experimentally reduced hip abductor muscle function on frontal plane mechanics. *Clin J Sport Med* 2013;23(1):45-51.
29. Hardcastle P, Nade S: The significance of the Trendelenburg test. *J Bone Joint Surg Br* 1985;67-B(5):741-746.
30. Martin HD, Kelly BT, Leunig M, et al: The pattern and technique in the clinical evaluation of the adult hip: The common physical examination tests of hip specialists. *Arthroscopy* 2010;26(2):161-172.
31. Blum A, Raymond A, Teixeira P: Strategy and optimization of diagnostic imaging in painful hip in adults. *Orthop Traumatol Surg Res* 2015;101(suppl 1):S85-S99.
32. Troum OM, Crues JV: The young adult with hip pain: Diagnosis and medical treatment, circa 2004. *Clin Orthop Relat Res* 2004;418:9-17.
33. Byrd JT, Jones KS: Diagnostic accuracy of clinical assessment, magnetic resonance imaging, magentic resonance arthrography, and intra-articular injection in hip arthroscopy patients. *Am J Sports Med* 2004;32(7):1668-1674.
34. Keeney JA, Peelle MW, Jackson J, Rubin D, Maloney WJ, Clohisy JC: Magnetic resonance arthrography versus arthroscopy in the evaluation of articular hip pathology. *Clin Orthop Relat Res* 2004;429:163-169.
35. Sutter R, Zanetti M, Pfirrmann CW: New developments in hip imaging. *Radiology* 2012;264(3):651-667.
36. Domayer SE, Mamisch TC, Kress I, Chan J, Kim YJ: Radial dGEMRIC in developmental dysplasia of the hip and in femoroacetabular impingement: Preliminary results. *Osteoarthritis Cartilage* 2010;18(11):1421-1428.
37. Murphy RJ, Subhawong TK, Chhabra A, Carrino JA, Armand M, Hungerford M: A quantitative method to assess focal acetabular overcoverage resulting from pincer deformity using CT data. *Clin Orthop Relat Res* 2011;469(10):2846-2854.
38. Martinoli C, Garello I, Marchetti A, et al: Hip ultrasound. *Eur J Radiol* 2012;81(12):3824-3831.
39. Wagner F, Negrao J, Campos J, et al: Capsular ligaments of the hip: Anatomic, histologic, and positional study in cadaveric specimens with MR arthrography. *Radiology* 2012;263(1):189-198.
40. Myers CA, Register BC, Lertwanich P, et al: Role of the acetabular labrum and the iliofemoral ligament in hip stability: An in vitro biplane fluoroscopy study. *Am J Sports Med* 2011;39:85S-91S.
41. Domb B, Philipon M, Giordano B: Arthroscopic capsulotomy, capsular repair, and capsular plication of the hip: Relation to atraumatic instability. *Arthroscopy* 2013;29(1):162-173.
42. Bergmann G, Graichen F, Rohlmann A: Hip joint loading during walking and running, measured in two patients. *J Biomech* 1993;26(8):969-990.
43. Bergmann G, Graichen F, Rohlmann A: Hip joint contact forces during stumbling. *Langenbeck's Arch Surg* 2004;389(1):53-59.
44. Correa TA, Crossley KM, Kim HJ, Pandy MG: Contributions of individual muscles to hip joint contact force in normal walking. *J Biomech* 2010;43(8):1618-1622.
45. Valente G, Taddei F, Jonkers I: Influence of weak hip abductor muscles on joint contact forces during normal walking: Probabilistic modeling analysis. *J Biomech* 2013;46(13):2186-2193.
46. Lewis CL, Sahrmann SA, Moran DW: Anterior hip joint force increases with hip extension, decreased gluteal force, or decreased iliopsoas force. *J Biomech* 2007;40:3725-3731.
47. Burnett SJ, Della Rocca GJ, Prather H, Curry M, Maloney WJ, Clohisy JC: Clinical presentation of patients with tears of acetabular labrum. *J Bone Joint Surg Am* 2006;88:1448-1457.

Anterior acetabular coverage (ACEA) is typically less than 20° in those with acetabular dysplasia. The Tönnis angle is typically greater than 10° to 14° in patients with acetabular dysplasia.[33]

Clinical Examination

The surgeon should apply a methodical approach during each evaluation. Observation of the patient standing is followed by a gait analysis, monitoring the pelvis, knees, and feet for antalgia, Trendelenburg sign, and dynamic internal rotation. A standing assessment of abductor strength can identify a Trendelenburg sign and abductor weakness. With the patient supine, a log-roll test and dial test can be performed with gentle internal and external rotation. A positive dial test correlates with capsular laxity.[34] Range of motion should then be assessed, documenting flexion, internal and external rotation in flexion (90°) and extension (prone), as well as abduction and adduction. Patients with dysplasia frequently exhibit greater ranges of motion than those with hip impingement possibly resulting from shallow coverage, soft-tissue laxity, or excessive femoral anteversion.[4,35] Abductor or trochanteric tenderness is frequent and can be palpated in the lateral decubitus position. Hip flexion, abduction, and adduction strength should also be assessed. Additional provocative testing, including impingement and FABER testing, should be performed with the patient supine. Instability testing should also be performed, evaluating both anterior (apprehension test) and posterior instability. A thorough neurovascular examination completes the full hip examination.

Treatments

A trial of conservative management should be attempted prior to considering surgical management. Anti-inflammatory medications, activity modification, physical therapy, and intra-articular injections may alleviate symptoms and should be the first line of treatment. Unfortunately, conservative means are unable to adequately correct osseous abnormalities, and surgical correction may often be necessary. Prior randomized studies have demonstrated benefit with physical therapy, but high crossover rates were seen, and additional investigation is needed.[36] Ultimately surgical intervention has shown favorable results as surgery effectively corrects the causes of chondrolabral injury resulting from impingement, dysplasia, and abnormal femoral version.

Hip Arthroscopy

First attempted in 1931, it was not until the early 2000s that hip arthroscopy saw technical advancement that allowed for proper treatment of FAI. Modern surgical techniques and instrumentation provide extensive access to the central compartment and peripheral compartments (**Figure 4**). Labral repair, débridement, and near-circumferential labral reconstruction are possible, along with extensive osseous resection including acetabuloplasty, femoroplasty, subspine resection, and heterotopic ossification excision, with additional cartilage restoration techniques including microfracture, abrasion chondroplasty, and cartilage transplantation. Recent anatomic, biomechanic, and clinical studies have highlighted the role of the capsule to confer stability to the hip, and a trend to close the hip capsule has surfaced in recent years.[37,38]

Hip arthroscopy is performed on a traction table by carefully distracting the joint with the minimum force required, as traction injuries are known complications.[39] The vast majority of intra- and extra-articular procedures are performed using two or three common portals. Fluoroscopy facilitates joint access for guidance and for proper osseous resection during acetabuloplasty or femoroplasty.

The overall outcomes after hip arthroscopy are consistently very good, with pain relief, functional improvement, and return to prior level of activity or play on par with surgeries for other joints in similar patient populations.[40-42] Subjective patient reported outcomes continue to support hip arthroscopy as the treatment of choice for properly selected patients with FAI who have previously failed nonsurgical treatment. The leading cause of failure after hip arthroscopy is inadequate bony resection of cam (majority) or pincer deformities.[43] Conversely, excessive resection has recently been proposed as a potential reason for failure as well.[44] Thus, diligent and meticulous osseous resection is required to properly correct and remove the cause of FAI and restore the labral seal. While arthroscopy provides a minimally invasive approach to the central and peripheral compartments, without an osteotomy and with less restrictive rehabilitation, arthroscopy does have limits. When bony deformity is excessive, difficult to access, or multiple procedures are to be performed, the surgical hip dislocation becomes the procedure of choice.[45]

Open Hip Preservation

Developed by Dr. Reinhold Ganz and colleagues in Switzerland, surgical dislocation of the hip (SDH) provides near 360° access to the acetabulum and femoral head without compromising the blood supply to the femoral head, and was the primary means of treating FAI prior to hip arthroscopy.[46] Surgery is performed in the lateral decubitus position using a Gibson approach

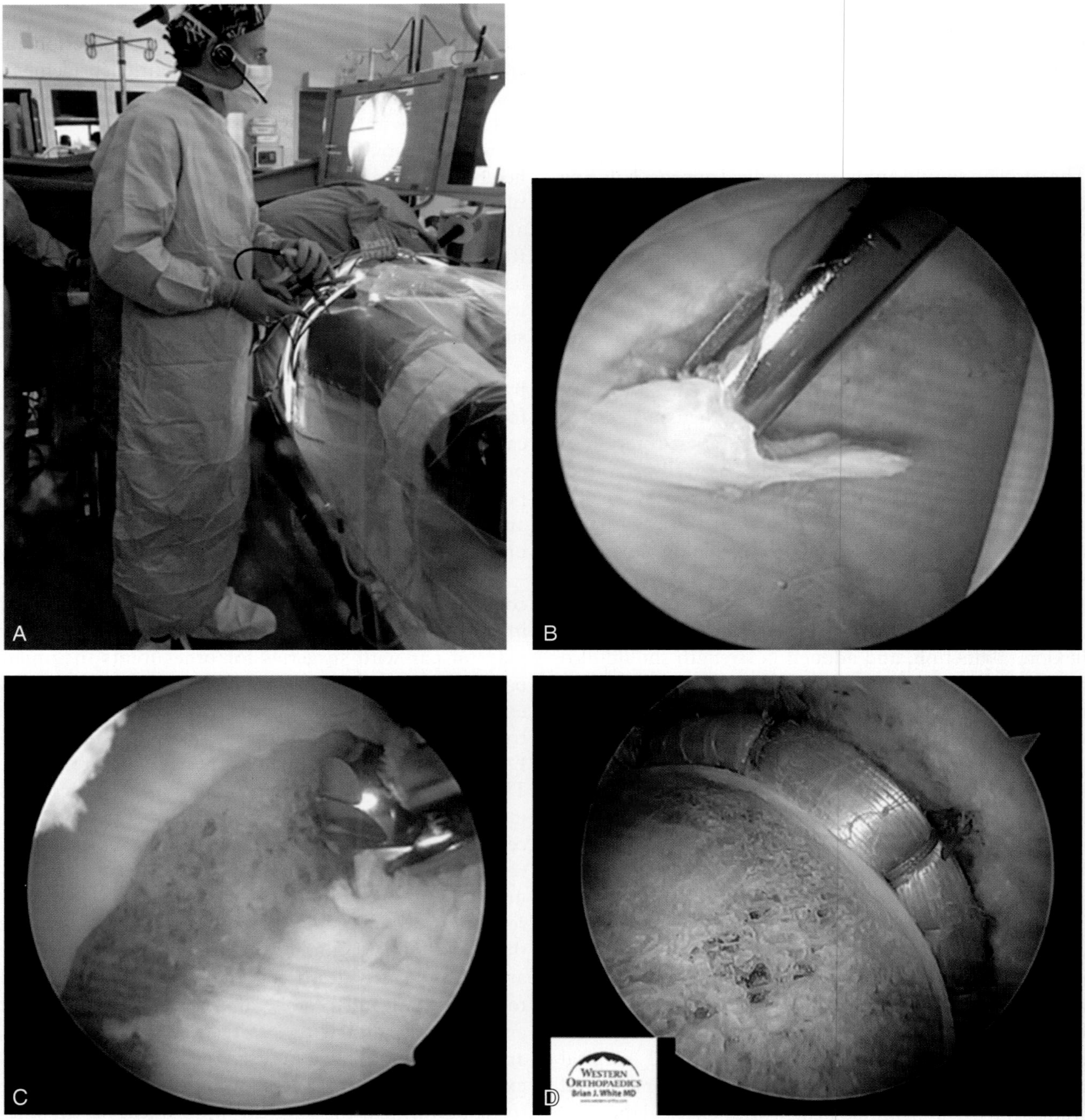

Figure 4 **A**, Photograph of hip arthroscopy set-up on a traction table with surgeon standing on the operative side using viewing and working portals to evaluate and treat hip pathology. **B**, Arthroscopic tool demonstrating a labral tear and associated chondrolabral delamination. **C**, Peripheral compartment view demonstrating the view through the capsulotomy as an arthroscopic burr is used to perform a femoroplasty. **D**, Peripheral compartment view of a circumferential labral reconstruction with fascia lata allograft demonstrating anatomic restoration of the labral seal against the femoral head. (Courtesy of and with permission from Brian J White, MD: Western Orthopaedics, Denver, CO, 2018.)

to separate the tensor fascia lata and gluteus maximus. A digastric osteotomy of the greater trochanter provides access to the anterior hip capsule, where a Z-capsulotomy exposes the joint without compromising the perforating vessels of the deep branch of the medial femoral circumflex artery.[46] Transection of the ligamentum teres is allows for anterior dislocation and complete access to the acetabulum, femoral head, neck and trochanteric region (**Figure 5**). The benefits of the SDH over arthroscopy include greater

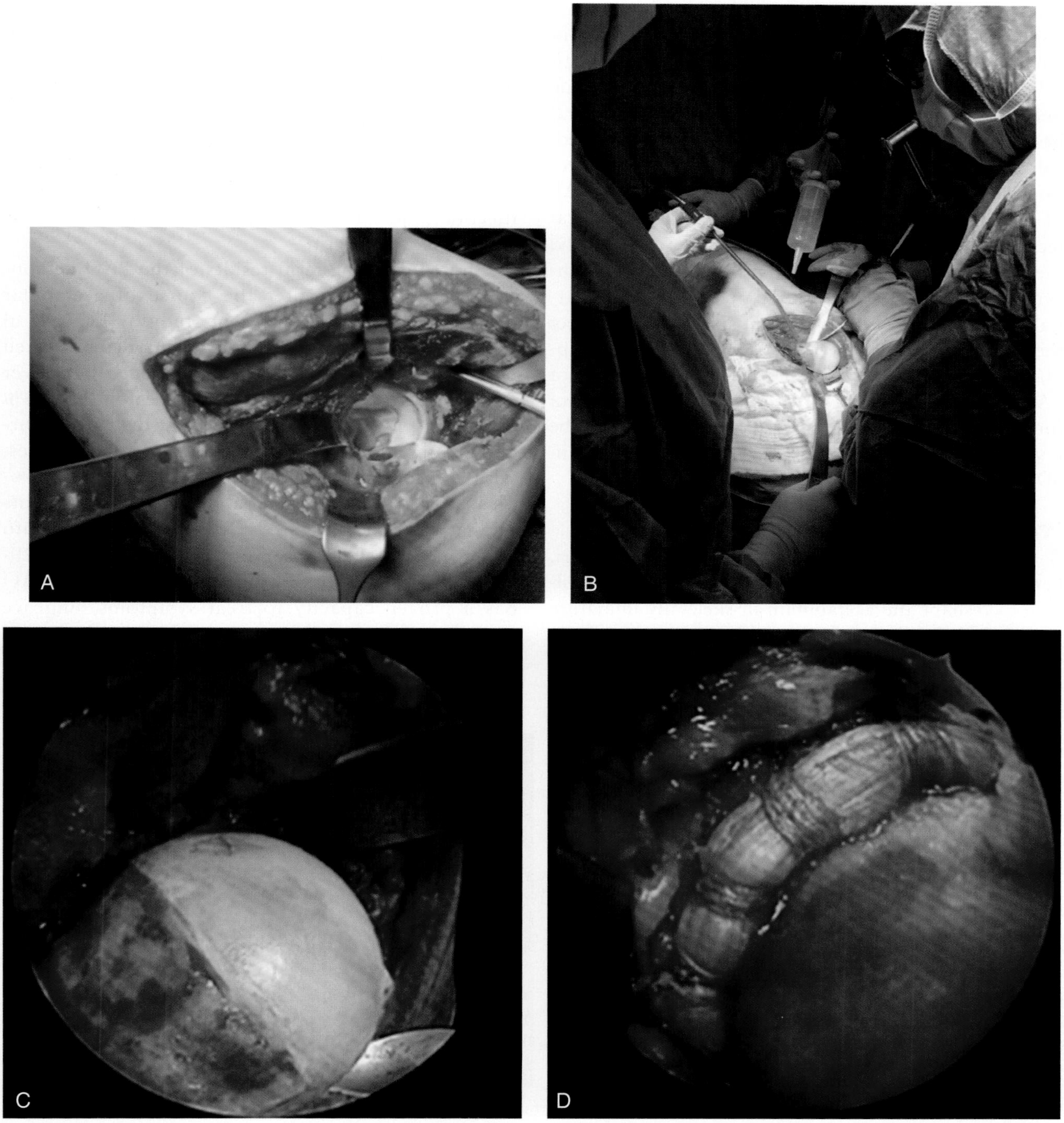

Figure 5 Clinical photograph demonstrating that surgical hip dislocation provides near-360° access to the (**A**) acetabulum and (**B**) femoral head. **C**, Arthroscopic view demonstrating that extensive femoroplasty for large and extensive cam deformities can be performed. **D**, Arthroscopic view of labral reconstruction. (A and B, Courtesy of Prof. Dr. med. Klaus Siebenrock and Prof. Dr. med. Moritz Tannast, Bern Switzerland, 2017.)

visualization, better access to global deformity, a thorough dynamic examination, treatment extra-articular impingement through the same approach, the ability to perform osteochondral transplantation, and the treatment of rare, complex deformities seen with Legg-Calvé-Perthes, slipped capital femoral epiphysis, and trauma.[46] Similar to hip arthroscopy, patient-reported outcomes demonstrate significant improvements in pain, function, and activity level.[46] However, surgical dislocation of the hip bears its own risks. While uncommon, iatrogenic osteonecrosis of the femoral head can occur if the perforator vessels are injured. Additionally, trochanteric nonunion, fracture, infection, and heterotopic ossification have been seen. All of these risks are minimized with meticulous surgical technique and proper patient selection. Additionally, the postoperative rehabilitation protocol differs significantly and requires trochanteric precautions and partial weight-bearing during the first six weeks to protect the osteotomy. While hip arthroscopy has largely supplanted surgical dislocation of the hip for treatment of FAI in the United States, it remains a highly useful tool for treatment of complex hip pathology but should be reserved for those with extensive surgical training in SDH.

Periacetabular Osteotomy

A variety of surgeries, including the Salter, Chiari, Pemberton, Steel and Triple osteotomies, are available to reshape the acetabulum in skeletally immature patients. Skeletally mature patients with symptomatic acetabular dysplasia have one surgical option—the eponymous Ganz osteotomy, which is a periacetabular osteotomy (PAO) developed by Reinhold Ganz for treatment of acetabular dysplasia.[47] The PAO is a complex pelvic osteotomy performed via a modified Smith-Peterson anterior approach that includes cuts of the ischium, superior pubic ramus, and innominate bones, completely freeing the acetabular fragment while maintaining the integrity of the posterior column (**Figure 6**). This complex osteotomy provides the ability to completely reposition the acetabulum and weight-bearing dome, balance the anterior, lateral, and posterior acetabular coverage, while simultaneously allowing partial weight bearing postoperatively. The PAO increases the stability of the hip joint, significantly improves joint kinematics and contact forces, reduces pain, improves function, and ultimately prevents degeneration in the long term.[48]

Short- and long-term results of the PAO demonstrate its ability to alter the course of acetabular dysplasia, described in a recent study by Lerch et al which indicated that 30% of patients demonstrated no radiographic signs of joint degeneration over 30 years after PAO. Subanalysis revealed that 50% of patients with a Tönnis grade <1 at the time of surgery exhibited no radiographic degenerative changes, with 40% eventually undergoing total hip arthroplasty (THA).[48] While generally reserved for patients with an LCEA less than 20, recent investigations into hip instability with borderline dysplasia (LCEA 20-25) suggest a potential role for the PAO.[49] The PAO has a proven capacity to treat symptoms, improve function, and alter the course of hip dysplasia and potentially has a greater role for treating our evolving understanding of hip instability.

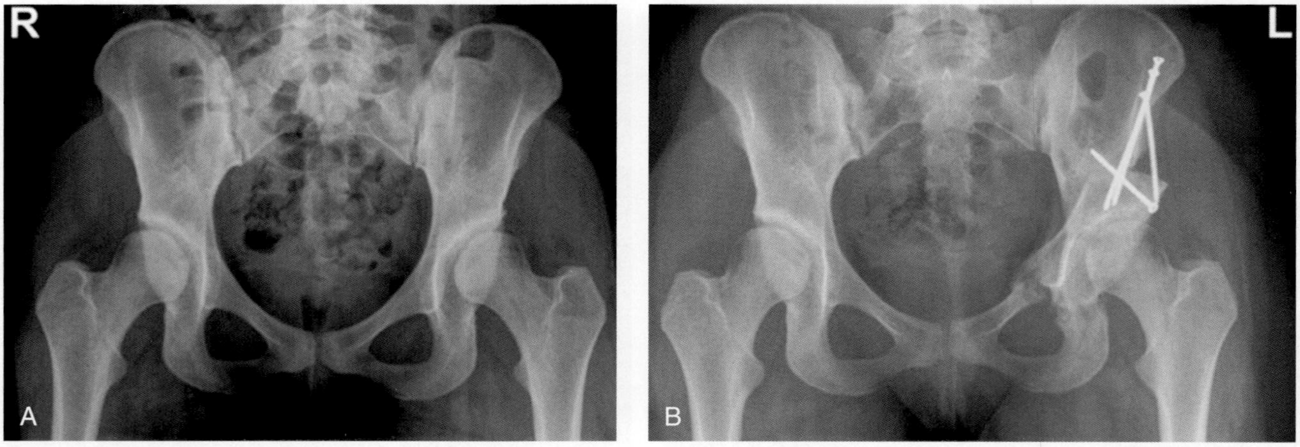

Figure 6 AP pelvis radiographs (**A**) before and (**B**) after a periacetabular osteotomy (PAO) in a young, athletic female demonstrating improvement of femoral head coverage and restoration of Shenton line.

Femoral Rotational Osteotomy

While historically used to treat hip or knee pain in children with excessive femoral antetorsion, Tönnis' femoral rotational osteotomy may have a role in treating adult hip pathology. Recent studies have demonstrated abnormal femoral torsion may be more common than previously thought.[8] Femoral torsion may be assessed clinically based on internal and external rotation in flexion and extension but is most accurately measured using CT or MRI.[11] Patients with excessive femoral antetorsion or retrotorsion frequently exhibit corresponding extremes of internal and external rotation, respectively. Excessive femoral antetorsion can lead to posterior ischiofemoral impingement, in which the femur (greater or lesser trochanter) contacts the ischium in external rotation, causing the femoral head to lever and subluxate anteriorly.[50] Conversely, excessive femoral retrotorsion causes impingement much earlier during internal rotation. Without proper correction of a rotational deformity, simple surgical treatment of the FAI may fail.

Proper correction of excessive femoral ante- or retroversion requires a femoral rotational osteotomy. A standard femoral rotational osteotomy can be performed open with a lateral incision and a compression plate or using an intramedullary nail, both of which use a subtrochanteric osteotomy. Occasionally, if the femoral neck demonstrates coxa valga, with a neck-shaft angle greater than 140°, a varus derotational osteotomy can be performed using a lateral approach and a plate to correct both the rotational and coronal deformities.

Summary

Our understanding of structural abnormalities of the acetabulum and femur and their role in chondrolabral damage and eventual joint degeneration has evolved significantly and, in tandem, so has the ability to treat a multitude of hip pathologies in the young adult. A thorough history and physical examination are essential to delineate the subtle differences among cam and pincer impingement, dysplasia and femoral version abnormalities. Diagnosed and treated properly, hip arthroscopy, surgical hip dislocation, periacetabular osteotomy, and/or femoral osteotomy have been shown to significantly improve pain and function and, in many cases, have the ability to alter the course of young adult hip pathology, potentially preventing early degenerative changes of the hip.

Key Study Points

- Osseous abnormalities of the acetabulum and proximal femur, including cam and pincer deformities, hip dysplasia, and abnormal femoral version, have been shown to cause pain, functional limitation, and eventual joint degeneration in young prearthritic hips.
- Hip impingement consists of cam, pincer, and combined deformities, each of which induce chondrolabral damage in distinct ways, ultimately leading to continued degeneration if not treated.
- Hip dysplasia is characterized by a shallow acetabulum with inadequate coverage of the femoral head and resultant abnormal contact mechanics, which cause accelerated degeneration of the articular surface at an early age.
- Femoral rotational abnormalities are relatively common and should be considered as a cause of extra-articular hip impingement.
- Hip arthroscopy, surgical hip dislocation, periacetabular osteotomy, and femoral rotational osteotomy have the ability to effectively treat hip pain and functional limitation in patients with prearthritic hip pain and ultimately have the potential to change the course of patients with hip impingement, dysplasia, and abnormal femoral version.

Annotated References

1. McCarthy JC, Noble PC, Schuck MR, Wright J, Lee J: The Otto E. Aufranc Award: The role of labral lesions to development of early degenerative hip disease. *Clin Orthop Relat Res* 2001:25-37.

2. Tanzer M, Noiseux N: Osseous abnormalities and early osteoarthritis: The role of hip impingement. *Clin Orthop Relat Res* 2004:170-177.

3. Philippon MJ, Nepple JJ, Campbell KJ, et al: The hip fluid seal—Part I: The effect of an acetabular labral tear, repair, resection, and reconstruction on hip fluid pressurization. *Knee Surg Sports Traumatol Arthrosc* 2014;22:722-729.

4. Wyles CC, Norambuena GA, Howe BM, et al: Cam deformities and limited hip range of motion are associated with early osteoarthritic changes in adolescent athletes: A prospective matched cohort study. *Am J Sports Med* 2017;45(13):3036-3043. doi:10.1177/0363546517719460.

This prospective matched cohort demonstrated progressive degenerative changes on MRI in young athletes after five years in those with limited internal rotation in flexion (<10°) and radiographic findings of FAI, compared with those with normal internal rotation, with the majority being asymptomatic at final follow-up. Chondrolabral changes progress in young athletes with FAI and limited IR without symptoms. Level II study.

5. Tresch F, Dietrich TJ, Pfirrmann CWA, Sutter R: Hip MRI: Prevalence of articular cartilage defects and labral tears in asymptomatic volunteers. A comparison with a matched population of patients with femoroacetabular impingement. *J Magn Reson Imaging* 2017;46:440-451.

   A prospective study comparing asymptomatic volunteers and symptomatic patients with FAI demonstrated chondrolabral damage in 80% and 57% of patients, respectively, indicating degenerative changes exist in the absence of symptoms. Not all chondrolabral injury is symptomatic. Level II study.

6. Wylie JD, Beckmann JT, Maak TG, Aoki SK: Arthroscopic treatment of mild to moderate deformity after slipped capital femoral epiphysis: Intra-operative findings and functional outcomes. *Arthroscopy* 2015;31:247-253.

7. Sankar WN, Duncan ST, Baca GR, et al: Descriptive epidemiology of acetabular dysplasia: The Academic Network of Conservational Hip Outcomes Research (ANCHOR) Periacetabular Osteotomy. *J Am Acad Orthop Surg* 2017;25:150-159.

   This descriptive study of 950 consecutive patients who underwent a PAO described demographics, disease characteristics, and functional outcomes. Patients were predominantly female (83%), young (25), white (87%), borderline overweight (body mass index [BMI] 25), and experienced significant functional limitations.

8. Lerch TD, Todorski IAS, Steppacher SD, et al: Prevalence of femoral and acetabular version abnormalities in patients with symptomatic hip disease: A controlled study of 538 hips. *Am J Sports Med* 2018;46:122-134.

   This cross-sectional study compared 462 symptomatic patients with a control group using CT and MRI to assess acetabular and femoral version. Abnormal femoral version (<10° or >25°) was found in 52% (severe in 17%) of symptomatic patients. Level III study.

9. Clohisy JC, Carlisle JC, Beaule PE, et al: A systematic approach to the plain radiographic evaluation of the young adult hip. *J Bone Joint Surg Am* 2008;90(suppl 4):47-66.

10. Nötzli HP, Wyss TF, Stoecklin CH, Schmid MR, Treiber K, Hodler J: The contour of the femoral head-neck junction as a predictor for the risk of anterior impingement. *J Bone Joint Surg Br* 2002;84:556-560.

11. Murphy SB, Simon SR, Kijewski PK, Wilkinson RH, Griscom NT: Femoral anteversion. *J Bone Joint Surg Am* 1987;69:1169-1176.

12. Smith-Petersen MN: The classic: Treatment of malum coxae senilis, old slipped upper femoral epiphysis, intrapelvic protrusion of the acetabulum, and coxa plana by means of acetabuloplasty (1936). *Clin Orthop Relat Res* 2009;467:608-615.

13. Ganz R, Parvizi J, Beck M, Leunig M, Nötzli H, Siebenrock KA: Femoroacetabular impingement: A cause for osteoarthritis of the hip. *Clin Orthop Relat Res* 2003:112-120. doi:10.1097/01.blo.0000096804.78689.c2.

14. Clohisy JC, Dobson MA, Robison JF, et al: Radiographic structural abnormalities associated with premature, natural hip-joint failure. *J Bone Joint Surg Am* 2011;93(suppl 2):3-9.

15. Tannast M, Goricki D, Beck M, Murphy SB, Siebenrock KA: Hip damage occurs at the zone of femoroacetabular impingement. *Clin Orthop Relat Res* 2008;466:273-280.

16. Beck M, Kalhor M, Leunig M, Ganz R: Hip morphology influences the pattern of damage to the acetabular cartilage: Femoroacetabular impingement as a cause of early osteoarthritis of the hip. *J Bone Joint Surg Br* 2005;87:1012-1018.

17. Nepple JJ, Vigdorchik JM, Clohisy JC: What is the association between sports participation and the development of proximal femoral cam deformity? A systematic review and meta-analysis. *Am J Sports Med* 2015;43:2833-2840.

18. Morris WZ, Li RT, Liu RW, Salata MJ, Voos JE: Origin of cam morphology in femoroacetabular impingement. *Am J Sports Med* 2018;46:478-486.

    This clinical update reviews the literature concerning cam deformities and proposed causes. Recent evidence suggests cams may result from epiphyseal extension as an adaptive response to provide stability to an open physis during vigorous sporting activity during youth.

19. Packer JD, Safran MR: The etiology of primary femoroacetabular impingement: Genetics or acquired deformity? *J Hip Preserv Surg* 2015;2:249-257.

20. Han J, Won S-H, Kim J-T, Hahn M-H, Won Y-Y: Prevalence of cam deformity with associated femoroacetabular impingement syndrome in hip joint computed tomography of asymptomatic adults. *Hip Pelvis* 2018;30:5-11.

    This retrospective review evaluated the prevalence of cam deformities in asymptomatic patients with no history of prior hip pathology using pelvic CT scans obtained during trauma evaluation. Cam deformities above 55° were found in only 31% of hips.

21. Frank JM, Harris JD, Erickson BJ, et al: Prevalence of femoroacetabular impingement imaging findings in asymptomatic volunteers: A systematic review. *Arthroscopy* 2015;31:1199-1204.

22. Clohisy JC, Baca G, Beaulé PE, et al: Descriptive epidemiology of femoroacetabular impingement: A North American cohort of patients undergoing surgery. *Am J Sports Med* 2013;41:1348-1356.

23. Reynolds D, Lucas J, Klaue K: Retroversion of the acetabulum. A cause of hip pain. *J Bone Joint Surg Br* 1999;81:281-288.

24. Seldes RM, Tan V, Hunt J, Katz M, Winiarsky R, Fitzgerald RH Jr: Anatomy, histologic features, and vascularity of the adult acetabular labrum. *Clin Orthop Relat Res* 2001:232-240.

25. Cross MB, Fabricant PD, Maak TG, Kelly BT: Impingement (acetabular side). *Clin Sports Med* 2011;30:379-390.

26. Corten K, Ganz R, Chosa E, Leunig M: Bone apposition of the acetabular rim in deep hips: A distinct finding of global pincer impingement. *J Bone Joint Surg Am* 2011;93(suppl 2):10-16.

27. Thomas GER, Palmer AJ, Batra RN, et al: Subclinical deformities of the hip are significant predictors of radiographic osteoarthritis and joint replacement in women. A 20 year longitudinal cohort study. *Osteoarthr Cartil* 2014;22:1504-1510.

28. Wedge JH, Wasylenko MJ: The natural history of congenital dislocation of the hip: A critical review. *Clin Orthop Relat Res* 1978:154-162.

29. Abraham CL, Knight SJ, Peters CL, Weiss JA, Anderson AE: Patient-specific chondrolabral contact mechanics in patients with acetabular dysplasia following treatment with periacetabular osteotomy. *Osteoarthr Cartil* 2017;25:676-684.

    This case-controlled prospective study used 3D computer modeling of CT scans of five patients before and after PAO to assess joint contact mechanics. Overall contact area increased and overall peak and average contact stresses decreased after PAO, indicating a positive change in joint contact mechanics after PAO.

30. Matsuda DK, Wolff AB, Nho SJ, et al: Hip dysplasia: Prevalence, associated findings, and procedures from large multicenter arthroscopy study group. *Arthroscopy* 2018;34:444-453.

    This large, multicenter comparative case series identified 13% of patients undergoing isolated hip arthroscopy to have acetabular dysplasia (LCEA <25°). Patients with dysplasia demonstrated hypertrophic labra and greater internal rotation compared with those without dysplasia. Level III study.

31. Sankar WN, Beaule PE, Clohisy JC, et al: Labral morphologic characteristics in patients with symptomatic acetabular dysplasia. *Am J Sports Med* 2015;43:2152-2156.

32. Babst D, Steppacher SD, Ganz R, Siebenrock KA, Tannast M: The iliocapsularis muscle: An important stabilizer in the dysplastic hip. *Clin Orthop Relat Res* 2011;469:1728-1734.

33. Tannast M, Hanke MS, Zheng G, Steppacher SD, Siebenrock KA: What are the radiographic reference values for acetabular under- and overcoverage? *Clin Orthop Relat Res* 2015;473:1234-1246.

34. Philippon MJ, Zehms CT, Briggs KK, Manchester DJ, Kuppersmith DA: Hip instability in the athlete. *Oper Tech Sport Med* 2007;15:189-194.

35. Chadayammuri V, Garabekyan T, Bedi A, et al: Passive hip range of motion predicts femoral torsion and acetabular version. *J Bone Joint Surg Am* 2016;98:127-134.

    This cohort study of 221 symptomatic patients with FAI used preoperative clinical examinations and CT scans to correlate passive motion and combined acetabular and femoral version. Passive motion of the hip strongly predicts femoral and acetabular version.

36. Wall PDH, Fernandez M, Griffin DR, Foster NE: Nonoperative treatment for femoroacetabular impingement: A systematic review of the literature. *PM R* 2013;5:418-426.

37. Chahla J, Mikula JD, Schon JM, et al: Hip capsular closure: A biomechanical analysis of failure torque. *Am J Sports Med* 2017;45:434-439.

    Nine cadaveric pelvis specimens were used to simulate a standard anterior capsulotomy used during hip arthrosocpy. Repair techniques using one, two, or three sutures were compared to assess torque to failure. All repairs failed at 36° of external rotation, but the two and three suture repairs were significantly stronger than the one suture repair.

38. Domb BG, Chaharbakhshi EO, Perets I, Walsh JP, Yuen LC, Ashberg LJ: Patient-reported outcomes of capsular repair versus capsulotomy in patients undergoing hip arthroscopy: Minimum 5-year follow-up-A matched comparison study. *Arthroscopy* 2018;34:853-863,e1.

    This 5-year retrospective comparative study evaluated patients with and without capsular repair after hip arthroscopy. At final follow-up those without capsule repair had deterioration in subjective scores and a higher conversion to arthroplasty compared to those with repair. Level III study.

39. Habib A, Haldane CE, Ekhtiari S, et al: Pudendal nerve injury is a relatively common but transient complication of hip arthroscopy. *Knee Surg Sports Traumatol Arthrosc* 2018;26:969-975.

    This systematic review of nerve injury complications related to hip arthroscopy demonstrated a 1.8% rate of pudendal nerve injury. Pudendal nerve injury was more common when a perineal post was used and when traction time was longer; all resolved within 3 months. Level IV study.

40. Domb BG, Chaharbakhshi EO, Rybalko D, Close MR, Litrenta J, Perets I: Outcomes of hip arthroscopic surgery in patients with tönnis grade 1 osteoarthritis at a minimum 5-year follow-up: A matched-pair comparison with a tönnis grade 0 control group. *Am J Sports Med* 2017;45:2294-2302.

    This retrospective cohort compared patients with Tönnis grade 0 to those with Tönnis grade 1 radiographs at 5-years after hip arthroscopy. Both groups significantly improved, but the survival rate for grade 1 group was lower than the grade 0 group (69% versus 88%). Level III study.

41. Perets I, Rybalko D, Chaharbakhshi EO, Mu BH, Chen AW, Domb BG: Minimum five-year outcomes of hip arthroscopy for the treatment of femoroacetabular impingement and labral tears in patients with obesity: A match-controlled study. *J Bone Joint Surg Am* 2018;100:965-973.

    This retrospective cohort evaluated obese and normal weight patients 5 years after hip arthroscopy. Both groups demonstrated significant improvements in mean outcome scores, but the obese group demonstrated a higher conversion to arthroplasty (30% versus 15%). Level III study.

42. Menge TJ, Briggs KK, Dornan GJ, McNamara SC, Philippon MJ: Survivorship and outcomes 10 years following hip arthroscopy for femoroacetabular impingement: Labral debridement compared with labral repair. *J Bone Joint Surg Am* 2017;99:997-1004.

This retrospective cohort compared labral repair with debridement 10 years after hip arthroscopy. Both demonstrated significant improvements in outcome scores, but 34% of patients converted to arthroplasty. Conversions were typically older, had <3 mm of joint space, and underwent acetabular microfracture. Level III study.

43. Clohisy JC, Nepple JJ, Larson CM, et al: Persistent structural disease is the most common cause of repeat hip preservation surgery. *Clin Orthop Relat Res* 2013;471:3788-3794.

44. Mansor Y, Perets I, Close MR, Mu BH, Domb BG: In search of the spherical femoroplasty: Cam overresection leads to inferior functional scores before and after revision hip arthroscopic surgery. *Am J Sports Med* 2018;46:2061-2071.

A retrospective radiographic and clinical outcome review comparing the quality of femoroplasty performed during hip arthroscopy. Overresection demonstrated inferior outcomes at 3 years, with higher conversion to arthroplasty compared with neural or underresection. Level III study.

45. Ganz R, Gill TJ, Gautier E, Ganz K, Krügel N, Berlemann U: Surgical dislocation of the adult hip a technique with full access to the femoral head and acetabulum without the risk of avascular necrosis. *J Bone Joint Surg Br* 2001;83:1119-1124.

46. Steppacher SD, Anwander H, Zurmühle CA, Tannast M, Siebenrock KA: Eighty percent of patients with surgical hip dislocation for femoroacetabular impingement have a good clinical result without osteoarthritis progression at 10 years. *Clin Orthop Relat Res* 2015;473:1333-1341.

47. Ganz R, Klaue K, Vinh TS, Mast JW: A new periacetabular osteotomy for the treatment of hip dysplasias. Technique and preliminary results. *Clin Orthop Relat Res* 1988:26-36.

48. Lerch TD, Steppacher SD, Liechti EF, Tannast M, Siebenrock KA: One-third of hips after periacetabular osteotomy survive 30 years with good clinical results, no progression of arthritis, or conversion to THA. *Clin Orthop Relat Res* 2017;475:1154-1168.

This long-term retrospective cohort evaluated 30-year outcomes after PAO. 30% of hips demonstrated no radiographic evidence of degeneration, while 70% required arthroplasty. Those older than 40 years, with a Tönnis grade >1 and poor preoperative outcome scores had worse outcomes.

49. Wyatt MC, Beck M: The management of the painful borderline dysplastic hip. *J Hip Preserv Surg* 2018;5:105-112.

This review evaluates current literature regarding borderline hips with instability based on clinical and radiographic assessment and provides suggestions for potential treatment and future areas of investigation.

50. Siebenrock KA, Steppacher SD, Haefeli PC, Schwab JM, Tannast M: Valgus hip with high antetorsion causes pain through posterior extraarticular FAI. *Clin Orthop Relat Res* 2013;471:3774-3780.

Chapter 36

Muscular, Neurovascular, and Soft-Tissue Conditions of the Hip

Brett R. Levine, MD, MS

ABSTRACT

Pathological conditions about the native hip are not uncommon and range from simple tendinitis, muscular injuries to various neurovascular issues. Sports injuries, overuse conditions, local nerve compression, and vascular abnormalities occur at various rates about the hip. Depending on the etiology various treatment options are available. Similar conditions can occur around total hip arthroplasty and may be related to the surgical procedure, the implants themselves, or the local soft tissues. The following chapter reviews recent updates to the muscular, neurovascular, and soft-tissue conditions regarding the hip.

Keywords: hip; meralgia paresthetica; snapping hip syndrome; trochanteric bursitis

Introduction

The complex soft tissue, muscular, bony, and neurovascular anatomy about the hip lend itself to outstanding function as well as the potential for substantial pain and dysfunction associated with numerous conditions. While most orthopaedic surgeons are facile at treating hip joint disorders, it is important to be able diagnose and manage the soft-tissue ailments surrounding the hip joint. A substantial portion of office visits will be related to these conditions, including trochanteric bursitis, gluteal muscle/tendon injuries, iliopsoas tendinitis, snapping hip, labral injuries, and neurovascular syndromes.

Dr. Levine or an immediate family member serves as a paid consultant to or is an employee of DJ Orthopaedics, Exactech, Inc., Link Orthopaedics, Medacta, and Merete; has received research support or institutional support from Artelon, Biomet, and Zimmer; and serves as a board member, owner, officer, or committee member of American Association of Hip and Knee Surgeons and CORD.

Muscular Conditions About the Hip

Abductor Complex Injuries/Disorders

The abductor complex is composed of the gluteus medius, gluteus minimus, and the tensor fascia lata muscles. As a group, they aid in support of the pelvis and stability of the hip and provide the strength for a normal gait pattern. In turn, they may be subjected to traumatic injuries and systemic processes that may lead to partial or complete rupture. This complex has often been deemed the "rotator cuff of the hip." The overall incidence of gluteus medius tears in those undergoing primary total hip arthroplasty (THA) or for treatment of femoral neck fractures has been estimated to be ~20%.[1,2] Associated conditions that have been thought to contribute to the pathogenesis of abductor muscle tears include anatomic variants, such as genu valgum, limb-length discrepancies, and pelvic morphology leading to a predilection for iliotibial band (ITB) tightness and abrasion of the gluteal muscles against the greater trochanter. Systemic conditions found in association with hip "rotator-cuff" injuries include gout, diabetes, anabolic steroid use, chondrocalcinosis, obesity, Paget disease, and inflammatory arthropathy.[2] Tears of the tendon gluteal tendons often start anteriorly and propagate posteriorly and superficially.

Presenting symptoms typically include some element of atraumatic pain in the buttock, lateral hip or groin. Patients may report some early fatigue with walking, difficulty climbing stairs, and pain with sleeping or direct palpation on the side of the affected hip. These injuries are often misdiagnosed as trochanteric bursitis, degenerative joint disease of the hip, or referred lumbar spine pathology. Standard radiographs including AP, lateral, shoot through lateral, and AP pelvis are often obtained after the physical examination to assess the local bony anatomy. Greater trochanteric fractures and surface irregularities can be found, with the latter suggestive of gluteus medius tears. MRI and ultrasonography afford a better picture of the soft tissues about the hip when searching for the appropriate diagnosis. Historic studies favor MRI as the diagnostic modality of choice (91% accurate and 95% specific) in the diagnosis of gluteal muscle injuries.[3-5] Sutter et al found that patients with abductor tendon tears more often displayed hypertrophy of the tensor fascia lata (TFL) on MRI, which likely represents muscular recruitment to accommodate for the dysfunction of the damaged gluteal muscles.[6]

The majority of these injuries (partial-thickness tears) are successfully managed nonsurgically with unloading of the affected hip, medications (nonsteroidal anti-inflammatory agents or acetaminophen), topical agents, and/or physical therapy (home exercises or formal outpatient physical therapy). When symptoms are refractory to the aforementioned measures or there is a complete tear, then surgical management may be favored based on the health, activity level, and physiologic condition of the patient. Surgical management ranges from endoscopic techniques to open repair (similar to the rotator cuff, with many of the surgical principles being the same).[2,4] Anatomic repair is vital to the success of a repair and restoration of function. Recognizing the four facets of the greater trochanter (superoposterior, lateral, anterior, and posterior) is important as is distinguishing between the distinct insertion sites of the gluteus medius and minimus. The medius attaches to the superoposterior (posterior fibers) and lateral (anterior and middle fibers) facets while the minimus attaches to the lateral facet and the joint capsule with a "bald spot" between the attachment sites.[5]

Partial-thickness tears can be successfully managed with suture anchors and endoscopic management with substantial clinical benefit.[7] Large (both anterior and posterior portions of the tendon), and full-thickness tears are best treated with open management reconstructing the anatomic tendon footprint with the reconstruction.[3] Makridis reported on 67 patients treated with an open double-row technique to repair gluteal tendon injuries with 85% good clinical results and 11 failures at an average of 4.6 years follow-up.[4] Additionally, he noted that muscular atrophy on preoperative MRI had a negative impact on functional outcomes. This has been confirmed more recently by Thaunat et al in a study on functional outcomes after endoscopic gluteus medius repair.[8] They found that fatty degeneration of the gluteus medius and minimus had a negative impact on functional and clinical outcomes after tendon repair.

During the reconstruction of the gluteal tendons, some have recommended local decortication of the greater trochanter to aid in healing; however, recently Putnam et al have called this practice into question.[9] In a cadaveric study, they found decreased pullout strength of suture anchors when cortical bone was removed or the bone density was poor and encouraged surgeons to consider these factors during the repair process. In the past, gluteal repairs have failed in up to 35% of cases; while modern techniques have improved upon these rates, there have been reports of using adjuncts such as acellular human dermal grafts to aid in such repairs.[10] With increasing success of these repairs (reduction in prior complication rates as highs as 19% of cases[5]) and expanding indications for endoscopic reconstructions, a significant amount of research has been focused on improving the outcomes for our patients with gluteal tendon injuries.

Postoperative rehabilitation and restrictions are vital to the success of these repairs. Most suggest an abduction brace with crutches and protected weight bearing for 4 to 6 weeks after surgery. Progressive return to activity is allowed at 3 months and strengthening programs will commence moving forward.

Hip Bursitis

Lateral-sided hip pain is a common condition that has been reported to be as debilitating as end-stage degenerative joint disease and is now more commonly recognized as a conglomerate of conditions (snapping hip, trochanteric bursitis, and gluteal tendinopathy) lumped together as greater trochanteric pain syndrome (GTPS).[11,12] In patients between 50 and 79 years of age, GTPS was found in 15% of women and 6.6% of men in one hip.[13] Lateral hip anatomy is more complex than it seems with most people having three to four bursae surrounding the side of their hips. The bursae allow improved muscle mechanics over the lateral part of the proximal femur. The largest bursa is found between the gluteus maximus muscle and the gluteus medius tendon, which is located directly lateral to the greater trochanter. Coupled with the bursa the muscular sheaths and tendinous attachments of the gluteus maximus, ITB, tensor fascia lata, gluteus medius, and gluteus minimus contribute to a complex local environment that is susceptible to overuse injuries, direct trauma, and gait alterations.[11] Despite being a common diagnosis, trochanteric bursitis is often related to the other conditions of GTPS and not true inflammation of the local bursa.[14] In making the correct diagnosis, there are many conditions that should be considered and thorough differential diagnosis can be found in **Table 1**. A thorough history and physical will help narrow down the differential and plain radiography, ultrasonography and MRI are adjuncts to confirm the diagnosis.

Trochanteric Bursitis

GTPS is commonly found with a valgus deformity of the lower extremity and is often relayed as a single traumatic episode by the patient or a more chronic condition (likely representing inflammation secondary

Table 1

Differential Diagnosis of Soft Tissue and Neuromuscular Hip Conditions of the Native and Replaced Hip

Soft Tissue	Bone-Related Conditions	Extra-Articular Conditions	Vascular Conditions	Nerve Conditions
Acute muscular injuries • Iliopsoas • Rectus femoris • Adductors • Abductors • Hamstring	*Femoral-acetabular impingement* • with labral injury • without labral injury	*Gynecologic disorders* • Ovarian conditions • Uterine fibroids • Malignancy • Infection	*Claudication*	*Meralgia paresthetica*
Acute tendon injuries • Iliopsoas • Rectus femoris • Adductor • Proximal hamstring • Gluteus medius • Gluteus maximus	*Fractures* • Femoral neck • Intertrochanteric • Subtrochanteric • Pubic rami • Sacrum • Iliac Wing	*Gastrointestinal* • Hernia • Appendicitis • Inflammatory bowel disease • Diverticulitis • Malignancy	*Osteonecrosis*	*Neuralgias* • Pudendal • Genitofemoral • Obturator • Femoral • Sciatic
Chronic injuries • Iliopsoas impingement • Labral tear • Adductor • Proximal hamstring • Gluteus medius • Gluteus maximus	*Osteitis pubis (athletic pubalgia)*	*Genitourinary* • Stones • Infection • Malignancy		*Lumbosacral spine conditions* • Spinal stenosis • Herniated disk • Vertebral fractures • SI joint disorders • Facet disorders
Other conditions • Piriformis syndrome • Trochanteric bursitis • Instability	*Childhood conditions* • Hip dysplasia • Perthes disease • Epiphyseal dysplasias • PFFD • SCFE			*Post-THA conditions* • Sciatic nerve injury • Lateral femoral cutaneous nerve injury • Superior gluteal nerve injury
Post-THA Conditions • Trochanteric bursitis • Iliopsoas tendinitis • Instability/abductor deficiency				

PFFD = proximal focal femoral deficiency, SCFE = slipped capital femoral epiphysis, SI = sacroiliac, THA = total hip arthroplasty

to local microtrauma). This diagnosis can often be confirmed with a local diagnostic injection and/or clinical examination. Radiographs are usually normal with GTPS; however, a trochanter protruding more lateral than the iliac crest, enthesophytes, and peritrochanteric calcifications are nonspecific findings that have are commonly seen.[11,15] Ultrasonography can be successfully used to determine the diagnosis of GTPS with a sensitivity of 79% to 100%.[16] MRI is typically the benchmark to help clarify a diagnosis. Treatment for GTPS starts with nonsurgical management in the form of rest, nonsteroidal anti-inflammatory agents, physical therapy, and other modalities (ie, extracorporeal shock wave therapy—ESWT).[17,18] Rompe et al reported on 229 patients in a randomized trial of ESWT (78 patients), corticosteroid injection (75 patients), or physical therapy (76 patients) to treat GTPS. Early on corticosteroid injections appeared to be the most successful option; however, by 15 months both ESWT and physical therapy were more successful in providing sustained pain relief.[18] When conservative management does not provide satisfactory relief, then surgical options can be considered after a trial of a minimum of 6 to 12 months. Surgical options include open versus endoscopic débridement of the bursa and ITB release. Overall satisfaction and success rates have been reported to be quite high with limited recurrence of the GTPS in the future.

External Snapping Hip Syndrome

Also known as external coxa saltans, typically occurs secondary to friction over the greater trochanter from the ITB rubbing over it. Patients (common in athletes that test the extreme ranges of hip motion) often state they can dislocate and relocate their own hip with minimal pain but shifting their leg around. Stair climbing, exercising, and squatting can lead to this snapping phenomenon as well. On physical examination as you test the hip moving it from extension (often with adduction and internal rotation) to flexion (with abduction and external rotation), the ITB may "snap" over the greater trochanter from posterior to anterior. This condition can be asymptomatic, but also can become painful and lead to overlying trochanteric bursitis and a thickened ITB.[11] Conservative management is the same as for GTPS and should be continued for at least 6 to 12 months before considering surgical management. Surgical management involves open versus arthroscopic release of the ITB (can be standard release or a Z-plasty) and often a bursectomy, similar to the options discussed above.

Hip Flexor Problems

Internal Snapping Hip Syndrome (Medial Coxa Saltans or Iliopsoas Syndrome)

Internal snapping occurs when the iliopsoas tendon catches over the iliopectineal eminence or the anterior femoral head.[19] An alternative pathological condition that has been proposed to create the snap of the hip to include movement by the iliacus muscle and the iliopsoas tendon.[20] Similar to external snapping of the hip, this syndrome is often asymptomatic and can occur in up to 10% of the population as a normal variant.[2] It may even be more prevalent in athletes whose sport requires extreme hip range of motion, such as, soccer players, weight lifters, runners, offensive lineman in football, and elite dancers.[19,21] On examination, it is reproducible when taking the hip into extension from a flexed position (like when getting in and out of a car, arising from a chair or going up and down stairs). Typically, radiographs are negative although a cam lesion may be present. AP and shoot through lateral radiographs may help assess the anatomy to include acetabular anteversion, cox vara, or developmental dysplasia.[19] Psoas bursography and ultrasonography are dynamic studies that may be able to capture the snapping as it is happening.[22] Approximately 50% of patients with an internal snapping hip syndrome will have associated intra-articular hip pathology that is best diagnosed with magnetic resonance arthrography (MRA). Treatment options (ie, physical therapy, deep massage, NSAIDs, injections, and myofascial release) typically involve a prolonged course of nonsurgical management similar to external snapping hip syndrome (pain relief through tendon stretching/lengthening). Modern efforts with eccentric-biased exercises and a gradual tendon loading program have shown some promise with the rehabilitation of iliopsoas tendinopathy.[23] Open and endoscopic releases have been performed and typically involve tendon release. Anatomic studies have shown that the iliopsoas tendon insertion (dual insertion of iliacus and psoas muscles) is typically on the anteromedial tip of the lesser trochanter and can be accessed at this location or anywhere along its path for an open release procedure.[24] There has been some debate regarding which location provides a more complete and consistent release of the tendon as at the level of the labrum the iliopsoas tendon consists of 40% tendon and 60% muscle versus the opposite percentages at the lesser trochanter.[25] With arthroscopic procedures, portals allow for the joint to be visualized and assessed for associated pathology. Additional portals can then be created to treat the conditions that are present. The iliopsoas tendon can be released from the lesser trochanter or via an anterior capsulotomy (transcapsular approach) to access the tendon between the anterior labrum and zona orbicularis.[19] Hwang et al reported 88% good to excellent results in 25 patients treated with an arthroscopic transcapsular release of the iliopsoas tendon.[26] Another option is to perform a fractional lengthening of the tendon which is associated with a higher rate of recurrence (18%) and 82% good to excellent clinical results.[27] Heterotopic ossification is not an uncommon complication, and prophylaxis may be required in select cases. Additionally, it is important to note that in 64.2% of cases, Philippon et al found two iliopsoas tendons in a cadaveric anatomy study.[28] In some cases, failure to recognize the second tendon can lead to recurrence of symptoms. When releasing the iliopsoas tendon, all patients will have some element of iliopsoas atrophy, although the clinical significance of this remains largely undetermined.

Iliopsoas Tendinitis

Very similar condition to the snapping hip with the noise or snapping sensation. Inflammation of the tendon is treated in a similar manner as above. Conservative management is the mainstay with arthroscopic débridement, release, or lengthening occurring in only refractory conditions.

Labral Pathology Associated With Iliopsoas Impingement

A characteristic labral lesion is found at the iliopsoas notch in the 3-o'clock position. Oftentimes, selective injection is useful in making this diagnosis.[29]

Other Conditions

Hamstring Injuries

Most commonly occur with indirect trauma resulting from overuse injury, eccentric muscle contracture, or excessive stretching.[30] Tears, avulsion, and tendinitis are not uncommon conditions; with chronic hamstring pain, it is important to look for posterior hip impingement processes. Furthermore, due to the intimate relationship between the hamstring origin at the ischium and the sciatic nerve, hamstring injuries can be often associated with sciatic nerve irritation as part of a condition termed, hamstring syndrome.

Adductor Muscle Strains

Often occur in sports like hockey, soccer, or any activity that may involve eccentric contracture of the adductor musculature. The adductor longus is the most likely muscle to be injured with this condition and typically presents as groin pain/strain. Balancing the strength between the abductor and adductor muscles may help prevent and/or treat these injuries with an emphasis on stretching and strengthening.[21]

Deep Gluteal Syndrome (Piriformis Syndrome)

Often associated with hamstring syndrome and ischiofemoral impingement.

Ischiofemoral Impingement

Refers to a pathological process of entrapment of the quadratus femoris (QF) muscle between the lesser trochanter and the ischial tuberosity, leading to the generation of pain.[31] Often presents as groin pain that radiates down through the inner thigh and knee, when the limb is placed in adduction, extension, and external rotation. Palpation just lateral to the ischial tuberosity often illicits pain with the patient in the prone or seated position.[32] This condition is more common in women and is associated with any process that leads to a reduction in the distance between the lesser trochanter and the ischium. Often diagnosed on MRI (+edema in the QF muscle and reduced distance between lesser trochanter and the ischium) or with a therapeutic injection of the quadratus femoris muscle/ischiofemoral space under ultrasonography guidance. Treatment typically involves standard nonsurgical measures, such as NSAIDs, physical therapy, and local injections. Surgical management is targeted at decompressing the ischiofemoral space via lesser trochanterplasty, ischioplasty, or both.[24,32,33]

Subspine Impingement

This describes the contact that can occur between a hypertrophic or malpositioned anterior inferior iliac spine (AIIS) and the anterior femoral neck when the hip is in flexion. Soft-tissue structures implicated in the impingement process include the rectus femoris (direct head), anterior hip capsule, and the iliocapsularis muscles.[31] Thought to occur with the following conditions: pelvic osteotomies, valgus and anteverted proximal femoral anatomy, apophyseal/rectus avulsions, and developmental conditions (such as acetabular retroversion).[31] Commonly found in conjunction with femoral acetabular impingement (FAI), the two conditions present and are treated similarly. Physical examination findings consistent with subspine impingement (SSI) include a "grinding" sensation within the hip, pain with kicking or sprinting motions, and local AIIS tenderness.[31,34] Typically can be diagnosed with plan radiography (AP pelvis and false-profile views) or a CT scan. Obtaining an MR arthrogram can rule out intra-articular pathology as well.[31,34] Treatment involves traditional nonsurgical measures, followed by arthroscopic resection of the impinging AIIS ("spinoplasty[35]") in refractory cases. Rarely treated as an isolated condition, outcomes often hinge on the management of the concomitant FAI-related problems.

Pectineofoveal Impingement

This is a lesser known disorder involving impingement of abnormally shaped medial synovial folds against adjacent soft tissues, commonly the zona orbicularis.[31] Pectineofoveal impingement (PFI) often presents with vague symptomatology of an irritable hip, and the definitive diagnosis is made via arthroscope. Small case series have described good success with arthroscopic débridement of the synovial fold.

Piriformis syndrome—Pain and symptoms originate from the piriformis muscle and sciatic nerve.[36] This syndrome is exacerbated by prolonged sitting or lying on the side that hurts. Oftentimes, ambulation will actually improve these symptoms. Can often be confused with lumbar spine pathology, and this needs to be ruled out prior to confirming the diagnosis of piriformis syndrome. Nonsurgical treatment is the mainstay with refractory cases requiring piriformis release or resection.[37]

Neurovascular Issues

Vascular Conditions About the Hip

A detailed description of the vascular supply to the hip is beyond the scope of this chapter; however, suffice it to say the majority of the blood supply to the mature femoral head is via the profunda femoris artery and its contributory branches of the medial femoral circumflex artery. Injury to these arteries or its branches during surgery, trauma, or external compression sources can contribute to osteonecrosis of the femoral head.[38] Certainly, vascular claudication can lead to hip and thigh pain and weakness and can be associated with aneurysm or arterial disease/stenosis. Gluteus maximus claudication can occur with stenosis of the gluteal arteries and as with typical vascular claudication the symptoms are relieved with rest.[30]

Neurological conditions specific to the hip region itself are relatively uncommon and can be associated with low back pathology, sciatica/sciatic nerve dysfunction, injury to local nerves during surgery (sciatic, femoral, lateral femoral cutaneous, superior/inferior gluteal), compressive disorders, and meralgia paresthetica. Electromyography and nerve conduction studies can be useful in making the diagnosis and the prognosis of these conditions.[30] Nerve entrapment syndromes can involve any of the nerves passing through the anatomical hip region (**Table 2**).[39]

Meralgia paresthetica is an uncommon nerve condition involving compression or entrapment of the lateral femoral cutaneous nerve as it passes under the inguinal ligament.[40] The nerve supplies the sensation to the anterolateral thigh and when compromised can result in numbness or pain in this dermatomal

Table 2

Nerve Entrapment Syndromes of the Hip

Nerve Involved	Sites of Entrapment	Signs and Symptoms
Posterior Nerve Entrapment Syndromes		
Sciatic	• Piriformis and obturator/gemelli complex • Proximal hamstring • Lesser trochanter and ischium	• (+) Seated piriformis stretch and active piriformis tests • Ischial tenderness • Posterior thigh pain worse with running in the popliteus fossa • (+) Ischial femoral impingement test
Pudendal	• Ischial spine, sacrospinous ligament and lesser sciatic notch • Greater sciatic notch and piriformis • Alcock's canal and obturator internus	• (+) Pain medial to ischium • Sciatic notch and piriformis pain • Obturator internus spasm and pain
Anterior Nerve Entrapment Syndromes		
Obturator	• Obturator canal • Adductor muscle fascia	• Medial thigh pain • Pain increase with abduction
Femoral	• Iliopsoas tendon • Inguinal ligament • Adductor canal	• Painful Thomas test • Quadriceps weakness • Anteromedial knee, leg, and foot pain
Lateral femoral cutaneous	• Inguinal ligament	• (+) Pelvic compression test

Adapted from Martin R, Martin HD, Kivlan BR: Nerve entrapment in the hip region: Current concepts review. *Int J Sports Phys Ther* 2017;12[7]:1163-1173, used with permission of The International Journal of Sports Physical Therapy.

distribution. Iatrogenic injury of the lateral femoral cutaneous nerve can occur with surgery (Smith Petersen approach to the hips). Additionally spontaneous etiologies include pregnancy, conditions causing increased intra-abdominal pressure, wearing belts or constrictive articles of clothing, and pelvic masses.[40] There is a predilection for males, obesity and diabetic patients.[41] Typically relieving the external pressure on the nerve helps resolve the symptoms (neuropathology is similar to carpal tunnel syndrome); however, in refractory cases, surgical decompression or neurolysis may be necessary. Alternative options to treat this condition include corticosteroid injections, alcohol neurolysis, and radiofrequency treatments. Ahmed et al found good success in six patients using ultrasonography-guided alcohol neurolysis of the lateral femoral cutaneous nerve.[40]

Deep gluteal syndrome involves entrapment of the sciatic nerve in the deep gluteal space.[30] Numerous conditions and anatomical structures can lead to compression of the nerve in this space and include gluteal muscles, hamstring muscles, short external rotator complex, fibrous bands, and space-occupying lesions/tumors/masses. Patients will often present with the inability to sit for greater than a half an hour with pain that radiates down the sciatic nerve distribution. Abnormal reflexes or distal weakness can occur as the nerve is persistently compressed, representing sciatic nerve dysfunction.[30] Recently, Martin et al found that using the combination of the seated piriformis stretch test and the piriformis active test lead to 91% sensitivity and 80% specificity of finding sciatic nerve entrapment during arthroscopy.[42]

Pudendal Nerve Entrapment

Pudendal neuralgia is the result of pudendal nerve entrapment or direct injury. The most common sites of nerve compression include between the sacrotuberous and sacrospinous ligaments. This often falls in the canal of Alcock, hence the pseudonym Alcock canal syndrome.[43] The most common causes of pudendal nerve entrapment include mechanical injuries, trauma during childbirth, and iatrogenic damage during surgery.[43] Habib et al reported a 1.8% incidence in reviewing 24 studies for a meta-analysis.[44] Risk factors include the use of a perineal post and extended traction times for the surgery. All reported nerve injuries resolved within 3 months of the surgery. Pain is often located in the perineum but can be perceived in the groin and buttocks leading to some crossover with classic hip pain generators (**Table 1**). MRI and diagnostic injections are helpful to confirm the diagnosis. Conservative measures are often successful in providing pain relief, including NSAIDs, antidepressants, antiepileptics, activity modification, corticosteroid injections, and physical therapy (neural and soft-tissue mobilization).[39,43] Pulsed radiofrequency ablation has been proposed to help in refractory cases.[43] Surgical decompression and neurolysis are rarely indicated but at times may be a necessary intervention.

Soft-Tissue Conditions Associated With Total Hip Arthroplasty

Trochanteric Bursitis

Associated with increasing the offset of the native hip after total hip arthroplasty. High-offset femoral necks and longer femoral heads may contribute to this condition. Typically presents similar to the native GTPS discussed above with lateral hip pain. The pain may radiate to the buttock, groin, or lower back and is typically exacerbated by ambulation, uphill walking, stair climbing, and rising from a chair.[45] If the diagnosis is not apparent, a metal artifact reduction sequence (MARS) MRI can be used to confirm this condition. The mainstay of treatment is nonsurgical management to include NSAIDs, topical agents, physical therapy, and corticosteroid injections as a last resort. Surgical management is rarely necessary, but overall hip offset may need to be altered to treat the underlying source generator of the pain. In rare cases, the abductor muscles may require a transfer procedure, and in instances of associated abductor deficiency, gluteus maximus transfer has been proposed as a solution to this difficult problem.[46,47]

Abductor Tears/Insufficiency

Occurs more commonly with anterolateral or direct lateral approaches that directly dissect around or through the abductor musculature, although can result from any approach to the hip.

Treatment Options

Direct repair for acute injuries or tears is possible. Reconstruction via a direct repair of the gluteus medius tendon with adjunctive fixation with an allograft tendon or advancement of the vastus lateralis can be a successful treatment option.[48]

In those with weak, damaged, or absent gluteus medius muscle or tendon, there has been a transfer of the gluteus maximus and tensor fascia lata to the greater trochanter procedure described by Whiteside.

Hip and Femur

This technique was found to be successful in 80% of the five reported cases, with one recurrent injury.[46,47]

Iliopsoas Tendinitis

Iliopsoas tendinitis can occur with impingement of the iliopsoas tendon over a THA femoral head or prominent edge (oversized or retroverted cup) of the acetabular cup.[5] Less common THA-related causes include excessive offset, limb-length discrepancy, cement extrusion with a cemented acetabular implant, anterior acetabular screw protrusion, and large femoral heads (metal-on-metal and dual mobility).[49] Reported to occur in up to 4.3% of THA cases.[49] Patel et al suggest iliopsoas tendon release at the lesser trochanter to treat refractory cases after THA for several reasons, including ease of approach as there is limited scarring in this area after THA, it involves an extra-articular approach, and there is a higher proportion of tendon to release anatomically. While some weakness is anticipated post release, this represents a safe, reproducible method to treat refractory iliopsoas tendinitis after THA.[49] Most recently, Chalmers et al reported on 49 patients treated for iliopsoas impingement after primary THA.[50] Their mean follow-up was 4 years with 21 undergoing acetabular revision, 8 an iliopsoas tenotomy, and 20 with nonsurgical management. Overall, they found that greater than or equal to 8 mm of acetabular overhang was found to be an appropriate threshold to recommend revision of the component. In those with a lesser extent of overhang, nonsurgical management and tenotomy were successful in managing this condition.[50]

Ischiofemoral Impingement

Can occur when the offset is reduced and the lesser trochanter moves closer to the ischium. Lesser trochanter excision to treat this condition can lead to joint instability, and it is preferred to revise the appropriate implant(s) to achieve greater hip offset.[31]

Conclusion

Muscular, neurovascular, and soft-tissue conditions around the hip joint are frequent causes for orthopaedic consultation. A thorough knowledge of the anatomy surrounding the hip is paramount to aid in the diagnosis and treatment of these conditions. While nonsurgical management is the mainstay of treatment, understanding surgical indications and options is important in this growing area of orthopaedic surgery.

Key Study Points

- Muscular, neurovascular, and soft-tissue conditions about the hip are extremely common causes for consultation. The abductor musculature complex is considered the "rotator cuff of the hip".
- The majority of these conditions about the hip can be managed with conservative measures, such as nonsteroidal anti-inflammatory agents, stretching exercises (physical therapy), and injections. After a prolonged attempt of nonsurgical management, surgical options come into play with arthroscopic treatments gaining recent popularity.
- Iliopsoas tendinitis can occur in up to 4% of THA cases. Revision surgery is the treatment of choice when cup overhang is 8 mm or more.
- Neurologic impingement around the hip is relatively uncommon, with the three most common conditions being meralgia paresthetica, deep gluteal syndrome, and pudendal nerve entrapment.

Annotated References

1. Bunker TD, Esler CN, Leach WJ: Rotator-cuff tear of the hip. *J Bone Joint Surg Br* 1997;79(4):618-620.
2. Ilizaliturri VM Jr, Camacho-Galindo J, Evia Ramirez AN, Gonzalez Ibarra YL, McMillan S, Busconi BD: Soft tissue pathology around the hip. *Clin Sports Med* 2011;30(2):391-415.
3. Harrasser N, Banke I, Gollwitzer H, et al: Gluteal insufficiency: Pathogenesis, diagnosis and therapy. *Z Orthop Unfall* 2016;154(2):140-147.

   The authors prepared a review article on the challenging task of determining the etiology, diagnosis and managing gluteal insufficiency and dysfunction. Physical exam findings, imaging modalities and various therapeutic options are reviewed in detail. They ultimately conclude that gluteal tendon reconstruction is often the solution for treating chronic muscle dysfunction with good reduction in pain and improvement in muscle power at mid-term follow-up. Level of evidence: IV.
4. Makridis KG, Lequesne M, Bard H, Djian P: Clinical and MRI results in 67 patients operated for gluteus medius and minimus tendon tears with a median follow-up of 4.6 years. *Orthop Traumatol Surg Res* 2014;100(8):849-853.
5. Mosier BA, Quinlan NJ, Martin SD: Peritrochanteric endoscopy. *Clin Sports Med* 2016;35(3):449-467.

   Mosier et al completed a well-balanced review article describing some of the advances in arthroscopic management of disorders of the hip. Peritrochanteric disorder management is described including coxa saltans. Level of evidence: V (Review article).

6. Sutter R, Kalberer F, Binkert CA, Graf N, Pfirrmann CW, Gutzeit A: Abductor tendon tears are associated with hypertrophy of the tensor fasciae latae muscle. *Skeletal Radiol* 2013;42(5):627-633.

7. Hartigan DE, Perets I, Ho SW, Walsh JP, Yuen LC, Domb BG: Endoscopic repair of partial-thickness undersurface tears of the abductor tendon: Clinical outcomes with minimum 2-year follow-up. *Arthroscopy* 2018;34(4):1193-1199.

   A minimum 2-year outcome report of 25 patients undergoing endoscopic transtendinous gluteus medius repair is described. Of 14 patients with a preoperative Trendelenburg gait, 12 displayed a normal gait at latest follow-up. The average patient satisfaction was 7.5, and there were no revisions or complications reported. Level of evidence: IV (Case series).

8. Thaunat M, Clowez G, Desseaux A, et al: Influence of muscle fatty degeneration on functional outcomes after endoscopic gluteus medius repair. *Arthroscopy* 2018;34(6): 1816-1824.

   Twenty-two hips were retrospectively reviewed to determine if fatty degeneration of the muscle impacted outcomes when endoscopically repairing tears of the gluteus medius tendon. At a mean of ~32 months, they found that an increase in the preoperative fatty degeneration index of the gluteus medius muscle correlated with decreasing levels of functional outcomes (hip scores). Otherwise, endoscopic repair, if performed prior to degeneration, was noted to be a successful procedure. Level of evidence: IV (Therapeutic case series).

9. Putnam JG, Chhabra A, Castaneda P, et al: Does greater trochanter decortication affect suture anchor pullout strength in abductor tendon repairs? A biomechanical study. *Am J Sports Med* 2018;46(7):1668-1673.

   This group utilized 19 cadaveric proximal femurs and randomized the specimens to receive no decortication or 2 mm of bone decortication prior insertion of a suture anchor. Decorticating the bone led to lower loads to failure, which held up under a multivariate analysis, as did bone density. These factors should be considered when performing a repair of the glutues medius tendon. Level of evidence: III (Controlled lab study).

10. Laskovski J, Urchek R: Endoscopic gluteus medius and minimus repair with allograft augmentation using acellular human dermis. *Arthrosc Tech* 2018;7(3):e225-e230.

    In this technical note, endoscopic repair of the gluteus medius and minimus was performed using an acellular human dermal allograft to augment the reconstruction. This has been used in rotator cuff repairs, and the authors are hoping to improve upon the up to 35% failure rate of gluteal tendon repairs. Level of evidence: V (Technical note).

11. Redmond JM, Chen AW, Domb BG: Greater trochanteric pain syndrome. *J Am Acad Orthop Surg* 2016;24(4): 231-240.

    This is a classic review style article covering the diagnosis and nonsurgical and surgical treatments for greater trochanteric pain syndrome. Open and arthroscopic procedures are described for when nonsurgical management is no longer providing adequate relief. Level of evidence: V (Review article).

12. Fearon AM, Cook JL, Scarvell JM, Neeman T, Cormick W, Smith PN: Greater trochanteric pain syndrome negatively affects work, physical activity and quality of life: A case control study. *J Arthroplasty* 2014;29(2):383-386.

13. Segal NA, Felson DT, Torner JC, et al: Greater trochanteric pain syndrome: Epidemiology and associated factors. *Arch Phys Med Rehabil* 2007;88(8):988-992.

14. Long SS, Surrey DE, Nazarian LN: Sonography of greater trochanteric pain syndrome and the rarity of primary bursitis. *Am J Roentgenol* 2013;201(5):1083-1086.

15. Viradia NK, Berger AA, Dahners LE: Relationship between width of greater trochanters and width of iliac wings in tronchanteric bursitis. *Am J Orthop (Belle Mead NJ)* 2011;40(9): E159-E162.

16. Westacott DJ, Minns JI, Foguet P: The diagnostic accuracy of magnetic resonance imaging and ultrasonography in gluteal tendon tears–a systematic review. *Hip Int* 2011;21(6):637-645.

17. Mani-Babu S, Morrissey D, Waugh C, Screen H, Barton C: The effectiveness of extracorporeal shock wave therapy in lower limb tendinopathy: A systematic review. *Am J Sports Med* 2015;43(3):752-761.

18. Rompe JD, Segal NA, Cacchio A, Furia JP, Morral A, Maffulli N: Home training, local corticosteroid injection, or radial shock wave therapy for greater trochanter pain syndrome. *Am J Sports Med* 2009;37(10):1981-1990.

19. Via AG, Basile A, Wainer M, Musa C, Padulo J, Mardones R: Endoscopic release of internal snapping hip: A review of literature. *Muscles Ligaments Tendons J* 2016;6(3): 372-377.

    The breadth of literature is reviewed regarding the management of internal snapping hip (tendon snapping over the anterior femoral head or iliopectineal ridge). Endoscopic tendon release was found to have less complications and a decreased failure rate compared to open procedures. However, it was noted that most cases of internal snapping hip will resolve with conservative management. If surgery is needed, patients should be counseled that they may have some loss of hip flexion strength after a tendon release. Level of evidence: II (Systematic review).

20. Deslandes M, Guillin R, Cardinal E, Hobden R, Bureau NJ: The snapping iliopsoas tendon: New mechanisms using dynamic sonography. *Am J Roentgenol* 2008;190(3):576-581.

21. Tyler TF, Fukunaga T, Gellert J: Rehabilitation of soft tissue injuries of the hip and pelvis. *Int J Sports Phys Ther* 2014;9(6):785-797.

22. Piechota M, Maczuch J, Skupinski J, Kukawska-Sysio K, Wawrzynek W: Internal snapping hip syndrome in dynamic ultrasonography. *J Ultrason* 2016;16(66):296-303.

    A technical note on performing dynamic ultrasonography for making the diagnosis of internal, extra-articular snapping hip syndrome is described. When performed in real time, this gives excellent visualization of the abnormal friction associated with the snapping of the tendon. Level of evidence: V (Technical note).

23. Rauseo C: The rehabilitation of a runner with iliopsoas tendinopathy using an eccentric-biased exercise-A case report. *Int J Sports Phys Ther* 2017;12(7):1150-1162.

This case report highlights the condition of iliopsoas tendinopathy and in particular describes an interesting eccentric-biased technique to treat this condition in a runner. After 12 weeks of intervention, this 39-year-old runner completed a successful course of rehabilitation using this eccentric-biased exercise program. Level of evidence: V (Case report).

24. Gomez-Hoyos J, Schroder R, Palmer IJ, Reddy M, Khoury A, Martin HD: Iliopsoas tendon insertion footprint with surgical implications in lesser trochanterplasty for treating ischiofemoral impingement: An anatomic study. *J Hip Preserv Surg* 2015;2(4):385-391.

25. Blomberg JR, Zellner BS, Keene JS: Cross-sectional analysis of iliopsoas muscle-tendon units at the sites of arthroscopic tenotomies: An anatomic study. *Am J Sports Med* 2011;39 suppl:58S-63S.

26. Hwang DS, Hwang JM, Kim PS, et al: Arthroscopic treatment of symptomatic internal snapping hip with combined pathologies. *Clin Orthop Surg* 2015;7(2):158-163.

27. El Bitar YF, Stake CE, Dunne KF, Botser IB, Domb BG: Arthroscopic iliopsoas fractional lengthening for internal snapping of the hip: Clinical outcomes with a minimum 2-year follow-up. *Am J Sports Med* 2014;42(7):1696-1703.

28. Philippon MJ, Devitt BM, Campbell KJ, et al: Anatomic variance of the iliopsoas tendon. *Am J Sports Med* 2014;42(4): 807-811.

29. Spiker AM, Degen RM, Camp CL, Coleman SH: Arthroscopic psoas management: Techniques for psoas preservation and psoas tenotomy. *Arthrosc Tech* 2016;5(6):e1487-e1492.

This technique paper addresses the iliopsoas tendon in relation to treatment for a snapping hip or refractory tendinitis. They describe a technique to identify and preserve the tendon during routine arthroscopy, with a particular focus on deepening the psoas tunnel to relieve impingement. Secondarily, they report on another technique to release the tendon for cases in which this is the desired outcome. Level of evidence: V (Technique paper).

30. Gomez-Hoyos J, Martin RL, Martin HD: Current concepts review: Evaluation and management of posterior hip pain. *J Am Acad Orthop Surg* 2018;26(17):597-609.

This review looks at diagnosing and managing the numerous etiologies of posterior hip pain that may occur. The review breaks the sources of pain down into intrapelvic and extrapelvic, covering imaging modalities and findings to differentiate between the various conditions. Level of evidence: V (Review paper).

31. Bardakos NV: Hip impingement: Beyond femoroacetabular. *J Hip Preserv Surg* 2015;2(3):206-223.

32. Wilson MD, Keene JS: Treatment of ischiofemoral impingement: Results of diagnostic injections and arthroscopic resection of the lesser trochanter. *J Hip Preserv Surg* 2016;3(2):146-153.

This is a seven-patient case series that looks at an imaging protocol and arthroscopic treatment regimen to treat ischiofemoral impingement. This process starts with documented ischiofemoral impingement on MRI and is followed by a confirmatory ultrasound-guided injection of local anesthetic and corticosteroid. They found that the combination of arthroscopic iliopsoas tendon release and resection of the lesser trochanter yielded complete pain relief in the groin and buttock caused by ischiofemoral impingement. Level of evidence: IV (Case series—imaging protocol).

33. Hatem MA, Palmer IJ, Martin HD: Diagnosis and 2-year outcomes of endoscopic treatment for ischiofemoral impingement. *Arthroscopy* 2015;31(2):239-246.

34. Hammoud S, Bedi A, Voos JE, Mauro CS, Kelly BT: The recognition and evaluation of patterns of compensatory injury in patients with mechanical hip pain. *Sports Health* 2014;6(2):108-118.

35. Matsuda DK, Calipusan CP: Adolescent femoroacetabular impingement from malunion of the anteroinferior iliac spine apophysis treated with arthroscopic spinoplasty. *Orthopedics* 2012;35(3):e460-e463.

36. Siddiq MAB: Piriformis syndrome and wallet neuritis: Are they the same? *Cureus* 2018;10(5):e2606.

This editorial focuses on distinguishing the terms piriformis syndrome and wallet neuritis as they are different entities with distinct treatments. Overall, the necessary workup is quite different between the two conditions and therefore should be separated to avoid unnecessary tests (a thorough history and physical may be enough to distinguish piriformis syndrome from wallet neuritis) and treatments when one or the other processes are suspected. Level of evidence: V (Editorial).

37. Ro TH, Edmonds L: Diagnosis and management of piriformis syndrome: A rare anatomic variant analyzed by magnetic resonance imaging. *J Clin Imaging Sci* 2018; 8:6.

This is a case report describing a rare anatomic variant found on MRI in a patient with left-sided lower back and buttock pain. It is important to be aware of variations and to be able to diagnose piriformis syndrome as this will lead to appropriate treatment of the condition. Level of evidence: V (Case report).

38. Seeley MA, Georgiadis AG, Sankar WN: Hip vascularity: A review of the anatomy and clinical implications. *J Am Acad Orthop Surg* 2016;24(8):515-526.

This paper describes the vascular anatomy to the proximal femur and acetabulum as we develop into adults. The clinical implications of vascular anatomy, pathology, and variants are thoroughly reviewed. This anatomy is critical to understand for surgeons treating conditions around the hip and pelvis. Level of evidence: V (Review article).

39. Martin R, Martin HD, Kivlan BR: Nerve entrapment in the hip region: Current concepts review. *Int J Sports Phys Ther* 2017;12(7):1163-1173.

This commentary reviews the anatomy, etiology, and evaluation of the numerous nerve entrapment conditions that may occur about the hip and pelvis. Nerves often involved include the sciatic, pudendal, obturator, femoral, and lateral femoral cutaneous. Impingement of these nerves in athletes often has distinct symptoms to identify the source, with treatment typically involving manual therapy, stretching/strengthening, aerobic condition, education, and potential office/surgical interventions. Level of evidence: V (Clinical commentary).

40. Ahmed A, Arora D, Kochhar AK: Ultrasound-guided alcohol neurolysis of lateral femoral cutaneous nerve for intractable meralgia paresthetica: A case series. *Br J Pain* 2016;10(4):232-237.

    This is a case series of six patients with refractory meralgia paresthetica. Confirmatory injections were completed as was prescription, oral antineuropathic medications without sustained relief. Ultimately, ultrasound-guided alcohol neurolysis of the nerve was performed with prolonged relief in these cases of intractable meralgia paresthetica. Level of evidence: V (Case series).

41. Payne RA, Harbaugh K, Specht CS, Rizk E: Correlation of histopathology and clinical symptoms in meralgia paresthetica. *Cureus* 2017;9(10):e1789.

    The clinical and histopathological findings of a case of refractory meralgia paresthetica are reviewed in this paper. They found a moderate loss of myelinated axons with atrophy as well as moderate perineurial thickening. This highlights the pathophysiology of meralgia paresthetica as well as role of surgical treatment in refractory or intractable cases. Level of evidence: V (Case report).

42. Martin HD, Kivlan BR, Palmer IJ, Martin RL: Diagnostic accuracy of clinical tests for sciatic nerve entrapment in the gluteal region. *Knee Surg Sports Traumatol Arthrosc* 2014;22(4):882-888.

43. Petrov-Kondratov V, Chhabra A, Jones S: Pulsed radiofrequency ablation of pudendal nerve for treatment of a case of refractory pelvic pain. *Pain Physician* 2017;20(3):E451-E454.

    This is a case report of the management of pudendal neuralgia, or nerve entrapment (Alcock syndrome). This led to chronic pelvic pain that was treated with pulsed radiofrequency ablation for 240 seconds at 42° C. The patient reported greater than 50% pain relief at over 6 weeks follow-up.

44. Habib A, Haldane CE, Ekhtiari S, et al: Pudendal nerve injury is a relatively common but transient complication of hip arthroscopy. *Knee Surg Sports Traumatol Arthrosc* 2018;26(3):969-975.

    For this systematic review, 24 studies were included to identify the rate of pudendal nerve injury after arthroscopy and the specific factors leading to this condition. They reported a 1.8% incidence of pudendal nerve injury with all having resolved by 3 months. Potential risk factors include the length of traction time for surgery and the use of a perineal post. Sexual and urinary dysfunctions are symptoms that can occur post-arthroscopy but will typically resolve by 3 months post-procedure. Level of evidence: IV (Systematic review of level I-IV studies).

45. Aaron DL, Patel A, Kayiaros S, Calfee R: Four common types of bursitis: Diagnosis and management. *J Am Acad Orthop Surg* 2011;19(6):359-367.

46. Whiteside LA: Surgical technique: Transfer of the anterior portion of the gluteus maximus muscle for abductor deficiency of the hip. *Clin Orthop Relat Res* 2012;470(2):503-510.

47. Jang SA, Cho YH, Byun YS, Gu TH: Abductor reconstruction with gluteus maximus transfer in primary abductor deficiency during total hip arthroplasty. *Hip Pelvis* 2016;28(3):178-181.

    This is a description of the glutues maximus transfer for managing abductor deficiency in the setting of a total hip arthroplasty. A review of the literature and technique description is included. Level of evidence: V (Surgical technique and literature review).

48. Betz M, Zingg PO, Peirrmann CW, Dora C: Advancement of the vastus lateralis muscle for irreparable hip abductor tears: Clinical and morphological results. *Acta Orthop Belg* 2012;78(3):337-343.

49. Patel KA, Chhabra A, Goodwin JA, Brown JC, Hartigan DE: Arthroscopic iliopsoas release at the level of the lesser trochanter following total hip arthroplasty. *Arthrosc Tech* 2017;6(4):e1421-e1426.

    This paper describes the procedure for an arthroscopic release of the iliopsoas tendon at the level of the lesser trochanter after a total hip arthroplasty. This is a reasonable procedure after nonsurgical management has been attempted and fails. Level of evidence: V (Technical note).

50. Chalmers BP, Sculco PK, Sierra RJ, Trousdale RT, Berry DJ: Iliopsoas impingement after primary total hip arthroplasty: Operative and nonoperative treatment outcomes. *J Bone Joint Surg Am* 2017;99(7):557-564.

    Forty-nine patients treated for iliopsoas impingement after a primary total hip arthroplasty were reviewed. Acetabular revision, tenotomy, and nonsurgical management were utilized in 21, 8, and 20 patients, respectively. At latest follow-up, 50% of the nonsurgical patients had pain relief compared with 76% in the surgical cohort. They found that patients with minimal cup overhang had a high rate of success with iliopsoas release, but that acetabular revision was indicated when there was greater than or equal to 8mm of overhang. Level of evidence: III (Therapeutic review).

joint infection (PJI) calculator based on multivariate analysis of 42 different risk factors, which was subsequently validated at an external institution using another database of almost 30,000 patients.[23] Using this PJI calculator, the risk of PJI can vary from as low as 0.5% to greater than 20% depending on patient-specific comorbidities and surgical factors. Using these new tools in a patient shared decision-making manner may help to further lower complication rates in the future.

Perioperative Total Hip Arthroplasty Protocols

The past decade has brought a dramatic shift in perioperative protocols surrounding THA. Tranexamic acid (TXA) has now become standard-of-care at most institutions performing hip arthroplasty given its well-established benefit in reducing surgical blood loss and subsequent transfusions, an important consideration given the mounting evidence that there is a dose-dependent relationship between blood transfusions and subsequent development of PJI.[24] There have been numerous studies comparing efficacy of different dosing intravenous, oral, and topical dosing regimens. Several have demonstrated that TXA is equally effective when dosed intravenously at a variety of different doses, and a 2017 RCT demonstrated that oral TXA was equally effective as IV administration, but at a greatly reduced cost.[25] A 2016 RCT found that perhaps the most effective way to reduce blood loss is a combined IV and topical application, which reduced total blood loss by an additional 200 mL compared with the single IV dose group.[26] Importantly, no orthopaedic study has yet to demonstrate concern for an increase in venous thromboembolic (VTE) events in the setting of TXA administration, and at present there are very few contraindications to its use on a routine basis, even in patients thought to be at high risk for VTE.[27] Aspirin continues to increase in popularity for VTE prophylaxis following THA, as it is inexpensive and readily available, is generally well-tolerated, requires no monitoring, and has an excellent safety profile with lower risks of major and minor bleeding complications and lower rates of incisional complications compared with alternative means of chemoprophylaxis. The most recent guidelines from the American College of Chest Physicians directly endorse aspirin as an effective agent for prophylaxis, and there is now sufficient published evidence demonstrating its efficacy in the prevention of VTE in THA patients.[28] More potent chemoprophylaxis, such as use of a novel oral anticoagulant (NOAC) or low-molecular-weight heparin (LMWH), should still be considered in patients thought to be at higher risk for the development of VTE, for example, in those with a personal history of a prior unprovoked venous thromboembolic event. The final decision for the proper mode of VTE prophylaxis should still, however, be left to the treating orthopaedic surgeon based on all of the pertinent clinical risk factors.

The recent practice of discharging the majority of THA patients from the hospital to an inpatient rehabilitation facility has undergone a drastic change, and the majority of patients are now discharged directly home from the hospital. The reasons for this shift are multifactorial, but it has happened rapidly in large part due to concerns of increased postdischarge morbidity[29] and increased costs[30] incurred with utilization of inpatient rehabilitation facilities. Improved perioperative protocols, surgical techniques, and pain control are largely responsible for allowing the majority of patients to be discharged directly home. Furthermore, length of hospital stay has decreased year-over-year, and so-called "rapid recovery protocols" are now commonly utilized without any increase in perioperative complications.[31] As these pathways have further evolved, selected patients are now often considered candidates for outpatient THA, which has increased in popularity without an increase in complications in either randomized controlled trials[32] or large national database studies.[33] Routine use of postoperative physical therapy has also been questioned, with a 2017 RCT of 120 patients undergoing unilateral THA reporting no significant difference in functional outcomes between patients receiving formal physical therapy and those participating in unsupervised home exercise; authors of this study concluded that formal physical therapy may not be required following THA.[34]

Surgical Techniques for Hip Arthroplasty

There continues to be a shift toward less invasive approaches to hip surgery. Though the pendulum of "MIS" (minimally invasive surgery) techniques has shifted again, more primary hip arthroplasties are being performed via an anterior approach, with the direct anterior approach (DAA) now utilized by more than 25% of US surgeons. Early adoption of the technique was often thought to be driven by the market influences, but recent studies add to a growing body of evidence to support less pain, a shorter length of stay, and an earlier return of function with anterior approach surgery.[35] Concerns remain about an increase in early complications with anterior approach surgery, particularly femoral complications such as periprosthetic fracture, subsidence, and failure of osteointegration, but several large registry and multi-institution studies have shown it can be performed safely without an increase in complications in experienced hands. In addition, abductor sparing approaches through the Watson Jones muscle interval has also gained in popularity as an alternative to the DAA approach with similar lower pain levels and faster recovery.

The past several years have also brought a much greater understanding about the influence of the lumbar spine and how alterations in spinopelvic mobility can change the orientation of the acetabular implant throughout a range of functional positions. Patients with spinal deformity, those who have undergone spinal fusion, or those with a fixed spinopelvic alignment have been shown to have a marked increase in the risk of instability, likely related to the influence of the spine on the functional position of the acetabular implant. With this additional insight, the previously well-accepted notion of a consistent or fixed "safe zone" for acetabular cup positioning has been questioned,[36] and there is an increased acceptance that a true safe zone might be much more patient-specific than previously thought, taking into account factors such as the pelvic tilt, spinopelvic relationships, and rigidity versus flexibility of the lumbar spine throughout a functional range of motion.

Bearing surfaces used in primary THA have changed tremendously in the past decade (**Table 2**), as detailed in a 2017 study that reviewed a data set of 28,504 primary THA performed between 2007 and 2015.[37] Over this time, utilization of metal-on-metal bearings decreased from 39.2% to 5.5% while the utilization of ceramic-on-polyethylene bearings increased from 6.4% to 52.0%. In 2015, over 90% of acetabular liners used in primary THA were made of cross-linked polyethylene (XLPE). The confidence in this bearing surface continues to increase as more long-term data support a marked decrease in wear, osteolysis, and revision surgery beyond 15 years with XLPE when compared with conventional polyethylene.[38]

Table 2

Change in Bearing Surface Utilization in Among Primary Total Hip Arthroplasty Patients From 2007 to 2015

Bearing Couple	2007	2015
Metal-on-polyethylene	48%	40%
Ceramic-on-polyethylene	6%	52%
Ceramic-on-ceramic	7%	3%
Metal-on-metal	39%	5%

Data from Bedard NA, Burnett RA, DeMik DE, Gao Y, Liu SS, Callaghan JJ: Are trends in total hip arthroplasty bearing surface continuing to change? 2007 to 2015 usage in a large database cohort. *J Arthroplasty* 2017;32(12):3777-3781.

Economics of Primary Total Hip Arthroplasty

Patients undergoing THA have clearly benefited from improved perioperative protocols and surgical techniques; however, more focus is now being turned to the cost of care. Because total joint arthroplasty contributes to over 5% of Medicare expenditures, the increasing prevalence of these procedures have placed a substantial financial burden on the US healthcare system, particularly as the costs of performing the procedure have also increased. A 2017 study of the US Nationwide Inpatient Sample (NIS) found an increase in mean hospital costs of THA from $15,792 in 2002 to $23,650 in 2013, representing a 49.8% increase over that time.[39] The increase in cost would have been even greater if not for a concurrent decrease in length of stay from 4.1 to 2.8 days over that same interval. The increasing prevalence combined with the increased per case costs have recently focused significant national attention on cost-containment strategies. Subsequently, the economics of THA are now a major concern for many US orthopedic surgeons. The most notable programs to be introduced are various types of alternative payment models, the largest of which has become episode of care payments. These bundled-payment programs have primarily been designed and implemented by the Centers for Medicare and Medicaid Services to replace fee-for-services reimbursement in these patient groups. These payment models have been proposed as a method to decrease costs, improve coordination of care, and improve quality and are expected to spread across various payers in years ahead.

Complex Primary and Conversion Total Hip Arthroplasty

Primary or conversion THA performed for conditions such as developmental dysplasia and other childhood hip disorders, osteonecrosis, PTOA, and other less-common hip conditions can add significant complexity to the surgical procedure and risk of complications. For instance, a 2018 study documented approximately 20% greater direct costs in patients undergoing conversion THA when compared with a matched group of patients undergoing primary THA.[40] These patients also faced significantly greater surgical times, estimated blood loss, length of stay, intraoperative complications, and postoperative complications. While some of these increased risks are unavoidable in this patient population, femoral and acetabular complications may be decreased with the advent of more modern types of implants specifically designed for more complex scenarios, such as dual mobility acetabular implants (discussed below) or versatile, conical femoral implants that can address challenging femoral anatomy.[41]

Revision Total Hip Arthroplasty

The epidemiology of revision THA has changed significantly over the past decade. A 2018 study of 320,496 revision THAs performed from the NIS (2007 to 2013) found a 30% increase in the adjusted revision rate among patients 45 to 64 years of age, but a simultaneous decrease in the adjusted revision rate in all other age groups.[42] Other significant findings in that study were a 14% decrease in the revision rate for instability across the overall cohort, as well as decreases in length of stay, hospital costs, and likelihood of discharge to an inpatient rehabilitation facility. Similar to trends seen in primary THA patients, most postoperative complications following revision THA also significantly decreased over this period, including VTE, myocardial infarction, transfusion, pneumonia, urinary tract infection, and mortality.

Instability Following Total Hip Arthroplasty

Despite the recent reduction in the revision rate for instability, recurrent dislocation still remains among the most common indications for revision THA. Increasing adoption of dual mobility bearings in the United States, which have been widely used in Europe for decades, may be responsible for the recent decrease in revision rates for instability.[42] Dual mobility bearings have shown benefit in reducing dislocation rates in high-risk primary THA cases, such as patients undergoing surgery for femoral neck fractures, patients with neuromuscular disorders, patients with osteonecrosis or dysplasia, and patients with spinopelvic disorders or lumbar fusions. In addition, dual mobility bearings have been associated with low rates of dislocation in revision THA cases, specifically in patients undergoing revision for instability. A 2018 systematic review reported a 1.6% combined rate of intraprosthetic and extraarticular dislocation in high-risk primary THA patients, and a 1.7% combined rate of dislocation among revision THA patients.[43] There is still a role for using constrained acetabular liners in unstable patients with well-positioned and well-fixed acetabular components, particularly those with deficiency of the abductor mechanism, but dual mobility liners offer a different and potentially more effective manner of addressing many patients at high risk for instability. Furthermore, dual mobility liners avoid the risk of specific failure modes unique to constrained liners, which may occur at higher rates than previously appreciated.

Fixation

Though there has been renewed interest in the United States for cemented femoral fixation, noncemented biologic fixation remains the benchmark for revision THA. Advances in implant design, fixation surfaces, and surgical techniques have improved options for noncemented fixation during revision THA, particularly in cases with deficient bone stock. On the femoral side, both modular and nonmodular fluted tapered stems continue to offer reliable fixation even in cases where bone stock is significantly compromised (**Figure 4**). A 2017 single-institution study reported a 96% 10-year survivorship among 519 aseptic femoral revisions where a modular fluted tapered stem was utilized; in this series, the implants achieved a high rate of fixation across all categories of preoperative bone loss.[44] Nonmodular fluted tapered stems, available from more implant manufacturers in recent years, may function equally well in most revision scenarios but potentially with lower cost and without the added complexity of modular junction assembly.[45]

On the acetabular side, construct rigidity is critical for achieving long-term biologic fixation in noncemented implants with advanced fixation surfaces. Noncemented hemispherical highly porous acetabular cups with supplemental screw fixation are sufficient for most acetabular revisions. Porous tantalum acetabular cup and augment construct (**Figure 4**), a commonly employed strategy for addressing major acetabular bone loss, offer the potential for excellent long-term fixation. A 2017 study reported 97% survivorship at 5 years among 85 hips revised with significant acetabular bone loss at a single institution.[46] For more complex acetabular defects, another 2017 study from the same institution reported excellent short-term

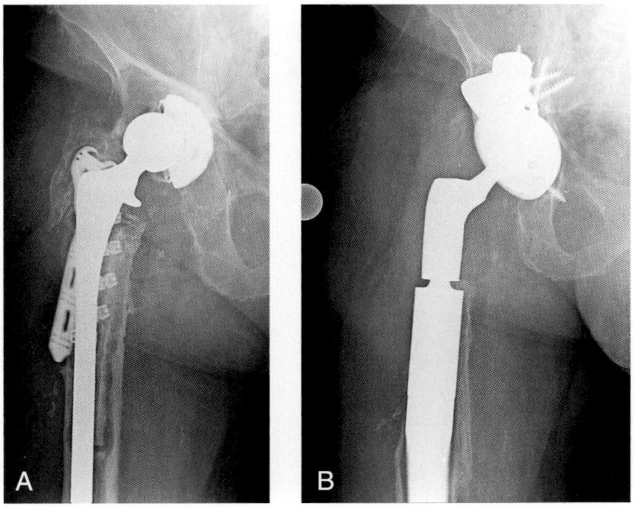

Figure 4 AP radiographs of a 64-year-old male with (**A**) massive bony defects of both the femur and acetabulum prior to revision in the setting of chronic periprosthetic joint infection. After an interval antibiotic-impregnated cement spacer, (**B**) reconstruction was performed utilizing a modular fluted tapered femoral stem and a noncemented acetabular shell with tantalum augments and a dual mobility bearing.

results using a cup-cage construct in 57 patients, 60% of whom had a concurrent pelvic discontinuity.[47] Custom triflange constructs, developed from preoperative CT scans, as well as pelvic distraction remain a good option for these complex defects as well.

Trunnionosis

The first case series describing adverse local tissue reactions (ALTR) arising secondary to corrosion at the modular head-neck taper in THA was published in 2012. Since that time, there have been dozens of studies published attempting to explain the etiology of the condition that has been commonly been referred to as "trunnionosis," whereby a process of mechanically assisted crevice corrosion (MACC) releases cobalt and chromium debris from the modular head-neck junction, which can subsequently lead to an inflammatory soft-tissue reaction frequently referred to as a pseudotumor or ALTR (adverse local tissue reaction). In addition to corrosion at the modular head-neck junction, ALTR can also occur from MACC at the modular neck-body junction in dual-modular femoral stems with an exchangeable cobalt chromium neck, and several implants in this category have been voluntarily recalled from the market. A 2018 study reported the prevalence of revision for ALTR among 2409 metal-on-polyethylene THAs was 0.5% at 7 years,[48] while the prevalence of ALTR has been reported to be markedly higher with specific dual-modular stem designs.

Trunnionosis should be considered in the differential diagnosis of most patients with a failed or painful THA and typically manifests as pain (around 2 to 5 years after index surgery) or soft-tissue destruction that can lead to instability. Serum metal ion levels and metal artifact reduction sequencing MRI remain diagnostic modalities of choice; however, the ability of these diagnostic tests to guide the decision for revision surgery has been questioned in recent studies. Revision surgery for ALTR continues to have a high risk of major orthopedic complications, with instability and PJI most prevalent, greater than 10% in many series.

Periprosthetic Joint Infection

The Musculoskeletal Infection Society (MSIS) revised their definition of periprosthetic joint infection in 2018

Table 3

2018 Musculoskeletal Infection Society Criteria for Periprosthetic Joint Infection

Major Criteria (At Least One of the Following)				**Decision**
Two positive cultures of the same organism				Infected
Sinus tract with evidence of communication to the joint or visualization of the prosthesis				
Preoperative Diagnosis	**Minor Criteria**		**Score**	**Decision**
	Serum	Elevated CRP or D-Dimer	2	≥6 infected
		Elevated ESR	1	2-5 possibly infected[a]
	Synovial	Elevated synovial *WBC count* or *LE*	3	0-1 not infected
		Positive alpha-defensin	3	
		Elevated synovial PMN (%)	2	
		Elevated synovial CRP	1	
Intraoperative Diagnosis		**Inconclusive Pre-op Score or Dry Tap**	**Score**	**Decision**
		Preoperative score	—	≥6 infected
		Positive histology	3	4-5 inconclusive[b]
		Positive purulence	3	≤3 not infected
		Single positive culture	2	

[a]For patients with inconclusive minor criteria, surgical criteria can also be used to fulfill definition for prosthetic joint infection (PJI).

[b]Consider further molecular diagnostics such as next-generation sequencing.

CRP = C-reactive protein, ESR = erythrocyte sedimentation rate, LE = leukocyte esterase, PMN = polymorphonuclear, WBC = white blood cell

Reprinted from Parvizi J, Tan TL, Goswami K, et al: The 2018 definition of periprosthetic hip and knee infection: An evidence-based and validated criteria. *J Arthroplasty* 2018;33(5):1309-1314.e2, Copyright 2018, with permission from Elsevier.

(**Table 3**),[49] acknowledging the role that several new tests such as alpha defensin, D-dimer, leukocyte esterase, and synovial CRP have come to play in helping to establish what at times still remains an elusive diagnosis. There have been many recent studies on these specific biomarkers demonstrating added utility in the diagnosis of PJI. The 2018 MSIS definition of PJI may continue to be refined in the future as new synovial fluid biomarkers are investigated. Optimal treatment strategies for PJI following THA are still debated and have yet to be fully defined. The benchmark remains two-stage exchange arthroplasty; however, there is a renewed interest in one-stage exchange for known susceptible organisms in properly selected patients. Additionally, a 2017 study reported a higher success rate of irrigation and débridement (I&D) for acute infection following THA, particularly in good hosts (92% success of I&D in McPherson host grade A) and in those treated with chronic antibiotic suppression (97% success when chronic suppression was used in patients still infection-free at 6 weeks after I&D).[50]

Summary

There is an approximate 25% lifetime risk of hip arthritis. Its development is associated with a number of genetic and environmental influences, more common in some populations than others. Hip arthritis can take a substantial toll on the physical, mental, and emotional well-being of patients that deal with its symptoms on a daily basis. THA continues to be an excellent, reliable option for patients with end-stage hip arthritis. Over the past decade THA has become a safer and easier procedure for most patients, with year-over-year improvements in mortality and perioperative complication rates. Over this time, there have been several major advances which may contribute to these improved outcomes, related to blood management, VTE prophylaxis, rapid recovery protocols, and evolving surgical techniques. Revision THA has undergone a similar transformation, with lower complication rates and improved surgical techniques and implants to address challenges such as instability, bone defects, and periprosthetic joint infection. Among the major challenges facing THA in the United States is its long-term economic viability in the setting of increased cost containment pressures. Bundled care programs have recently been introduced to decrease costs while improving coordination of care and quality and will likely become more common given early positive returns of these programs.

Key Study Points

- Hip osteoarthritis is a major public health issue with an average lifetime risk of 25% and can severely affect quality of life, mobility, activity level, and interfere with sleep, mood, or personality predispositions.
- When nonsurgical modalities fail, THA is a reliable surgical intervention for end-stage disease and has become safer over the past decade. Success has also been improved with increased attention to preoperative risk-stratification and optimization of modifiable risk factors. Evolution of perioperative protocols, led by widespread adoption of tranexamic acid and multimodal pain control, has significantly changed the delivery of THA. These changes have helped facilitate a shorter hospitalization and greater likelihood of home discharge through rapid-recovery protocols and more recently, adaptation of outpatient THA for the properly indicated patient.
- A major focus on THA currently is decreasing costs and achieving greater value, spurred by the increasing adoption of bundled-payment programs.

Annotated References

1. Jafarzadeh SR, Felson DT: Updated estimates suggest a much higher prevalence of arthritis in United States adults than previous ones. *Arthritis Rheumatol* 2017;70:185-192.

   Using different assumptions and Bayesian models, the authors conclude that previous assumptions of arthritis epidemiology have been low.

2. Murphy LB, Cisternas MG, Pasta DJ, Helmick CG, Yelin EH: Medical expenditures and earnings losses among US adults with arthritis in 2013. *Arthritis Care Res* 2018;70:869-876.

   The authors estimate the economic impact of arthritis using 2013 US Medical Expenditure Panel Survey (MEPS) data. Level of evidence: II (Economic).

3. Murphy LB, Helmick CG, Schwartz TA, et al: One in four people may develop symptomatic hip osteoarthritis in his or her lifetime. *Osteoarthr Cartil* 2010;11:1372-1379.

4. 2017 Annual Report of the American Joint Replacement Registry. Available at: http://www.ajrr.net/publications-data/annual-reports. Accessed August 31, 2018.

5. Koenig L, Zhang Q, Austin MS, et al: Estimating the societal benefits of THA after accounting for work status and productivity: A Markov model approach. *Clin Orthop Relat Res* 2016;474:2645-2654.

   The authors determine the cost effectiveness of THA compared to nonsurgical treatments and the increased productivity after THA per patient. Level of evidence: III (Economic and decision analysis).

6. Wyles CC, Heidenreich MJ, Jeng J, Larson DR, Trousdale RT, Sierra RJ: The John Charnley award: Redefining the natural history of osteoarthritis in patients with hip dysplasia and impingement. *Clin Orthop Relat Res* 2017;475:336-350.

Average 20-year follow-up of 162 patients with Tönnis grade 0 were studied, with degenerative changes and time to THA compared. Level of evidence: III (Prognostic).

7. Amstutz HC, Le Duff MJ: The natural history of osteoarthritis: What happens to the other hip? *Clin Orthop Relat Res* 2016;474:1802-1809.

This study had an average 11-year radiographic follow-up of 367 patients undergoing THA without contralateral hip symptoms and examined radiographic features associated with the development of OA. Level of evidence: IV (Prognostic).

8. Moreta J, Foruria X, Sánchez A, Aguirre U: Prognostic factors after a traumatic hip dislocation. A long-term retrospective study. *Rev Esp Cir Ortop Traumatol* 2017;61:367-374.

A review of 30 native hip dislocations was performed at 11 years to determine factors leading to OA or AVN. Level of evidence: IV (Prognostic).

9. Hess SR, O'Connell RS, Bednarz CP, Waligora AC IV, Golladay GJ, Jiranek WA: Association of rapidly destructive osteoarthritis of the hip with intra-articular steroid injections. *Arthroplast Today* 2018;4:205-209.

This report of 129 corticosteroid injections in 109 patients found 23 (21%) cases of rapidly destructive OA of the hip. Level of evidence: IV (Therapeutic).

10. Oh C, Slover JD, Bosco JA, Iorio R, Gold HT: Time trends in characteristics of patients undergoing primary total hip and knee arthroplasty in California, 2007-2010. *J Arthroplasty* 2018;33:2376-2380.

A state-wide database study examining demographic trends in primary hip and knee arthroplasty.

11. Goodman SM, Bykerk VP, DiCarlo E, et al: Flares in patients with rheumatoid arthritis after total hip and total knee arthroplasty: Rates, characteristics, and risk factors. *J Rheumatol* 2018;45:604-611.

This review of 120 patients with RA evaluated the incidence of flares after arthroplasty. Level of evidence: IV (prognostic).

12. Fehring TK, Odum SM, Curtin BM, Mason JB, Fehring KA, Springer BD: Should depression be treated before lower extremity arthroplasty? *J Arthroplasty* 2018;33(10):3143-3146 [Epub ahead of print].

Depression improved following arthroplasty; therefore, surgery need not wait for treatment of depression first. Level of evidence: IV (Therapeutic).

13. Taylor SS, Hughes JM, Coffman CJ, et al: Prevalence of and characteristics associated with insomnia and obstructive sleep apnea among veterans with knee and hip osteoarthritis. *BMC Musculoskelet Disord* 2018;19:79.

A study of 300 veterans found 53% and 66% prevalence of insomnia and OSA associated with arthritis. Level of evidence: III (Prognostic).

14. Jung JH, Seok H, Choi SJ, et al: The association between osteoarthritis and sleep duration in Koreans: A nationwide cross-sectional observational study. *Clin Rheumatol* 2018;37:1653-1659.

In 11,540 Korean patients, those sleeping fewer than 6 hours were more likely to have symptomatic OA. Level of evidence: III (Prognostic).

15. Parmelee PA, Tighe CA, Dautovich ND: Sleep disturbance in osteoarthritis: Linkages with pain, disability, and depressive symptoms. *Arthritis Care Res* 2018;67:358-365.

This study evaluates cross-sectional relationships between sleep, pain, and depression in OA.

16. Innes KE, Sambamoorthi U: The association of perceived memory loss with osteoarthritis and related joint pain in a large appalachian population. *Pain Med* 2018;19:1340-1356.

Patients with OA were three times as likely to report memory loss. Level of evidence: III (Prognostic).

17. Clauw DJ, Hassett AL: The role of centralised pain in osteoarthritis. *Clin Exp Rheumatol* 2017;107:79-84.

This reviews pain of OA and the mechanisms of different pharmacological treatments in OA.

18. da Costa BR, Nüesch E, Kasteler R, et al: Opioids for osteoarthritis. *Cochrane Rev* 2014.

19. Krebs EE, Gravely A, Nugent S, et al: Effect of opioid vs nonopioid medications on pain-related function in patients with chronic back pain or hip or knee osteoarthritis pain. The SPACE randomized clinical trial. *J Am Med Assoc* 2018;319:872-882.

Randomized comparison of opioids versus nonopioids and showing nonsuperiority of opioids in treating OA. Level of evidence: I (Therapeutic).

20. Maradit Kremers H, Larson DR, Crowson CS, et al: Prevalence of total hip and knee replacement in the United States. *J Bone Joint Surg Am* 2015;97(17):1386-1397.

21. Sanders TL, Maradit Kremers H, Schleck CD, Larson DR, Berry DJ: Subsequent total joint arthroplasty after primary total knee or hip arthroplasty: A 40-year population-based study. *J Bone Joint Surg Am* 2017;99(5):396-401.

Historical cohort study examining 1933 THA and 2139 TKA performed between 1969 and 2008, which assess the likelihood of undergoing a subsequent TJA as 30% to 45% in a contralateral cognate joint and 5% in noncognate joints within 20 years. Level of evidence: IV (Therapeutic).

22. Partridge T, Jameson S, Baker P, Deehan D, Mason J, Reed MR: Ten-year trends in medical complications following 540,623 primary total hip replacements from a national database. *J Bone Joint Surg Am* 2018;100(5):360-367.

Large database study examining patients undergoing primary THA 2005 to 2014, which found the 90-day mortality dropped steadily from 0.60% in 2005 to 0.15% in 2014. Most other indicators of quality of care also improved, despite an increasing level of comorbidity Level of evidence: IV (Therapeutic).

23. Tan TL, Maltenfort MG, Chen AF, et al: Development and evaluation of a preoperative risk calculator for periprosthetic joint infection following total joint arthroplasty. *J Bone Joint Surg Am* 2018;100(9):777-785.

Risk calculator for PJI developed using 42 individual risk factors, based on a retrospective review of 27,717 patients who underwent TJA at a single institution, which was then externally validated at another institution against a dataset of 29,252 patients. Level of evidence: IV (Prognostic).

24. Everhart JS, Sojka JH, Mayerson JL, Glassman AH, Scharschmidt TJ: Perioperative allogeneic red blood-cell transfusion associated with surgical site infection after total hip and knee arthroplasty. *J Bone Joint Surg Am* 2018;100(4):288-294.

Single-institution study of nearly 7000 patients undergoing TJA between 2000 and 2011, which found a dose-dependent relationship between allogeneic transfusion and SSI risk. Level of evidence: III (Therapeutic).

25. Kayupov E, Fillingham YA, Okroj K, et al: Oral and intravenous tranexamic acid are equivalent at reducing blood loss following total hip arthroplasty: A randomized controlled trial. *J Bone Joint Surg Am* 2017;99(5):373-378.

Double-blinded RCT of 89 patients undergoing primary THA, randomized to oral versus IV perioperative TXA, which found equivalent reductions in blood loss at a greatly reduced cost when using the oral formulation. Level of evidence: I (Therapeutic).

26. Yi Z, Bin S, Jing Y, Zongke Z, Pengde K, Fuxing P: Tranexamic acid administration in primary total hip arthroplasty: A randomized controlled trial of intravenous combined with topical versus single-dose intravenous administration. *J Bone Joint Surg Am* 2016;98(12):983-991.

Prospective RCT of 150 patients divided into (1) combined IV + topical, (2) IV alone, and (3) placebo groups for TXA dosing. The combined group had lower EBL compared to IV alone, which in turn outperformed placebo Level of evidence: I (Therapeutic).

27. Whiting DR, Gillette BP, Duncan C, Smith H, Pagnano MW, Sierra RJ: Preliminary results suggest tranexamic acid is safe and effective in arthroplasty patients with severe comorbidities. *Clin Orthop Relat Res* 2014;472(1): 66-72.

28. Parvizi J, Ceylan HH, Kucukdurmaz F, Merli G, Tuncay I, Beverland D: Venous thromboembolism following hip and knee arthroplasty: The role of aspirin. *J Bone Joint Surg Am* 2017;99(11):961-972.

Review article focusing on the increasingly recognized benefits of aspirin as an agent-of-choice for prophylaxis against venous thromboembolic disease. Level of evidence: V (Therapeutic).

29. Fu MC, Samuel AM, Sculco PK, MacLean CH, Padgett DE, McLawhorn AS: Discharge to inpatient facilities after total hip arthroplasty is associated with increased postdischarge morbidity. *J Arthroplasty* 2017;32(9S):S144-S149.e1.

NSQIP study of 54,837 THAs (2011 to 2014) documenting increased rates of postdischarge morbidity and unplanned readmission, after propensity matching, in the 26% of patient discharged to an inpatient facility compared to the 74% of patients discharged home. Level of evidence: II (Prognostic).

30. Sabeh KG, Rosas S, Buller LT, Roche MW, Hernandez VH: The impact of discharge disposition on episode-of-care reimbursement after primary total hip arthroplasty. *J Arthroplasty* 2017;32(10):2969-2973.

Large database study that found postdischarge costs represent a sizeable portion of the overall THA expense and that patients who went home as compared to an inpatient rehabilitation facility cost significantly less.

31. Sutton JC III, Antoniou J, Epure LM, Huk OL, Zukor DJ, Bergeron SG: Hospital discharge within 2 days following total hip or knee arthroplasty does not increase major-complication and readmission rates. *J Bone Joint Surg Am* 2016;98(17):1419-1428.

NSQIP database study of 19,909 patients who underwent primary unilateral THA 2011 to 2012 and found that early (POD 0-2) discharge was not an independent risk factor for 30-day major complications or readmission. Level of evidence: III (Prognostic).

32. Goyal N, Chen AF, Padgett SE, et al: Otto Aufranc award: A multicenter, randomized study of outpatient versus inpatient total hip arthroplasty. *Clin Orthop Relat Res* 2017;475(2):364-372.

Prospective RCT of 220 patients meeting specific inclusion criteria who were randomized to outpatient versus inpatient THA, documenting no significant differences in pain, reoperations, or readmissions, but with a 24% rate of crossover. Level of evidence: I (Therapeutic).

33. Basques BA, Tetreault MW, Della Valle CJ: Same-day discharge compared with inpatient hospitalization following hip and knee arthroplasty. *J Bone Joint Surg Am* 2017;99(23):1969-1977.

NSQIP database study of 1,236 patients who underwent THA between 2005 and 2014 who were discharged from the hospital same day (0.70% of the overall THA population), with no significant differences in overall complications or readmission. (Level of evidence: III (Therapeutic).

34. Austin MS, Urbani BT, Fleischman AN, et al: Formal physical therapy after total hip arthroplasty is not required: A randomized controlled trial. *J Bone Joint Surg Am* 2017;99(8):648-655.

Prospective RCT of 120 patients undergoing primary unilateral THA, randomized to formal PT or an unsupervised, self-directed program. There were no differences in any measured functional outcomes between patients at any time point. Level of evidence: I (Therapeutic).

35. Zhao HY, Kang PD, Xia YY, Shi XJ, Nie Y, Pei FX: Comparison of early functional recovery after total hip arthroplasty using a direct anterior or posterolateral approach: A randomized controlled trial. *J Arthroplasty* 2017;32(11):3421-3428.

Prospective RCT of 120 patients randomized to DAA versus posterolateral approach, that found the DAA group had significantly shorter hospital stays, lower pain scores, lower serum inflammatory and muscle damage markers, lower variance in cup inclination and anteversion, and better HHS scores, UCLA scores, and gait analysis at 3 months. Level of evidence: I (Therapeutic).

36. Seagrave KG, Troelsen A, Malchau H, Husted H, Gromov K: Acetabular cup position and risk of dislocation in primary total hip arthroplasty: A systematic review of the literature. *Acta Orthop* 2017;88(1):10-17. doi:10.1080/17453674.2016.1251255.

    A systematic review of 28 articles comparing acetabular cup position and risk of dislocation, that concluded the Lewinnek safe zone could not be justified and it is difficult to identify a definitive target zone for positioning. Level of evidence: III (Prognostic).

37. Bedard NA, Burnett RA, DeMik DE, Gao Y, Liu SS, Callaghan JJ: Are trends in total hip arthroplasty bearing surface continuing to change? 2007 to 2015 usage in a large database cohort. *J Arthroplasty* 2017;32(12):3777-3781.

    Review of the 2007 to 2015 Humana dataset, documenting a tremendous change in bearing surface choice over this time.

38. de Steiger R, Lorimer M, Graves SE: Cross-linked polyethylene for total hip arthroplasty markedly reduces revision surgery at 16 years. *J Bone Joint Surg Am* 2018;100(15):1281-1288.

    Review of the Australian National Registry from 1999 to 2016, which found a markedly lower revision rate when using cross-linked polyethylene compared with conventional polyethylene. Level of evidence: III (Therapeutic).

39. Molloy IB, Martin BI, Moschetti WE, Jevsevar DS: Effects of the length of stay on the cost of total knee and total hip arthroplasty from 2002 to 2013. *J Bone Joint Surg Am* 2017;99(5):402-407.

    Large database study of 2.8 million admissions following THA from 2002 to 2013 using the National Inpatient Sample, which found average costs increased over this period but were attenuated by reduced length of stay.

40. Ryan SP, DiLallo M, Attarian DE, Jiranek WA, Seyler TM: Conversion vs primary total hip arthroplasty: Increased cost of care and perioperative complications. *J Arthroplasty* 2018;33(8):2405-2411.

    Single-institution study of 163 conversion THAs performed 2012 to 2015, that documented greater costs, increased OR time, and greater perioperative complications when compared to primary THA. Level of evidence: III (Therapeutic).

41. Zhang Q, Goodman SB, Maloney WJ, Huddleston JI: Can a conical implant successfully address complex anatomy in primary THA? Radiographs and hip scores at early followup. *Clin Orthop Relat Res* 2016;474(2):459-464.

    Single-center, retrospective review of 59 complex primary THA, documenting a conical femoral stem provides reproducible improvements in hip scores at mean 4-year follow-up as well as promising short-term radiographic results in complex femoral anatomy. Level of evidence: IV (Therapeutic).

42. Rajaee SS, Campbell JC, Mirocha J, Paiement GD: Increasing burden of total hip arthroplasty revisions in patients between 45 and 64 years of age. *J Bone Joint Surg Am* 2018;100(6):449-458.

    Large database study (2007 to 2013 NIS) of 320,496 THAs that found revision rate has significantly increased in patients aged 45 to 64 years, but the rate of surgically treated dislocations has decreased significantly along with rate of complications of revision THA. Level of evidence: IV (Therapeutic).

43. Darrith B, Courtney PM, Della Valle CJ: Outcomes of dual mobility components in total hip arthroplasty: A systematic review of the literature. *Bone Joint Lett J* 2018;100-B(1):11-19.

    Systematic review of 54 articles that concluded dual mobility articulations are a viable bearing with low rates of complication, offering low rates of instability and good overall survivorship. Level of evidence: III (Therapeutic).

44. Abdel MP, Cottino U, Larson DR, Hanssen AD, Lewallen DG, Berry DJ: Modular fluted tapered stems in aseptic revision total hip arthroplasty. *J Bone Joint Surg Am* 2017;99(10):873-881.

    Retrospective, single-center review of 519 aseptic femoral revisions that used a modular fluted tapered stem, documenting a 10-year survivorship of 96% with revision for any reason as the end point, and 90% with any reoperation as the end point. Level of evidence: IV (Therapeutic).

45. Huang Y, Zhou Y, Shao H, Gu J, Tang H, Tang Q: What is the difference between modular and nonmodular tapered fluted titanium stems in revision total hip arthroplasty. *J Arthroplasty* 2017;32(10):3108-3113.

    Retrospective review of 289 revision THAs demonstrating both modular and nonmodular stem designs provide satisfactory midterm results. Level of evidence: III (Therapautic).

46. Jenkins DR, Odland AN, Sierra RJ, Hanssen AD, Lewallen DG: Minimum five-year outcomes with porous tantalum acetabular cup and augment construct in complex revision total hip arthroplasty. *J Bone Joint Surg Am* 2017;99(10):e49.

    Retrospective, single-center review of 85 THAs revised using porous tantalum augments, documenting 97% survivorship at minimum 5 years (with failure defined as aseptic loosening requiring repeat revision surgery). Level of evidence: IV (Therapeutic).

47. Sculco PK, Ledford CK, Hanssen AD, Abdel MP, Lewallen DG: The evolution of the cup-cage technique for major acetabular defects: Full and half cup-cage reconstruction. *J Bone Joint Surg Am* 2017;99(13):1104-1110.

    Retrospective, single-center review of 57 patients treated with a cup-cage for major acetabular bone loss, which found both full and half cup-cage constructs demonstrated successful outcomes at a mean 5-year follow-up. Level of evidence: III (Therapeutic).

48. Persson A, Eisler T, Bodén H, Krupic F, Sköldenberg O, Muren O: Revision for symptomatic pseudotumor after primary metal-on-polyethylene total hip arthroplasty with a standard femoral stem. *J Bone Joint Surg Am* 2018;100(11):942-949.

Prospective observational cohort of 2469 THAs performed with the same femoral stem, documenting a 0.5% prevalence of revision for symptomatic pseudotumor formation at mean 7-year follow-up. Level of evidence: IV (Therapeutic).

49. Parvizi J, Tan TL, Goswami K, et al: The 2018 definition of periprosthetic hip and knee infection: An evidence-based and validated criteria. *J Arthroplasty* 2018;33(5):1309-1314.e2.

Multiinstitution study that updated the prior 2011 MSIS definition of PJI, using an evidence-based and validated updated version incorporating new diagnostic tests and lessons learned from the prior version. Level of evidence: II (Diagnostic).

50. Bryan AJ, Abdel MP, Sanders TL, Fitzgerald SF, Hanssen AD, Berry DJ: Irrigation and debridement with component retention for acute infection after hip arthroplasty: Improved results with contemporary management. *J Bone Joint Surg Am* 2017;99(23):2011-2018.

Single-institution retrospective review of 90 hips treated with I&D and component retention for strictly-defined acute PJI between 2000 to 2012, reporting an 83% success rate following a defined protocol. Level of evidence: IV (Therapeutic).

Section 8
Knee

EDITOR

Antonia F. Chen, MD

Chapter 38

Knee Anatomy

Wolfgang Fitz, MD • Jeffrey Lange, MD

ABSTRACT

The anatomy of the knee has been described in depth, with the addition of the newly recognized anterolateral ligament. Knee kinematics is discussed, clarifying aspects of modern dynamic motion analysis. Advancements in knee imaging focus on simplifying routine radiographs by implementing fixed flexion series and introducing weight-bearing MRI, which is not currently available for routine clinical use. Future imaging improvements may assist in the diagnosis of unstable meniscal injuries and painful activities of the patellofemoral joint. Better three-dimensional imaging techniques may replace stress views for a more accurate assessment of all three parts of the knee joint when planning surgical treatment, such as high tibial osteotomies or unicompartmental knee arthroplasties.

Keywords: anatomy; knee kinematics and imaging; physical examination

Introduction

The human knee is composed of three articular compartments surrounded by a robust soft-tissue envelope, including synovium, joint capsule, muscle, tendon, bursa, subcutaneous tissue, and skin. The complex dynamic relationship between these structures confers the knee's function as a major weight-bearing joint of the body, allowing for great flexibility, pivoting, and high-impact activities. The anatomy of the human knee could be a topic of an entire textbook in and of itself. We offer a brief overview below as a basis for understanding the clinically and orthopaedically relevant anatomy of the human knee.

Dr. Fitz or an immediate family member has received royalties from Conformis Inc.; serves as a paid consultant to or is an employee of Conformis Inc.; has stock or stock options held in Conformis Inc.; and has received research or institutional support from IGB. Neither Dr. Lange nor any immediate family member has received anything of value from or has stock or stock options held in a commercial company or institution related directly or indirectly to the subject of this chapter.

General Knee Anatomy

Bone

The knee consists of articulations among three bones: the tibia, the femur, and the patella. The tibiofemoral articulation has two compartments, medial and lateral. Each of these two compartments houses the interaction between its respective tibial and femoral condyles. The patellofemoral compartment houses the interaction between the patella and the femur's trochlear groove. In each articular compartment, the bone serves as a weight-bearing surface and scaffold for the overlying articular cartilage. Each articulation and the relevant bony anatomy are reviewed in the "Knee kinematics" section below.

Articular Cartilage

All articular surfaces of the knee joint consist of an articular cartilage cap that is supported by underlying bone. Articular cartilage is highly resistant to wear and allows for low-friction gliding motions under normal knee conditions.[1] Articular cartilage is composed of chondrocytes and extracellular matrix. Extracellular matrix is largely composed of water, proteoglycans, and collagen (predominantly type II), with much smaller amounts of noncollagenous proteins and glycoproteins.[2] Articular cartilage is avascular and receives its nutrition by diffusion through the extracellular matrix. It is a highly organized structure, consisting of four major zones: superficial zone, middle (transitional) zone, deep zone, and calcified zone (**Figure 1**). Each zone performs a unique function in the development and maintenance of the articular cartilage layer.

Synovium

The knee joint cavity is lined by tissue called synovium. The synovium has two layers—the intima, adjacent to the knee joint itself, and the subintima, which adheres to the joint capsule just superficial to it. The synovium

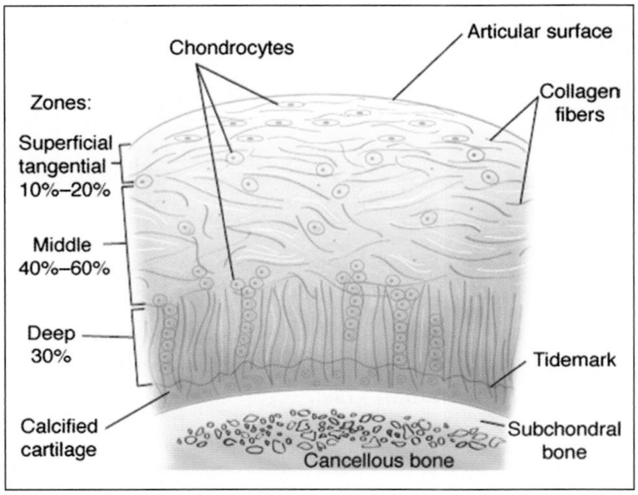

Figure 1 Illustration demonstrating articular cartilage architecture. The four zones of articular cartilage are depicted, with the underlying subchondral bone beneath. The arrangement of collagen fibers throughout the articular cartilage layer is demonstrated schematically. (Reprinted from Buckwalter JA, Mow VC, Ratcliffe A: Restoration of injured or degenerated articular cartilage. *J Am Acad Orthop Surg* 1994;2[4]:192-201.)

contributes to the production of synovial fluid, which provides joint lubrication and diffusion of nutrients to the articular cartilage. The intimal layer contains two types of specialized cells, or synoviocytes, that are responsible for production and maintenance of synovial fluid. Type A cells are macrophage-like cells that clear the joint of excess material or pathogens. Type B cells produce vital components of synovial fluid. The subintimal layer contains numerous cell types and acts as a conduit to the overlying joint capsule. This layer exhibits a rich vascular and nerve supply, which may be related to its function in both joint nutrition and biomechanical optimization.[3,4]

Meniscus

The knee has two menisci—medial and lateral. Each is composed of multiple collagen types and extracellular matrix.[5] The meniscus functions as both a load distributor during weight bearing and as a secondary stabilizer of the knee joint throughout range of motion. The medial meniscus is bound more tightly to the joint capsule via the deep medial collateral ligament (MCL) and the meniscotibial and meniscofemoral ligaments. The medial meniscus demonstrates relatively little excursion during range of motion, while the lateral meniscus demonstrates relatively great excursion during range of motion. Each has anterior and posterior roots tethered to the anterior and posterior tibia, respectively. The posterior root of the lateral meniscus attaches to the posteromedial femoral condyle via the anterior and posterior meniscofemoral ligaments, otherwise known as the ligaments of Humphrey (anterior to posterior cruciate ligament) and Wrisberg (posterior to posterior cruciate ligament).[5] The properties of the menisci contribute to the knee's effective pivot on the medial side, as the medial femoral condyle remains relatively centered on the tibial plateau, while the lateral femoral condyle moves about more freely on the lateral tibial plateau during range of motion (see "Knee kinematics" section below).

Ligaments

There are four major ligaments of the knee and multiple lesser ligaments. The four major ligaments are the anterior cruciate ligament (ACL), the posterior cruciate ligament (PCL), the medial collateral ligament (MCL), and the lateral collateral ligament (LCL). The ACL is an intra-articular structure, finding its attachments on the tibial eminence anteriorly, as well as the lateral aspect of the femoral notch of the lateral femoral condyle. The PCL finds its attachments on the medial aspect of the femoral notch and the midportion of the posterior tibial plateau. The superficial portion of the MCL originates at the medial femoral epicondyle and inserts on the proximal medial tibia, arising deep to the quadriceps' aponeurosis and superficial to the knee's joint capsule. The deep portion of the MCL, located in the midsagittal plane, is a confluence of the meniscofemoral ligament extensions, meniscotibial ligament extensions, and the knee capsule on the medial side. The LCL originates at the lateral femoral epicondyle and inserts on the fibular head.[6,7]

Recently, the anterolateral ligament (ALL) has been recognized as a distinct structure separate to the LCL.[8] Originally described by Segond in 1879 as a "pearly, resistant, fibrous band," the ALL has not been fully recognized as a distinct structure until recently.[8] In their cadaveric dissection analysis, Claes et al. identified the ALL as a distinct structure in 97% of specimens.[8] Brockmeyer et al corroborated these findings in a separate dissection analysis of 23 knees, identifying a distinct ALL structure in 100% of specimens.[9] The authors describe a reproducible course of the ALL from its femoral insertion overlapping the LCL slightly proximal and posterior to the lateral femoral epicondyle, and coursing distal and anterior, inserting on the tibia between Gerdy tubercle and the fibular head.[9] Others have noted similar findings after dissection in separate cadaveric cohorts.[10,11]

There are several other ligaments that surround the knee joint and contribute to its stability throughout range of motion. These ligaments can be visualized in **Figure 2**.

MRI

Limitations of radiographs have identified MRI as the most appropriate imaging modality to assess joint status specifically in osteoarthritis research studies.[39] MRIs detect abnormalities in the articular cartilage, subchondral bone quality, and meniscal and ligament integrity and provide good cartilage visualization to assess thickness and volume of articular cartilage. Standard clinical knee MRI protocols consist of 2D fluid-sensitive T2-weighted and intermediate-weighted fast spin-echo (FSE) sequences acquired in three anatomical planes and provide excellent tissue contrast for the diagnosis of internal knee derangement. There are some disadvantages, such as high-resolution formatting, volume averaging artifacts, and increased scan time for multiplanar acquisition.[41-43] Currently, 3D FSE requires longer acquisition times and has no proven diagnostic advantage.[44] For most protocols, 1.5-Tesla scanners provide sufficient image quality.[45]

Weight-bearing MRIs are currently not available for routine clinical use, but is an area of active research and may provide future improvements for the diagnosis of unstable meniscal injuries and may have the potential to elucidate patellofemoral kinematics during painful activities to improve treatment for patellofemoral pain.[46]

CT Arthrography

CT arthrography is widely available and relatively inexpensive, but it is invasive and increases radiation exposure. Iodinated contrast is injected into the knee before a high-resolution CT is performed. It has high sensitivity for detecting meniscal and ligament tears, cartilage loss, subchondral cysts, sclerosis, and osteophyte formation[47] and has been used in routine practice where MRI is less available. With the introduction of patient-specific cutting blocks[48] and patient-specific unicompartmental arthroplasty,[49] routine cartilage imaging may improve patient selection and may at least be equal to quality stress views.[39] Weight-bearing cone beam CT scanners provide advantages, such as shorter acquisition times in natural standing positions, and are relatively portable with low radiation and lower costs compared with systems currently implemented in clinical practice.[50,51]

Summary

It is important to understand basic knee anatomy, as it is the underlying basis of clinical physical examination and imaging. Knee kinematics utilizing modern dynamic motion analysis has provided additional insight into aspects of individual and activity-specific kinematics. Weight-bearing MRIs and CT may be available for future routine clinical use, which may elucidate more information about kinematics to improve surgical interventions.

Key Study Points

- The anterolateral ligament (ALL) is a distinct ligamentous structure of the knee.
- In vivo knee kinematics are an active area of study and may differ based on dynamic knee positioning.
- Advancements in knee imaging include (1) the simplification of routine radiographs by implementing fixed flexion views and (2) the introduction of weight-bearing MRI, which is currently not available for routine clinical use.

Knee

Annotated References

1. Bhosale AM, Richardson JB: Articular cartilage: Structure, injuries and review of management. *Br Med Bull* 2008;87:77-95. doi:10.1093/bmb/ldn025.
2. Sophia Fox AJ, Bedi A, Rodeo SA: The basic science of articular cartilage: Structure, composition, and function. *Sports Health* 2009;1:461-468. doi:10.1177/1941738109350438.
3. Monemdjou R, Fahmi H, Kapoor M: Synovium in the pathophysiology of osteoarthritis. *Therapy* 2010;7:661-668. doi:10.2217/thy.10.72.
4. Smith MD: The normal synovium. *Open Rheumatol J* 2011;5:100-106. doi:10.2174/1874312901105010100.
5. Makris EA, Hadidi P, Athanasiou KA: The knee meniscus: Structure–function, pathophysiology, current repair techniques, and prospects for regeneration. *Biomaterials* 2011;32:7411-7431. doi:10.1016/j.biomaterials.2011.06.037.
6. Flandry F, Hommel G: Normal anatomy and biomechanics of the knee. *Sports Med Arthrosc Rev* 2011;19:82-92. doi:10.1097/JSA.0b013e318210c0aa.
7. De Maeseneer M, Van Roy F, Lenchik L, Barbaix E, De Ridder F, Osteaux M: Three layers of the medial capsular and supporting structures of the knee: MR imaging—anatomic correlation. *Radiographics* 2000;20:S83-S89. doi:10.1148/radiographics.20.suppl_1.g00oc05s83.
8. Claes S, Vereecke E, Maes M, Victor J, Verdonk P, Bellemans J: Anatomy of the anterolateral ligament of the knee. *J Anat* 2013;223:321-328. doi:10.1111/joa.12087.
9. Brockmeyer M, Orth P, Hofer D, et al: The anatomy of the anterolateral structures of the knee—A histologic and macroscopic approach. *Knee* 2019;26:636-646. doi:10.1016/j.knee.2019.02.017 [Epub ahead of print].

The authors performed a dissection of 23 human cadaveric knees and demonstrated the presence of a distinct structure, the anterolateral ligament (ALL), in 100% of specimens. This distinction was demonstrated by gross inspection, as well as histologic compositional differences between the ALL, iliotibial band, and anterolateral knee joint capsule. Level of evidence: II (Descriptive anatomic study).

10. Daggett M, Busch K, Sonnery-Cottet B: Surgical dissection of the anterolateral ligament. *Arthrosc Tech* 2016;5(1):e185-e188.

The authors describe a dissection technique aimed at isolating the anterolateral ligament (ALL). The three major steps described include iliotibial band reflection, followed by posterior capsulectomy and identification of the ALL, and subsequently followed by anterior capsulectomy for full visualization of the ALL. Level of evidence: VI (Description of dissection technique).

11. Parker M, Smith HF: Anatomical variation in the anterolateral ligament of the knee and a new dissection technique for embalmed cadaveric specimens. *Ant Sci Int* 2018;93(2):177-187.

The authors performed dissection of 53 human cadaveric knees, and described a novel dissection technique that can be performed when flexion of the knee is not possible due to stiffness. They describe anatomic variations among specimens, including 30% of specimens with more laterally based tibial insertions, and 7.5% of specimens with more proximal, superior, and lateral origins on the femur. Level of evidence: II (Descriptive anatomic study).

12. DePhilip RM: Atlas of human anatomy, fourth edition, by Frank H. Netter and edited by Jennifer K. Brueckner, et al. *Clin Anat* 2008;21:735-736. doi:10.1002/ca.20682.
13. Leyvraz PF, Rakotomanana L: The anatomy and function of the knee–the quest for the holy grail? *J Bone Joint Surg Br* 2000;82:1093-1094.
14. Hollister AM, Jatana S, Singh AK, Sullivan WW, Lupichuk AG: The axes of rotation of the knee. *Clin Orthop Relat Res* 1993:259-268.
15. Komistek RD, Dennis DA, Mahfouz M: In vivo fluoroscopic analysis of the normal human knee. *Clin Orthop Relat Res* 2003;410:69-81. doi:10.1097/01.blo.0000062384.79828.3b.
16. Moro-oka T-A, Hamai S, Miura H, et al: Dynamic activity dependence of in vivo normal knee kinematics. *J Orthop Res* 2008;26:428-434. doi:10.1002/jor.20488.
17. Tanifuji O, Sato T, Kobayashi K, et al: Three-dimensional in vivo motion analysis of normal knees using single-plane fluoroscopy. *J Orthop Sci* 2011;16:710-718. doi:10.1007/s00776-011-0149-9.
18. Goodfellow J, O'Connor J: The mechanics of the knee and prosthesis design. *J Bone Joint Surg Br* 1978;60-B:358-369.
19. Rajendran K: Mechanism of locking at the knee joint. *J Anat* 1985;143:189-194.
20. Barnett CH: Locking at the knee joint. *J Anat* 1953;87:91-95.
21. Menschik A: Mechanik des Kniegelenkes. *Z Orthop* 1974;112:481-495.
22. Hirschmann MT, Müller W: Complex function of the knee joint: The current understanding of the knee. *Knee Surg Sport Traumatol Arthrosc* 2015;23:2780-2788.
23. Gasparutto X, Moissenet F, Lafon Y, Chèze L, Dumas R: Kinematics of the normal knee during dynamic activities: A synthesis of data from intracortical pins and biplane imaging. *Appl Bionics Biomech* 2017;2017:1908618-1908619. doi:10.1155/2017/1908618.

The authors attempted to synthesize a large of amount of data described in the literature regarding in vivo human knee kinematics. They created their own model based on averages from 17 studies and 126 subjects across all studies. Two main clusters emerged with regard to knee motion and kinematics among the queried studies. The authors propose that their work may serve as a reference for normal in vivo knee kinematics. Level of evidence: IV.

24. Rossi R, Dettoni F, Bruzzone M, Cottino U, D'Elicio DG, Bonasia DE: Clinical examination of the knee: Know your tools for diagnosis of knee injuries. *Sport Med Arthrosc Rehabil Ther Technol* 2011;3:25.
25. Szebenyi B, Dieppe PA, Buckland-Wright JC: Une position radio-anatomique pour la radiographie de profil de l'articulation fémoro-patellaire humaine. *Surg Radiol Anat* 1995;17:79-81. doi:10.1007/BF01629506.
26. Bhatnagar S, Carey-Smith R, Darrah C, Bhatnagar P, Glasgow MM: Evidence-based practice in the utilization of knee radiographs–a survey of all members of the British Orthopaedic Association. *Int Orthop* 2006;30:409-411.
27. Ravaud P, Auleley GR, Chastang C, et al: Knee joint space width measurement: An experimental study of the influence of radiographic procedure and joint positioning. *Rheumatology* 1996;35:761-766. doi:10.1093/rheumatology/35.8.761.
28. Petersson IF, Boegard T, Saxne T, Silman AJ, Svensson B: Radiographic osteoarthritis of the knee classified by the Ahlback and Kellgren & Lawrence systems for the tibiofemoral joint in people aged 35-54 years with chronic knee pain. *Ann Rheum Dis* 1997;56:493-496. doi:10.1136/ard.56.8.493.
29. Kellgren JH, Lawrence JS: Radiological assessment of osteoarthrosis. *Ann Rheum Dis* 1957;16:494-502.
30. Rosenberg TD, Paulos LE, Parker RD, Coward DB, Scott SM: The forty-five-degree posteroanterior flexion weight-bearing radiograph of the knee. *J Bone Joint Surg Am* 1988;70:1479-1483.
31. Peterfy C, Li J, Zaim S, et al: Comparison of fixed-flexion positioning with fluoroscopic semi-flexed positioning for quantifying radiographic joint-space width in the knee: Test-retest reproducibility. *Skeletal Radiol* 2003;32:128-132. doi:10.1007/s00256-002-0603-z.
32. Niinimäki T, Ojala R, Niinimäki J, Leppilahti J: The standing fixed flexion view detects narrowing of the joint space better than the standing extended view in patients with moderate osteoarthritis of the knee. *Acta Orthop* 2010;81:344-346. doi:10.3109/17453674.2010.483989.

33. Buckland-Wright C: Review of the anatomical and radiological differences between fluoroscopic and non-fluoroscopic positioning of osteoarthritic knees. *Osteoarthr Cartil* 2006;14:19-31. doi:10.1016/j.joca.2003.09.012.

34. Kan H, Arai Y, Kobayashi M, et al: Radiographic measurement of joint space width using the fixed flexion view in 1,102 knees of Japanese patients with osteoarthritis in comparison with the standing extended view. *Knee Surg Relat Res* 2017;29:63-68. doi:10.5792/ksrr.16.046.

The authors retrospectively reviewed the radiographs of 567 patients (1,102 knees) who had undergone radiography for knee pain and were diagnosed with knee osteoarthritis by radiograph. All subjects underwent both fixed flexion views (FEV) and standing extended views (SEV). Medial joint space width was statistically signifcantly smaller on FEV than on SEV (3.02 ± 1.55 mm versus 4.31 ± 1.30 mm; $P < 0.001$). Knee osteoarthritis was graded the same or worse on FEV as compared to SEV. Level of evidence: IV (Retrospective cohort study).

35. Conrozier T, Mathieu P, Piperno M, et al: Lyon Schuss radiographic view of the knee. Utility of fluoroscopy for the quality of tibial plateau alignment. *J Rheumatol* 2004;31:584-590.

36. Mazzuca SA, Hellio Le Graverand MP, Vignon E, et al: Performance of a non-fluoroscopically assisted substitute for the Lyon Schuss knee radiograph: Quality and reproducibility of positioning and sensitivity to joint space narrowing in osteoarthritic knees. *Osteoarthr Cartil* 2008;16:1555-1559. doi:10.1016/j.joca.2008.04.010.

37. Kraus VB, Vail TP, Worrell T, McDaniel G: A comparative assessment of alignment angle of the knee by radiographic and physical examination methods. *Arthritis Rheum* 2005;52:1730-1735. doi:10.1002/art.21100.

38. Gibson PH, Goodfellow JW: Stress radiography in degenerative arthritis of the knee. *J Bone Joint Surg Br* 1986;68-B:608-609. doi:10.1302/0301-620X.68B4.3733839.

39. Waldstein W, Monsef JB, Buckup J, Boettner F: The value of valgus stress radiographs in the workup for medial unicompartmental arthritis. *Clin Orthop Relat Res* 2013;471:3998-4003. doi:10.1007/s11999-013-3212-3.

40. Thienpont E, Schwab P-E, Omoumi P: Wear patterns in anteromedial osteoarthritis of the knee evaluated with CT-arthrography. *Knee* 2014;21(suppl 1):S15-S19. doi:10.1016/S0968-0160(14)50004-X.

41. Peterfy C, Woodworth T, Altman R: Workshop for consensus on osteoarthritis imaging. *Osteoarthr Cartil* 2006;14:1. doi:10.1016/j.joca.2006.02.018.

42. Kijowski R, Davis KW, Woods MA, et al: Knee joint: Comprehensive assessment with 3D isotropic resolution fast spin-echo MR imaging–diagnostic performance compared with that of conventional MR imaging at 3.0 T. *Radiology* 2009;252:486-495. doi:10.1148/radiol.2523090028.

43. Kijowski R, Gold GE: Routine 3D magnetic resonance imaging of joints. *J Magn Reson Imaging* 2011;33:758-771. doi:10.1002/jmri.22342.

44. Garwood ER, Recht MP, White LM: Advanced imaging techniques in the knee: Benefits and limitations of new rapid acquisition strategies for routine knee MRI. *Am J Roentgenol* 2017;209:552-560. doi:10.2214/AJR.17.18228.

The authors performed a review of multiple studies concerning conventional and novel MRI sequencing techniques. They reviewed the pros and cons of each approach, which including three-dimensional fast-spin echo protocols, parallel imaging, compressed sensing, simultaneous multislice, and machine-learning techniques. They noted that current standard clinical knee MRI protocols remain closely tied to two- and three-dimensional fast-spin echo techniques. Level of evidence: IV (Review).

45. Hunter DJ, Altman RD, Cicuttini F, et al: OARSI Clinical Trials Recommendations: Knee imaging in clinical trials in osteoarthritis. *Osteoarthr Cartil* 2015;23:698-715. doi:10.1016/j.joca.2015.03.012.

46. Bruno F, Barile A, Arrigoni F, et al: Weight-bearing MRI of the knee: A review of advantages and limits. *Acta Biomed* 2018;89:78-88. doi:10.23750/abm.v89i1-S.7011.

The authors performed a review of multiple studies concerning weight-bearing MRI of the knee. Configurations include standing and sitting MRIs with load applied in either position. While still an active area of research, weight-bearing MRI may help to identify unstable meniscal tears, latent instability, and patellofemoral maltracking. Level of evidence: IV (Review).

47. Omoumi P, Mercier GA, Lecouvet F, Simoni P, Vande Berg BC: CT arthrography, MR arthrography, PET, and scintigraphy in osteoarthritis. *Radiol Clin North Am* 2009;47:595-615. doi:10.1016/j.rcl.2009.04.005.

48. Hafez MA, Chelule KL, Seedhom BB, Sherman KP: Computer-assisted total knee arthroplasty using patient-specific templating. *Clin Orthop Relat Res* 2006;443:184-192.

The authors used CT-based planning and rapid prototyping technology to create distal femoral and proximal tibial cutting templates for 16 cadaveric and 29 plastic knees. Mean error of six random CT showed a mean error for alignment and bone resection within 1.7° and 0.8 mm and concluded that patient specific jigs are a practical alternative to conventional instrumentation. Level of evidence: IV (Cadaveric study).

49. Demange MK, Keudell Von A, Probst C, Yoshioka H, Gomoll AH: Patient-specific implants for lateral unicompartmental knee arthroplasty. *Int Orthop* 2015;39:1519-1526. doi:10.1007/s00264-015-2678-x.

50. Tuominen EKJ, Kankare J, Koskinen SK, Mattila KT: Weight-bearing CT imaging of the lower extremity. *Am J Roentgenol* 2013;200:146-148. doi:10.2214/AJR.12.8481.

51. Ristow O, Steinbach L, Sabo G, et al: Isotropic 3D fast spin-echo imaging versus standard 2D imaging at 3.0 T of the knee–image quality and diagnostic performance. *Eur Radiol* 2009;19:1263-1272. doi:10.1007/s00330-008-1260-y.

Chapter 39

Degenerative Conditions of the Knee

Brian A. Klatt, MD • Michael J. O'Malley, MD

ABSTRACT

Degenerative joint disease of the knee is one of the most common orthopaedic conditions. Various disease processes can lead to degeneration of the knee. All orthopaedic surgeons should have a grasp of the various disease processes, the diagnosis, and the treatment options. Research continues on the pathology and treatment of these diseases. Understanding the American Academy of Orthopaedic Surgeons (AAOS) guidelines and new treatments is critical to providing evidenced-based care.

Keywords: degenerative disease; knee; lupus arthritis; osteoarthritis; post-traumatic arthritis; psoriatic arthritis; rheumatoid arthritis; septic arthritis

Introduction

A recent publication by the Centers for Disease Control and Prevention estimates doctor-diagnosed arthritis affected an estimated 23% of adults (54 million) in the United States from 2013 to 2015.[1] Arthritis limits the activities of 24 million adults, is associated with severe joint pain among 15 million adults, and is projected to affect 78.4 million adults by 2040. In 2013, total national medical care expenditures and earnings losses attributable to arthritis were $303.5 billion.[1] Approximately 16.9 million of US adults (7.9%) reported arthritis-attributable activity limitations in 2003.[2] This was projected to increase to 17.6 million by 2005 and to 25 million (9.3% of the US adult population) by 2030[2] (**Table 1**). Projections are based on increases in the number of patients who will suffer from arthritis because of an aging population and an obesity epidemic.

Arthritis develops when the cartilage of the knee becomes damaged and loses its function through a variety of processes. Traditional classifications have divided knee cartilage disorders into osteoarthritis (OA, noninflammatory) or inflammatory arthritis. Noninflammatory causes discussed in this chapter include osteoarthritis and posttraumatic arthritis. It should be noted that there is an inflammatory component to OA as well. Debate continues as to whether the inflammatory component of OA is part of the progression of the disease or the initiating event. The prototype inflammatory arthritis is rheumatoid arthritis, but there are numerous other types of inflammatory processes that result in arthritis. This chapter will also discuss psoriatic arthritis, lupus arthritis, and septic arthritis.

Understanding of the various types of knee arthritis will enable healthcare providers to properly care for these patients.

Osteoarthritis

Osteoarthritis (OA) is the most common cartilage disorder and continues to be the leading cause of disability and impaired quality of life in developed countries.[3] OA is defined as the progressive loss of cartilage structure and function, and it is also known as degenerative joint disease (DJD). Primary OA is an idiopathic process of cartilage degeneration that occurs with normal use. It involves "wear and tear" of the joint and becomes more prevalent with advancing age. Secondary OA is the development of OA due to an insult or injury that initiates and accelerates the degenerative process of OA. The age of incidence of secondary OA depends on the disease process that initiates cartilage degeneration. It can be the result of infection, traumatic joint injury, osteonecrosis, and a variety of hereditary, developmental, metabolic, and neurological disorders. An extensive list of causes of secondary OA is shown in **Table 2**.

Dr. Klatt or an immediate family member serves as a board member, owner, officer, or committee member of the American Academy of Orthopedic Surgeons, AAOSAAHKS Abstract Review Committee, the American Association of Hip and Knee Surgeons, and MSIS. Neither Dr. O'Malley nor any immediate family member has received anything of value from or has stock or stock options held in a commercial company or institution related directly or indirectly to the subject of this chapter.

Knee

Table 1

Recommendations for Management of RA Drugs at the Time of Knee Replacement Surgery

DMARDs: CONTINUE these medications through surgery.	**Dosing Interval**	**Continue/Withhold**
Methotrexate	Weekly	Continue
Sulfasalazine	Once or twice daily	Continue
Hydroxychloroquine	Once or twice daily	Continue
Leflunomide (Arava)	Daily	Continue
Doxycycline	Daily	Continue
BIOLOGIC AGENTS: STOP these medications before surgery and schedule surgery at the end of the dosing cycle. Resume medications at minimum 14 d after surgery in the absence of wound healing problems, surgical site infection, or systemic infection.	**Dosing Interval**	**Schedule Surgery (relative to last biologic agent dose administered) during**
Adalimumab (Humira)	Weekly or every 2 wk	Week 2 or 3
Etanercept (Enbrel)	Weekly or twice weekly	Week 2
Golimumab (Simponi)	Every 4 wk (SQ) or every 8 wk (IV)	Week 5 or 9
Infliximab (Remicade)	Every 4, 6, or 8 wk	Week 5, 7, or 9
Abatacept (Orencia)	Monthly (IV) or weekly (SQ)	Week 2 or 5
Certolizumab (Cimzia)	Every 2 or 4 wk	Week 3 or 5
Rituximab (Rituxan)	2 doses 2 wk apart every 4-6 mo	Month 7
Tocilizumab (Actemra)	Every week (SQ) or every 4 wk (IV)	Week 2 or 5
Anakinra (Kineret)	Daily	Day 2
Secukinumab (Cosentyx)	Every 4 wk	Week 5
Ustekinumab (Stelara)	Every 12 wk	Week 13
Belimumab (Benlysta)	Every 4 wk	Week 5
Tofacitinib (Xeljanz): Stop this medication 7 d before surgery	Daily or twice daily	7 d after last dose
SEVERE SLE-SPECIFIC MEDICATIONS: CONTINUE these medications in the perioperative period.	**Dosing Interval**	**Continue/Withhold**
Mycophenolate mofetil	Twice daily	Continue
Azathioprine	Daily or twice daily	Continue
Cyclosporine	Twice daily	Continue
Tacrolimus	Twice daily (IV and PO)	Continue
NOT-SEVERE SLE: DISCONTINUE these medications 1 wk before surgery.	**Dosing Interval**	**Continue/Withhold**
Mycophenolate mofetil	Twice daily	Withhold
Azathioprine	Daily or twice daily	Withhold
Cyclosporine	Twice daily	Withhold
Tacrolimus	Twice daily (IV and PO)	Withhold

DMARDs = disease-modifying antirheumatic drugs, IV = intravenous, PO = oral, SLE = systemic lupus erythematosus, SQ = subcutaneous

Reproduced with permission from Goodman SM, Springer B, Guyatt G, et al: 2017 American College of Rheumatology/American Association of Hip and Knee Surgeons guideline for the perioperative management of antirheumatic medication in patients with rheumatic diseases undergoing elective total hip or total knee arthroplasty. *Arthritis Rheumatol* 2017;69(8):1538-1551. © 2017, American College of Rheumatology.

Table 2

Known Causes of Joint Degeneration (Secondary Osteoarthrosis)

Cause	Presumed Mechanism
Intra-articular fracture	Damage to articular cartilage or incongruity of joint or both
High-intensity-impact joint loading	Damage to articular cartilage or subchondral bone or both
Ligament injuries	Instability of the joint
Dysplasia of joint and cartilage (developmental and hereditary)	Abnormal shape of joint or abnormal articular cartilage or both
Aseptic necrosis	Bone necrosis leads to collapse of articular surface and incongruity of joint
Acromegaly	Overgrowth of articular cartilage produces incongruity or joint or abnormal cartilage or both
Paget disease	Distortion or incongruity of joint as a result of bone remodeling
Ehlers-Danlos syndrome	Instability of joint
Gaucher disease (hereditary deficiency of enzyme glucocerebrosidase, leading to accumulation of glucocerebroside)	Bone necrosis or pathological fracture leads to incongruity of joint
Stickler syndrome (progressive, hereditary arthro-ophthalmopathy)	Abnormal development of joint or articular cartilage or both
Infection of joint (inflammation)	Destruction of articular cartilage
Hemophilia	Multiple joint hemorrhages
Hemochromatosis (excess deposition of iron in multiple tissues)	Mechanism unknown
Ochronosis (hereditary deficiency of enzyme homogentisic acid oxidase leading to accumulation of homogentisic acid)	Deposition of homogentisic acid polymers in articular cartilage
Calcium pyrophosphate deposition disease	Accumulation of calcium pyrophosphate crystals in articular cartilage
Neuropathic arthropathy (Charcot joints due to syphilis, diabetes mellitus, syringomyelia, myelomeningocele, leprosy, congenital insensitivity to pain, amyloidosis)	Loss of proprioception and joint sensation results in increased impact loading and torsion, instability of joint, and intra-articular fracture

Reproduced from Buckwalter JA: Mankin HJ: Instructional Course Lectures, The American Academy of Orthopaedic Surgeons - Articular Cartilage. Part II: Degeneration and Osteoarthrosis, Repair, Regeneration, and Transplantation Articular cartilage II: Degeneration and osteoarthrosis, repair, regeneration, and transplantation. *JBJS Am* 1997;79(4):612-632.

Osteoarthritis Disease Progression

Changes to Cartilage

The progressive loss of cartilage is a process that involves three overlapping stages: cartilage matrix damage or alteration, chondrocyte response to tissue damage, and decline of the chondrocyte synthetic response with progressive loss of tissue.

The first phase can result from a mechanical insult, such as a traumatic high energy impact. There is loss of proteoglycan content, and proteoglycans are found in an unaggregated form that is not bound to hyaluronate. This disrupts the matrix macromolecular framework, which makes the extracellular matrix (ECM) more permeable. The water content of the cartilage matrix increases, which decreases matrix stiffness. This softening of the cartilage is clinically identified as chondromalacia. These changes cause the cartilage surface to fray and fibrillate, which increase the vulnerability of the joint to further mechanical insult.[4]

The second phase involves the cellular response of the chondrocytes to mechanical changes. When the chondrocytes recognize tissue damage and changes to the ECM, they release or upregulate mediators that initiate a cellular response. Static and dynamic loading of cartilage results in an increase in the reactive oxygen species nitric oxide (NO), which increases chondrocyte apoptosis and premature senescence. Premature senescence is a pathological process characterized by shortened telomeres, decreased amount of mitochondria adenosine triphosphate (ATP) produced by the mitochondria, and increased β-galactosidase.[5] NO also inhibits collagen and proteoglycan synthesis by inducing production of the cytokines interleukin-1 (IL-1) and tumor necrosis factor-α (TNF-α), which stimulates the production of matrix metalloproteinases (MMPs) that further degrade the matrix macromolecules. As the collagen network degrades, upregulation of molecules such as aggrecan, aggrecanase-2 (ADAMTS-5), c-fos, c-jun, and fibronectin occur, which further weakens the mechanical properties of cartilage by destabilizing the type II collagen fiber network.[6] To combat this cartilage degradation, there is a small repair component associated with the second stage of OA that stimulates chondrocytes to synthesize macromolecules and proliferate. The repair can counteract some of the effects of the inflammatory response, although chondrocytes have minimal capability to reproduce.

The third stage of OA occurs when cartilage is unable to respond to and recover from the mechanical and chemical insult of catabolic factors, including other inflammatory mediators such as IL-6, IL-8, and prostaglandin E2.[7] Age leads to a decline in the anabolic response of chondrocytes, and thus OA is seen more commonly in the elderly.[7]

Changes to Bone

As the cartilage degenerates, there is increased exposure of the subchondral bone. As the pressure of cyclical joint loading impacts the subchondral bone, the subchondral bone increases in density and becomes sclerotic. With the exposed subchondral bone, cysts may form in the bone that can contain myxoid, fibroid, or cartilaginous tissues. Because cartilage tissue does not easily regenerate, the joint may form osteophytes from mesenchymal stem cells from periosteal tissue that are fibrous, bony, and cartilaginous outgrowths.[8] These osteophytes can restrict knee motion and cause contractures, as they can be a source of pain leading to limitations of joint motion.

Changes to Periarticular Tissues

The soft tissues of the joint react to the changes and loss of cartilage. The synovium can become inflamed from the release of inflammatory factors from chondrocytes and release further chemokines and MMPs. Synovium can release collagenase and hydrolytic enzymes to further break down cartilage and stimulate vascular hyperplasia.[9] With chronic OA, the joint capsule and ligaments become tightened and contracted, which decreases range of motion. Muscle can also undergo atrophy with the relative inactivity of the joint from the pain.

Changes to Alignment

It has been shown that abnormal hip-knee-ankle alignment can accelerate structural changes in osteoarthritic knees, as varus malalignment increases medial compartment disease fourfold and valgus malalignment increases lateral compartment disease twofold.[10] Alignment is affected by multiple factors in the joint, including meniscal degeneration or previous menisectomy, incompetent anterior cruciate ligament, osteophytes, and incongruous tibiofemoral contact. Whether malalignment is associated with the development of OA or if malalignment is a result of OA is still a topic of debate. However, it has been demonstrated that malalignment can affect more than cartilage, as malalignment predisposes OA patients to bone marrow lesions.[11] A study by Felson et al demonstrated that greater bone marrow edema was correlated with increased pain with OA.[12]

Diagnosis of Osteoarthritis

OA is classically diagnosed by clinical examination and with plain radiographs. Physical examination of a joint with OA reveals joint pain, loss of motion, crepitance, joint effusion, and deformity. Findings of OA on radiographs include joint-space narrowing, osteophytes, subchondral sclerosis, and bone cysts (**Table 3**). The severity of symptoms does not always correlate well with radiographic findings.

Patients in the early stages of OA usually have minimal signs and symptoms, as there may be soreness and pain after excessive activity that resolves with several days of rest or a short course of anti-inflammatory medication. As the disease progresses, the symptoms can become quite life altering. Joints will be stiff with initial motion, and there will be pain with activities of daily living, such as walking up and down stairs.

Much of the research effort today to treat OA revolves around early diagnosis and treatment. Research has been focused on means to identify early OA, and some experimental techniques may gain clinical use in the evaluation of cartilage. Several new MRI techniques have been used for assessing the biochemical integrity of articular cartilage, including T1Rho, T2 mapping, sodium MRI, and delayed gadolinium-enhanced MRI of cartilage (dGEMRIC).[13] T2 mapping and dGEMRIC have become the most commonly used imaging modalities in the clinical setting. T2 mapping is useful in the evaluation of cartilage after reparative procedures, because it can determine

Table 3

Kellgren Scale of Osteoarthritis

Radiograph	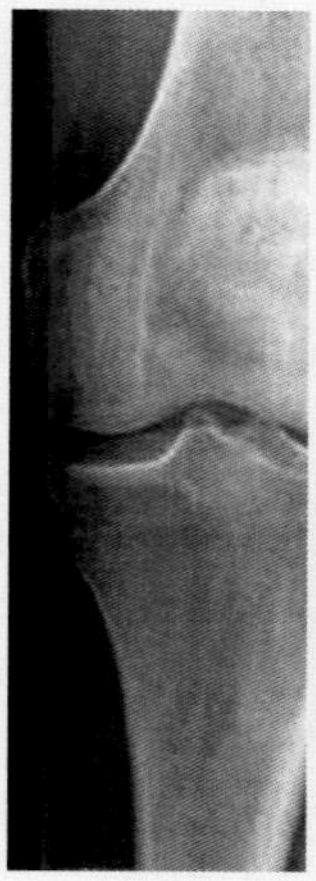	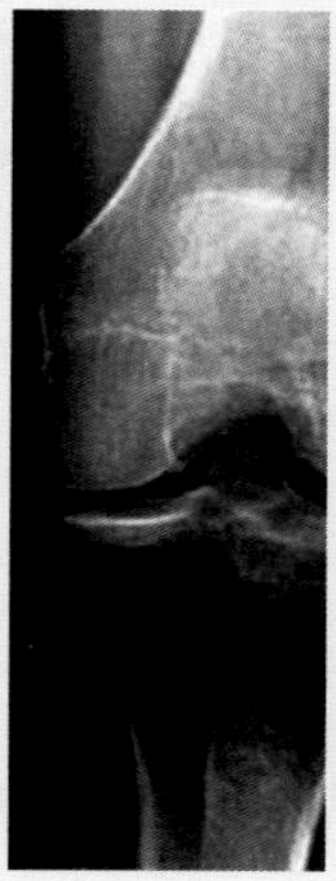	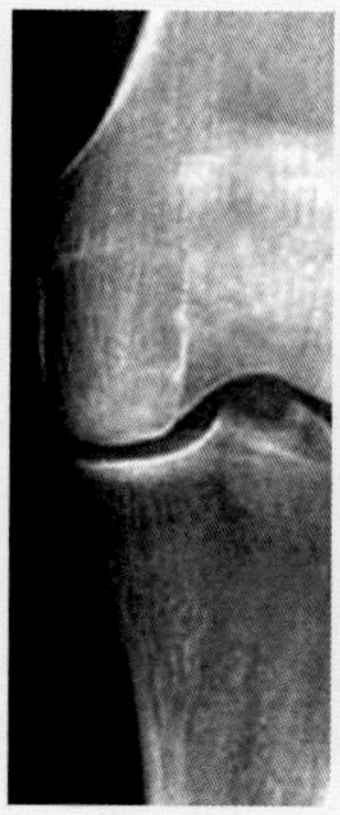	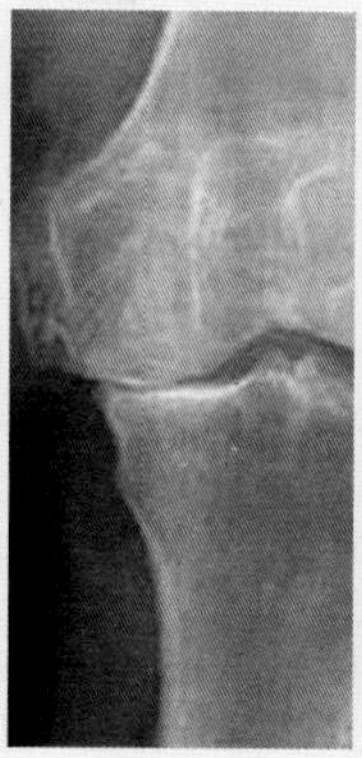	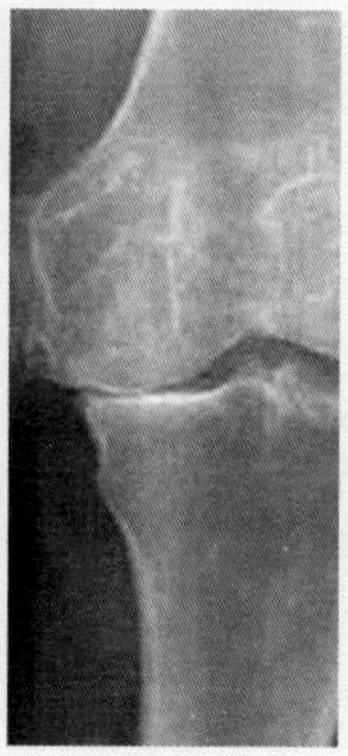
Grade	0	I	II	III	IV
Classification	Normal	Doubtful	Definite	Moderate	Severe
Description	No osteoarthritis	Minimal joint space narrowing and minute osteophytes	Possible mild joint space narrowing and definite osteophytes	Moderate joint space narrowing, moderate multiple osteophytes, some sclerosis	Severe joint space narrowing, large osteophytes, severe sclerosis, deformity of bone contour

Reproduced from Klatt, Chen, Tuan. Arthritis and other cartilage disorders, in Cannada LK, ed: *Orthopaedic Knowledge Update 11*. Rosemont, IL, American Academy of Orthopaedic Surgeons, 2014, pp 207-223.

if the expected normal zonal variations in healthy articular cartilage have been restored. dGEMRIC requires high doses of gadolinium contrast, but has been able to show the glycosaminoglycan (GAG) concentration of cartilage. Owman et al found that changes seen on dGEMRIC correlated well with the development of knee OA in the future.[14] In addition to MRI techniques, optical coherence tomography (OCT) may allow arthroscopic evaluation of cartilage by performing microscopic cross-sectional imaging of articular cartilage.[15,16]

Treatment of Osteoarthritis

The treatment of OA is multifaceted and can be divided into seven main categories: patient education and lifestyle modification, rehabilitation, complementary and alternative therapy, pain relievers, intra-articular injections, needle lavage, and surgical intervention. The literature for categories was evaluated in depth by a workgroup of specialists and was compiled into the clinical practice guidelines for the treatment of knee OA by AAOS.[17] Levels of evidence of studies were evaluated, and recommendations were graded Strong, Moderate, Limited, Inconclusive, and Consensus.

Lifestyle Modification

For early arthritis, symptoms can be treated with patient lifestyle modification, including participation in self-management programs, strengthening, low-impact aerobic exercises, and neuromuscular education. This received a strong recommendation in the AAOS clinical practice guidelines. Additionally, weight loss for patients with symptomatic osteoarthritis of the knee and a BMI ≥25 received a moderate recommendation.

In terms of mechanical intervention, there is inconclusive advice on the use of offloading knee braces (Strength of Recommendation: Inconclusive), and lateral heel wedges are not recommended for treating medial unicompartmental OA (Strength of Recommendation: Moderate).

The AAOS guidelines did not comment on assistive devices or patellar taping. Studies have shown that patellar taping may be beneficial for short-term relief of pain associated with knee OA.[18]

Pharmacological

None of the pharmacological methods of treatment restore or regenerate cartilage. Medications that are used to treat OA patients are aimed at treating symptoms. Acetaminophen is a good pain control medication. Acetaminophen is only an analgesic, and it does not possess any anti-inflammatory effects. AAOS guidelines were unable to recommend for or against the use of acetaminophen, opioids, or pain patches for patients with symptomatic OA of the knee (Strength of Recommendation: Inconclusive). Nonsteroidal anti-inflammatory drugs (NSAIDs) can provide good pain relief for the inflammation from OA. However, the side effects of NSAIDs can make them challenging for treating elderly patients. The gastrointestinal (GI) effects are the most significant, as NSAIDs are associated with the development of ulcers. Although selective cyclooxygenase-2 inhibitors may have less GI and bleeding side effects, they have been associated with increased cardiovascular events. The use of NSAIDs or tramadol is recommended by the AAOS workgroup (Strength of recommendation: Strong). Oral steroid medications are not routinely used to treat OA. Oral glucosamine and oral chondroitin have not demonstrated any effect in restoring cartilage, and the AAOS workgroup strongly recommends against prescribing them (Strength of recommendation: Strong).

Injections of glucocorticoids and hyaluronic acid (HA) are sometimes used to mitigate the symptoms of OA. The AAOS workgroup was unable to recommend for or against the use of intra-articular (IA) corticosteroids for patients with symptomatic OA of the knee (Strength of Recommendation: Inconclusive). The AAOS workgroup did not recommend using hyaluronic acid for patients with symptomatic OA of the knee (Strength of Recommendation: Strong). In theory, the use of viscosupplementation, such as HA, may increase the viscosity of the existing synovial fluid and may reduce the degradation of hyaluronan in synovium and cartilage. However, the use of HA can cause a localized joint reaction, including erythema, effusion, swelling, infection, and pain.[19] The therapeutic benefit of HA injections remains somewhat controversial.[20] In theory, exogenous HA reduces proinflammatory mediators and MMPs, as well as stimulates chondrocytes to synthesize endogenous HA and proteoglycans.[21] However, there is a common misperception among patients that hyaluronic acid injections restore cartilage.

Cartilage Regeneration and Stem Cell Therapy

Biologic solutions through cartilage regeneration may be the future treatment for OA. Research is underway to find the appropriate cell source, the scaffold to support and organize these cells, bioactive factors, and bioreactors to support cartilage growth.

Tissue scaffolds are biomaterials that establish a three-dimensional structure to retain the cells and provide mechanical support to enable cartilage development over time. There are four main groups of scaffolding that may be applied for cartilage tissue engineering: (1) protein-based polymers, (2) carbohydrate-based polymers, (3) synthetic polymers, and (4) composite polymers, that combine biomaterials from the other three categories.[22]

To stimulate cells to grow within scaffolds, bioactive factors are endogenous polypeptide molecules that can be applied to constructs. Transforming growth factor-β (TGF-β) is the most common growth factor used to stimulate chondrogenesis, ECM production, and mesenchymal stem cells.[23] Other members of the TGF superfamily are also responsible for stimulating cartilage repair, including TGF-β1, bone morphogenetic (BMP)-2, and BMP-7, TGF-β3, and cartilage-derived morphogenetic proteins (CDMP-1 and CDMP-2). TGF-β or BMP-7 can be used with insulin growth factor-1 (IGF-1) to stimulate anabolic cartilage pathways and decrease catabolic pathways. Fibroblast growth factors (FGFs), specifically FGF-2 and FGF-18, bind to cell surface receptors to promote anabolic pathways and downregulate aggrecanase. Platelet-derived growth factor (PDGF) attracts mesenchymal stem cells and can stimulate proteoglycan production and chondrocyte proliferation. Platelet-rich plasma (PRP) contains growth factors that may serve as an adjunct to treating OA, but very few studies have been conducted to make any meaningful conclusions in OA patients.[24]

Gene Therapy

The use of gene therapy was first proposed to treat rheumatoid arthritis.[25] For OA, five gene therapeutic targets that enhance chondrogenesis have been extensively studied: (1) growth factors—including TGF-β, BMP, FGF, IGF-1β, and epidermal growth factor (EGF); (2) transcription factors—SOX9; (3) signal transduction molecules—SMADS; (4) proinflammatory cytokine inhibition—TNF-α and IL-1; and (5) apoptosis or senescence inhibition—Bcl-2, Bcl-XL, and inducible nitric oxide synthase (iNOS).[26] TNF- β1 has been studied in a phase II clinical trial examining the efficacy of a cell-mediated gene therapy system, TissueGene-C (TG-C, TissueGene Inc.), that contains allogeneic chondrocytes that express TGF-β1.[27] The safety of this product was established, and further studies seek to determine the usefulness of the product in the treatment of OA.

There are multiple vectors that can be used to deliver genes, and they are divided into viral and nonviral vectors. Nonviral vectors include plasmids, liposomes, naked DNA, and complexed DNA. Unfortunately, these vectors are transient, but they are noninfectious. Viral vectors, such as adenovirus, adeno-associated virus, lentivirus, herpes simplex virus, and foamy virus, deliver the genes directly into DNA and provide stable gene expression. However, host DNA is altered, the host can react to the infectious proteins, and there can be insertional mutagenesis.

Posttraumatic Arthritis

Introduction

The pathophysiology of posttraumatic osteoarthritis (PTOA) is similar to that of degenerative OA; however, it develops following a precipitating joint trauma such as articular fracture, ligament injury, articular cartilage, or meniscus injury. The common end result is articular cartilage degeneration that results in pain, stiffness, joint destruction, and disability. The articular cartilage damage can occur from the injury itself or overtime due to residual joint malalignment, incongruity, or instability.[28]

Incidence

Accurate total population incidence is difficult to assess; however, it is estimated that PTOA accounts for 12% of the overall prevalence of symptomatic arthritis, corresponding to 5.6 million individuals in the United States.[28] PTOA affects patients at a younger age, developing an estimated 10 years earlier than degenerative OA of the knee.

Risk Factors

ACL injuries are very common with 80,000 to 250,000 injuries per year in the United States alone.[29] The annual incidence of reconstruction in 50,000 to 105,000 per year.[29] History of ACL injury is a well-recognized cause of PTOA with several studies showing >40% incidence of PTOA 5 to 15 years after injury.[30] Additionally, patients who have a concomitant meniscus tear at the time of injury are at further increased risk for the development of PTOA.[31] There is debate in the literature regarding the effectiveness of ACL reconstruction to decrease the risk of PTOA.[31] Although the precise contribution of these factors to the development of PTOA is unknown, accumulating evidence suggests that the cartilage damage at the time of injury rather than persistent joint instability is the incipient cause of eventual joint degeneration. As support of this theory, there is little difference in the development of PTOA in patients who have undergone ACL reconstruction and those treated conservatively.[32]

It has been suggested that meniscus injuries predispose patients to subsequent PTOA. The meniscus is an important structure that provides knee stability, shock absorption, and force distribution across the knee joint.[33] Meniscus injury or dysfunction results in altered joint loading, which is postulated to result in articular cartilage injury and early joint degeneration.[16] Meniscus injury is a risk factor for the development of OA.[34] The results published by Badlani et al in the OA initiative noted that patients with meniscus extrusion and radial tears were more likely to develop radiographic signs of OA.[34] Menisectomy, partial or total, was a common treatment for symptomatic meniscus tears. 48% of patients developed advanced radiographic changes (Kellgren Lawrence ≥ 2) 21 years following total menisectomy. Total menisectomy has been calculated to increase the contact stress in the joint by 235%.[33]

Intra-articular fractures are a known cause of PTOA, as 44% of intra-articular fractures of the knee will progress to PTOA 7.5 years after injury.[35] Intra-articular distal femur and tibial plateau fractures are rare in comparison to ligament injuries of the knee; however, their damage can be catastrophic. Intra-articular fractures often create articular step-offs or gaps at the articular surface. There is debate as to whether or not anatomic restoration of the joint surface reduces the risk of PTOA formation. Animal studies have demonstrated that anatomic restoration of articular fragments with compression can result in hyaline-like repair tissue.[36] However, there is little support in the literature for the assertion that anatomic restoration of the articular surface (≤2 mm) results in a clinical outcome benefit.[37,38]

Pathophysiology

Damage to the articular cartilage can occur without visible disruptions of the surface, such as following ACL disruption or a traumatic meniscus tear.[39] Abnormal joint loading during trauma can result in disruptions of the ECM. Chondrocytes are not able to restore the ECM, leaving them vulnerable to excessive force leading to eventual cell death and further cartilage degeneration.[39]

In articular fractures, the subchondral bone is violated, which permits blood to enter the defect and bring inflammatory cells that quickly form a hematoma. The hematoma is remodeled into a fibrin clot. The platelets within the clot release inflammatory cytokines and growth factors, including TGF-β, BMPs, PDGF, and insulinlike growth factor (IGF) that further influence repair cell functions. Mesenchymal stem cells infiltrate and synthesize a collagen matrix and proteoglycans. Early repair cartilage is mainly composed of type-II hyaline and type-I fibrocartilage; however, after several weeks to months, the tissue is remodeled and is mainly composed of mechanically inferior type-I fibrocartilage and fibroblast-like cells.[40]

Treatment

PTOA is a burden on society as it often affects younger individuals.[28] As with OA, nonoperative treatment options available include nonsteroidal anti-inflammatories, maintenance of a healthy body weight, activity modifications, and low-impact exercise. Ultimately, surgery may be recommended if the degeneration progresses and symptoms of arthritis become recalcitrant to nonoperative means. Existing surgical options for PTOA include fusion and arthroplasty. Fusion is less common, as surgeons have become more confident in newer implant technology lasting for younger patients.

When compared with patients with OA, total knee arthroplasty (TKA) for PTOA is often more complex and are at increased risk for complication following TKA.[41] Surgeons may need to contend with severe deformity, hardware, and bone stock deficiencies. A systematic review concluded that patients undergoing TKA for PTOA is an effective treatment as it improves function, alleviates pain and improves range of motion; however, there was increased complication risk including infection, stiffness, wound complications, and ligament damage.[42]

A potential novel treatment avenue is to protect the cartilage from further damage at the time of injury to limit downstream affects. Common targets for gene therapy are the inflammatory cytokines, particularly IL-1, and growth factors IGF-1 and TGF-B1. The ability to intervene early in the disease process requires identification of the factors associated with articular cartilage injury and arthritis progression.[25]

Inflammatory Arthritis

Inflammatory arthritis is a large collection of different diseases that cause inflammation in the joints. The diagnosis requires a complete review of the disease process profile. There are no simple clinical tests that can be used to diagnose these diseases, thus the rheumatologic history and physical examination plays a critical role in diagnosis and treatment. The location of the problems and symmetry of presentation are important disease features. For example, rheumatoid arthritis (RA) has a predilection for the wrists and the proximal joints of the hands and feet, whereas psoriatic arthritis involves the distal interphalangeal joint of the hands. The physical findings with RA tend to be symmetrical, but other inflammatory arthritis conditions are not. Onset and chronology of the disease are important features, as well. The onset of RA tends to present in a subacute manner, whereas septic arthritis has a rapid onset in several hours. Age, gender, and precipitating factors can also aid in diagnosis. The medical treatment of all of these diseases should involve the interdisciplinary care of rheumatologists and infectious disease specialists.

Rheumatoid Arthritis

Rheumatoid arthritis is the most common inflammatory arthritis. The incidence of RA in the United States is 25 per 100,000 for men and 54 per 100,000 for women. The definitive cause of this disease has not been determined, but the most common theory is that it is an autoimmune disease that can be stimulated in genetically susceptible individuals. Environmental antigens, such as smoking or periodontal disease, have been postulated as potential initiators of the autoimmune response.[43]

Rheumatoid factor (RF), a set of self-reactive anti-immunoglobulin (IgM) antibodies and autoantibodies against citrullinated peptides (ACPAs), are the characteristic antibodies in blood that are detected in 80% of those suffering with RA.[44] These patients are described as having seropositive RA. Joint destruction in RA begins with leukocyte infiltration of the synovium resulting from immune activation.[45] This then activates transcription pathways NF-κB, signal transducers and activators of transcription (STATs), and mitogen-activated protein kinases (MAPKs), which enable the upregulation of cytokines, such as TNF-α, IL-1, IL-6, and IL-17. In response to this cytokine release, multiple destructive enzymes, including MMPs (eg, collagenase and gelatinase), cathepsins, and serine proteases (eg, trypsin), act to destroy cartilage. Bone destruction is also activated by the same cytokines (TNF-α, IL-1, and IL-17) that upregulate receptor activator of NF-κB ligand (RANKL). With increased expression of RANKL on T cells and fibroblast-like cells, more osteoclasts are activated, which lead to bony erosions. This inflammation and invasion of the synovial pannus into articular cartilage and bone leads to the destruction of joints and causes pain and deformity.[46]

2. Hootman JM, Helmick CG: Projections of US prevalence of arthritis and associated activity limitations. *Arthritis Rheum* 2006;54(1):226-229. doi:10.1002/art.21562.
3. Centers for Disease Control and Prevention (CDC): Prevealence of disabilities and associated health conditions among adults. *MMMWR Morb Mortal Wkly Rep* 2001;50(7):120-125.
4. Uccioli L, Sinistro A, Almerighi C, et al: Proinflammatory modulation of the surface and cytokine phenotype of monocytes in patients with acute Charcot foot. *Diabetes Care* 2010;33(2):350-355. doi:10.2337/dc09-1141.
5. Witzke KA, Vinik AI, Grant LM, et al: Loss of RAGE defense: A cause of Charcot neuroarthropathy? *Diabetes Care* 2011;34(7):1617-1621. doi:10.2337/dc10-2315.
6. Lee JH, Fitzgerald JB, DiMicco MA, Grodzinsky AJ: Mechanical injury of cartilage explants causes specific time-dependent changes in chondrocyte gene expression. *Arthritis Rheum* 2005;52(8):2386-2395. doi:10.1002/art.21215.
7. Buckwalter JA, Mankin HJ, Grodzinsky AJ: Articular cartilage and osteoarthritis, in Einhorn T, Buckwalter JA, eds: *Orthopaedic Basic Science*, ed 3. Rosemont, IL, American Academy of Orthopaedic Surgeons, 2007, pp 161-174.
8. van der Kraan PM, van den Berg WB: Osteophytes: Relevance and biology. *Osteoarthr Cartil* 2007;15(3):237-244. doi:10.1016/j.joca.2006.11.006.
9. Krasnokutsky S, Attur M, Palmer G, Samuels J, Abramson SB: Current concepts in the pathogenesis of osteoarthritis. *Osteoarthr Cartil* 2008;16 suppl 3:S1-S3. doi:10.1016/j.joca.2008.06.025.
10. Cerejo R, Dunlop DD, Cahue S, Channin D, Song J, Sharma L: The influence of alignment on risk of knee osteoarthritis progression according to baseline stage of disease. *Arthritis Rheum* 2002;46(10):2632-2636. doi:10.1002/art.10530.
11. Hunter DJ, Zhang Y, Niu J, et al: Increase in bone marrow lesions associated with cartilage loss: A longitudinal magnetic resonance imaging study of knee osteoarthritis. *Arthritis Rheum* 2006;54(5):1529-1535. doi:10.1002/art.21789.
12. Felson DT, McLaughlin S, Goggins J, et al: Bone marrow edema and its relation to progression of knee osteoarthritis. *Ann Intern Med* 2003;139(5 pt 1):330-336. doi:10.7326/0003-4819-139-5_Part_1-200309020-00008.
13. Jazrawi LM, Alaia MJ, Chang G, Fitzgerald EF, Recht MP: Advances in magnetic resonance imaging of articular cartilage. *J Am Acad Orthop Surg* 2011;19(7):420-429. doi:10.1007/s003300100911.
14. Owman H, Tiderius CJ, Neuman P, Nyquist F, Dahlberg LE: Association between findings on delayed gadolinium-enhanced magnetic resonance imaging of cartilage and future knee osteoarthritis. *Arthritis Rheum* 2008;58(6):1727-1730. doi:10.1002/art.23459.
15. Chu CR: Arthroscopic microscopy of articular cartilage using optical coherence tomography. *Am J Sports Med* 2004;32(3):699-709. doi:10.1177/0363546503261736.
16. Chu CR, Williams A, Tolliver D, Kwoh CK, Bruno S, Irrgang JJ: Clinical optical coherence tomography of early articular cartilage degeneration in patients with degenerative meniscal tears. *Arthritis Rheum* 2010;62(5):1412-1420. doi:10.1002/art.27378.
17. Jevsevar DS, Brown GA, Jones DL, et al: The American Academy of Orthopaedic Surgeons evidence-based guideline on: Treatment of osteoarthritis of the knee, 2nd edition. *J Bone Joint Surg Am* 2013;95(20):1885-1886. doi:10.1016/S0021-9355(13)73858-X.
18. Hochberg MC, Altman RD, April KT, et al: American College of Rheumatology 2012 recommendations for the use of nonpharmacologic and pharmacologic therapies in osteoarthritis of the hand, hip, and knee. *Arthritis Care Res* 2012;64(4):465-474. doi:10.1002/acr.21596.
19. Webber TA, Webber AE, Matzkin E: Rate of adverse reactions to more than 1 series of viscosupplementation. *Orthopedics* 2012;35(4):e514-e519. doi:10.3928/01477447-20120327-26.
20. Lo GH, LaValley M, McAlindon T, Felson DT. Intra-articular hyaluronic acid in treatment of knee osteoarthritis: A meta-analysis. *J Am Med Assoc* 2003;290(23):3115-3121.
21. Moreland LW: Intra-articular hyaluronan (hyaluronic acid) and hylans for the treatment of osteoarthritis: Mechanisms of action. *Arthritis Res Ther* 2003;5(2):54-67. doi:10.1186/ar623.
22. Safran MR, Kim H, Zaffagnini S: The use of scaffolds in the management of articular cartilage injury. *J Am Acad Orthop Surg* 2008;16(6):306-311. doi:10.5435/00124635-200806000-00002.
23. Fortier LA, Barker JU, Strauss EJ, McCarrel TM, Cole BJ: The role of growth factors in cartilage repair. *Clin Orthop Relat Res* 2011;469(10):2706-2715. doi:10.1007/s11999-011-1857-3.
24. Levy DM, Petersen KA, Scalley Vaught M, Christian DR, Cole BJ: Injections for knee osteoarthritis: Corticosteroids, viscosupplementation, platelet-rich plasma, and autologous stem cells. *Arthroscopy* 2018;34(5):1730-1743. doi:10.1016/j.arthro.2018.02.022.

    This is a review article discussing the benefits of corticosteroid, viscosupplementation, platelet-rich plasma, and autologous mesenchymal stem cell injections for the treatment of patients with knee osteoarthritis. Level of evidence: V.
25. Evans C: Gene transfer to human joints: Progress toward a gene therapy of arthritis. *Proc Natl Acad Sci* 2005;102(24):8698-8703.
26. Evans CH, Gouze JN, Gouze E, Robbins PD, Ghivizzani SC: Osteoarthritis gene therapy. *Gene Ther* 2004;11(4):379-389. doi:10.1038/sj.gt.3302196.
27. Lee B, Parvizi J, Bramlet D, et al: Results of a phase II study to determine the efficacy and safety of genetically engineered allogeneic human chondrocytes expressing TGF-β1. *J Knee Surg* 2019. doi:10.1055/s-0038-1676803. [Epub ahead of print].

Phase II study evaluating 24-months results of treated Kellgren-Lawrence (K-L) grade III osteoarthritis with genetically engineered chondrocytes virally transduced with a transforming growth factor (TGF)-β1 expression vector TissueGene_C (TG-C). 102 patients were randomized (2:1) to treatment or placebo. Patients who received TG-C had significant improvements in International Knee Documentation Committee (IKDC) and VAS scores. Level of evidence: I.

28. Brown T, Johnston R, Saltzman C, Marsh JL: Posttraumatic osteoarthritis a first estimate of incidence. *J Orthop Trauma* 2006;20(10):739-744.

29. Griffin LY, Albohm MJ, Arendt EA, et al: Understanding and preventing noncontact anterior cruciate ligament injuries: A review of the Hunt Valley II Meeting, January 2005. *Am J Sports Med* 2006;34(9):1512-1532. doi:10.1177/0363546506286866.

30. Lohmander LS, Östenberg A, Englund M, Roos H: High prevalence of knee osteoarthritis, pain, and functional limitations in female soccer players twelve years after anterior cruciate ligament injury. *Arthritis Rheum* 2004;50(10):3145-3152. doi:10.1002/art.20589.

31. Risberg MA, Oiestad BE, Gunderson R, et al: Changes in knee osteoarthritis, symptoms, and function after anterior cruciate ligament reconstruction. *Am J Sports Med* 2016;44(5): 1215-1224. doi:10.1177/0363546515626539.

The purpose of this study was to evaluate the development of both radiographic and symptomatic knee OA in patients with isolated and combined (ACL/meniscus) injuries to the ACL 15 to 20 years after ACL reconstruction. This is a prospective cohort study. The reported prevalence of radiographic knee OA was 42% in tibiofemoral (TF) joint and 21% in patellofemoral (PF) joint. Additionally 25% of those with TF OA and 14% of patients with PF OA were symptomatic. Patients with combined injuries had more significant progression and symptoms than those with isolated injuries. Level of evidence: II.

32. Luc B, Gribble PA, Pietrosimone BG: Osteoarthritis prevalence following anterior cruciate ligament reconstruction: A systematic review and numbers-needed-to-treat analysis. *J Athl Train* 2014;49(6):806-819. doi:10.4085/1062-6050-49.3.35.

33. Baratz ME, Fu FH, Mengato R: Meniscal tears: The effect of meniscectomy and of repair on intraarticular contact areas and stress in the human knee. A preliminary report. *Am J Sports Med* 1986;14(4):270-275. doi:10.1177/036354658601400405.

34. Badlani JT, Borrero C, Golla S, Harner CD, Irrgang JJ: The effects of meniscus injury on the development of knee osteoarthritis: Data from the osteoarthritis initiative. *Am J Sports Med* 2013;41(6):1238-1244. doi:10.1177/0363546513490276.

35. Honkonen S: Degenerative arthritis after tibial plateau fractures. *J Orthop Trauma* 1995;9(4):273-277. doi:10.1097/00005131-199509040-00001.

36. Mitchell N, Shepard N: Healing of articular cartilage in intra-articular fractures in rabbits. *J Bone Joint Surg Am* 1980;62(4):628-634. doi:10.2106/00004623-198062040-00018.

37. Buckwalter JA, Brown TD: Joint injury, repair, and remodeling. *Clin Orthop Relat Res* 2004;423(423):7-16. doi:10.1097/01.blo.0000131638.81519.de.

38. Rasmussen PS: Tibial condylar fractures. Impairment of knee joint stability as an indication for surgical treatment. *J Bone Joint Surg Am* 1973;55(7):1331-1350. doi:10.2106/00004623-197355070-00001.

39. Bear DM, Szczodry M, Kramer S, Coyle CH, Smolinski P, Chu CR: Optical coherence tomography (OCT) detection of subclinical traumatic cartilage injury. *J Orthop Trauma* 2011;24(9):577-582. doi:10.1097/BOT.0b013e3181f17a3b. Optical.

40. Uccioli L, Sinistro A, Almerighi C, et al: Proinflammatory modulation of the surface and cytokine phenotype of monocytes in patients with acute Charcot foot. *Diabetes Care* 2010;33(2):350-355. doi:10.2337/dc09-1141.

41. Weiss NG, Parvizi J, Hanssen AD, Trousdale RT, Lewallen DG: Total knee arthroplasty in post-traumatic arthrosis of the knee. *J Arthroplasty* 2003;18(3 suppl 1):23-26. doi:10.1054/arth.2003.50068.

42. Saleh H, Yu S, Vigdorchik J, Schwarzkopf R: Total knee arthroplasty for treatment of post-traumatic arthritis: Systematic review. *World J Orthop* 2016;7(9):584-591. doi:10.5312/wjo.v7.i9.584.

Systematic review to report the functional outcomes, complications, and survivorship following TKA in patients with post-traumatic OA. Authors reported that knee ROM and outcome studies improved in PTOA patients. However, complication rates were significantly higher in PTOA patients. Most frequent complications reported include, infection, stiffness, wound complications, instability, and loosening. Level of evidence: IV.

43. Silman AJ, Newman J, MacGregor AJ: Cigarette smoking increases the risk of rheumatoid arthritis: Results from a nationwide study of disease-discordant twins. *Arthritis Rheum* 1996;39(5):732-735. doi:10.1002/art.1780390504.

44. Barra L, Pope J, Bessette L, Haraoui B, Bykerk V: Lack of seroconversion of rheumatoid factor and anti-cyclic citrullinated peptide in patients with early inflammatory arthritis: A systematic literature review. *Rheumatology* 2011;50(2): 311-316. doi:10.1093/rheumatology/keq190.

45. Smolen JS, Aletaha D, McInnes IB: Rheumatoid arthritis. *Lancet* 2016;388:2023-2038. doi:10.1016/S0140-6736(16)30173-8.

Comprehensive review of rheumatoid arthritis that describes the current research on genetics, etiology, pathophysiology, and treatment of patients with RA. Level of evidence: V.

46. Rutherford A, Nikiphorou E, Galloway J: Rheumatoid arthritis. *Comorbidity Rheum Dis* 2017;388(10055):53-79. doi:10.1007/978-3-319-59963-2_3.

47. Cohen SB, Moreland LW, Cush JJ, et al: A multicentre, double blind, randomised, placebo controlled trial of anakinra (Kineret), a recombinant interleukin 1 receptor antagonist, in patients with rheumatoid arthritis treated with background methotrexate. *Ann Rheum Dis* 2004;63(9):1062-1068. doi:10.1136/ard.2003.016014.

48. Bresnihan B, Newmark R, Robbins S, Genant HK: Effects of anakinra monotherapy on joint damage in patients with rheumatoid arthritis. Extension of a 24-Week randomized, placebo-controlled trial. *J Rheumatol* 2004;31(6):1103-1111.

49. Klippel J: *Primer on the Rheumatic Diseases*. New York, NY, Springer, 2008.

50. Goodman SM, Springer B, Guyatt G, et al: 2017 American College of Rheumatology/American Association of Hip and Knee Surgeons guideline for the perioperative management of antirheumatic medication in patients with rheumatic diseases undergoing elective total hip or total knee arthroplasty. *J Arthroplasty* 2017;32(9):2628-2638. doi:10.1016/j.arth.2017.05.001.

The collaboration between the American College of Rheumatology and the American Association of Hip and Knee Surgeons developed an evidence-based guideline for the perioperative management of antirheumatic drug therapy. Level of evidence: V.

51. Taylor W, Gladman D, Helliwell P, Marchesoni A, Mease P, Mielants H: Classification criteria for psoriatic arthritis: Development of new criteria from a large international study. *Arthritis Rheum* 2006;54(8):2665-2673. doi:10.1002/art.21972.

52. Ogdie A, Weiss P: The epidemiology of psoriatic arthritis. *Rheum Dis Clin North Am* 2015;41(4):545-568. doi:10.1016/j.rdc.2015.07.001.

53. de Vlam K, Gottlieb AB, Mease PJ: Current concepts in psoriatic arthritis: Pathogenesis and management. *Acta Derm Venereol* 2014;94(6):627-634. doi:10.2340/00015555-1833.

54. Cancienne JM, Werner BC, Browne JA: Complications of primary total knee arthroplasty among patients with rheumatoid arthritis, psoriatic arthritis, ankylosing spondylitis, and osteoarthritis. *J Am Acad Orthop Surg* 2016;24(8):567-574. doi:10.5435/JAAOS-D-15-00501.

Case-control study using a national database to evaluate 90-day postoperative complication rates, readmission rates, and revision rates after TKA in patients with inflammatory arthritis. Authors found increased perioperative complication rates, revision rates, and 90-day readmission rates after primary TKA. Level of evidence: III.

55. Yu C, Gershwin ME, Chang C: Diagnostic criteria for systemic lupus erythematosus: A critical review. *J Autoimmun* 2014;48-49:10-13. doi:10.1016/j.jaut.2014.01.004.

56. Mukherjee S, Culliford D, Arden N, Edwards C: What is the risk of having a total hip or knee replacement for patients with lupus? *Lupus* 2015;24(2):198-202. doi:10.1177/0961203314547894.

57. Domsic RT, Lingala B, Krishnan E: Systemic lupus erythematosus, rheumatoid arthritis, and postarthroplasty mortality: A cross-sectional analysis from the nationwide inpatient sample. *J Rheumatol* 2010;37(7):1467-1472. doi:10.3899/jrheum.091371.

58. Fein AW, Figgie CA, Dodds TR, et al: Systemic lupus erythematosus does not increase risk of adverse events in the first 6 months after total knee arthroplasty. *J Clin Rheumatol* 2016;22(7):355-359. doi:10.1097/RHU.0000000000000435.

Case-control study performed at a single institution comparing postoperative complications following TKA in SLE patients and those in osteoarthritis patients. The authors found no difference in postoperative adverse events between groups. Level of evidence: III.

59. Brennan MB, Hsu JL: Septic arthritis in the native joint. *Curr Infect Dis Rep* 2012;14(5):558-565. doi:10.1007/s11908-012-0285-1.

60. Kennedy N, Chambers ST, Nolan I, et al: Native joint septic arthritis: Epidemiology, clinical features, and microbiological causes in a New Zealand population. *J Rheumatol* 2015;42(12):2392-2397. doi:10.3899/jrheum.150434.

61. Fitzgerald RH. Infected total hip arthroplasty: Diagnosis and treatment. *J Am Acad Orthop Surg* 1995;3(5):249-262. http://www.ncbi.nlm.nih.gov/pubmed/10795031.

62. Shirtliff ME, Mader JT: Acute septic arthritis. *Clin Microbiol Rev* 2002;15(4):527-544. doi:10.1128/CMR.15.4.527-544.2002.

63. Sultan AA, Mahmood B, Samuel LT, et al: Patients with a history of treated septic arthritis are at high risk of periprosthetic joint infection after total joint arthroplasty. *Clin Orthop Relat Res* 2019;477(7):1605-1612. doi:10.1097/corr.0000000000000688.

This is retrospective multicenter study investigating the risk of PJI in patients with previously treated same-joint native arthritis, and identification of potential risk factors. The authors reported an 8% risk of PJI in this patient population. Total knee arthroplasty appeared more susceptible than hips. The authors found smoking (HR, 8.06; 95% CI, 1.33 to 48.67; $P = 0.023$) to be associated with increased risk for PJI. Level of evidence: IV.

64. Puius YA, Kalish RA: Lyme arthritis: Pathogenesis, clinical presentation, and management. *Infect Dis Clin North Am* 2008;22(2):289-300. doi:10.1016/j.idc.2007.12.014.

65. Baldwin KD, Brusalis CM, Nduaguba AM, Sankar WN: Predictive factors for differentiating between septic arthritis and lyme disease of the knee in children. *J Bone Joint Surg Am* 2016;98(9):721-728. doi:10.2106/JBJS.14.01331.

The objective of this study was to identify predictors to differentiate septic arthritis from Lyme arthritis. A retrospective review of patients younger than 18 years who underwent aspiration of effusions at a single institution between 2005 and 2013 was performed. Historical, clinical, and laboratory data were compared and reported between groups to identify independent predictive variables. Level of evidence: III.

66. McCutchan HJ, Fisher RC: Synovial leukocytosis in infectious arthritis. *Clin Orthop Relat Res* 1990 (257): 226-230.

67. Bovonratwet P, Nelson SJ, Bellamkonda K, et al: Similar 30-day complications for septic knee arthritis treated with arthrotomy or arthroscopy: An American College of surgeons national surgical quality improvement program analysis. *Arthroscopy* 2018;34(1):213-219. doi:10.1016/j.arthro.2017.06.046.

Knee

Retrospective study using the American College of Surgeons National Surgical Quality Improvement Program (NSQIP) to evaluate differences in 30-day perioperative complications between open arthrotomy and arthroscopy for the treatment of septic knees. Two groups, 168 patients undergoing knee arthrotomy and 216 patients undergoing knee arthroscopy for septic knee were identified. In conclusion no difference in perioperative complications, rate of return to the operating room, and rate of readmission were found after open and arthroscopic debridement for septic knees. Level of evidence: III.

68. Wormser GP, Dattwyler RJ, Shapiro ED, et al: The clinical assessment, treatment, and prevention of lyme disease, human granulocytic anaplasmosis, and babesiosis: Clinical practice guidelines by the infectious diseases society of America. *Clin Infect Dis* 2006;43(9):1089-1134. doi:10.1086/508667.

Chapter 40

Soft-Tissue Injuries About the Knee

Carola F. van Eck, MD, PhD • Freddie H. Fu, MD, DSc (Hon), DPs (Hon)

ABSTRACT

Soft-tissue injuries about the knee are common and are frequently the results of sports participation. These injuries can include the menisci, cruciates, collateral ligament as well as the patellar and quadriceps tendon. This chapter outlines these different injuries and their corresponding anatomy, history, physical examination, imaging studies, and treatment options.

Keywords: ACL; LCL; MCL; meniscus; patellar tendon; PCL; PLC; quadriceps tendon

Introduction

Soft-tissue injuries about the knee are common in the athletic population. Anatomic structures involved in these injuries include the medial and lateral meniscus, the anterior and posterior cruciates (ACL and PCL), lateral collateral ligament (LCL), posterolateral corner (PLC), medial collateral ligament (MCL), and quadriceps and patellar tendon. In this chapter, the anatomy and the types of injuries involving these structures are described, along with associated history and physical examination findings. Appropriate imaging studies that should be ordered and their corresponding findings are explained. Lastly, conservative and surgical treatment options are discussed.

Dr. Fu or an immediate family member serves as a paid consultant to or is an employee of Medicrea - son Gordon; serves as an unpaid consultant to Smith & Nephew; and serves as a board member, owner, officer, or committee member of the American Orthopaedic Society for Sports Medicine, the International Society of Arthroscopy, Knee Surgery, and Orthopaedic Sports Medicine, and the World Endoscopy Doctors Association. Neither Dr. van Eck nor any immediate family member has received anything of value from or has stock or stock options held in a commercial company or institution related directly or indirectly to the subject of this chapter.

Meniscus

Anatomy

The menisci are composed of fibroelastic cartilage, consisting of an interlacing network of mostly type I collagen, proteoglycans, glycoproteins, and cellular elements. They contain 65% to 75% water. There are longitudinally and radially oriented fibers, which help the meniscus to expand under compressive forces and increase the contact area of the joint.[1] The meniscus is C-shaped with a triangular cross section. The average width of the medial meniscus is 9 to 10 mm, and average thickness is 3 to 5 mm. The lateral meniscus is more circular with a smaller distance between the anterior and posterior horns and covers a larger portion of the articular surface of the tibial plateau. Its average width is 10 to 12 mm and thickness 4 to 5 mm. The transverse intermeniscal ligament connects the medial and lateral meniscus anteriorly. The coronary ligament connects the meniscus peripherally. The medial meniscus has less mobility with more rigid peripheral fixation than the lateral meniscus.[1] The meniscofemoral ligament connects the posterior horn lateral meniscus to the substance of the posterior cruciate ligament (PCL). There are two components: Humphrey ligament is more anterior and the ligament of Wrisberg is more posterior.

The meniscus receives its blood supply from various sources. The medial inferior geniculate artery supplies the peripheral 20% to 30% of the medial meniscus. The lateral inferior geniculate artery supplies the peripheral 10% to 25% of the lateral meniscus. The more central portion of the menisci receives blood supply through diffusion (**Figure 1**).[2] This is why tears in the peripheral 25%, also referred to as the red zone, have the highest healing potential. More central tears have limited (red-white zone) to no (white zone) intrinsic healing ability.[3] Nerve innervation is through type I and II nerve endings. The posterior horns have the highest concentration of mechanoreceptors.[4]

The main function of the menisci is to optimize force transmission across the knee. It does this by increasing the congruency and contact area, therefore decreasing point loading and improving shock absorption. It

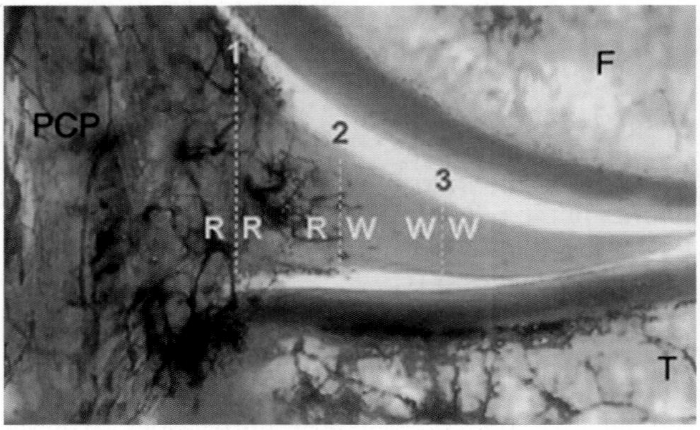

Figure 1 Illustration showing the frontal section of medial compartment. Branching radial vessels from the perimeniscal capillary plexus (PCP) can be observed penetrating the peripheral border of the medial meniscus. Three zones are seen: (1) RR, red-red area is fully vascularized; (2) RW, red-white is at the border of the vascular area; and (3) WW, white-white is within the avascular area of the meniscus. F = femur, PCP = perimeniscal capillary plexus, T = tibia. (Reprinted with permission from Fox AJ, Wanivenhaus F, Burge AJ, Warren RF, Rodeo SA: The human meniscus: A review of anatomy, function, injury, and advances in treatment. *Clin Anat* 2015;28[2]:269-287.)

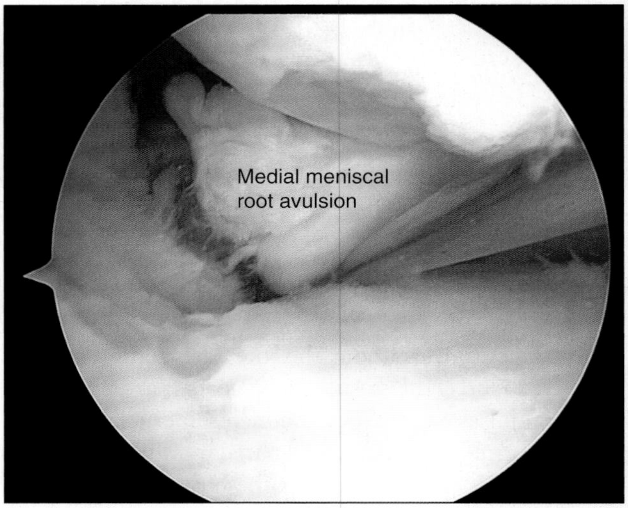

Figure 2 Arthroscopy of a right knee showing a medial meniscal root tear.

transmits 50% of the weight-bearing load in extension and 85% in flexion.[1] In addition, the menisci act as secondary stabilizers to the cruciate ligaments by deepening the tibial surface. The posterior horn of the medial meniscus is the main secondary stabilizer to anterior tibial translation, whereas the ACL is the primary stabilizer.[5] The lateral meniscus is less stabilizing than the medial meniscus because it has twice the excursion.[1]

Injury

Injury to the meniscus is the most common indication for knee surgery. Medial meniscal tears are more common than lateral tears. Lateral meniscus tears are most common with an acute ACL injury, whereas medial meniscus injuries occur more commonly in the setting of chronic ACL deficiency. Posterior horn medial meniscus tears are the most common in older patients with arthritis. Tears are classified based on size and orientation: vertical/longitudinal, bucket-handle tear which may displace into the notch, oblique/flap/parrot beak tears which can cause mechanical symptoms, radial, horizontal, root, and complex tears (**Figure 2**).

History and Physical Examination

Patients may present after an injury to the knee with pain localized to the medial or lateral joint line and/or mechanical symptoms such as locking and clicking and swelling of the knee. Physical examination should include inspection for an effusion, palpation for joint line tenderness, as well as several provocative tests. The McMurray test can be performed for both the medial and lateral meniscus. For the medial meniscus, the patient is supine; the knee is flexed; and a hand is placed on the medial side of the knee while the leg is externally rotated and brought into extension. A positive test is when there is a palpable pop or click. For the lateral meniscus, the knee is held by one hand, which is placed along the lateral joint line, and flexed to complete flexion. The examiner then rotates the leg internally while extending the knee to 90° of flexion. If a pop or click is felt along with pain, this constitutes a positive test. The Apley test is performed with the patient lying prone on an examination table. The knee is flexed to a 90° angle. The examiner then places his or her own knee across the posterior aspect of the patient's thigh. The tibia is then compressed onto the knee joint while being externally rotated. If this maneuver produces pain, this constitutes a positive test.

Imaging

Plain radiographs should be performed in young patients after an injury to rule out fractures. In older patients, radiographs can be helpful to assess the degree of arthritis. Meniscal calcifications can be seen in the setting of crystalline arthropathies. MRI is diagnostic but has a high false-positive rate. Criteria for a tear are a linear signal which extends to either the superior or inferior surface of the meniscus. A displaced bucket-handle tear can give a "double PCL" sign, where the displaced fragment runs parallel with the PCL in the notch. Similarly, a "double anterior horn" sign can be seen (**Figure 3**).

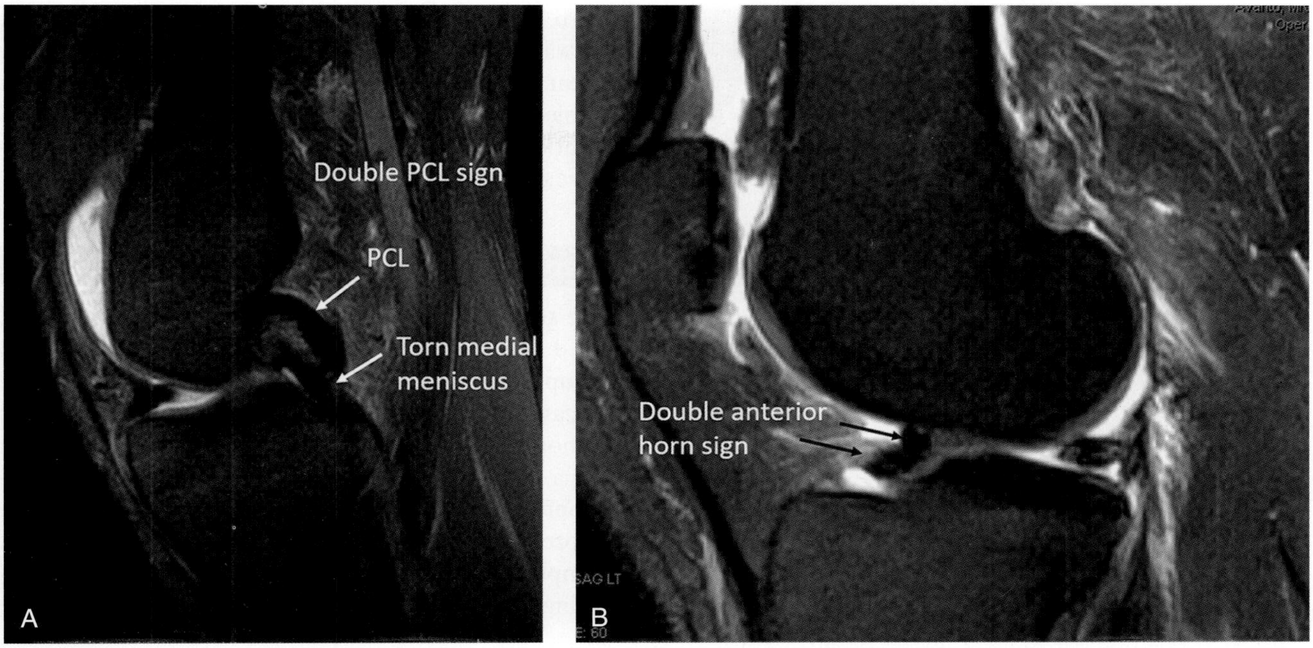

Figure 3 Sagittal T2 MRI of a right knee. **A**, Bucket-handle medial meniscus tear with double posterior cruciate ligament (PCL) sign. **B**, Bucket-handle lateral meniscus tear resulting in a double anterior horn sign.

Treatment

Treatment for meniscal tears can be nonsurgical or surgical depending on the type and severity of the tear. Surgical management should be considered for mechanical symptoms, such as locking of the knee. However, surgery is generally not found to be beneficial in the setting of advances arthritic changes.[6]

Conservative management includes rest, anti-inflammatory pain medication and physical therapy. Surgery options include partial menisectomy, meniscal repair, and meniscal transplantation. Total meniscectomy should be avoided as it has been shown that >70% of patients who underwent this procedure developed advanced arthritic changes within three years after surgery with 100% having arthritis at 20 years.[7]

Partial meniscectomy should be performed for tear types not amendable to repair or those with poor healing potential (ie, tears in the white zone, complex, degenerative, and radial tear patterns). Postoperative rehabilitation should focus on early mobilization and range of motion. The short-term outcomes are >80% satisfactory at short-term follow-up, but 50% have radiographic evidence of arthritis at mid- to long-term follow-up.

Meniscal repair is better for chondroprotection in the long-term but requires a longer recovery time.[8] A review article[9] (Level of evidence: III) addressed the decision making for meniscectomy versus repair, and the authors presented evidence that partial meniscectomy may be beneficial, for managing degenerative meniscus tears in knees with mild preexisting arthritis and mechanical symptoms. In younger patients, partial meniscectomy may provide equal long-term symptom relief, earlier return to play, and lower revision surgery rate compared with meniscal repair. However, this might result in earlier development of osteoarthritis.[9] Tear types with good outcome after repair are peripheral tears in the red-red zone, bucket-handle tears at the menisco-capsular junction, vertical/longitudinal tears, and root avulsions (**Figure 4**).[10] There are several different repair techniques, and the choice for which technique to use depends mostly on the location of the tear.[11] Inside-out repair is done through a medial or lateral approach to the capsule. It provides access to the posterior body and horn of the menisci. Complications include injury to the saphenous nerve and vein, peroneal nerve, and popliteus vessels. Outside-in provides the best access to the anterior horn and body. All-inside repair techniques are newer, but they have a higher risk of device breakage and iatrogenic chondral injury.[12] Weight bearing is protected to 50% partial weight bearing for the first 5 weeks. Range of motion is limited to 0° to 90° of flexion for the same duration. The success rate of meniscal repair is 70% to 95% and is the highest when done in conjunction with an ACL reconstruction.

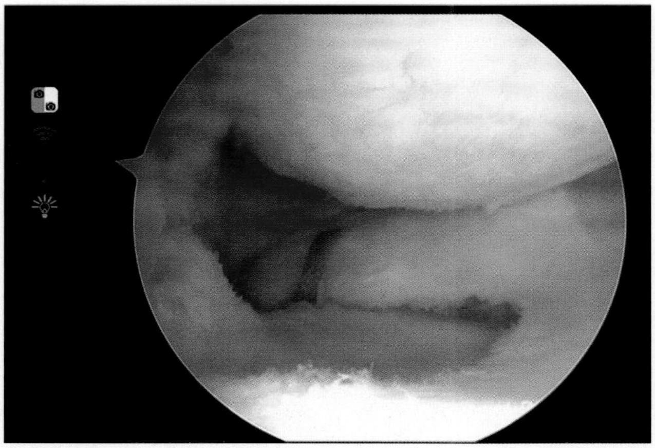

Figure 4 Arthroscopy of a right knee showing the end result after medial meniscal root repair.

Meniscal transplantation can be considered in young patients with prior near-total meniscectomy.[13] Contraindications are inflammatory arthritis, instability, obesity, malalignment (if not addressed concurrently), greater than grade II chondrosis of that compartment, or diffuse knee arthritis. The transplant can be held in place with bone plugs/block or sutures alone. Correct donor sizing is important and is done based on MRI measurements of the patient (**Figure 5**). Weight bearing and range of motion are restricted for the first 5 weeks, similar to after meniscus repair. Return to sports usually takes place at 6 to 9 months, but total healing time for the graft is 8 to 12 months. At 10-year follow-up, most patients report improvement in subjective pain and function, but it is not uncommon for patients to have radiographic progression of degenerative changes and retear.[13]

Discoid Meniscus

Three to five percent of the population has a discoid shaped meniscus. This is thought to be due to abnormal development and usually involves the lateral meniscus. This can lead to pain, clicking, and locking, which most commonly presents in adolescence. Radiographs can show a widened joint space with squaring of the femoral condyle, and MRI is diagnostic when there are three or more 5 mm sagittal images with meniscal continuity. If symptomatic, the meniscus can be saucerized by performing an arthroscopic partial meniscectomy.

Lateral Collateral Ligament and Posterolateral Corner

Anatomy

The lateral collateral ligament (LCL) is also referred to as the fibular collateral ligament (FCL). It originates from the lateral femoral epicondyle posterior and

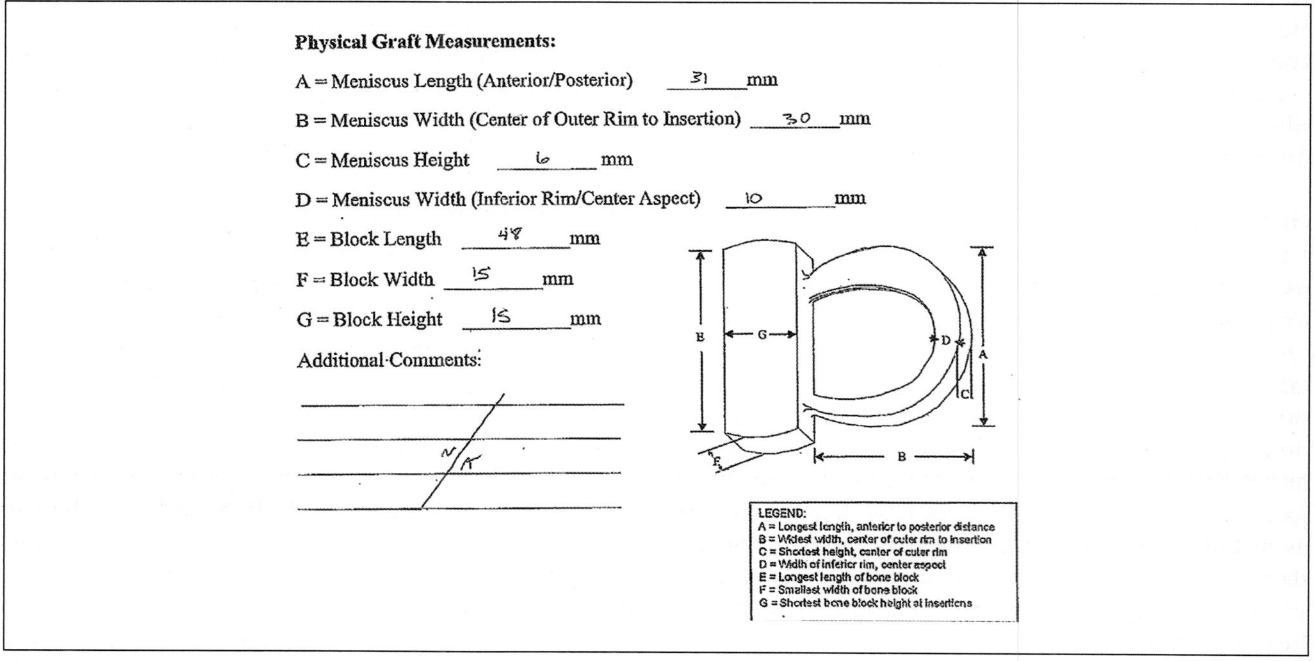

Physical Graft Measurements:

A = Meniscus Length (Anterior/Posterior) 31 mm

B = Meniscus Width (Center of Outer Rim to Insertion) 30 mm

C = Meniscus Height 6 mm

D = Meniscus Width (Inferior Rim/Center Aspect) 10 mm

E = Block Length 48 mm

F = Block Width 15 mm

G = Block Height 15 mm

Additional Comments:

N/A

Figure 5 Example photograph of a tissue company form showing the dimensions of a meniscal allograft as to allow matching of the donor to the recipient.

proximal to the insertion of the popliteus and inserts onto the anterolateral fibular head. It measures about 3 to 4 mm in diameter and 66 mm in length. It receives its blood supply from the superolateral and inferolateral geniculate arteries. The LCL is tight in extension and lax in flexion. It is the primary restraint to varus stress at 5° and 25° of knee flexion, and it is the secondary restraint to posterolateral rotation in low knee flexion angles. It works very closely with other lateral structures of the knee, and this entire complex is also referred to as the posterolateral corner (PLC).[14]

Structures of the PLC include the LCL, popliteus tendon and popliteofibular ligament, but also the lateral capsule, arcuate ligament, fabellofibular ligament, biceps femoris, popliteus muscle, iliotibial band (ITB), and lateral head of the gastrocnemius. The popliteus works synergistically with the PCL to control external rotation, varus and posterior translation. The popliteus and popliteofibular ligament function maximally in knee flexion to resist external rotation. The lateral structures of the knee are described in three layers: **layer 1**: ITB, biceps; **layer 2**: retinaculum, patellofemoral ligament; and **layer 3**: LCL, fabellofibular ligament and deep to this are the arcuate ligament, coronary ligament, popliteus tendon, and popliteofibular ligament and capsule. The common peroneal nerve lies between layer I and II. The lateral geniculate artery runs between deep and superficial layer.[15]

Injury

Approximately 7% to 16% of all knee ligament injuries involve the lateral ligamentous complex. The most common mechanisms are athletic injury and motor vehicle accidents causing excessive varus stress, external tibial rotation, and/or hyperextension as well as knee dislocations.

History and Physical Examination

Patients present with complaints of instability, difficulty ascending and descending stairs, difficulty with cutting or pivoting sports, lateral joint line pain, and swelling. On physical examination, there can be ecchymosis, lateral joint line tenderness, opening on varus stress at 30° (isolated LCL) and 0° (combined LCL and cruciate injury), increased tibial external rotation at 30° (PLC) and 90° (PLC and PCL), recurvatum, and a varus thrust gait. This is done both at 30° of knee flexion, as well as in full extension. Opening to varus stress at 30° of flexion only points toward isolated collateral injury, whereas opening at both 30° of flexion and full extension is concerning for a concomitant cruciate injury. Other tests include the posterolateral drawer test performed by applying a posterolateral force to the tibia with the hip flexed 45°, the knee flexed 80°, and the foot in 15° of external rotation. The reverse pivot shift is performed by placing the knee at 90° of flexion and an external rotation and valgus force is applied to the tibia as the knee is extended. The tibia will reduce with a palpable clunk if there is a PLC injury.[16]

A neurovascular examination should be performed, as the common peroneal nerve is often involved in the injury (15% to 29%). In addition, a vascular injury may be present in the setting of a knee dislocation mechanism. The popliteal artery can become occluded as the result from direct compression when the knee is dislocated. If the knee is dislocated on presentation, this should be reduced promptly. Distal pulses should be palpated, and the ankle-brachial index (ABI) should be assessed.[17,18]

Imaging

Radiographs should include AP and lateral views. An avulsion fracture of the fibula (arcuate fracture) or femoral condyle may be seen. Varus stress views may be helpful when the physical examination alone is inconclusive. MRI is the imaging modality of choice to determine the grade and location of the ligamentous injuries (**Figure 6**). MRI grading is based on the amount of ligamentous disruption: grade I is minimal; grade II is partial; grade III is complete. However, the interpretation of these structures can be challenging when first attempted. A recent radiology article (no Level of evidence) provided a comprehensive review of the normal anatomy and pathology of the PLC. The authors also highlighted potential pitfalls of image interpretation and detail.[19] When there is concern for a vascular injury, such as no palpable pulses or ABI < 0.9, a CT-angiogram should be considered.[20]

Treatment

Nonsurgical management is reserved for lower grade and isolated LCL injuries, which includes limited immobilization, progressive range of motion, and functional rehabilitation. Return to sports is expected at 6 to 8 weeks. Surgical treatment is generally indicated for high-grade LCL injuries with instability, injury to the PLC, or those combined with ACL and PCL injury. The outcome is improved if surgery is performed when the injuries are acute versus chronic. If the LCL is avulsed off the fibula, acute repair (<2 weeks) with suture anchors into the fibular head, either with or without graft augmentation, can be performed. A lateral approach to the knee using the interval between the ITB (innervation: superior gluteal nerve) and biceps femoris (innervation: sciatic nerve) is used to exposed the LCL insertion on

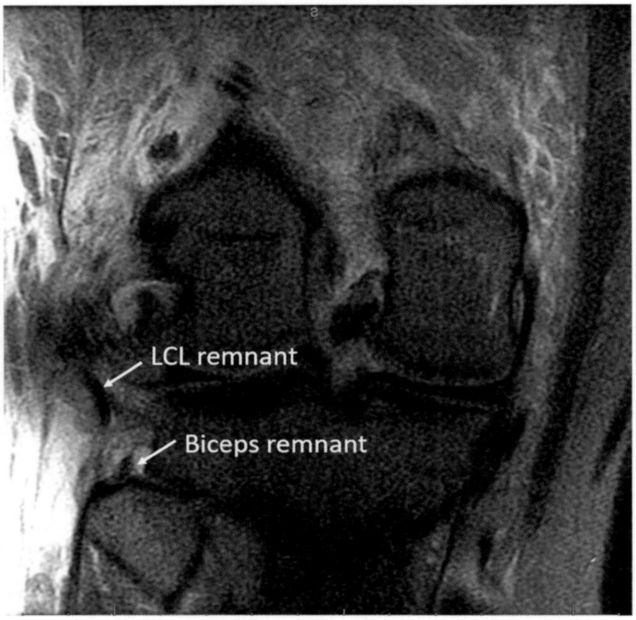

Figure 6 Coronal T2 MRI of a right knee with a complete distal avulsion of the posterolateral corner structures. LCL = lateral collateral ligament.

the fibular head. A window in the ITB is used to expose the lateral femoral epicondyle. The same can be done for the remainder of the PLC structures. Repair has a higher failure rate than reconstruction.[21]

Reconstruction of the LCL and PLC is done through the same approach. Surgical techniques include a single-stranded graft for isolated LCL reconstruction, a fibular-based reconstruction (Larson technique) for combined LCL and popliteofibular ligament reconstruction, or an anatomic reconstruction of the PLC. With the modified Larson technique, a single graft is passed through a fibular bone tunnel and the limbs are crossed to create a figure-of-8 fixed to the lateral femur. In the anatomic technique, the graft is passed through the fibular bone tunnel and the anterior limb is placed into the lateral femoral epicondyle to reconstruct the LCL. The posterior limb is first placed into the posterior tibial tunnel, and the remaining graft limb is placed at the femoral attachment of the popliteus to reconstruct both the popliteus and popliteofibular ligament. An osteotomy should be considered if there is malalignment. Failure to correct this malalignment results in a high failure rate. Complications include arthrofibrosis and peroneal nerve injury. Postoperative rehabilitation includes immobilization with a brace to prevent varus and external rotation and a period of protected weight bearing, early passive ROM, and avoidance of active hamstring exercises.[21]

Medial Collateral Ligament

Anatomy

The medial collateral ligament (MCL) is both the primary and secondary restraint to valgus stress. The superficial MCL is primary restraint to valgus stress and the deep MCL and posterior oblique ligaments (POL) form the secondary restraints to valgus stress. In addition, the semimembranosus, vastus medialis, medial retinaculum, sartorius, semimembranosus, and gracilis all act as dynamic stabilizers. Combined, these are also referred to as the posteromedial corner.[22] The medial side of the knee has also been described in layers: **layer 1** is the deep fascia; **layer 2**, the superficial MCL; and **layer 3**, the joint capsule and deep MCL. The MCL receives its blood supply from the superior medial and inferior medial geniculate arteries.

Injury

The MCL is the most commonly injured ligament in the knee. The mechanism is a valgus and external rotation force to the lateral knee.[22] The most common injury location is the femoral insertion, and this location has great healing potential. Distal ruptures are less common and more often lead to residual valgus laxity. Injuries are classified based on the amount of laxity and the integrity of the ligament. **Grade I** involves minimal torn fibers and 1 to 4 mm opening on valgus stress at 30°; **grade II** is partial tearing of the fibers, but they remain opposed with 5 to 10 mm laxity at 30° with a firm end point; and **grade III** is a complete tear with >10 mm opening without an end point. Associated injuries can include injuries of the ACL, medial patellofemoral ligament (MPFL), and meniscus.[23]

History and Physical Examination

Patient may present after a contact or noncontact valgus injury and report feeling a "pop." Symptoms include medial-sided knee pain, difficulty ambulating, and instability. Physical examination may reveal medial ecchymosis and/or tenderness along the proximal or distal attachment of the MCL. An effusion may indicate associated intra-articular pathology. Valgus stress should be applied at both 0° and 30°. Opening at 0° indicates a posteromedial capsular or associated cruciate (ACL/PCL) injury.

Imaging

Plain radiographs should be performed to rule out fracture. A Pellegrini-Stieda lesion can be seen, which is a calcification at the medial femoral insertion site

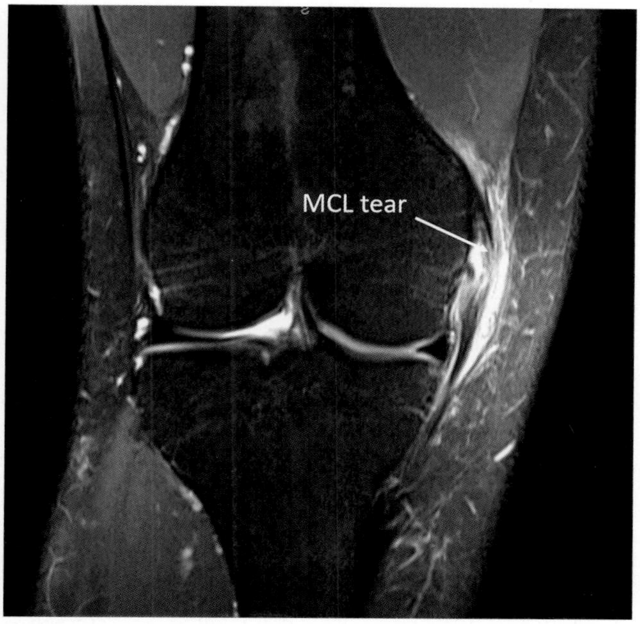

Figure 7 Coronal T2 MRI of a right knee with a proximal medial collateral ligament (MCL) tear.

resulting from chronic MCL deficiency. MRI is not routinely necessary unless concomitant injuries are suspected (**Figure 7**).[23]

Treatment

Most MCL injuries can be managed nonsurgically with rest, ice, anti-inflammatories, bracing treatment, and physical therapy, while focusing on quadriceps sets, straight leg raises, hip adduction, cycling, and progressive return to full activity. Return to play depends on the injury and ranges from 5 to 7 days for grade I injuries to 4 to 8 weeks for grade III injuries. There is some evidence to suggest that functional bracing treatment can prevent MCL injury in football players, specifically linemen.[24] Return to play rates after an MCL injury alone are usually good; however, when combined with ACL and meniscal injuries, this changes significantly. A study (Level of evidence: III) on 272 athletes with an ACL injury revealed that when patients had combined ACL and MCL injuries, they were much less likely to return to sports at 1 years, compared with those who did not have an MCL injury (odds ratio [OR] 7.61; 95% confidence interval [CI], 1.42 to 40.87; $P = 0.018$).[25]

Surgical treatment is usually reserved for distal avulsion fracture with a Stener lesion where the torn end of the ligament gets trapped in the medial compartment, as well as in the setting of the multiligament injured knee. Repair with suture anchors can be attempted in acute and subacute avulsions. Reconstruction is indicated for chronic or unrepairable tears. A diagnostic arthroscopy can be considered at the time of reconstruction to rule out associate injuries. In some cases, reconstruction of the POL using a separate graft is necessary to restore normal laxity when the posteromedial corner structures are compromised. The surgery is performing through a medial approach to the knee and often hamstring, achilles, or tibialis allograft is used. Complications include arthrofibrosis, injury to the saphenous nerve, and residual laxity.

Anterior Cruciate Ligament

Anatomy

The ACL is the main restraint against anterior tibial translation relative to the femur. In addition, it prevents tibial rotation and varus/valgus rotation. The ACL is approximately 32 mm in length and 7 to 12 mm wide. The ligament is composed of 90% type I collagen and 10% type III collagen, and its strength is 2,200 N. It consists of two functional bundles: the anteromedial (AM) and posterolateral (PL) bundle, named after the location of their insertion site on the tibia (**Figure 8**). The AM bundle is tightest in flexion and is primarily responsible for restraining anterior tibial translation, while the PL is tightest in extension and looser in midflexion, which allows for rotation. On the femoral side, the lateral intercondylar ridge demarcates the anterior edge of the ACL where the bifurcate ridge separates the two bundles.[26] The ACL receives its blood supply from the middle geniculate artery and its innervation from the posterior articular nerve, which is a branch of the tibial nerve.[27]

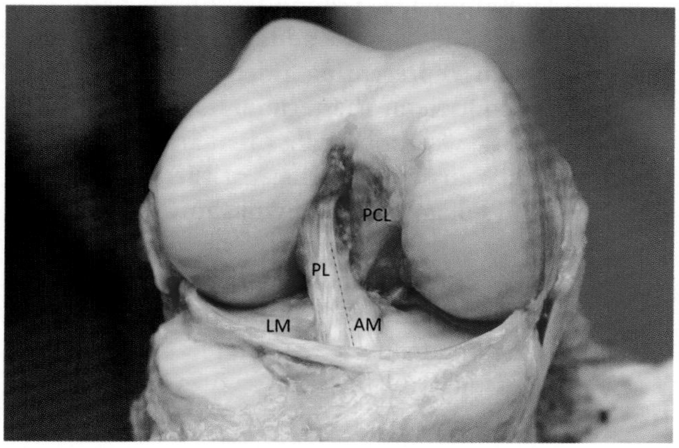

Figure 8 Photograph demonstrating dissection of a right knee showing the two bundles of the anterior cruciate ligament (ACL): anteromedial (AM) and posterolateral (PL) named after their location on the tibia. The posterior cruciate ligament (PCL) and anterior horn of the lateral meniscus (LM) are also shown.

Knee

Injury

An ACL injury usually is the result of a noncontact pivoting injury during sports. It is 4.5 times more common in female athletes compared with males, which is thought to be due to landing biomechanics and neuromuscular patterns.[28] Associated injuries can include the lateral meniscus, medial meniscus, MCL, and cartilage.[27]

History and Physical Examination

Patients may sustain an ACL injury after a twisting injury and report feeling a "pop" followed by immediate swelling. Physical examination may reveal an effusion, usually representing hemarthrosis. They walk with a quadriceps avoidance gait. Provocative testing includes the Lachman test, an anteriorly directed force on the tibia with the knee in 20° to 30° of flexion. This is the most sensitive test.[29] It is graded from 1 to 3 based on the amount of anterior translation (grade 1 = 0 to 5 mm, grade 2 = 6 to 10 mm, grade 3 = 11 to 15 mm difference with the contralateral side), followed by an A for firm end point and B for soft end point.[29] An arthrometer is a device that can be used to measure the exact amount (mm) of translation during this test. The pivot shift test is performing by moving the knee from extension to flexion while applying a valgus and internal rotation load to the tibia. The tibia will reduce with a clunk, but often the patient will guard their leg when performing this test unless they are completely relaxed or under anesthesia.[29]

Imaging

Plain radiographs are most often normal but can sometimes show a Segond fracture, which is an avulsion fracture of the anterolateral knee capsule from the proximal lateral tibia. A Segond fracture is pathognomonic for an ACL tear. In addition, it may show a deep sulcus sign, representing a depression on the lateral femoral condyle at the terminal sulcus, the junction between the weight bearing tibial articular surface and the patellar articular surface of the femoral condyle. An MRI is diagnostic and will show the ACL tear location and severity along with concomitant injuries. A typical bone bruising includes the middle third of the lateral femoral condyle and the posterior third of the lateral tibial plateau.

Treatment

The treatment for an ACL injury depends on the activity level of the patient. Nonsurgical treatment is usually reserved for those patients with low demand or few instability complaints. This includes physical therapy to regain range of motion and strength, bracing treatment, and lifestyle modification. However, chronic ACL deficiency has been down to increase the risk for meniscal and cartilage pathology.[30]

Surgical treatment is indicated in young patients and those involved in jumping, cutting, and pivoting sports as well as manual laborers and patients with concomitant injuries requiring surgery. Surgical repair of the ACL historically has high failure rates; however, newer methods for structural augmentation of the repair have shown promising results.[31] A systematic review (Level of evidence: III) on ACL repair identified 89 papers describing preclinical and clinical studies. The authors found that proximal ACL tear patterns showed better healing potential with primary repair than distal or midsubstance tears. Some form of internal support of the repair with sutures or scaffolds increased the success rate of ACL repair. Biological characteristics of the repair could be improved by bone marrow access by drilling tunnels or microfracture. Augmentation with platelet-rich plasma was beneficial only in combination with a structural scaffold. Lastly, skeletally immature patients had the best outcomes along with patients where the repair was performed in the acute setting.[31] The standard of care is anatomic reconstruction using either the patellar tendon, hamstring or quadriceps autograft or allograft tissue (**Figure 9**). Autograft has a faster healing time, less immune reaction, and no risk for disease transmission, but is associated with increased postoperative pain. The patellar tendon autograft has the advantage of bone to bone healing and is often considered the benchmark, but has the highest incidence of anterior knee pain. Hamstring autograft uses a smaller incision, but can result in permanent decreased hamstring strength which is a risk factor for graft rupture. Allograft has less donor site morbidity, but a higher failure rate in the young athletic population. However, the most common reason for graft failure is tunnel malpositioning. The tunnels for the graft should be placed in the center of anatomic ACL femoral and tibial footprint (**Figure 10**). The physis needs to be taken into consideration in pediatric patients by using a physeal sparing method of tunnel drilling, such as all epiphyseal or over the top. An osteotomy should be considered if there is evidence of malalignment.

Reconstruction can be done as a single- or double-bundle technique.[32-34] Double-bundle reconstruction is technically more demanding but may result in improved stability.[32] In a Swedish National Knee Ligament Registry (Level of evidence: III) study, 22,460 patients undergoing either single- or double-bundle ACL reconstruction with hamstring tendon autograft were included and followed over time using surveys.

Patellar Tendon Rupture

Patellar tendon ruptures are most common in the third and fourth decades of life and more common in males than females. They are less prevalent than quadriceps tendon ruptures. Risk factors include systemic lupus erythematous, rheumatoid arthritis, chronic renal disease, diabetes mellitus, steroid injection, and preexisting patellar tendinopathy. Rupture is usually the result of end stage or long-standing chronic tendon degeneration. The mechanism of injury is tensile overload of the extensor mechanism. Most ruptures occur with the knee in a flexed position. The most common injury pattern is a proximal sided rupture. However, midsubstance ruptures or distal avulsions are also possible.

The patellar tendon receives its blood supply from the infrapatellar fat pad and from the retinaculum through the medial and lateral inferior geniculate arteries. It routinely sees forces of 3 times body weight when ascending stairs, and it take over 17 times body weight to rupture a normal tendon.

Patients typically present after a sudden popping sensation during quadriceps contraction with the knee in a flexed position or a fall with a flexed knee. They complain of pain inferior to the patella and difficulty ambulating. On physical examination, there is patella alta, ecchymosis, tenderness to palpation, and a palpable gap. The patient cannot perform a straight leg raise or maintain a passively extended knee. If the retinaculum is intact, they will be able to actively extend, but there will be an extensor lag of several degrees.

Plain radiographs will show patella alta as evidenced by an increase Insall-Salvati ratio >1.2. Ultrasonography or MRI can be used to confirm the diagnosis and will reveal associated injuries.

Partial tears with an intact extensor mechanism may be managed conservatively with immobilization in full extension, followed by progressive weight bearing and range of motion. However, in cases of complete ruptures with dysfunction of the extensor mechanism, surgery is indicated. Repair is performed through a midline incision using sutures end to end, sutures into bone tunnels, or suture anchors. In cases with poor tissue quality or chronic tears, augmentation with autograft or allograft tissue may be necessary. Postoperative rehabilitation includes early weight bearing with the knee braced in extension, exercises to optimize range of motion with passive extension, active closed chain flexion, and prone open chain flexion.[44,45] Full return to sports is usually achieved at 6 months. The outcome largely depends on the timing of the surgery, as acute repairs often do better than those performed in the chronic setting.[51] Complications include arthrofibrosis, decreased quadriceps strength, and quadriceps atrophy.[52]

Summary

Soft-tissue injuries about the knee are common. Injuries can involve the menisci, cruciates, collateral ligament, and patellar and quadriceps tendon. Anatomic knowledge, history and physical examination findings, necessary imaging studies, and treatment options are important to know to provide patients with the best potential for a successful recovery.

Key Study Points

- Injury to the meniscus is the most common indication for knee surgery, and the MCL is the most commonly injured ligament in the knee.
- Structures of the PLC include the LCL, popliteus tendon, and popliteofibular ligament, along with the lateral capsule, arcuate ligament, fabellofibular ligament, biceps femoris, popliteus muscle, iliotibial band, and lateral head of the gastrocnemius.
- Opening to valgus stress at 0° indicates an injury of the MCL combined with either the posteromedial capsular or a cruciate (ACL or PCL).
- The Lachman test is the most sensitive physical examination test to diagnose an ACL tear in the office.
- Chronic PCL deficiency results in altered joint contact pressures leading to medial and patellofemoral compartment arthrosis.

Annotated References

1. Bylski-Austrow DI, Ciarelli MJ, Kayner DC, Matthews LS, Goldstein SA: Displacements of the menisci under joint load: An in vitro study in human knees. *J Biomech* 1994;27(4):421-431.

2. Scapinelli R: Vascular anatomy of the human cruciate ligaments and surrounding structures. *Clin Anat* 1997;10(3):151-162.

3. Henning CE, Lynch MA, Clark JR: Vascularity for healing of meniscus repairs. *Arthroscopy* 1987;3(1):13-18.

4. Fox AJ, Wanivenhaus F, Burge AJ, Warren RF, Rodeo SA: The human meniscus: A review of anatomy, function, injury, and advances in treatment. *Clin Anat* 2015;28(2):269-287.

5. Musahl V, Citak M, O'Loughlin PF, Choi D, Bedi A, Pearle AD: The effect of medial versus lateral meniscectomy on the stability of the anterior cruciate ligament-deficient knee. *Am J Sports Med* 2010;38(8):1591-1597.
6. AAOS CPG on Surgical Management of Osteoarthritis of the Knee. Available at: http://www.orthoguidelines.org/topic?id=1019.
7. Han SB, Shetty GM, Lee DH, et al: Unfavorable results of partial meniscectomy for complete posterior medial meniscus root tear with early osteoarthritis: A 5- to 8-year follow-up study. *Arthroscopy* 2010;26(10):1326-1332.
8. LaPrade CM, Jansson KS, Dornan G, Smith SD, Wijdicks CA, LaPrade RF: Altered tibiofemoral contact mechanics due to lateral meniscus posterior horn root avulsions and radial tears can be restored with in situ pull-out suture repairs. *J Bone Joint Surg Am* 2014;96(6):471-479.
9. Feeley BT, Lau BC: Biomechanics and clinical outcomes of partial meniscectomy. *J Am Acad Orthop Surg* 2018;15(26):853-863.

   In this review paper, the authors state that use of partial meniscectomy to manage degenerative meniscus tears in knees with mild preexisting arthritis and mechanical symptoms may be beneficial; however, its routine use in the degenerative knee over physical therapy alone is not supported. In younger populations, partial meniscectomy may provide equal long-term symptom relief, earlier return to play, and lower revision surgery rate compared with meniscal repair. Partial meniscectomy may result in earlier development of osteoarthritis. Treatment should be patient specific in a shared decision-making process with the patient after discussion about known outcomes. Level of evidence: NA (Review paper).
10. Ahn JH, Kwon OJ, Nam TS: Arthroscopic repair of horizontal meniscal cleavage tears with marrow-stimulating technique. *Arthroscopy* 2015;31(1):92-98.
11. Rankin CC, Lintner DM, Noble PC, Paravic V, Greer E: A biomechanical analysis of meniscal repair techniques. *Am J Sports Med* 2002;30(4):492-497.
12. Espejo-Baena A, Golano P, Meschian S, Garcia-Herrera JM, Serrano Jimenez JM. Complications in medial meniscus suture: A cadaveric study. *Knee Surg Sports Traumatol Arthrosc* 2007;15(6):811-816.
13. Lee AS, Kang RW, Kroin E, Verma NN, Cole BJ: Allograft meniscus transplantation. *Sports Med Arthrosc Rev* 2012;20(2):106-114.
14. James EW, LaPrade CM, LaPrade RF: Anatomy and biomechanics of the lateral side of the knee and surgical implications. *Sports Med Arthrosc Rev* 2015;23(1):2-9.
15. LaPrade RF, Ly TV, Wentorf FA, Engebretsen L: The posterolateral attachments of the knee: A qualitative and quantitative morphologic analysis of the fibular collateral ligament, popliteus tendon, popliteofibular ligament, and lateral gastrocnemius tendon. *Am J Sports Med* 2003;31(6):854-860.
16. Lubowitz JH, Bernardini BJ, Reid JB III: Current concepts review: Comprehensive physical examination for instability of the knee. *Am J Sports Med* 2008;36(3):577-594.
17. Fanelli GC: Multiple ligament injured knee: Initial assessment and treatment. *Clin Sports Med* 2019;38(2):193-198.

    This article presents the author's approach and experience to the initial assessment and treatment of the multiple ligament injured (dislocated) knee. Level of evidence: NA (Review paper).
18. Johnson JP, Kleiner J, Klinge SA, McClure PK, Hayda RA, Born CT: Increased incidence of vascular injury in obese patients with knee dislocations. *J Orthop Trauma* 2018;32(2):82-87.

    In this cohort study on knee dislocation, the authors found significant increases in costs of stay with obese patients sustaining knee dislocations when compared with normal weight knee dislocation patients. Vascular injuries were found to be far more common in obese and morbidly obese patient groups than nonobese patients. Providers should be on high alert when managing knee dislocations in obese patients because a significant number require prompt vascular intervention. Level of evidence: III.
19. Porrino J, Sharp JW, Ashimolowo T, Dunham G: An update and comprehensive review of the posterolateral corner of the knee. *Radiol Clin North Am* 2018;56(6):935-951.

    This is a review paper on the posterolateral corner. It presents a comprehensive review of the normal anatomy and pathology of the PLC. We highlight potential pitfalls of image interpretation and detail what the referring physician needs to know. Level of evidence: NA (Review paper).
20. Fanelli GC, Orcutt DR, Edson CJ: The multiple-ligament injured knee: Evaluation, treatment, and results. *Arthroscopy* 2005;21(4):471-486.
21. Stannard JP, Brown SL, Farris RC, McGwin G Jr, Volgas DA: The posterolateral corner of the knee: Repair versus reconstruction. *Am J Sports Med* 2005;33(6):881-888.
22. Wijdicks CA, Griffith CJ, Johansen S, Engebretsen L, LaPrade RF: Injuries to the medial collateral ligament and associated medial structures of the knee. *J Bone Joint Surg Am* 2010;92(5):1266-1280.
23. Shelbourne KD, Carr DR: Combined anterior and posterior cruciate and medial collateral ligament injury: Nonsurgical and delayed surgical treatment. *Instr Course Lect* 2003;52:413-418.
24. Pietrosimone BG, Grindstaff TL, Linens SW, Uczekaj E, Hertel J: A systematic review of prophylactic braces in the prevention of knee ligament injuries in collegiate football players. *J Athl Train* 2008;43(4):409-415.
25. Hamrin Senorski E, Svantesson E, Beischer S, et al: Low 1-year return-to-sport rate after anterior cruciate ligament reconstruction regardless of patient and surgical factors: A prospective Cohort study of 272 patients. *Am J Sports Med* 2018;46(7):1551-1558.

    In this cohort study on return to sports after ACL reconstruction, the authors found that positive predictors of a return to knee-strenuous sport were male sex, younger age, a high preinjury level of physical activity, and the absence of concomitant injuries to the medial collateral ligament and meniscus. Level of evidence: III.

26. Fu FH, Jordan SS: The lateral intercondylar ridge–a key to anatomic anterior cruciate ligament reconstruction. *J Bone Joint Surg Am* 2007;89(10):2103-2104.

27. Zantop T, Petersen W, Sekiya JK, Musahl V, Fu FH: Anterior cruciate ligament anatomy and function relating to anatomical reconstruction. *Knee Surg Sports Traumatol Arthrosc* 2006;14-10:982-992.

28. Vairo GL, Myers JB, Sell TC, Fu FH, Harner CD, Lephart SM: Neuromuscular and biomechanical landing performance subsequent to ipsilateral semitendinosus and gracilis autograft anterior cruciate ligament reconstruction. *Knee Surg Sports Traumatol Arthrosc* 2008;16(1):2-14.

29. van Eck CF, van den Bekerom MP, Fu FH, Poolman RW, Kerkhoffs GM: Methods to diagnose acute anterior cruciate ligament rupture: A meta-analysis of physical examinations with and without anaesthesia. *Knee Surg Sports Traumatol Arthrosc* 2013;21(8):1895-1903.

30. Magnussen RA, Duthon V, Servien E, Neyret P: Anterior cruciate ligament reconstruction and osteoarthritis: Evidence from long-term follow-up and potential solutions. *Cartilage* 2013;4(3 suppl):22S-26S.

31. van Eck CF, Limpisvasti O, ElAttrache NS: Is there a role for internal bracing and repair of the anterior cruciate ligament? A systematic literature review. *Am J Sports Med* 2018;46(9):2291-2298.

    In this systematic review on ACL repair, the authors found that proximal ACL tear patterns showed a better healing potential with primary repair than distal or midsubstance tears. Some form of internal bracing increased the success rate of ACL repair. Improvement in the biological characteristics of the repair was obtained by bone marrow access by drilling tunnels or microfracture. Augmentation with platelet-rich plasma was beneficial only in combination with a structural scaffold. Skeletally immature patients had the best outcomes. Acute repair offered improved outcomes with regard to load, stiffness, laxity, and rerupture. Level of evidence: III.

32. Svantesson E, Sundemo D, Hamrin Senorski E, et al: Double-bundle anterior cruciate ligament reconstruction is superior to single-bundle reconstruction in terms of revision frequency: A study of 22,460 patients from the Swedish National Knee Ligament Register. *Knee Surg Sports Traumatol Arthrosc* 2017;25(12):3884-3891.

    In this Swedish Register study, the authors found that double-bundle ACL reconstruction is associated with a lower risk of revision surgery than single-bundle ACL reconstruction. Single-bundle procedures performed using transportal femoral drilling technique had significantly higher risk of revision surgery compared with double-bundle. However, a reference reconstruction with transportal drilling defined as a more complete anatomic reconstruction reduces the risk of revision surgery considerably. Level of evidence: III.

33. Hussein M, van Eck CF, Cretnik A, Dinevski D, Fu FH: Prospective randomized clinical evaluation of conventional single-bundle, anatomic single-bundle, and anatomic double-bundle anterior cruciate ligament reconstruction: 281 cases with 3- to 5-year follow-up. *Am J Sports Med* 2012;40(3):512-520.

34. Hussein M, van Eck CF, Cretnik A, Dinevski D, Fu FH: Individualized anterior cruciate ligament surgery: A prospective study comparing anatomic single- and double-bundle reconstruction. *Am J Sports Med* 2012;40(8):1781-1788.

35. MARS Group: Rehabilitation predictors of clinical outcome following revision ACL reconstruction in the MARS Cohort. *J Bone Joint Surg Am* 2019;101(9):779-786.

    This multicenter study on revision ACL surgery showed that rehabilitation-related factors that the physician can control at the time of an ACL reconstruction have the ability to influence clinical outcomes at 2 years. Weight bearing and motion can be initiated immediately postoperatively. Bracing during the early postoperative period is not helpful. Use of a functional brace early in the postoperative period was associated with an increased risk of a reoperation. Use of a functional brace for a return to sports improved the knee injury and osteoarthritis outcome score on the sports/recreation subscale. Level of evidence: I.

36. Margheritini F, Rihn J, Musahl V, Mariani PP, Harner C: Posterior cruciate ligament injuries in the athlete: An anatomical, biomechanical and clinical review. *Sports Med* 2002;32(6):393-408.

37. Garofalo R, Fanelli GC, Cikes A, et al: Stress radiography and posterior pathological laxity of knee: Comparison between two different techniques. *Knee* 2009;16(4):251-255.

38. Strobel MJ, Weiler A, Schulz MS, Russe K, Eichhorn HJ: Arthroscopic evaluation of articular cartilage lesions in posterior-cruciate-ligament-deficient knees. *Arthroscopy* 2003;19(3):262-268.

39. Song EK, Park HW, Ahn YS, Seon JK: Transtibial versus tibial inlay techniques for posterior cruciate ligament reconstruction: Long-term follow-up study. *Am J Sports Med* 2014;42(12):2964-2971.

40. Giffin JR, Stabile KJ, Zantop T, Vogrin TM, Woo SL, Harner CD: Importance of tibial slope for stability of the posterior cruciate ligament deficient knee. *Am J Sports Med* 2007;35(9):1443-1449.

41. Kaufman KR, An KN, Litchy WJ, Morrey BF, Chao EY: Dynamic joint forces during knee isokinetic exercise. *Am J Sports Med* 1991;19(3):305-316.

42. Maffulli N, Del Buono A, Spiezia F, Longo UG, Denaro V: Light microscopic histology of quadriceps tendon ruptures. *Int Orthop* 2012;36(11):2367-2371.

43. Garner MR, Gausden E, Berkes MB, Nguyen JT, Lorich DG: Extensor mechanism injuries of the knee: Demographic characteristics and comorbidities from a review of 726 patient records. *J Bone Joint Surg Am* 2015;97(19):1592-1596.

44. West JL, Keene JS, Kaplan LD: Early motion after quadriceps and patellar tendon repairs: Outcomes with single-suture augmentation. *Am J Sports Med* 2008;36(2):316-323.

45. Stuart MJ, Meglan DA, Lutz GE, Growney ES, An KN: Comparison of intersegmental tibiofemoral joint forces and muscle activity during various closed kinetic chain exercises. *Am J Sports Med* 1996;24(6):792-799.

46. Zwerver J, Bredeweg SW, van den Akker-Scheek I: Prevalence of Jumper's knee among nonelite athletes from different sports: A cross-sectional survey. *Am J Sports Med* 2011;39(9):1984-1988.

47. Witvrouw E, Bellemans J, Lysens R, Danneels L, Cambier D: Intrinsic risk factors for the development of patellar tendinitis in an athletic population. A two-year prospective study. *Am J Sports Med* 2001;29(2):190-195.

48. Bahr R, Fossan B, Loken S, Engebretsen L: Surgical treatment compared with eccentric training for patellar tendinopathy (Jumper's Knee). A randomized, controlled trial. *J Bone Joint Surg Am* 2006;88(8):1689-1698.

49. Horstmann H, Clausen JD, Krettek C, Weber-Spickschen TS: Evidence-based therapy for tendinopathy of the knee joint: Which forms of therapy are scientifically proven? *Unfallchirurg* 2017;120(3):199-204.

In this review of literature on treatments for tendinopathy about the knee, the authors found that treatment with platelet-rich plasma showed a significantly better outcome when used correctly. Treatment with shock waves, surgical treatment, and sclerotherapy have also shown positive effects. Treatment with corticosteroid injections and with oral NSAIDs showed positive short-term effects (follow-up ±4 weeks). No reasonable data are available for the treatment of tendinopathy in the knee region by acupuncture, fascial therapy, or cryotherapy. The use of kinesio taping showed no significant relief from complaints compared with standard conservative treatment. Level of evidence: III.

50. Al-Duri ZA, Aichroth PM: Surgical aspects of patellar tendonitis: Technique and results. *Am J Knee Surg* 2001;14(1):43-50.

51. Casey MT Jr, Tietjens BR: Neglected ruptures of the patellar tendon. A case series of four patients. *Am J Sports Med* 2001;29(4):457-460.

52. Volk WR, Yagnik GP, Uribe JW: Complications in brief: Quadriceps and patellar tendon tears. *Clin Orthop Relat Res* 2014;472(3):1050-1057.

Chapter 41

Knee Arthroscopy and Preservation, Knee Reconstruction

Caitlin C. Chambers, MD • Derek Ward, MD • C. Benjamin Ma, MD

ABSTRACT

Articular cartilage injury in the knee can impact a focal area, a single joint compartment, or the entire knee. Surgical options for knee cartilage injury include arthroscopic débridement, cartilage restoration procedures, meniscal preservation procedures, realignment osteotomy, and unicompartmental or total knee arthroplasty. Multiple implant designs and assistive technologies, such as patient-specific instrumentation, computer navigation, and robotic assistance, have been developed with the goal of improving unicompartmental and total knee arthroplasty outcomes. Choosing the correct intervention is dependent upon careful analysis of the patient's physical examination, activity levels, plain radiographs, and advanced imaging findings.

Keywords: arthritis; cartilage injury; knee arthroplasty; knee arthroscopy; knee cartilage; osteochondral defect

Introduction

Articular cartilage injuries within the knee can be seen as a result of age-related degenerative changes, previous trauma or injury, congenital osteochondral defects, inflammatory conditions, infection, and other causes. The chronicity, severity, and focal versus generalized nature of a patient's cartilage injury guides treatment, with surgical options including arthroscopic débridement, osteochondral grafting, realignment osteotomy, or knee arthroplasty. Physical examination along with radiographic or advanced imaging findings must be used concomitantly to determine the source of each patient's symptoms, and to determine appropriate surgical intervention when nonsurgical measures such as activity modification, weight loss, nonsteroidal anti-inflammatory drugs (NSAIDs), corticosteroid injections, and physical therapy have failed.

This chapter summarizes the range of surgical options available to treat articular cartilage injuries in the knee, beginning with a review of indicated radiographic and advanced imaging modalities. The indications, surgical approach, and outcomes of knee arthroscopy for cartilage injury will then be discussed. Knee preservation techniques including cartilage restoration, meniscal preservation or transplantation, and realignment osteotomies are detailed followed by a summary of arthroplasty techniques, including recent advances in the design of unicompartmental and total knee arthroplasty.

Imaging

Weight-bearing flexion posterior-anterior, lateral, and merchant or sunrise view radiographs (**Figure 1**) allow for multiplanar assessment of joint space narrowing, subchondral bone defect or sclerosis, ossified loose bodies, and osteophyte formation that may guide treatment recommendations in the case of cartilage injury. The weight-bearing flexion posterior-anterior view allows for visualization of the entire tibial articular surface by accounting for the posterior tibial slope. Standard plain radiographs of the knee should be obtained along with long-standing cassette radiographs for evaluation of limb alignment when there is clinical concern for malalignment that may place increased load on the affected joint compartment (**Figure 2**). Any identified malalignment should be addressed before or concurrent with cartilage procedures to ensure that the region of interest is appropriately off-loaded. Coronal plane malalignment can be identified using the measurements described in **Table 1**.

MRI without contrast should be obtained in cases where patients report a mechanical block to motion, large effusion, or significant locking or catching in the knee. MRI allows for identification of loose bodies and meniscal, ligamentous, or focal articular cartilage injury that can contribute to such mechanical complaints that may be remedied with surgical intervention (**Figure 3**).

None of the following authors or any immediate family member has received anything of value from or has stock or stock options held in a commercial company or institution related directly or indirectly to the subject of this chapter: Dr. Chambers, Dr. Ward, and Dr. Ma.

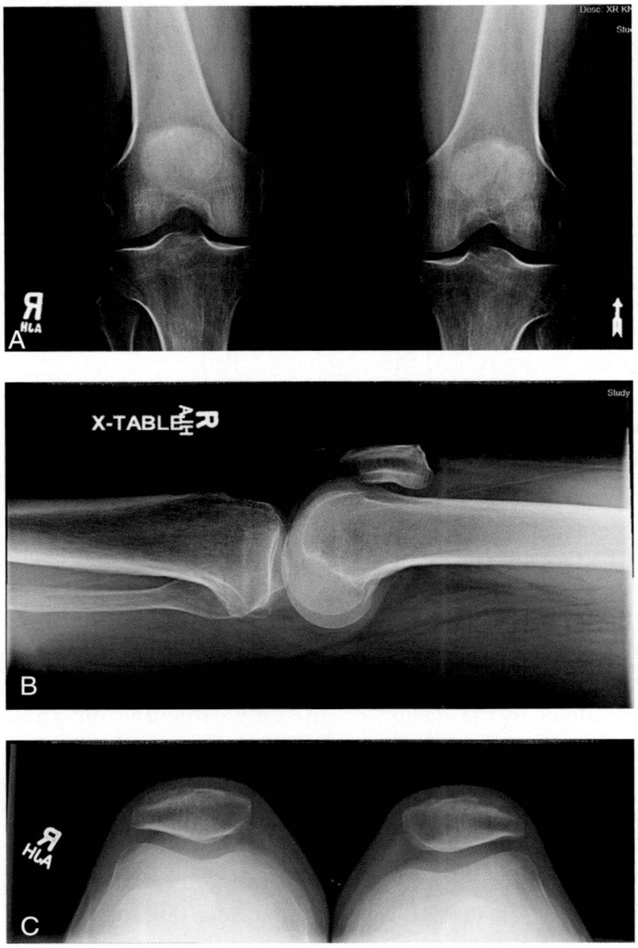

Figure 1 Radiographs of the knee: weight-bearing flexion posterior-anterior (**A**), lateral (**B**), and merchant view (**C**).

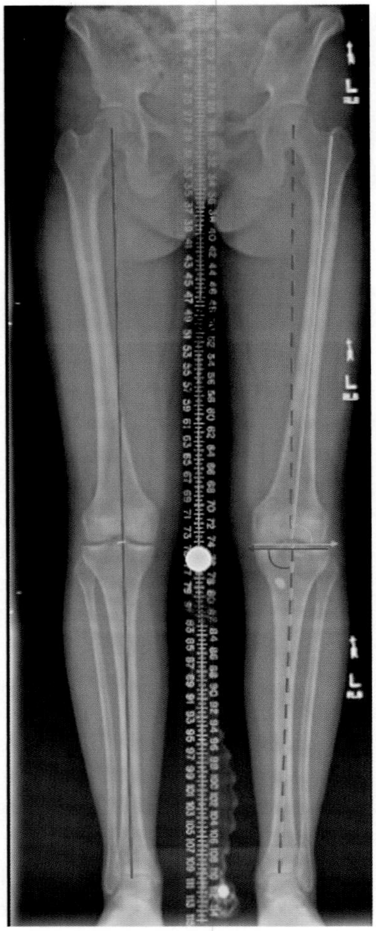

Figure 2 Long-standing cassette alignment radiographs demonstrating: solid red line: mechanical axis of the limb; dashed red line: mechanical axes of the femur and tibia; green line: anatomic axes of the femur and tibia; blue arrow: tangent to the most distal part of the femoral condyles; the lateral angle between this line and the femur mechanical axis (dashed red line) is the mechanical lateral distal femoral angle (mLDFA). Purple arrow: tangent to the proximal tibial plateau; the medial angle between this line and the tibia mechanical axis (dashed red line) is the medial proximal tibial angle (MPTA); yellow line (right knee): mechanical axis deviation.

MRI is 78% to 89% sensitive and 88% to 95% specific for meniscal injury, and 83% sensitive and 94% specific for the detection of chondral injury.[1,2]

Although not currently practical for routine clinical use, there are multiple MRI compositional sequences that allow for evaluation of articular cartilage quality. These sequences focus on the collagen network and water content of cartilage (T2 mapping, T2* mapping) or changes in cartilage extracellular matrix and proteoglycan or glycosaminoglycan content (T1ρ, dGEMRIC, gagCEST).[3] These specialized sequences have the potential to identify cartilage degeneration at an earlier stage than is possible with current morphologic MRI sequences. Increased T1ρ signal in the area of impaction laterally after anterior cruciate ligament (ACL) injury has been correlated with significantly worse postinjury and postreconstruction pain and functional outcomes, providing a valuable tool for identifying otherwise subtle cartilage injury and allowing for better prediction of patient outcomes[4] (**Figure 4**). As feasibility studies are ongoing, these sequences are now most commonly used for research rather than clinical purposes.

Knee Arthroscopy

Indications

Knee arthroscopy with procedures including débridement, chondroplasty, loose body removal, microfracture, and partial meniscectomy is an acceptable treatment for appropriately indicated patients after

Table 1

Measurements of Lower Extremity Coronal Alignment

Measurement	How to Measure	Normal	Abnormal
Mechanical axis	Limb: A line drawn from the center of the femoral head to the center of the talar dome Femur: A line drawn from the center of the femoral head to the center of the knee Tibia: A line drawn from the center of the talar dome to the center of the knee	Limb mechanical axis passes immediately medial to the center of the knee, near medial tibial spine	Lateral location = genu valgum Medial location = genu varum
Anatomic axis	Line bisecting the medullary canal of the femur or tibia	Tibia: anatomic axis = mechanical axis Femur: anatomic axis is in 5°-7° valgus relative to mechanical axis	
Mechanical lateral distal femoral angle (mLDFA)	Lateral angle between the mechanical axis of the femur and a line tangent to the most distal point on the femoral condyles	85°-90°	Increased mLDFA = genu varum
Medial proximal tibial angle (MPTA)	Medial angle between the tibial mechanical axis and a line tangent to the proximal tibial plateau	85°-90°	Increased MPTA = genu valgum
Tibiofemoral angle	Angle between anatomic axis of tibia and femur	6°-7° valgus	
Mechanical axis deviation	Perpendicular distance between the limb's mechanical axis and center of the intercondylar notch	1-15 mm medial of midline	Medial deviation = genu varum Lateral deviation = genu valgum

Data from Paley D: *Principles of Deformity Correction*, ed 2. Berlin, Germany, Springer-Verlag, 2002.

failure of nonsurgical care. In the setting of nonfocal cartilage loss, arthroscopic intervention may be considered for alleviation of mechanical symptoms or significant effusion related to meniscal pathology, articular cartilage flaps, or loose bodies. These patients will typically present with complaints of knee swelling, locking, catching, or sudden giving way. Physical examination often reveals an effusion, joint line tenderness and positive meniscal signs including pain or palpable click with McMurray's test, pain with Thessaly's test or Apley's test, or pain while performing a deep squat. Importantly, patients should be made to understand that while alleviation of mechanical symptoms is relatively consistent, they may continue to have pain related to existing chondral wear.[5] In all cases, imaging findings should be diligently reviewed to determine the appropriate potential for improvement in each patient.

Surgical Approach

Palpable surface landmarks including the inferior pole of the patella, patellar tendon, and tibial plateau guide proper placement of arthroscopy portals. The anterolateral portal is established first, located directly adjacent to the lateral patellar tendon edge at the level of the joint line (below the inferior pole of the patella and proximal to the lateral tibial plateau). This primarily serves as a viewing portal. An anteromedial portal is established under direct visualization, first using a spinal needle to determine appropriate portal position and trajectory. Most basic arthroscopic procedures can be completed with these two portals, but occasionally, posteromedial and/or posterolateral portals may be necessary to retrieve loose bodies behind the cruciate ligaments or to treat injuries of the meniscal roots. Posteromedial and posterolateral portals should be placed under direct arthroscopic visualization using a spinal needle for localization, entering

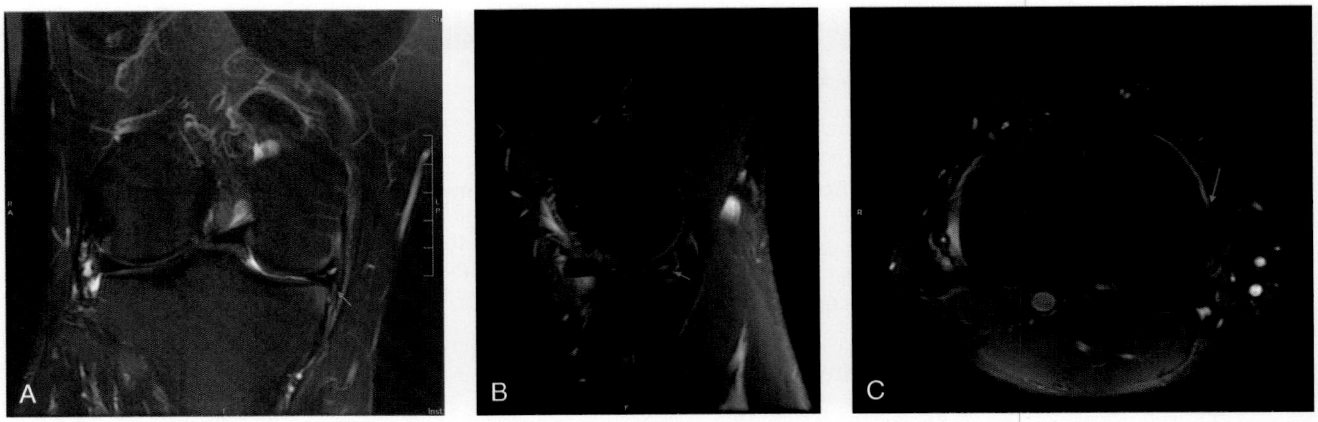

Figure 3 Magnetic resonance image of a displaced medial meniscus flap tear (arrows) abutting the medial collateral ligament in the following planes: coronal (**A**), sagittal (**B**), and axial(**C**).

the skin 1 cm proximal to the joint line and just posterior to the medial collateral ligament or lateral collateral ligament, respectively.

Outcomes

A landmark study by Moseley et al comparing arthroscopic débridement with sham surgery in patients with knee arthritis found no difference in postoperative pain or functional outcomes between groups.[6] Several subsequent studies specifically assessing outcomes after partial meniscectomy versus physical therapy for patients with knee osteoarthritis (OA) and a meniscal tear similarly have demonstrated no significant difference in outcomes between groups. However, about 30% of patients randomized to the physical therapy group crossed over and choose to undergo surgery because of continued pain, and good outcomes were achieved in patients who crossed over.[7,8] This suggests that while surgery should not be the initial recommendation for most patients with arthritis, even in the presence of meniscal tear, those who fail to improve with conservative measures can have good outcomes with delayed meniscectomy. Patients with mechanical symptoms in particular may benefit from arthroscopic débridement including partial meniscectomy and chondroplasty after failure of nonsurgical care.[5]

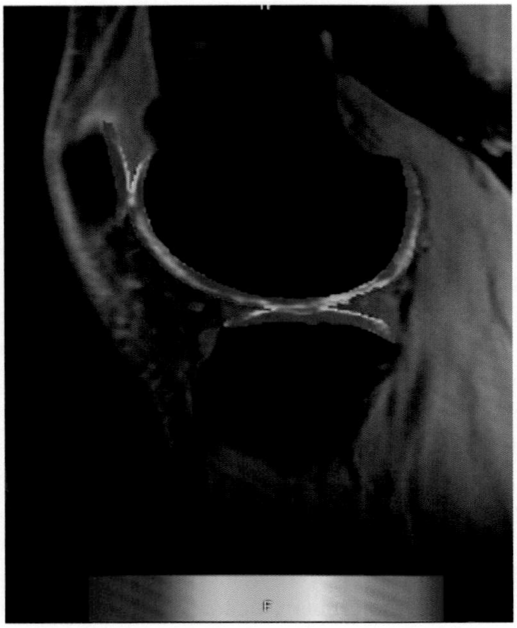

Figure 4 Select sagittal cuts of a T1ρ magnetic resonance image sequence showing focal cartilage breakdown over the posterior medial femoral condyle (red shading).

Knee Preservation

Cartilage Restoration Procedures

Patients with symptoms and physical examination findings localized to the site of focal full-thickness cartilage loss in the knee are candidates for cartilage restoration procedures. These procedures are not appropriate in the setting of multifocal cartilage loss, diffuse arthritis, or inflammatory arthropathy. Additionally, patients with unaddressed ligamentous instability, malalignment, or meniscal deficiency are not candidates for cartilage restoration procedures. Cartilage restoration procedures can be generally classified as bone marrow stimulation techniques, osteochondral autograft or allograft transplantation, and autologous or allogeneic cell-based therapies (**Table 2**).

Bone marrow stimulation techniques include abrasion chondroplasty and microfracture, which represent the most simple and cost-effective techniques. These are single-stage arthroscopic surgeries that fill the defect with nonhyaline fibrocartilaginous tissue and

Table 2

Cartilage Restoration Techniques

Category	Examples	Summary	Pros	Cons
Bone marrow stimulation techniques	• Abrasion chondroplasty • Microfracture	Subchondral bone is perforated to recruit mesenchymal stem cells (MSCs) from bone marrow into the cartilage defect, creating a fibrocartilaginous defect fill	• Technically easy • Cost-effective	• Osseous overgrowth[9] • Low MSC concentration with age[10] • Deterioration in clinical benefit over time[11]
Whole tissue transplantation	• Osteochondral autograft transfer • Osteochondral allograft transplantation	Osteochondral plugs from either allograft or autograft sources are used to replace areas of articular cartilage ± subchondral bone loss. Autologous grafts are harvested from a non–weight-bearing area of the knee (commonly superomedial/ superolateral trochlea or intercondylar notch)	• Single-stage surgery • Fills subchondral bone defects • Hyaline cartilage • Good revision and large defects • Precise surface contour matching (allograft)	• Donor site morbidity (autograft) • Risk of immunological rejection or disease transmission (allograft) • Expensive • Technically demanding
Autologous cell-based therapy	• ACI (autologous chondrocyte implantation) • MACI (autologous cultured chondrocytes on porcine collagen membrane)	Autologous chondrocytes are harvested and expanded in a laboratory, then reimplanted ± collagen scaffold	• Hyaline cartilage • Good outcomes in bipolar defects and patellofemoral joint[12] • Good outcomes in large lesions[13]	• Two-stage procedure • Expensive • Requires intact subchondral bone
Allograft cell-based therapy	• Particulated juvenile cartilage • Biocartilage	Fragmented cartilage allograft used to fill defect ± biologic adjuvant (ie, platelet-rich plasma), heals with hyaline-like cartilage[14,15]	• Single-stage surgery • Technically easy	• Cost • Lacking long-term outcome data

Data from Brown WE, Potter HG, Marx RG, Wickiewicz TL, Warren RF: Magnetic resonance imaging appearance of cartilage repair in the knee. *Clin Orthop Relat Res* 2004:214-223; Tran-Khanh N, Hoemann CD, McKee MD, Henderson JE, Buschmann MD: Aged bovine chondrocytes display a diminished capacity to produce a collagen-rich, mechanically functional cartilage extracellular matrix. *J Orthop Res* 2005;23:1354-1362; Kreuz PC, Erggelet C, Steinwachs MR, et al: Is microfracture of chondral defects in the knee associated with different results in patients aged 40 years or younger? *Arthroscopy* 2006;22:1180-1186; Gomoll AH, Gillogly SD, Cole BJ, et al: Autologous chondrocyte implantation in the patella: A multicenter experience. *Am J Sports Med* 2014;42:1074-1081; Rosenberger RE, Gomoll AH, Bryant T, Minas T: Repair of large chondral defects of the knee with autologous chondrocyte implantation in patients 45 years or older. *Am J Sports Med* 2008;36:2336-2344; Hirahara AM, Mueller KW Jr: BioCartilage: A New biomaterial to treat chondral lesions. *Sports Med Arthrosc Rev* 2015;23:143-148; and Yanke AB, Tilton AK, Wetters NG, Merkow DB, Cole BJ: DeNovo NT particulated juvenile cartilage implant. *Sports Med Arthrosc Rev* 2015;23:125-129.

present the risk of osseous overgrowth that can result in increased joint contact pressures.[9] There are also worse outcomes with larger cartilage defects or in patients with high body mass indexes. Additionally, mesenchymal stem cell (MSC) concentration decreases with age, which may render these procedures less efficacious in older patients, and despite promising short-term improvements, clinical deterioration has been shown across patients of all ages with long-term follow-up after knee microfracture.[10,11]

Autologous and allogeneic cell-based therapies allow for fill of cartilage-only defects (lesions with intact subchondral bone) with hyaline or hyaline-like cartilage, respectively. Autologous cell-based therapies, such as autologous chondrocyte implantation (ACI) and autologous cultured chondrocytes on porcine collagen membrane otherwise known as matrix-induced ACI (MACI), have demonstrated good clinical outcomes for treatment of large and even bipolar (abutting) lesions in the tibiofemoral and patellofemoral joints, with histology-proven hyaline cartilage fill.[12,13] These are both two-stage procedures, as they require initial chondrocyte biopsy with subsequent in vitro cell proliferation before final implantation. Alternatively, allograft-based therapies such as particulated juvenile cartilage (DeNovo, Zimmer-Biomet, Warsaw, IN, USA) or acellular extracellular matrix (Biocartilage, Arthrex, Naples, FL, USA) allow for single-stage treatment of cartilage-only defects using fragmented cartilage allograft with or without a biologic adjuvant such as platelet-rich plasma.[14,15] These have been shown to heal with cartilage that is histologically similar to hyaline cartilage, but long-term clinical data are not yet available.[15]

Osteochondral autograft transfer and osteochondral allograft transplantation are ideal options for large osteochondral lesions and revision cases. They are also the preferred method to address lesions that include bone loss in addition to cartilage loss. Both are single-stage procedures. Osteochondral autograft transfer utilizes a bone and cartilage plug harvested from the superomedial or superolateral trochlea or the intercondylar notch of the knee. These donor sites provide viable hyaline surfaces, but an imprecise contour match. Use of autograft is generally limited by the size of the defect and availability of good articular cartilage from the donor sites. On the the hand, osteochondral allograft transplantation allows surgeons to address very large defects with precise contour matching, but size-matched donors take a variable time to become available, and the allograft is expensive (**Figure 5**). Additionally, while donor site morbidity is avoided with use of allograft, the risks of immunological response and disease transmission are introduced.[16]

Meniscal Preservation

Meniscal injury is identified on MRI in 31% of asymptomatic athletes and 91% of patients with knee osteoarthritis.[17,18] Consideration of treatment for meniscal tears therefore relies heavily on patient history and clinical examination. In nonarthritic knees, focal joint line tenderness, effusion, and positive meniscal signs on physical examination may indicate meniscal pathology as a symptomatic source worthy of surgical intervention. In the presence of OA, mechanical symptoms such as locking or catching in combination with unstable meniscal tears on MRI warrant intervention, but débridement of stable meniscal tears is unlikely to provide lasting relief.[5-8] Historically, it was common to perform total menisectomies, but the procedure is now rarely performed, as the relative risk of OA after undergoing total meniscectomy is 14.0, with 4% cartilage loss per year.[19,20] Whenever possible, meniscal repair is preferred to partial meniscectomy, as the extent of subsequent joint degeneration is directly proportional to the amount of meniscal tissue removed.[21] The benefit of meniscal repair is balanced with an increased risk of revision surgery after meniscal repair (20.7%) as compared with partial meniscectomy (3.9%).[22]

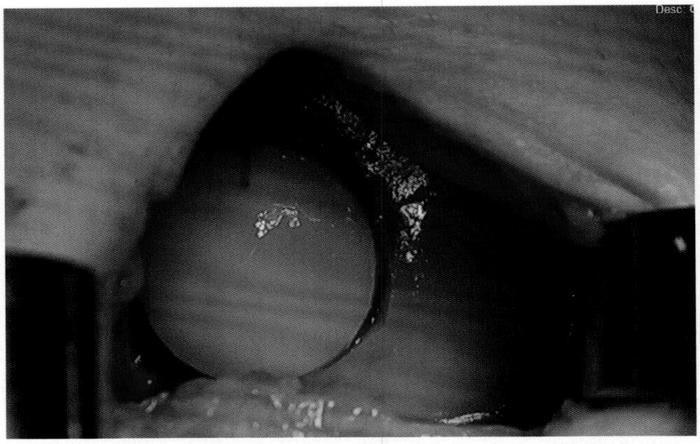

Figure 5 Intraoperative photograph showing osteochondral allograft transplantation of a large, unstable medial femoral condyle osteochondral defect.

Despite best efforts, large meniscal tears are occasionally not salvageable, most often in the setting of chronic injury. In patients who have undergone total or subtotal meniscectomy and develop symptomatic meniscal deficiency, meniscal allograft transplantation affords a reconstructive opportunity. Meniscal transplantation is contraindicated in knees with diffuse arthritic changes, morbid obesity, age over 50 years, or unaddressed ligamentous instability, limb malalignment, or chondral defects.[23] Allografts may be implanted with the meniscal soft tissue only, secured to the capsule and root attachment sites through standard repair techniques, or with a bone block including the bony insertion of the anterior and posterior meniscal roots inserted into a prepared bone trough in the recipient's knee. Use of an allograft with a bone block is more common for lateral meniscus transplantation because of the minimal distance between anterior and posterior root attachments making soft-tissue fixation more difficult (**Figure 6**).

Both medial and lateral meniscal allograft transplantation result in significant improvements in pain, quality of life, and functional outcomes compared with preoperative scores, even despite progressive joint space narrowing at long-term follow-up.[24] Meniscal transplantation allows patients to return to the same level of athletic competition 75% to 85% of the time.[25] Overall failure rate (conversion to total knee arthroplasty) ranges from 10% to 29% in long-term follow-up.[25] Although the survivorship of meniscal

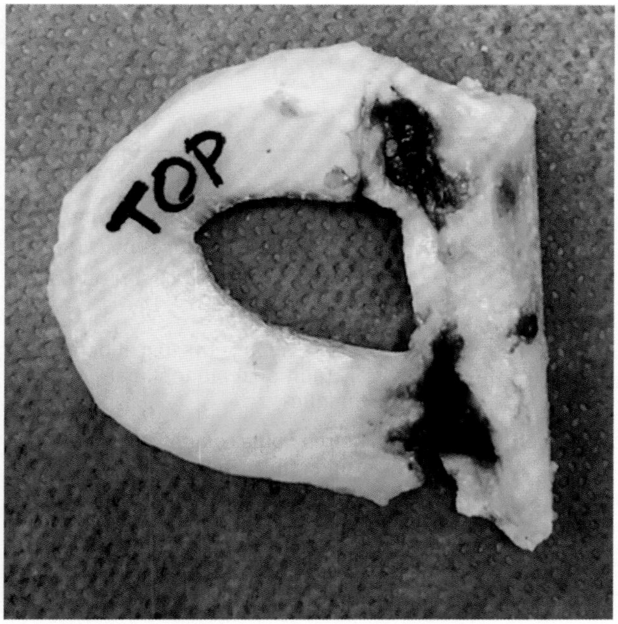

Figure 6 Photograph of lateral meniscus allograft with bone block. Note the close proximity of the anterior and posterior roots of the meniscus, marked with purple on the bone block.

transplantation is imperfect, the procedure provides patients the ability to improve quality of life and delay arthroplasty.

Realignment Osteotomies About the Knee

Lower extremity malalignment may occur physiologically or as a result of trauma, growth disturbance, or age-related degenerative changes. Small changes in limb alignment can result in significant increases in compartment peak pressures.[26] Correction of malalignment and offloading of the affected compartment can be obtained with osteotomy of the proximal tibia (high tibial osteotomy, HTO) or distal femur (distal femoral osteotomy, DFO). For the purposes of knee preservation, these osteotomies are most commonly done for correction of coronal plane malalignment (**Table 3**). Opening and closing wedge osteotomies are most common, although dome and chevron osteotomies can also be considered. Contraindications to osteotomy include multicompartmental degenerative changes, inflammatory arthritis, arc of motion less than 120°, more than 5° flexion contracture, extreme deformities with tibial subluxation, and age over 65 years.[27]

Genu varum is associated with increased contact stress on the medial compartment of the knee and can be corrected with lateral closing wedge or medial opening wedge HTO. Lateral closing wedge HTO has more inherent stability, but requires fibular osteotomy with disruption of the proximal tibiofibular joint, risks peroneal nerve injury, and results in distal tibia bone stock loss, which can increase the difficulty of subsequent knee arthroplasty.[28] Medial opening wedge techniques allow for precise correction of malalignment with the use of wedged plates, bone graft, or bone graft substitutes of a defined size to accommodate the desired correction. The downsides of opening wedge HTO include the need to be non-weight bearing for approximately 6 weeks postoperatively because of the risk of collapse with loss of correction, and the risk of patella baja, which may increase patellofemoral contact pressures and make future knee arthroplasty more challenging. Although most surgeons prefer medial opening wedge HTOs, both techniques provide excellent improvement in knee pain and function.[28]

Medial opening wedge HTO can also be performed in a biplanar fashion using a retrotubercle cut. By preferentially opening the medial wedge cut posteriorly, the tibial slope can be decreased to account for ACL deficiency or to correct for excessive native tibial slope, which has been correlated with increased risk for ACL reconstruction failure, particularly when in excess of 12°.[29] As compared with traditional monoplanar medial opening wedge HTO, the biplanar technique can prevent patella baja when the cut leaves the tubercle attached to the proximal tibial segment and has more inherent stability, thus lowering the risk of subsequent loss of angular correction.[30,31] Literature comparing clinical outcomes of biplanar with traditional monoplanar medial opening wedge HTO is lacking, and given its increased complexity, most surgeons continue to use monoplanar medial opening wedge HTO techniques.

Lateral joint compartment stresses are increased with valgus malalignment of the knee and can be improved with a lateral opening wedge DFO, medial closing wedge DFO, or a medial closing wedge HTO. HTO for the treatment of genu valgum has the added benefit of offloading the lateral compartment in both flexion and extension, whereas DFO only affects joint forces in knee extension due to articulation of the posterior rather than distal femur with the tibia during knee flexion. On the other hand, HTO creates obliquity of the knee joint line, resulting in shear forces across the knee and eventual tibial subluxation.[32] Although medial closing wedge HTO (varus-producing) was historically the benchmark for offloading the lateral compartment, these patients experienced signicantly worse outcomes than either varus-producing DFO or valgus-producing HTO.[33,34] This led surgeons to favor DFO for correction of large valgus deformity. Lateral opening wedge and medial closing wedge DFOs both result in significant improvements in pain and function postoperatively and have similar

Knee

Table 3

Correctional Osteotomies About the Knee

Deformity	Osteotomy	Pros	Cons
Genu varum (medial compartment overload)	Monoplanar medial opening wedge high tibial osteotomy (HTO)	• Precise correction	• Patella baja • Requires limited weight bearing • Requires bone graft or substitute • Risk of collapse, loss of correction
	Biplanar medial opening wedge HTO	• Avoids patella baja • Can correct tibial slope • Inherent stability after cut	• Complex technique • Lacking evidence of clinical benefit over traditional monoplanar technique
	Lateral closing wedge HTO	• Inherent stability after cut	• Requires fibular osteotomy (disrupts proximal tibia-fibula joint) • Peroneal nerve injury • Distal bone stock loss
Genu valgum (lateral compartment overload)	Lateral opening wedge distal femoral osteotomy (DFO)	• Lateral approach to femur • No limb shortening • No joint line alteration	• Traction neurapraxia • Does not offload in flexion • Requires bone graft or substitute • Requires limited weight bearing
	Medial closing wedge DFO	• Inherent stability after cut • No joint line alteration	• Medial approach to femur • Limb shortening • Does not offload in flexion
	Medial closing wedge HTO	• Offloads lateral compartment in extension AND flexion	• Oblique joint line • Worse clinical outcomes than DFO[25,34]

Data from Samitier G, Alentorn-Geli E, Taylor DC, et al: Meniscal allograft transplantation. Part 2: systematic review of transplant timing, outcomes, return to competition, associated procedures, and prevention of osteoarthritis. *Knee Surg Sport Traumatol Arthrosc*: official journal of the ESSKA 2015;23:323-333; and Maquet P. The treatment of choice in osteoarthritis of the knee. *Clin Orthop Relat Res* 1985:108-112.

nonunion rates, complication rates, and survivorship.[35] Closing wedge DFO offers the advantage of improved stability after osteotomy, but by removing bone, it both shortens the limb and alters distal bone stock for future arthroplasty. Opening wedge DFO utilizes the more familiar lateral approach to the distal femur and offers precise angular correction. By lengthening the limb, lateral opening wedge DFO can result in traction neurapraxia with large corrections, and also requires the use of bone graft or substitute along with a period of protected weight bearing because of decreased stability.

Knee Reconstruction

Unicompartmental Knee Arthroplasty

Unicompartmental knee arthroplasty (UKA) is another option for patients with OA limited to a single tibiofemoral compartment. The classic indications for UKA described by Kozinn and Scott in 1989 have been expanded, as newer studies have demonstrated good outcomes in both young and obese patients.[36,37] Modern indications for UKA include unicompartmental OA, at least 90° arc of motion, flexion contracture less than 15°, and minimal pain at rest.[36] Exclusion criteria include inflammatory arthritis, hemochromatosis, hemophilia, chondrocalcinosis, severe lateral patella facet disease, and ligamentous instability.[38] The decision between UKA and HTO or DFO is often made based on surgeon preference, given the significant overlap in surgical indications. Although UKA is more commonly performed for medial compartment OA, equally good results are seen at short- and long-term follow-up in lateral UKA.[39] Although some modern UKA studies report 10-year survivorship exceeding 90%, registry data do not bear this out, as studies have shown higher long-term revision rates for UKA, particularly for surgeons with UKA comprising 5% or less of their arthroplasty practice.[40] This may depend significantly on surgeon volume, which could account for the higher success in smaller studies. Additionally, later revision to TKA yields functional outcomes similar to revision TKA in some studies, as opposed to primary TKA.[41]

Patellofemoral arthroplasty (PFA) is indicated in patients with symptomatic isolated patellofemoral arthritis that has failed to improve with conservative treatment. Contraindications to PFA include tibiofemoral OA, unaddressed coronal malalignment or ligamentous instability, inflammatory arthropathy, or infection.[42] Anterior knee pain may persist in 7% to 19% of patients after PFA, but second-generation implants with improved trochlear designs now yield good to excellent outcomes in 66% to 100% of patients at both short- and long-term follow-up.[43] Early PFA implants were associated with significantly increased rates of revision surgery (odds ratio [OR] 4.33) and revision arthroplasty (OR 3.60), but second-generation PFA designs now yield no difference in rates of revision surgery, revision, complications, mechanical complaints, or pain when compared with TKA. However, some studies continue to report lower patient satisfaction rates.[44,45] The most common cause of PFA failure is progression of tibiofemoral OA.[46] Although PFA is a good option for select patients, the indications make it a relatively rare procedure.

Total Knee Arthroplasty

After failure of conservative care for knee OA, total knee arthroplasty (TKA) consistently provides substantial improvements in pain, function, and patient satisfaction with excellent survivorship.[47] TKA is a highly cost-effective surgical treatment and is the mainstay of surgical approaches for addressing advanced arthritis. Controversy remains with regard to alignment and surgical technique. Many studies have compared gap balancing versus measured resection techniques, and cruciate retaining (CR) versus posterior stabilized (PS) implants with essentially equivalent outcomes in terms of pain, function, and survivorship.[48] All of these techniques are well-studied and viable options for performing TKA. However, debate remains over treatment of the patella, with studies showing good outcomes with and without patellar resurfacing.[49] Importantly, no studies have convincingly shown that minimally invasive techniques or newer technologies, such as patient-specific instrumentation (PSI), can lead to improved outcomes or decreased complications.[50-52]

Surgical Technique and Implant Choice in TKA

When performing TKA, limb alignment remains an area of controversy, with studies advocating for both mechanical and kinematic alignment. There are limited data with direct comparison between techniques, but a recent randomized controlled trial showed no significant difference in functional outcomes at 2 years when comparing both alignment techniques.[53]

Cruciate ligament management during TKA is another area of continued debate. CR, which preserves the posterior cruciate ligament (PCL), and PS, where both the ACL and PCL are removed, TKA techniques both provide good results with no difference in surgical complications, range of motion, patient-reported outcome scores, or implant survivorship.[48] Bicruciate retaining (BCR) knee arthroplasty, where both the ACL and PCL are retained, has been proposed to preserve intra-articular proprioception and native joint kinematics. Single-surgeon studies have shown good outcomes after BCR TKA, but it is a technically demanding surgery. Because some studies have shown high early failure rates, adoption of BCR TKA has been limited.[54,55]

Although traditional fixed-bearing TKA implants have excellent long-term survival, mobile bearing implants are also a viable option. Mobile bearing TKA implants were developed to allow for increased tibiofemoral contact area with reduced polyethylene contact stress and wear.[56] However, studies have not demonstrated improved survivorship in mobile bearing TKA.[56] Careful attention must be paid to gap balancing when using mobile bearing implants, as bearing spin-out can occur in the presence of a loose flexion gap. Both implant types provide significant improvements in pain and function, with no significant differences in pain, function, quality of life, complication, or revision rates between implant designs.[56] All-polyethylene or metal-backed monoblock tibial components have also shown good long-term outcomes and are reasonable options for implant choice.

As TKA is increasingly performed in younger patients, there has been a resurgence of interest in noncemented TKA, with improved implant design and instrumentation. Outcome studies of modern noncemented TKA implants show survivorship and functional outcomes equivalent to cemented prostheses.[57] Long-term studies will determine if these designs are indeed better for younger patients with good bone stock.

New Technologies in TKA

PSI utilizes custom cutting jigs created based on preoperative magnetic resonance or CT scans. The goal behind developing this technology was to potentially improve bone cut accuracy and resultant postoperative limb alignment, decrease surgical times, and improve operating room efficiency by decreasing the number of instrument trays needed per case. There is conflicting evidence, as some studies have reported shorter surgical and turnover times, with improved alignment accuracy with PSI TKAs as compared with conventional TKA techniques.[48] However, other studies report no improvement or even worsening of these variables when using PSI.[50]

Computer-assisted navigation is another tool aimed at improving component positioning by using markers affixed to defined bony landmarks that are tracked in three dimensions. These landmarks are then integrated into a software that determines appropriate bony cuts and can also assist with soft-tissue gap balancing. Overall, current literature reports improved component positioning but increased surgical time with use of navigation technology for TKA.[58] There is insufficient evidence to determine whether the improved component alignment with computer-assisted navigation leads to improved functional outcomes postoperatively.

Robotic systems have also been introduced for use in TKA and can be described as either passive, semiactive, or active.[51] Each system utilizes imaging-based preoperative planning software to determine appropriate component size and position. In passive systems, the robot holds a cutting guide in a location determined by the preoperative planning software while the surgeon controls and completes all bone cuts with manual instruments. Semiactive systems provide haptic feedback that augments the surgeon's control of manual cutting tools by limiting their reach within space. Active robotic systems autonomously perform the surgical procedure without direct input from the surgeon. The cost of robotic systems is significant up front and for single-use materials for each surgery. Robots are also imperfect, and problems such as registration failure, software issues, and patellar tendon damage have been reported.[59] Current literature endorses a reduction in outliers of limb alignment with robotic-assisted TKA, but no significant difference in clinical outcome sores as compared with conventional TKA.[51,52] More studies are needed to determine if PSI, navigation, and robotics will lead to improved survivorship and better long-term outcomes, especially given the added costs and time.

Summary

Cartilage injury in the knee can be focal, isolated to one joint compartment, or diffuse. Assessment of the joint must combine physical examination along with radiographic (including full-length alignment views) and MRI findings. In some cases, arthroscopy can be beneficial for patients with OA and mechanical symptoms recalcitrant to conservative care, but this should not be the first-line intervention. Arthroscopic treatment is indicated for the following procedures: débridement, chondroplasty, loose body removal, microfracture, and partial menisectomy. Treatment for focal cartilage lesions depends upon the lesion size, lesion location, and the status of the underlying subchondral bone. These treatment options include bone marrow stimulation techniques, osteochondral autograft or allograft transplantation, autologous cell-based therapy, and allograft cell-based therapies. In the case of symptomatic meniscal deficiency, allograft meniscal transplantation can provide significant symptomatic relief and improvements in quality of life, although radiographic OA may still progress.

Significant cartilage damage isolated to one joint compartment can be effectively treated with an offloading HTO or UKA. TKA is effective at improving pain and function in patients with tricompartmental OA using various surgical techniques leading to good outcomes. Implant options include CR, PS; fixed or mobile bearing; and cemented or noncemented. PSI, computer navigation, and robotic-assisted technologies may marginally improve component position and limb alignment, but require further studies of long-term clinical benefit and cost-effectiveness to determine their optimal role in TKA.

Key Study Points

- Arthroscopic knee débridement may provide relief from mechanical symptoms in carefully selected osteoarthritis (OA) patients, but should not be offered as a first-line treatment in lieu of nonsurgical measures. Patients may continue to have pain because of underlying OA, but mechanical symptoms are more reliably improved.
- Correction of ligamentous instability and limb malalignment is paramount to success of cartilage restoration procedures and meniscal transplantation.
- Surgical options for treatment of focal cartilage injury include bone marrow stimulation techniques (microfracture, abrasion chondroplasty), osteochondral autograft or allograft transplantation, autologous cell-based therapy (autologous chondrocyte implantation ± collagen membrane), and allograft therapies (particulated juvenile cartilage or acellular extracellular matrix).
- For isolated medial compartment degeneration, surgical options include medial opening wedge high tibial osteotomy (HTO), lateral closing wedge HTO, or unicompartmental knee arthroplasty (UKA). Lateral compartment OA can be treated with lateral closing wedge distal femoral osteotomy (DFO), medial opening wedge DFO, medial closing wedge HTO, or UKA.
- Multiple TKA implant designs (cruciate retaining [CR], posterior stabilized [PS], or bicruciate retaining [BCR]; fixed or mobile bearing, cemented or noncemented) and surgical techniques (conventional, patient-specific instrumentation [PSI], computer navigated, or robot-assisted) have been successful in improving patient pain and function without any overwhelming evidence favoring one over the other.

Annotated References

1. Phelan N, Rowland P, Galvin R, O'Byrne JM: A systematic review and meta-analysis of the diagnostic accuracy of MRI for suspected ACL and meniscal tears of the knee. *Knee Surg Sport Traumatol Arthrosc* 2016;24:1525-1539.

   A systematic review quantifying the accuracy of MRI for detection of meniscal injury and ACL tear. Level of evidence: III.

2. Galea A, Giuffre B, Dimmick S, Coolican MR, Parker DA: The accuracy of magnetic resonance imaging scanning and its influence on management decisions in knee surgery. *Arthroscopy* 2009;25:473-480.
3. Guermazi A, Alizai H, Crema MD, Trattnig S, Regatte RR, Roemer FW: Compositional MRI techniques for evaluation of cartilage degeneration in osteoarthritis. *Osteoarthritis Cartilage* 2015;23:1639-1653.
4. Wang A, Pedoia V, Su F, et al: MR T1ρ and T2 of meniscus after acute anterior cruciate ligament injuries. *Osteoarthritis Cartilage* 2016;24:631-639.

   The authors present a summary of compositional MRI techniques (ie, T1ρ, T2*, dGEMRIC, gagCEST) used for early recognition of cartilage degeneration. Level of evidence: IV.

5. Buldu MT, Marsh JL, Arbuthnot J: Mechanical symptoms of osteoarthritis in the knee and arthroscopy. *J Knee Surg* 2016;29:396-402.

   A retrospective analysis of consecutive patients with knee osteoarthritis undergoing knee arthroscopy for treatment of mechanical symptoms, which found significant improvements in patient-reported outcome scores, pain, and mechanical symptoms. Level of evidence: III.

6. Moseley JB, O'Malley K, Petersen NJ, et al: A controlled trial of arthroscopic surgery for osteoarthritis of the knee. *N Engl J Med* 2002;347:81-88.
7. Herrlin SV, Wange PO, Lapidus G, Hallander M, Werner S, Weidenhielm L: Is arthroscopic surgery beneficial in treating non-traumatic, degenerative medial meniscal tears? A five year follow-up. *Knee Surg Sport Traumatol Arthrosc* 2013;21:358-364.
8. Katz JN, Brophy RH, Chaisson CE, et al: Surgery versus physical therapy for a meniscal tear and osteoarthritis. *N Engl J Med* 2013;368:1675-1684.
9. Brown WE, Potter HG, Marx RG, Wickiewicz TL, Warren RF: Magnetic resonance imaging appearance of cartilage repair in the knee. *Clin Orthop Relat Res* 2004:214-223.
10. Tran-Khanh N, Hoemann CD, McKee MD, Henderson JE, Buschmann MD: Aged bovine chondrocytes display a diminished capacity to produce a collagen-rich, mechanically functional cartilage extracellular matrix. *J Orthop Res* 2005;23:1354-1362.
11. Kreuz PC, Erggelet C, Steinwachs MR, et al: Is microfracture of chondral defects in the knee associated with different results in patients aged 40 years or younger? *Arthroscopy* 2006;22:1180-1186.
12. Gomoll AH, Gillogly SD, Cole BJ, et al: Autologous chondrocyte implantation in the patella: A multicenter experience. *Am J Sports Med* 2014;42:1074-1081.
13. Rosenberger RE, Gomoll AH, Bryant T, Minas T: Repair of large chondral defects of the knee with autologous chondrocyte implantation in patients 45 years or older. *Am J Sports Med* 2008;36:2336-2344.
14. Hirahara AM, Mueller KW Jr: BioCartilage: A New biomaterial to treat chondral lesions. *Sports Med Arthrosc Rev* 2015;23:143-148.
15. Yanke AB, Tilton AK, Wetters NG, Merkow DB, Cole BJ: DeNovo NT particulated juvenile cartilage implant. *Sports Med Arthrosc Rev* 2015;23:125-129.
16. Getgood A, Bollen S: What tissue bankers should know about the use of allograft tendons and cartilage in orthopaedics. *Cell Tissue Bank* 2010;11(1):87-97.
17. Bhattacharyya T, Gale D, Dewire P, et al: The clinical importance of meniscal tears demonstrated by magnetic resonance imaging in osteoarthritis of the knee. *J Bone Joint Surg Am* 2003;85-a:4-9.
18. Beals CT, Magnussen RA, Graham WC, Flanigan DC: The prevalence of meniscal pathology in asymptomatic athletes. *Sport Med* 2016;46:1517-1524.

   A systematic review of asymptomatic meniscal pathology in athletes which describes isolated meniscal pathology (including intrasubstance meniscal signal) in 31% and frank meniscal tear in 3.9%. Level of evidence: IV.

19. Roos H, Lauren M, Adalberth T, Roos EM, Jonsson K, Lohmander LS: Knee osteoarthritis after meniscectomy: Prevalence of radiographic changes after twenty-one years, compared with matched controls. *Arthritis Rheum* 1998;41:687-693.
20. Cicuttini FM, Forbes A, Yuanyuan W, Rush G, Stuckey SL: Rate of knee cartilage loss after partial meniscectomy. *J Rheumatol* 2002;29:1954-1956.
21. Hede A, Larsen E, Sandberg H: The long term outcome of open total and partial meniscectomy related to the quantity and site of the meniscus removed. *Int Orthop* 1992;16:122-125.
22. Paxton ES, Stock MV, Brophy RH: Meniscal repair versus partial meniscectomy: A systematic review comparing reoperation rates and clinical outcomes. *Arthroscopy* 2011;27:1275-1288.
23. Brophy RH, Matava MJ: Surgical options for meniscal replacement. *J Am Acad Orthop Surg* 2012;20:265-272.
24. Vundelinckx B, Vanlauwe J, Bellemans J: Long-term subjective, clinical, and radiographic outcome evaluation of meniscal allograft transplantation in the knee. *Am J Sports Med* 2014;42:1592-1599.
25. Samitier G, Alentorn-Geli E, Taylor DC, et al: Meniscal allograft transplantation. Part 2: Systematic review of transplant timing, outcomes, return to competition, associated procedures, and prevention of osteoarthritis. *Knee Surg Sport Traumatol Arthrosc* 2015;23:323-333.

26. Hsu RW, Himeno S, Coventry MB, Chao EY: Normal axial alignment of the lower extremity and load-bearing distribution at the knee. *Clin Orthop Relat Res* 1990:215-227.

27. Uquillas C, Rossy W, Nathasingh CK, Strauss E, Jazrawi L, Gonzalez-Lomas G: Osteotomies about the knee: AAOS exhibit selection. *J Bone Joint Surg Am* 2014;96:e199.

28. Rossi R, Bonasia DE, Amendola A: The role of high tibial osteotomy in the varus knee. *J Am Acad Orthop Surg* 2011;19:590-599.

29. Tischer T, Paul J, Pape D, et al: The impact of osseous malalignment and realignment procedures in knee ligament surgery: A systematic review of the clinical evidence. *Orthop J Sports Med* 2017;5.

A systematic review summarizing the impact of three-dimensional knee osseous malalignment on the outcome of knee ligament reconstruction. Level of evidence: IV.

30. Elmali N, Esenkaya I, Can M, Karakaplan M: Monoplanar versus biplanar medial open-wedge proximal tibial osteotomy for varus gonarthrosis: A comparison of clinical and radiological outcomes. *Knee Surg Sport Traumatol Arthrosc* 2013;21:2689-2695.

31. Pape D, Lorbach O, Schmitz C, et al: Effect of a biplanar osteotomy on primary stability following high tibial osteotomy: A biomechanical cadaver study. *Knee Surg Sport Traumatol Arthrosc* 2010;18:204-211.

32. Coventry MB: Osteotomy about the knee for degenerative and rheumatoid arthritis. *J Bone Joint Surg Am* 1973;55:23-48.

33. Sherman SL, Thompson SF, Clohisy JCF: Distal femoral varus osteotomy for the management of valgus deformity of the knee. *J Am Acad Orthop Surg* 2018;26:313-324.

A review article summarizing the history, indications, technique, and outcomes of distal femoral varus-producing osteotomy for treatment of genu valgum. Level of evidence: IV.

34. Maquet P: The treatment of choice in osteoarthritis of the knee. *Clin Orthop Relat Res* 1985:108-112.

35. Chahla J, Mitchell JJ, Liechti DJ, et al: Opening- and closing-wedge distal femoral osteotomy: A systematic review of outcomes for isolated lateral compartment osteoarthritis. *Orthop J Sports Med* 2016;4:2325967116649901.

A systematic review describing the outcomes of both medial closing and lateral opening wedge distal femoral osteotomies for treatment of lateral compartment knee OA. Level of evidence: IV.

36. Thompson SA, Liabaud B, Nellans KW, Geller JA: Factors associated with poor outcomes following unicompartmental knee arthroplasty: Redefining the "classic" indications for surgery. *J Arthroplasty* 2013;28:1561-1564.

37. Kozinn SC, Scott R: Unicondylar knee arthroplasty. *J Bone Joint Surg Am* 1989;71:145-150.

38. Berger RA, Meneghini RM, Jacobs JJ, et al: Results of unicompartmental knee arthroplasty at a minimum of ten years of follow-up. *J Bone Joint Surg Am* 2005;87:999-1006.

39. van der List JP, McDonald LS, Pearle AD: Systematic review of medial versus lateral survivorship in unicompartmental knee arthroplasty. *Knee* 2015;22:454-460.

40. Liddle AD, Pandit H, Judge A, Murray DW: Optimal usage of unicompartmental knee arthroplasty: A study of 41,986 cases from the National Joint Registry for England and Wales. *Bone Joint J* 2015;97-B:1506-1511.

41. Leta TH, Lygre SH, Skredderstuen A, et al: Outcomes of unicompartmental knee arthroplasty after aseptic revision to total knee arthroplasty: A comparative study of 768 TKAs and 578 UKAs revised to TKAs from the Norwegian Arthroplasty Register (1994 to 2011). *J Bone Joint Surg* 2016;98:431-440.

A large registry-based study comparing the outcomes of revision UKA → TKA and revision TKA → TKA. Level of evidence: III.

42. Pisanu G, Rosso F, Bertolo C, et al: Patellofemoral arthroplasty: Current concepts and review of the literature. *Joints* 2017;5:237-245.

A review of the history, implant design improvements, indications, techniques, and outcomes of patellofemoral arthroplasty. Level of evidence: IV.

43. Walker T, Perkinson B, Mihalko WM: Patellofemoral arthroplasty: The other unicompartmental knee replacement. *J Bone Joint Surg Am* 2012;94:1712-1720.

44. Dy CJ, Franco N, Ma Y, Mazumdar M, McCarthy MM, Gonzalez Della Valle A: Complications after patello-femoral versus total knee replacement in the treatment of isolated patello-femoral osteoarthritis. A meta-analysis. *Knee Surg Sport Traumatol Arthrosc* 2012;20:2174-2190.

45. Kazarian GS, Tarity TD, Hansen EN, Cai J, Lonner JH: Significant functional improvement at 2 years after isolated patellofemoral arthroplasty with an onlay trochlear implant, but low mental health scores predispose to dissatisfaction. *J Arthroplasty* 2016;31:389-394.

A retrospective cohort analysis defining the impact of low mental health scores on patient satisfaction after patellofemoral arthroplasty despite satisfactory radiographic and clinical outcomes. Level of evidence: III.

46. van der List JP, Chawla H, Villa JC, Pearle AD: Why do patellofemoral arthroplasties fail today? A systematic review. *Knee* 2017;24:2-8.

A review comparing older (before 2000) and more recent (after 2000) literature describing failure of patellofemoral arthroplasty, aimed at identifying causes for failure of PFA with modern implant design. Level of evidence: III.

47. Jauregui JJ, Cherian JJ, Pierce TP, Beaver WB, Issa K, Mont MA: Long-term survivorship and clinical outcomes following total knee arthroplasty. *J Arthroplasty* 2015;30:2164-2166.

48. Li N, Tan Y, Deng Y, Chen L: Posterior cruciate-retaining versus posterior stabilized total knee arthroplasty: A meta-analysis of randomized controlled trials. *Knee Surg Sport Traumatol Arthrosc* 2014;22:556-564.

49. He JY, Jiang LS, Dai LY: Is patellar resurfacing superior than nonresurfacing in total knee arthroplasty? A meta-analysis of randomized trials. *Knee* 2011;18:137-144.

50. Voleti PB, Hamula MJ, Baldwin KD, Lee GC: Current data do not support routine use of patient-specific instrumentation in total knee arthroplasty. *J Arthroplasty* 2014;29:1709-1712.

51. Banerjee S, Cherian JJ, Elmallah RK, Jauregui JJ, Pierce TP, Mont MA: Robotic-assisted knee arthroplasty. *Expert Rev Med Devices* 2015;12:727-735.

52. Liow MH, Xia Z, Wong MK, Tay KJ, Yeo SJ, Chin PL: Robot-assisted total knee arthroplasty accurately restores the joint line and mechanical axis. A prospective randomised study. *J Arthroplasty* 2014;29:2373-2377.

53. Young SW, Walker ML, Bayan A, Briant-Evans T, Pavlou P, Farrington B: The Chitranjan S. Ranawat Award: No difference in 2-year functional outcomes using kinematic versus mechanical alignment in TKA: A randomized controlled clinical trial. *Clin Orthop Relat Res* 2017;475:9-20.

    An impactful randomized controlled trial demonstrating no difference in outcomes with utilization of either kinematic alignment, which aims to match the patient's prearthritic anatomy, or neutral mechanical alignment. Level of evidence: I.

54. Christensen JC, Brothers J, Stoddard GJ, et al: Higher frequency of reoperation with a new bicruciate-retaining total knee arthroplasty. *Clin Orthop Relat Res* 2017;475:62-69.

    A prospective study of patients undergoing bicruciate-retaining TKA specifically focused on revision rates. Level of evidence: III.

55. Pritchett JW: Bicruciate-retaining total knee replacement provides satisfactory function and implant survivorship at 23 years. *Clin Orthop Relat Res* 2015;473:2327-2333.

56. Hofstede SN, Nouta KA, Jacobs W, et al: Mobile bearing vs fixed bearing prostheses for posterior cruciate retaining total knee arthroplasty for postoperative functional status in patients with osteoarthritis and rheumatoid arthritis. *Cochrane Database Syst Rev* 2015:CD003130.

57. Cherian JJ, Banerjee S, Kapadia BH, Jauregui JJ, Harwin SF, Mont MA: Cementless total knee arthroplasty: A review. *J Knee Surg* 2014;27:193-197.

58. Alcelik IA, Blomfield MI, Diana G, Gibbon AJ, Carrington N, Burr S: A comparison of short-term outcomes of minimally invasive computer-assisted vs minimally invasive conventional instrumentation for primary total knee arthroplasty: A systematic review and meta-analysis. *J Arthroplasty* 2016;31:410-418.

    A meta-analysis of literature describing outcomes after computer-assisted versus traditional minimally invasive TKA. Level of evidence: II.

59. Netravali NA, Shen F, Park Y, Bargar WL: A perspective on robotic assistance for knee arthroplasty. *Adv Orthop* 2013;2013.

60. Paley D: *Principles of Deformity Correction*, ed 2. Berlin, Germany, Springer-Verlag, 2002.

Section 9

Foot and Ankle

EDITOR

Brian S. Winters, MD

Chapter 42

Foot and Ankle Anatomy and Biomechanics

Adam G. Miller, MD • Benjamin E. Stein, MD

ABSTRACT

This chapter examines the recent advances in anatomy and biomechanics of the foot and ankle. Achieving anatomic syndesmotic reduction has been a focus of recent literature. Appropriate radiographs are the first line of imaging a surgeon obtains. Ankle reconstruction and total ankle arthroplasty continue to be explored as an alternative to fusion. Gait analysis is a useful tool in research to identify patient outcomes.

Keywords: anatomy; biomechanics; gait; imaging; syndesmosis; total ankle

Introduction

An understanding of the structure of the foot and ankle is imperative to treat it successfully. The forces applied to these structures and how the foot and ankle move give us insight to normal function and treating pathology. This chapter examines the recent advances in anatomy and biomechanics of the foot and ankle.

Anatomy: Osseous

Twenty-eight bones make up the foot, creating a support for the ankle and rest of the lower extremity. One can think of the foot as a tripod where the calcaneus, first metatarsal head, and lesser metatarsal heads act as three pillars of support. Deviation from this creates uneven stress to the foot resulting in pathology. There is inherent stability and flexibility to the foot. With eversion, the chopart joints unlock and become parallel to allow for accommodation to the ground. When the foot inverts and prepares for impact (such as during running), the chopart joints are not parallel and stiffen the foot. The ankle has inherent bony stability due to the mortise and tenon joint design. The talus acts as the tenon fitting into the mortise comprised of the tibia and fibula.

The syndesmosis stabilizes the mortise while still allowing for rotation and translation of the fibula. Syndesmotic reduction and fixation techniques are still evolving. One concern is achieving anatomic reduction. A report of the bony anatomy of the incisura at the level of the syndesmosis may shed light to reasons for malreduction of syndesmotic injuries. In a series of postreduction ankle CT scans, malreduction was thought to be associated with native anatomy. A deep incisura was at risk for too much compression with a clamp resulting in overreduction (**Figure 1**). Anteverted and retroverted incisuras predisposed reductions to fail in those associated directions.[1] This information could give surgeons assistance in reduction techniques by identifying landmarks on CT.

Anatomy: Ligamentous

Ankle ligaments ensure the bony anatomy remain congruent through articulation. Lateral collateral ligamentous structures including the anterior talofibular and calcaneofibular ligaments are the most commonly repaired or reconstructed ligaments of the ankle.

Minimally invasive surgery relies on palpable and visual landmarks to assess accurate incisional placement. Lateral ankle instability surgery performed with a minimally invasive technique has gained popularity. The fibular obscure tubercle is a component of the distal fibula's surface anatomy. It can be manually detected in 57% of patients and allows a surgeon identification of appropriate anterior talofibular ligament (ATFL) and calcaneofibular ligament (CFL) origins. The tubercle occurs "1.3 mm proximal to the articular tip of the fibula, 2.7 mm to the intersection of the ATFL and CFL, and 3.7 mm distal to the ATFL."[2] Detailed understanding of surface anatomy may make minimally invasive surgery more accepted.

Neither of the following authors nor any immediate family member has received anything of value from or has stock or stock options held in a commercial company or institution related directly or indirectly to the subject of this chapter: Dr. Miller and Dr. Stein.

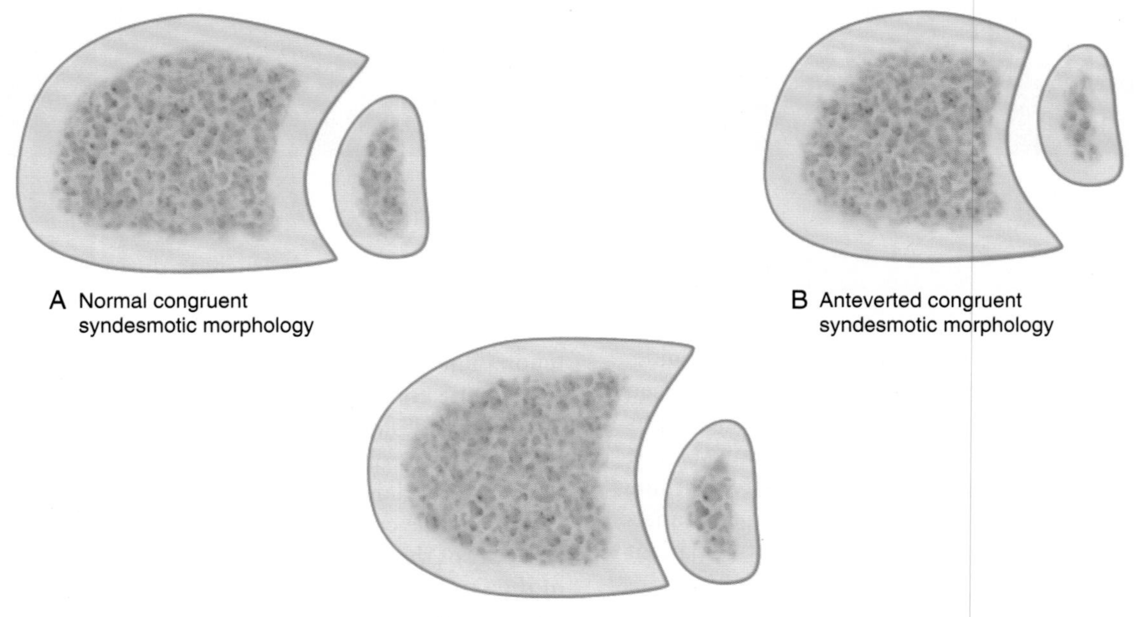

Figure 1 Axial depiction of tibiofibular bony relationship. (**A**) Normal congruent syndesmotic morphology. (**B**) Anteverted syndesmotic morphology. (**C**) Retroverted syndesmotic morphology.

Concurrent pathology with ankle instability is common, and therefore, ankle arthroscopy can be used to identify and treat osteochondral lesions and loose bodies. In addition, arthroscopy may be used to identify instability. Arthroscopic visualization of the ankle is utilized during minimally invasive Brostrom techniques. A feasibility study confirmed that one can see the ATFL and CFL safely through arthroscopy of the ankle.[3]

While bony anatomy in the midfoot is responsible for adding the stability of the midfoot, the Lisfranc ligament is crucial to maintaining articular relationships and ultimately the contour of the arch in the coronal and sagittal planes. Injury to the Lisfranc ligament—if determined to be unstable—requires surgical intervention. Although open reduction and internal fixation and fusion are both acceptable options established in literature, no clear treatment guidelines exist in choosing which option is best for which patient.

Anatomy: Tendinous

With bony tripod of the foot stabilized by ligamentous structures, tendons move and accommodate this tripod to surfaces. Pathology in a tendon not only creates pain and possibly weakness but also imbalance to the foot. The peroneal brevis tendon is a primary evertor of the foot balanced by the posterior tibial tendon's inversion pull. Injury may disrupt this. A relatively new fixation technique uses fibular fixation with a retrograde intramedullary nail. This puts the brevis tendon at risk coursing in the retrofibular groove. With insertion of the nail, the peroneus brevis is most at risk for injury. In an anatomical study, on average, the brevis tendon was 5 mm from the nail path. The superficial peroneal nerve was also at risk variably with anterior to posterior screws placed through the nail.[4]

Tendon imbalance can also be in the sagittal plane with dorsiflexion and plantarflexion of the ankle. The Achilles tendon originating with the soleus and gastrocnemius muscle bellies provides a strength and pull that may result in equinus position of the ankle. Gastrocnemius release is common, and several methods exist. A proximal medial head release depending on location of incision can encroach upon several structures. A proximal medial gastrocnemius release brought semimembranosus tendon, popliteus artery, and tibial nerve all within 11 mm of the incision in 100% of specimens in one study. A more distal alternative medial gastrocnemius release incision encountered only saphenous vein and nerve with a large variability in distances (5 to 18.6 mm).[5]

Tendon transfers may help to balance a foot and ankle. The flexor halluces longus (FHL) tendon is often transferred for Achilles support and sometimes to the lateral foot in patients with deficient peroneal tendons. The flexor digitorum longus (FDL) is commonly used to replace or augment the posterior tibial tendon when reconstructions are performed. Plantar tendon harvest often encounters chiasma plantare between the flexor halluces longus and flexor digitorum longus. In a series of 50 cadaveric dissections, 61% of FHL tendons provided one or more attachments to the FDL (second and third being most common). Thirty nine percent of specimens had direct intertendon connections. Overall, the FHL is involved in 97% of second tendons and 53% of third tendons.[6]

Anatomy: Neurovascular

With any intervention, intimate knowledge of nerve location is essential. The superficial peroneal nerve has variability in its exit location from lower leg fascia proximally to distally requiring caution during dissections. This nerve is protected during creation of the anterolateral arthroscopy portal and can be encountered in lateral ankle approaches. Recently, location of the nerve in relation to the ankle was reviewed. The mean distance from the fibular head to the emergence of the SPN is 24.6 cm in a study of 10 cadaveric specimens (**Figure 2**). The mean distance from the lateral malleolus to the nerve at the level of the ankle was 4.68 cm.[7]

Another anatomic study evaluated SPN location in relation to the distal fibula. When performing minimally invasive techniques one can palpate the distal fibula and determine relative safe zones for dissection. Lateral ankle instability performed minimally invasive should not dissect 22 mm past the distal fibula anteriorly in an effort to protect against superficial peroneal nerve injury.[8]

The posterior tibial nerve lies underneath the laciniate ligament in the tarsal tunnel and arborizes into the calcaneal, medial plantar, and lateral plantar branches. The cause of tarsal tunnel syndrome is incompletely understood. In 2016, an anatomical study evaluated the neurovascular relationships in the tunnel. Their conclusion was that an extensive vascular supply to the posterior tibial nerve in the tarsal tunnel may cause vascular congestion and leave the nerve susceptible to symptomatic compression more than other nerve compression relationships.[9]

Imaging

As in many of the orthopaedic specialties, diagnostic imaging is an essential component of the medical workup for much of the pathology encountered by the

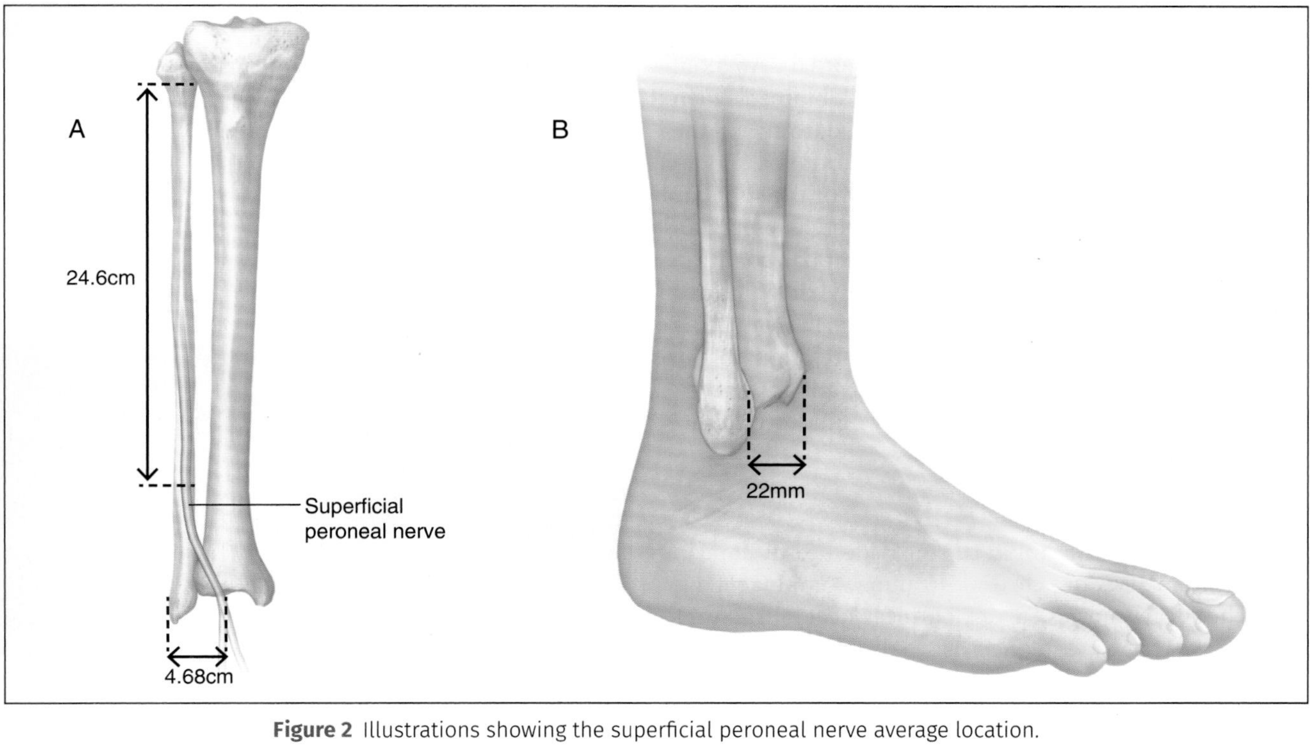

Figure 2 Illustrations showing the superficial peroneal nerve average location.

foot and ankle specialist. In an era of multiple imaging modalities, it is incumbent on the treating physician to understand the intricacies of these various modalities and to utilize them when appropriately indicated.

Plain Radiographs

Plain radiographs of the foot and ankle serve a critical role in the accurate assessment and diagnostics of foot and ankle pathology. In most clinical scenarios, plain radiographs are the initial study of choice in imaging workup. These studies are low-cost and easily obtainable in the office setting and provide important diagnostic data with regard to assessing alignment, trauma, degenerative, and potential neoplastic conditions. Weight-bearing radiographs are particularly useful and are strongly preferred with the exception of postoperative or traumatic situations that may warrant non–weight-bearing radiographs.

A standard series of weight-bearing radiographs of the foot includes AP, lateral, and oblique radiographs (**Figure 3**). Depending on the clinical context, additional "special views" may also be indicated. These may include dedicated radiographs of the toes, sesamoids (**Figure 4**), and possible stress radiographs of the foot when indicated (ie, suspected unstable Lisfranc injury).

A standard series of weight-bearing radiographs of the hindfoot and ankle includes AP, lateral, and mortise radiographs (**Figure 5**). As with the foot, there are additional views that may be obtained depending on the context. Stress radiographs of the ankle are performed in determining stability of certain ankle fracture patterns as well as in assessing competency of ligamentous structures in more chronic scenarios (**Figure 6**). An axial or Harris view of the calcaneus can be obtained when indicated to better visualize the bony anatomy of the calcaneus. The Broden view of the hindfoot is a special view used in assessing the posterior facet of the subtalar joint. This can be particularly useful when assessing an intra-articular calcaneal fracture or a subtalar coalition (**Figure 7**). The hindfoot alignment view or Saltzman view is now also commonly obtained when evaluating the axial alignment of the hindfoot in relation to the ankle above. This is particularly important for preoperative planning purposes in corrective hindfoot deformity surgery (**Figure 8**).

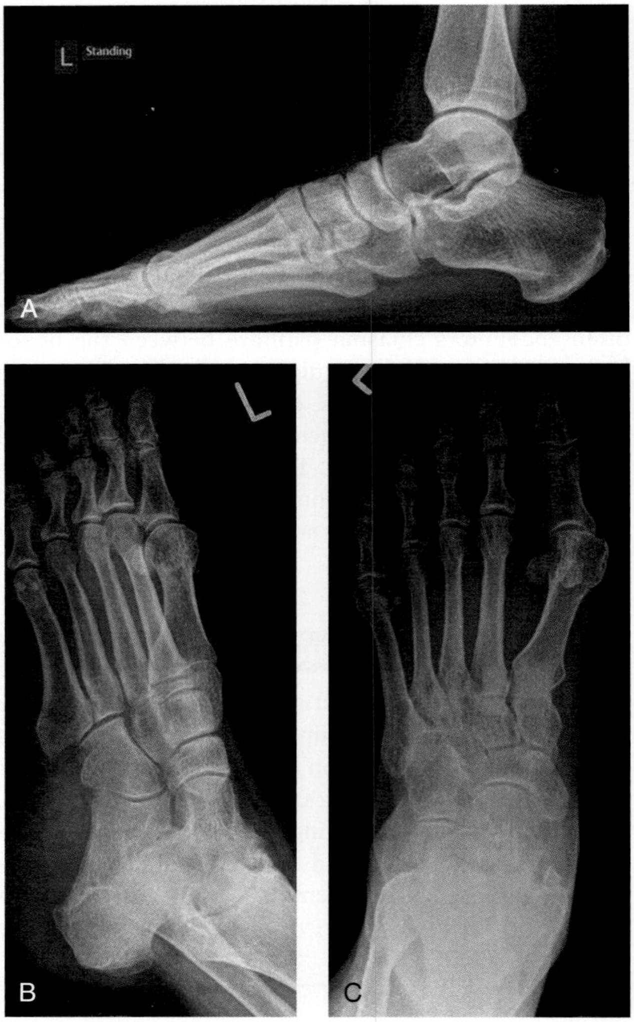

Figure 3 AP, lateral, and oblique plain weight-bearing radiographs of the foot.

MRI

MRI of the foot and ankle can provide useful data in evaluating acute or chronic trauma, impingement, osteochondral injuries, arthropathies, occult fractures or stress reactions, osteonecrosis, soft-tissue and osseous tumors, infection, nerve entrapment syndromes, and tendon pathology. When indicated, it can be a critical part of determining the diagnosis and guiding appropriate treatment. There are a variety of MRI systems available, but most commonly, midfield (1.5-T)

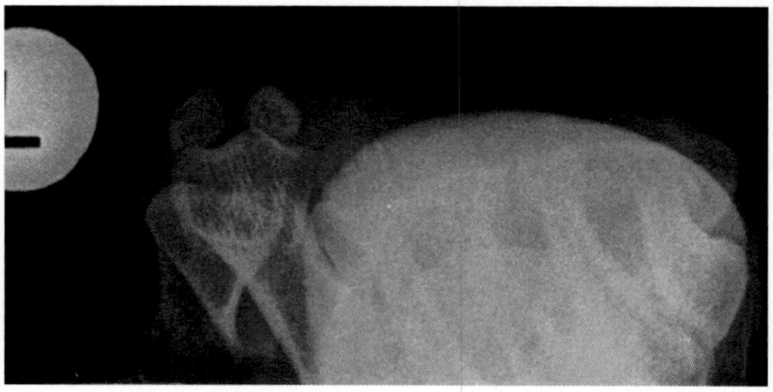

Figure 4 Sesamoid view radiograph.

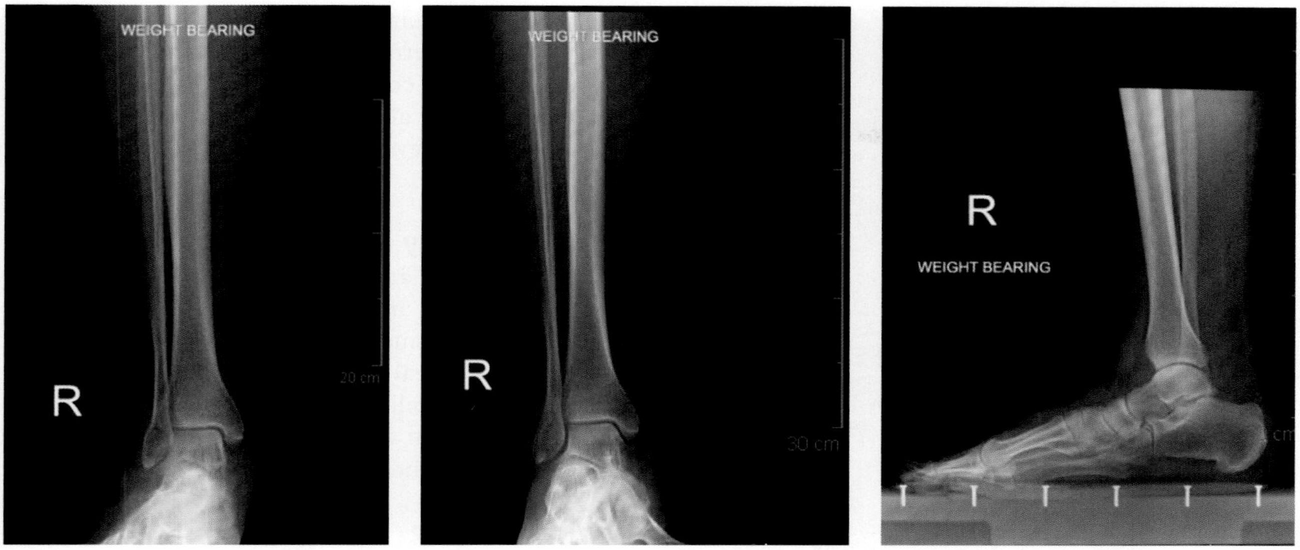

Figure 5 AP, lateral, and mortise plain weight-bearing radiographs of the ankle.

and high-field (3-T) systems are used in the evaluation of the foot and ankle.[10] The higher field systems allow for higher resolution and are thus preferable in most circumstances for the foot and ankle specialist. There are specific scenarios such as when previous internal fixation is present that a midfield (1.5-T) MRI system would be preferable.

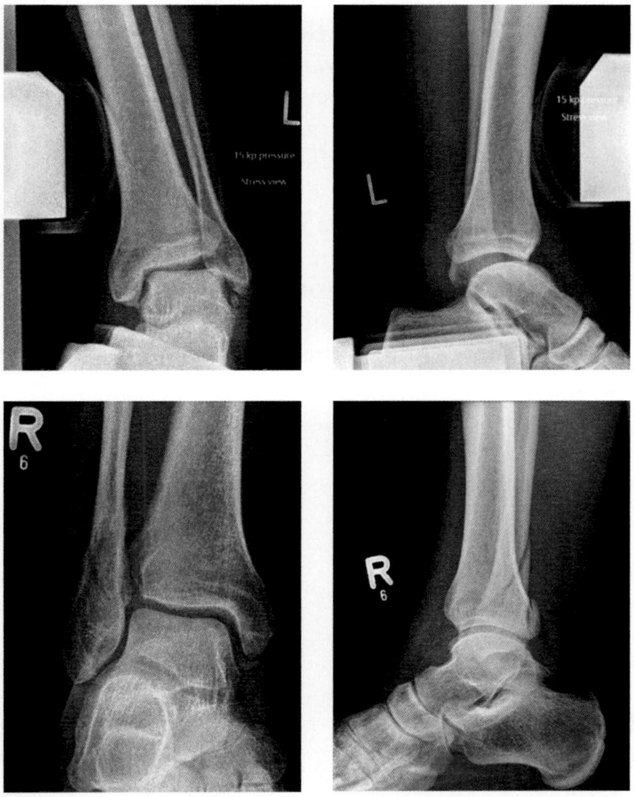

Figure 6 Stress radiographs of the ankle are performed in determining stability of certain ankle fracture patterns as well as in assessing competency of ligamentous structures in more chronic scenarios.

Standard sequences that are obtained in the foot and ankle include T1-weighted and T2-weighted axial, sagittal, and coronal images. Frequently, sagittal and coronal proton-density (PD)–weighted sequences are also obtained to allow for better evaluation of

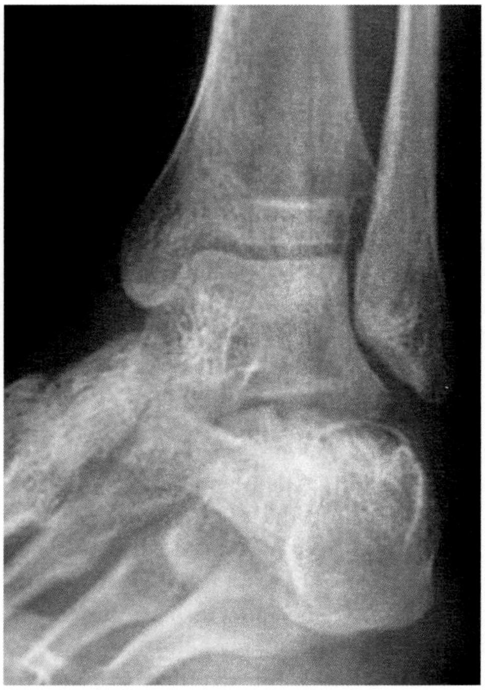

Figure 7 Broden view radiograph.

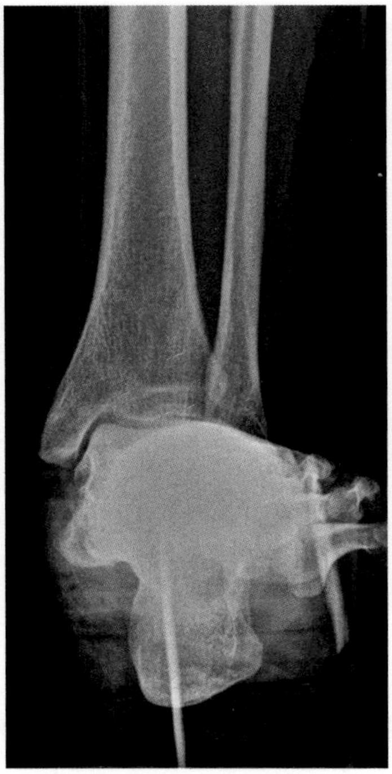

Figure 8 Hindfoot alignment view (Saltzman view) radiograph.

chondral surfaces. Special sequences can also be utilized such as oblique sagittal and axial PD-weighted images to evaluate the syndesmosis or axial oblique T-1 images to evaluate soft-tissue injuries in the hindfoot and midfoot. The use of IV contrast medium can be helpful in the evaluation of infection and tumor. It is important to determine the patient's renal function prior to administration. In certain clinical scenarios, magnetic resonance (MR) arthrography may have a role such as when evaluating an osteochondral lesion of the talus or when evaluating anterior ankle soft-tissue impingement.

Newer MRI imaging techniques are being developed to allow for improved visualization and assessment of articular cartilage.[11] These include delayed gadolinium-enhanced MRI of Cartilage (dGEMRIC), T2 mapping, and T1 Rho mapping.

CT

Multidetector CT imaging of the foot and ankle provides excellent bony detail and is very useful in the realm of foot and ankle. Standard axial imaging sequences in addition to sagittal and coronal reconstructions are routinely obtained. Depending on the scenario, obtaining specialized three-dimensional (3D) reconstructions can also be helpful for the surgeon. This modality allows for detailed evaluation of the osseous structures and is very important to the foot and ankle surgeon in the preoperative workup of complex fracture patterns, osteochondral injuries, osteoarthritis, congenital coalitions (**Figure 9**), foreign bodies, and neoplasms. It also importantly allows for postoperative follow-up evaluation of fracture, osteotomy, or arthrodesis union.

Ultrasonography

In the foot and ankle diagnostics, ultrasonography imaging provides an easily accessibly means of low-cost clinical assessment. It can provide the experienced examiner with real-time ability to assess soft-tissue dynamics and stability; power Doppler modes can provide useful data on vascularity, as well as the ability to guide diagnostic and therapeutic injections.

Nuclear Imaging

The use of nuclear imaging scans has certainly diminished in an era now dominated by the use of MRI; however, there remain certain scenarios where its use can aid in diagnostics. Bone scans provide a map of osteoblastic activity and can be a sensitive tool in the evaluation of osseous stress injuries, metabolic bone disorders, neoplastic diseases, infection, complex regional pain syndrome, and musculoskeletal pain of unknown origin (**Figure 10**). More advanced scans such as tagged white blood cell or leukocyte scans have allowed for an additional method for assessing infection and can be particularly useful in difficult scenarios such as periprosthetic infection or the diabetic foot. Single-photon emission CT or SPECT is a newer tool that is a hybrid of CT imaging and a gamma camera.[12] This allows for improved localization of abnormal bone function, which has been used as a diagnostic aid in the evaluation of midfoot arthritis and osteochondral lesions of the talus.

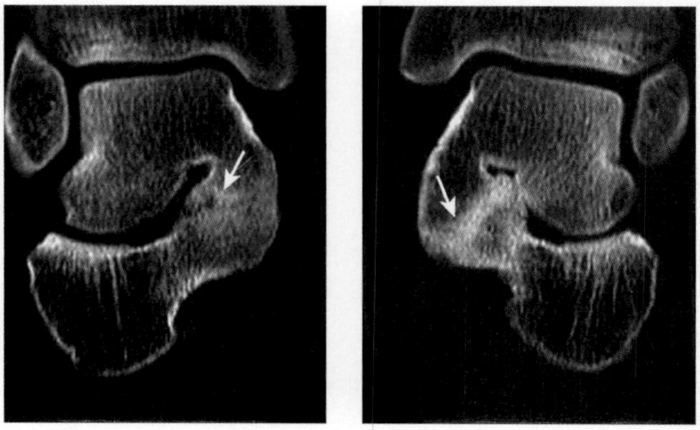

Figure 9 CT imaging demonstrating bilateral osseous coalitions of the middle subtalar joints (arrows).

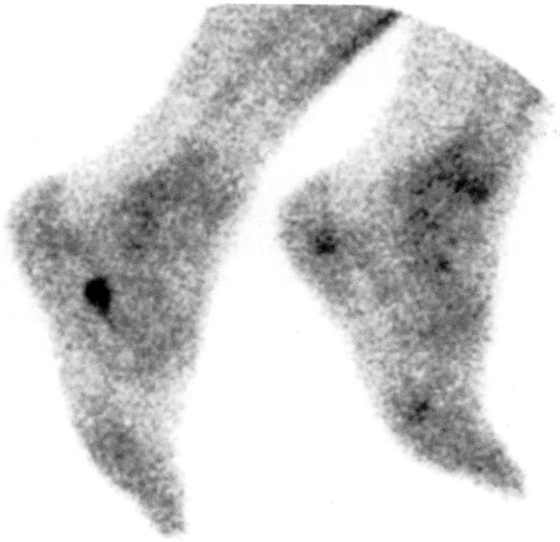

Figure 10 Nuclear bone scan demonstrating increased activity and bone uptake in a symptomatic os peroneum.

Biomechanics

Biomechanics of the foot and ankle is the study of kinetics (forces) and kinematics (motion and velocity) with regard to the lower extremity. While clinical studies ultimately guide treatment, many biomechanics studies utilize bench research and cadaveric models to simulate treatment and pathology. This assists clinicians in identifying further clinical studies and current treatment methods.

Ankle

Ankle biomechanics are more complex than other lower extremity joints (knee, hip) due to the multiplanar motion at the talocrural joint. The ankle joint is a constrained joint made up of the tibia fibula and talus. If this constraint is compromised, then arthritis can occur. For example, in a cadaveric study evaluating syndesmotic injury, syndesmotic disruption decreased tibial plafond contact area and force. Syndesmotic reduction did not restore ankle loading mechanics to values measured in the intact condition.[13] This demonstrates how syndesmotic instability may lead in posttraumatic arthrosis.

The talus architecture allows for internal rotation during plantar flexion and external rotation during dorsiflexion. During gait, forces exceed five times body weight and shear forces approach three times body weight. This stress on a relatively small surface area, multiplanar motion, and poor biomechanical knowledge likely led to poor outcomes in total ankle replacements in early models. Correcting alignment to achieve neutrality and more natural biomechanics is paramount in total ankle arthroplasty surgery. At 24 months out from a replacement, patients with preexisting valgus or varus deformity corrected at the time of surgery have been shown to have similar results to normally aligned patients.[14] Overall viability of total ankle replacements today in midterm results approaches 80% retained replacement at 10 years.

Currently ankle fusion and ankle replacement are both viable options for treatment of ankle arthritis. One concern with ankle fusion surgery is adjacent joint degeneration due to increased motion over time. This was recently shown in a cadaveric study measuring subtalar and talonavicular motion showing increased kinematics after tibiotalar arthrodesis.[15] This shows concern for potential degeneration of these joints over time. Although ankle replacement is generally thought of as the more natural gait, it has been shown that ankle fusion does improve preoperative biomechanics of the ankle. Although those changes are not normal, they demonstrate better motion than prior to surgery.[16] Range of motion of adjacent joints increased as well as step length and velocity.

Supramalleolar osteotomies provide an option to relatively young patients to realign an incongruent arthritic ankle and provide pain relief. Stability of these osteotomies is a concern, particularly in opening wedge osteotomies due to graft incorporation and fixation. However, it seems that stability is more dependent on an intact cortex where the wedge hinges for stability instead of the plate and screw construct chosen.[17]

Beside bony alignment and mechanics, stability of soft tissue is integral to normal articulation. It is important to assess instability on examination. Examination of ankle instability relies on drawer examination. In a cadaveric study, allowing for internal rotation while performing an anterolateral drawer test was to help the examiner detect instability more easily.[18] Athletes often use a stability brace or taping of the ankle when returning to sports. In one evaluation of ankle taping, ankle and knee range of motion were reduced with application of the tape. Internal rotation was particularly affected. While this may provide the desired result of ankle protection, it may also limit the knee motion.[19]

In syndesmotic injuries, rotation occurs and several anatomic structures can be damaged. Anatomic reduction with surgical treatment can be challenging, and the ideal treatment is debated. In a cadaveric test, sectioning of components of the syndesmosis was performed. The study demonstrated more instability with each structure that was sectioned. In addition, isolated sectioning of the anterior-inferior tibiofibular ligament was enough to demonstrate rotation consistent with instability.[20] In

Foot and Ankle

a separate study, fixation techniques were compared: solitary 3.5 mm screw, solitary suture-button construct, and two divergent suture-buttons. The conclusion was a solitary suture-button construct might not create enough stability in the sagittal plane. Screw and divergent suture-buttons were comparable in this study.[21] In addition, it has also been shown that solitary suture-button does not re-create normal motion.[22]

Hindfoot

The hindfoot is composed of the calcaneus and talus articulating at the chopart joints with the cuboid and navicular. The kinematics of these joints is mostly inversion/eversion. With eversion the foot accommodates to ground; however, with inversion the chopart joints articulate obliquely to each other, thereby locking the foot. Injury or pathology to this region is often treated with fusion. Subtalar hindfoot arthrodesis is associated with changes of the ankle tibiotalar joint when performed in isolation. In one study after subtalar fusion, the ankle showed decreased contact area and total force but increase in external rotation at the tibiotalar joint.[23]

Tibiotalocalcaneal arthrodesis success relies on many factors including preparation, alignment, patient factors, and construct stability. How to best perform this surgery with optimized biomechanics is unclear. When comparing lateral plate, nail, and isolated screw constructs in a cadaver model, plate application was shown to have a higher compressive force than screws alone at the ankle and subtalar joints. Nail application provided more compression than screws alone but less than plate. These results were not statistically significant.[24]

Tendons surrounding the hindfoot affect the foot kinetics. Imbalance may lead to deformity if left unchecked. The Achilles tendon may create equinus contracture or accentuate varus/valgus deformities. Achilles tendon is the longest and strongest tendon in the body. At the calcaneal insertion, pathology is common with tendinopathy, calcaneal exostosis, and Haglund deformity. Resection of this bony pathology and repair of the tendon has a deleterious effect on the pullout strength of the tendon. In one recent cadaveric study using an isolated two-anchor repair, the pullout strength was 740 N compared with 1300 N in normal subjects.[25]

Midfoot

Within the midfoot the most concerning injury requiring surgery is tarsometatarsal instability due to fracture and/or ligament tear of the Lisfranc ligament. The plantar component of the Lisfranc ligament is the most important when determining tears. Loss of Lisfranc ligament integrity results in loss of stability of the midfoot. Over time the foot collapses and abducts resulting in a predictable arthritis. Midfoot open reduction and internal fixation surgery can be achieved with transarticular screws or plate application with the ultimate goal being no residual instability. A cadaver model to compare fixation stability between plate and screw construct stabilizing the first and second tarsometatarsal joints demonstrated no significant differences under cyclic loading.[26] There is no consensus in current treatment.

Forefoot

The forefoot under normal conditions distributes pressure over 50% into the first ray and the rest into the lesser metatarsals. Imbalance of forces results in undo pressure with stress fractures or pathology along the metatarsophalangeal joints. There is increased attention to plantar plate tears as a fixable deformity and pathology. Reducing forefoot plantar pressure is a necessary goal in ulcer healing in diabetics. Total contact casts are meant to help offload areas of ulceration and improve healing. In a study measuring plantar pressures using total contact orthosis, peak plantar pressures were significantly decreased.[27] While casting remains the benchmark, this study suggests orthosis may help in some patients.

Increased forces along the lateral foot—particularly in the varus foot—lead to stress fractures and acute fractures in the fifth metatarsal. These forces in the recovery period following fixation can delay complete bony fusion. In addition technique can affect outcome. If an intramedullary screw is applied, the screw achieves best compression and fixation when centered in the intramedullary canal (**Figure 11**). Optimal starting point for Jones fracture fixation of the fifth metatarsal is just adjacent and lateral to the cartilage of the fifth base, at the center of the canal.[28]

Gait Analysis

The human gait cycle and its analysis can provide very useful data regarding the impact of certain foot and ankle pathology and surgical interventions upon locomotion. A single cycle is often defined as the motion between the heel strike of one step and the heel strike of the same foot on the subsequent step. The analysis of this complex and coordinated cycle has evolved over time and is accomplished by utilization of force plates to determine ground reaction forces in conjunction with other tools such as high-speed cameras with

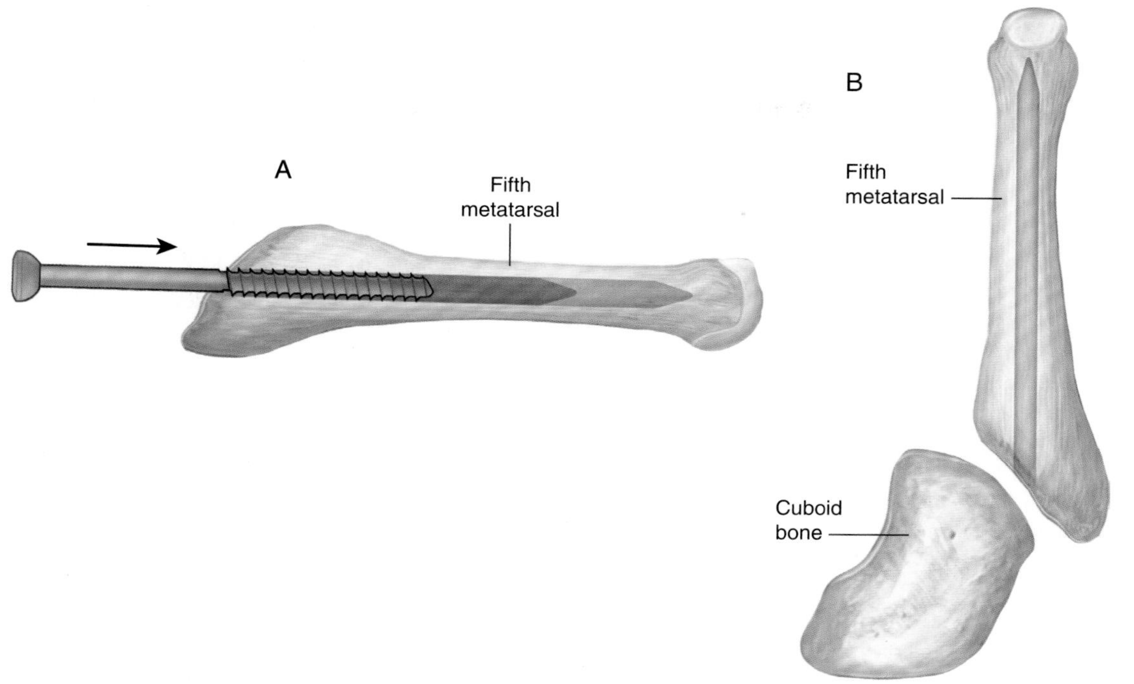

Figure 11 Illustration showing fifth metatarsal screw placement.

motion sensing equipment, electrogoniometers, and electromyography devices. These data can aid the foot and ankle specialist in better assessing the functional impact of certain conditions on their patients' ability to walk and also how the treatment ultimately provided can improve their function.

Summary

Recent advances have focused on understanding total ankle arthroplasty longevity, syndesmotic ligament treatment, and optimizing current treatment regimens. Imaging will continue to evolve to provide more consistent and detailed information. Gait assessment as it becomes more advanced may help quantify outcomes for patients.

Key Study Points

- Preexisting syndesmotic anatomy may affect reduction outcome from surgery, and currently no best treatment method exists.
- Total ankle arthroplasty attempts to re-create native kinetics and kinematics.
- Advanced MRI sequencing and SPECT imaging will allow for improved functional visualization of articular cartilage and associated pathology.

Annotated References

1. Boszczyk A, Kwapisz S, Krummel M, Grass R, Rammelt S: Correlation of incisura anatomy with syndesmotic malreduction. *Foot Ankle Int* 2018;39(3):369-375. [Epub 2017/12/20].

   The syndesmoses with a deep incisura and the fibula not engaged into the tibial incisura were at risk of overcompression, anteverted incisuras at risk of anterior fibular translation, and retroverted incisuras at risk of posterior fibular translation. Level of evidence: III.

2. Matsui K, Oliva XM, Takao M, et al: Bony landmarks available for minimally invasive lateral ankle stabilization surgery: A cadaveric anatomical study. *Knee Surg Sports Traumatol Arthrosc* 2017;25(6):1916-1924. [Epub 2016/06/29].

   The present study describes the utility of clinically relevant bony landmarks that may assist in identifying the origins and insertions of the ATFL and CFL to facilitate minimally invasive ankle stabilization surgery. Level of evidence: V.

3. Thes A, Klouche S, Ferrand M, Hardy P, Bauer T: Assessment of the feasibility of arthroscopic visualization of the lateral ligament of the ankle: A cadaveric study. *Knee Surg Sports Traumatol Arthrosc* 2016;24(4):985-990. [Epub 2015/09/28].

   Arthroscopic identification of the ATFL, CFL, and their corresponding footprints can be considered safe and reliable. Tunnels entrances, in preparation for arthroscopic ligament reconstruction, are precisely positioned. Level of evidence: V.

4. Goss DA Jr, Reb CW, Philbin TM: Anatomic structures at risk when utilizing an intramedullary nail for distal fibular fractures: A cadaveric study. *Foot Ankle Int* 2017;38(8):916-920. [Epub 2017/05/26].

The peroneal tendons and superficial peroneal nerve were at the highest risk; however, no structures were injured during instrumentation. Strict adherence to sound percutaneous technique is needed in order to minimize iatrogenic damage to neighboring structures when performing retrograde locked intramedullary fibular nail insertion. This includes making skin-only incisions, blunt dissection down to bone, and maintaining close approximation between tissue protection sleeves and bone at all times. Level of evidence: V.

5. Kaplan N, Fowler X, Maqsoodi N, DiGiovanni B, Oh I: Operative anatomy of the medial gastrocnemius recession vs the proximal medial gastrocnemius recession. *Foot Ankle Int* 2017;38(4):424-429. [Epub 2017/04/04].

   The article identified the major structures at risk when performing the proximal medial gastrocnemius release and propose a novel, possibly safer alternative for the medial gastrocnemius release. Level of evidence: V.

6. Pretterklieber B: The high variability of the chiasma plantare and the long flexor tendons: Anatomical aspects of tendon transfer in foot surgery. *Ann Anat* 2017;211:21-32. [Epub 2017/02/07].

   The aim of the study was to reinvestigate the formation of the chiasma plantare and the composition of the long flexor tendons in order to clarify the inexact and partly contradictory descriptions published from 1865 onward. Level of evidence: V.

7. Ribak S, Fonseca JR, Tietzmann A, Gama SA, Hirata HH: The anatomy and morphology of the superficial peroneal nerve. *J Reconstr Microsurg* 2016;32(4):271-275. [Epub 2015/12/18].

   This study describes the location of the superficial peroneal nerve in relation to compartments and the ankle which is useful for safety in approaches. Level of evidence: V.

8. Jorge JT, Gomes TM, Oliva XM: An anatomical study about the arthroscopic repair of the lateral ligament of the ankle. *Foot Ankle Surg* 2018;24(2):143-148. [Epub 2018/02/08].

   This discusses the superficial peroneal nerve in relation to minimally invasive surgery. An accessory incision to include the inferior extensor retinaculum in the repair should not surpass the 22 mm distance from the lateral malleolus in the anterior direction, due to the risk of damaging the nerve. Level of evidence: V.

9. Manske MC, McKeon KE, McCormick JJ, Johnson JE, Klein SE: Arterial anatomy of the posterior tibial nerve in the tarsal tunnel. *J Bone Joint Surg Am* 2016;98(6):499-504. [Epub 2016/03/18].

   Vascular supply to the posterior tibial nerve was reviewed. Advancing the understanding of the arterial anatomy supplying the nerve and its branches may provide insight into the cause and treatment of tarsal tunnel syndrome. Level of evidence: V.

10. Bruno F, Arrigoni F, Palumbo P, et al: New advances in MRI diagnosis of degenerative osteoarthropathy of the peripheral joints. *Radiol Med* 2019;124(11):1121-1127.

    Discussion of limb MRI evaluation. Level of evidence: V.

11. Guermazi A, Alizai H, Crema MD, et al: Compositional MRI techniques for evaluation of cartilage degeneration in osteoarthritis. *Osteoarthr Cartil* 2015;23(10):1639-1653.

    Describes compositional MRI techniques for cartilage evaluation.

12. Tamam C, Tamam M, Yildirim D, Mulazimoglu M: Diagnostic value of single-photon emission computed tomography combined with computed tomography in relation to MRI on osteochondral lesions of the talus. *Nucl Med Commun* 2015;36(8):808-814.

    Discussion of osteochondral lesions with SPECT.

13. LaMothe J, Baxter JR, Gilbert S, Murphy CI, Karnovsky SC, Drakos MC: Effect of complete syndesmotic disruption and deltoid injuries and different reduction methods on ankle joint contact mechanics. *Foot Ankle Int* 2017;38(6):694-700. [Epub 2017/03/17].

    The study examines motion of native and repaired syndesmosis. Fixation of a syndesmotic injury with a single suture-button construct did not restore physiological fibular motion, which may have implications for postoperative care and clinical outcomes. Level of evidence: V.

14. Grier AJ, Schmitt AC, Adams SB, Queen RM: The effect of tibiotalar alignment on coronal plane mechanics following total ankle replacement. *Gait Posture* 2016;48:13-18. [Epub 2016/08/02].

    The study investigated whether preoperative tibiotalar alignment (varus, valgus, or neutral) resulted in significantly different coronal plane mechanics or ground reaction forces post-total ankle replacement. Restoration of alignment demonstrated similar outcomes at 24 months. Level of evidence: III.

15. Sturnick DR, Demetracopoulos CA, Ellis SJ, et al: Adjacent joint kinematics after ankle arthrodesis during cadaveric gait simulation. *Foot Ankle Int* 2017;38(11):1249-1259. [Epub 2017/08/25].

    The objective of this study was to identify the isolated effect of ankle arthrodesis on adjacent joint kinematics during simulated walking. Increased motion of the adjacent joints caused by ankle arthrodesis may explain the articular degeneration observed clinically. Level of evidence: V.

16. Brodsky JW, Kane JM, Coleman S, Bariteau J, Tenenbaum S: Abnormalities of gait caused by ankle arthritis are improved by ankle arthrodesis. *Bone Joint J* 2016;98-B(10):1369-1375. [Epub 2016/10/04].

    The purpose of this study was to assess postoperative gait function with gait before arthrodesis. The purpose of this study was to assess postoperative gait function with gait before arthrodesis. Compared with the preoperative analysis there was improvement in numerous temporal-spatial, kinematic, and kinetic measures. Level of evidence: III.

17. Ettinger S, Schwarze M, Yao D, et al: Stability of supramalleolar osteotomies using different implants in a sawbone model. *Arch Orthop Trauma Surg* 2018;138(10):1359-1363. [Epub 2018/06/24].

This study was performed to analyze the stability of different implants and their appropriateness for supramalleolar osteotomies. The intact hinge apparently provides enough support to compensate for lower moment of inertia of some plates. Level of evidence: V.

18. Miller AG, Myers SH, Parks BG, Guyton GP: Anterolateral drawer versus anterior drawer test for ankle instability: A biomechanical model. *Foot Ankle Int* 2016;37(4):407-410. [Epub 2015/12/15].

    A cadaveric test to measure drawer testing displacement. Anterolateral drawer testing provides a more sensitive clinical test than anterior drawer. Level of evidence: V.

19. Williams SA, Ng L, Stephens N, Klem N, Wild C: Effect of prophylactic ankle taping on ankle and knee biomechanics during basketball-specific tasks in females. *Phys Ther Sport* 2018;32:200-206. [Epub 2018/05/29].

    This study investigate the effects of ankle taping on ankle and knee joint biomechanics during cutting and rebound activities in females. The taping restricted motion. Level of evidence: IV.

20. Clanton TO, Williams BT, Backus JD, et al: Biomechanical analysis of the individual ligament contributions to syndesmotic stability. *Foot Ankle Int* 2017;38(1):66-75. [Epub 2016/09/30].

    This study defined normal motion of the syndesmosis and the biomechanical consequences of injury. The degree of instability was increased with each additional injured structure; however, isolated injuries to the AITFL alone may lead to significant external rotary instability. Level of evidence: V.

21. Clanton TO, Whitlow SR, Williams BT, et al: Biomechanical comparison of 3 current ankle syndesmosis repair techniques. *Foot Ankle Int* 2017;38(2):200-207.

    Three separate constructs were evaluated for syndesmotic stability following repair. Screw and two suture button techniques created the most stability in the saggital plane. Level of evidence: V.

22. LaMothe JM, Baxter JR, Murphy C, Gilbert S, DeSandis B, Drakos MC: Three-dimensional analysis of fibular motion after fixation of syndesmotic injuries with a screw or suture-button construct. *Foot Ankle Int* 2016;37(12):1350-1356.

    The purpose of this study was to characterize the effects of a syndesmotic injury and reduction techniques on ankle joint contact mechanics in a biomechanical model. Level of evidence: V.

23. Hutchinson ID, Baxter JR, Gilbert S, et al: How do hindfoot fusions affect ankle biomechanics: A cadaver model. *Clin Orthop Relat Res* 2016;474(4):1008-1016. [Epub 2015/12/23].

    Loss or deficit in function of the subtalar joint may be sufficient to alter ankle loading. These findings warrant consideration in the treatment of the arthritic hindfoot and also toward defining biomechanical goals for ankle arthroplasty in the setting of concomitant hindfoot degeneration or arthrodesis. Level of evidence: V.

24. Hamid KS, Glisson RR, Morash JG, Matson AP, DeOrio JK: Simultaneous intraoperative measurement of cadaver ankle and subtalar joint compression during arthrodesis with intramedullary nail, screws, and tibiotalocalcaneal plate. *Foot Ankle Int* 2018;39(9):1128-1132. doi:10.1177/1071100718774271. [Epub 2018/05/17].

    The study examines whether the hindfoot nail and lateral plate options should be strongly considered when aiming to maximize compression in patients undergoing tibiotalar calcaneal arthrodesis. Level of evidence: V.

25. Pfeffer G, Gonzalez T, Zapf M, Nelson TJ, Metzger MF: Achilles pullout strength after open calcaneoplasty for Haglund's syndrome. *Foot Ankle Int* 2018;39(8):966-969. [Epub 2018/04/14].

    This study assessed Achilles tendon pullout strength after an open calcaneoplasty for Haglund syndrome. The purpose of this study was to investigate those changes in a cadaveric model and provide objective data upon which to base post-operative recovery. Level of evidence: V.

26. Ho NC, Sangiorgio SN, Cassinelli S, et al: Biomechanical comparison of fixation stability using a Lisfranc plate versus transarticular screws. *Foot Ankle Surg* 2017;25(1):71-78. [Epub 2018/02/08].

    Diastasis at the Lisfranc joint following fixation with a novel plate or transarticular screw fixation were comparable. Therefore, the Lisfranc plate may provide adequate support without risk of iatrogenic injury to the articular cartilage. Level of evidence: V.

27. Nouman M, Leelasamran W, Chatpun S: Effectiveness of total contact orthosis for plantar pressure redistribution in neuropathic diabetic patients during different walking activities. *Foot Ankle Int* 2017;38(8):901-908. [Epub 2017/05/02].

    The aim of this study was to investigate the plantar pressure from four regions of the foot during different walking activities (level walking, ramp ascending, ramp descending, stair ascending, and stair descending) in neuropathic diabetic patients with and without a total contact cast. Level of evidence: IV.

28. Watson GI, Karnovsky SC, Konin G, Drakos MC: Optimal starting point for fifth metatarsal zone II fractures: A cadaveric study. *Foot Ankle Int* 2017;38(7):802-807. [Epub 2017/05/10].

    This study evaluated the ideal starting position for screw placement of zone II base of the fifth metatarsal fractures, which should be considered when performing internal fixation for these fractures. Level of evidence: V.

Foot and Ankle

radiographic alignment.[30] The bone block wedge helps to restore the native talus alignment. A recent study demonstrated that although patient-reported outcome scores were low compared with a reference population, 90% of patients undergoing subtalar arthrodesis after calcaneus fracture would recommend the procedure to others and 76% of patients experienced pain relief.[31]

Talonavicular Joint

Isolated talonavicular arthritis typically occurs in the setting of rheumatoid arthritis or Mueller-Weiss disease. Favorable fusion rates of near 95% and improvement in patient-reported outcomes scores have been reported with this procedure.[32,33] However, hardware fixation in this relatively small joint is a concern. Plate and screws versus screws alone for the fixation of the talonavicular joint provided equivalent stability in a cadaver model.[34] However, another study reported that one retrograde screw and a dorsal locked compression plate was more effective at limiting motion across the talonavicular joint than two retrograde screws.[35]

Midfoot

Midfoot arthritis, which is a "grab-bag" term for deformity and arthritis of the midtarsal and tarsometatarsal joints, occurs from ligamentous insufficiency, trauma, neuropathic arthropathy, autoimmune arthritis, among others. Posttraumatic degeneration is the most common cause. As with arthritis of other joints, symptoms of arthritis without deformity can be treated nonsurgically with full-length rigid inserts, stiff inserts, rocker bottom shoes, and steroid injections, although none of these treatments remove the arthritis. However, surgery should not be taken lightly as it can be difficult to identify the specific joints for arthrodesis and union is not guaranteed.

For nonneuropathic midfoot deformity and arthritis, arthrodesis using internal fixation has demonstrated reasonable results. A series of 30 patients with symptomatic midfoot arthritis and deformity were treated with internal fixation.[36] Union occurred in 93% of the patients. In addition, 90% of patients rated their result as good or excellent. However, the authors cautioned that although most patients were satisfied, the feet were not perceived as normal and had residual pain, deformity, and the need for orthotic use. Corroborating these results, Nemec et al[37] published on a series of 104 feet that underwent midfoot arthrodesis with internal fixation for primary midfoot arthritis. Union was achieved in 92% of the feet. There was significant improvement in pain and functional outcomes. Often, there is abduction and dorsiflexion deformity with long-standing midfoot arthritis. Achieving an anatomic reduction has been identified as the most important predictor of a good outcome.[38]

Midfoot arthritis in the neuropathic foot without infection can be treated with a custom walker boot. This treatment has demonstrated improved patient-reported outcomes and maintenance of foot alignment.[39] However, inadequate symptom relief or deformity with actual or impending skin compromise requires surgical intervention. Open reduction of the deformity and arthrodesis of the neuropathic midfoot collapse using multiple axially placed intramedullary screws has demonstrated significantly improved foot alignment and a stable foot with either total or partial union achieved in 95% of patients.[40] In addition to internal fixation, midfoot realignment and arthrodesis with external fixation has also been described for neuropathic deformities. A comparison review study found that external fixation was eight times more likely to develop radiographic nonunion.[41] Moreover, internal fixation was 1.5 times more likely to result in amputation, 2 times more likely to result in deep infection, and a 20% increase in the need for unplanned additional surgery. With inconclusive results, internal versus external fixation should be chosen on an individual basis.

First Metatarsophalangeal Joint

Hallux rigidus refers to arthritis of the great toe metatarsophalangeal (MTP) joint. Arthritis of the foot is the most common in this location. Unlike other locations of arthritis in the foot where trauma is the most common cause, the cause of hallux rigidus is unclear. Most commonly the cause is considered to be idiopathic. Some additional causes include family history, metatarsal head shape, metatarsus adductus, and hallux valgus interphalangeus. Nonsurgical treatment consists of NSAIDs, steroid injections, and a rigid orthotic with a Morton's extension.

Surgical treatment is divided into joint-sparing (cheilectomy, interpositional arthroplasty, synthetic implant, metallic arthroplasty) and joint-sacrificing (arthrodesis) procedures, traditionally based on arthritis severity. Arthritis severity is based on radiographic characteristics and examination findings. The most commonly used classification was proposed by Coughlin.[42] It is based on pain with motion, the amount of motion, and radiographic osteophytes and joint space narrowing. Unfortunately, classification systems do not always maintain a high level of clinical importance. A recent study by Baumhauer et al[43] compared the Coughlin grade to motion, pain, and intraoperative arthritis in 202 patients. They found no correlation with active peak dorsiflexion and pain, and a small correlation to

Foot and Ankle

intraoperative cartilage loss. They concluded that clinical symptoms and signs should be used to guide treatment rather than a grade. We typically use the presence or absence of midrange motion pain to guide our surgical treatment. The absence of midrange motion indicates that joint-sparing procedures will likely be effective. Midrange motion pain indicates more widespread disease and therefore joint-sacrificing or joint-sparing procedures that address the entire joint are needed.

Cheilectomy with joint débridement is the benchmark and provides excellent results for mild hallux rigidus.[44] However, recently the indication for cheilectomy has increased to advanced hallux rigidus with 85% patient satisfaction and significant improvement in patient-reported outcomes.[45] Interpositional arthroplasty is an additional joint-sparing alternative to arthrodesis for advanced hallux rigidus. One study reported on 10 patients who received capsular interpositional arthroplasty as compared with 12 patients who underwent first metatarsophalangeal arthrodesis.[46] The interpositional arthroplasty group had significantly higher postoperative patient-reported scores, greater range of motion, and significantly less plantar pressure under the great toe.

Metallic arthroplasty has been proposed to treat end-stage hallux rigidus. Although some studies support favorable results with short-term follow-up, at least one study reports long-term results and compares these patients to arthrodesis. Stone et al[47] reported that at 15 years, patients who underwent arthrodesis experienced less pain and were more satisfied compared with those who had a metallic arthroplasty. There were no functional differences between the groups but there were more revision procedures in the arthroplasty group.

A modern synthetic implant has been employed for advanced hallux rigidus with excellent results. A prospective randomized trial of a synthetic cartilage implant or first metatarsophalangeal joint arthrodesis was performed. At 24 months, there was equivalent pain relief and functional outcomes.[48] Another study compared arthrodesis to a synthetic implant. They found no difference in success between the two when stratified by grade.[43]

Arthrodesis of the first MTP joint remains the benchmark treatment for severe arthritis. In fact, an evidenced-based analysis of surgical treatments for hallux rigidus, there was fair evidence (grade B) to support arthrodesis and poor evidence to support all other surgical treatment modalities.[49] It is the only procedure that can also address deformities such concomitant hallux valgus or varus or those from neuromuscular causes. Alignment is critical. Optimal position of the great toe should be in neutral rotation, which can be assessed by looking at the nail plates of the other toes, 5° to 15° of valgus, and 10° to 15° of dorsiflexion relative to the floor. Valgus malalignment can cause rubbing on the second toe and varus or plantar flexion or dorsiflexion malalignment can cause rubbing on shoe wear. The joint is secured with either crossed screws, a dorsal plate, or a combination of a crossed screw and a dorsal plate. Similar to ankle arthrodesis, a crossed screw and dorsal plate is the strongest biomechanical construct and has shown good clinical results and 93% to 98% fusion rate[50,51] (**Figure 3**).

Osteonecrosis

Osteonecrosis typically presents in the talus or navicular and can result from multiple conditions including trauma (fracture and/or dislocation), chronic corticosteroid use, alcohol abuse, sickle cell disease, immunosuppression, hemoglobinopathies, and idiopathic causes.[52-55] Osteonecrosis is likely more common in the talus and navicular because of the tenuous blood supply to these bones.

Talus

Osteonecrosis of the talus causes pain and decreased function through the development of tibiotalar and/or subtalar joint arthritis. The majority of talus osteonecrosis is from talar neck fractures and/or subtalar dislocations (**Figure 4**). In fact, traumatic osteonecrosis accounts for 75% of the cases with increasing incidence with higher Hawkins grades of talar neck fractures.[56] Sequelae of talus osteonecrosis include talar collapse leading to arthritis of the ankle joint, subtalar joint, or both. Nonsurgical and surgical treatments exist, but as the osteonecrosis and arthritis progress, surgical treatments are warranted. Surgical techniques can be divided into joint-sparing (core decompression) and joint-sacrificing (arthrodesis) techniques.

Arthrodesis

The majority of literature regarding the treatment of this pathology focuses on tibiotalar arthrodesis or combined tibiotalocalcaneal (TTC) arthrodesis with minimal reports on isolated subtalar arthrodesis (discussed later). Obviously, the avascular talus does not provide healthy bone. However, fusions have been performed with the avascular talus, complete talectomy, cadaver bone, and even metal implants. To make interpretation of the literature more complicated, fusion constructs have consisted of external fixators, internal plate and screw fixation, and intramedullary nail fixation. Therefore, it is difficult to compare results across

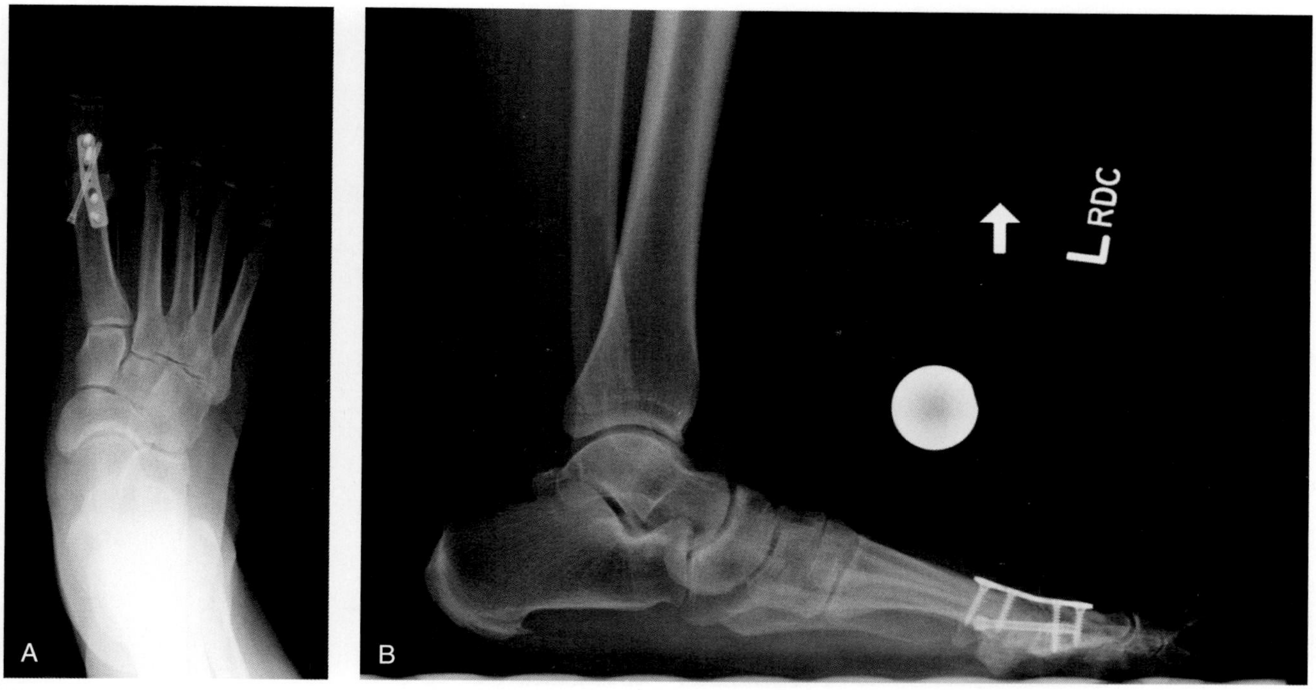

Figure 3 A successful first metatarsophalangeal joint arthrodesis with a crossed screw and dorsal plate demonstrated in AP (**A**) and lateral (**B**) radiographs.

studies. Moreover, the outcomes are not promising. Gross et al,[57] in a systematic review, concluded lengthy times to fusion and a high rate of complications make arthrodesis an unattractive option, at least for early osteonecrosis of the talus.

The authors of a recent study reported on 14 patients who underwent retrograde intramedullary nail arthrodesis for talus osteonecrosis.[58] Most of the necrosed tali were left in place with variable treatment techniques regarding biologic augmentation. Thirteen patients went on to union and the remaining patient had a pseudarthrosis accommodative to a brace. Similarly, another group reported their experience with mainly using the avascular talus in 14 TTC arthrodeses.[59] They did have to completely resect the avascular talus in four cases. All cases used some type of biologic supplementation, including autograft (majority). Arthrodesis was achieved in all cases. These studies support the use of the avascular talus.

Another option is the use of bulk autograft. In a series of talus osteonecrosis secondary to talar fracture nonunion, a recent report focused on removal of the avascular talus and replacing it with iliac crest autograft.[60] At a mean of 23 months, solid osseous fusion was achieved in only 8/12 of the patients (67%). The authors concluded that this is a reasonable treatment option. The authors of this study chose autograft over allograft because of biological superiority.

However, the results of bulk allograft are not much different. Jeng et al[61] reported on the results of 32 patients who underwent TTC arthrodesis using bulk femoral head allograft to fill large bony voids. The defects were the result of talar osteonecrosis, failed total ankle arthroplasty, trauma, osteomyelitis, Charcot or failed reconstructive surgery. Sixteen patients healed their fusion for an overall success rate of 50%. Diabetes mellitus was a predictive factor for failure. All nine patients with diabetes developed a nonunion. As previously mentioned, the avascular talus can be completely excised and not replaced with any graft. Dennison et al[62] reported on six cases of talar osteonecrosis treated with complete talectomy and shortening using Ilizarov ringed-external fixator arthrodesis. Five of six patients reported good results and all six patients went on to union. However, the long-term results of shortening are not known but will likely result in gait abnormalities.

A subset of patients with talus osteonecrosis develop isolated or primarily symptomatic subtalar arthritis and may benefit from isolated subtalar arthrodesis instead of ankle or TTC arthrodesis. In a series of 148 isolated subtalar arthrodeses for various pathologies,[26] the authors reported that all nonunions developed in patients who were found to have 2 mm of avascular subchondral bone at the time of surgery (although the preoperative diagnosis of osteonecrosis was not specified).

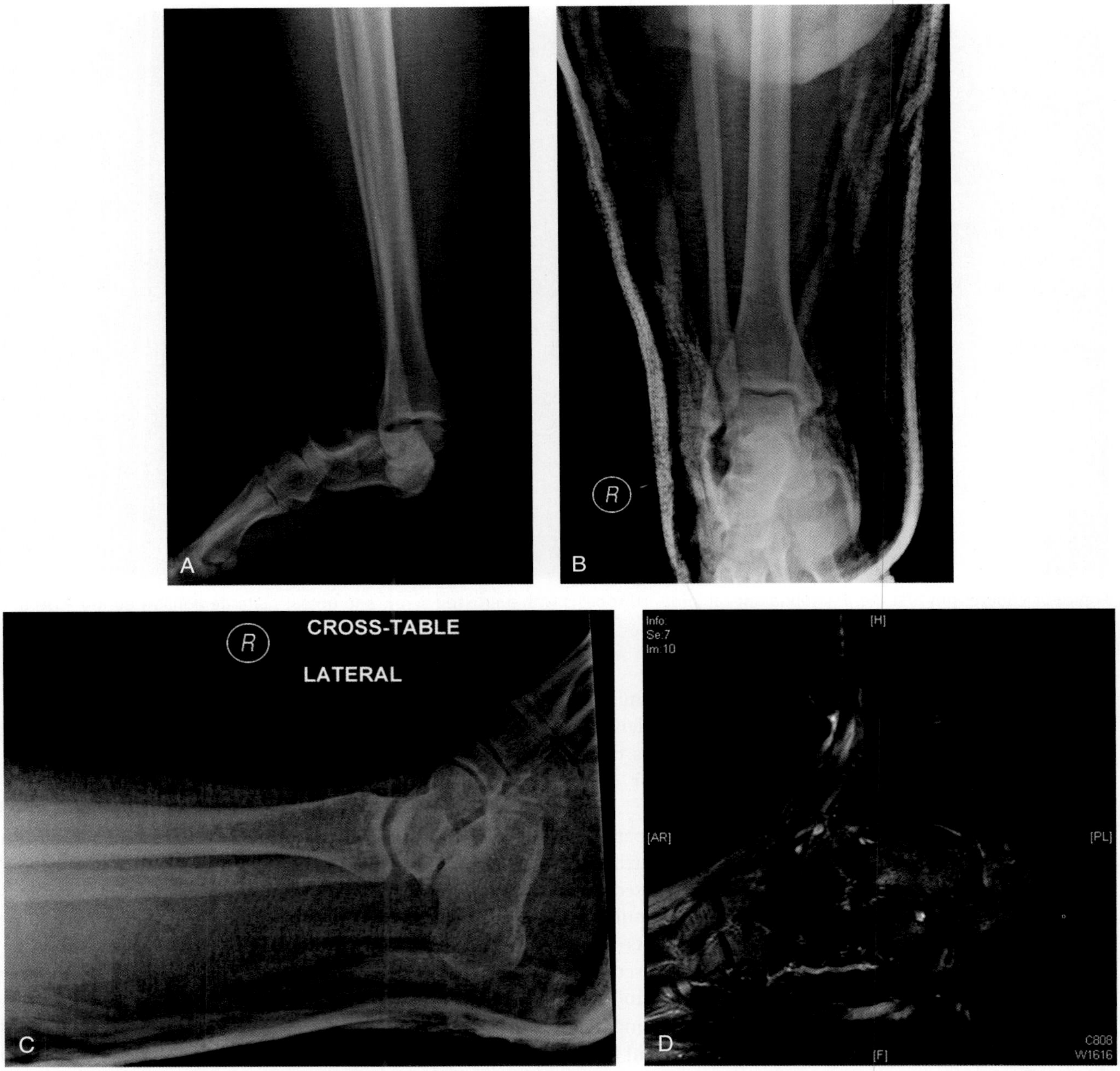

Figure 4 Osteonecrosis after a subtalar dislocation. Emergency department spot radiograph demonstrating a subtalar dislocation (**A**). AP (**B**) and lateral (**C**) radiographs demonstrating reduction of the dislocation. Sagittal magnetic resonance image of the same patient demonstrating osteonecrosis of the talus and subtalar arthritis (**D**).

Joint-Sparing Techniques

Joint-sparing techniques include core decompression and partial or total talus replacement. Joint-sparing techniques are appropriate for symptomatic osteonecrosis with minimal to no arthritis in the ankle, subtalar, or talonavicular joints. Core decompression should be reserved for cases where there is no associated arthritis on the tibia, calcaneus, or navicular. Core decompression has demonstrated some success. A recent systematic review found three studies totaling 85 ankles that underwent core decompression for largely atraumatic osteonecrosis.[57] There was improvement in AOFAS scores as well as other functional outcome scores. Decompression was found to be an appropriate treatment for early and late stage atraumatic osteonecrosis.

The avascular talus does not always have to be replaced with bone. The use of alumina-ceramic talar body replacement in 22 patients has recently been reported on.[63] The prosthesis had a peg design to attach to the talar neck, but the authors found that there were signs of loosening around the peg and therefore the design was changed to be peg-less. At a mean of 98 months of follow-up, the results were mixed. Some patients were improved, but the authors concluded that they cannot recommend the use of a talar body replacement and recommend in favor of total talus replacement. Another study with ceramic total talar replacements was performed in 55 ankles.[64] There was improvement in pain, function, and alignment. However, at final follow-up, 44% of the tibiae and 9% of the naviculae demonstrated radiographic evidence of joint degeneration.

With the advent of 3D printing, total talus replacement is becoming more common, but it must be stressed that the long-term outcomes are not known (**Figure 5**). It is also important to understand that removal of the entire talus makes revision surgery more complicated in that subsequent arthrodesis must address the talonavicular joint.

Navicular

Trauma and spontaneous osteonecrosis are the most common causes of navicular osteonecrosis. Based on the Sangeorzan classification, type 1 (navicular divided into anterior and posterior fragments) and type 3 (comminution in the middle and lateral sections of the navicular) are most commonly associated with navicular osteonecrosis.[65] Mueller-Weiss syndrome is spontaneous osteonecrosis of the navicular of unknown etiology in adults. This is

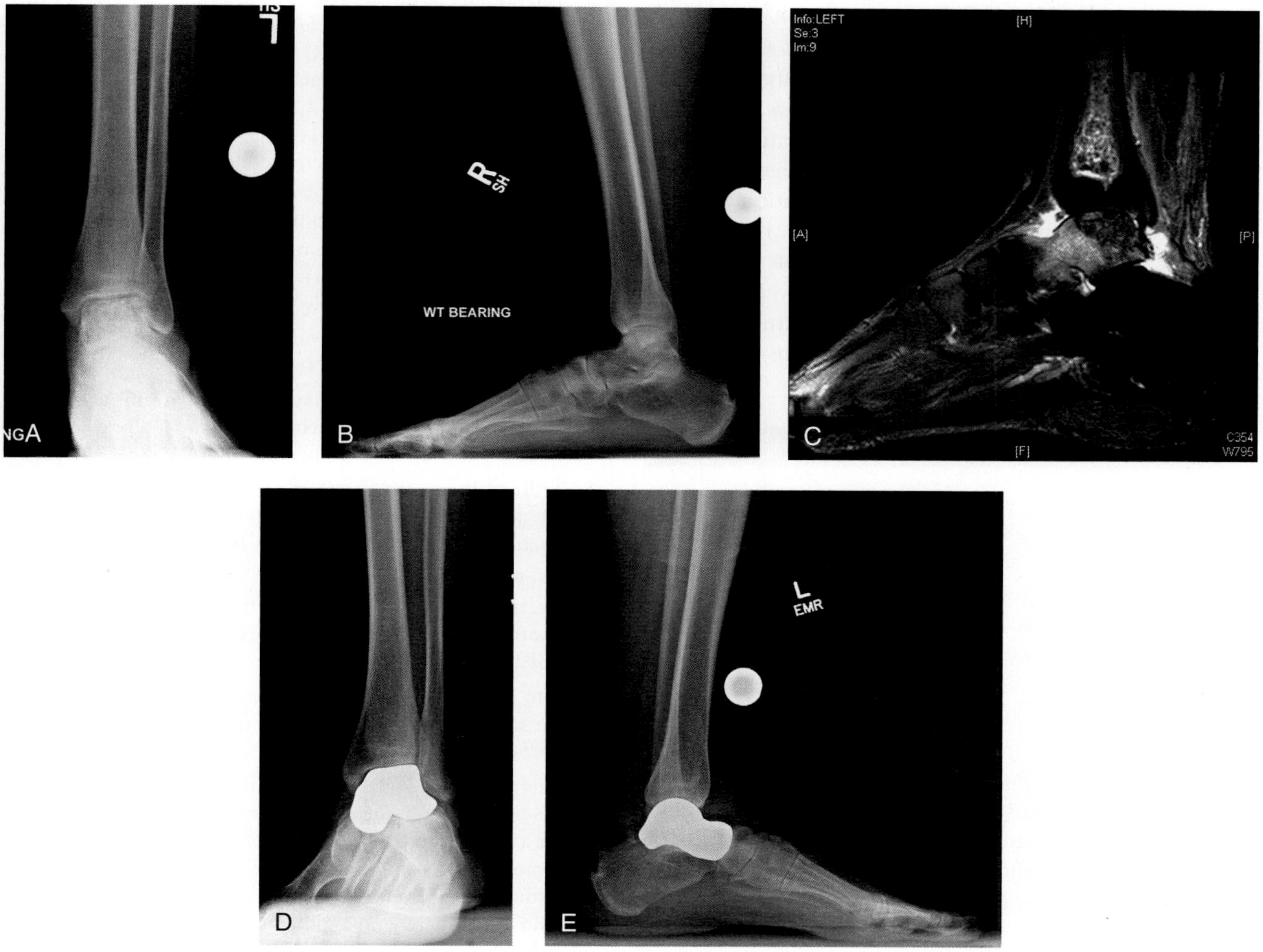

Figure 5 AP (**A**) and lateral (**B**) radiographs of a 67-year-old man with osteonecrosis of the talus. Sagittal magnetic resonance image demonstrating osteonecrosis of the talus (**C**). Oblique (**D**) and lateral (**E**) radiographs of an example of a 3D printed total talus for osteonecrosis of the talus.

different from Kohler's disease, which is osteochondrosis of the tarsal navicular in children. Leading theories are primary osteonecrosis, trauma, congenital malformations, or biomechanical causes.[66] With osteonecrosis of the navicular, it can be difficult to determine if isolated talonavicular arthrodesis or more involved talonavicular-cuneiform (TNC) arthrodesis is needed. In a recent study addressing this concern, the authors performed preoperative MRIs to assess the location of perinavicular arthritis.[66] Sixteen patients underwent isolated talonavicular arthrodesis and 14 underwent TNC arthrodesis. Both groups improved and there were no nonunions. The authors concluded that based on MRI evaluation of the extent of perinavicular arthritis, both isolated talnovicular and TNC arthrodeses have good clinical outcomes.

Summary

Degenerative conditions of the foot and ankle, although varied in etiology, are treated similarly. Most arthritic and avascular conditions can be treated nonsurgically with NSAIDs, altered footwear including orthotics, and corticosteroid injections. However, these treatment modalities only help with pain control and do not alter the underlying pathology. Surgical treatment varies by location but universally relies on arthrodesis as the mainstay. Fusion rates also vary by location, but once a solid fusion is obtained patient satisfaction is generally improved over preoperative levels. Fusion is not guaranteed and future research will likely focus on optimizing the fusion state or developing or improving replacement options.

Key Study Points

- Nonsurgical management of arthritis and osteonecrosis of the foot and ankle includes anti-inflammatories, steroid injections, and bracing treatment.
- Arthritis affects nearly every joint of the foot and ankle. Arthrodesis remains the preferred treatment for end-stage disease in most of these joints. However, ankle replacement has demonstrated equivocal if not better results for the treatment of ankle arthritis and will likely eventually replace arthrodesis as the preferred treatment modality.
- Osteonecrosis most commonly affects the talus or navicular bones as a result of trauma (fracture and/or dislocation), chronic corticosteroid use, alcohol abuse, sickle cell disease, immunosuppression, hemoglobinopathies, or idiopathic causes. Osteonecrosis is likely more common in the talus and navicular because of the tenuous blood supply to these bones.

Annotated References

1. Segal AD, Shofer J, Hahn ME, Orendurff MS, Ledoux WR, Sangeorzan BJ: Functional limitations associated with end-stage ankle arthritis. *J Bone Joint Surg Am Vol* 2012;94(9):777-783.

2. Sun SF, Hsu CW, Sun HP, Chou YJ, Li HJ, Wang JL: The effect of three weekly intra-articular injections of hyaluronate on pain, function, and balance in patients with unilateral ankle arthritis. *J Bone Joint Surg Am Vol* 2011;93(18):1720-1726.

3. DeGroot H III, Uzunishvili S, Weir R, Al-omari A, Gomes B: Intra-articular injection of hyaluronic acid is not superior to saline solution injection for ankle arthritis: A randomized, double-blind, placebo-controlled study. *J Bone Joint Surg Am Vol* 2012;94(1):2-8.

4. Fukawa T, Yamaguchi S, Akatsu Y, Yamamoto Y, Akagi R, Sasho T: Safety and efficacy of intra-articular injection of platelet-rich plasma in patients with ankle osteoarthritis. *Foot Ankle Int* 2017;38(6):596-604.

   The purpose of this study was to determine the efficacy of platelet-rich plasma (PRP) for the treatment of ankle OA. Twenty ankles with varus OA received three injections of PRP at 2-week intervals. Pain and functional outcomes significantly decreased at 4, 12, and 24 weeks after injection. There were no adverse effects. The authors determined that PRP can be a safe and effective option in the treatment of ankle OA. Level of evidence: IV.

5. Knupp M, Stufkens SA, Bolliger L, Barg A, Hintermann B: Classification and treatment of supramalleolar deformities. *Foot Ankle Int* 2011;32(11):1023-1031.

6. Pagenstert G, Knupp M, Valderrabano V, Hintermann B: Realignment surgery for valgus ankle osteoarthritis. *Oper Orthop Traumatol* 2009;21(1):77-87.

7. Tanaka Y, Takakura Y, Hayashi K, Taniguchi A, Kumai T, Sugimoto K: Low tibial osteotomy for varus-type osteoarthritis of the ankle. *J Bone Joint Surg Br* 2006;88(7):909-913.

8. Tellisi N, Fragomen AT, Kleinman D, O'Malley MJ, Rozbruch SR: Joint preservation of the osteoarthritic ankle using distraction arthroplasty. *Foot Ankle Int* 2009;30(4):318-325.

9. Nguyen MP, Pedersen DR, Gao Y, Saltzman CL, Amendola A: Intermediate-term follow-up after ankle distraction for treatment of end-stage osteoarthritis. *J Bone Joint Surg Am Vol* 2015;97(7):590-596.

10. Kim JG, Ha DJ, Gwak HC, et al: Ankle arthrodesis: A comparison of anterior approach and transfibular approach. *Clin Orthop Surg* 2018;10(3):368-373.

    This study retrospectively compared the anterior approach (38 patients) with the transfibular (22 patients) approach for ankle arthrodesis. Patients from both approaches demonstrated significant improvement in the American Orthopaedic Foot and Ankle Society score at most recent follow-up. There was no difference between groups. Ankle arthrodesis by the anterior approach and the transfibular approach showed comparably good clinical results. Level of evidence: IV.

11. Jones CR, Wong E, Applegate GR, Ferkel RD: Arthroscopic ankle arthrodesis: A 2-15 year follow-up study. *Arthroscopy* 2018;34(5):1641-1649.

Retrospective case series evaluating the results of arthroscopic ankle arthrodesis. One-hundred one ankles underwent AAA and were included in the study. Ninety-four percent of ankles achieved fusion. Seventy-five percent reports "good/excellent" results according to the AOS scoring system. Eighty-five percent of ankles had no changes in the talonavicular joint and 69% of ankles had no changes in the subtalar joint in regard to progression of arthritis at a mean follow-up of 86 months. No cases of deep infection or serious adverse events were reported. Level of evidence: IV.

12. Mitchell PM, Douleh DG, Thomson AB: Comparison of ankle fusion rates with and without anterior plate Augmentation. *Foot Ankle Int* 2017;38(4):419-423.

Retrospective cohort study comparing ankle arthrodesis utilizing a compression screw construct with or without anterior plate augmentation. Twenty-six ankles had the screw only construct and 39 ankles had the screw and plate construct. There was no statistically significant difference between the groups in regard to nonunion rate and revision rate, although the numbers trended toward improvement with anterior plate augmentation. There was also a trend toward higher numbers of deep wound infection with anterior plate use; however, this was also not supported statistically. Level of evidence: III.

13. Zwipp H, Rammelt S, Endres T, Heineck J: High union rates and function scores at midterm followup with ankle arthrodesis using a four screw technique. *Clin Orthop Relat Res* 2010;468(4):958-968.

14. Hendrickx RP, Stufkens SA, de Bruijn EE, Sierevelt IN, van Dijk CN, Kerkhoffs GM: Medium- to long-term outcome of ankle arthrodesis. *Foot Ankle Int* 2011;32(10):940-947.

15. Chalayon O, Wang B, Blankenhorn B, et al: Factors affecting the outcomes of uncomplicated primary open ankle arthrodesis. *Foot Ankle Int* 2015;36(10):1170-1179.

16. Coester LM, Saltzman CL, Leupold J, Pontarelli W: Long-term results following ankle arthrodesis for post-traumatic arthritis. *J Bone Joint Surg Am Vol* 2001;83-A(2):219-228.

17. Adams SB Jr, Demetracopoulos CA, Queen RM, Easley ME, DeOrio JK, Nunley JA: Early to mid-term results of fixed-bearing total ankle arthroplasty with a modular intramedullary tibial component. *J Bone Joint Surg Am Vol* 2014;96(23):1983-1989.

18. Stavrakis AI, SooHoo NF: Trends in complication rates following ankle arthrodesis and total ankle replacement. *J Bone Joint Surg Am Vol* 2016;98(17):1453-1458.

Retrospective cohort study using a large state-wide database comparing total ankle replacement to ankle arthrodesis, in regard to utilization rates and complication rates. In total, 8,491 ankle arthrodesis and 1,290 ankle replacements were reviewed. TAR patients had lower rates of readmission and periprosthetic joint infection/wound infections. Over a 15-year period, total ankle replacement utilization increased, whereas ankle arthrodesis utilization stayed similar. Level of evidence: III.

19. Daniels TR, Younger AS, Penner M, et al: Intermediate-term results of total ankle replacement and ankle arthrodesis: A COFAS multicenter study. *J Bone Joint Surg Am Vol* 2014;96(2):135-142.

20. Harston A, Lazarides AL, Adams SB Jr, DeOrio JK, Easley ME, Nunley JA II. Midterm outcomes of a fixed-bearing total ankle arthroplasty with deformity analysis. *Foot Ankle Int* 2017;38(12):1295-1300.

Retrospective cohort study evaluating the outcomes of INBONE I total ankle arthroplasty, specifically in regard to preoperative deformity (<10° or >10°). One-hundred forty-nine patients were reviewed at an average of 5.9 years. Overall survivorship was 90.6%. When comparing groups in regard to preoperative deformity, there were no statistically significant differences in outcome scores (VAS, AOFAS, SF-36, SMFA) or revision rates; however, there was statistically significant difference in reoperation rates (22.2% with >10° versus 37.7% in <10°). Level of evidence: III.

21. Daniels TR, Mayich DJ, Penner MJ: Intermediate to long-term outcomes of total ankle replacement with the Scandinavian Total Ankle Replacement (STAR). *J Bone Joint Surg Am Vol* 2015;97(11):895-903.

22. Barg A, Zwicky L, Knupp M, Henninger HB, Hintermann B: HINTEGRA total ankle replacement: Survivorship analysis in 684 patients. *J Bone Joint Surg Am Vol* 2013;95(13):1175-1183.

23. Koivu H, Kohonen I, Mattila K, Loyttyniemi E, Tiusanen H: Long-term results of Scandinavian Total Ankle Replacement. *Foot Ankle Int* 2017;38(7):723-731.

Retrospective case series evaluating the long-term results of the Scandinavian Total Ankle Replacement (STAR). Thirty-four ankles were included in the study with a median follow-up of 13.3 years. Implant survival rate was 93.9% at 5 years, 86.7% at 10 years, and 63.6% at 15 years. Forty-four percent of ankles had undergone some form of revision surgery. Subjective patient outcome scores were improved at every follow-up interval compared with preoperative values. Level of evidence: IV.

24. Ellington JK, Gupta S, Myerson MS: Management of failures of total ankle replacement with the agility total ankle arthroplasty. *J Bone Joint Surg Am Vol* 2013;95(23):2112-2118.

25. Hintermann B, Zwicky L, Knupp M, Henninger HB, Barg A: HINTEGRA revision arthroplasty for failed total ankle prostheses. *J Bone Joint Surg Am Vol* 2013;95(13):1166-1174.

26. Easley ME, Trnka HJ, Schon LC, Myerson MS: Isolated subtalar arthrodesis. *J Bone Joint Surg Am Vol* 2000;82(5):613-624.

27. Rungprai C, Phisitkul P, Femino JE, et al Open versus posterior arthroscopic subtalar arthrodesis in 121 patients. *J Bone Joint Surg Am Vol* 2016;98(8):636-646.

Retrospective cohort study comparing open subtalar arthrodesis (129 feet) with arthroscopic subtalar arthrodesis (60 feet). The arthroscopic group had statistically significant shorter time to union (11.6 weeks compared with 15.5 weeks), as well as earlier return to activities of daily living,

Foot and Ankle

return to sports, and release to work. Otherwise, the union rate, overall hindfoot alignment, and all functional outcome scores at 1 and 2 years were similar between groups. There were no statistically significant differences in complications between the two groups. Level of evidence: III.

28. Ziegler P, Friederichs J, Hungerer S: Fusion of the subtalar joint for post-traumatic arthrosis: A study of functional outcomes and non-unions. *Int Orthop* 2017;41(7):1387-1393.

    Prospective cohort study evaluating patients who had ungergone subtalar arthrodesis for posttraumatic arthritis, specifically the rate of nonunion, associated risk factors for nonunion, and functional outcomes. Two-hundred fifty-four patients underwent screw fixation and 13 patients underwent external fixation for arthrodesis technique. Risk factors included in the study were infection, smoking, obesity, diabetes, and alcohol abuse. Overall fusion rate for the cohort was 76.2%. Patients with zero risk factors had a fusion rate 88%, one risk factor 75%, two risk factors 72%, and three risk factors 57%. Functional outcome scores were relatively poor in both the primary and the revision cohorts according to AOFAS hindfoot score and VAS score. Level of evidence: II.

29. Zanolli DH, Nunley JA II, Easley ME: Subtalar fusion rate in patients with previous ipsilateral ankle arthrodesis. *Foot Ankle Int* 2015;36(9):1025-1028.

30. Garras DN, Santangelo JR, Wang DW, Easley ME: Subtalar distraction arthrodesis using interpositional frozen structural allograft. *Foot Ankle Int* 2008;29(6):561-567.

31. Hollman EJ, van der Vliet QMJ, Alexandridis G, Hietbrink F, Leenen LPH: Functional outcomes and quality of life in patients with subtalar arthrodesis for posttraumatic arthritis. *Injury* 2017;48(7):1696-1700.

    Retrospective cohort study evaluating patients who had undergone subtalar arthrodesis for posttraumatic arthritis. The main goal was to evaluate these patients in regard to functional outcome scores in the form of a questionnaire. Forty-patients underwent this procedure; however, only 30 patients responded the questionnaire. The median interval between the trauma and the arthrodesis procedure was 23 months. The median interval between the arthrodesis procedure and the patient outcome score collection was 6.8 years. Fusion rate was 94%. Ninety-percent would "recommend this procedure to a friend in a similar situation," 76% had less pain, and 69% had improved walking ability. Level of evidence: III.

32. Chiodo CP, Martin T, Wilson MG: A technique for isolated arthrodesis for inflammatory arthritis of the talonavicular joint. *Foot Ankle Int* 2000;21(4):307-310.

33. Chen CH, Huang PJ, Chen TB, et al: Isolated talonavicular arthrodesis for talonavicular arthritis. *Foot Ankle Int* 2001;22(8):633-636.

34. Jarrell SE III, Owen JR, Wayne JS, Adelaar RS: Biomechanical comparison of screw versus plate/screw construct for talonavicular fusion. *Foot Ankle Int* 2009;30(2):150-156.

35. Granata JD, Berlet GC, Ghotge R, Li Y, Kelly B, DiAngelo D: Talonavicular joint fixation: A biomechanical comparison of locking compression plates and lag screws. *Foot Ankle Spec* 2014;7(1):20-31.

36. Gougoulias N, Lampridis V: Midfoot arthrodesis. *Foot Ankle Surg* 2016;22(1):17-25.

    Case series evaluating 30 patients with symptomatic midfoot arthritis and deformity who underwent arthrodesis. Twenty-eight patients (93.3%) went on to union. Average time to union was 12.9 weeks. Five patients (20%) had postoperative complications including nonunion, metal hardware reaction, Achilles tendon rupture, and superficial peroneal nerve neuropraxia. There were no wound issues or deep wound infection. Fourteen patients (47%) rated their outcome as "excellent," 13 (43%) as "good," and 3 (10%) as "fair or poor." Level of evidence: IV.

37. Nemec SA, Habbu RA, Anderson JG, Bohay DR: Outcomes following midfoot arthrodesis for primary arthritis. *Foot Ankle Int* 2011;32(4):355-361.

38. Sangeorzan BJ, Veith RG, Hansen ST Jr: Salvage of Lisfranc's tarsometatarsal joint by arthrodesis. *Foot Ankle* 1990;10(4):193-200.

39. Parisi MC, Godoy-Santos AL, Ortiz RT, et al: Radiographic and functional results in the treatment of early stages of Charcot neuroarthropathy with a walker boot and immediate weight bearing. *Diabet Foot Ankle* 2013;4. doi:10.3402/dfa.v4i0.22487. eCollection 2013.

40. Sammarco VJ, Sammarco GJ, Walker EW Jr, Guiao RP: Midtarsal arthrodesis in the treatment of Charcot midfoot arthropathy. *J Bone Joint Surg Am Vol* 2009;91(1):80-91.

41. Lee DJ, Schaffer J, Chen T, Oh I: Internal versus external fixation of Charcot midfoot deformity realignment. *Orthopedics* 2016;39(4):e595-601.

    Systematic review of 11 studies (10 case series and 1 case report) evaluating either internal fixation or external fixation for Charcot midfoot deformity. Eight of the studies (88 feet) evaluated internal fixation and three of the studies (38 feet) evaluated external fixation. The internal fixation group had a 25% higher odds of returning to functional ambulation and a 42% reduced rate of ulcer occurrence; however, they also had a 1.5-fold increase in extremity amputation and 2-fold increase in deep infection, and a 3.4-fold increase in wound healing complications. The external fixation group was eight times more likely to develop radiographic nonunion. Level of evidence: IV.

42. Coughlin MJ, Shurnas PS: Hallux rigidus. Grading and long-term results of operative treatment. *J Bone Joint Surg Am Vol* 2003;85-A(11):2072-2088.

43. Baumhauer JF, Singh D, Glazebrook M, et al: Correlation of hallux rigidus grade with motion, VAS pain, intraoperative cartilage loss, and treatment success for first MTP joint arthrodesis and synthetic cartilage implant. *Foot Ankle Int* 2017;38(11):1175-1182.

    Retrospective study evaluating patients who were previously prospectively, randomized to receive either a synthetic cartilage implant (Cartiva) or arthrodesis for hallux valgus. The goal of this study was to see if there was any correlation between range of motion, subjective pain score, preoperative arthritis grading, and intraoperative extent of arthritis. In 202 patients, there was statistically significant correlation between preoperative

Foot and Ankle

grade and intraoperative severity of arthritis; however, there was no correlation between preoperative grade and ROM and subjective pain scores. Level of evidence: II.

44. Bussewitz BW, Dyment MM, Hyer CF: Intermediate-term results following first metatarsal cheilectomy. *Foot Ankle Spec* 2013;6(3):191-195.

45. O'Malley MJ, Basran HS, Gu Y, Sayres S, Deland JT: Treatment of advanced stages of hallux rigidus with cheilectomy and phalangeal osteotomy. *J Bone Joint Surg Am Vol* 2013;95(7):606-610.

46. Mackey RB, Thomson AB, Kwon O, Mueller MJ, Johnson JE: The modified oblique keller capsular interpositional arthroplasty for hallux rigidus. *J Bone Joint Surg Am Vol* 2010;92(10):1938-1946.

47. Stone OD, Ray R, Thomson CE, Gibson JN: Long-term follow-up of arthrodesis vs total joint arthroplasty for hallux rigidus. *Foot Ankle Int* 2017;38(4):375-380.

Randomized, controlled study comparing arthroplasty (unconstrained) versus arthrodesis for hallux rigidus. Thirty arthrodeses and 36 arthroplasties were included in the final study. Mean follow-up was 15.2 years. Subjective outcome measures showed that the arthrodesis group had statistically significant less pain and were more satisfied than the arthroplasty group. The arthrodesis group also has statistically significant less revision rates. Nine arthroplasties underwent revision and the most common reasoning being aseptic loosening of the phalangeal component. Level of evidence: I.

48. Baumhauer JF, Singh D, Glazebrook M, et al: Prospective, randomized, multi-centered clinical trial assessing safety and efficacy of a synthetic cartilage implant versus first metatarsophalangeal arthrodesis in advanced hallux rigidus. *Foot Ankle Int* 2016;37(5):457-469.

Prospective, randomized, multicenter study comparing a synthetic cartilage implant (Cartiva) to arthrodesis for advanced hallux rigidus. There were 152 patients in the synthetic implant group and 50 patients in the arthrodesis group. Both groups had similar improvement in subjective outcome scores (FAAM, VAS). The synthetic implant group also has improved first MTP active dorsiflexion movement (6.2°). Secondary surgical procedures were also similar between groups. Level of evidence: I.

49. McNeil DS, Baumhauer JF, Glazebrook MA: Evidence-based analysis of the efficacy for operative treatment of hallux rigidus. *Foot Ankle Int* 2013;34(1):15-32.

50. Hyer CF, Scott RT, Swiatek M: A retrospective comparison of first metatarsophalangeal joint arthrodesis using a locked plate and compression screw technique. *Foot Ankle Spec* 2012;5(5):289-292.

51. Doty J, Coughlin M, Hirose C, Kemp T: Hallux metatarsophalangeal joint arthrodesis with a hybrid locking plate and a plantar neutralization screw: A prospective study. *Foot Ankle Int* 2013;34(11):1535-1540.

52. Issa K, Naziri Q, Kapadia BH, Lamm BM, Jones LC, Mont MA: Clinical characteristics of early-stage osteonecrosis of the ankle and treatment outcomes. *J Bone Joint Surg Am Vol* 2014;96(9):e73.

53. Chiodo CP, Herbst SA: Osteonecrosis of the talus. *Foot Ankle Clin* 2004;9(4):745-755, vi.

54. Delanois RE, Mont MA, Yoon TR, Mizell M, Hungerford DS: Atraumatic osteonecrosis of the talus. *J Bone Joint Surg Am Vol* 1998;80(4):529-536.

55. Kemnitz S, Moens P, Peerlinck K, Fabry G: Avascular necrosis of the talus in children with haemophilia. *J Pediatr Orthop B* 2002;11(1):73-78.

56. Gross CE, Sershon RA, Frank JM, Easley ME, Holmes GB Jr: Treatment of osteonecrosis of the talus. *JBJS Rev* 2016;4(7). doi: 10.3402/dfa.v4i0.22487. eCollection 2013.

Review article discussing the etiology, diagnosis, and current management of osteonecrosis of the talus. Level of evidence: V.

57. Gross CE, Haughom B, Chahal J, Holmes GB Jr: Treatments for avascular necrosis of the talus: A systematic review. *Foot Ankle Spec* 2014;7(5):387-397.

58. Devries JG, Philbin TM, Hyer CF: Retrograde intramedullary nail arthrodesis for avascular necrosis of the talus. *Foot Ankle Int* 2010;31(11):965-972.

59. Tenenbaum S, Stockton KG, Bariteau JT, Brodsky JW: Salvage of avascular necrosis of the talus by combined ankle and hindfoot arthrodesis without structural bone graft. *Foot Ankle Int* 2015;36(3):282-287.

60. Abd-Ella MM, Galhoum A, Abdelrahman AF, Walther M: Management of nonunited talar fractures with avascular necrosis by resection of necrotic bone, bone grafting, and fusion with an intramedullary nail. *Foot Ankle Int* 2017;38(8):879-884.

This case series evaluated 12 patients after talus fractures who went on to develop a nonunion and avascular necrosis. The authors performed resection of the necrotic bone regions, bone grafting with autologous iliac crest, and then used a tibiotalocalcaneal intramedullary nail for fixation. Mean follow-up was 23 months, solid bone fusion was achieved in 8 patients, stable fibrous union in 1 patient, and 3 patients required reoperation and went on to fusion. All patients scored "good" or "excellent" at final follow-up according their AOFAS score. Level of evidence: IV.

61. Jeng CL, Campbell JT, Tang EY, Cerrato RA, Myerson MS: Tibiotalocalcaneal arthrodesis with bulk femoral head allograft for salvage of large defects in the ankle. *Foot Ankle Int* 2013;34(9):1256-1266.

62. Dennison MG, Pool RD, Simonis RB, Singh BS: Tibiocalcaneal fusion for avascular necrosis of the talus. *J Bone Joint Surg Br* 2001;83(2):199-203.

63. Taniguchi A, Takakura Y, Sugimoto K, et al: The use of a ceramic talar body prosthesis in patients with aseptic necrosis of the talus. *J Bone Joint Surg Br* 2012;94(11): 1529-1533.

64. Taniguchi A, Takakura Y, Tanaka Y, et al: An alumina ceramic total talar prosthesis for osteonecrosis of the talus. *J Bone Joint Surg Am Vol* 2015;97(16):1348-1353.

65. DiGiovanni CW, Patel A, Calfee R, Nickisch F: Osteonecrosis in the foot. *J Am Acad Orthop Surg* 2007;15(4):208-217.

66. Cao HH, Lu WZ, Tang KL: Isolated talonavicular arthrodesis and talonavicular-cuneiform arthrodesis for the Muller-Weiss disease. *J Orthop Surg Res* 2017;12(1):83.

Thirty patients of stage III and IV Müller-Weiss disease were divided into the talonavicular (TN) arthrodesis group and the talonavicular-cuneiform (TNC) arthrodesis group according to the perinavicular osteoarthritis by MRI scans. According to MRI evaluation, either TN or TNC arthrodesis for stage III or IV Müller-Weiss disease have the good clinical outcomes with solid fusion rate and obvious improvement of the quality of life of patients. Level of evidence: III.

Chapter 44

The Diabetic Foot

Michael S. Pinzur, MD

ABSTRACT

Foot morbidity affecting patients with diabetes consumes a substantial partial of healthcare resources, leading to over 70,000 lower extremity amputations yearly in the United States. One-third of these patients will die during the first 2 years following a transtibial amputation. This chapter will discuss the pathophysiology leading to diabetic foot morbidity, discuss the various expressions of the disease process, and highlight the modern approach to lessening the impact of this multiple organ system disease process.

Keywords: Charcot foot; diabetic foot; neuropathic foot

Introduction

The United States Centers for Disease Control now estimates that there are over 29 million diabetics in the United States alone, or almost 10% of the population. One of the most important resource-consuming comorbidities of diabetes is foot infection, which now leads to more than 70,000 lower extremity amputations yearly in the United States.[1] Although not appreciably decreasing mortality from peripheral vascular disease, our vascular surgery colleagues have used endovascular surgical techniques to decrease the risk for amputation in diabetics with peripheral vascular disease. Our efforts to address diabetic foot ulcer and infection have not been as successful, as the amputation rate due to infection has not substantially changed over the past 10 years[2,3] (**Figure 1**). This becomes even more important when we appreciate that the 2-year mortality rate following amputation in the diabetic population has not improved during the same period.[1-4]

Dr. Pinzur or an immediate family member is a member of a speakers' bureau or has made paid presentations on behalf of Stryker; serves as a paid consultant to or is an employee of Stryker; and serves as a board member, owner, officer, or committee member of the American Academy of Orthopaedic Surgeons and the American Orthopaedic Foot and Ankle Society.

Pathophysiology of Diabetic Organ System Morbidity

It appears that there is a common pathophysiologic pathway that leads to multiple organ system pathology, as each affected organ system appears to be affected at a similar magnitude and rate. It is likely that this pathologic process stems from the disease impact on the vascular system. Advanced glycation end products (AGEs) appear to accumulate in the walls of blood vessels. These AGEs impact on local perfusion and appear to trigger specific cytokine release. The combination of impaired perfusion and cytokine release leads to dysfunction of targeted organs and organ systems.[5]

Diabetic Peripheral Neuropathy

One of the major pathologic end organ responses is the development of peripheral neuropathy. The most obvious expression of peripheral neuropathy is the loss of protective sensation, most easily diagnosed with insensitivity to the Semmes-Weinstein 5.07 (10 g) monofilament (**Figure 2**). Motor and vasomotor neuropathy will be discussed relative to the development of Charcot foot arthropathy.

Immune Deficiency

Associated with this long-standing organ system pathology is an important concomitant associated immune system deficiency, making patients more prone to deep infection associated with an acquired deformity. Contrary to the falsely held belief that this pathologic sensory neuropathy is painless, patients will often have pain with or without an accompanied fracture or deformity.

Diabetic Foot Ulcers and Foot Infection

Risk Factors

Diabetics who have previously had a foot ulcer or infection, or have undergone a partial or whole foot amputation, are at the greatest risk for developing a foot ulcer

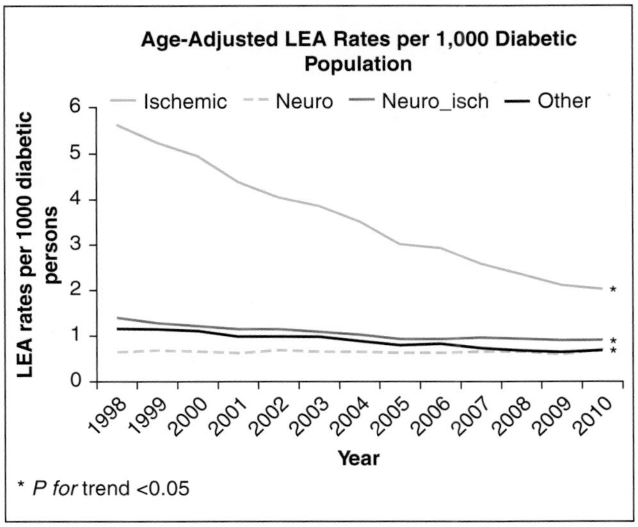

Figure 1 Illustration showing differential trends for ischemic and neuropathic lower extremity amputation (LEA) rates in the United States, 1998-2010. (From the Division of Diabetes Translation, Centers for Disease Control and Prevention.)

or foot infection. Risk factors for those who have never had a foot ulcer or infection are peripheral neuropathy, as measured by insensitivity to the Semmes-Weinstein 5.07 (10 g) monofilament, or peripheral vascular disease (see **Figure 2**). The final modifiable risk factor is bony deformity, as diabetic foot ulcers are most likely to occur secondary to external shearing forces, most commonly footwear, to skin overlying bony prominences.[5-8]

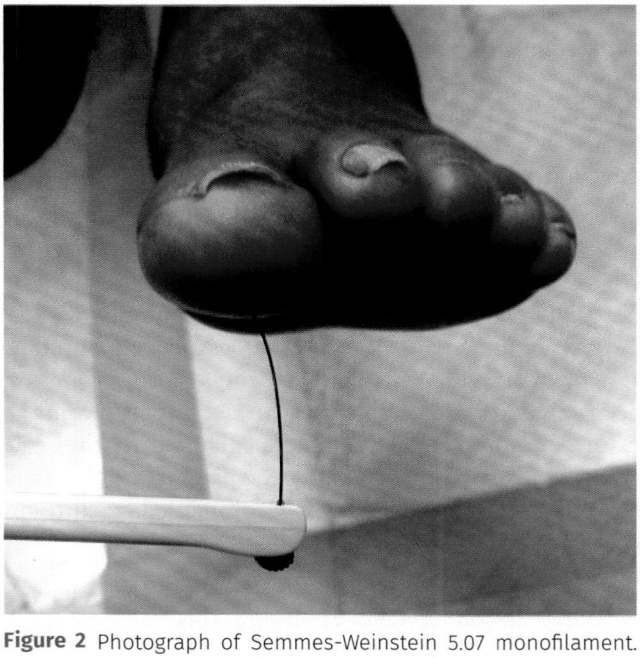

Figure 2 Photograph of Semmes-Weinstein 5.07 monofilament. When applied to the plantar surface of the foot, the monofilament imparts 10 g of pressure. This amount of pressure appears to be a reasonable threshold for protective sensation in the diabetic population. This tool becomes an excellent method for screening for risk status in the diabetic.

Many grading systems have been developed to categorize risk. Most are cumbersome and not predictive. Understanding the spectrum of risk is a simple methodology to assign risk. At the low end of risk stratification is the diabetic patient with no structural deformity, protective sensation (as measured by the Semmes-Weinstein 5.07, 10 g monofilament), and normal palpable pedal pulses. The opposite end of the spectrum is the patient with structural deformity (hallux valgus, hammer toes, or Charcot-associated deformity), peripheral neuropathy (insensitivity to the monofilament), and absent pedal pulses.

Grading of Diabetic Foot Ulcers

The Meggitt-Wagner grading system for the classification of diabetic foot ulcers is a validated tool that can be used to both risk stratify and determine treatment strategy[9-14] (**Figure 3**). Wagner grade 0 patients have either had a previous foot ulcer or infection or are "at risk" to develop an ulcer or infection. Grade I (superficial ulcer) or grade II (deep wound without abscess or bony involvement) can be treated as an outpatient with local débridement, empiric oral first-generation cephalosporin antibiotic therapy, and either a commercially available offloading device or total contact cast. Once resolved, these patients are managed longitudinally with ongoing patient education, periodic monitoring, and therapeutic footwear. Grade III ulcers are defined by the presence of an abscess or osteomyelitis. These patients will require a minimum of surgical débridement, culture-specific antibiotic therapy, and longitudinal care.

Outpatient Treatment of Diabetic Foot Ulcers

The desired optimal clinical outcome of any patient with diabetic foot morbidity is an ulcer- and infection-free limb that can be managed longitudinally with commercially available depth-inlay therapeutic footwear and custom accommodative foot orthoses/insoles[6,14-16] (**Figure 4**). It has been demonstrated that a proactive program combining foot-specific patient education, ongoing clinical monitoring, and accommodative footwear can be very successful in decreasing the incidence of diabetic foot ulceration, infection, and amputation. Foot-specific patient education includes instruction on daily foot inspection, appropriate footwear, and instruction on nail and callus care.[1,6,8,14,15] The Medicare Therapeutic Shoe Bill of 1993 provides one pair of appropriate depth-inlay shoes and three insoles per year for Medicare-entitled

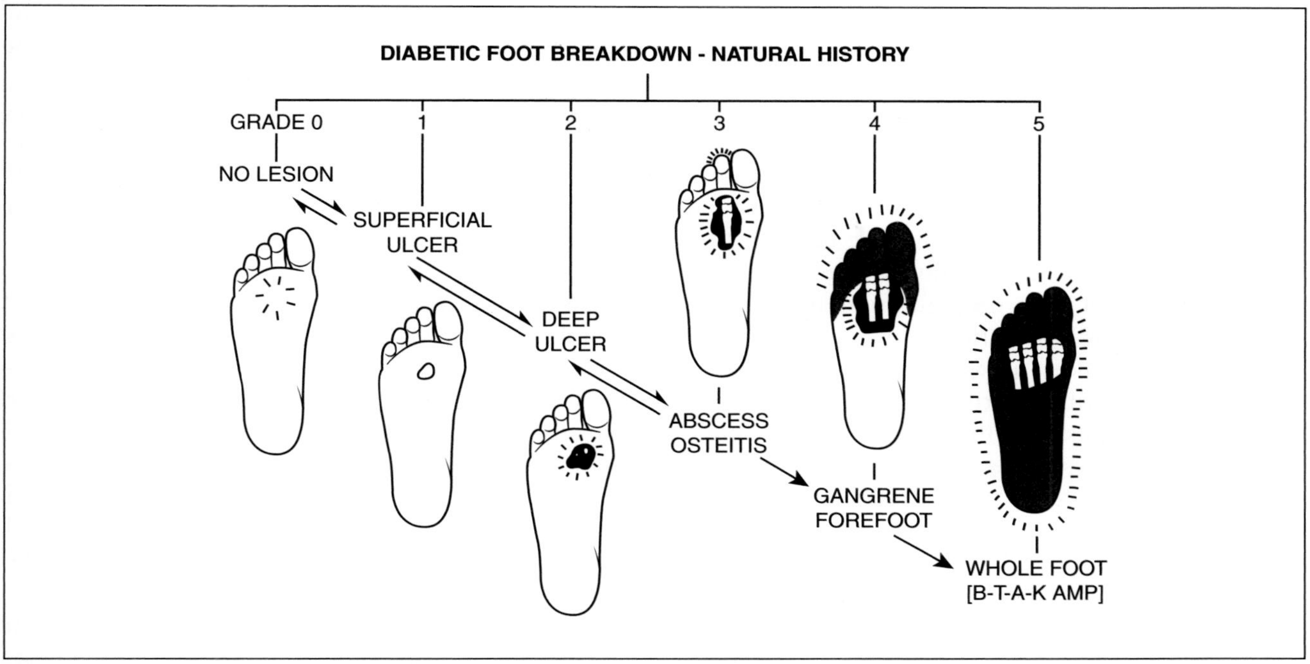

Figure 3 Illustration showing Wagner-Meggitt classification system for diabetic foot wounds. (Reprinted with permission from Wagner FW Jr: The dysvascular foot: A system for diagnosis and treatment. *Foot Ankle* 1981;2:64-122.)

individuals.[17] Most insurance-providers in the United States follow these well-thought-out guidelines. Such is not the case for patients with silent vascular disease (ie, diminished or absent pulses) as the vascular surgeon does not consider intervention until the patient has a nonhealing wound or ischemic pain at rest.

Using the prognostic value of the Wagner-Meggitt risk stratification tool, the grade 0 patient simply requires foot-specific patient education, ongoing clinical monitoring, and appropriate footwear. Patients with grade I and II wounds are managed as outpatients. Because of their sensory neuropathy, necrotic or infected tissue can be excised, and calluses removed in an office or wound care clinic setting. Longitudinal care of the wound can be managed with simple dressings. Patients are allowed to bear weight in either a total contact cast or various commercially available "offloading" devices. "Offloading" the wound is accomplished by distributing weight-bearing pressure over a large surface area with either a healing shoe, custom orthotic, commercially available fracture foot with pressure-dissipating insole, or a total contact cast.[6,8,10,11,14]

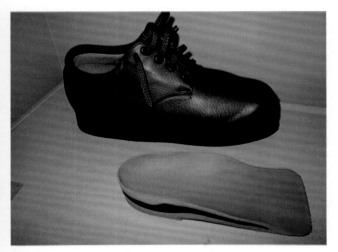

Figure 4 Photograph of depth-inlay shoe with custom accommodative foot orthosis.

Inpatient Management of Diabetic Foot Infection

A Wagner-Meggitt grade III wound is defined by deep wound or abscess. It is differentiated from a grade IV wound which has bony involvement (eg, osteomyelitis). The grade III wound crosses a threshold that will require inpatient care, extensive surgical débridement, and/or amputation and parenteral antibiotic therapy. Diabetic patients with an abscess will often present with clinical signs of sepsis characterized by fever, chills, hypotension, and hyperglycemia. A foot abscess and sepsis is often the first sign that the patient is diabetic. Unfortunately, diabetic patients with infection can be challenging to make an appropriate diagnosis because of the associated immune impairment that often complicates long-standing diabetes. This type of presentation in the outpatient clinic might be swelling and erythema with or without a wound. When questioned, long-standing diabetics might have noticed prodromal elevated blood glucose or difficulty controlling blood glucose.[18]

It is highly unusual for a diabetic foot abscess to develop in the absence of an ulcer, open wound, infected ingrown toenail, or skin crack between toes. Hematogenous source of infection is rare. The most accurate test to identify a deep infection and the need for surgical intervention is the "probe-to-bone" test[18] (**Figure 5**). Every ulcer or wound in a diabetic foot should be probed with a sterile applicator stick. A positive test is accomplished if the "probe" contacts bone, defining the wound as a Wagner-Meggitt grade III or IV wound. A positive test virtually assures deep infection and the need for surgery. Unfortunately, a negative test does not rule out deep infection.

All patients in should have weight-bearing plain radiographs both to characterize bony deformity and to act as a baseline for diagnosing osteomyelitis. Bony lucency can be suggestive of osteomyelitis or may well represent osteoporosis. Bony destruction with

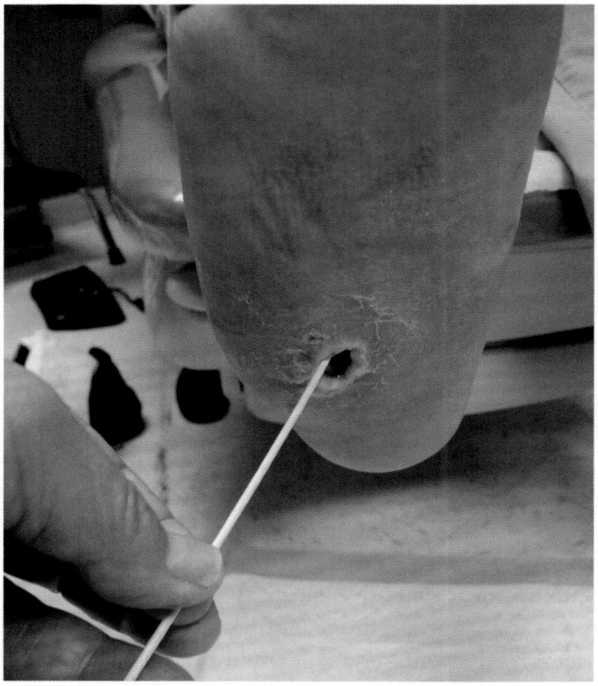

Figure 5 Photograph showing the "probe-to-bone" test. When an applicator stick (eg, probe) is placed into a diabetic foot wound and contacts the bone, there is a high likelihood that the bone is infected. A negative test does not assure absence of deep infection.

a break in the cortex is a late finding, making plain radiographs very difficult to interpret. Treatment should not be delayed pending advanced imaging. Radionucleotide imaging with or without labels has a high false-positive and false-negative rate. The same can be said for MRI. Thus, the diagnosis of deep infection and the need for surgery is primarily a clinical decision.[8,12,18-20]

Vascular Evaluation

Palpation of dorsals pedis and posterior tibial pulses should be part of the initial evaluation. An ankle-brachial index (ABI) should be obtained if pulses are not palpable and "normal." Patients are unlikely to heal a surgical wound or an amputation if the ABI is less than 0.5.[12] The ABI will not be adequately measured in up to 15% of diabetic patients because of calcified noncompressible vessels. Doppler toe pressures will be necessary to determine inflow in such affected patients. Vascular surgery consultation should be obtained in patients with impaired inflow, following surgical resolution of the infection.[14,21]

Nutritional Support

Diabetic patients with infection are often malnourished and have a high potential for wound failure. A serum albumin of 3.0 g/dL appears to be necessary to support wound healing in this highly comorbid patient population. Following surgical resolution of the acute infection, nutritional support is necessary to support wound healing. Patients with renal failure and low serum albumin levels are unlikely to achieve successful healing of surgical débridement wounds or distal amputation levels. Initial results and long-term clinical outcomes would suggest that these patients are often better served with amputation at the transtibial or knee disarticulation levels.[22-24]

Surgical Treatment of Diabetic Foot Infections

Cultures should be taken at the time of the positive "probe-to-bone" test. Empiric antibiotic therapy should be initiated with a first-generation cephalosporin pending obtaining aerobic and anaerobic tissue cultures at the time of surgery.[8,18] Localized infections can be treated with longitudinal incisions and complete excision of all infected tissue. Aerobic and anaerobic tissue cultures should be taken from the base of the wound. If adequate surgical margins cannot be achieved with longitudinal incisions, then a transverse amputation should be performed, retaining as much viable tissue as possible. Vacuum-assisted wound closure is a valuable adjunct to be used following completed excision of infected tissue.[25]

Wound closure should be delayed until the "zone of injury/infection" has recovered, culture-specific antibiotic therapy has been initiated, sepsis has been resolved, and tissue nutrition has been improved (serum albumin approaching 3.0 g/dL). Failure to achieve early wound healing should prompt the surgeon to consider more proximal amputation.

Functional Amputation Levels

Hallux Amputation

Retention of the insertion of the flexor hallucis brevis at the level of the proximal metaphysis retains medial column stability. The optimal soft-tissue envelope for hallux amputation is accomplished with a long plantar flap. Patients with perceived weakness or instability at terminal stance phase of gait can use a carbon graphite "Morton's extension" foot orthosis to substitute for absent flexor hallucis.

Lesser Toe Amputation

With the exception of the second toe, there is little functional loss from lesser toe amputation. A severe hallux valgus with prominence of the medial border of the first metatarsal can be avoided by retaining the proximal metaphysis of the second toe.

Ray Resection

First or fifth ray resection is generally indicated for osteomyelitis of an involved outer metatarsal. It is rarely indicated in dysvascular disease because of the geographic nature of the disease process. First ray resection should be avoided, when possible, in active individuals, because of the likelihood of developing an apropulsive gait pattern due to loss of the flexor hallucis tendons. A severe late varus deformity can be avoided following fifth ray resection by retaining the base of the metatarsal with the attachment of the peroneus brevis tendon. Oblique osteotomy of the metatarsal will allow maintenance of a smooth lateral border of the residual foot.

Central ray resection is best used for initial débridement of infection. Once the infection is resolved and the patient is medically optimized, transmetatarsal or tarsal-metatarsal amputation is a very reasonable clinical outcome.[26]

Midfoot Amputation

A reasonable platform for weight-bearing amputation can be achieved with amputation at the transmetatarsal or tarsal-metatarsal levels. The most durable soft-tissue envelope is accomplished with a plantar-based flap. This flap will generally require performing the bony transection at the level of the proximal metaphysis of each of the metatarsals. Late varus or equinus deformity can be avoided by performing a percutaneous tendon Achilles or gastrocnemius muscle lengthening and application of a short leg walking cast with the ankle positioned at 90° for 1 month.[22]

Hindfoot Amputation

Hindfoot amputation has a high likelihood to result in a severe equinus deformity, even with tendon Achilles release. Even when successful, the residual limb provides no lever arm for walking propulsion. These patients are functionally far better served with the Syme's ankle disarticulation.

Syme's Ankle Disarticulation Amputation

The Syme's ankle disarticulation is an end-bearing amputation that retains the weight-bearing surface of the distal tibia and the normal soft-tissue envelope of the retained heel pad.

The apices of the fish-mouth incision are placed at the anterior midpoints of the medial and lateral malleoli. The incision is taken down to the bone, followed by removal of the talus and calcaneus via sharp dissection. Care is taken to protect the posterior tibial artery, which is the primary blood supply of the flap. The malleoli are removed flush with the articular surface of the retained tibia and the metaphysical flares of the distal tibia and fibula are removed with a small power saw. The heel pad is then secured to the retained tibia with a nonabsorbable suture placed through a drill hole in the anterior corner of the residual tibia.[23,24]

Charcot Foot Arthropathy

Charcot neuropathic osteoarthropathy (CN), commonly referred to as Charcot foot, is a relatively common pathologic condition of the foot that occurs in patients with long-standing peripheral neuropathy, most commonly diabetic associated. Once thought to be rare, the incidence is likely as high as 0.3 per thousand per year.[27] Trauma, often trivial, initiates a cytokine-mediated inflammatory process in patients with long-standing peripheral neuropathy. Many patients are incorrectly diagnosed as cellulitis, gout, or tenosynovitis. Following a short period of disability, most heal with, at most, a small amount of residual deformity. A small number of patients progress through the three-stage process that we have come to know as Charcot foot.[28-30]

There is no single cause for the development of Charcot foot. The predisposing factors are long-standing peripheral neuropathy, most commonly associated with diabetes. Trauma appears to initiate a cytokine pathway characterized by acute and chronic inflammation, osteoclastic bone resorption, and mechanical bony failure (eg, fracture). This process is followed by an impaired healing response, leading to a resultant deformity. The resultant deformity can be characterized by bony union with deformity or deformity with characteristics similar to a nonunion.[28-30]

One should also appreciate the role of associated motor and autonomic neuropathies. Neuropathy affects smaller nerves and, associated, muscles earlier than the impact on larger nerves and muscles. The impact on the development of Charcot foot is the resultant motor imbalance between the relatively weakened ankle dorsiflexors and overpowering plantar flexors. This motor imbalance leads to a relative dynamic ankle equinus loading during terminal stance phase of gait. Loading of prepositioned dynamic equinus osteoporotic bone, which is universally present in the long-standing diabetic, creates a bending moment. This mechanical overloading creates a situation akin to a "stress fracture." The patient continues to load the bone because of the loss of protective sensation. This leads to mechanical failure of the bone which is dependent on the direction of the loading. Not surprisingly, morbidly obese patients are more likely to present with acquired deformity.

The final complicating factor of peripheral neuropathy is the autonomic peripheral neuropathy that is expressed as loss of autonomic vascular tone, with resulting venous swelling. Swollen tissues have less resistance to repetitive trauma, making tissue breakdown overlying bony deformity more likely.[6,21,30]

Eichenholtz described a time-line of a destructive disease process that was arbitrarily divided into three phases. The active phase (stage I) is characterized by swelling and no structural deformity or radiographic abnormality. This evolves to an active destructive phase (stage II) characterized by peri-articular fracture or dislocation. A healing phase (stage III) is characterized by healing with a residual deformity.[28]

Classically, treatment has involved non–weight-bearing immobilization during the active phase of the disease process, followed by accommodative bracing treatment of the residual deformity. This approach was based on observation and has not been supported by modern evidentiary standards. An observational investigation of the American Orthopaedic Foot and Ankle Society Charcot Study group demonstrated that the health-related quality of life of patients successfully treated with this paradigm was roughly equivalent to similar patients with a transtibial amputation.[31-33] A recent corroborating investigation was performed as a benchmark for patients undergoing an attempt at surgical reconstruction.[34] These observations have led to the modern paradigm of treatment.

Treatment

It has been demonstrated that immobilization appears to turn off the destructive process. Patients are now immobilized in a weight-bearing total contact cast or commercially available fracture boot during the active phase (Eichenholtz stage I) of the disease process.[31,32] Patients will then progress to the healing phase (Eichenholtz stage III) with, or without, deformity. Patients with residual deformity that allows weight-bearing on the normal plantar surface of the foot are considered clinically plantigrade and are managed longitudinally with commercially available depth-inlay shoes and custom accommodative foot orthoses[35,36] (**Figure 6**, A).

The historic indications for surgery were osteomyelitis and wounds that did not heal with accommodative treatment with a total contact cast or custom orthotic device. Surgical correction of the acquired deformity is now well accepted when patients are either clinically or radiographically nonplantigrade, as these individuals are far more likely to develop tissue breakdown and ulceration[37-40] (**Figure 6**, B). A relatively new indication for surgery is for pain at the site of an unstable Charcot arthropathy deformity. A large retrospective case series has established a new deformity stratification with implications on clinical outcomes following surgical correction of the acquired deformity.[41]

Reconstruction of Nonplantigrade Deformity

The first step in treatment is a percutaneous tenon Achilles lengthening or gastrocnemius muscle lengthening to achieve muscle balance. The next step is a wedge-resection of bone at the apex of the deformity. Immobilization is best accomplished with either intramedullary bolts or external fixation[39-41] (**Figure 7**).

Amputation for Charcot Foot

Amputation should generally be part of the discussion as an alternative to reconstruction for Charcot foot deformity, especially in the presence of osteomyelitis. Amputation level decision-making should

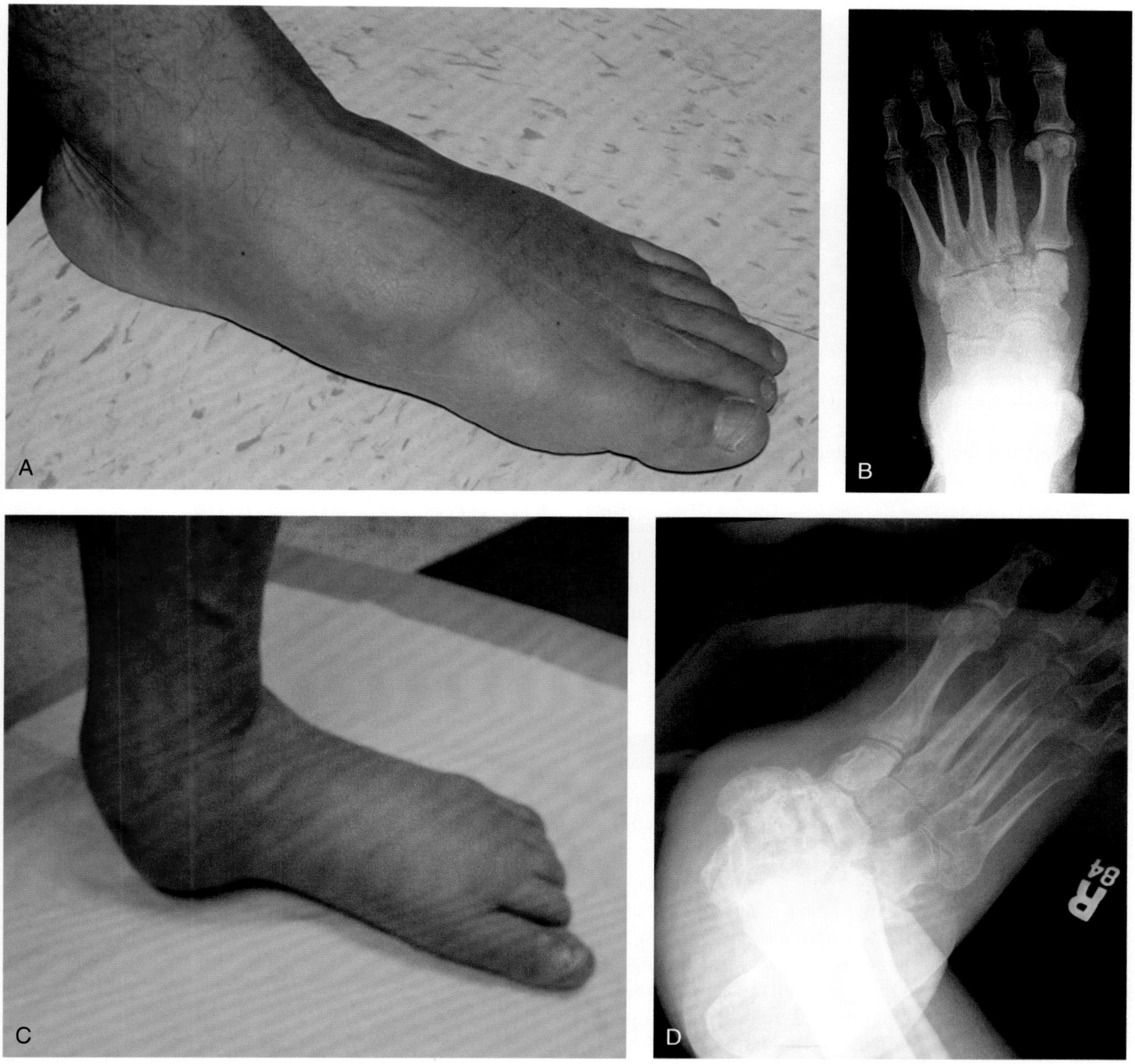

Figure 6 Surgical correction of the acquired deformity associated with Charcot foot arthropathy is currently advised when patients are clinically or radiographically nonplantigrade. Photograph (**A**) and weight-bearing AP radiograph (**B**) of a patient who is both clinically and radiographically plantigrade. Patients are considered clinically plantigrade when they weightbear through the plantar tissue of the involved foot. Patients are considered radiographically plantigrade when a line drawn through the axis of the talus, representing the axis of the hindfoot (talus), is reasonably colinear with a line drawn through the axis of the first metatarsal, representing the axis of the forefoot. Photograph (**C**) and weight-bearing AP radiograph (**D**) of a patient with a nonplantigrade Charcot foot deformity. Note that he is weightbearing on nonplantar skin of the medial foot overlying the head of the talus. It is likely that the skin overlying the talar head will break down and ulcerate. Surgical correction of this deformity is advised.

be carefully correlated with outcome expectations. It should be appreciated that morbidly obese diabetics with renal failure are difficult to fit with a prosthetic socket because of residual limb volume fluctuation. Knee disarticulation should be considered in these patients.

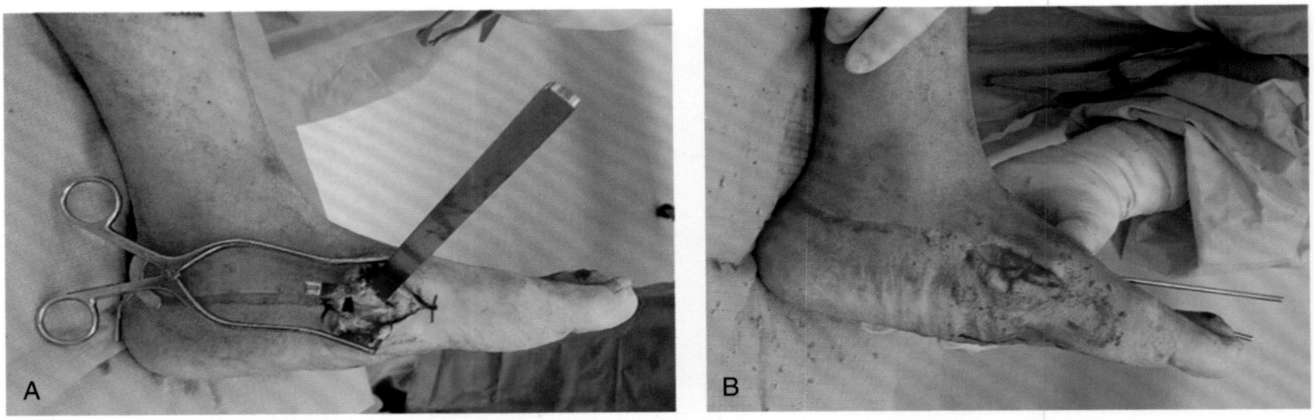

Figure 7 Intraoperative photographs showing surgical correction of deformity. A wedge of bone is removed from the apex of the deformity. **A**, This wedge is created by making an osteotomy perpendicular to the axis of the proximal segment, and perpendicular to the axis of the distal segment. The resulting wedge will be larger medial and plantar. **B**, When removed, the alignment of the forefoot becomes colinear with hindfoot, thus reestablishing a clinically plantigrade foot.

Summary

Diabetic foot morbidity leads to over 100,000 lower extremity amputations and early death yearly in the United States. Optimal diabetic management and a foot-specific patient education program are essential to avoid diabetic foot morbidity, amputation, and early death in this very complex patient population.

Key Study Points

There are currently several key issues on treatment of diabetic foot morbidity that affect the orthopaedic surgeon:

- The incidence of lower extremity amputation in the diabetic secondary to ischemic disease has been positively influenced by our Vascular Surgery colleagues, likely because of proliferation of endovascular surgery. Although death rates have not been radically improved, it is likely that the proliferation of endovascular surgery has allowed these affected patients to die without undergoing an amputation.
- The same cannot be said for the treatment of diabetic foot infection, where amputation rates have not drastically improved over the past decade. Our challenge going forward, is to improve our ability to identify and treat diabetic foot ulcers and infection, with a goal of preventing amputation and prolonging life.
- There is an increasing interest in the surgical correction of acquired deformity associated with Charcot Foot. Recent investigations have better characterized the deformities and provided better guidance in successful surgical correction of deformity and limb salvage.

Annotated References

1. https://www.cdc.gov/diabetes/pdfs/data/statistics/national-diabetes-statistics-report.pdf.
2. Wang J, Geiss L, Cheng YJ, Li Y, Gregg E: *Differential Trends for Ischemic and Neuropathic Lower Extremity Amputation Rates, United States, 1998-2010*. 73rd Scientific Session. Chicago, IL, June, 2013.
3. Gregg EW, Li Y, Wang J, et al: Changes in diabetes related complications in the United States, 1990-2010. *N Engl J Med* 2014;370(16):1514-1523.
4. Pinzur MS, Gottschalk F, Smith D, et al: Functional outcome of below-knee amputation in peripheral vascular insufficiency. *Clin Orthop* 1993;286:247-249.
5. Cooper ME, Bonnet F, Oldfield M, Jandeleit-Dahm K: Mechanisms of diabetic vasculopathy: An overview. *Am J Hypertens* 2001;14:475-486.
6. This is the website of the International Working Group on the Diabetic Foot. It is a good resource for the reader. Available at: http://iwgdf.org/. Accessed 14.23.2018.
7. This is also a valuable resource – it is the educational website from the National Institutes of Health. Available at: http://ndep.nih.gov/publications/PublicationDetail.aspx?PubId=116. Accessed 4.23.2018.
8. Lipsky BA, Berendt AR, Cornia P, et al: 2012 Infectious Diseases Society of America clinical practice guidelines for the diagnosis and treatment of diabetic foot infections. *Clin Infect Dis* 2012;54:132-173. PMID:22619242.
9. Meggitt B: Surgical management of the diabetic foot. *Br J Hosp Med* 1976;16:227-332.
10. Wagner FW Jr: The dysvascular foot: A system for diagnosis and treatment. *Foot Ankle* 1981;2:64-122.
11. Lipsky BA, Polis AB, Lantz KC, Norquist JM, Abramson MA: The value of a wound score for diabetic foot infections in predicting treatment outcome: A prospective analysis from the SIDESTEP trial. *Wound Repair Regen* 2009;17:671-677.

12. Lipsky BA, Berendt AR, Deery HG, et al: Diagnosis and treatment of diabetic foot infections. *Clin Infect Dis* 2004;39:885-910.

13. Schaper NC: Diabetic foot ulcer classification system for research purposes: A progress report on criteria for including patients in research studies. *Diabetes Metab Res Rev* 2004;20(suppl 1):S90-S95.

14. Pinzur MS, Cavanah Dart H, Hershberger RC, Lomasney LM, O'Keefe P, Slade DH: Team Approach: Treatment of diabetic foot ulcer. *JBJS Rev* 2016;4(7). doi:10.2106/JBJS.RVW.15.00080. PMID:27509330.

15. https://www.niddk.nih.gov/-/media/4ADA36507AD94759BA05E15986328A6D.ashx. Accessed May 8, 2018.

16. Pinzur MS, Slovenkai MP, Trepman E: American Orthopaedic Foot & Ankle Society guidelines for diabetic foot care. *Foot Ankle Int* 1999;20:695-702. PMID:10582844.

17. https://www.medicare.gov/coverage/therapeutic-shoes-or-inserts.html. Accessed May 8, 2018.

18. Wukich DK, Armstrong DG, Attinger CE, et al: Inpatient management of diabetic foot disorders: A clinical guide. *Diabetes Care* 2013;36(9):2862-2871. doi:10.2337/dc12-2712. PubMed PMID:23970716.

19. Cavanagh PR, Lipsky BA, Bradbury AW, Botek G: Treatment for diabetic foot ulcers. *Lancet* 2015;366:1725-1735.

20. Jeffcoate WJ, Vileikyte L, Boyko E, Armstrong DG, Boulton AJM: Current challenges and opportunities in the prevention and management of diabetic foot ulcers. *Diabetes Care* 2018;41:645-652.

21. https://www.jvascsurg.org/issue/S0741-5214%2815%29X0005-X. Accessed 5.10.2018.

22. Pinzur MS, Kaminsky M, Sage R, Cronin R, Osterman H: Amputations at the middle level of the foot. *J Bone Joint Surg* 1986;68A:1061-1064.

23. Pinzur MS, Stuck R, Sage R, Hunt N, Rabinovich Z: Syme's ankle disarticulation in patients with diabetes. *J Bone Joint Surg* 2003;85A:1667-1672. PMID:12954823.

24. Finkler ES, Marchwiany DA, Schiff AP, Pinzur MS: Long term outcomes following Syme's amputation. *Foot Ankle Int* 2017;38(7):732-735.

25. Eneroth M1, van Houtum WH: The value of debridement and Vacuum-Assisted Closure (V.A.C.) Therapy in diabetic foot ulcers. *Diabetes Metab Res Rev* 2008;24 suppl 1:S76-S80. doi:10.1002/dmrr.852.

26. Pinzur MS, Sage R, Schwaegler P: Ray resection in the dysvascular foot. *Clin Orthop* 1984;191:232-234.

27. Fabrin J, Larsen K, Holstein PE: Long-term follow-up in diabetic Charcot feet with spontaneous onset. *Diabetes Care* 2000;23:796-800.

28. Eichenholtz SN: *Charcot Joints*. Springfield, Illinois, Charles C. Thomas Publisher, 1966.

29. Strotman P, Reif TJ, Pinzur MS: Current concepts: Charcot arthropathy of the foot and ankle. *Foot Ankle Int* 2016;37(11):1255-1263.

30. Rogers LC, Frykberg RG, Armstrong DG, et al: The diabetic Charcot foot syndrome: A report of the joint task force on the Charcot foot by the American Diabetes Association and the American Podiatric Medical Association. *Diabetes Care* 2011;34:2123-2129. PMID:21868781.

31. Dhawan V, Spratt KF, Pinzur MS, Baumhauer J, Rudicel S, Saltzman CL: Reliability of AOFAS Diabetic Foot Questionnaire in Charcot Arthropathy: Stability, internal consistency and measurable difference. *Foot Ank Int* 2005;26(9):717-731. PMID:16174503.

32. Pinzur MS, Evans A: Health related quality of life in patients with Charcot foot. *Amer J Ortho* 2003;32:492-496.

33. Raspovic KR, Wukich DK: Self-reported quality of life in patients with diabetes: A comparison of patients with and without Charcot neuroarthropathy. *Foot Ankle Int* 2014;35(10):195-200. PMID:24351658.

34. Kroin E, Schiff AP, Pinzur MS, Davis ES, Chaharbakhshi E, DiSilvio FA JR: Functional impairment of patients undergoing surgical correction for Charcot foot arthropathy. *Foot Ankle Int* 2017;38(7):705-709.

35. deSouza L: Charcot arthropathy and immobilization in a weight-bearing total contact cast. *J Bone Joint Surg* 2008;90A:754-759.

36. Pinzur MS, Lio T, Posner M: Treatment of Eichenholtz stage I Charcot foot arthropathy with a weight bearing total contact cast. *Foot Ank Int* 2006;27:324-329.

37. Jones C, McCormick J, Pinzur MS: Surgical treatment of Charcot foot. *Diabetes Metab Res Rev* 2018;67:255-267.

38. Bevan WP, Tomlinson MP: Radiographic measure as a predictor of ulcer formation in diabetic Charcot midfoot. *Foot Ank Int* 2008;29:568-573.

39. Sammarco VJ, Sammarco GJ, Walker EW, Guiao RP: Midtarsal arthrodesis in treatment of Charcot midfoot arthropathy. *J Bone Joint Surg* 2009;91(1):80-91. PMID:19122082.

40. Pinzur MS: Neutral ring fixation for high risk non-plantigrade Charcot midfoot de-formity. *Foot Ank Int* 2007;28(9):961-966. PMID:17880868.

41. Pinzur MS, Schiff AP: Deformity and clinical outcomes following surgical correction of Charcot foot: A new classification with implications for treatment. *Foot Ankle Int* 2018;39(3):265-270.

Chapter 45

Foot and Ankle Reconstruction

Rachel J. Shakked, MD • Daniel J. Fuchs, MD • Steven M. Raikin, MD

ABSTRACT

Hallux valgus may be associated with pain and can be corrected with a variety of surgical techniques. Lesser toe deformity is often seen in the setting of hallux valgus and can be managed with or without surgery. Adult acquired flatfoot deformity is typically progressive and associated with pain and dysfunction. Nonsurgical treatment includes bracing treatment and physical therapy, whereas surgical treatment includes reconstruction with osteotomies and tendon transfers or selective arthrodesis. Cavovarus deformity is similarly treated with bracing treatment or surgical reconstruction. Lisfranc injuries are commonly missed and may lead to midfoot arthritis when not treated appropriately. Surgery is often recommended when any instability of the midfoot is noted. Achilles tendinopathy may be treated nonsurgically with eccentric training of the tendon or with open débridement of the tendon. Ankle sprains have an excellent prognosis, but some patients go on to develop chronic instability, which may benefit from physical therapy or surgical reconstruction of the ankle ligaments.

Keywords: achilles tendinopathy; cavovarus; hallux valgus; hammer toe; pes planus.

Introduction

Deformity can affect all portions of the foot, including the forefoot, midfoot, and hindfoot. When associated with pain, nonsurgical treatment is always attempted. When surgical treatment is indicated, the mechanical structure and function of the foot and ankle are considered. In low-energy trauma resulting in ligamentous injuries, ankle sprains are typically treated nonsurgically at first, although midfoot sprains associated with instability may require acute surgery.

None of the following authors or any immediate family member has received anything of value from or has stock or stock options held in a commercial company or institution related directly or indirectly to the subject of this chapter: Dr. Shakked, Dr. Fuchs, and Dr. Raikin.

Hallux Valgus

Hallux valgus (HV) deformity is defined as the lateral deviation of the proximal phalanx of the first metatarsophalangeal joint (MTP). The etiology is a combination of intrinsic factors such as genetic predisposition, or a hypermobile first tarsometatarsal joint, and extrinsic factors, predominantly related to high-heeled shoes with a narrow toe box. Other predisposing factors include rheumatoid or inflammatory arthritis, generalized ligamentous laxity, and dysmorphism of the first metatarsal (MT). The deformity is usually progressive, although the rate and degree of progression is often nonlinear. HV is most commonly seen in female patients in their fourth or fifth decades of life.

The pathoanatomy of HV involves gradual failure of the medial supportive structures (medial collateral ligament and tibial sesamoid) resulting in a varus position of the first metatarsal. Valgus deviation at the MTP joint of the proximal phalanx subsequently develops. As the deformity progresses, the alignment of the flexor and extensor hallucis longus tendons shifts laterally relative to the MTP joint, further exacerbating the deformity. The first MT varus results in a prominent first MT head medially which is the bump or "bunion" of which the patient reports. This prominent medial eminence is a common source of pain related to shoe wear. Secondary pathology and deformity can develop in the lesser toes, such as hammertoes and claw toes, which may be symptomatic.

The severity of the hallux valgus deformity and any associated pes planus can be best assessed while the patient is standing. While seated, the first MTP joint area is evaluated for signs of local irritation and bursal hypertrophy secondary to shoe wear, tenderness over the medial eminence, and range of motion of the first MTP joint. Any pain with motion may suggest arthritis within the joint. Numbness can occur in the dorsal medial cutaneous nerve distribution because of external pressure from a shoe. The first tarsometatarsal joint is evaluated for hypermobility, which remains a diagnostic challenge with poor reproducibility.[1]

Diagnostic confirmation of HV is made with the use of standard AP and lateral weight-bearing radiographs, as non–weight-bearing radiographs tend to underestimate the deformity.[2] Radiographs should be assessed for presence of arthritis at the first MTP joint, severity of the deformity as determined by the intermetatarsal angle between the first and second metatarsals (IMA), sesamoid subluxation, and the hallux valgus angle (HVA) (**Figure 1**). Radiographs are also assessed for first tarsometatarsal hypermobility (**Figure 2**, **A** and **B**) and congruency of the MTP joint, which is assessed by measuring the distal metatarsal articular angle (DMAA) of the first MT head (**Figure 3**). This metatarsal dysmorphism may be present more often in patients with juvenile onset of HV and in males.

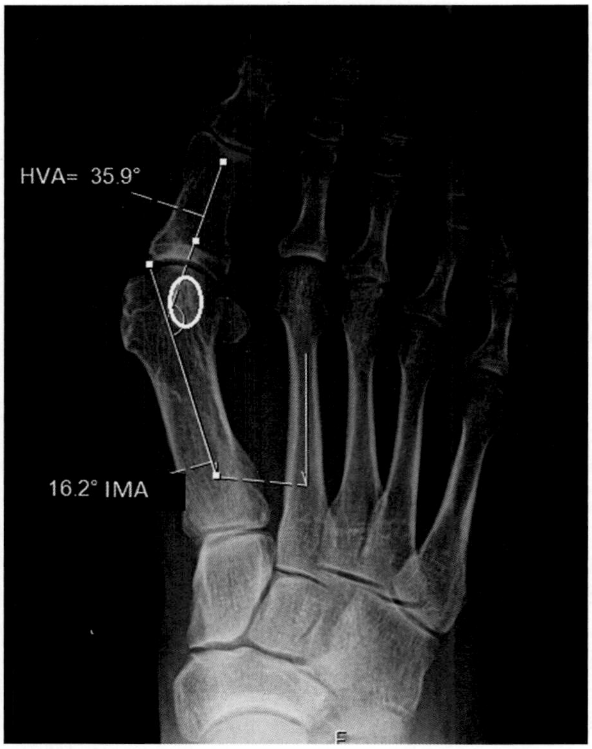

Figure 1 AP weight-bearing image of the foot demonstrating the appropriate way to measure the first-second intermetatarsal angle (IMA, normal ≤ 9°); and hallux valgus angle (HVA, normal ≤ 15°).

Treatment of hallux valgus deformity should initially include wearing a wider toe-boxed shoe to accommodate the deformity. There are a number of orthotic devices including pads, spacers, arch supports, and night splints available, but none of these have been demonstrated to be successful.

The major indication for surgery following failure of the above modalities is pain; there is no indication for cosmetic surgery. More than 100 surgical procedures have been described to correct HV deformities, with no single procedure indicated for all HV varieties. **Figure 4** outlines a suggested algorithm for managing patients with recalcitrant HV deformities and pain. The presence of degenerative arthritis within the first MTP joint typically requires a fusion of the first MTP joint. In the absence of arthritis, joint-sparing procedures can usually be performed using osteotomies for deformity correction. However, if hypermobility or arthritis of the first tarsometatarsal joint is present, a first tarsometatarsal fusion with correction of the intermetatarsal angle (Lapidus procedure) should be undertaken. The Lapidus procedure should always be performed together with a medial eminence resection and a distal soft-tissue rebalancing procedure at the first MTP joint (modified McBride procedure).

If there is concern about an abnormally high DMAA (usually greater than 15°), a double osteotomy is required to correct both the joint angulation and the intermetatarsal deformity which typically involves a medial closing wedge osteotomy of the distal first MT.

In the absence of the above concerns, focus of the correction is dependent on the severity of the deformity.[3] In mild deformities with a normal IMA (<9°), no osteotomy is required. The medial eminence is resected, the medial capsule is reefed, and a modified McBride procedure is performed to release the contracted lateral structures preventing deformity correction. These structures include the following:

- Second MT to lateral sesamoid "intermetatarsal" ligament
- Adductor hallucis muscle inserting into the lateral base of the proximal phalanx
- Lateral sesamoid suspensory ligament
- Lateral MTP joint capsule

Moderate deformities (IMA 10° to 14°) may undergo a chevron osteotomy, which is a distal osteotomy of the first MT followed by translation of the metatarsal head laterally. Fixation is maintained with a temporary Kirschner wire or a bone screw.

In severe deformities characterized by an IMA greater than 14°, a proximal metatarsal osteotomy is required for a more powerful correction. There are a number of described procedures for this including the

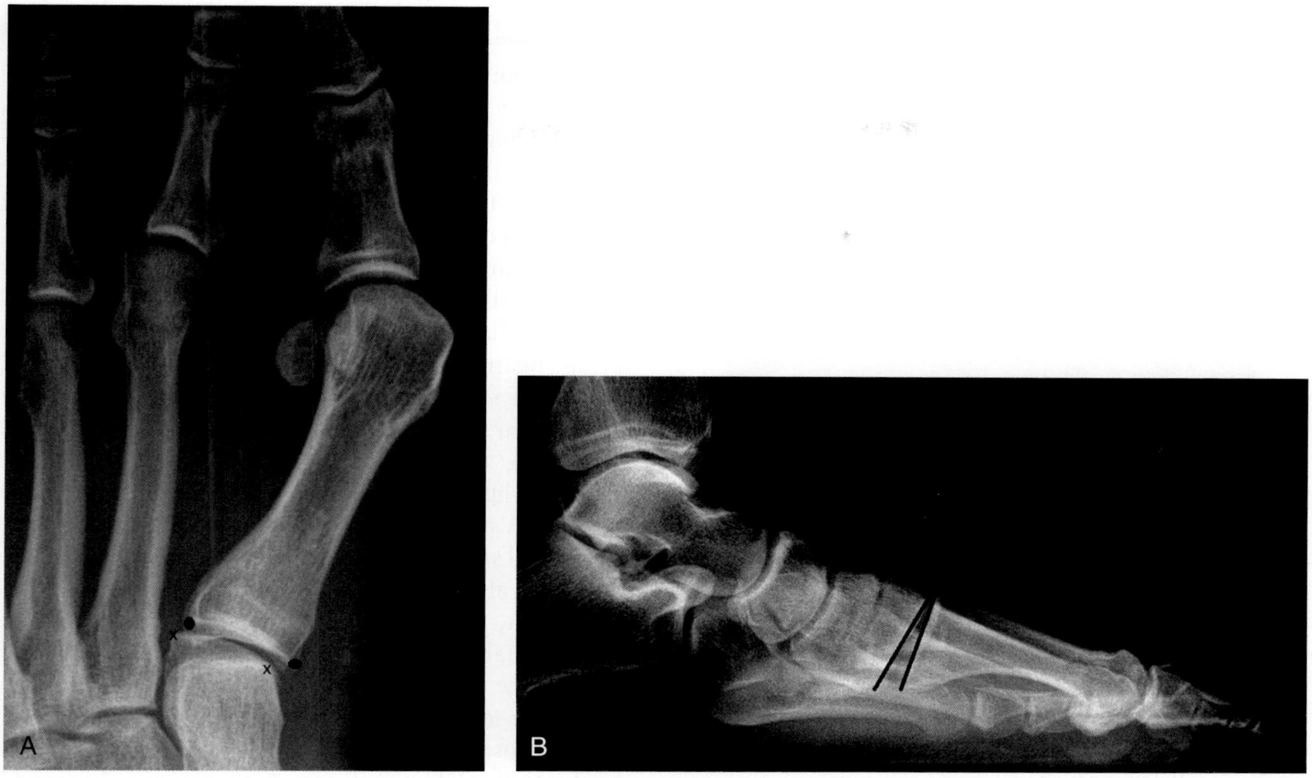

Figure 2 AP weight-bearing radiograph (**A**) demonstrating medial subluxation and incongruency of the first tarsometatarsal joint, with lateral radiograph (**B**) demonstrating dorsal subluxation of the joint with plantar gapping at the tarsometatarsal joint suggestive of tarsometatarsal hypermobility.

scarf, Ludloff oblique, proximal chevron, and crescentic osteotomies. No procedure has been proven superior to another, so long as adequate correction is attained. These procedures should always be combined with a modified McBride procedure.

A variation of hallux valgus is hallux valgus interphalangeus in which the angular abnormality is between the proximal and distal phalanges of the hallux. This is corrected with a medial closing wedge osteotomy of the proximal phalanx (Akin procedure).[4] Inadequate reduction of the sesamoids back to their anatomic position under the first MT head is the greatest predictor of procedure failure and recurrent deformity.[5,6]

Lesser Toe Deformity

Lesser toe deformities develop as a result of tendinous imbalance between the toe flexors and extensors. Extrinsic forces may contribute such as high-heeled shoes, associated HV deformity, long metatarsals, cortisone injections, and inflammatory arthritic conditions.

Nonsurgical treatment includes high toe box shoe wear, inserts including metatarsal pads, Budin splints, and stiff-soled shoes. Steroid injections should be used judiciously as they may result in progression of the deformity.

Flexion contracture at the distal interphalangeal joint (DIPJ) with neutral alignment of the proximal IPJ and MTP joint is called a mallet toe (**Figure 5**, A). Pain can occur at the dorsum of the DIPJ as this rubs against the shoe, or at the tip of the toe which impacts the floor. In flexible deformities correction can be obtained through percutaneous release of the flexor digitorum longus tendon at the DIPJ. Fixed deformities are managed with a resection arthroplasty with or without arthrodesis of the DIPJ.

Hammer toe deformity is a flexion contracture of the proximal IPJ of the lesser toe, with a stable MTP joint (**Figure 5**, B). Pain and callus formation usually occurs at the dorsum of the proximal IPJ. Flexible deformities are treated with a flexor to extensor tendon transfer, whereas fixed deformities require an excision arthroplasty of the proximal IPJ with or without arthrodesis (hammer toe correction).

Chronic and severe hammer toe deformities may result in synovitis at the MTP joint leading to secondary instability of the joint. As the plantar plate gets stretched

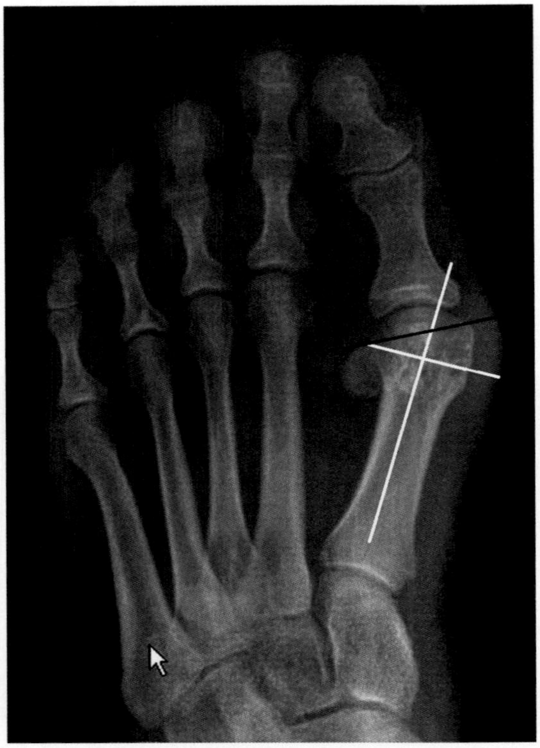

Figure 3 AP weight-bearing radiograph of the foot demonstrating the distal metatarsal articular angle (DMAA, normal ≤ 15°). This is the angle created by the black line connecting the ends of the articular surface and the line perpendicular to the long axis of the first metatarsal.

out or tears, an extension deformity will develop at the MTP joint.[7] In combination with the proximal IPJ flexion, the deformity is considered a claw toe (**Figure 5**, C). Claw toes can also develop secondary to intrinsic muscle weakness often associated with neuromuscular conditions. If concomitant pathology develops within the collateral ligaments of the MTP joint, medial or lateral deviation will occur resulting in a crossover toe deformity. These conditions are frequently associated with metatarsalgia as the plantar fat pad atrophies or displaces distally as the proximal phalanx extends. Surgical treatment for claw toes usually includes a shortening distal oblique osteotomy of the metatarsal to unload the MTP joint, combined with a hammer toe correction. The osteotomy also rebalances the metatarsal cascade in the setting of a long metatarsal. Newer procedures include repairing the plantar plate to the proximal phalanx insertion with strong nonabsorbable suture.[8] If there is a crossover component to the deformity, the damaged collateral ligament needs to be repaired with nonabsorbable sutures to balance the coronal alignment of the toe.

Adult Acquired Flatfoot Deformity

Adult acquired flatfoot deformity (AAFD) is characterized by collapse of the medial longitudinal arch, hindfoot valgus, and midfoot abduction related to dysfunction of the posterior tibial tendon (PTT).

The PTT inverts the hindfoot, which locks the transverse tarsal joint, providing a stable platform for push-off during gait. When the PTT degenerates, the hindfoot falls into valgus, which stresses the medial static stabilizers of the ankle and foot, including the spring ligament. The navicular translates laterally, because of spring ligament incompetence, resulting in medial talar head uncoverage and midfoot abduction. Progressive valgus stress through the ankle may result in deltoid ligament incompetence, talar tilt, and ankle arthritis. A gastrocnemius contracture develops as the axis of pull shifts laterally, which can further exacerbate the valgus alignment. AAFD is most commonly seen in overweight, middle-aged females. Risk factors include obesity, diabetes, hypertension, trauma, and history of cortisone injections.[9] Subtalar joint orientation may predispose some patients to developing AAFD.[10]

The most common classification system is based on the degree of deformity[11] (see **Table 1**). Stage I is tendinopathy of the posterior tibial tendon in the absence of significant deformity. Stage II is characterized by a flexible deformity with talar head uncoverage seen on the weight-bearing AP foot radiograph. Talar head uncoverage of greater than 30% differentiates between a stage IIa and IIb deformity. Stage III is a rigid deformity due to arthritis in the hindfoot, and stage IV indicates ankle joint involvement.

Clinically, the patients present with medial ankle pain and gait dysfunction related to deformity. With progressive disease, lateral ankle pain may develop because of subfibular impingement. On examination, there is tenderness over the PTT. Standing evaluation from behind the patient demonstrates valgus alignment. If the patient is able to perform a single-limb heel rise and the hindfoot inverts as the heel elevates, the PTT remains functional and the deformity is considered flexible. If the hindfoot does not invert, the deformity is considered rigid. The presence of a gastrocnemius contracture is assessed with the Silfverskiold test, making sure to invert the hindfoot out of valgus during examination.[12]

Weight-bearing radiographs of the foot and ankle are evaluated for degree of deformity and degenerative changes. Arch collapse is quantified by measuring Meary's angle on the lateral view (see **Figure 6**, A), and percentage uncoverage of the talar head on the AP

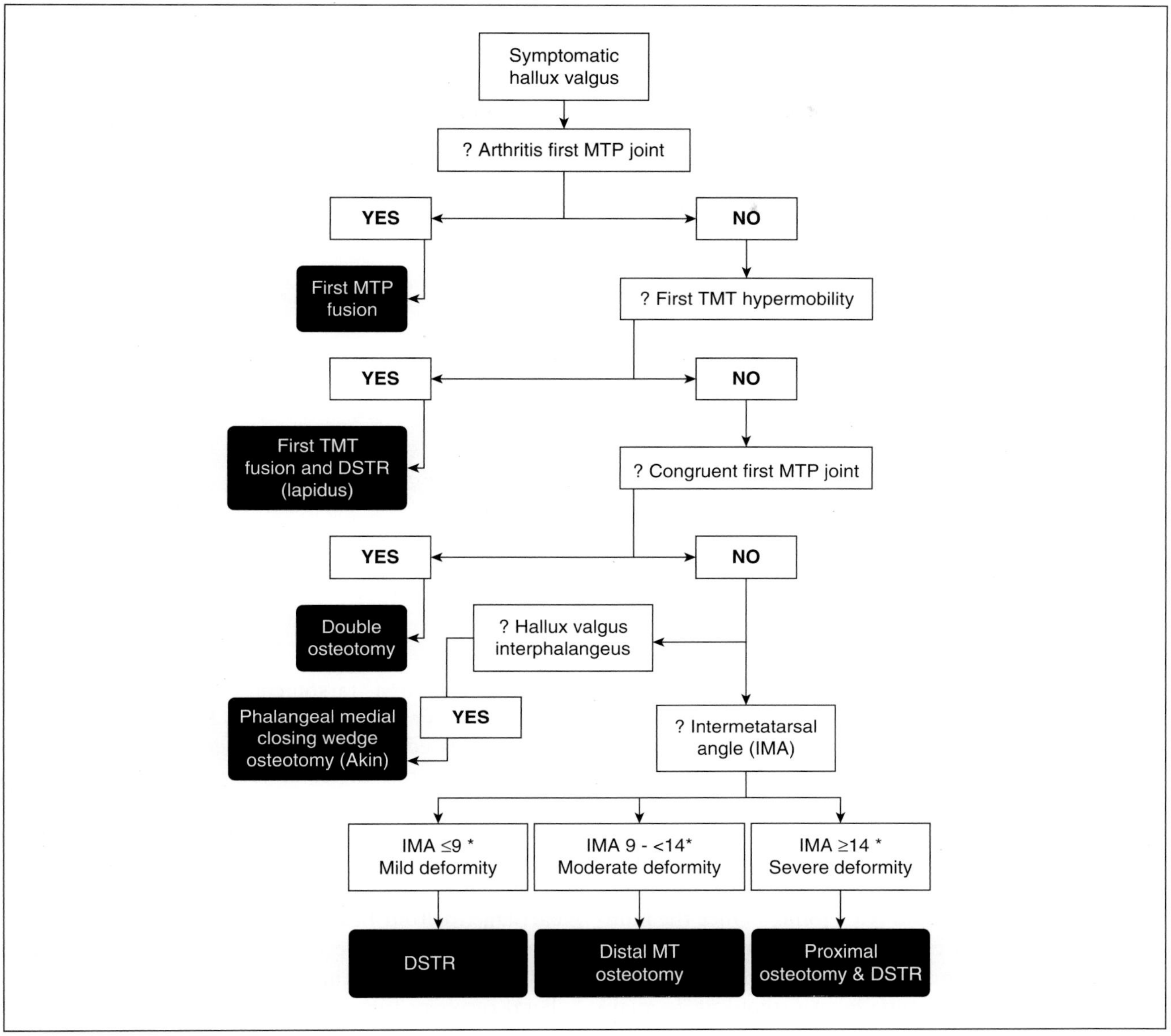

Figure 4 Recommended algorithm for the selection of the appropriate surgical treatment for patients with symptomatic hallux valgus.

foot radiograph is measured (see **Figure 6**, B). A hindfoot alignment radiograph may be useful to measure hindfoot moment arm, which can predict the amount of intraoperative deformity correction required[13] (see **Figure 6**, C). Ankle radiographs should always be performed to assess for valgus talar tilt (see **Figure 6**, D). MRI may demonstrate degeneration in the PTT and spring ligament injury; however, it is not a requisite preoperative study in the presence of significant deformity.

Nonsurgical treatment is recommended before considering surgery. Anti-inflammatory medications, rest, and immobilization should be used initially, especially in the setting of an acute exacerbation of pain. Custom orthotics including arch support with medial heel posting may help with alignment in milder cases, together with physical therapy to work on gastrocnemius stretching and eccentric strengthening of the PTT. In the setting of more severe deformity, a custom-molded ankle-foot orthosis (AFO) or Arizona brace may help to mitigate symptoms.

Flatfoot reconstruction in the setting of a flexible deformity involves a combination of flexor digitorum longus (FDL) tendon transfers and realignment osteotomies, usually combined with a lengthening of the Achilles tendon. While exposing the PTT and FDL, the

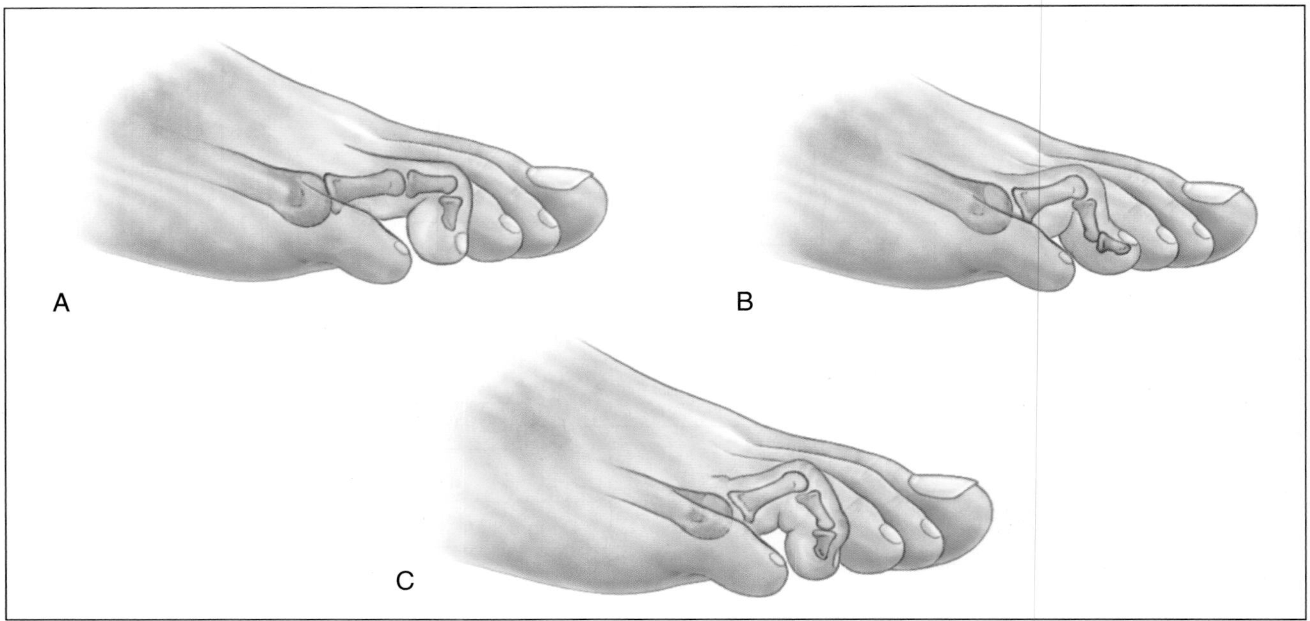

Figure 5 Illustration of a mallet toe (**A**), hammer toe (**B**), and claw toe (**C**). (Reprinted from *The Foot: Examination and Diagnosis*, ed 2. edited by Alexander IJ. Lesser Toe Deformities, p 83-87, Copyright Elsevier 1997.)

spring ligament overlying the talar head is assessed for tear. Direct repair or reconstruction of the spring ligament may improve midfoot abduction.[14] To improve hindfoot valgus, a medializing calcaneal osteotomy (MCO) is performed. Abduction can be further corrected by performing a lateral column lengthening (LCL), which involves placing bone graft or a metal wedge along the lateral aspect of the calcaneus, proximal to the calcaneocuboid (CC) joint.[15] Once the hindfoot and midfoot are corrected, the forefoot is assessed for residual supination, which can be corrected with a dorsal opening wedge cuneiform osteotomy to plantarflex the first ray.[16] If there is arthritis or instability through the first tarsometatarsal (TMT) joint, an arthrodesis can be performed. Rigid flatfoot deformity is treated with a realignment arthrodesis of the subtalar and talonavicular joints. The CC joint may also be fused if arthritis is present. In the setting of AAFD with talar tilt, the presence of arthritic changes in the ankle is an indication for ankle arthrodesis or arthroplasty. If there is talar tilt and preserved ankle cartilage, deltoid ligament reconstruction can be considered.[17] Flatfoot reconstruction is associated with sustained improvement in functional scores and pain.[18] Total recovery time may take up to 2 years, and pain relief is sustained thereafter.[18-20]

Table 1

Commonly Used Classification System Considering Deformity Severity and Flexibility

Posterior Tibial Tendon Dysfunction Classification		
Stage I	Posterior tibial tendinopathy with minimal underlying deformity	
Stage II	Flexible deformity. Variable degree of midfoot abduction measured as percentage talonavicular (TN) uncoverage on weight-bearing AP foot XR	Stage IIa: <30% TN uncoverage Stage IIb: >30% TN uncoverage
Stage III	Rigid deformity: no hindfoot inversion with single-limb heel rise and deformity is not passively correctable	
Stage IV	Ankle involvement: talar tilt ± valgus ankle arthritis due to long-standing foot deformity	

Data from Nair P, Deland JT, Ellis SJ: Current concepts in adult acquired flatfoot deformity. *Curr Orthop Pract* 2015;26(2):160-168.

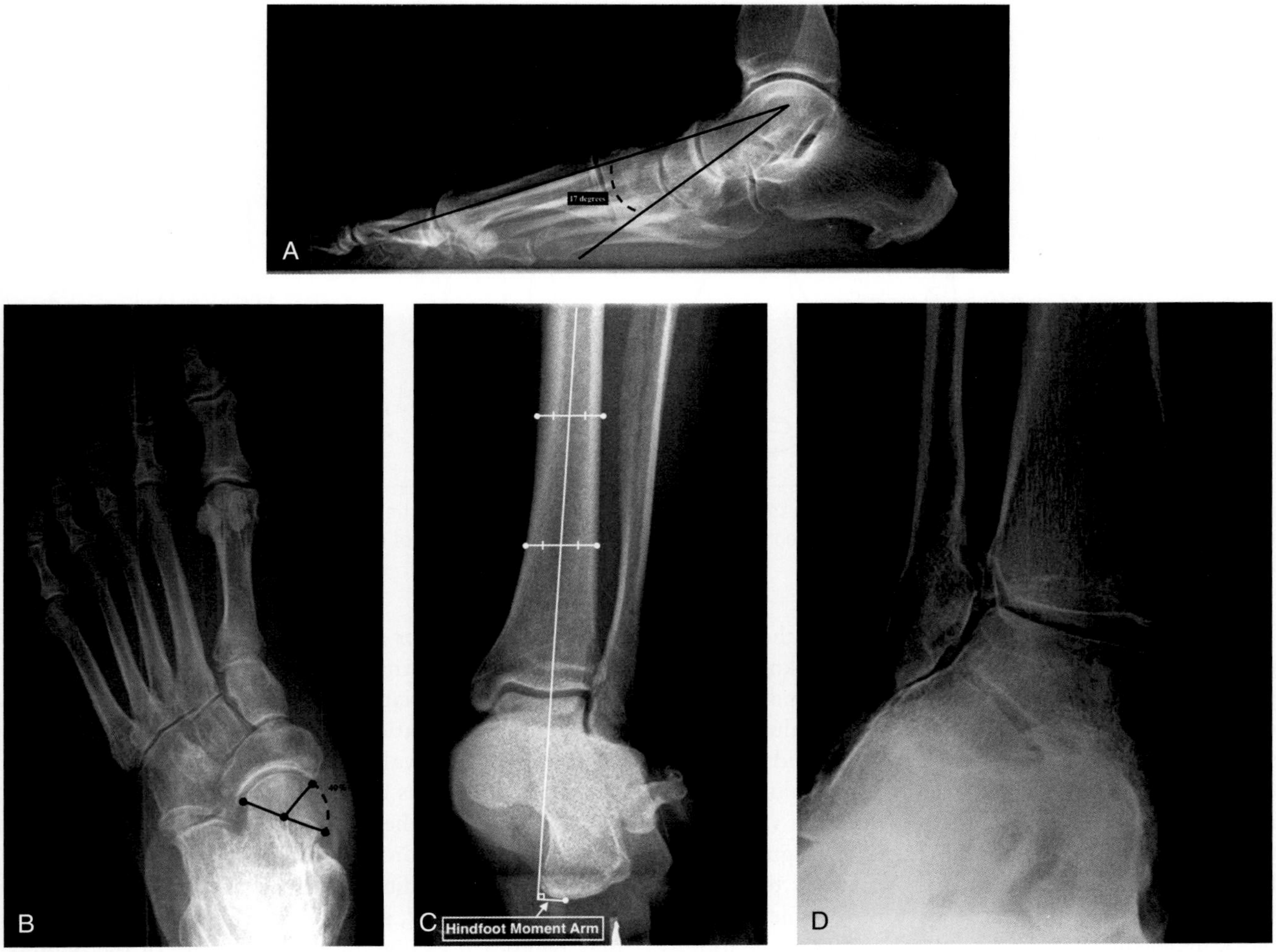

Figure 6 Lateral (**A**) and AP (**B**) weight-bearing radiographs of the left foot demonstrate abnormal Meary's angle of 17° (normal zero to 10°) and talar head uncoverage (normal zero to 30%). Hindfoot moment arm can be measured on the hindfoot alignment view to determine severity of hindfoot valgus (**C**). AP ankle radiograph demonstrates talar tilt, which may occur because of long-standing deformity and deltoid ligament insufficiency (**D**). (C, Reproduced with permission from Williamson ER, Chan JY, Burket JC, Deland JT, Ellis SJ: New radiographic parameter assessing hindfoot alignment in stage II adult-acquired flatfoot deformity. *Foot Ankle Int* 2015;36[4]:417-423.)

Cavovarus Foot

A cavus foot is one with a high medial longitudinal arch. Approximately 10% of skeletally mature individuals have cavovarus (CV) foot alignment,[21] with most of these individuals being asymptomatic. Unlike planovalgus deformity, which is usually degenerative in origin, many patients with a cavovarus foot deformity have underlying neurologic/neuromuscular disorder. The most common disorder is Charcot-Marie-Tooth disease (hereditary motor sensory neuropathy type I), a progressive condition which affects 50% of patients with a neuromuscular cavovarus foot. A neurologic/neuromuscular etiology should be expected when there is a family history of cavus feet, rapid onset and progression of a cavus foot deformity, marked asymmetry in foot shape, very severe deformity especially with marked clawing of the toes, focal wasting (anterior or lateral compartments) or spasticity (deep posterior compartment), or other neurologic findings. Nonneurologic causes include congenital clubfoot, posttraumatic (calcaneus or talar neck fracture with varus malunion), missed compartment syndrome, burn contractures, and idiopathic etiology.

Neuromuscular imbalance between a nonfunctioning peroneus brevis muscle and its antagonist, the posterior tibialis muscle, pulls the hindfoot into varus. Similarly, forefoot-driven varus can occur when a relatively weak anterior tibialis muscle is overpowered by its antagonist, the peroneus longus muscle, plantarflexing the first ray resulting in a cavus arch.

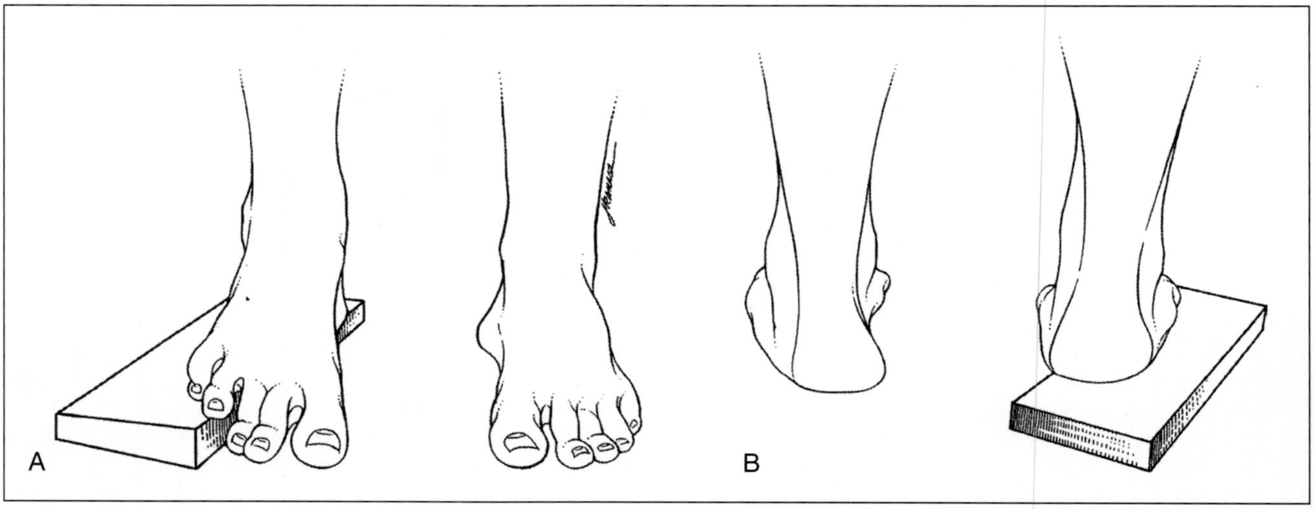

Figure 7 Illustration of Coleman block test. As seen from the front (**A**) and from behind (**B**) the patient. (Reproduced from Alexander IJ: Pes cavus, in Nunley JA, Pferrer GB, Sanders RW, Trepman E, eds: *Advanced Reconstruction of the Foot and Ankle*. Rosemont, IL, AAOS, 2004, pp 495-502.)

Clinical evaluation starts with observing the patient's gait for subtle footdrop (anterior tibialis weakness), compensatory toe clawing, ankle instability, and peroneal weakness. The patient's foot should be evaluated both standing and sitting, and viewed from behind and from the front of the foot. When alignment is evaluated from behind the patient, the calcaneus is seen in a varus position rather than the natural 3° to 5° of valgus. To differentiate if the hindfoot varus is secondary to forefoot varus, a Coleman block test is performed which places a block under the heel and the lateral border of the foot to "elevate" the floor. This allows the plantarflexed first ray to drop down without hitting the floor and supinating the hindfoot. If the hindfoot varus corrects, the deformity is considered forefoot-driven varus or flexible varus[22] (**Figure 7**). The hindfoot flexibility can additionally be evaluated with the patient sitting with the physician passively manipulating the hindfoot into valgus. If the hindfoot deformity does not correct with passive manipulation or the Coleman block test, the deformity is considered hindfoot-driven varus or fixed varus. Fixed varus should not be confused with arthritic involvement and does not require a surgical fusion for correction. Fixed deformity indicates that the Chopart joints are locked in varus and that a hindfoot corrective osteotomy is required.

When the patient is standing, the foot will have a bean-shaped appearance because of the combined hindfoot varus and forefoot adductus. Clawing of the hallux and lesser toes are often seen in neuromuscular CV. The medial heel pad, which is usually not visible, will be seen from behind the patient because of the hindfoot varus and is referred to as a "peek-a-boo" heel[23] (**Figure 8**).

A detailed motor and sensory neurologic evaluation also must be performed to evaluate for neurologic etiology and differentiate between upper and lower motor neuron lesion causation.

Radiographic evaluation is undertaken with weight-bearing radiographs of the foot and ankle. On the lateral radiographs, the fibula often is located posterior to the posterior border of the distal tibia at the level of the ankle. In addition, the calcaneal pitch angle may be greater than 20°, and the talar first metatarsal angle may be apex dorsally angulated because of the plantar flexion of the first ray.

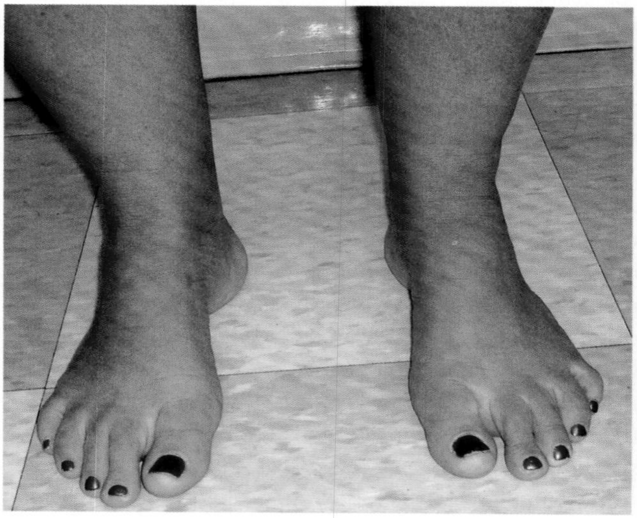

Figure 8 Photograph showing a peek-a-boo heel as viewed from the front of the patient.

In the AP radiographs of the foot, the metatarsals often are adducted and the forefoot is rotated into supination. In the AP radiographs of the ankle the talus may tilt into varus as a result of lateral ankle ligament insufficiency. Hindfoot alignment radiographs can be obtained to assess the degree of varus and overall tibiocalcaneal alignment. Tertiary imaging studies, such as an MRI, are usually not required, unless an evaluation for concomitant tendon damage or arthritis is needed.

Nonsurgical treatment for CV deformity include utilization of laterally posted custom orthotic inserts with the posting extended to the midfoot to simulate a Coleman block test, combined with physical therapy to optimize peroneal muscle strength and function. Additionally, a custom AFO can be considered for more severe deformities involving the hindfoot or ankle.

Cavovarus foot deformity can result from a spectrum of different disorders, and therefore each patient needs to be evaluated individually to plan a surgical correction that fully balances the foot. Whenever possible, deformity correction should be accomplished with joint-sparing osteotomies and tendon transfers. Arthrodesis should be reserved for salvage procedures or in combination with tendon transfers in patients with severe deformity in whom joint-sparing surgery would fail or has failed.[24] Undercorrection is the leading causes of poor outcomes in patients who undergo CV reconstruction.[25]

In forefoot-driven CV, the mainstay of surgical correction is cutting the peroneus longus tendon and transferring it to the adjacent peroneus brevis tendon.[26] This decreases the plantar flexion of the first ray and increases the valgus pull on the hindfoot. In most cases this is accompanied by a dorsal closing wedge osteotomy of the base of the first metatarsal to physically elevate the ray. The plantar fascia may need to be lengthened to allow the first ray to elevate. In cases of clawing of the hallux, the extensor hallucis longus tendon is released from its insertion in the distal phalanx and transferred to a bone tunnel in the first MT neck, changing its deforming force to become an additional elevator of the first ray. To prevent flexion contracture of the hallux interphalangeal (IP) joint, IP fusion is performed (Jones suspension).

In cases of hindfoot-driven or fixed deformities, a Dwyer closing wedge osteotomy can be performed with the use of a lateral slide and/or internal rotation of the posterior tuberosity.[27] Additionally, the calcaneal tuberosity can be translated proximally to decrease the calcaneal pitch angle and functionally lengthen the Achilles tendon. The tendon transfer for hindfoot-driven CV transects the posterior tibial tendon (which pulls the hindfoot into varus) and transfers the tendon through the interosseous membrane to the lateral cuneiform, so as to act as an ankle dorsiflexor and evertor. Many patients with more advanced or complex deformities will require additional procedures including a transtarsal midfoot closing wedge osteotomy and fusion, a lateral ligament reconstruction, split anterior tibial tendon transfer, and even an ankle or triple arthrodesis.[28]

Subtle CV may be associated with lateral ankle ligament instability, peroneal pathology, and fifth metatarsal fracture. Failure to correct the CV in these patients may result in failure of any procedure performed to treat their primary pathology.[23]

Lisfranc Injuries

Injury to the Lisfranc joint complex may be primarily bony or ligamentous, subtle or profound with obvious dislocation through the TMT joints, and associated with low-impact or high-impact trauma. The typical mechanism of injury involves abduction and direct axial impact to the forefoot while in an equinus position.[29] Lisfranc injuries are reportedly missed up to 20% of the time, which can result in posttraumatic arthritis, progressive deformity, and pain.[30]

The plantar Lisfranc ligament links the base of the second metatarsal to the medial cuneiform and is known to be the strongest and most important ligament in this region of the foot.[31] Bony anatomy contributes to the stability of this region; the second metatarsal base is considered the keystone of the transverse arch of the foot and is recessed proximally between the medial and lateral cuneiforms.

Lisfranc injuries are classified into three main categories (see **Figure 9**):

- Type A: incongruity of the entire TMT joint
- Type B: incongruity of a portion of the TMT joint
- Type C: medial and lateral displacement at the TMT joint[32]

Patients presenting with a Lisfranc injury have substantial swelling throughout the foot, limited ability to weightbear, and may have plantar ecchymosis, which is pathognomonic for midfoot injury. A gross deformity may be visible with midfoot abduction and loss of the transverse arch. Passive pronation and abduction will elicit increased pain. Careful neurovascular examination is important as injury to the deep peroneal nerve and artery may occur. Compartment syndrome of the foot may occur in high-energy cases.

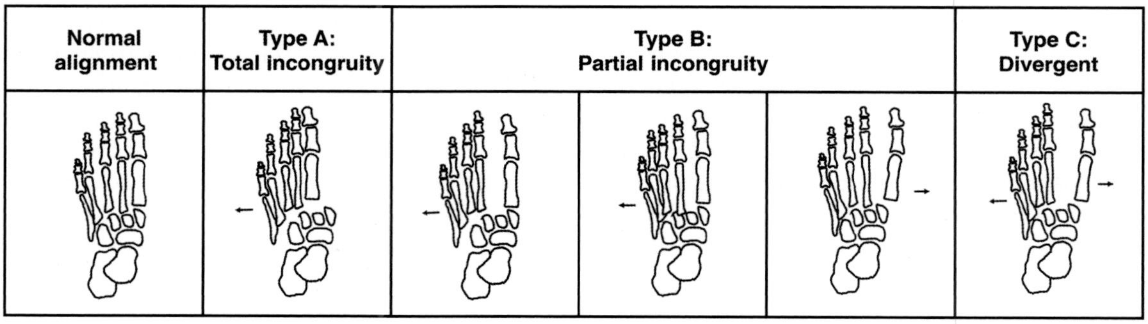

Figure 9 Illustration of Lisfranc injury classification described by Hardcastle et al.

Weight-bearing foot radiographs are performed; a comparison AP view of the contralateral side is useful in subtle cases. Radiographs should be assessed for anatomic alignment (see **Figure 10**):

- AP: medial border of second metatarsal lines up with medial aspect of middle cuneiform and <2 mm between first and second metatarsal bases[33]
- Oblique: medial border of fourth metatarsal lines up with medial border of cuboid
- Lateral: dorsal cortex of first metatarsal lines up with medial cuneiform

An avulsion fracture is occasionally seen between the second metatarsal base and medial cuneiform. If other fractures are thought to be present, a CT scan is obtained to better assess the degree of displacement and articular involvement. MRI is beneficial in more subtle cases to evaluate the status of the Lisfranc ligament and presence of occult fractures. If true weight-bearing radiographs are not possible and advanced imaging is equivocal, there is a role for stress examination under anesthesia to evaluate midfoot stability in the setting of suspected Lisfranc injury.

Lisfranc injuries with anatomic alignment and no significant instability on weight-bearing radiographs may be treated nonsurgically with restricted weight bearing for 6 weeks followed by gradual return to previous activity. Any joint subluxation noted on preoperative imaging is indicated for surgical fixation. Nonsurgical treatment in the setting of instability is associated with poor outcomes with up to 30% developing arthritis over time.[32,34] Open reduction and internal fixation (ORIF) of the midfoot and midfoot arthrodesis are both associated with good outcomes and return to activity.[35-39] The most important factor for excellent clinical results is quality of the reduction.[34,40,41] In the subtle ligamentous Lisfranc injury related to a low-energy mechanism, open or percutaneous reduction and internal fixation with one or two screws is successful.[42-44] In higher energy injuries that destabilize multiple joints with or without fractures of the metatarsal bases/cuneiforms, a formal open approach with two dorsal incisions is necessary to restore native alignment of the midfoot.

There is ongoing debate as to whether ORIF or arthrodesis is associated with better outcomes.[41,45] ORIF preserves the joints of the midfoot although requires a second surgery for removal of hardware. Unrecognized chondrocyte injury from the trauma may predispose patients to midfoot arthritis, despite anatomic alignment. Midfoot arthrodesis eliminates motion in the involved joints and precludes the risk of posttraumatic arthritis, although patients may develop adjacent joint arthritis. A prospective, randomized study by Ly and Coetzee found that high-energy ligamentous injuries fared better with midfoot arthrodesis than ORIF.[37]After arthrodesis, patients returned to 92% of their previous activity level versus 65% after ORIF. However, a single screw was used in the ORIF group and most patients developed loss of reduction. A subsequent prospective, randomized study failed to demonstrate any functional outcome difference between ORIF versus arthrodesis, although this study was underpowered, had limited follow-up, and included bony and ligamentous injuries.[36] Many retrospective studies have been performed and most show similar results among patients who underwent ORIF and those who underwent primary arthrodesis.[35,41,45,46] Further study is necessary to determine optimal treatment after high-energy Lisfranc. In cases of ORIF, hardware may be removed at 4 to 6 months, and gradual return to sports is permitted at approximately 6 to 8 months postoperatively.[47,48]

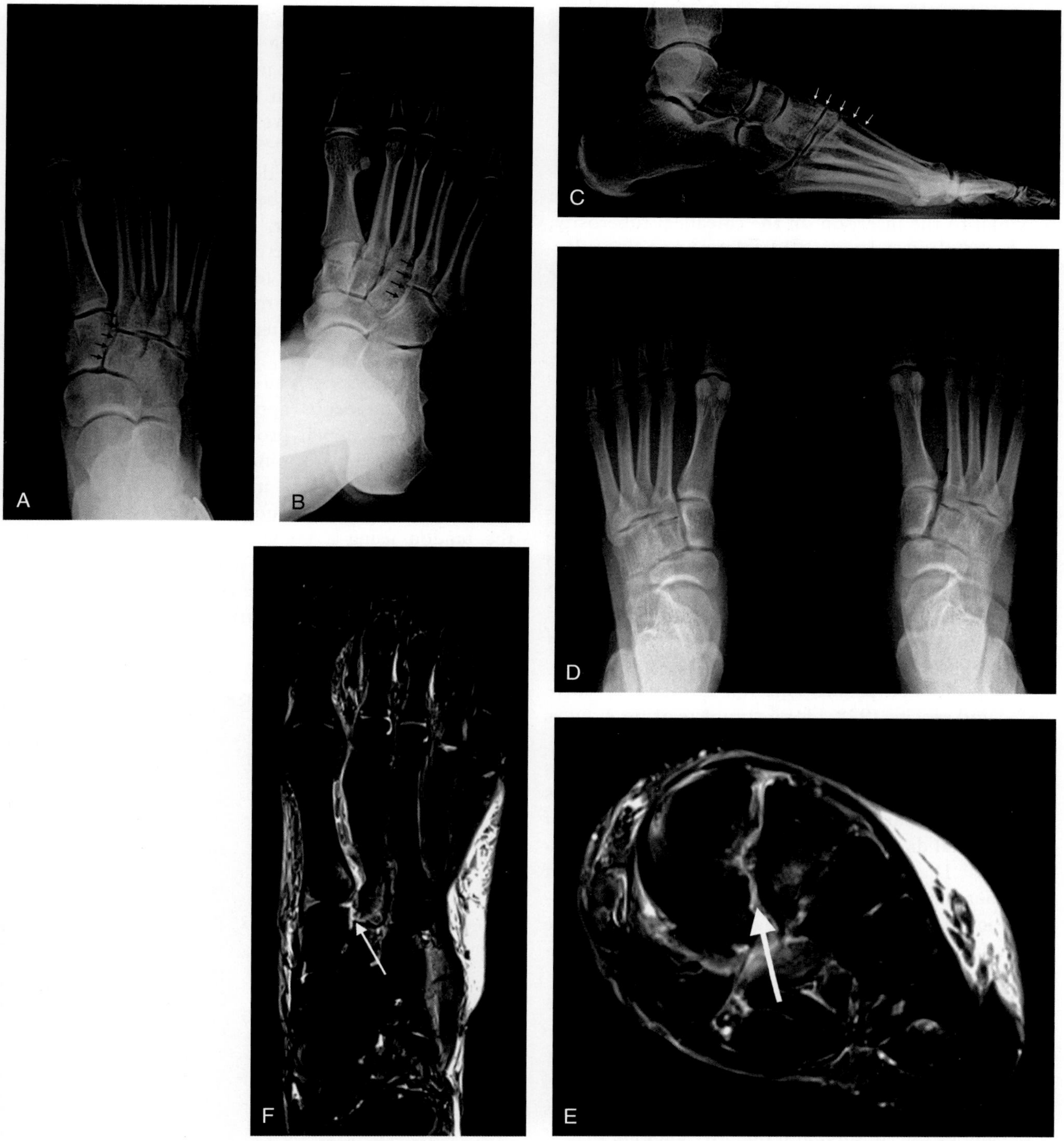

Figure 10 Normal AP, oblique, and lateral weight-bearing radiographs of the right foot in an asymptomatic patient (**A** to **C**). Arrows indicate normal alignment of the medial second metatarsal base with the middle cuneiform (**A**), the medial fourth metatarsal base with the cuboid (**B**), and the dorsal first metatarsal base with the medial cuneiform (**C**). AP bilateral foot XR in a different patient with right Lisfranc injury (**D**). Arrow indicates diastasis between the medial cuneiform and second metatarsal base, as well as intercuneiform diastasis. Axial (**E**) and coronal (**F**) T2 magnetic resonance images demonstrate injury to the Lisfranc ligament as indicated by the arrows.

Achilles Tendon Rupture

Ruptures of the Achilles tendon are common injuries and occur most frequently in recreational male athletes in the third to fifth decades.

Most ruptures occur as an indirect loading mechanism during eccentric muscle contracture. Seventy-five percent of ruptures occur between 5 and 6 cm proximal to the insertion on the calcaneal tuberosity, which correlates to a zone of relative hypovascularity. A subgroup of patients with an acute rupture have antecedent pain at the Achilles and these tendons frequently show degenerative changes on histopathologic evaluation.[49]

The diagnosis of a suspected Achilles rupture is based largely on history and physical examination. Most injuries occur during sports participation with the patients typically reporting a sensation of being kicked or shot in the leg despite no contact occurring to the tendon. Physical examination reveals a decreased resting tension compared with the contralateral side, plantar flexion weakness with recruitment of toe flexors to substitute for the power of the gastrocnemius-soleus complex, and a palpable gap at the site of the rupture. Thompson testing is positive indicating the absence of passive ankle plantar flexion upon calf squeeze with the patient positioned prone. This test is highly sensitive (96%) and specific (93%) for a complete acute Achilles rupture.[50,51]

Achilles ruptures must be divided into acute versus chronic; the distinction is most commonly described as 4 to 6 weeks. Chronic ruptures are often the result of missed initial diagnosis, which can occur in up to 25% of cases.[51] Diagnostic imaging is not needed in most cases, but can be useful to rule out alternative or additional injuries, confirm the diagnosis, or better define the injury for preoperative planning purposes, especially in cases of delayed or unclear diagnosis.

MRI and ultrasonography can both be used to confirm an Achilles tendon rupture in the case of ambiguous physical examination findings but are not routinely necessary. They may also be helpful to localize the level of an acute rupture, identify any underlying tendinosis at the site of the rupture, and quantify gapping of tendon ends, which may influence treatment (**Figure 11**).

Acute Achilles tendon ruptures can be treated with either surgical repair or nonsurgical functional immobilization and rehabilitation. Historical studies which compared surgical to nonsurgical treatment implemented cast immobilization for 6 to 8 weeks as the nonsurgical treatment. These studies showed higher rates of re-rupture with nonsurgical treatment, which were as high as 12%.[52] However, multiple newer randomized-controlled trials have been performed using functional rehabilitation with early initiation of weight bearing and active plantar flexion for both surgical and nonsurgical treatment and have shown no significant difference in re-rupture rates.[53,54] For the most part, studies have also been unable to detect differences in strength and functional outcomes between surgical and nonsurgical treatment. However, one randomized-controlled trial showed a 14% increased peak plantar flexion torque at 1 and 2 years following surgical treatment and a meta-analysis of randomized-controlled trials found that surgically treated patients returned to work 19 days faster.[53,54]

Surgical treatment can be performed through an open or percutaneous approach. Minimally invasive or percutaneous repair procedures have gained popularity in an attempt to minimize complications related to wound healing and infection. Current methods involve passing multiple nonabsorbable sutures across the tendon using a guide system. Generally, studies have shown fewer wound complications without a corresponding increase in re-rupture rates, and possibly a faster return to preinjury activities when repair is

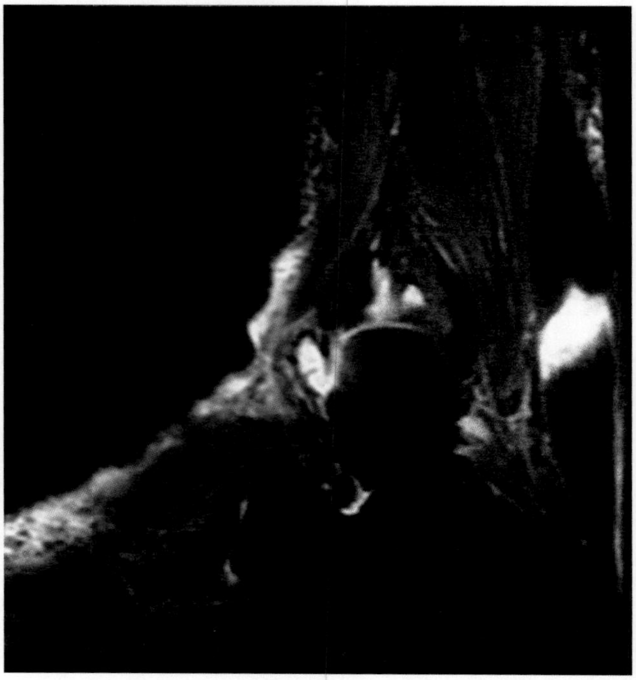

Figure 11 T2 sagittal magnetic resonance image demonstrating subacute Achilles rupture in setting of noninsertional Achilles tendinosis. Rounded tendon ends indicate chronicity of rupture. Severe tendon thickening at site of rupture indicates underlying tendinosis.

performed percutaneously.[55,56] There has been concern for increased rates of sural nerve injury using percutaneous techniques for repair in some studies,[57] whereas others have shown rates similar to open repair.[56]

Chronic Achilles ruptures typically require surgical treatment to optimize strength and function. Functional rehabilitation has not been shown to be effective in these cases, with nonsurgical treatment requiring a long-term AFO for support and ambulatory assistance. Several techniques for surgical reconstruction of chronic Achilles ruptures have been described and evidence to support these techniques is mostly limited to case series. Defects less than 2 cm may be treated with excision of the fibrous tissue and direct repair of the proximal and distal tendon ends. Defects between 2 and 5 cm can be treated with a V-Y lengthening with or without a tendon transfer. Finally, defects greater than 5 cm should be treated with tendon transfer alone versus tendon transfer with V-Y advancement or gastrocnemius-soleus complex turndown.[58] Proposed tendon transfer procedures include flexor hallucis longus (FHL), flexor digitorum longus (FDL), and peroneus brevis transfers. Interposition autografts options include gracilis and fascia lata, although Achilles tendon allograft has been used as well.

Achilles Tendinopathy

Achilles tendinopathy is characterized by pain and dysfunction of the Achilles tendon. Histopathology typically does not show markers of inflammation within the tendon and the term "tendinitis" is a misnomer. The most clinically useful classification of these conditions distinguishes between insertional (at the calcaneal tuberosity) and noninsertional Achilles tendinopathy (2 to 6 cm proximal to the insertion). Achilles tendinopathy is a degenerative condition that is thought to be related to overuse. Patients present with pain at the Achilles tendon that correlates with increased activity. Examination reveals tenderness and swelling at the level of the tendinosis. Patients with noninsertional Achilles tendinopathy typically have fusiform thickening or nodularity of the tendon 4 to 6 cm proximal to the insertion and associated tenderness to palpation. A contracture of the gastrocnemius-soleus complex is often observed. Weight-bearing ankle radiographs may demonstrate intratendinous calcification at the affected level; in the case of insertional tendinopathy, there may be an insertional osteophyte and/or Haglund deformity, representing a prominence at the superior, posterolateral aspect of the calcaneal tuberosity (**Figure 12**, A). MRI or ultrasonography evaluation are useful for presurgical planning and can detect the degree of tendon degeneration (**Figure 12**, **B** and **C**).

Initial nonsurgical treatment consists of a period of rest, activity modification, use of heel lifts with or without immobilization in a walking boot. Physical therapy with a focus on eccentric strengthening has shown efficacy for the nonsurgical treatment of insertional and noninsertional Achilles tendinopathy.[59,60] Extracorporeal shock wave therapy can be considered, and some studies show benefit over eccentric physical therapy.[61,62] Long-term use of an ankle-foot orthosis to neutralize the Achilles tendon can be considered as an alternative to surgery if other nonsurgical treatments have been ineffective.

Surgical Treatment of Insertional Achilles Tendinopathy

Surgical treatment should be considered following 3 to 6 months of failed nonsurgical treatment. A variety of surgical procedures have been proposed; however, the principles involve resection of the Haglund deformity and insertional osteophytes, débridement of degenerative Achilles tendon, and repair of the tendon to the calcaneal tuberosity, with or without a flexor hallucis longus transfer. Surgical exposure can be via the lateral or medial border of the Achilles tendon or a midline incision with splitting of the tendon to access the Haglund exostosis. If symptoms are localized to the Haglund deformity and retrocalcaneal bursa without significant tendon degeneration or insertional pain, one can consider a lateral exposure with calcaneal exostectomy and minimal tendon detachment. With more significant tendon involvement, detachment of the tendon is required for adequate débridement. Repair is performed using multiple suture anchors, and a double row repair can be used to better appose the distal aspect of the tendon to the cut surface of the calcaneal tuberosity. If greater than 50% of the Achilles tendon cross-sectional area is débrided, the repair should be augmented with an FHL transfer. The FHL transfer can also be considered for elderly or obese patients even with preservation of greater than 50% of the tendon.[63]

Surgical Treatment of Noninsertional Achilles Tendinopathy

A variety of techniques have been described for this condition. Several minimally invasive procedures have been proposed including ultrasonography guided percutaneous tenotomy, mini-open scraping of hypervascular peritendinous tissue, and endoscopic débridement of the paratenon and degenerative

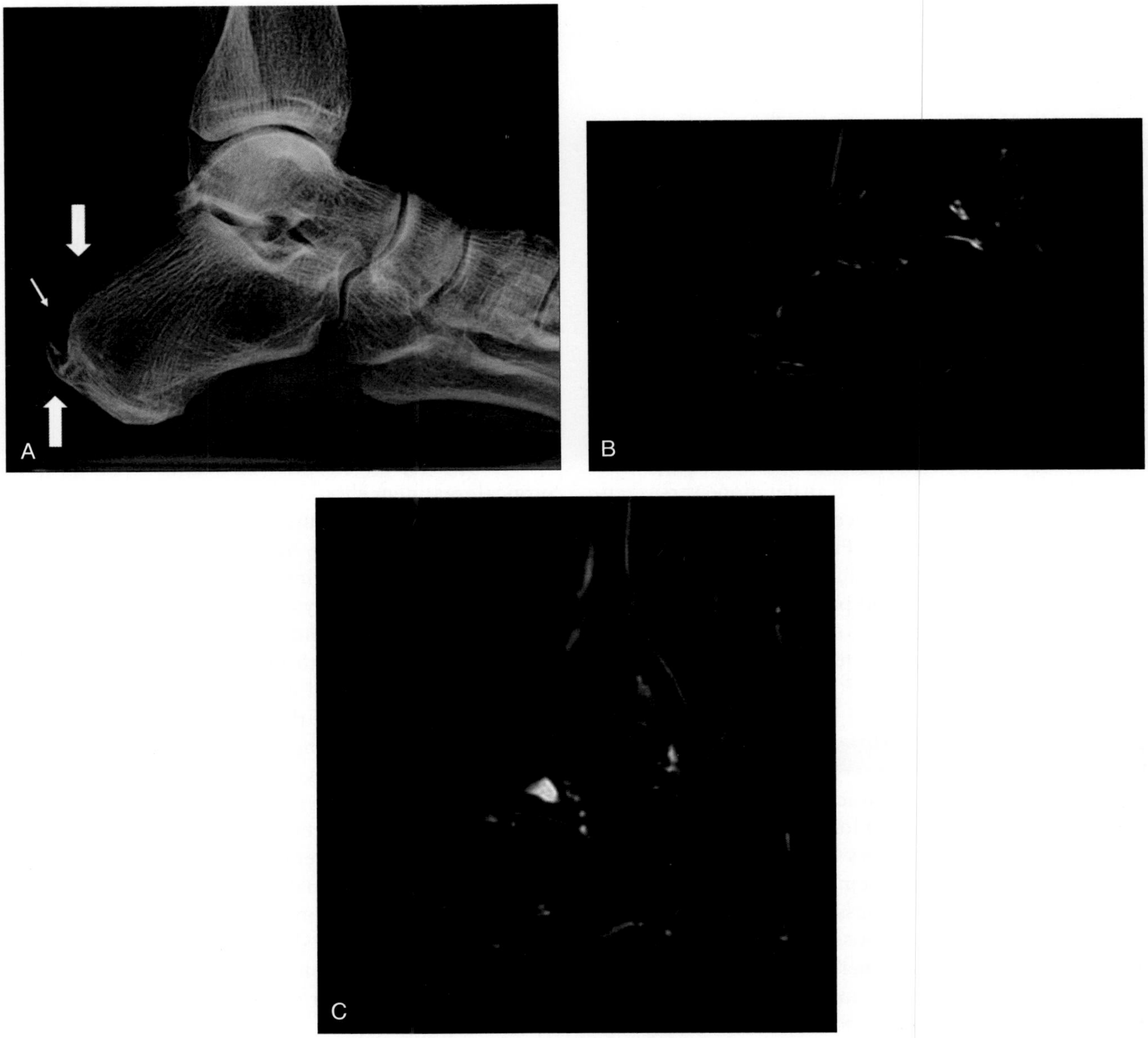

Figure 12 **A**, Lateral radiograph of a patient with insertional Achilles tendinopathy. Demonstrates Haglund deformity (thick downward arrow), insertional osteophyte (thick upward arrow), and intratendinous calcification (thin arrow). **B**, Sagittal T2 magnetic resonance image of a patient with insertional Achilles tendinopathy demonstrating insertional bone marrow edema, tendon thickening, intrasubstance hyperintense signal. **C**, Sagittal T2 magnetic resonance image of a patient with noninsertional Achilles tendinosis demonstrating severe tendon thickening and intrasubstance hyperintense signal indicating partial thickness interstitial tearing.

tendon. Alternatively, an isolated gastrocnemius recession has been proposed to address pathology indirectly by neutralizing the contracture that is a contributing factor in the pathogenesis.

More diffuse tendon involvement requires a standard open exposure to perform an adequate débridement. A posteromedial approach to the tendon is performed and adhesions between the tendon and paratenon can be released. If the paratenon is severely thickened and inflamed, portions can be excised. Areas of degenerative tendon should be incised and débrided back to the level of healthy tendon. If the cross-sectional area of involvement is less than 50%, the remaining tendon can be tubularized. However, if greater than 50% of the tendon is involved, the repair should be augmented with an FHL tendon transfer.

Chronic Ankle Instability

Lateral Ankle Instability

Lateral ankle sprains are one of the most common injuries encountered during sports activity and during normal activities of daily living. These occur with an inversion force to the ankle and result in partial or complete tearing of the lateral ankle ligaments, which include the anterior talofibular ligament (ATFL), calcaneofibular ligament (CFL), and posterior talofibular ligament. The ATFL is most commonly involved in isolation, followed by a combined injury to the ATFL and CFL. The majority of patients are adequately treated with functional rehabilitation; however, 10% to 20% of patients go on to have chronic ankle instability.[64]

The development of chronic lateral ankle instability is multifactorial and can involve a patient's abnormal neuromuscular response and proprioception, abnormal gait mechanics, global ligamentous laxity, increased body weight, and anatomic features of the hindfoot and ankle including cavus alignment and hindfoot stiffness. Patients present with the sensation of instability, often with recurrent and frequent inversion injuries. Symptoms occur with walking on uneven ground or participating in athletic activity. On examination, an ankle effusion may be present because of chronic instability and synovitis or from an associated osteochondral lesion or loose body. Anterior drawer testing and talar tilt stress are performed to evaluate competency of the ATFL and CFL, respectively. Patients should be assessed for evidence of global ligamentous laxity and weight-bearing hindfoot alignment.

AP, mortise, and lateral weight-bearing radiographs of the ankle are performed. Additionally, stress radiographs can be used to confirm instability; a lateral radiograph is obtained while performing the anterior drawer test and a mortise radiograph while performing the talar tilt test. MRI is useful in evaluating for associated pathology to the peroneal tendons or talar articular surface. Although it will confirm the abnormal appearance of the affected ligaments which may be thickened or indistinct, MRI does not help determine functional instability.

Conservative treatment focuses on functional rehabilitation with peroneal strengthening and proprioceptive training. Additional modalities include bracing treatment and consideration of an orthotic with a lateral based wedge, especially in the presence of hindfoot varus foot alignment.

Surgical treatment involves reconstruction of the lateral ligaments, and numerous techniques have been described including anatomic and nonanatomic reconstructions. Anatomic procedures involve the repair or reconstruction of the ATFL and CFL ligaments, whereas nonanatomic procedures most commonly involve the rerouting of part or all of the peroneus brevis through bone tunnels in the fibula to restore ankle stability. Anatomic procedures have the advantage of more closely recreating the native anatomy and preserving motion at the ankle and subtalar joints, whereas nonanatomic tenodesis procedures may provide additional stability in patients at high risk of failure such as those with ligamentous laxity, obesity, or prior stabilization procedures. Recently, additional procedures have been described to incorporate free tendon grafts (allograft or autograft) in a more anatomic fashion to provide the additional stability of historical nonanatomic tenodesis procedures while avoiding the associated stiffness and weakening of the peroneal tendons.

The most commonly used anatomic repair technique is the Gould modification of the Broström repair.[65] This procedure involves imbrication of the ATFL and CFL ligaments with additional reinforcement with the lateral talocalcaneal ligament and inferior extensor retinaculum. This repair was initially described as a midsubstance imbrication but can also be performed with drill holes or suture anchors in the distal fibula. Numerous studies have reported greater than 85% excellent results using these types of anatomic repairs at short-, intermediate-, and long-term follow-up.[66] Newer adaptations of this procedure include performing the technique arthroscopically. This minimally invasive approach may reduce postoperative pain and swelling and allow for concomitant arthroscopic evaluation of the ankle to assess for impingement and osteochondral lesions of the talus. Finally, another popular modification of the modified Broström-Gould technique is to supplement the ligament repair with suture tape affixed to the fibula and talus with knotless anchors. This provides increased stability in patients with poor native tissue or other risk factors for failure.[67] It may also allow for a more rapid and aggressive rehabilitation protocol.

Summary

Foot and ankle reconstruction relies on an understanding of alignment and function of key structures. Pain related to foot deformities such as hallux valgus, planovalgus alignment, or cavovarus foot deformities require bony and soft-tissue realignment procedures to restore balance to a patient's extremity. Ligament injury may result in chronic disability and appropriate diagnosis and treatment is paramount.

Key Study Points

- Surgical treatment of hallux valgus deformity typically involves osteotomy of the first metatarsal to correct the intermetatarsal angle, release of the contracted structures at the lateral first MTP joint (modified McBride), and imbrication of the medial joint capsule.
- Fixed hammer toe correction typically requires resection arthroplasty of PIP joint and temporary Kirschner wire fixation. Hyperextension is commonly seen at the MTP joint, which may require shortening osteotomy of the metatarsal with or without lengthening of the extensor tendon.
- Adult acquired flatfoot deformity (AAFD) occurs as a progressive loss of function of the posterior tibial tendon; ultimately, the hindfoot progresses to valgus alignment, the midfoot abducts, and the forefoot supinates.
- Cavovarus foot alignment may be associated with underlying neuropathic conditions such as Charcot-Marie-Tooth disease (hereditary motor sensory neuropathy type I).
- Ankle instability is treated with functional rehabilitation for a period of 3 to 6 months; surgical treatment with direct ligament repair versus ligament reconstruction with autograft or allograft can successfully stabilize the ankle.

Annotated References

1. Klaue K, Hansen ST, Masquelet AC: Clinical, quantitative assessment of first tarsometatarsal mobility in the sagittal plane and its relation to hallux valgus deformity. *Foot Ankle Int* 1994;15(1):9-13.
2. Welck MJ, Al-Khudairi N: Imaging of hallux valgus: How to approach the deformity. *Foot Ankle Clin* 2018;23(2):183-192.

   This article describes the pathogenesis of hallux valgus (HV) and the traditional ways to image the deformities. It also discusses up-to-date advances and research in the field of imaging in HV. Level of evidence: NA.
3. Matthews M, Klein E, Youssef A, et al: Correlation of radiographic measurements with patient-centered outcomes in hallux valgus surgery. *Foot Ankle Int* 2018;39(12):1416-1422. doi:10.1177/1071100718790255.

   Retrospective analysis examining whether patient-reported outcomes (PROs) after bunion surgery correlated with radiographic parameters in hallux valgus deformity. No radiographic measurement achieved anything more than a weak correlation with any of the PROs. Study conclude that radiographic angles were not well correlated with patient-centered outcomes in hallux valgus surgery. Level of evidence: III.
4. Martinelli N, Giacalone A, Bianchi A, Hosseinzadeh M, Bonifacini C, Malerba F: Distal Akin osteotomy for hallux valgus interphalangeus. *Foot Ankle Surg* 2018;24(3):205-207.

   Study assess clinical and radiological outcomes in patients who underwent distal Akin osteotomy for hallux valgus interphalangeus (HVI). 52.9% were "very satisfied," 41.2% "satisfied," and just a 5.9% was "not satisfied." The mean HVI value decreased from 24.9° ± 7.8° preoperatively to 13.1° ± 5.8° postoperatively ($P < 0.05$). Level of evidence: IV.
5. Chen JY, Rikhraj K, Gatot C, Lee JY, Singh Rikhraj I: Tibial sesamoid position influence on functional outcome and satisfaction after hallux valgus surgery. *Foot Ankle Int* 2016;37(11):1178-1182.

   This retrospective review of 250 patients undergoing hallux valgus correction followed up at 2 years postsurgery. The authors demonstrated that reduction of the tibial sesamoid to an anatomic position medial to the crista of the metatarsal head resulted in greatest improvement in pain and function following hallux valgus correction. Level of evidence: III.
6. Okuda R, Kinoshita M, Yasuda T, Jotoku T, Kitano N, Shima H: Postoperative incomplete reduction of the sesamoids as a risk factor for recurrence of hallux valgus. *J Bone Joint Surg Am* 2009;91(7):1637-1645.
7. Doty JF, Coughlin MJ: Metatarsophalangeal joint instability of the lesser toes and plantar plate deficiency. *J Am Acad Orthop Surg* 2014;22(4):235-245.
8. Flint WW, Macias DM, Jastifer JR, Doty JF, Hirose CB, Coughlin MJ: Plantar plate repair for lesser metatarsophalangeal joint instability. *Foot Ankle Int* 2017;38(3):234-242.

   Study evaluated the subjective, functional, and radiographic outcomes of plantar plate repair from a dorsal approach. Eighty percent of patients scored "good" to "excellent" satisfaction. They concluded that the plantar plate could be repaired through a dorsal approach with reliable outcomes. Level of evidence: IV.
9. Holmes GB Jr, Mann RA: Possible epidemiological factors associated with rupture of the posterior tibial tendon. *Foot Ankle* 1992;13(2):70-79.
10. Apostle KL, Coleman NW, Sangeorzan BJ: Subtalar joint axis in patients with symptomatic peritalar subluxation compared to normal controls. *Foot Ankle Int* 2014;35(11):1153-1158.
11. Myerson MS: Adult acquired flatfoot deformity: Treatment of dysfunction of the posterior tibial tendon. *Instr Course Lect* 1997;46:393-405.
12. Silfverskold N: Reduction of the uncrossed two-joints muscles of the leg to one-joint muscles in spastic conditions. *Acta Chir Scand* 1924;56:315-330.
13. Williamson ER, Chan JY, Burket JC, Deland JT, Ellis SJ: New radiographic parameter assessing hindfoot alignment in stage II adult-acquired flatfoot deformity. *Foot Ankle Int* 2015;36(4):417-423.
14. Baxter JR, LaMothe JM, Walls RJ, Prado MP, Gilbert SL, Deland JT: Reconstruction of the medial talonavicular joint in simulated flatfoot deformity. *Foot Ankle Int* 2015;36(4):424-429.

15. Chan JY, Greenfield ST, Soukup DS, Do HT, Deland JT, Ellis SJ: Contribution of lateral column lengthening to correction of forefoot abduction in stage IIb adult acquired flatfoot deformity reconstruction. *Foot Ankle Int* 2015;36(12):1400-1411.

16. Lutz M, Myerson M: Radiographic analysis of an opening wedge osteotomy of the medial cuneiform. *Foot Ankle Int* 2011;32(3):278-287.

17. Ellis SJ, Williams BR, Wagshul AD, Pavlov H, Deland JT: Deltoid ligament reconstruction with peroneus longus autograft in flatfoot deformity. *Foot Ankle Int* 2010;31(9):781-789.

18. Coster MC, Rosengren BE, Bremander A, Karlsson MK: Surgery for adult acquired flatfoot due to posterior tibial tendon dysfunction reduces pain, improves function and health related quality of life. *Foot Ankle Surg* 2015;21(4):286-289.

19. Chadwick C, Whitehouse SL, Saxby TS: Long-term follow-up of flexor digitorum longus transfer and calcaneal osteotomy for stage II posterior tibial tendon dysfunction. *Bone Joint J* 2015;97-B(3):346-352.

20. Rohm J, Zwicky L, Horn Lang T, Salentiny Y, Hintermann B, Knupp M: Mid- to long-term outcome of 96 corrective hindfoot fusions in 84 patients with rigid flatfoot deformity. *Bone Joint J* 2015;97-B(5):668-674.

21. Sachithanandam V, Joseph B: The influence of footwear on the prevalence of flat foot. A survey of 1846 skeletally mature persons. *J Bone Joint Surg Br* 1995;77(2):254-257.

22. Coleman SS, Chesnut WJ: A simple test for hindfoot flexibility in the cavovarus foot. *Clin Orthop Relat Res* 1977;(123):60-62.

23. Deben SE, Pomeroy GC: Subtle cavus foot: Diagnosis and management. *J Am Acad Orthop Surg* 2014;22(8):512-520.

24. Zide JR, Myerson MS: Arthrodesis for the cavus foot: When, where, and how? *Foot Ankle Clin* 2013;18(4):755-767.

25. Raikin SM, Parek S: Avoiding failure and complications in cavovarus foot deformity reconstruction. *Instr Course Lect* 2018;67:269-274.

    Paper delivers a comprehensive approach to cavovarus deformity, including clinical evaluation, radiographic studies, and treatment. Through demonstrating the biomechanics of the imbalance leading to the deformity, a algorithmic approach to surgical management is created, allowing the reader to avoid potential complications and failure of treatment. Level of evidence: NA.

26. Ortiz C, Wagner E: Tendon transfers in cavovarus foot. *Foot Ankle Clin* 2014;19(1):49-58.

27. An TW, Michalski M, Jansson K, Pfeffer G: Comparison of lateralizing calcaneal osteotomies for varus hindfoot correction. *Foot Ankle Int* 2018;39(10):1229-1236. doi:10.1177/1071100718781572.

    This comparative study evaluated the ability of four lateralizing calcaneal osteotomies, with and without Dwyer wedge resection and coronal rotation of the posterior tuberosity, to correct severe heel varus using a 3D computer printed calcaneal model. The Dwyer wedge osteotomy significantly improved lateralization (effect = 8.0 mm), valgus hindfoot angle (effect = 6.1°), and coronal calcaneal tilt (effect = −17.6°) compared with the oblique osteotomy. Internal rotation of the posterior tuberosity further improved lateralization valgus hindfoot angle and coronal calcaneal tilt. Lateralization, combined with Dwyer osteotomy and coronal plane internal rotation, achieved the greatest correction of varus heel. Level of evidence: NA.

28. Kaplan JR, Myerson MS: The failed cavovarus foot: What went wrong and why? *Instr Course Lect* 2016;65:331-342.

    Paper reviews the spectrum of the adult cavovarus foot and describes the evaluation to determine the extent of the deformity and then choose from a multitude of surgical procedures to achieve correction. Treatment should include an algorithmic approach to adequately achieve a stable, balanced, and plantigrade foot. Level of evidence: NA.

29. Myerson MS, Cerrato RA: Current management of tarsometatarsal injuries in the athlete. *J Bone Joint Surg Am* 2008;90(11):2522-2533.

30. Renninger CH, Cochran G, Tompane T, Bellamy J, Kuhn K: Injury characteristics of low-energy Lisfranc injuries compared with high-energy injuries. *Foot Ankle Int* 2017;38(9):964-969.

    Retrospective case series characterizing Lisfranc injury patterns in low-energy versus high-energy mechanisms of injury. Level of evidence: III.

31. Solan MC, Moorman CT 3rd, Miyamoto RG, Jasper LE, Belkoff SM: Ligamentous restraints of the second tarsometatarsal joint: A biomechanical evaluation. *Foot Ankle Int* 2001;22(8):637-641.

32. Hardcastle PH, Reschauer R, Kutscha-Lissberg E, Schoffmann W: Injuries to the tarsometatarsal joint. Incidence, classification and treatment. *J Bone Joint Surg Br* 1982;64(3):349-356.

33. Shakked RJ: Lisfranc injury in the athlete. *JBJS Rev* 2017;5(9):e4.

    Current review article focusing on low-energy and subtle Lisfranc injuries including diagnosis and management. Level of evidence: NA.

34. Kuo RS, Tejwani NC, Digiovanni CW, et al: Outcome after open reduction and internal fixation of Lisfranc joint injuries. *J Bone Joint Surg Am* 2000;82-A(11):1609-1618.

35. Abbasian MR, Paradies F, Weber M, Krause F: Temporary internal fixation for ligamentous and osseous Lisfranc injuries: Outcome and technical tip. *Foot Ankle Int* 2015;36(8):976-983.

36. Henning JA, Jones CB, Sietsema DL, Bohay DR, Anderson JG: Open reduction internal fixation versus primary arthrodesis for Lisfranc injuries: A prospective randomized study. *Foot Ankle Int* 2009;30(10):913-922.

37. Ly TV, Coetzee JC: Treatment of primarily ligamentous Lisfranc joint injuries: Primary arthrodesis compared with open reduction and internal fixation. A prospective, randomized study. *J Bone Joint Surg Am* 2006;88(3):514-520.

38. Reinhardt KR, Oh LS, Schottel P, Roberts MM, Levine D: Treatment of Lisfranc fracture-dislocations with primary partial arthrodesis. *Foot Ankle Int* 2012;33(1):50-56.

39. MacMahon A, Kim P, Levine DS, et al: Return to sports and physical activities after primary partial arthrodesis for Lisfranc injuries in young patients. *Foot Ankle Int* 2016;37(4):355-362.

Retrospective case series evaluating return to sports after partial primary arthrodesis for Lisfranc injury. Level of evidence: IV.

40. Lau S, Guest C, Hall M, Tacey M, Joseph S, Oppy A: Functional outcomes post Lisfranc injury—Transarticular screws, dorsal bridge plating or combination treatment? *J Orthop Trauma* 2017;31(8):447-452.

Retrospective case series comparing fixation method for Lisfranc injury. Level of evidence: III.

41. Hawkinson MP, Tennent DJ, Belisle J, Osborn P: Outcomes of Lisfranc injuries in an active duty military population. *Foot Ankle Int* 2017;38(10):1115-1119.

Retrospective database review of military population evaluating return to active duty after ORIF versus partial arthrodesis. Level of evidence: III.

42. Wagner E, Ortiz C, Villalon IE, Keller A, Wagner P: Early weight-bearing after percutaneous reduction and screw fixation for low-energy Lisfranc injury. *Foot Ankle Int* 2013;34(7):978-983.

43. Deol RS, Roche A, Calder JD: Return to training and playing after acute Lisfranc injuries in elite professional soccer and rugby players. *Am J Sports Med* 2016;44(1):166-170.

Prospective case series assessing return to play after ORIF Lisfranc injury in professional soccer and rugby players. Level of evidence: IV.

44. Vosbikian M, O'Neil JT, Piper C, Huang R, Raikin SM: Outcomes after percutaneous reduction and fixation of low-energy Lisfranc injuries. *Foot Ankle Int* 2017;38(7):710-715.

Retrospective case series evaluating clinical and radiographic outcome after percutaneous ORIF Lisfranc injury. Level of evidence: IV.

45. Smith N, Stone C, Furey A: Does open reduction and internal fixation versus primary arthrodesis improve patient outcomes for Lisfranc trauma? A systematic review and meta-analysis. *Clin Orthop Relat Res* 2016;474(6):1445-1452.

Systematic review performed to compare primary partial arthrodesis with ORIF for acute Lisfranc injury. Level of evidence: I.

46. Cochran G, Renninger C, Tompane T, Bellamy J, Kuhn K: Primary arthrodesis versus open reduction and internal fixation for low-energy Lisfranc injuries in a young athletic population. *Foot Ankle Int* 2017;38(9):957-963.

Retrospective case series in a military population evaluating return to full duty after ORIF versus primary partial arthrodesis for Lisfranc injury. Level of evidence: III.

47. Lewis JS Jr, Anderson RB: Lisfranc injuries in the athlete. *Foot Ankle Int* 2016;37(12):1374-1380.

Review of athletic Lisfranc injuries including presentation, management, and outcomes. Level of evidence: NA.

48. Hsu AR, Anderson RB: Foot and ankle injuries in American Football. *Am J Orthop* 2016;45(6):358-367.

Review of lower extremity athletic injuries in American Football players. Level of evidence: NA.

49. Fox JM, Blazina ME, Jobe FW, et al: Degeneration and rupture of the Achilles tendon. *Clin Orthop Relat Res* 1975;(107):221-224.

50. Maffulli N: The clinical diagnosis of subcutaneous tear of the Achilles tendon. A prospective study in 174 patients. *Am J Sports Med* 1998;26(2):266-270.

51. Raikin SM, Garras DN, Krapchev PV: Achilles tendon injuries in a United States population. *Foot Ankle Int* 2013;34(4):475-480.

52. Khan RJ, Fick D, Keogh A, Crawford J, Brammar T, Parker M: Treatment of acute Achilles tendon ruptures: A meta-analysis of randomized, controlled trials. *J Bone Joint Surg Am* 2005;87(10):2202-2210.

53. Soroceanu A, Sidhwa F, Aarabi S, Kaufman A, Glazebrook M: Surgical versus nonsurgical treatment of acute Achilles tendon rupture: A meta-analysis of randomized trials. *J Bone Joint Surg Am* 2012;94(23):2136-2143.

54. Willits K, Amendola A, Bryant D, et al: Operative versus nonoperative treatment of acute Achilles tendon ruptures: A multicenter randomized trial using accelerated functional rehabilitation. *J Bone Joint Surg Am* 2010;92(17):2767-2775.

55. Hsu AR, Jones CP, Cohen BE, Davis WH, Ellington JK, Anderson RB: Clinical outcomes and complications of percutaneous Achilles repair system versus open technique for acute Achilles tendon ruptures. *Foot Ankle Int* 2015;36(11):1279-1286.

56. Lim J, Dalai R, Waseem M: Percutaneous vs. open repair of the ruptured Achilles tendon—A prospective randomized controlled study. *Foot Ankle Int* 2001;22(7):559-568.

57. Maes R, Copin G, Averous C: Is percutaneous repair of the Achilles tendon a safe technique? A study of 124 cases. *Acta Orthop Belg* 2006;72(2):179-183.

58. Myerson M: Achilles tendon ruptures. *Instr Course Lect* 1999;48:219-230.

59. Alfredson H, Pietilä T, Jonsson P, Lorentzon R: Heavy-load eccentric calf muscle training for the treatment of chronic Achilles tendinosis. *Am J Sports Med* 1998;26(3):360-366.

60. Jonsson P, Alfredson H, Sunding K, Fahlström M, Cook J: New regimen for eccentric calf muscle training in patients with chronic insertional Achilles tendinopathy: Results of a pilot study. *Br J Sports Med* 2008;42:746-749.

61. Rompe JD, Furia J, Maffulli N: Eccentric loading compared with shock wave treatment for chronic insertional Achilles tendinopathy. A randomized, controlled trial. *J Bone Joint Surg Am* 2008;90(1):52-61.

62. Rompe JD, Furia J, Maffulli N: Eccentric loading versus eccentric loading plus shock-wave treatment for midportion Achilles tendinopathy: A randomized controlled trial. *Am J Sports Med* 2009;37(3):463-470.

63. Shakked RJ, Raikin SM: Insertional tendinopathy of the Achilles: Debridement, primary repair, and when to augment. *Foot Ankle Clin* 2017;22(4):761-780.

A review of insertional Achilles tendinopathy was performed including diagnosis and surgical and nonsurgical treatment methods. Reviewed surgical treatment options include medial versus midline versus lateral approach, single versus double row repair, and whether to augment the repair with an FHL transfer. Level of evidence: NA.

64. Karlsson J, Lansinger O: Lateral instability of the ankle joint. *Clin Orthop Relat Res* 1992;(276):253-261.

65. Gould N, Seligson D, Gassman J: Early and late repair of lateral ligament of the ankle. *Foot Ankle* 1980;1(2):84-89.

66. DiGiovanni CW, Brodsky A: Current concepts: Lateral ankle instability. *Foot Ankle Int* 2006;27(10):854-866.

67. Cho B-K, Park K-J, Park J-K, SooHoo NF: Outcomes of the modified Broström procedure augmented with suture-tape for ankle instability in patients with generalized ligamentous laxity. *Foot Ankle Int* 2017;38(4):405-411.

A case series was performed on the modified Broström lateral ligament repair with suture tape augmentation for 28 patients with generalized ligamentous laxity. FAOS and FAAM clinical outcome scores were significantly improved at 2 years and there was only one case of recurrent instability. Level of evidence: IV.

Section 10

Spine

EDITOR

Arya Nick Shamie, MD

Chapter 46

Spinal Anatomy

Scott D. Daffner, MD

ABSTRACT

The vertebral column consists of 33 bones (7 cervical, 12 thoracic, 5 lumbar, 5 sacral, and 4 to 5 coccygeal segments). The stability of the spinal column is maintained by the paraspinal muscles as well as a complex ligamentous structure. The anterior longitudinal ligament, posterior longitudinal ligament, supraspinous ligament, intraspinous ligaments, and ligamentum flavum run the length of the spine. The ligamentous anatomy of the craniocervical junction is specialized and provides stability while facilitating the complex range of motion of this region of the spine. The spinal cord runs through this protective barrier and gives off 31 pairs of spinal nerves (8 cervical, 12 thoracic, 5 lumbar, 5 sacral, 1 coccygeal). The majority of the blood supply of the spinal cord derives from medullary branches of the segmental arteries which merge to form the anterior spinal artery. The anatomic structures of the spine contribute to and facilitate its complex biomechanics. A thorough understanding of the anatomic relationships within the spine is integral to understanding spinal pathology. The purpose of this chapter is to review the basic boney, ligamentous, neural, and vascular anatomy of the spine.

Keywords: intervertebral disk; spinal anatomy; spinal cord; spinal ligaments; vertebrae

Dr. Daffner or an immediate family member serves as a paid consultant to or is an employee of Bioventus; has stock or stock options held in Amgen Co. and Pfizer; has received research or institutional support from Bioventus, Orthopedic & Muscular System, Pfizer, and Spinal Kinetics; and serves as a board member, owner, officer, or committee member of the Lumbar Spine Research Society and the North American Spine Society.

Introduction

Spinal anatomy represents a complex mix of musculoskeletal, ligamentous, vascular, and nervous structures. A thorough understanding of the complex anatomic relationships in the spine is paramount to understanding the various pathologic conditions that affect the spine. Unlike other chapters in this text, this chapter is not a review of recent literature per se, but rather provides a background for the understanding of subsequent chapters within this section.

Embryology and Development

Starting around the third week of gestation, the primitive streak deepens, forming the primitive groove (**Figure 1**). In turn, this groove deepens within the ectoderm, and as it folds onto itself, it forms the neural tube. The neural crest forms dorsally and the notochord forms ventrally. The neural crest ultimately forms the peripheral nervous system, spinal ganglia, and the sympathetic trunk. The neural tube goes on to become the spinal cord, and the notochord develops into the spinal column (vertebral bodies and disks). The vertebrae develop from somites, which surround the notochord and neural tube. The somites differentiate into sclerotomes, which divide horizontally. Each vertebra forms from the caudal portion of one sclerotome and the rostral portion of the subjacent level (**Figure 2**). The space between the segments eventually forms the intervertebral disk.[1] Vertebrae have three primary ossification centers: the centrum forms the anterior vertebral body, the neural arch forms the lamina, pedicles, and a portion of the vertebral body, and the costal center forms the anterior portion of the lateral mass, transverse process, or rib. Around the fifth week, the intervertebral disks form from different cells. The nucleus pulposus derives from notochordal cells, whereas the anulus fibrosus develops from sclerotomal cells, mesenchymal stem cells surrounding the notochord.[2]

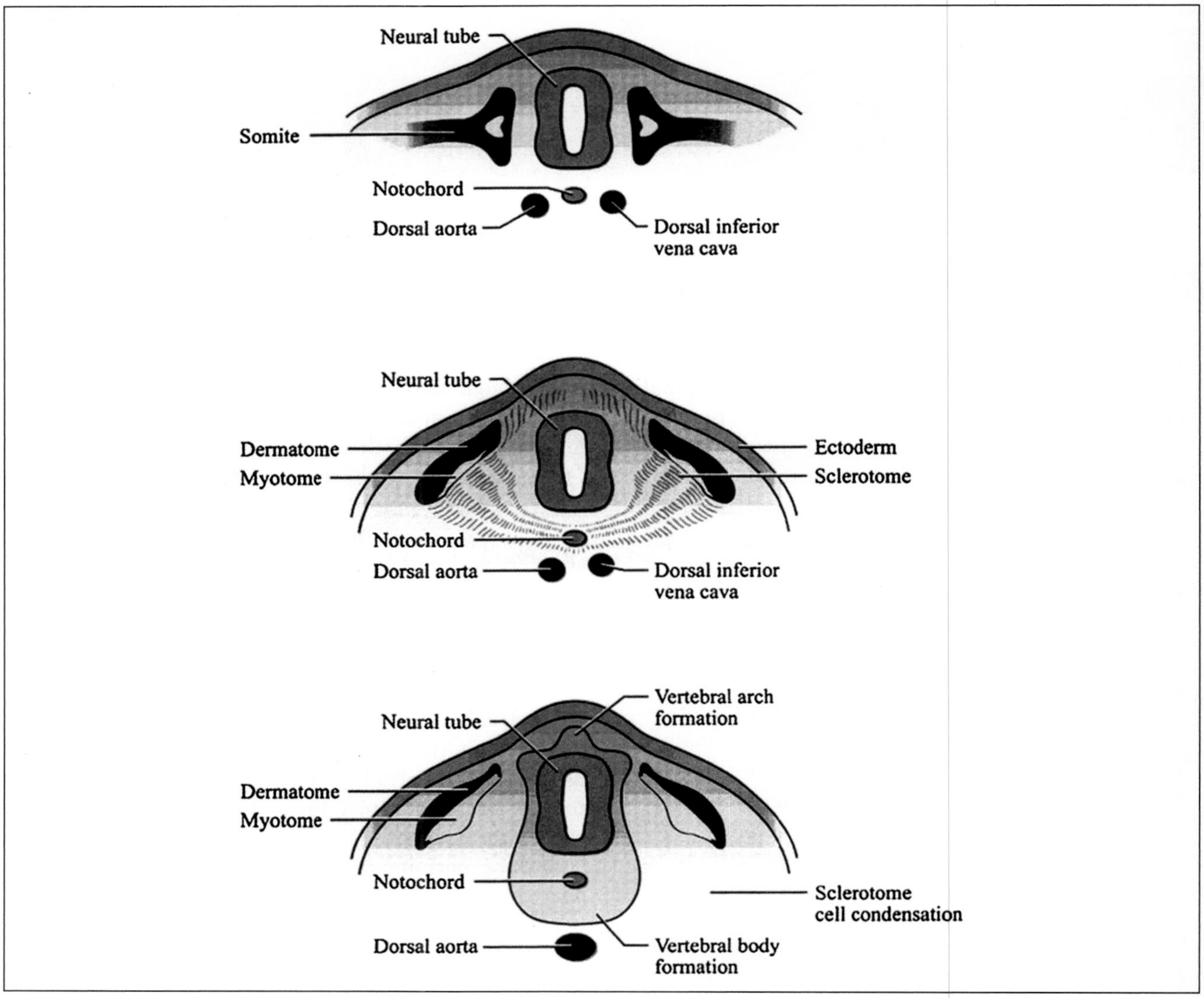

Figure 1 Illustration shows early embryonic development of the spine. The midsagittal groove deepens within the ectoderm and begins to fold onto itself, creating the neural tube. (Reproduced from Rinella A: Human embryology emphasizing spinal and neural development, in Spivak JM, Connolly PJ, eds: *Orthopaedic Knowledge Update Spine 3*. Rosemont, IL, American Academy of Orthopaedic Surgeons, 2006, pp 3-13.)

Failure of any of the above development can lead to congenital spinal anomalies.[1] Failure of the neural tube to close can cause anencephaly if it occurs cranially. If it occurs caudally, it can cause spina bifida, meningocele, or myelomeningocele. Failure of segmentation of somites may result in block vertebrae or unsegmented bars. Failure of formation can lead to congenital hemivertebrae.

Osseous Anatomy

The bony anatomy of the spine consists of 7 cervical vertebrae, 12 thoracic vertebrae, 5 lumbar vertebrae, 5 fused sacral vertebrae, and 4 or 5 fused coccygeal vertebrae (**Figure 3**). There are regional differences between the vertebrae, but the basic anatomy is fairly consistent. The vertebral body consists of a fairly cylindrical mass of bone. It is connected by the pedicles to the posterior arch of the vertebra, which consists of the lamina and spinous process. These structures create the spinal canal (body anteriorly, lamina posteriorly, pedicles laterally) through which the spinal cord passes. The regional anatomic differences in the vertebrae are reflective of the motion and biomechanical forces within a particular portion of the spine. The structure of the spinal column provides support and protection for the spinal cord and nerve roots. The vertebral bodies function

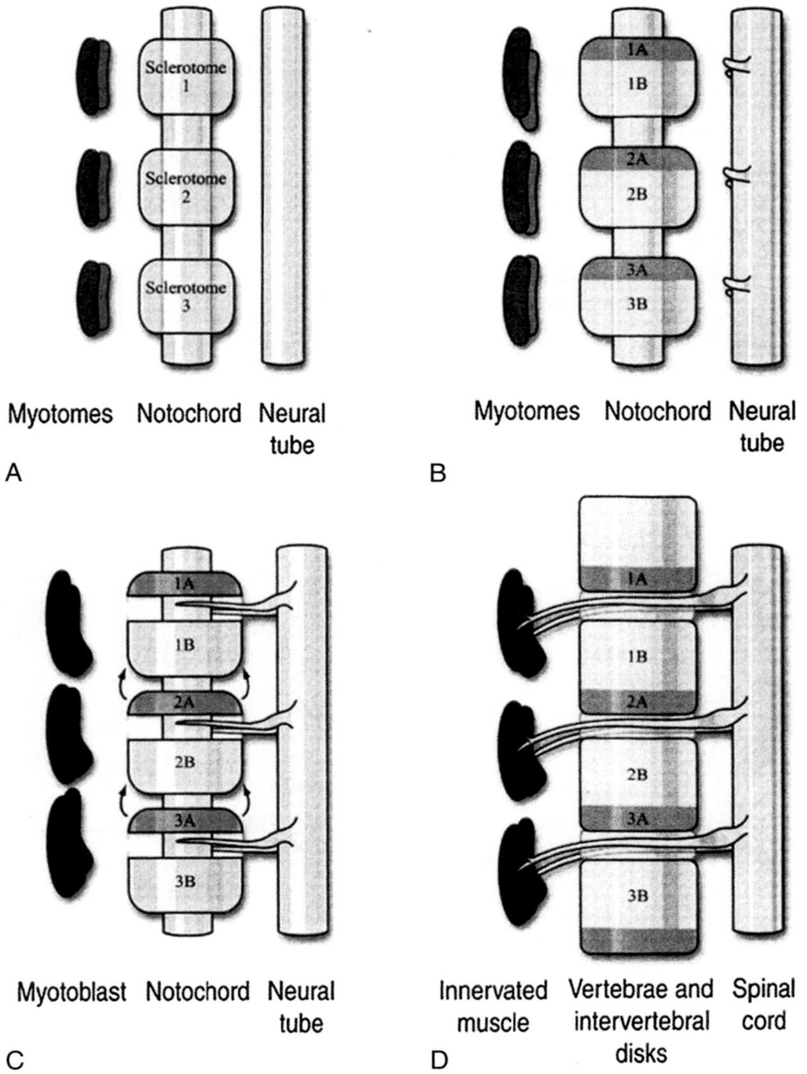

Figure 2 Illustrations demonstrating vertebral development. **A**, Somite differentiation: the somites differentiate into sclerotomes overlying the notochord and dermal myoblasts. **B**, Metameric shift: the sclerotomes begin to divide into two components. **C**, Each sclerotome divides, forming an intervertebral disk between the two segments. **D**, Formation of vertebral bodies and innervation of the dermatomes and myotomes. (Reproduced from Rinella A: Human embryology emphasizing spinal and neural development, in Spivak JM, Connolly PJ, eds: *Orthopaedic Knowledge Update Spine 3*. Rosemont, IL, American Academy of Orthopaedic Surgeons, 2006, pp 3-13.)

primarily to bear weight and transfer forces to the pelvis and hips; the posterior elements provide protection to the neural structures and also function as a tension band.[1-3]

Craniocervical Junction and Upper Cervical Spine

The craniocervical junction represents the most specialized bony anatomy of the spine. The occiput-C1 and C1-C2 articulations account for approximately 50% of the motion of the cervical spine.[1] The C1 vertebra (atlas) lacks a true vertebral body ventrally. The weight of the cranium is supported by the two saddle-shaped superior articular processes which sit atop the relatively robust lateral masses. The occipital condyles sit snugly within the articular processes. This orientation allows substantial flexion and extension.

The axis (C2) articulates with the C1 ring at the atlantoaxial joint (superior C2 articular process, inferior C1 articular process). The odontoid process (or

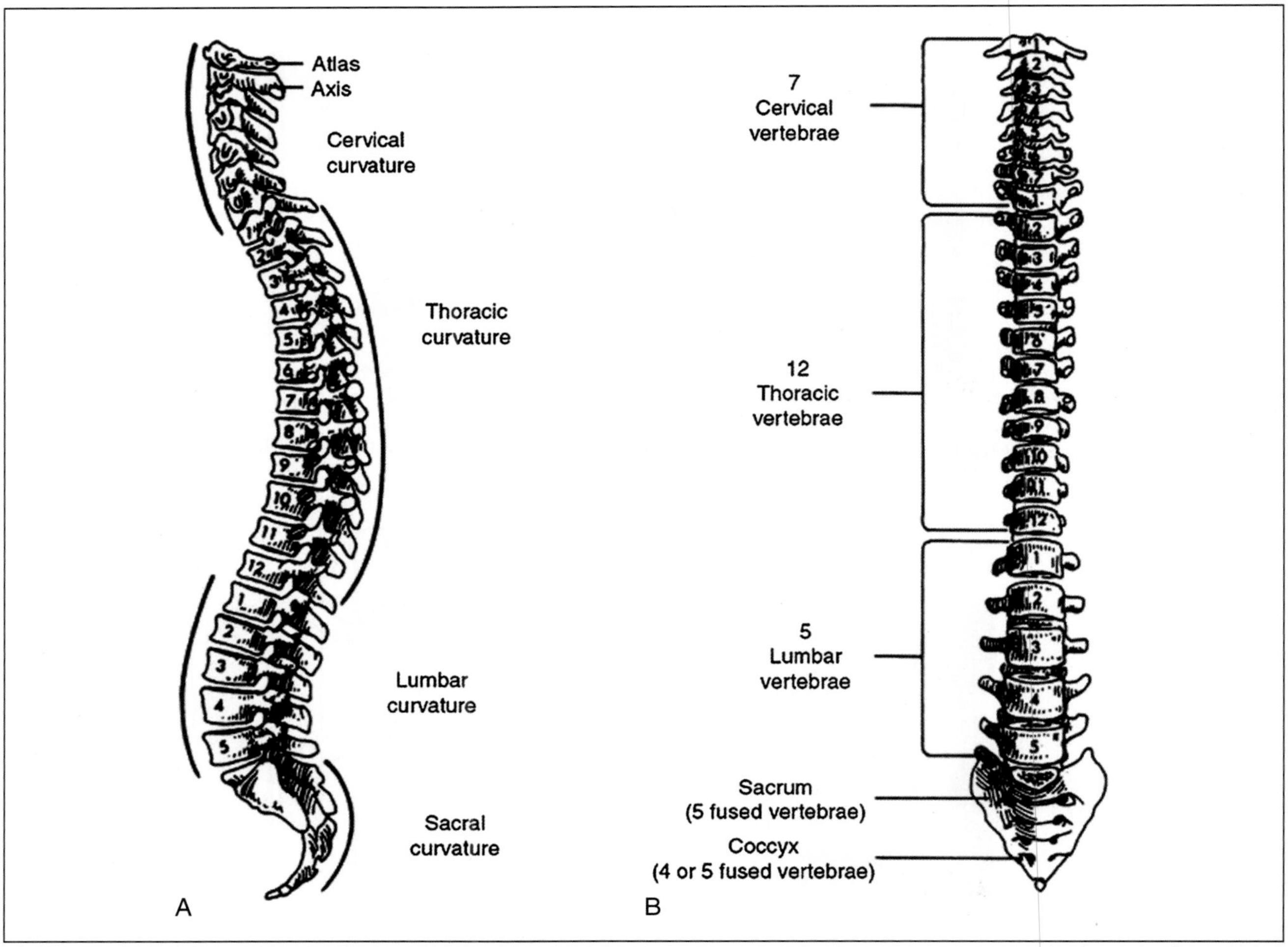

Figure 3 Illustrations show sagittal (**A**) and coronal (**B**) views of the spine.

dens) projects cranially from the C2 vertebral body and acts as a post about which the C1 ring can rotate. This arrangement is stabilized by the ligamentous attachments in the region, particularly the cruciate ligament, which prevents anterior translation of C1 on C2.[1-3]

Subaxial Cervical Spine

From C3 to C7 the vertebrae more closely resemble one another. Of all the vertebrae in the spine, the cervical vertebrae, due to the need to support less of an anatomic load, are the smallest in size. The size of vertebrae increases moving from cranial to caudal. The superior end plate of the vertebral body is a little concave. As one moves laterally, the end plate curves upward along the lateral border forming the uncinated process, which runs the entire anterior-posterior dimension of the vertebra. These form the uncovertebral joints, also known as the joints of Luschka. The posterior portion of the uncinate process forms the ventral aspect of the vertebral foramen, through which the nerve root passes. Hypertrophy or osteophyte formation here can cause nerve root impingement.

Cervical pedicles are short and angulate substantially from dorsolateral to ventromedial. The laminae are relatively thin. The spinous processes are often bifid (although C7 is usually an exception to this rule). The transverse processes are thin and contain the transverse foramen, through which the vertebral artery passes (typically from C6 to C1, although anatomic variants are not uncommon). The lateral masses essentially constitute the pars interarticularis, connecting the superior and inferior facet articular surfaces. The orientation of the facet joints in the cervical spine is more horizontal than other regions, facilitating a large degree of freedom in flexion, extension, axial rotation, and lateral bending.[1-3]

Thoracic Vertebrae

Although it contains the largest number of vertebrae, the thoracic spine has the most variable anatomy. It represents two transitional zones: first, from the highly mobile cervical spine into the more rigid thoracic region, then back to the more mobile lumbar spine. As such, the upper thoracic vertebrae share some similar features as cervical vertebrae, and the lower thoracic levels share some features with the lumbar vertebrae. The outstanding characteristic of the thoracic spine is its rigidity. In conjunction with the ribs and the sternum, this region essentially forms a bony "cube," which is an inherently stable structure, providing protection to the heart and lungs.

The vertebral bodies of the thoracic spine are larger than those of the cervical spine, but smaller than the lumbar vertebrae. The pedicles arise more superiorly from the posterior vertebral body than in the cervical or lumbar spine and project more obliquely from superodorsal to inferoventral. Similar to cervical vertebrae, the pedicles of T1 and to a lesser degree T2 have a more medial trajectory. Moving caudally, the remaining thoracic pedicles have significantly less medial angulation, projecting almost straight forward. The upper thoracic pedicles (T1 and T2) have fairly generous cross-sectional area. Moving caudally, the pedicles narrow in diameter until the midthoracic spine and then increase again toward the most caudal levels. The posterior arch of thoracic vertebrae encloses the spinal canal, which is narrowest in this region of the spine. The spinous processes of the upper four thoracic vertebrae project more horizontally, with only slight inferior angulation, similar to cervical levels. In the midthoracic spine, the spinous processes project sharply obliquely, overlapping the lamina and spinous processes inferiorly. From T10 to T12, the spinous processes again transition to a more horizontal projection, consistent with lumbar vertebrae. Similar to the spinous processes, the laminae of the midthoracic spine overlap considerably. The superior articular facets project cranially from the junction of the laminae and pedicles. They are oriented coronally. The inferior articular facets are essentially contiguous with the ventral aspect of the lamina. The orientation of the facets permits only a small arc of motion.[1-3]

The rib heads articulate with the lateral aspect of the vertebral bodies. There is a shared articulation at the level of the disk space with the rib head articulating with the superolateral aspect of the vertebral body for which it is named and the inferior aspect of the level above, with the articulation referred to as a demifacet, as it is partially on each vertebra. The first, eleventh, and twelfth vertebral bodies have only a single articulation for the same-numbered rib head. The transverse processes project obliquely superolaterally. Along the ventral aspect of the transverse process is the costotransverse joint, the point at which the rib articulates with the same-numbered transverse process. There is no costotransverse articulation at T11 or T12. These levels represent a transitional zone to the lumbar spine, and their transverse processes are shorter and project more laterally than the levels above.[2]

Lumbar Vertebrae

The vertebral bodies of the lumbar spine are large, with a transverse diameter greater than the anterior-posterior diameter. The pedicles arise from the superior aspect of the vertebral bodies and project more horizontally than thoracic pedicles. The L1 pedicles are only minimally medially angled (from dorsal to ventral), but as one progresses down the lumbar spine the orientation becomes more medial, particularly at L5. The transverse processes project more perpendicular relative to the vertebral body, and in the upper lumbar spine, they are large and flat. The L4 and L5 transverse processes are often smaller. The spinous processes are thick and project straight dorsally. The superior articular facet arises at the junction of the pedicle and lamina. It is oriented such that the articular surface faces dorsomedially. The inferior facet extends down from the lamina and nestles snugly on the medial side of the superior facet. The sagittal orientation of the lumbar facet joints allows flexion and extension, while providing resistance to axial rotation and translation.[1-3]

Sacrum and Coccyx

The sacrum forms the posterior aspect of the pelvis and, through its articulations with the ilea via the sacroiliac joints, acts to transfer forces from the upper body and spine to the pelvis and ultimately to the hips and lower extremities. It is comprised of five fused vertebrae and is roughly triangular in shape, with a concave ventral surface and convex dorsal surface.[1-3] Transverse lines, representing the remnants of the intervertebral disks separate the bodies of the sacrum. The sacral alae represent fused anterior costal processes and posterior transverse processes.[2] The articular surface of the sacroiliac joint is comprised of the lateral aspect of the S1 through S3 alae. Large dorsal and ventral neuroforamina lie lateral to the sacral bodies. The fused spinous processes comprise the middle sacral crest, a shallow dorsal projection from the posterior sacrum.[2] The medial sacral crest or articular crest runs the length of the sacrum just medial to the dorsal foramina and represents the fused articular processes.[2] On the cranial end of the sacrum, the crest projects superiorly as the S1 articular facet. Unlike lumbar facets, it is oriented coronally, resisting translation of the L5 vertebra.

The coccyx consists of four or five rudimentary vertebrae projecting inferiorly in the same arc as the curvature of the sacrum. The first coccygeal segment is often separate with the remaining segments fused. The coccygeal segments have no dorsal elements and serve primarily as an attachment site for pelvic muscles and the gluteus maximus.[1-3]

Intervertebral Disk

The intervertebral disks run between vertebral bodies from C2 to S1 and function to resist loads on the spine and provide stability. The disks contribute up to one-third of the height of the spinal column. The disk consists of the cartilaginous end plates of the vertebral bodies, the outer anulus fibrosus, and the inner nucleus pulposus. The end plate serves as a point of attachment of the disk to the superior and inferior surfaces of the vertebral bodies. It is a thin layer of hyaline cartilage. The adult intervertebral disk is avascular and derives its nutrition through diffusion from terminal capillaries in the vertebral bodies just below the end plates.[2]

The nucleus pulposus is the remnant of the embryonic notochord and comprises the gelatinous center of the intervertebral disk. Its extracellular matrix (ECM) is composed of primarily type II collagen and aggrecan, which makes it relatively hydrophilic. The nucleus pulposus serves to resist axial loads as well as provide height to the intervertebral disk.[2-5] The anulus fibrosus consists of concentrically layered fibrous cartilage lamellae (primarily type I collagen), which surrounds the nucleus pulposus. The fibers run in alternating oblique trajectories. The anulus fibrosus resists tensile forces within the spine, including those due to the compression of the nucleus pulposus (**Figure 4**).[2-5]

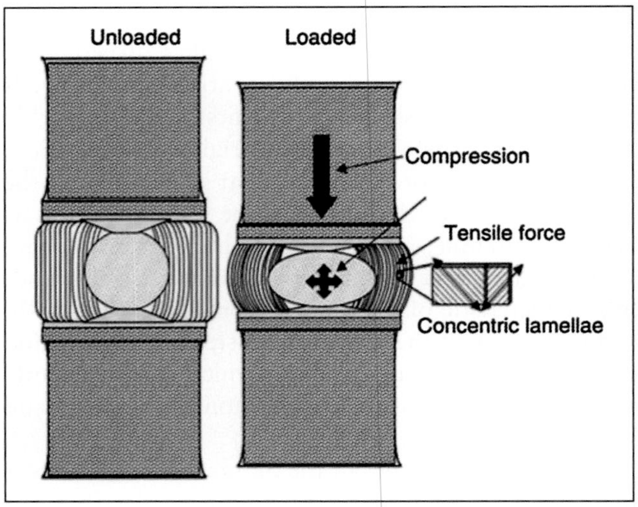

Figure 4 Illustration showing the biomechanics of an intact intervertebral disk. The biomechanical functions of the intervertebral disk are directly related to the extracellular matrix (ECM) components. Aggrecans present in the nucleus pulposus are highly hydrophilic, imbibing water and establishing an internal hydrostatic pressure in the intervertebral disk. This hydrostatic pressure (swelling pressure) is generated by the resistance provided by the anulus fibrosus and end plates to fluid transport. The swelling pressure in the nucleus pulposus also provides resistance to compressive forces. In addition to facilitating the maintenance of the swelling pressure, collagen fibrils run at an angle of about 60 (alternating between adjacent lamellae), ensuring tension of the anulus fibrosus structures during rotational movements. The composite nature of the end plates provides resilience and prevents fractures in the motion segment during load transmission. (Reproduced from Martin JA, Ramakrishnan PS, Lim TH, Thedens D, Buckwalter JA: Articular cartilage and intervertebral disk, in Flynn JM, ed: *Orthopaedic Knowledge Update 10.* Rosemont, IL, American Academy of Orthopaedic Surgeons, 2011, pp 23-36.)

Ligamentous Anatomy

Ligaments of the spine are crucial in facilitating normal physiologic function, while conferring stability and restricting pathological degrees of motion. These structures consist primarily of the anterior longitudinal ligament (ALL), posterior longitudinal ligament (PLL), ligamentum flavum, interspinous ligament, and supraspinous ligament (**Figure 5**).[3] The capsules around the facet joints also confer added stability. Although fairly consistently located throughout the spine, there are several localized specializations of these ligaments, particularly at the upper cervical spine and craniocervical junction.

Anterior Longitudinal Ligament

The ALL runs essentially the entire length of the vertebral column, extending from the ventral aspect of the clivus to the sacrum. At its most cranial end, it is referred to as the anterior atlanto-occipital membrane. It runs along the ventral aspect of the vertebrae, spanning one-quarter to one-third of the width of the body. It integrates with the bone of the vertebral bodies as well as the anulus fibrosus of the intervertebral disks. The ALL functions to prevent hyperextension of the spine.

Posterior Longitudinal Ligament

The PLL also runs the length of the spinal column along the dorsal aspect of the vertebrae within the spinal

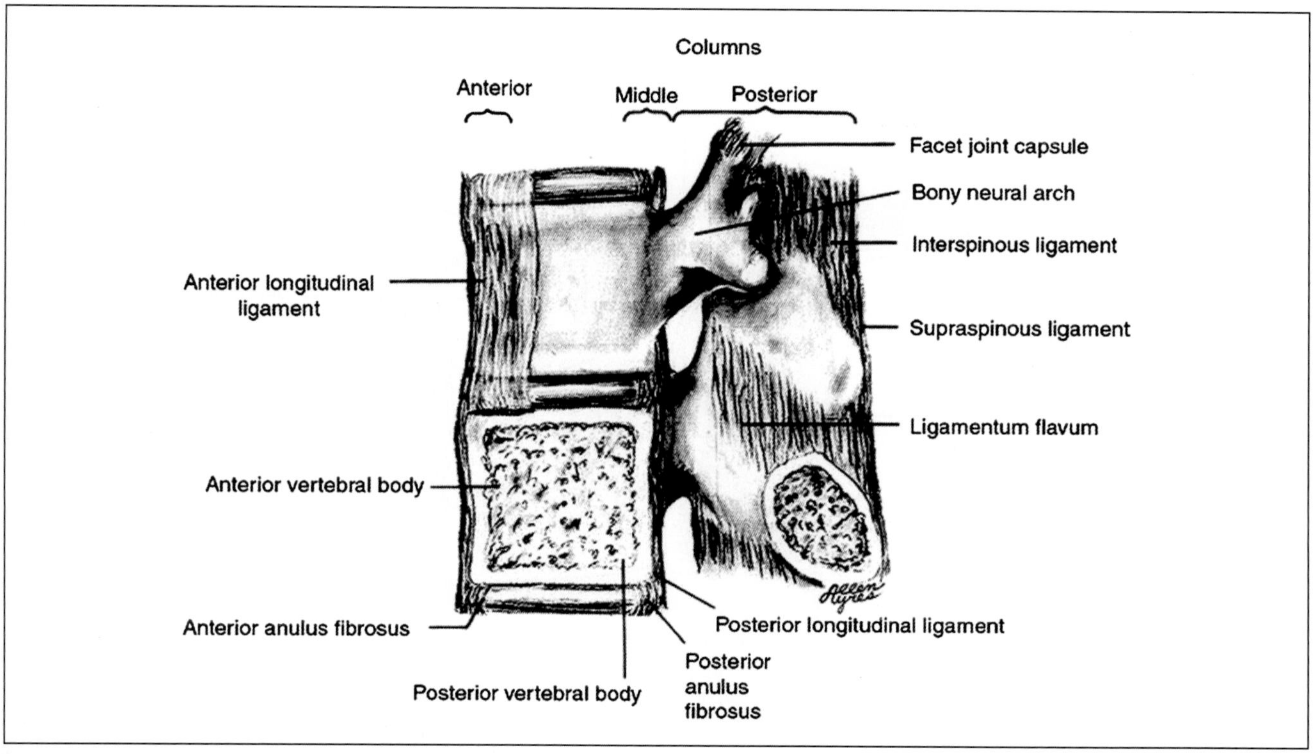

Figure 5 Illustration demonstrates the anatomic structures comprising the three longitudinal columns of stability in the thoracolumbar spine: the anterior column (anterior two-thirds of the vertebral body, anterior part of the anulus fibrosus, and anterior longitudinal ligament), the middle column (posterior third of the vertebral body, posterior part of the anulus fibrosus, and posterior longitudinal ligament), and the posterior column (facet joint capsules, ligamentum flavum, bony neural arch, supraspinous ligament, interspinous ligament, and articular processes). (Adapted with permission from McAfee P, Yuan H, Fredrickson BE, Lubicky JP: The value of CT in thoracolumbar fractures: an analysis of one hundred consecutive cases and a new classification. *J Bone Joint Surg Am* 1983;65[4]:461-473.)

canal. Cranially, it begins as the tectorial membrane, running from the posterior basion (at the ventral aspect of the foramen magnum) to the dorsal aspect of the dens. It continues along the dorsal aspect of the vertebral bodies and disks to the sacrum. Similar to the ALL, it integrates with the posterior annulus of the intervertebral disks. The primary function of the PLL is to limit hyperflexion.

Interspinous and Supraspinous Ligaments

The interspinous ligaments run vertically from the superior aspect of the spinous process of one vertebra to the inferior aspect of the spinous process of the level above. Unlike the ALL and PLL, the interspinous ligaments are discrete entities at each level. The supraspinous ligament runs continuously along the most dorsal aspect of the spinous processes from the sacrum to approximately the C6-C7 level, at which point it remains elevated from the tips of the spinous processes, becoming the ligamentum nuchae, inserting onto the occiput. Together, the intraspinous and supraspinous ligaments primarily restrict flexion, contributing to stability of the posterior elements.

Ligamentum Flavum

The ligamentum flavum originates along the leading edge of the lower lamina (both dorsally and ventrally) and inserts along the ventral surface of the lamina above it. The insertion point is about half way up the ventral surface of the lamina.[6] Laterally, the ligamentum flavum integrates with the medial aspect of the facet capsule. Typically, at each level, there are two ligamenta flava, one on either side of the laminae which meet in the midline, but usually do not fuse. This creates a raphe in the midline which can be utilized to help elevate the ligamentum from the dura, which lies just ventral to it within the spinal canal.

Craniocervical Junction

The ligamentous anatomy of the craniocervical junction is complex and facilitates stability in a highly mobile portion of the spine (**Figure 6**).[2] The apical ligament runs from the tip of the dens to the basion. The alar ligaments attach on the lateral side of the tip of the dens and run horizontally to the anteromedial aspect of the occipital condyles. The cruciate ligament is comprised of both a

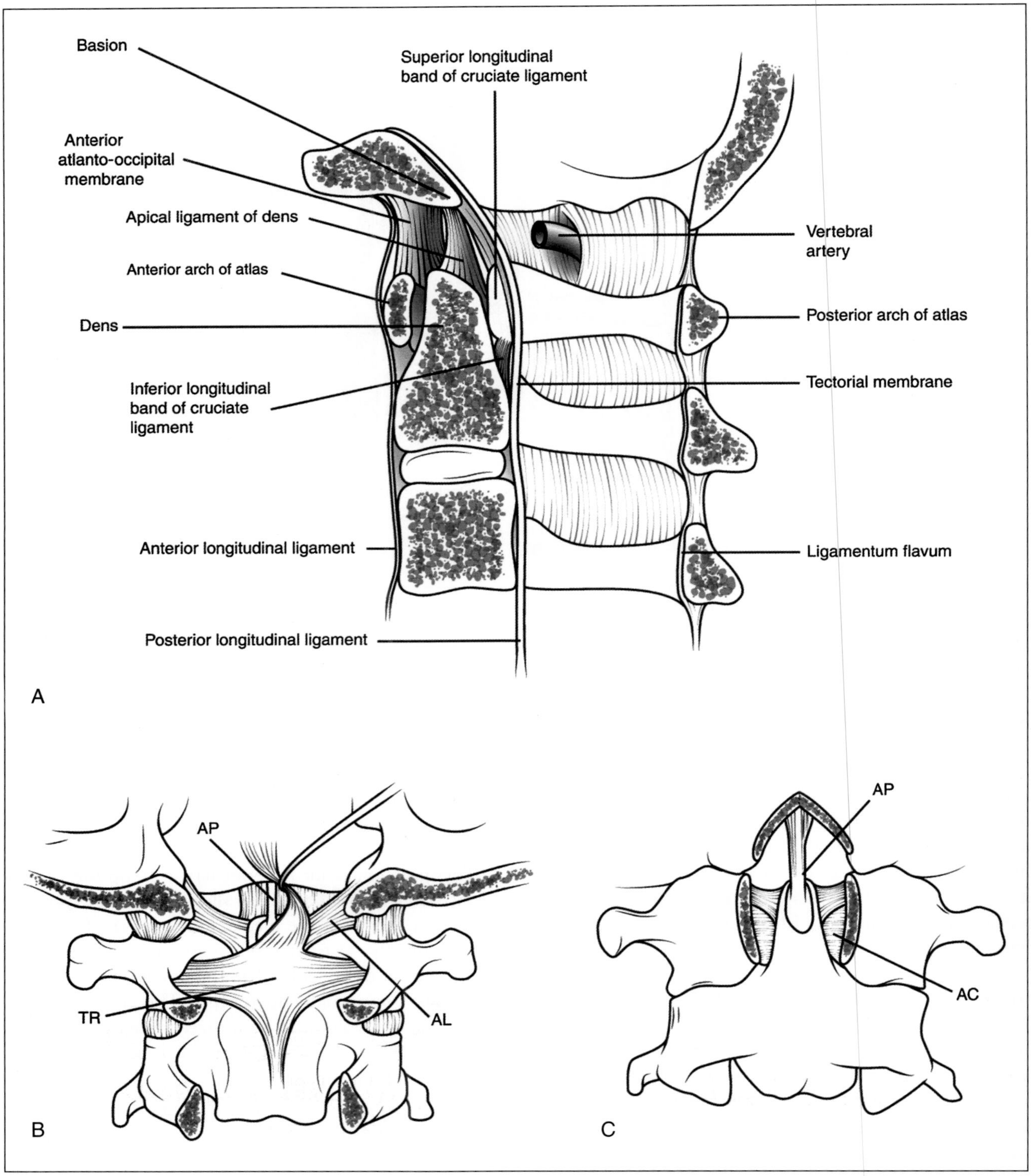

Figure 6 **A**, Illustration demonstrating sagittal view of the occipitocervical articulation. Posterior (**B**) and anterior (**C**) illustrations of the atlantoaxial articulation. AC = accessory ligament, AL = alar ligament, AP = apical ligament, TR = transverse atlantal ligament. (Reproduced with permission from Louis-Ugbo J, Pedlow FX Jr., Heller JG: Anatomy of the cervical spine, in Benzel EC, ed: The Cervical Spine, ed 5. Philadelphia, PA, WK Health, 2012, pp 1-33. © Cervical Spine Research Society.)

transverse and craniocaudal component. The transverse ligament spans from the lateral masses of C1, running just dorsal to the dens; the craniocaudal component of the cruciate ligament runs in the midline from the transverse ligament cranially to the basion and caudally to the C2 vertebral body. The posterior occipito-atlantal membrane runs from the posterior arch of C1 to the posterior aspect of the foramen magnum (opisthion), with a gap laterally for the vertebral arteries.[1,2]

Spinal Cord

Within the spinal cord, dorsal cells are primarily sensory and ventral cells are primarily motor (**Figure 7**). The dorsal columns are responsible for transfer of vibration, deep pressure, and proprioception. The lateral spinothalamic tract lies anterolaterally and transmits pain and temperature sensation. The ventral spinothalamic tract transmits light touch. Efferent voluntary motor function is transmitted along the lateral corticospinal tracts.[1,3] The arrangement of cells within these tracts is such that fibers of the upper extremities are located deeper within the spinal column, with those related to the torso and lower extremities located sequentially more superficially.[1] At each level of the spinal cord, anterior and posterior roots leave the cord separately then unite to form a common segmental nerve root with both motor and sensory components. The dorsal root ganglion lies along the posterior root and is the point at which peripheral sensory nerves synapse with afferent spinal nerves.[2]

The spinal cord changes position within the spinal canal with growth; at birth the conus medullaris lies around the L3 level, but by adulthood it lies around the L1-L2 level.[2] Because of this, the neurologic level of the spinal cord does not necessarily correspond with the vertebral level. The 31 pairs of spinal nerves (8 cervical, 12 thoracic, 5 lumbar, 5 sacral, and 1 coccygeal) leave the spinal cord at the corresponding level of the cord, although this may be several levels higher than the corresponding vertebral level. For example, because the conus medullaris ends at approximately the L1-L2 level, the lumbar, sacral, and coccygeal roots exit the cord at the levels corresponding to the lower thoracic or upper lumbar vertebrae and then form the cauda equina within the canal before exiting the spine. Once nerve roots leave the spinal cord, they exit the canal through the neuroforamen, formed by the pedicles superiorly and inferiorly, the intervertebral disk anteriorly, and the facet joint and capsule posteriorly. In the cervical spine, the roots exit above the same-numbered pedicle (ie, C5 root runs superior to the C5 pedicle). The exception to this is the eighth nerve root which exits under the C7 pedicle. From T1 distally, the nerve roots exit the spine below the same-numbered pedicle.

Vascular Anatomy

The vascular anatomy of the spine is complex and intricate, but a few generalizations are possible. The thoracic and lumbar levels are supplied by paired segmental arteries which originate directly from the aorta along its posterior surface, then run posteriorly along the midportion of the vertebral body.[6] Branches of the segmental arteries supply the vertebral body, the paraspinal musculature, and the spinal cord.

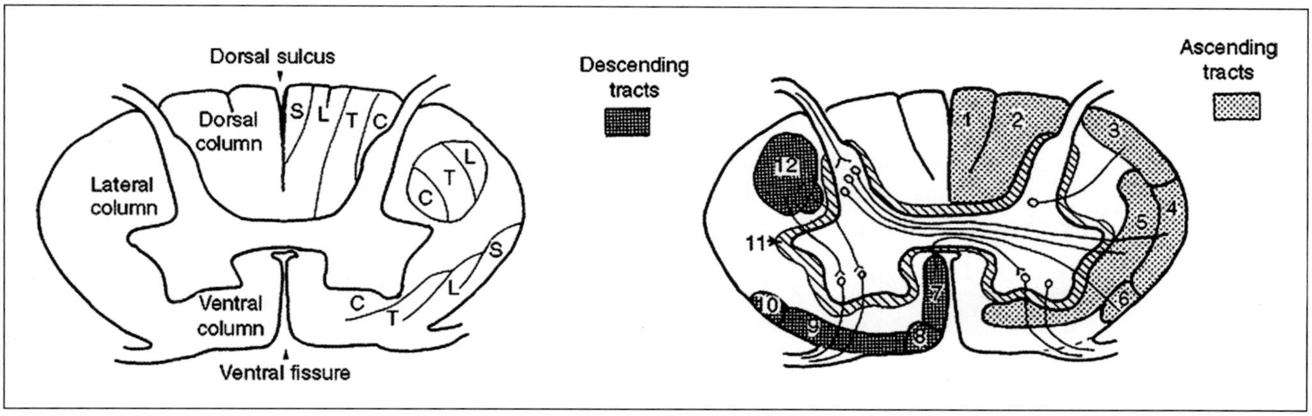

Figure 7 Drawings of the cross-sectional anatomy of the cervical spinal cord. C = cervical, L = lumbar, S = sacral, T = thoracic, 1 = fasciculus gracilis, 2 = fasciculus cuneatus, 3 = dorsal spinocerebellar tract, 4 = ventral spinocerebellar tract, 5 = lateral spinothalamic tract, 6 = spino-olivary tract, 7 = ventral corticospinal tract, 8 = tectospinal tract, 9 = vestibulospinal tract, 10 = olivospinal tract, 11 = propriospinal tract, 12 = lateral corticospinal tract. (Reproduced with permission from Louis-Ugbo J Pedlow FX Jr Heller JG: Anatomy of the cervical spine, in Benzel EC, ed: *The Cervical Spine*, ed 5. Philadelphia, PA, WK Health, 2012, pp 1-33. © Cervical Spine Research Society.)

The cervical spine derives its circulation primarily from the vertebral arteries.[2] The vertebral arteries arise from the subclavian arteries on either side, coursing superiorly. They typically enter the transverse foramen at the C6 level and run proximally thorough the transverse foramina to C1, then course posteriorly over the superior aspect of the C1 ring before turning proximally again and entering the foramen magnum, where they merge to form the basilar artery. Segmental branches to each cervical vertebra arise from the vertebral artery and the deep cervical branch of the costocervical trunk. There is a great deal of variability in the anatomy of the vertebral artery. Typically one side is more dominant, having a larger diameter than the other. Occasionally, the vertebral artery enters through the transverse foramen of C7 rather than C6. In addition, it is not uncommon to see anomalous courses of the artery where, for example, the vessel loops through a cervical vertebral body before returning to its longitudinal course through the transverse foramen. Because of these inconsistencies, care must be taken when planning cervical procedures such as corpectomy or instrumentation to evaluate the course of the vertebral artery.

The vascular supply of the spinal cord is primarily from the medullary branches of the segmental spinal arteries.[2] These merge to feed the anterior spinal artery, which is responsible for supplying approximately 80% of the vascular supply to the spinal cord. Typically, three anterior medullary arteries supply the cervical region, one or two supply the thoracic region, and one supplies the lumbosacral spinal cord, which creates several watershed areas within the spinal cord at the distal ends of these vascular trees. This latter artery is known as the arteria medullaris magna (AMM), arteria radicularis magna, or the artery of Adamkiewicz. The AMM is the largest anterior segmental artery and typically arises on the left side anywhere between the T8 and L1 level, although right-sided origins are not uncommon.[2] As with the vertebral artery, careful evaluation of the AMM is necessary for any planned anterior procedures at the thoracolumbar junction, as ligation or injury to this artery could have disastrous consequences.

Biomechanics

Alignment

The alignment of the spine varies by region (**Figure 3**). Normal cervical alignment is approximately 15° of lordosis. The thoracic spine generally ranges from 20° to 40° of kyphosis, and the lumbar spine has approximately 40° to 50° of lordosis. The sacrum is again kyphotic. These values are general estimates, and a wide degree of variability exists. The curvatures of the spine function to keep the head balanced over the pelvis and to transmit axial forces through the spine to the pelvis.[4] Kyphotic segments (thoracic, sacral) are considered "primary" curvatures as they are already present in utero and at birth; the lordotic curvatures of the cervical and lumbar spine develop secondarily later in life to allow the growing child to develop an upright posture.[3,5] The center of gravity of the spinal column runs from the odontoid process proximally through the sacral promontory caudally.[3] Changes in sagittal balance (whether degenerative, traumatic, developmental, or iatrogenic), particularly those that shift the center of gravity too far ventrally can result in significant pain and disability.

Functional Spinal Unit

The basic motion segment of the spine consists of the "functional spinal unit." This is comprised of two vertebrae, the disk between them, and the facet joints (and their capsules).[2,4] It is also helpful to consider this segment in the context of the adjacent ligamentous and neural structures. The functional spinal unit serves to limit motion of the spine within the confines of protecting the neural structures contained therein. The degree to which the spinal motion segment accomplishes this varies depending on the level or region of the spine, the direction of motion, the vector of force applied to the spine, and the duration of exposure to such forces.

Load Bearing

Vertebral bodies are loaded in series; the more caudal levels must support more weight than more cranial segments. The vertebral bodies bear 70% to 90% of the static axial load of the spine. The facet joints support 10% to 20% of axial load in a standing, neutral alignment.[5] Changes in posture, however, alter the loads on the facets. In extension, they may bare up to 30% of the axial load, whereas in flexion, they may be burdened with up to 50% of the anterior shear load.[5] The intervertebral disk helps absorb axial loads. As compressive forces are applied to the disk, the nucleus pulposus deforms, redistributing axial forces radially. This radial pressure is then resisted by the tensile properties of the alternating bands of fibers within the anulus fibrosus (**Figure 4**).[2,4,5] The spinous processes and transverse processes act as lever arms, providing mechanical advantage for the muscles that insert along their surfaces.

Summary

The unique bony, ligamentous, neural, and vascular anatomy of the spine contribute to and facilitate its multiple biologic and biomechanical functions. The spine provides axial support for the head and upper body yet allows significant flexibility and range of motion, all while protecting the neural structures as they run from the skull to the sacrum. A thorough understanding of the anatomy, and in particular the anatomic relationships of different structures, is required to appreciate both the biomechanical function of the spine and the various pathologic conditions that affect it.

Key Study Points

- The peripheral nervous system derives from the neural crest, the spinal cord develops from the neural tube, and the spinal column (vertebrae and intervertebral disks) develop from the notochord.
- Ligamentous stability at the craniocervical junction and upper cervical spine is conferred by the transverse atlantal ligament (running horizontally behind the dens), the apical ligament (running vertically from the tip of the dens to the basion), and the paired alar ligaments (running obliquely from the lateral aspect of the dens to the occipital condyles).
- The nucleus pulposus is hydrophilic, is composed of type II collagen, and functions to maintain disk space height and resist compressive loads; the anulus fibrosus is composed of lamina of obliquely oriented type I collagen fibrils and functions to resist tensile loads.
- Within the spinal cord, nerve fibers destined for the upper extremities are located deeper, and those related to the torso and lower extremities are located sequentially more superficially.
- The artery of Adamkiewicz or arteria medullaris magna (AMM) is a large segmental artery usually found on the left side of the spine at a variable level between T8 and L1 and is the primary blood supply to the lumbosacral spinal cord. Injury to it can result in spinal cord infarction.

Annotated References

1. Cain CMJ: Anatomy, in Patel VV, Patel A, Harrop JS, Burger E, eds: *Spine Surgery Basics*. Heidelberg, Springer, 2014, pp 3-12.
2. Parke WW, Bono CM, Garfin SR: Applied anatomy of the spine, in Herkowitz HN, Grafin SR, Eismont FJ, Bell GR, Balderston RA, eds: *Rothman-Simeone: The Spine*, ed 6. Philadelphia, Elsevier Saunders, 2011, pp 15-53.
3. Wardak Z, Lavelle ED, Kistler BJ, Lavelle WF: Functional anatomy of the spine, in Benzel EC, ed: *Spine Surgery Techniques, Complication Avoidance, and Management*, ed 3. Philadelphia, Elsevier Saunders, 2012, pp 55-62.
4. Marras WS: Biomechanics of the spinal motion segment, in Herkowitz HN, Grafin SR, Eismont FJ, Bell GR, Balderston RA, eds: *Rothman-Simeone: The Spine*, ed 6. Philadelphia, Elsevier Saunders, 2011, pp 109-128.
5. Steffen T: General biomechanics of the spinal motion segment and the spinal organ, in Aebi M, Arlet V, Webb JK, eds: *AOSpine Manual: Principles and Techniques*. Stuttgart, Thieme, 2007, vol 1, pp 33-51.
6. Hoppenfeld S, deBoer P: The spine, in Hoppenfeld S, deBoer P, eds: *Surgical Exposures in Orthopaedics: The Anatomic Approach*, ed 3. Philadelphia, Lippincott Williams & Wilkins, 2003, pp 247-342.

Chapter 47

Spine Evaluation, Clinical Examination, and Imaging

Brandon J. Rebholz, MD

ABSTRACT

The breadth of spinal pathology and conditions requires that practitioners be confident in obtaining a complete history and performing a comprehensive physical examination in different clinical settings. This is further supplemented by the use of safe and appropriate imaging to establish the diagnosis and augment intraoperative accuracy. Through the proper understanding and use of these techniques, providers can continue to improve on delivering safe, high-value care to patients with spinal conditions.

Keywords: spine differential diagnosis; spine imaging; spine physical examination

Introduction

Successful care of patients with neurologic and musculoskeletal problems begins with arriving at the proper diagnosis. The importance of developing an accurate and efficient process to arrive at these diagnoses cannot be overstated. It is through a thorough history, complete physical examination, and appropriate imaging modalities that the correct diagnoses can be made, and best practice treatment recommendations can be offered, optimizing safe, value-driven care.

Physical Examination

The comprehensive history and physical examination are the initial interactions set on delivering the correct diagnosis and subsequent treatment recommendations to patients. Symptoms can often be similar for spinal and appendicular musculoskeletal etiologies: cervical spine symptoms can often mimic shoulder problems, brachial plexopathies, and peripheral compressive neuropathies; lumbar spine symptoms are often very similar to those originating from the hip, sacroiliac joint, or even vascular insufficiencies; patients with myelopathy may present with vague symptoms that could be mistaken for other systemic or neurologic disorders. By having a thorough understanding of the entirety of the neurologic and musculoskeletal system, providers can guide patients through the most appropriate treatments, while limiting unnecessary workups or procedures.

The evaluation begins with elucidating an accurate history. The presenting symptoms should be described by the patient and additional history developed with the provider. This history should ultimately include the symptom location with or without associated radiation, severity, onset, duration, quality and character, aggravating or alleviating factors, and previous related treatments. Additional attention should be given to the patient's other medical diagnoses. Caution should be taken attributing symptoms to these underlying medical diagnoses as symptoms can often be multifactorial. In the acutely injured patient, specific attention should be given to the mechanism of injury and associated injuries. By completing a comprehensive history, the provider can often develop an appropriate differential diagnosis, which can be further narrowed by the examination.

The initial examination of the spine patient should include a complete neurologic and musculoskeletal examination. Attention is given to the specific myotomal and dermatomal distributions to determine potential level of pathology. Strength testing is graded on a scale of 0 to 5. In the upper extremities strength is described as it pertains to shoulder abduction (C5); elbow flexion and wrist extension (C6); elbow extension, wrist flexion, and digit extension (C7); digit flexion (C8); and the digit abduction (T1). Similarly, in the lower extremities strength is tested in hip flexion (L2), knee extension (L3), ankle dorsiflexion (L4), great toe extension (L5), and ankle plantar flexion (S1). The sensory examination is tested and described in dermatomal distributions for sensation to light touch or pressure, pin prick, and temperature. Utilization of the examination in conjunction with a knowledge of the somatotrophic organization of

Dr. Rebholz or an immediate family member serves as a paid consultant to or is an employee of Biomet and serves as an unpaid consultant to Ulrich Spine.

the spinal cord can help distinguish different incomplete spinal cord injury patterns in the acute or traumatic setting.

Sacral sparing is a defined as preservation of sensory or motor function of the most caudal aspect of the spinal cord. This includes sensation to light touch, pin prick, or deep anal pressure in the S4 and S5 nerve root distributions and voluntary contraction of the external anal sphincter as assessed by digital rectal examination. Complete spinal cord injury is defined as no sensory and/or motor function at the sacral segments, whereas incomplete spinal cord injury maintains some sacral sensory and/or motor function.[1] These components of sacral sparing can have some prognostic significance in that more components of sacral sparing present within the first 30 days, the greater the likelihood of improvement in American Spinal Injury Association (ASIA) Impairment Scale (AIS) at 1-year follow-up.[2] This improvement in AIS does not necessarily equate to meaningful functional improvement, so caution should be used when communicating potential prognostic information to patients and families.

Reflex examination is routinely performed in the upper and lower extremities. Deep tendon reflexes are tested about the biceps (C5/C6), triceps (C7), brachioradialis (C6), patellar (L4), and Achilles (L5/S1) tendons. Hyperreflexia is potentially consistent with upper motor neuron dysfunction, whereas hyporeflexia is consistent with lower motor neuron dysfunction. Additional reflex testing is elicited through the testing of the Hoffman sign, Trömner sign, abdominal reflexes, Babinski reflex, and bulbocavernosus reflex. These additional tests are used for specific purposes and may or may not be included depending on the clinical scenario.

Hoffman's sign is performed by flexion and release of the distal interphalangeal joint of the middle finger while observing the interphalangeal joints of the ipsilateral index finger and thumb. Reflexive flexion of the interphalangeal joint of both the thumb and index fingers indicates a possible central compressive pathology in the cervical spine. A recent systematic review was performed to determine the utility of the Hoffman's test as a screening tool for cervical spondylotic myelopathy. The presence of the Hoffman sign has a positive predictive value of 68% (LR of 2.6 with 95% CI 1.8 to 3.9) and negative predictive value of 70% (LR of 0.51 with 95% CI 0.3 to 0.6) as compared with the benchmark of MRI with associated spinal cord compression and loss of surrounding CSF with or without cord signal change.[3] There is a known incidence of positive Hoffman's sign in the asymptomatic population of approximately 0.3% to 2%.[4] As such, the authors conclude that a positive Hoffman's sign is useful only in the context of the complete history and physical examination. The presence of hyperreflexia, Hoffman and/or Trömner sign, upgoing toes for Babinski testing, and sustained ankle clonus can be used together to inform the possible diagnoses of myelopathy.[5,6]

The bulbocavernosus reflex is most commonly used in the acute posttraumatic setting. This reflex is elicited during the digital rectal examination by either gently pulling on an inserted Foley catheter or squeezing the glans penis. Subsequent involuntary contraction of the external anal sphincter is consistent with an intact reflex. In the setting of an acute spinal cord injury, this indicates the termination of spinal shock, at which time determination of spinal cord injury severity can be made according to the ASIA standards. The bulbocavernosus reflex can also distinguish between conus medullaris syndrome or lower thoracic cord compression/injury and cauda equina syndrome. Absence of the bulbocavernosus reflex outside the setting of spinal shock would be consistent with lower motor neuron dysfunction interrupting this reflex arc.

Inspection of the back allows for assessment of the skin and soft tissues. In the setting of acute trauma, significant ecchymosis would be indicative of a possible underlying fracture. If a spinal cord injury or spinal fracture is suspected, this examination should be performed only initially in conjunction with the rectal examination as described previously. Palpation for asymmetry and midline tenderness may be indicative of underlying fractures. In the routine clinical setting, percussion of the spine can distinguish between acute and chronic compression fractures.

Spinal deformity can best be assessed in the standing position. The pelvis and shoulders are examined for symmetry. Adam's forward bend test allows for evaluation of the rotatory component of scoliosis, and location of any notable prominence should be noted. If the patient has positive sagittal balance, then the forward gaze may be impacted. Additionally, lumbar lordosis may be compromised, and hip flexion contractures may develop as compensatory mechanisms in an attempt to maintain as upright a walking posture as possible.

Observation of gait is an important component of both the neurologic and musculoskeletal examinations. Initiating from a seated position will allow the practitioner to observe if there is a component of "start-up" pain consistent with potential hip pathology. If the patient demonstrates an antalgic gait, then this could be indicative of hip arthritis or a compressive radiculopathy. A Trendelenburg gait could be related to an L5 nerve root compression with subsequent hip abductor weakness. In this case the patient's pelvis will drop on the unaffected side as the patient leans her torso toward the affected side.

Distinguishing between spinal pathology, hip pathology, and sacroiliac joint (SIJ) dysfunction can be difficult as symptoms often have overlapping patterns. Radicular pain often begins in the buttocks, then radiates to the thigh and potentially to the leg and foot, typically in dermatomal patterns. Intra-articular hip pathology typically results in a referred pain pattern to the buttock, groin, thigh, knee, and low back. Sacroiliac joint pain similarly presents with pain in the low back, buttock, and thigh.

The diagnostic utility of individual physical examination tests in confirming lumbar radiculopathy has been shown to be somewhat equivocal.[7,8] As such, a combination of the aforementioned neurologic tests along with neural tension tests including the straight leg raise and femoral stretch tests can improve the sensitivity and specificity for radiculopathy. These should be performed in the supine and prone positions, respectively.

Testing of the hip joint is typically done in the supine position, with the examiner passively flexing the hip joint past 90° and providing an internal rotation force through the hip joint. Gentle circumduction can also be performed. Pain provocation in the groin, buttock, thigh, and potentially the knee would be consistent with intraarticular hip pathology. Hip range of motion is concomitantly assessed. This is also the best position to assess for hip flexion contractures as these can easily be overlooked in the seated position.

Sacroiliac joint dysfunction can present a significant diagnostic challenge. Specific testing of the SIJ is typically performed with six provocative maneuvers: hip flexion, abduction, and external rotation (FABER or Patrick test) (**Figure 1**, A), pelvic compression, pelvic distraction, thigh thrust, sacral thrust, and Gaenslen test (**Figure 1**, B). As with other physical examination tests, the utility of individual tests is limited; however, the sensitivity and specificity of these tests are improved when three or more provocative maneuvers reproduce symptoms.[9] Confirmation of the SIJ as the source of pain can be made by an intra-articular injection of local anesthetic with or without steroids. Based on pooled data from multiple studies, even with three provocative examination maneuvers being positive, the likelihood of at least 75% temporary improvement following an injection is not statistically significant compared with those who respond to the injection based on the location of the pain alone.[10]

There is additionally significant crossover in the presentation of cervical symptoms and upper extremity symptoms. Shoulder pain can overlap with C4, C5, and C6 radiculopathies, depending on the pattern. An examination of the shoulder should include provocative tests and strength testing, particularly of the rotator cuff musculature. Rotator cuff tears have been shown to be accurately diagnosed through a combination of physical examination tests. The Jobe or "empty can" test, performed with the arm resisted while abducted to 90° and internally rotated; the lift-off test, performed with the dorsum of the wrist and arm placed upon the lumbar region above the waist as the patient lifts the forearm posteriorly away from the back; and comparison of the external rotation strength of the affected to the unaffected side together allow for determination of the likelihood of a rotator cuff tear being present.[11] Additional tests should be performed for labral pathology, adhesive capsulitis, impingement, and biceps tendinopathy.

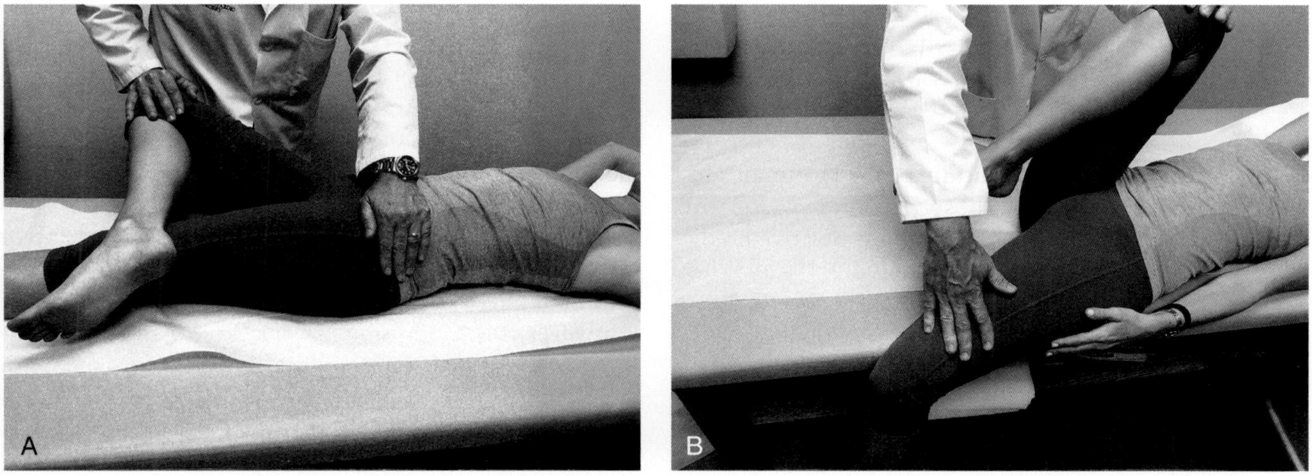

Figure 1 Examination maneuvers for the diagnosis of sacroiliac joint dysfunction. **A**, FABER or Patrick's test; **B**, Gaenslen test.

Peripheral compressive neuropathies can originate most commonly from the brachial plexus, cubital tunnel, carpal tunnel or Guyon's canal. Underlying systemic polyneuropathy may also be present. Reproduction of symptoms related to peripheral compression can be produced through various techniques, such as hyperflexion of the elbow, Phalen's test, and Tinel's test about the carpal or cubital tunnels. These physical examination techniques can then be combined with electrodiagnostic studies for conformation. When there is a suspected cervical radiculopathy and a concomitant peripheral neuropathy, there is recommendation for use of needle EMG in the diagnosis of cervical radiculopathy and nerve conduction studies in the assessment of entrapment neuropathies.[12]

Specific physical examination tests for cervical radiculopathy in the absence of sensory or motor neurologic deficits are limited. A recent systematic review evaluated various physical tests in relation to their ability to diagnose cervical radiculopathy. Spurling maneuver has a highly variable sensitivity of approximately 38% to 99%, but specificity of 85% to 100%.[13] Sensitivities are generally improved with the addition of advanced imaging consistent with radiculopathy.[14] Both the shoulder abduction relief test (escape sign) and the traction test for arm relief additionally have acceptably high sensitivities at approximately 85% and greater than 95%, respectively, and may help confirm the diagnosis. The more recently described arm squeeze test has the potential to be very useful in the ability of the examiner to distinguish between shoulder and cervical etiologies. This test is performed by the examiner applying a gentle squeezing force to the middle one-third of the arm with the thumb on the midtriceps and the remaining fingers on the midbiceps. An increase in arm pain of 3 points on a 0 to 10 pain scale with this maneuver indicates a positive test. The diagnostic sensitivity and specificity of this test for cervical radiculopathy relative to shoulder pathology are 96% (Positive LR: 10.5 to 48) and 91% to 100% (Negative LR: 0.04 to 0.44), respectively.[15]

Imaging

Optimal spinal imaging is important for the development of an accurate diagnosis and directing appropriate treatment recommendations. If imaging studies are chosen properly, the results should confirm or rule out a specific diagnostic question as much as possible. Ultimately, the working diagnosis is the synthesis of the history, physical examination, and diagnostic studies. The American College of Radiology has compounded Appropriateness Criteria (AC), evidence-based recommendations for imaging studies in specific circumstances. In addition, there is as increased focus on patient and provider safety and minimization of radiation exposure from diagnostic imaging. All of these factors should be considered when determining which imaging modalities are best used.

In the acute traumatic setting, guidelines have been developed following the National Emergency X-Radiography Utilization Study (NEXUS) and Canadian C-spine Rule study groups. In patients who meet NEXUS and CCR criteria, a CT scan of the cervical spine with sagittal and coronal reformatting is the initial imaging modality of choice, replacing conventional radiographs. The current resolution of CT scans in patients with suspected cervical spinal injury allows for a negative predictive value of 99.2% in patients with normal studies and a negative predictive value of 99.8% for cervical spine injuries requiring immobilization even in intoxicated patients.[16] Magnetic resonance scans of the cervical spine should be obtained when safe and feasible in patients with acute neurologic deficits, suspected myelopathy, or suspected ligamentous injury as it can provide complementary information to that provided by the CT scan alone. Patients who sustain blunt trauma to the head and/or neck with basilar skull fractures, occipitocervical dissociation, presence of ankylosing spondylitis/diffuse idiopathic spondylosis, or fractures extending into the foramen transversarium foramen with displacement >1 mm should additionally be considered for CT or MR angiography to assess for vertebral artery injury.[17]

In patients with acute blunt injuries suspected to the thoracic and/or lumbar spines, sagittal and coronal reconstructions can be created from the CT scans of the chest, abdomen, and pelvis. Indications for obtaining MRI imaging of the thoracic or lumbar spines are similar to those in the cervical spine mentioned previously.

In the ambulatory clinic setting, standard AP and lateral plain radiographs of the specific area of spine (cervical, thoracic, or lumbar) can easily be obtained and should be performed the upright position when possible. The addition of dynamic, lateral flexion and extension views are unlikely to change clinical decision making in the initial assessment of degenerative conditions and may no longer be considered routine.[18,19] However, these additional views can be useful in certain clinical situations and should be obtained with specific diagnostic goals in mind. Late instability of spinal fractures or ligamentous injuries treated nonoperatively may be assessed for translation with dynamic, flexion-extension radiographs.[20] Another useful clinical scenario is in assessment of patients who previously underwent anterior cervical diskectomy and fusion. The accuracy of a pseudarthrosis diagnosis following this procedure by lateral and dynamic flexion radiographs can approach that of CT scans by using measurements of interspinous motion measured at the fusion level (>1 mm) and the level superjacent to the fusion (>4 mm) with 150% imaging magnification.[21]

Imaging to assess spinal deformity should include standing PA and lateral scoliosis radiographs incorporating the entirety of the spine from the hip joints to the base of the skull to allow for measurements of appropriate radiographic spinal parameters. Alternatives to the convention radiographs have been developed to minimize radiation dose in patients with scoliosis. A biplanar, slot scanning imaging system has been commercially available for a number of years as an alternative to conventional radiographs. As these techniques have been further refined, microdose protocols have been developed for use with this system that can potentially limit ionizing radiation doses greater than 90% compared with conventional radiographs in adolescents.[22] The effect of cumulative lifetime ionizing radiation exposure and subsequent potential cancer risk for patients with routine surveillance of scoliosis is significantly higher for females compared with males and higher for patients with above average body size compared with normal body size with the same follow-up schedule. This holds true for standard radiographs, low-dose biplanar slot scanning, and microdose slot scanning techniques.[23-25]

Routine imaging for nonspecific back pain without red flag signs does not alter clinical decision making and is not recommended.[26] However, there is persistent pressure upon providers to obtain early imaging, particularly with the increased emphasis on patient satisfaction. Greater than 85% of patients with back pain report that they would choose to have radiographs if they were offered. Additionally, patients who underwent early imaging reported being significantly more satisfied than those who did not.[27] When assessing the value of early MRI compared with delayed selective MRI, there is higher value associated with delayed selective imaging; however, when patient factors are considered, early imaging remains more costly, but also more effective with an incremental cost per QALY of approximately $1500 (US 2017).[28] This highlights the importance of patient education in regard to appropriate imaging.

Specific clinical scenarios warrant specialized imaging. In adolescent patients with low back pain along with consistent history and physical examination findings, spondylolysis may be suspected. Plain radiographs do not improve the accuracy of this diagnosis significantly over a complete history and physical examination. CT scan is considered the most specific modality to assess for pars defects and potential bony healing; however, this exposes the patient to higher doses of radiation. SPECT has also fallen out of favor given the need for administration of a radioactive isotope and high radiation exposure. MRI has specific appeal as the preferred imaging modality in that it is readily available, can identify bony edema/stress reactions, fracture healing, and does not expose the patient to ionizing radiation.[29,30]

In patients with suspected compressive radiculopathy, myelopathy, neurologic deficits, infection, tumor, or occult fracture, MRI remains the modality of choice.[31] The use of MRI following gadolinium-based contrast agents (GBCAs) has been typically reserved for patients with suspected infection, known or suspected spinal tumors, and in postoperative patients to distinguish scar tissue from recurrent disk herniations. GBCAs are renally eliminated but known to accumulate in the brain and can have potential effects on the kidneys. Although there is no current recommendation to restrict use, providers should consider this when ordering these tests and additional information in the form of an FDA Medication Guide must be provided to the patient before administration.[32]

There has been recent promise for advanced MRI techniques that are attempting to provide additional diagnostic and functional information to imaging of the spinal cord. These include diffusion tensor imaging (DTI), magnetization transfer (MT), MR spectroscopy (MRS), and functional MRI (fMRI). Although these techniques may hold promise of improved diagnosis and prognosis in the future, particularly in the fields of myelopathy and spinal cord injury, the current evidence is lacking for routine clinical use.[33]

Innovations in intraoperative imaging have further advanced the practice of spine surgery, allowing for improved instrumentation accuracy and progression of minimally invasive techniques. Although fluoroscopy has been routinely used for years, there have been concerns about exposure to ionizing radiation, for both patients and operating room staff. Minimally invasive procedures can increase this exposure when compared with standard open techniques.[34] There are many intraoperative factors that can result in high variability in exposures including surgeon comfort and skill level, patient body habitus, location of beam source, and use of protective equipment. Intraoperative cone CT has been used in conjunction with navigated instrumentation to reduce occupational exposure to operating room staff but may expose patients to higher doses of ionizing radiation.[35] It is important to have a thorough understanding of the many variables as it relates to use of intraoperative imaging, so providers can limit doses of ionizing radiation to operating room personnel and patients while ensuring accuracy of instrumentation.

Summary

Through the use of a careful history and physical examination along with thoughtful and appropriate imaging techniques, providers can be well-equipped to provide safe, high-value care to their patients with spinal pathology.

Key Study Points

- The physical examination of spine patients can be appropriately tailored to the clinical scenario to achieve optimal diagnostic goals.
- Correlation of the neurologic examination with knowledge of spinal anatomy and spinal cord somatotrophic organization allows providers to make informed decisions on likely diagnosis, aid in obtaining appropriate diagnostic studies, and ultimately provide best evidence treatment recommendations.
- Considerations for diagnostic and intraoperative imaging modalities should be made based on appropriate use recommendations, imaging accuracy for different clinical scenarios, and potentially radiation safety to provide highest value spine care.

Annotated References

1. Waters RL, Adkins RH, Yakura JS: Definition of complete spinal cord injury. *Spinal Cord* 1991;29(9):573-581. doi:10.1038/sc.1991.85.
2. Kirshblum SC, Botticello AL, Dyson-Hudson TA, Byrne R, Marino RJ, Lammertse DP: Patterns of sacral sparing components on neurologic recovery in newly injured persons with traumatic spinal cord injury. *Arch Phys Med Rehabil* 2016;97(10):1647-1655. doi:10.1016/j.apmr.2016.02.012.

   Retrospective review of 1738 patients with spinal cord injury. The greater the number of components of sacral sparing at initial evaluation, the greater the potential for recovery and the greater the number of sacral components recovered, the greater the motor recovery at 1 year. Level of evidence: IV.
3. Fogarty A, Lenza E, Gupta G, Jarzem P, Dasgupta K, Radhakrishna M: A systematic review of the utility of the Hoffmann sign for the diagnosis of degenerative cervical myelopathy. *Spine* 2018;43(23):1664-1669. doi:10.1097/BRS.0000000000002697.

   Systematic review of Hoffman for DCM. Hoffman alone is unlikely to provide additional accuracy of diagnosis of myelopathy compared with MRI. Data are insufficient supporting Hoffman sign's independent ability to confirm or refute the diagnosis. Level of evidence: III.
4. Malanga GA, Landes P, Nadler SF: Provocative tests in cervical spine examination: Historical basis and scientific analyses. *Pain Physician* 2003;6(2):8.
5. Tejus MN, Singh V, Ramesh A, Kumar VRR, Maurya VP, Madhugiri VS: An evaluation of the finger flexion, Hoffman's and plantar reflexes as markers of cervical spinal cord compression – a comparative clinical study. *Clin Neurol Neurosurg* 2015;134:12-16. doi:10.1016/j.clineuro.2015.04.009.
6. Chikuda H, Seichi A, Takeshita K, et al: Correlation between pyramidal signs and the severity of cervical myelopathy. *Eur Spine J* 2010;19(10):1684-1689. doi:10.1007/s00586-010-1364-3.
7. van der Windt DA, Simons E, Riphagen II, et al: Physical examination for lumbar radiculopathy due to disc herniation in patients with low-back pain. Cochrane Back and Neck Group, ed. *Cochrane Database Syst Rev* 2010;(2):CD007431. doi:10.1002/14651858.CD007431.pub2.
8. Tawa N, Rhoda A, Diener I: Accuracy of clinical neurological examination in diagnosing lumbo-sacral radiculopathy: A systematic literature review. *BMC Musculoskelet Disord* 2017;18(1). doi:10.1186/s12891-016-1383-2.

   Systematic review of accuracy of sensory, motor, reflex, and neurodynamic exam tests in the ability to diagnose lumbar radiculopathy compared with MRI, CT, intraoperative findings, and neurodiagnostic studies. Combination of exam tests are best.
9. Laslett M, Aprill CN, McDonald B, Young SB: Diagnosis of sacroiliac joint pain: Validity of individual provocation tests and composites of tests. *Man Ther* 2005;10(3):207-218. doi:10.1016/j.math.2005.01.003.
10. Kennedy DJ, Engel A, Kreiner DS, Nampiaparampil D, Duszynski B, MacVicar J: Fluoroscopically guided diagnostic and therapeutic intra-articular sacroiliac joint injections: A systematic review. *Pain Med* 2015;16(8):1500-1518. doi:10.1111/pme.12833.
11. Jain NB, Fan R, Higgins LD, Kuhn JE, Ayers GD: Does my patient with shoulder pain have a rotator cuff tear? A predictive model from the ROW Cohort. *Orthop J Sports Med* 2018;6(7):232596711878489. doi:10.1177/2325967118784897.

    Cohort study of 301 patients with shoulder pain. Predictors of male sex, external rotation strength ratio, positive liftoff test, and positive Jobe test used to develop a nanogram for the diagnosis of rotator cuff tears. Level of evidence: II.

12. American Association of Electrodiagnostic Medicine: Practice parameter for needle electromyogrphic evaluation of patients with suspected cervical radiculopathy: Summary statement. *Muscle Nerve* 1999;22(suppl 8):S209-S211. *Muscle Nerve*. 1999;22(suppl 8):S209-S211.

13. Thoomes EJ, van Geest S, van der Windt DA, et al: Value of physical tests in diagnosing cervical radiculopathy: A systematic review. *Spine J* 2018;18(1):179-189. doi:10.1016/j.spinee.2017.08.241.

    Systematic review of studies for the diagnostic accuracy of diagnostic tests for cervical radiculopathy. Combination of Spurling's, axial traction, and arm squeeze tests increases likelihood of cervical radiculopathy, and combination of negative tests can rule out.

14. Rubinstein SM, Pool JJM, van Tulder MW, Riphagen II: A systematic review of the diagnostic accuracy of provocative tests of the neck for diagnosing cervical radiculopathy. *Eur Spine J* 2007:13.

15. Gumina S, Carbone S, Albino P, Gurzi M, Postacchini F: Arm squeeze test: A new clinical test to distinguish neck from shoulder pain. *Eur Spine J* 2013;22(7):1558-1563. doi:10.1007/s00586-013-2788-3.

16. Bush L, Brookshire R, Roche B, et al: Evaluation of cervical spine clearance by computed tomographic scan alone in intoxicated patients with blunt trauma. *JAMA Surg* 2016;151(9):807. doi:10.1001/jamasurg.2016.1248.

    Prospective observational study of 1668 patients with blunt trauma. CT scans of cervical spine had overall negative predictive value of 99.2% for patients with cervical spine injuries and negative predictive value of 99.8% for ruling out injuries requiring immobilization.

17. Lebl DR, Bono CM, Velmahos G, Metkar U, Nguyen J, Harris MB: Vertebral artery injury associated with blunt cervical spine trauma: A multivariate regression analysis. *Spine* 2013;38(16):1352-1361. doi:10.1097/BRS.0b013e318294bacb.

18. White AP, Biswas D, Smart LR, Haims A, Grauer JN: Utility of flexion-extension radiographs in evaluating the degenerative cervical spine: *Spine* 2007;32(9):975-979. doi:10.1097/01.brs.0000261409.45251.a2.

19. Hammouri QM, Haims AH, Simpson AK, Alqaqa A, Grauer JN: The utility of dynamic flexion-extension radiographs in the initial evaluation of the degenerative lumbar spine. *Spine* 2007;32(21):2361-2364. doi:10.1097/BRS.0b013e318155796e.

20. Aarabi B, Mirvis S, Shanmuganathan K, et al: Comparative effectiveness of surgical versus nonoperative management of unilateral, nondisplaced, subaxial cervical spine facet fractures without evidence of spinal cord injury: Clinical article. *J Neurosurg Spine* 2014;20(3):270-277. doi:10.3171/2013.11.SPINE13733.

21. Song K-S, Piyaskulkaew C, Chuntarapas T, et al: Dynamic radiographic criteria for detecting pseudarthrosis following anterior cervical arthrodesis: *J Bone Joint Surg Am Vol* 2014;96(7):557-563. doi:10.2106/JBJS.M.00167.

22. Pedersen PH, Petersen AG, Østgaard SE, Tvedebrink T, Eiskjær SP: EOS® micro-dose protocol: First full-spine radiation dose measurements in anthropomorphic phantoms and comparisons with EOS standard-dose and conventional digital radiology (CR). *Spine*. April 2018. doi:10.1097/BRS.0000000000002696.

    A comparative study of conventional diagnostic radiology (CR), standard dose EOS, and microdose EOS in anthropomorphic phantoms. Substantial reductions in ionizing radiation measured in microdose compared with standard dose and in both compared with CR.

23. Law M, Ma W-K, Lau D, Chan E, Yip L, Lam W: Cumulative radiation exposure and associated cancer risk estimates for scoliosis patients: Impact of repetitive full spine radiography. *Eur J Radiol* 2016;85(3):625-628. doi:10.1016/j.ejrad.2015.12.032.

    Computer model of cumulative radiation risk in scoliosis patients found that maximal dose radiation from standard radiographic follow-up from age 5 years to 30 years is equivalent to 7 years of background radiation. Lifetime attributable cancer risk is two times greater in females.

24. Law M, Ma W-K, Chan E, et al: Evaluation of cumulative effective dose and cancer risk from repetitive full spine imaging using EOS system: Impact to adolescent patients of different populations. *Eur J Radiol* 2017;96:1-5. doi:10.1016/j.ejrad.2017.09.006.

    Computer model of cumulative radiation risk in scoliosis patients followed with semi-annual EOS imaging from age 10 years to 18 years is equivalent to less than 1 year of background radiation. Lifetime attributable cancer risk is greater in females.

25. Law M, Ma W-K, Lau D, et al: Cumulative effective dose and cancer risk for pediatric population in repetitive full spine follow-up imaging: How micro dose is the EOS microdose protocol? *Eur J Radiol* 2018;101:87-91. doi:10.1016/j.ejrad.2018.02.015.

    Computer model of cumulative radiation risk in scoliosis patients followed with semi-annual EOS imaging using microdose protocol from age 5 years to 18 years is equivalent to approximately 14% of 1 year of background radiation.

26. Chou R, Fu R, Carrino JA, Deyo RA: Imaging strategies for low-back pain: Systematic review and meta-analysis 2009;373:10.

27. Kendrick D: Radiography of the lumbar spine in primary care patients with low back pain: Randomised controlled trial. *BMJ* 2001;322(7283):400-405. doi:10.1136/bmj.322.7283.400.

28. Gilbert F, Grant A, Gillan M, Vale M, Scott N: Does early magnetic resonance imaging influence management or improve outcome in patients referred to secondary care with low back pain? A pragmatic randomised controlled trial. *Health Technol Assess* 2004;8(17):1-131.

29. Ledonio CGT, Burton DC, Crawford CH, et al: Current evidence regarding diagnostic imaging methods for pediatric lumbar spondylolysis: A report from the Scoliosis Research Society Evidence-Based Medicine Committee. *Spine Deform* 2017;5(2):97-101. doi:10.1016/j.jspd.2016.10.006.

Literature review and consensus statement in regard to imaging of pediatric lumbar spondylolysis. CT scan remains benchmark for diagnosis; however, MRI may replace CT as definitive study given accuracy and that is does not expose patients to radiation.

30. Kobayashi A, Kobayashi T, Kato K, Higuchi H, Takagishi K: Diagnosis of radiographically occult lumbar spondylolysis in young athletes by magnetic resonance imaging. *Am J Sports Med* 2013;41(1):169-176. doi:10.1177/0363546512464946.

31. Wang B, Fintelmann FJ, Kamath RS, Kattapuram SV, Rosenthal DI: Limited magnetic resonance imaging of the lumbar spine has high sensitivity for detection of acute fractures, infection, and malignancy. *Skeletal Radiol* 2016;45(12):1687-1693. doi:10.1007/s00256-016-2493-5.

Case-control study of limited sequence MRI for evaluation of degenerative conditions versus acute fractures, infection, and malignancy demonstrates sensitivity of 96.9% and diagnostic accuracy of 96%. Level of evidence: III.

32. FDA warns that gadolinium-based contrast agents (GBCAs) are retained in the body; requires new class warnings. Available at: https://www.fda.gov/downloads/Drugs/DrugSafety/UCM589442.pdf. Accessed August 28, 2018.

33. Martin AR, Aleksanderek I, Cohen-Adad J, et al: Translating state-of-the-art spinal cord MRI techniques to clinical use: A systematic review of clinical studies utilizing DTI, MT, MWF, MRS, and fMRI. *NeuroImage Clin* 2016;10:192-238. doi:10.1016/j.nicl.2015.11.019.

Systematic review of advanced MRI spinal cord techniques. Although several of these techniques have shown promise, further study is necessary before standardization and validation allow for widespread clinical adaptation.

34. Yu E, Khan SN: Does less invasive spine surgery result in increased radiation exposure? A systematic review. *Clin Orthop Relat Res* 2014;472(6):1738-1748. doi:10.1007/s11999-014-3503-3.

35. Mendelsohn D, Strelzow J, Dea N, et al: Patient and surgeon radiation exposure during spinal instrumentation using intraoperative computed tomography-based navigation. *Spine J* 2016;16(3):343-354. doi:10.1016/j.spinee.2015.11.020.

Case-control study comparing intraoperative fluoroscopy to CT nagvigation. Radiation exposure higher for the patient but lower for the operating room personnel with the use of intraoperative CT with navigation compared with fluoroscopy.

Chapter 48

Cervical Degenerative Conditions

Yu-Po Lee, MD • Saif Aldeen Farhan, MD • Nitin Bhatia, MD

ABSTRACT

Degenerative disorders of the spine can present as a spectrum of disorders. In its mildest form degeneration of the cervical disks can cause mild neck pain and stiffness. However, advanced progression of the degenerative process can result in nerve root and spinal cord injury. Degeneration of the cervical spine can also lead to deformity of the cervical spine with spinal cord and nerve root impingement. The ability to recognize key signs and symptoms of progressive cervical degeneration and how to differentiate between the various ways that it can present is essential for physicians and surgeons who treat patients with cervical disorders.

This chapter will describe the evaluation and management of cervical degenerative disorders.

Keywords: cervical deformity; cervical spondylosis; cervical spondylotic myelopathy; cervical stenosis

Dr. Lee or an immediate family member serves as a paid consultant to or is an employee of DePuy, A Johnson & Johnson Company. Dr. Bhatia or an immediate family member has received royalties from Alphatec Spine, Biomet, Seaspine, Spineart, and Stryker; is a member of a speakers' bureau or has made paid presentations on behalf of Alphatec Spine, Biomet, Seaspine, Spineart, and Stryker; serves as a paid consultant to or is an employee of Alphatec Spine, Biomet, DiFusion, Seaspine, Spineart, Zimmer, and Stryker; has stock or stock options held in DiFusion; and serves as a board member, owner, officer, or committee member of the Cervical Spine Research Society, the North American Spine Society, and the Western Orthopaedic Association. Neither Dr. Farhan nor any immediate family member has received anything of value from or has stock or stock options held in a commercial company or institution related directly or indirectly to the subject of this chapter.

Introduction

Degenerative disorders of the spine can present as a spectrum of disorders. In its mildest form degeneration of the cervical disks can cause mild neck pain and stiffness, although it frequently is asymptomatic.[1-3] As the degenerative process advances, degeneration of the disks leads to protrusion of the disks and osteophyte formation. Bulging of the disks and osteophyte formation can compress the nerves and spinal cord and lead to pain and loss of function. This spinal degenerative process is also called spondylosis. Dysfunction of the nerve roots due to nerve root compression is termed radiculopathy, and dysfunction of the spinal cord due to spinal cord compression is termed myelopathy. Cervical spondylosis is the most common cause of cervical myelopathy in people aged 55 years and older, and the disorder is termed cervical spondylotic myelopathy (CSM).[4] The rate and degree of neurologic deterioration are variable. Early recognition and treatment of CSM is critical before the onset of spinal cord damage.

Cervical disk herniations can also be a source of severe pain and disability.[1-3] As the disk degenerates, a fragment of the nucleus pulposus or anulus fibrosus can break off and herniate into the canal. This can lead to symptoms of radiculopathy or myelopathy depending on if the disk compresses the nerve roots or spinal cord, respectively. At the end of the spectrum of cervical degenerative disorders is cervical deformity. This can present as cervical kyphosis (sagittal plane deformity) or scoliosis (coronal plane deformity). Progressive degeneration of the disks and weakening of the muscles and soft tissues leads to deformity of the cervical spine with spinal cord and nerve root impingement.

This chapter will describe the evaluation and management of cervical degenerative disorders.

Evaluation

Evaluation of cervical degenerative disorders starts with a careful history and physical examination. Questions that may provide clues to the cause of a patient's symptoms include whether the patient has pain, loss of sensation, or weakness.[5-7] The primary location of the symptoms is also important. Is the pain in the neck or does it radiate into their arms? Is there a loss of sensation and loss of coordination in the hands or is there any difficulty with balance and gait? Important factors include when the symptoms occurred, how long the symptoms were present, and if there was antecedent trauma. Other factors include if the symptoms have improved or worsened over time or if they have waxed and waned over time. Also, it is important to consider factors that alleviate and exacerbate the symptoms. Asking these questions can help in formulating a differential diagnosis.

Patients with disk degeneration may complain of axial neck pain. The pain will often be chronic and insidious in nature. Sometimes there is an inciting event that worsens their pain. The neurologic examination will be benign in most cases. Patients with a cervical disk herniation, however, will complain of a sudden and acute pain that is very intense. Depending on the level of the herniation they will have loss of sensation and motor weakness in a distribution that is consistent with the nerve root affected.

Myelopathy presents with a variety of subtle neurologic findings.[5-7] Characteristic signs and symptoms can present insidiously and include the loss of manual dexterity in the hands, weakness, stiffness, urinary symptoms, spasticity in their extremities, and gait disturbance including a stiff or spastic gait. Patients demonstrate a wide-based gait and report a history of loss of balance and falls. Sensory findings often include proprioceptive loss, and patients may report that they have difficulty with buttons, a change in their handwriting, or that they are dropping objects.

A comprehensive neurologic examination should be performed. The motor examination may be completely normal even in cases of nerve root or spinal cord compression. When upper extremity weakness is present, it often presents as diminished grip and/or intrinsic strength. The finding of severe weakness of major muscle groups in the upper or lower extremities is relatively uncommon. Sensory examination should also be performed, but the findings are often subtle. The neurologic examination should include an assessment for gait instability. Hyperreflexia may be present in the upper and/or lower extremities and is suggestive of spinal cord compression with upper motor neuron signs. These findings, however, can be masked or diminished in patients who have concomitant diabetes mellitus, peripheral neuropathy, or lumbar stenosis.

Spinal cord compression with myelopathy can manifest with abnormal upper motor neuron signs such as Hoffman's sign, inverted radial reflex, pathological clonus, and Babinski's sign.[5-7] The Hoffman's sign is described as quick flexion of both the thumb and index finger when the middle finger nail is snapped. Clonus is a series of abnormal reflex movements of the foot in plantar flexion, induced by sudden dorsiflexion. This finding is caused by alternate contraction and relaxation of the triceps surae muscle. The number of times the foot contracts in plantar flexion is recorded and may be a sign of spinal cord pathology. The Babinski reflex occurs after the sole of the foot has been firmly stroked. The big toe then moves upward or toward the top surface of the foot while the other toes fan out. The inverted radial reflex is noted by flexion of the fingers without flexion of the forearm when the distal end of the radius is tapped. Lhermitte's sign is an electric shock-like sensation that runs down the center of the patient's back and enters the limbs during flexion of the neck.

Myelopathy can often be accompanied by radicular findings in some patients. Myeloradiculopathy is associated with spinal stenosis with concurrent compression of the neuroforaminal contents, which produces lower motor neuron signs at the level of the cervical cord lesion and upper motor neuron signs caudal to the level of compression.

Differential Diagnosis

Once a careful history and physical examination have been performed, the surgeon can then start to formulate a differential diagnosis. There are many conditions that affect the central and peripheral nervous system that can mimic the signs and symptoms of cervical degenerative disorders. Some pathologies to include in the differential are a central nervous system disorders, demyelinating processes such a multiple sclerosis and transverse myelitis, stroke, tumor, trauma, infection, peripheral nerve compression disorders, nutritional myelopathy such as a vitamin B_{12} deficiency, and even shoulder pathology.[8,9]

Amyotrophic lateral sclerosis (ALS) is a neurodegenerative disorder that can be difficult to recognize because of overlapping demographics and clinical symptoms with cervical degenerative disorders. ALS can present with upper and lower motor neuron deficits, as well as cranial nerve deficits. An electromyography study (EMG) demonstrating a denervation pattern can serve as diagnostic evidence for ALS, although a muscle biopsy may be necessary during the diagnostic process. Guillain-Barré syndrome can present with a subacute onset of progressive weakness. This disorder occurs when the immune system attacks the peripheral nervous system. Multiple sclerosis is a demyelinating disorder that can cause progressive loss of sensation and weakness. While the cause is unclear, the underlying mechanism is thought to be either destruction by the immune system or failure of the myelin-producing cells. Gait and bladder dysfunction can be found in patients with normal pressure hydrocephalus. Additional cranial nerve abnormalities and/or a hyperactive jaw jerk reflex would suggest the presence of a brain stem or intracranial lesion. Cognitive dysfunction can help differentiate between normal pressure hydrocephalus and other central nervous disorders from CSM.

Peripheral nerve compression disorders should also be included in the differential diagnosis. Patients should be screened for possible carpal tunnel syndrome, cubital tunnel syndrome, and thoracic outlet syndrome if their signs and symptoms suggest such diagnoses. It is not uncommon for patients to have nerve compression in their spinal canal and at a distant site. This dual compression is called a double crush syndrome. Patients with rotator cuff tears and other shoulder pathology may also present with symptoms mimicking cervical degeneration, although examination of the shoulder may provide insight as to the underlying pathology.

Imaging

Plain radiographs are commonly used as the initial imaging of the spine as they are relatively inexpensive and easy to obtain. Radiographs can provide useful information regarding the specific location and severity of spinal degeneration. Spinal cord and/or nerve root impingement may be suspected if the clinical history and physical examination correlate with affected degenerated levels seen on radiographs. Radiographs can also show instability and deformity. Routine radiographs often include AP and lateral radiographs as well as flexion-extension views.

To confirm spinal cord compression, advanced imaging using MRI or CT myelography is preferred. MRI is noninvasive and provides visualization of the intervertebral disks, spinal cord, and nerve roots. MRI also provides good visualization of spinal cord and nerve root compression. Signal changes within the spinal cord seen on MRI are suggestive of severe compression and spinal cord injury.[10] Signal changes seen on T1- and T2-weighted MRI imaging of the spinal cord have also shown a moderate ability to predict outcomes after surgical intervention (**Figure 1**). In general, T2 weak signal hyperintensity (more intense than normal spinal cord but less intense than CSF) that appears diffuse without clear

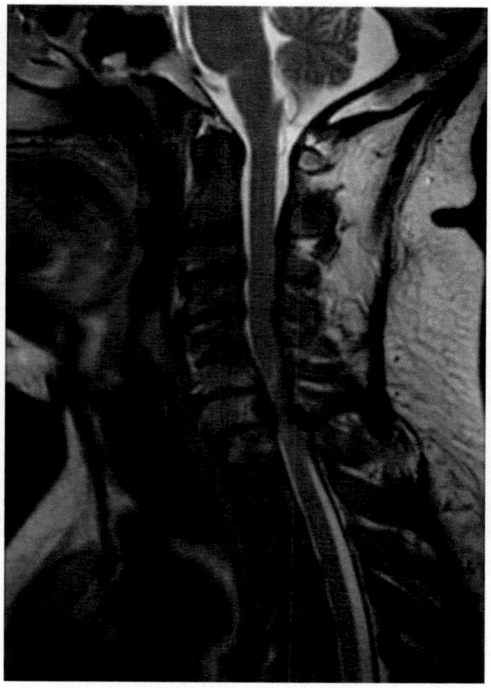

Figure 1 T2-weighted image showing severe central canal stenosis with myelomalacia.

bordering has been associated with potentially reversible changes such as edema, Wallerian degeneration, demyelination, and ischemia. T2 imaging showing substantial hyperintensity with sharp bordering and T1 hypointensity represent changes considered to be irreversible such as cavitation, neural tissue loss, myelomalacia, necrosis, and spongiform changes in gray matter. In addition, myelopathic signs as discussed previously have been shown to be significantly more common in patients with cord signal changes suggestive of myelomalacia.

If a patient cannot undergo MRI for medical reasons (such as the presence of cardiac pacemakers, aneurysm clips, or claustrophobia), or if metal or scar tissue from prior cervical surgery obscures visualization on MRI because of artifact, CT myelography is a good alternative. Plain CT is also a good adjunct to MRI in some cases. For example, a CT scan can be helpful if OPLL (ossification of posterior longitudinal ligament) (**Figure 2, A** and **B**) is suspected or to better visualize the vertebral artery if a corpectomy or C2 pedicle screws are planned.

Nonsurgical Management

The first line of treatment for cervical degenerative disorders is rest, lifestyle modifications, and even a short period of immobilization in a soft collar.[11-13] Cervical degenerative disorders can cause muscular strain and

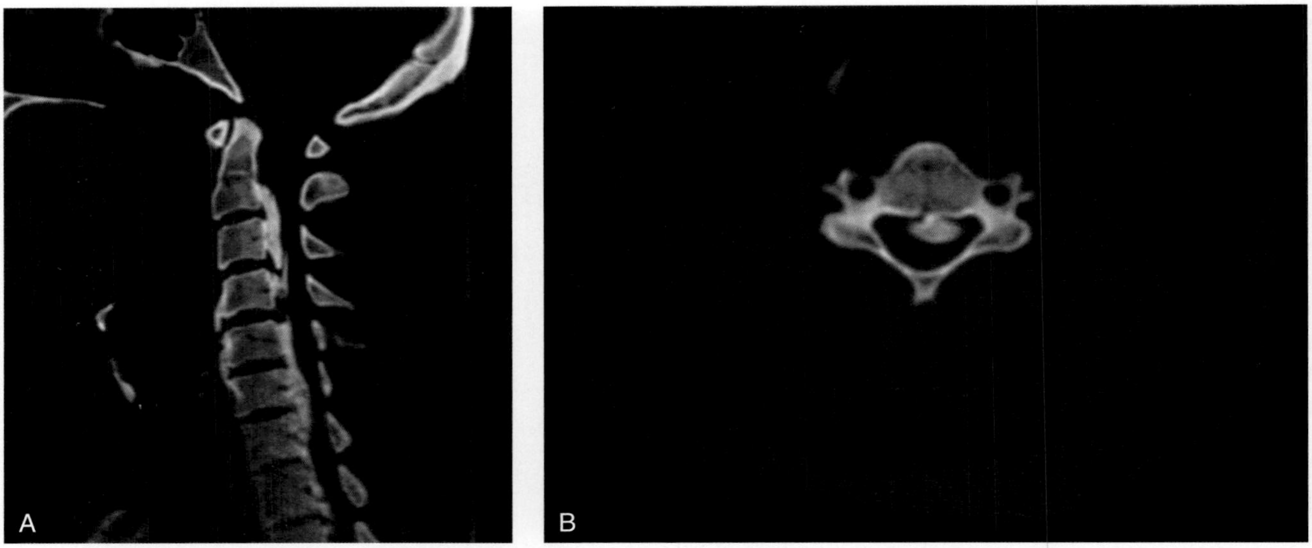

Figure 2 **A**, Sagittal CT showing ossification of posterior longitudinal ligament (OPLL). **B**, Axial view showing OPLL compressing the spinal cord.

inflammation to the disks and facet joints. Rest and avoidance of re-injuring the muscles and tendons can often result in good pain relief. People often use computers at work and even for recreation, but prolonged use of computers and poor ergonomics and can result in muscle strain and spasms from prolonged straining of the neck and shoulders to view the computer screen. Improving the ergonomics of a patient's work station include adjusting the height of the screen to eye level and making sure to get up periodically to stretch. Ice and massage can also be helpful in decreasing acute muscular pain and spasms. Immobilization in a soft collar can provide pain relief. The warmth of the collar and resting the muscles help decrease muscular pain and spasms, but a cervical collar should not be used for a prolonged period of time as the muscles can atrophy over time.

Further treatment may include the addition of pain relieving medications. Acetaminophen and nonsteroidal anti-inflammatory medications are the first line of medications in patients presenting with acute neck pain.[11-13] These medications can help reduce pain and inflammation. A short course of oral steroids may be beneficial if the pain and inflammation is severe. Muscle relaxers can help decrease pain by decreasing muscular pain and spasms. Gabapentin is also a good medication to help with nerve-related pain. Narcotics may be considered for a short period but should be monitored closely.

Physical therapy is another treatment option for cervical degenerative disorders. Strengthening the neck and shoulder muscles may help decrease muscle-related spasms and fatigue. Stronger cervical muscles will also help provide stability to the cervical spine and decrease inflammation and nerve root irritation. The therapist can also use gentle cervical traction, and massage and other modalities can be helpful to maximize the results of therapy.

Pain management can also be a useful adjunct in the treatment of cervical degenerative disorders. Treatment options include trigger point injections, epidural injections, medial branch blocks, and radiofrequency ablation, depending on the patient's presenting symptoms and imaging findings. The patient should have an MRI or CT myelogram to show that there is only mild to moderate stenosis before intraspinal injections to avoid potential neurologic injury.

There is a lack of high-level studies comparing these modalities to surgical intervention. Therefore, conservative therapies are often initiated based on a clinician's preference or past experiences. The nonsurgical treatment of axial neck pain, cervical radiculopathy, or mild CSM may be attempted safely without the risk of neurologic deterioration. Surgical intervention, however, may be more efficacious in patients with symptomatic moderate to severe nerve root or cord compression.

Relative indications for surgical intervention for cervical degenerative spondylosis include the progression of neurologic symptoms, presence of myelopathy for more than 6 months, compression ratio approaching 0.4 (measured as the ratio of the smallest sagittal cord diameter to the largest transverse cord diameter at the same level), and transverse area of the cord <40 mm. The presence of any of these factors can be an indication for surgical intervention.[11-13]

Surgery

Many factors play a role in the decision-making process for surgical intervention. These factors include duration of symptoms, degree of spinal cord dysfunction, general health of the patient, degree of functional deterioration, and radiographic findings.

Anterior Versus Posterior Surgery

The optimal surgical approach is not always clear and has been under investigation over the past several years. An anterior approach offers the following advantages: direct decompression of pathologies in the anterior cervical spine, a muscle-sparing dissection to minimize postoperative pain, lower infection rates, and the ability to decompress and correct cervical kyphosis.[14,15] Most spine surgeons prefer an anterior approach when one to two levels are involved. When three or more levels are involved, however, the complication rates with an anterior approach rise and a posterior approach may be more efficacious. If there is focal kyphosis and the compressive pathology is posterior, then a combined approach can also be considered. The posterior approach allows for a wider decompression and is dependent on the ability of the cord to drift away from anterior lesions. It is therefore important to take cervical sagittal alignment into consideration, as the cord may not drift posteriorly with significant cervical kyphosis.

The degree of kyphosis or lordosis can be quantitatively calculated by the sagittal cervical Cobb angle.[16] C2-C7 lordosis is measured as the angle of intersection between vertical lines drawn from lines parallel to the inferior end plates of C2 and C7. There is evidence that lordotic patients exhibited similar improvement when approached anteriorly or posteriorly, whereas kyphotic patients exhibited greater improvement when approached by an anterior or combined approach. More recently, the cervical sagittal alignment, as assessed by the C2-C7 sagittal vertical axis (SVA, in mm displacement) has also been shown to play a major role in clinical outcomes. The cervical (C2-C7) SVA is measured as the deviation of the C2 plumb line from the posterior superior end plate of C7, and the cervical SVA has previously been shown to correlate with postoperative disability scores. Studies suggest that a SVA ≥40 mm is associated with greater pain and disability.

The current evidence is not clear on whether an anterior or posterior approach is superior; rather the sagittal alignment, number of pathologic levels, and degree of anterior or posterior compression dictate what would be the most appropriate approach for the decompression.

Anterior Surgery

Methods of anterior decompression include anterior cervical diskectomy and fusion (ACDF) (**Figure 3**, **A** and **B**), anterior cervical corpectomy and fusion (ACCF), hybrid procedures, and cervical diskectomy with arthroplasty. Anterior approaches generally demonstrate lower perioperative complications and morbidity and tend to be performed on younger patients when compared with other approaches. Clinical series have demonstrated successful arthrodesis in most patients (92% to 96%) after single-level ACDF with satisfactory clinical outcomes. For compression at multiple levels, numerous options exist, including multilevel ACDF, corpectomy, and hybrid techniques. While the rate of neurologic improvement remains high for multilevel ACDFs, the incidence of nonunion increases with the number of levels being fused. Anterior cervical plating increases the fusion rates in patients undergoing multilevel surgery. An alternative method to improve fusion rates and provide a more extensive decompression would be to employ a corpectomy, which can also be combined with anterior diskectomy procedures. The addition of a posterior segmental fusion can increase the fusion rate and decrease the incidence of graft and implant-related problems in multilevel cases.

Complications of anterior procedures include postoperative dysphagia (2% to 48%), hoarseness

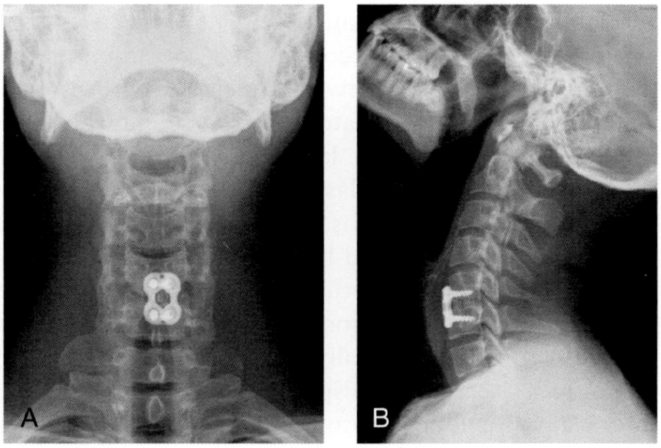

Figure 3 **A**, AP view of patient after C5-6 anterior cervical diskectomy and fusion. **B**, Lateral view of C5-6 anterior cervical diskectomy and fusion.

(temporary in 3% to 11%, permanent in 0.33%), and injury to the vertebral artery (0.03%) and carry an incidence of adjacent segment disease of 3% per year.

The literature on arthroplasty for patients with myelopathy is limited. Studies suggest that cervical arthroplasty has good rates of overall success, long-term functional outcomes, and a lower incidence of adjacent segment degeneration in comparison to anterior cervical fusion procedures.[17] However, patients with significant degenerative changes in the cervical spine may be better suited for a fusion procedure to prevent further degenerative changes at the affected levels. These patients may not be ideal candidates for cervical arthroplasty, as the increased motion can exacerbate the degenerative changes. Instead, cervical arthroplasty may be best reserved for patients with acute neurologic deficits due to a herniated disk without significant degenerative changes, especially in the facet joints.

Posterior Surgery

Posterior approaches offer the opportunity to avoid technical problems encountered with anterior approaches that result from obesity, a short neck, barrel chest, or previous anterior cervical surgery. Options for a posterior approach for spinal cord decompression include a laminoplasty or a laminectomy with or without fusion.

The laminoplasty technique is often ideal for the patient with spinal stability, good cervical lordosis, and minimal neck pain.[18] Laminoplasty technique offers the opportunity to preserve some of the natural cervical biomechanical motion without necessitating fusion. Variations in the laminoplasty technique include the open-door laminoplasty, the double-door laminoplasty, and various muscle-sparing laminoplasty alterations. The open-door laminoplasty involves a thinned hinge on one side of the lamina and a complete cut through the lamina on the opposite side. The laminae on the open side can then be reconstructed with mini-plates, anchored with a stitch between the spinous process and the hinged lamina, or plated open by fixing the open lamina with subsequent levels. The double-door or "French Door" laminoplasty expands the canal symmetrically as the opening is created in the midline. This technique is accomplished by splitting the spinous processes in the midline with the left and right hemilaminae hinging on the lamina-spinous process and ligamentum flavum complex bilaterally. Various muscle-sparing techniques (sparing semispinalis cervicis, multifidus, and C7 musculoligamentous attachments) have also been described with the aim to limit postoperative axial neck pain, kyphosis, and segmental instability.

Complications from the laminoplasty procedure can include delayed C5 nerve root injury (2% to 13.3%), neck pain (40% to 60%), loss of range of motion (20% to 50%), or new-onset kyphosis (2% to 15%).[18] Interestingly, C5 nerve palsy is classically correlated with laminoplasty, but more recent studies have shown the risk of C5 nerve palsy with various forms of cervical decompression including anterior decompression and laminectomy.

In the past, a laminectomy alone was regarded as the standard treatment for multilevel CSM. Many surgeons still perform laminectomy only, but the incidence of postoperative kyphosis (6% to 46%) and segmental instability (~18%) requiring additional stabilization has led many surgeons to add instrumentation and fusion to prevent against these potential problems. The differences in the range of postoperative kyphosis can be due to surgical sagittal alignment and directly related to the extent of the laminectomy procedure (amount of lateral dissection, facet capsule disruption, resection of more than 50% of the facet joint). Cervical laminectomy and fusion offers the advantage to stabilize and maintain the decompressed segment in a lordotic posture while preventing segmental instability, thereby allowing for a more expansive decompression. There is insufficient evidence to determine whether the addition of cervical fixation improves functional outcome, however. The addition of fixation also carries the risks of complications related to misplaced screws, long-term hardware failure, and the alteration of the natural cervical biomechanics distributed to adjacent levels.

When the clinical scenario allows the opportunity, these general techniques can be further tailored to be less invasive. For example, skip laminectomy can be used to limit the disruption of the posterior cervical tension band. By employing this method, decompression between C3-C7 can be accomplished by a C4 and C6 skip laminectomy to preserve the C3, C5, and C7 posterior arches as well as all the muscular attachments to those spinous processes. More recently, minimally invasive endoscopic approaches for posterior decompression have also been used for cervical degenerative conditions.

Cervical Deformity

The techniques for correcting cervical spine deformity are quite varied and depend on the pathology. If dynamic radiographs suggested a flexible deformity or if the deformity was reducible by traction,

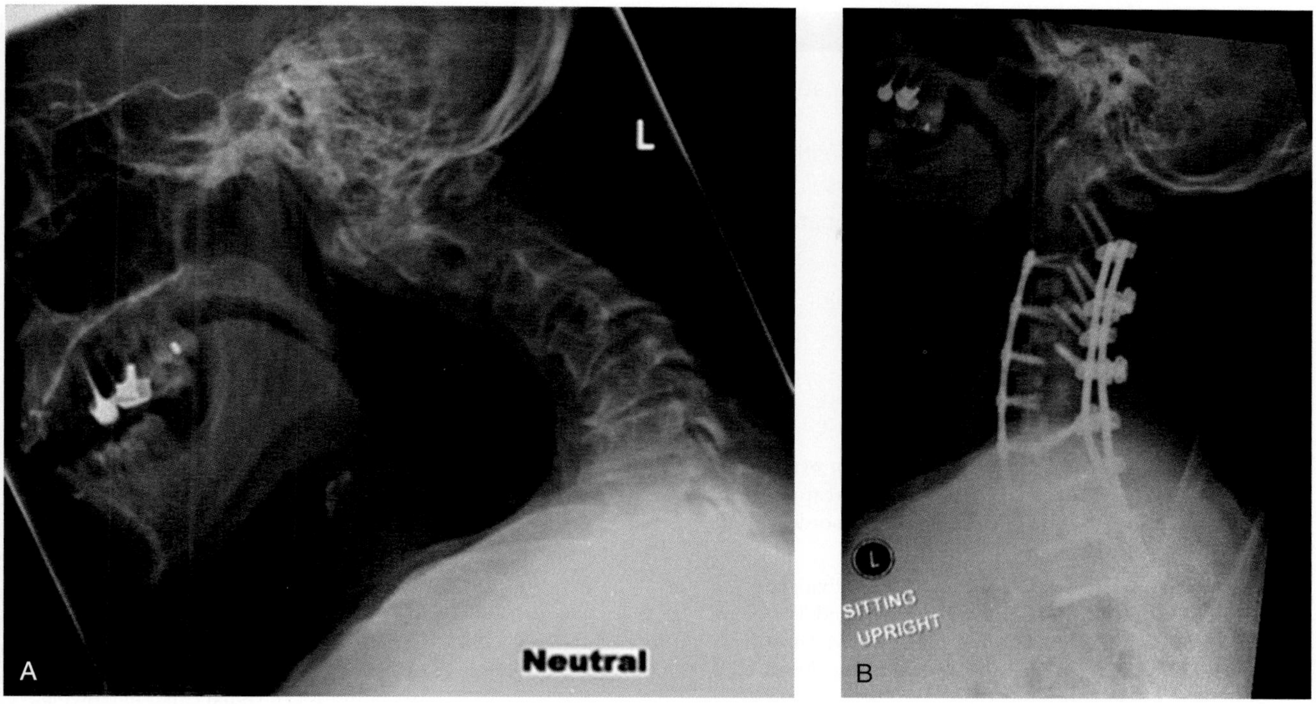

Figure 4 **A**, Preoperative lateral radiograph: Fixed cervical kyphosis following multilevel posterior cervical laminectomy for cervical myelopathy. **B**, Postoperative lateral radiograph: Correction of cervical deformity through anterior and posterior approach.

correction could be accomplished via an isolated posterior approach using a decompression and instrumented fusion. In patients with ventral compressive pathologies, compromised integrity of the ventral column, or a fixed kyphotic deformity, an anterior approach can be considered in conjunction with a posterior fusion (**Figure 4**). Decompression can be performed anteriorly or posteriorly as dictated by the pathology. An osteotomy can be used to correct severe kyphotic deformities. Posterior-based osteotomies are most commonly performed at C7 because the vertebral artery typically does not pass through the C7 transverse foramina, but it is advisable to verify the location of the vertebral artery with an MRI, CT, or CT angiogram before surgery. Osteotomy of C7 includes complete laminectomy of C-7, partial laminectomies of C-6 and T-1, partial pedicle osteotomy, osteoclasis of the ventral vertebral body, and finally correction of the deformity. The correction is maintained with instrumentation, and in severe cases a halo brace may be necessary. Preoperative traction may be used in some cases before surgery as well. There is risk of spinal cord injury, durotomy, and the C8 nerve root is at risk with closure of the osteotomy at C7, and patients should be counseled regarding this before surgery.

Summary

Cervical degenerative conditions can be a major cause of disability, particularly in elderly patients in whom these degenerative conditions tend to be more prevalent. The clinical presentation and natural history of cervical degenerative conditions are variable because of the many ways that these conditions can manifest. For mild degenerative conditions, nonsurgical options may be tried with careful observation. However, surgical intervention has shown to be superior for conditions where there is symptomatic moderate to severe spinal cord and nerve root compression. The success of surgical or conservative management of these conditions is multifactorial and high-quality studies are lacking. The optimal surgical approach is still under debate and can vary depending on the location of the spinal cord compression, number of levels involved, sagittal alignment, instability, and patient comorbidities. The goal of surgery is to decompress any spinal cord or nerve root compression, correct any deformity, and stabilization to maintain correction or prevent deformity. Further high-quality randomized clinical studies with long-term follow up are still needed to further define the natural history and help predict the most ideal surgical strategy.

Key Study Points

- To be able to evaluate and diagnose patients with degenerative cervical spine disorders.
- To appropriately order and read diagnostic imaging of degenerative cervical spine disorders.
- To be able to form a treatment plan for patients with degenerative cervical spine disorders.

Annotated References

1. Bono CM, Ghiselli G, Gilbert TJ, et al: An evidence-based clinical guideline for the diagnosis and treatment of cervical radiculopathy from degenerative disorders. *Spine J* 2011;11(1):64-72.

   The North American Spine Society (NASS) Evidence-Based Clinical Guideline on the Diagnosis and Treatment of Cervical Radiculopathy from Degenerative Disorders reviews the diagnosis and treatment of cervical radiculopathy from degenerative disorders. This guideline addresses these questions based on the highest quality clinical literature available on this subject as of May 2009. The guideline's recommendations assist the practitioner in delivering optimum efficacious treatment of and functional recovery from this common disorder.

2. Tetreault L, Goldstein CL, Arnold P, et al: Degenerative cervical myelopathy: A spectrum of related disorders affecting the aging spine. *Neurosurgery* 2015;77(suppl 4):S51-S67.

   In this article, the authors review the range of degenerative spinal disorders resulting in progressive cervical spinal cord compression. This review summarizes current knowledge of the pathophysiology of cervical disk degeneration and describes the cascade of events that occur after compression of the spinal cord, including ischemia, destruction of the blood–spinal cord barrier, demyelination, and neuronal apoptosis. Other topics of this review include epidemiology, the prevalence of degenerative changes in the asymptomatic population, the natural history and rates of progression, risk factors of diagnosis (clinical, imaging and genetic), and management strategies.

3. Nouri A, Tetreault L, Singh A, et al: Degenerative cervical myelopathy: Epidemiology, genetics, and pathogenesis. *Spine* 2015;40(12):E675-E693.

   The authors review the epidemiology, pathogenesis, and genetics of conditions causing cervical disk degeneration. Pathophysiologically, myelopathy results from static compression, spinal malalignment leading to altered cord tension and vascular supply, and dynamic injury mechanisms. Occupational hazards, including transportation of goods by weight bearing on top of the head, and other risk factors may accelerate cervical disk degeneration. Potential genetic factors include those related to MMP-2 and collagen IX for degenerative disk disease, and collagen VI and XI for ossification of the posterior longitudinal ligament. In addition, congenital anomalies including spinal stenosis, Down syndrome, and Klippel-Feil syndrome may predispose to the development of cervical disk degneration.

4. Buser Z, Ortega B, D'Oro A, et al: Spine degenerative conditions and their treatments: National trends in the United States of America. *Global Spine J* 2018;8(1):57-67.

   The authors perform a retrospective database study on degenerative cervical and lumbar disorders. Within the Medicare database there were 6,206,578 patients diagnosed with lumbar and 3,156,215 patients diagnosed with cervical degenerative conditions between 2006 and 2012, representing a 16.5% (lumbar) decrease and 11% (cervical) increase in the number of diagnosed patients. Level of evidence: IV.

5. Wilson JR, Barry S, Fischer DJ, et al: Frequency, timing, and predictors of neurological dysfunction in the nonmyelopathic patient with cervical spinal cord compression, canal stenosis, and/or ossification of the posterior longitudinal ligament. *Spine* 2013;38(22 suppl 1):S37-S54.

   The authors conducted a literature review and an international survey of spine surgeons to answer the following key questions in patients with radiographical evidence of cervical spinal cord compression, spinal canal narrowing, and/or OPLL but no symptoms of myelopathy: (1) What are the frequency and timing of symptom development? (2) What are the clinical, radiographical, and electrophysiological predictors of symptom development? (3) What clinical and/or radiographical features influence treatment decisions based on an international survey of spine care professionals? The authors concluded that patients with cervical canal stenosis and cord compression secondary to spondylosis, without clinical evidence of myelopathy, and who present with clinical or electrophysiological evidence of cervical radicular dysfunction or central conduction deficits seem to be at higher risk for developing myelopathy and should be counseled to consider surgical treatment.

6. Matsunaga S, Komiya S, Toyama Y: Risk factors for development of myelopathy in patients with cervical spondylotic cord compression. *Eur Spine J* 2015;24(suppl 2):142-149.

   The authors reviewed articles in which risk factors for the development of myelopathy in patients with cervical spondylotic cord compression were discussed. Cervical motion segment disorders are considered to be multifactorial, and developmental size of the canal and foramina, pathological encroachment, biomechanical effects, and circulatory deficiencies are always present to some degree. Static and dynamic factors should be considered for the development of myelopathy. To clarify the pathomechanism of the development of myelopathy in patients with cervical spondylotic spinal cord compression, the exact natural history of cervical spondylotic myelopathy should be understood.

7. Fehlings MG, Tetreault LA, Riew KD, Middleton JW, Wang JC: A clinical practice guideline for the management of degenerative cervical myelopathy: Introduction, rationale, and scope. *Global Spine J* 2017;7(3 suppl):21S-27S.

Degenerative cervical myelopathy (DCM) is a progressive spine disease and the most common cause of spinal cord dysfunction in adults worldwide. Patients with DCM may present with common signs and symptoms of neurological dysfunction, such as paresthesia, abnormal gait, decreased hand dexterity, hyperreflexia, increased tone, and sensory dysfunction. Clinicians across several specialties encounter patients with DCM, including primary care physicians, rehabilitation specialists, therapists, rheumatologists, neurologists, and spinal surgeons. Currently, there are no guidelines that outline how to best manage patients with mild (defined as a modified Japanese Orthopaedic Association [mJOA] score of 15 to 17), moderate (mJOA = 12 to 14), or severe (mJOA ≤ 11) myelopathy, or nonmyelopathic patients with evidence of cord compression. The authors discuss evidence-based recommendations to specify appropriate treatment strategies for these populations. Level of evidence: I.

8. Kuijper B, Tans JT, Schimsheimer RJ, et al: Degenerative cervical radiculopathy: Diagnosis and conservative treatment. A review. *Eur J Neurol* 2009;16(1):15-20.

   The authors discuss the diagnosis and nonsurgical treatment of degenerative cervical radiculopathy. They performed a literature search for studies on epidemiology, diagnosis including electrophysiological examination and imaging studies, and different types of conservative treatment. The most common causes of cervical root compression were spondyloarthrosis and disk herniation.

9. Woods BI, Hilibrand AS: Cervical radiculopathy: Epidemiology, etiology, diagnosis, and treatment. *J Spinal Disord Tech* 2015;28(5):E251-E259.

   Cervical radiculopathy can often be diagnosed with a thorough history and physical examination, but an magnetic resonance imaging or computed tomographic myelogram should be used to confirm the diagnosis. Because of the ubiquity of degenerative changes found on these imaging modalities, the patient's symptoms must correlate with pathology for a successful diagnosis. The authors discuss the different causes and treatments of cervical radiculopathy.

10. Karpova A, Arun R, Davis AM, et al: Reliability of quantitative magnetic resonance imaging methods in the assessment of spinal canal stenosis and cord compression in cervical myelopathy. *Spine* 2013;38(3):245-252.

    A prospective study to evaluate the intra- and interobserver reliability of commonly used quantitative MRI measures such as transverse area (TA) of spinal cord, compression ratio (CR), maximum canal compromise (MCC), and maximum spinal cord compression (MSCC). All four measurement techniques demonstrated a good to moderately high degree of intra- and interobserver reliability. Highest reliability was noted in the assessment of T2-weighted sequences and axial MRI. The results showed that the measurements of MCC, MSCC, and CR are sufficiently reliable and correlate well with clinical severity of cervical myelopathy.

11. Rhee JM, Shamji MF, Erwin WM, et al: Nonoperative management of cervical myelopathy: A systematic review. *Spine* 2013;38(22 suppl 1):S55-S67.

    A systematic search was conducted in PubMed and the Cochrane Collaboration Library for articles on the treatment of cervical myelopathy. The authors concluded that there is a paucity of evidence for nonsurgical treatment of cervical myelopathy, and further studies are needed to determine its role more definitively. Because myelopathy is known to be a typically progressive disorder and there is little evidence that nonsurgical treatment halts or reverses its progression, the authors recommended not routinely prescribing nonsurgical treatment as the primary modality in patients with moderate to severe myelopathy.

12. Fehlings MG, Tetreault LA, Riew KD, et al: A clinical practice guideline for the management of patients with degenerative cervical myelopathy: Recommendations for patients with mild, moderate, and severe disease and nonmyelopathic patients with evidence of cord compression. *Global Spine J* 2017;7(3 suppl):70S-83S.

    The authors discuss guidelines that outline how to best manage (1) patients with mild, moderate, and severe myelopathy and (2) nonmyelopathic patients with evidence of cord compression with or without clinical symptoms of radiculopathy. Five systematic reviews of the literature were conducted to synthesize evidence on disease natural history; risk factors of diseaseprogression; the efficacy, effectiveness, and safety of nonsurgical and surgical management; the impact of preoperative duration of symptoms and myelopathy severity on treatment outcomes; and the frequency, timing, and predictors of symptom development. A multidisciplinary guideline development group used this information, and their clinical expertise, to develop recommendations for the management of degenerative cervical myelopathy (DCM). Level of evidence: I.

13. Rhee J, Tetreault LA, Chapman JR, et al: Nonoperative versus operative management for the treatment degenerative cervical myelopathy: An updated systematic review. *Global Spine J* 2017;7(3 suppl):35S-41S.

    The authors performed a database study to determine the role of nonsurgical treatment in the management of DCM by updating a systematic review published by Rhee and colleagues in 2013. The updated search yielded two additional citations that met inclusion criteria and compared the efficacy of conservative management and surgical treatment. Based on a single retrospective cohort, there were no significant differences in posttreatment Japanese Orthopaedic Association (JOA) or Neck Disability Index scores or JOA recovery ratios between patients treated nonsurgically versus surgically. A second retrospective study indicated that the incidence rate of hospitalization for spinal cord injury was 13.9 per 1000 person-years in a nonsurgical group compared with 9.4 per 1000 person-years in a surgical group (adjusted hazard ratio = 1.57; 95% confidence interval = 1.11 to 2.22; $P = 0.011$). Nonsurgical management results in similar outcomes as surgical treatment in patients with a modified JOA ≥ 13, single-level myelopathy, and intramedullary signal change on T2-weighted magnetic resonance imaging. Furthermore, patients managed nonsurgically for DCM have higher rates of hospitalization for spinal cord injury than those treated surgically. The overall level of evidence for these findings was rated as low. Level of evidence: I.

14. Shamji MF, Massicotte EM, Traynelis VC, Norvell DC, Hermsmeyer JT, Fehlings MG: Comparison of anterior surgical options for the treatment of multilevel cervical spondylotic myelopathy: A systematic review. *Spine* 2013;38(22 suppl 1):S195-S209.

The authors performed a systematic search in MEDLINE and the Cochrane Collaboration Library for human studies regarding anterior surgical treatment of cervical spondylotic myelopathy. All three surgical approaches are effective strategies for the anterior surgical management of cervical spondylotic myelopathy. When the patient pathoanatomy permits, selection of multiple diskectomies is favored compared with corpectomy or diskectomy-corpectomy hybrid approaches.

15. Lawrence BD, Jacobs WB, Norvell DC, Hermsmeyer JT, Chapman JR, Brodke DS: Anterior versus posterior approach for treatment of cervical spondylotic myelopathy: A systematic review. *Spine* 2013;38(22 suppl 1):S173-S182.

The authors conducted a systematic search for literature published through September 2012. The authors determined that for both effectiveness and safety, there is no clear advantage to either an anterior surgical approach or a posterior surgical approach when treating patients with multilevel cervical spondylotic myelopathy. With that, a surgical strategy developed on a patient-to-patient basis should be used to achieve optimal patient outcomes.

16. Passias PG, Soroceanu A, Scheer J, et al: Magnitude of preoperative cervical lordotic compensation and C2-T3 angle are correlated to increased risk of postoperative sagittal spinal pelvic malalignment in adult thoracolumbar deformity patients at 2-year follow-up. *Spine J* 2015;15(8):1756-1763.

This was a retrospective review of a multicenter, prospective database. Patients were assessed for cervical deformity based on the following criteria: C2-C7 SVA greater than 4 cm, C2-C7 SVA less than 4 cm, cervical kyphosis (CL greater than 0), cervical lordosis (CL less than 0), any deformity (C2-C7 SVA greater than 4 cm or CL greater than 0), and both CD (C2-C7 SVA greater than 4 cm and CL greater than 0). Patients with sagittal spinal malalignment associated with significant cervical compensatory lordosis are at increased risk of realignment failure at 2-year follow-up. Assessment of the degree of cervical compensation may be helpful in pre-op evaluation to assist in realignment outcome prediction.

17. Findlay C, Ayis S, Demetriades AK: Total disc replacement versus anterior cervical discectomy and fusion. *Bone Joint Lett J* 2018;100-B(8):991-1001.

The authors performed a study using a systematic review and meta-analysis to determine how the short- and medium- to long-term outcome measures after total disk replacement (TDR) compared with those of anterior cervical diskectomy and fusion (ACDF). Databases including Medline, Embase, and Scopus were searched. Inclusion criteria involved prospective randomized control trials (RCTs) reporting the surgical treatment of patients with symptomatic degenerative cervical disk disease. Two independent investigators extracted the data. The strength of evidence was assessed using the Grading of Recommendations, Assessment, Development and Evaluation (GRADE) criteria. The primary outcome measures were overall and neurological success, and these were included in the meta-analysis. Standardized patient-reported outcomes, including the incidence of further surgery and adjacent segment disease, were summarized and discussed. A total of 22 papers published from 14 RCTs were included, representing 3160 patients with follow-up of up to 10 years. TDR is as effective as ACDF and superior for some outcomes. Disk replacement reduces the risk of adjacent segment disease. Continued uncertainty remains about degeneration of the prosthesis. Long-term surveillance of patients who undergo TDR may allow its routine use. Level of evidence: I.

18. Yoon ST, Hashimoto RE, Raich A, Shaffrey CI, Rhee JM, Riew KD: Outcomes after laminoplasty compared with laminectomy and fusion in patients with cervical myelopathy: A systematic review. *Spine* 2013;38(22 suppl 1):S183-S194.

The authors conducted a database search to identify studies that compared laminoplasty with laminectomy and fusion. For patients with CSM, there is low-quality evidence that suggests that laminoplasty and laminectomy and fusion procedures are similarly effective in treating CSM. For patients with ossification of the posterior longitudinal ligament, the evidence regarding the effectiveness of these procedures is insufficient. For both patient populations, the evidence as to whether one procedure is safer than the other is insufficient. Higher quality research is necessary to more clearly delineate when one procedure is preferred compared with the other.

compressing several nerves within the dura. Lateral recess stenosis results from superior articular process hypertrophy combined with disk bulging, causing compression of the traversing nerve root. Foraminal stenosis can be caused by multiple factors. Disk herniations or bulges into the foramen can decrease the AP dimension of the foramen resulting in exiting nerve root compression. Alternatively, loss of disk height decreases the superior-inferior dimension, causing nerve root compression between the pedicles and the adjacent pedicle, disk, or osteophyte. Other causes, although less common than degenerative etiologies, can also result in stenosis including congenital stenosis, achondroplasia (short and narrow pedicles), metabolic conditions such as osteopetrosis, neoplasm, infection, or postsurgical changes.

Presentation

Depending on the location of the stenosis, patients present with a combination of neurogenic claudication with decreased walking tolerance, radiculopathy, and low back pain. In a prospective trial analyzing patients with symptomatic LSS, 95% of patients endorsed some degree of lumbar pain, 91% endorsed claudication symptoms, and 70% reported sensory disturbance in the legs.[23]

Neurogenic claudication classically presents as bilateral buttock and proximal thigh heaviness, fatigue, and pain, and it tends to worsen with prolonged standing or walking. These symptoms should be differentiated from vascular claudication, which typically begins distally and causes predominantly calf pain and burning.

There is often a dynamic component to the symptoms. Because the spinal canal diameter changes between flexion and extension, patients notice exacerbation or relief of symptoms often based upon positioning. Leaning forward, such as walking uphill, can provide relief of symptoms, and thus patients frequently find using a walker or holding onto a stroller to be easier. Walking downhill and extension activities narrow the canal dimensions and therefore exacerbate symptoms. Lying down is frequently more comfortable than sitting or standing.

Diagnostic Workup

Physical examination is often normal in patients with lumbar spinal stenosis, and therefore, the history is crucial to the diagnosis. In SPORT, only 50% of patients had physical examination findings including depressed reflexes, sensory or motor deficits, or positive nerve tension signs.[24] Therefore, it is also crucial to perform an examination of the lower extremities to rule out alternative causes for pain, as lumbar spine pathology and lower extremity joint dysfunction, especially the hip, are common. AP and lateral radiographs of the lumbar spine, with consideration for dynamic radiographs are important to evaluate alignment and evidence of instability. MRI has become the benchmark for identifying spinal pathology. T2-weighted sagittal and axial images can demonstrate disk bulges, facet hypertrophy, ligamentum flavum hypertrophy, cysts, and other causes of stenosis, whereas sagittal T1-weighted images best show foraminal stenosis (**Figures 2** and **3**). Although imaging is an important modality, it cannot replace a history and physical examination, as radiographic findings of spinal stenosis increase with age, yet many patients never become symptomatic. In a study of asymptomatic individuals, one study found that over 20% of patients older than 60 years had MRI evidence of lumbar spinal stenosis.[4] For those patients who cannot undergo MRI, CT myelography can also demonstrate compression although with less detail than MRI. Electrodiagnostic studies can be used to help rule out a peripheral neuropathy; however, their role in diagnosis of spinal stenosis is unclear.

Nonsurgical Management

The first-line treatment for LSS remains a combination of nonsurgical modalities including medication, physical therapy, and injections. The true efficacy of any one of these modalities, however, remains to be proven. Medications including NSAIDs and neuromodulators,

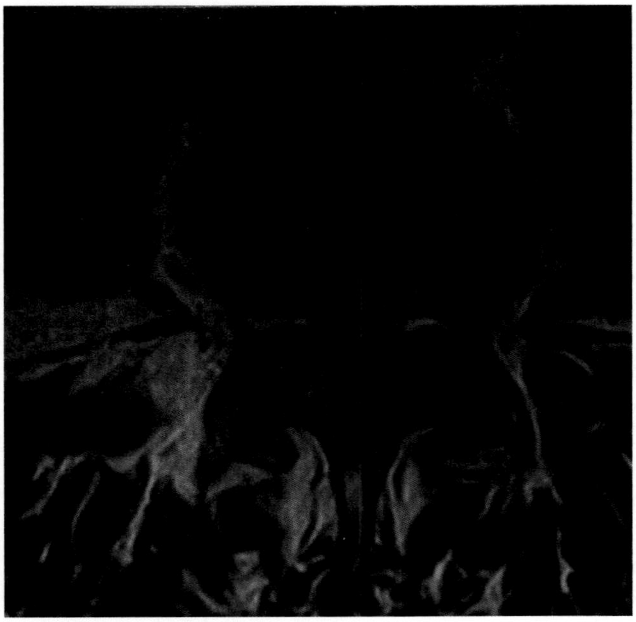

Figure 2 Axial T2 MRI scan demonstrating central and lateral recess stenosis.

Spine

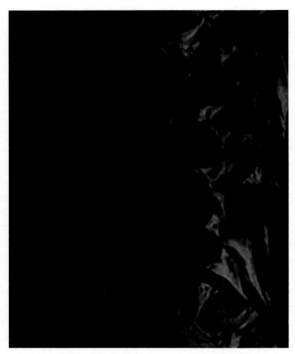

Figure 3 Sagittal T2 MRI scan demonstrating foraminal stenosis.

such as gabapentin and pregabalin, have been shown to improve symptoms of low back pain and radiculopathy. In a study evaluating patients with low back and leg pain refractory to NSAIDs, pregabalin was shown to improve visual analog scale scores for pain and sleep quality.[25] Structured physical therapy has also been shown to improve walking ability in patient with neurogenic claudication.[26] Several small studies support the use of epidural steroid injections for providing short- and medium-term relief of radiculopathy and neurogenic claudication; however, large randomized trials are lacking.

Surgical Management

Once the decision for surgery is made, the current benchmark remains a laminectomy. Traditionally this is performed through an open approach, where a central laminectomy is performed with bilateral medial facetectomies. Care must be taken to remove less than 50% of each facet and leave sufficient pars to decrease the possibility of iatrogenic instability. The decompression is performed from the cranial to the caudal pedicle to ensure decompression of the exiting and traversing nerve roots.

Several studies have demonstrated the benefit of surgery over nonsurgical treatment, the most rigorous of which remains SPORT. The SPORT enrolled 289 patients into a randomized cohort and 365 patients into an observational cohort comparing surgery and nonsurgical treatment. Although the study was limited by significant crossover, the randomized cohort demonstrated a significant difference in favor of surgery for Medical Outcomes Study 36-Item Short Form (SF-36) bodily pain scores, and the as-treated analysis favored surgery for all primary outcomes. These results were significant even at 2 years.[27] Follow-up studies demonstrated that the results remained significant at 4 years,[27] and at 8 years, the observational cohort still demonstrated a significant advantage for surgery over nonsurgical treatment.[28]

The role of fusion for spinal stenosis has also been discussed and is currently not indicated in patients without evidence of instability or in whom instability is not expected as part of the decompression. A recent prospective randomized controlled trial in the *New England Journal of Medicine* compared decompression with and without fusion in patients with LSS and found that there was no difference in patient-reported outcomes; however, the fusion cohort had a longer hospital stay, longer surgical time, increased bleeding, and increased surgical costs compared with the decompression-only group.[29] A meta-analysis similarly noted a 17% increase in revision surgery risk and double the risk of complications when decompression was accompanied with a fusion procedure.[30]

The results of less invasive strategies compared with traditional open laminectomy remains to be fully elucidated. A systematic review of 16 studies evaluating open versus minimally invasive decompression demonstrated no difference in terms of Oswestry Disability Index (ODI); however, it did note better visual analog scale scores for back pain and shorter hospital stay and blood loss with the minimally invasive surgery (MIS) cohort.[31] Another systematic review noted similar results potentially favoring the minimally invasive approach, but admitted that the literature contains several different "minimally invasive" strategies, making their comparison difficult. Although some results were statistically significant, blood loss, for example, was only 20 mL less in the MIS group, questioning the clinical relevance of these differences even when present.[32] Better high-quality studies need to be performed to truly determine whether the MIS approach offers a benefit in both the short and long term.

Degenerative Spondylolisthesis

Degenerative spondylolisthesis (DS) represents an acquired form of spondylolisthesis, where one vertebra subluxates relative to an adjacent vertebra. Given that degenerative spondylolisthesis frequently leads to lumbar spinal stenosis, there is significant overlap between the two pathologies.

Spine

Epidemiology and Pathophysiology

DS, unlike LSS, exhibits specific epidemiologic characteristics. In a recent cross-sectional survey, DS at L4-L5 demonstrated approximately a 5:1 ratio of female to male. Mean age of patients demonstrating L4-L5 DS was 68 years in male and 71 years in females, and DS was rarely found in patients younger than 40 years.[33] Unlike isthmic spondylolisthesis which most frequently occurs at L5-S1, DS is most commonly found at L4-L5.

The exact causes of DS remain unknown but is likely multifactorial. Studies have demonstrated an increased incidence in patients with sagittal orientation of facets, providing a biomechanical mechanism.[34] Additionally, given that DS occurs more frequently in females, there is likely a hormonal etiology, perhaps providing greater ligamentous laxity and resulting in instability, especially in the setting of disk degeneration, and facet arthritis.

Presentation

As DS progresses, symptoms of spinal stenosis develop as previously noted. These include a combination of neurogenic claudication and radiculopathy. At L4-L5, the most common location, patients generally present with L5 symptoms, including pain and sensory changes in the posterolateral thigh and leg and into the dorsum of the foot. Motor weakness can include great toe extension, inversion and eversion of the ankle, and hip abduction. Although it is commonly believed that back pain is a common report and caused by DS, the data do not necessarily support this. In the Copenhagen Osteoarthritis Study,[33] there was no statistically significant relationship between the presence of DS and back pain, and these results were similarly noted in SPORT.

Workup

Standing AP and lateral radiographs including flexion/extension radiographs are crucial for making the proper diagnosis. DS is classified according to the Meyerding classification, which grades the percentage of anterolisthesis according to the superior end plate of the inferior vertebra and giving a grade of I-V (0% to 25%, 26% to 50%, 51% to 75%, 76% to 100% and >100%) (**Figure 4**). Most DS remains grade I with only a small percentage presenting as grade II. As in patients with LSS, MRI demonstrates the areas of compression, generally showing central and lateral recess stenosis. It is also important to look at secondary markers of instability, such as the facet orientation and fluid within the facet (**Figure 5**). A study examining MRI findings found that a facet effusion >1.5 mm is predictive of the presence of DS,

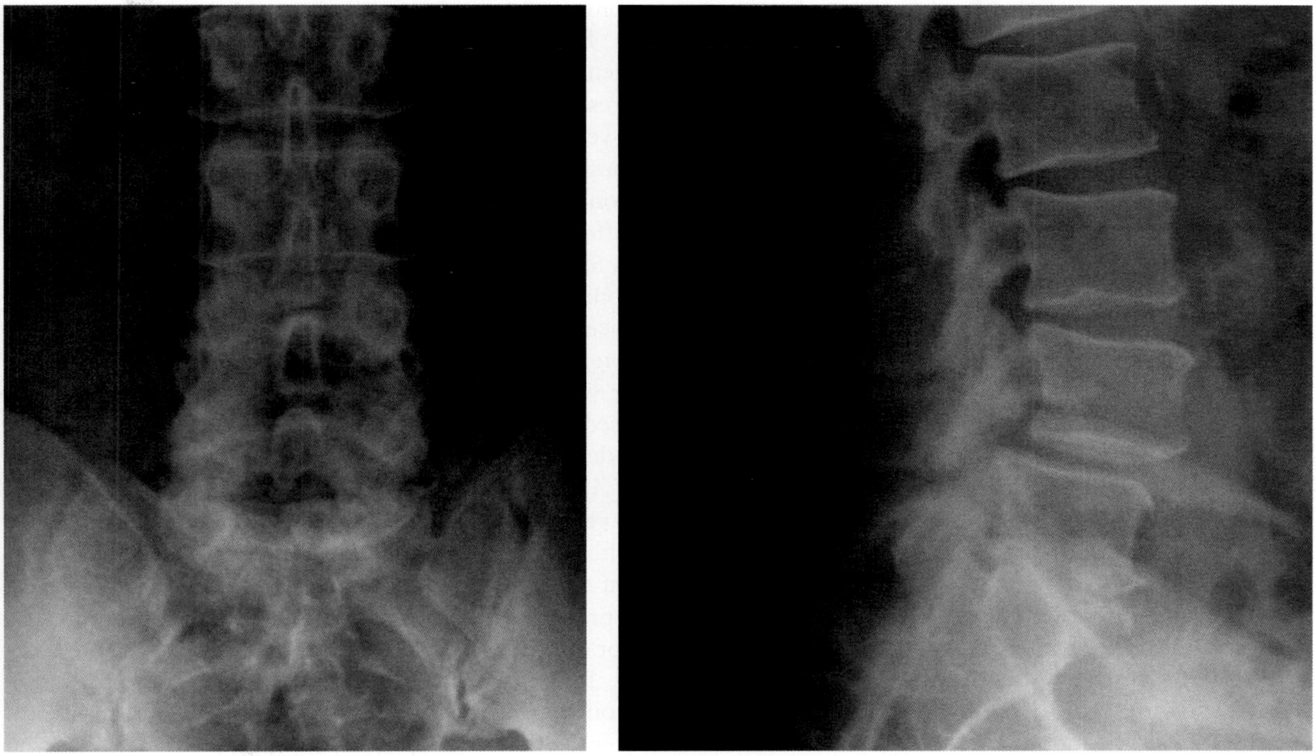

Figure 4 AP and lateral radiographs demonstrating L4-L5 grade 1 spondylolisthesis.

Spine

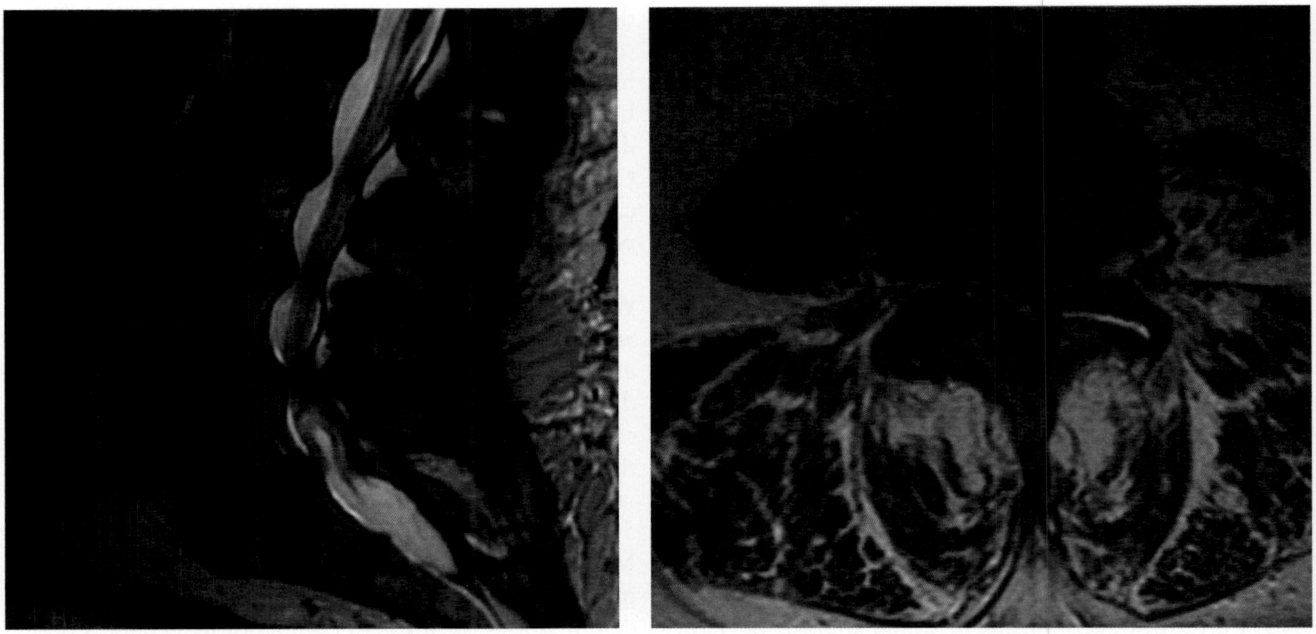

Figure 5 Sagittal and axial T2-weighted MRI scans demonstrating central and lateral recess stenosis associated with L4-L5 spondylolisthesis.

and the probability increases with increasing effusion size.[35] CT myelography remains an additional option for patients in whom MRI cannot be performed.

Nonsurgical Management

Similar to LSS, the nonsurgical modalities for DS include a combination of rest, physical therapy, medications, and injections. Although only a small percentage of patients ultimately require surgery, according to recent North American Spine Society guidelines, there remains a paucity of data to provide definitive recommendations on nonsurgical management including medical therapy and injections.[36]

Surgical Management

Surgery for DS is highly effective. Data from SPORT have demonstrated the advantage of surgery over nonsurgical management at intermediate and longer term follow-up. At 4 and 8 years, the surgical as-treated group had significant advantage in SF-36 scores and improved ODI when compared with the nonsurgical group.[37] When discussing the surgical options, several classic articles have been the foundation for recommending an open instrumented posterolateral fusion. In a prospective study of 50 patients undergoing decompression versus uninstrumented fusion, the intertransverse fusion group has significantly better back and leg pain scores.[38] A later prospective randomized study evaluating the use of instrumentation noted that the use of pedicle screws led to higher fusion rates, although the study did note no difference in clinical outcomes.[39] Follow-up of the patients in the previous two studies who underwent posterolateral uninstrumented fusion noted that the patients who achieved fusion had superior outcomes compared with those that had a nonunion.[40]

But there remains controversy over the optimal treatment for DS, and there are still proponents of decompression alone. A Canadian multicenter study analyzed 2-year outcomes in patients with a stable spondylolisthesis who underwent decompression or decompression with fusion and noted no statistically significant difference in the groups with respect to improvement in SF-36 physical component summary (PCS) score or ability to achieve minimal clinically important difference.[41] Additionally, another study described how *New England Journal of Medicine,* patients with LSS with or without DS were randomized to decompression or decompression with fusion. The fusion group had significantly higher blood loss, surgical cost, length of stay (7.4 versus 4.1 days), and longer operating time, yet at 5 years there was no difference in clinical outcome.[29] Although the authors argue that fusion confers no benefit for patients with LSS and DS, critics counter that it represents an oversimplification, because the authors do not distinguish between stable and unstable slips.

But while some data do support decompression alone in terms of equal or improved short-term outcomes, the need for revision surgery remains a concern. A retrospective study with over 10-year follow-up examining patients who underwent decompression or decompression with fusion for DS noted that revision surgery rate was significantly higher in the decompression group (28.0% versus 17.1%).[42] A recent randomized controlled trial also showed that not only did patients who underwent a fusion procedure have a clinically significant improvement in health-related quality of life (HRQOL) measures, but they had a significantly lower revision surgery rate over 4 years (34% versus 14%).[43] Of importance to note is that patients with instability (>3 mm motion) were excluded from this trial, so these were still considered relatively stable slips. At this time, the data likely still support a decompression and instrumented posterolateral fusion for the diagnosis of DS with stenosis; however, further studies need to be performed to elucidate which specific patients may benefit from decompression alone. Additionally, with an increase in minimally invasive surgical techniques and the use of interbody devices, their role in managing DS must also be further examined.

Sagittal Deformity and Degenerative Thoracolumbar Kyphosis

Adult spinal deformity (ASD) remains a challenging degenerative process that involves complex biomechanical interactions at the intersection of the rigid thoracic spine and mobile lumbar spine. Patients present with chronic back pain, spinal stenosis and neurogenic claudication, lumbar radiculopathy, and difficulty with standing upright and walking, all of which lead to major functional disability. Currently, ASD treatment begins with the assessment of pelvic parameters in conjunction with the thoracolumbar spine, representing global sagittal alignment. Sagittal imbalance is defined as a radiographic imbalance of greater than 5 cm in the sagittal plane. The major radiographic measurements evaluated for global sagittal alignment includes lumbar lordosis (LL), thoracic kyphosis (TK), sagittal vertical axis (SVA), pelvic tilt (PT), sacral slope (SS), and pelvic incidence (PI)[44] (**Figures 6** and **7**, **Table 1**).

Improving sagittal balance in ASD surgical correction is critical for achieving optimal outcomes. A recent retrospective review analyzed 47 patients 50 years of age or older with lumbar or thoracolumbar degenerative kyphosis treated with posterolateral spinal decompression and fusion with a mean follow-up of 6.4 years. They measured preoperative and postoperative PT, PI, SS, TK, LL, C7 SVA, and spinosacral angle (angle formed between the sacral tilt and C7 plumb line). There was a significant correlation with SF-36 physical component score and SS, LL, and spinosacral angle, and although ODI and Scoliosis Research Society (SRS) 30-Item Instrument were not significantly correlated, these values noted mild to moderate disability at final follow-up.[45]

Classification of Thoracolumbar Deformity in ASD

Given the multiple radiographic components that affect ASD, the classification of ASD requires assessment beyond LL and TK. The SRS-Schwab classification reliably describes the spinopelvic measurements and its importance in global sagittal alignment.

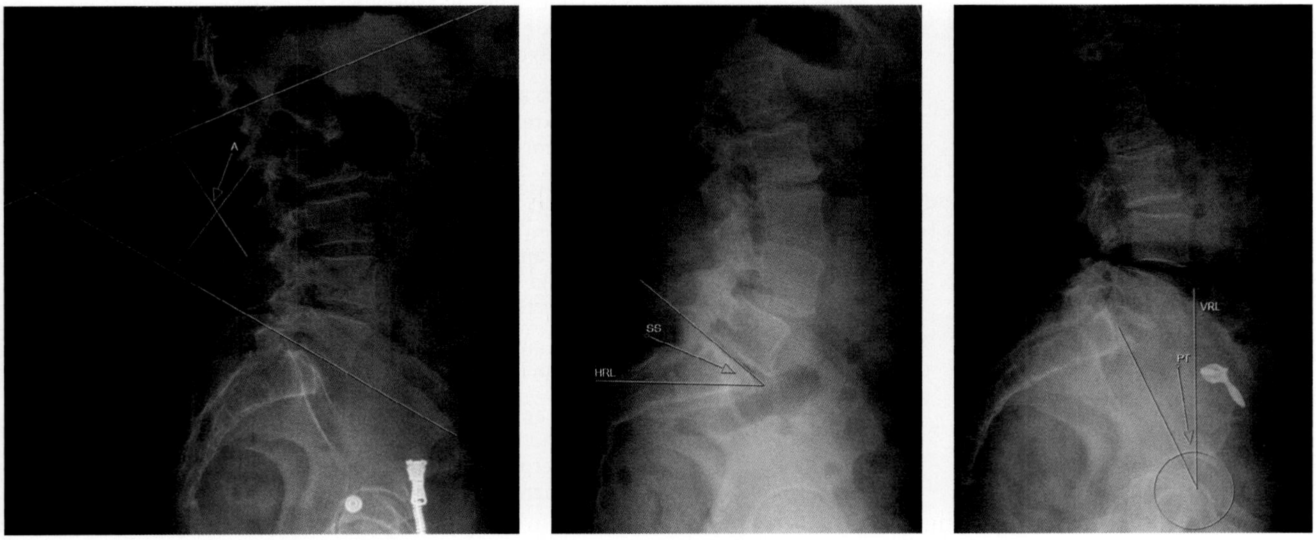

Figure 6 Radiographs of methods of calculating lumbar lordosis (left), sacral slope (middle), and pelvic tilt (right).

Spine

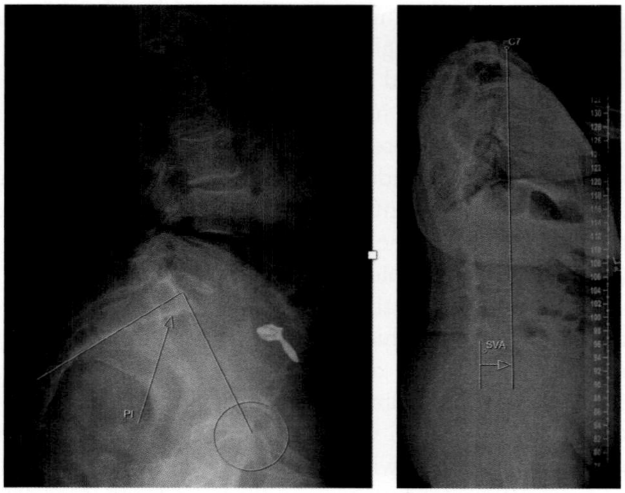

Figure 7 Radiographs of methods of calculating pelvic incidence (left) and sagittal vertical axis (right).

This schema requires full-length standing AP and lateral spine radiographs that include the femoral heads. The curve type is first defined based on Cobb angle measurement in the coronal plane. A sagittal modifier is added based upon the PI-LL mismatch. Global alignment is scored based upon the SVA. Finally, compensation is determined by calculating PT.[46]

The SRS-Schwab classification has shown significant value due to its reliability and clinical application.[47] Most important, a study prospectively compared 164 nonsurgical and 177 surgical patients with ASD utilizing the SRS-Schwab classification in assessment of baseline and 1-year follow-up radiographs and correlated parameters to HRQOL measures. Patients with improved sagittal modifiers were significantly more likely to achieve minimal clinically important difference for ODI, SF-36 physical component score (SVA and PI-LL only), SRS activity, and SRS pain (PI-LL only).[48]

Ankylosing Spondylitis in Thoracolumbar Deformity

Ankylosing spondylitis (AS) is a systemic inflammatory condition with spondyloarthropathy that affects the axial skeleton and can be a challenging disease process to manage in patients with ASD. The erosion of spinal apophyseal and sacroiliac joints with subsequent ossification of the surrounding soft tissues creates a rigid yet brittle spinal column.[49] With the progression of AS, the fixed rigidity of the thoracolumbar spine leads to severe kyphosis and a downward tilt of the head and neck, resulting in pain and difficulty with horizontal gaze.

Sagittal alignment in patients with AS with thoracolumbar kyphosis affects the quality of life and clinical outcomes following correction. One hundred seven patients with AS with thoracolumbar deformity were divided into two groups (moderate or severe deformity)

Table 1

Definition of Major Radiographic Measurements for Global Sagittal Alignment

Name	Abbreviation	Units of Measurement	Definition
Lumbar lordosis	LL	Degrees	Cobb angle measurement of the angle between extension line of boundary of the first and fifth lumbar vertebral body.
Thoracic kyphosis	TK	Degrees	Cobb angle measurement and the angle between extension line of boundary of the 1st and 12th thoracic vertebral body.
Sagittal vertical axis	SVA	Centimeters	Sagittal offset of a plumb line dropped from the C7 vertebral body from the posterosuperior corner of S1.
Pelvic tilt	PT	Degrees	The angle between the line joining the femoral heads and the center of the S1 end plate and the reference vertical line.
Sacral slope	SS	Degrees	The angle between the line along the S1 end plate and the reference horizontal line.
Pelvic incidence	PI	Degrees	The angle between the line joining the femoral heads and the center of the S1 end plate and the line perpendicular to the S1 end plate. The summation of sacral slope and pelvic tilt (SS + PT = PI).

based on a kyphosis cutoff of 70° and the authors correlated SVA, sacrospinal angle (SSA), and T1 pelvic angle (TPA) to ODI and SF-36 physical component and mental component summary scores. All of these parameters correlated significantly with ODI and SF-36 physical component summary scores, and they increased proportionally with increased degree of deformity.[50]

Management Considerations

Determining the appropriate management options for thoracolumbar deformity requires meticulous assessment of preoperative radiographs in conjunction with the presenting complaints. Accurate definition of ASD via SRS-Schwab classification has been shown to define thresholds for determining surgical and nonsurgical management. A prospective multicenter study looking at 492 consecutive ASD patients correlated PT, PI-LL mismatch, and SVA with HRQOL measures. The threshold values for severe disability by ODI (>40) correlated to a PT greater than 22, SVA greater than 4.7 cm, and PI-LL mismatch greater than 11° and helps guide treatment strategy.[51]

Complications

It is important to recognize that spinal deformity reconstruction can have major postoperative complications, including proximal junctional failure, instrumentation failure, and common perioperative problems including wound complications, neurologic dysfunction, and significant blood loss. In one review of 291 patients with ASD correction, there was a 52% overall complication rate, with the most common complications being implant failure (27.8%), neurologic (27.8%), cardiopulmonary (18.9%), and infectious/wound complications (14.8%) with age 65 years and older ($P = 0.009$), prior spinal fusion ($P < 0.007$), elevated BMI ($P < 0.031$), and three-column osteotomy ($P = 0.036$) as significant risk factors.[52]

Summary

Thoracolumbar degenerative conditions present with various patterns of patient disability. Although the surgical treatment of common pathologies, including lumbar spinal stenosis and degenerative spinal stenosis, result in predictable good outcomes, there remains much research to be done to further optimize outcomes and determine the best treatment strategy for individual patterns of instability. The role of novel minimally invasive strategies for decompression, fusion, and deformity correction remain to be fully elucidated, and better high-level studies are required.

Key Study Points

- Lumbar decompression remains the benchmark for patients with LSS, and there is no benefit to routinely performing fusion.
- The complication rate for patients undergoing adult spinal deformity surgery is high, and patients should be counseled on their risk for short- and long-term complications and need for potential revision surgery.
- Additional studies are required to elucidate which patients with degenerative spondylolisthesis can undergo a decompression only, which require a fusion, and which can benefit from interbody fusion.

Spine

Annotated References

1. Andersson GB: Epidemiological features of chronic low-back pain. *Lancet* 1999;354(9178):581-585.
2. Guo HR, Tenaka S, Haperin WE, Cameron LL: Back pain prevalence in US industry and estimates of lost workdays. *Am J Public Health* 1999;89(7):L1029-L1035.
3. Katz JN: Lumbar disc disorders and low-back pain: Socioeconomic factors and consequences. *J Bone Joint Surg Am* 2006;88(suppl 2):21-24.
4. Boden SD, Davis DO, Dina TS, Patronas NJ, Wiesel SW: Abnormal magnetic-resonance scans of the lumbar spine in asymptomatic subjects. A prospective investigation. *J Bone Joint Surg Am* 1990;72(3):403-408.
5. Borsenstein DG, O'Mara JW Jr, Boden SD, et al: The value of magnetic resonance imaging of the lumbar spine to predict low-back pain in asymptomatic subjects: A seven-year follow-up study. *J Bone Joint Surg Am* 2001;83-A(9):1306-1311.
6. Cuellar JM, Stauff MP, Herzog RJ, Carrino JA, Baker GA, Carragee EJ: Does provocative discography cause clinically important injury to the lumbar intervertebral disc? A 10-year matched cohort study. *Spine J* 2016;16(3):273-280.

   A prospective, 10-year matched cohort study evaluated the effects of lumbar diskography, related to surgical intervention, low back pain, disability, and medical visits.
7. Jacobs WC, van der Gaag NA, Kruyt MD, et al: Total disc replacement for chronic discogenic low back pain: A Cochrane review. *Spine* 2013;38(1):24-36.
8. Furunes H, Storheim K, Brox JI, et al: Total disc replacement versus multidisciplinary rehabilitation in patients with chronic low back pain and degenerative discs: 8-year follow-up of a randomized controlled multicenter trial. *Spine J* 2017;17(10):1480-1488.

   This multicenter, prospective randomized controlled trial evaluated outcomes of total disk replacement versus multidisciplinary rehabilitation for low back pain and disk degeneration.

9. Rihn JA, Radcliff K, Norvell DC, et al: Comparative effectiveness of treatments for chronic low back pain: A multiple treatment comparison analysis. *Clin Spine Surg* 2017;30(5):204-225.

   A systematic review of randomized controlled trials evaluating treatment options for chronic low back pain is presented. The studies included total disk replacement, fusion, and various forms of multimodal rehabilitation regimens. Outcomes were pre- and posttreatment ODI, back pain, additional surgeries, and complications.

10. Wu W, Liang J, Chen Y, Chen A, Wu B, Yang Z: Microstructural changes in compressed nerve roots treated by percutaneous transforaminal endoscopic discectomy in patients with lumbar disc herniation. *Medicine* 2016;95(40):e5106.

   This prospective cohort study used diffusion tensor imaging on MRI to evaluate molecular diffusion and microstructural changes in nerve roots affected by lumbar disk herniation.

11. Takahashi N, Kikuchi S, Shubayev VI, Campana WM, Myers RR: TNF-alpha and phosphorylation of ERK in DRG and spinal cord: Insights into mechanisms of sciatica. *Spine* 2006;31(5):523-529.
12. Saal JA, Saal JS. Nonoperative treatment of herniated lumbar intervertebral disc with radiculopathy. An outcome study. *Spine* 1989;14(4):431-437.
13. Weber H: Lumbar disc herniation. A controlled, prospective study with ten years of observation. *Spine* 1983;8(2):131-140.
14. Atlas SJ, Keller RB, Wu YA, Deyo RA, Singer DE: Long-term outcomes of surgical and nonsurgical management of sciatica secondary to a lumbar disc herniation: 10 year results from the maine lumbar spine study. *Spine* 2005;30(8):927-935.
15. Leven D, Passias PG, Errico TJ, et al: Risk factors for reoperation in patients treated surgically for intervertebral disc herniation: A subanalysis of eight-year SPORT data. *J Bone Joint Surg Am* 2015;97(16):1316-1325.
16. Pearson A, Lurie J, Tosteson T, et al: Who should have surgery for an intervertebral disc herniation? Comparative effectiveness evidence from the spine patient outcomes research trial. *Spine* 2012;37(2):140-149.
17. Koerner JD, Glaser J, Radcliff K: Which variables are associated with patient-reported outcomes after discectomy? Review of SPORT disc herniation studies. *Clin Orthop* 2015;473(6):2000-2006.
18. Schoenfeld AJ, Bono CM: Does surgical timing influence functional recovery after lumbar discectomy? A systematic review. *Clin Orthop* 2015;473(6):1963-1970.
19. Rihn JA, Hilibrand AS, Radcliff K, et al: Duration of symptoms resulting from lumbar disc herniation: Effect on treatment outcomes: Analysis of the spine patient outcomes research trial (SPORT). *J Bone Joint Surg Am* 2011;93(20):1906-1914.
20. Fritzell P, Knutsson B, Sanden B, Strömqvist B, Hägg O: Recurrent versus primary lumbar disc herniation surgery: Patient-reported outcomes in the Swedish Spine Register Swespine. *Clin Orthop* 2015;473(6):1978-1984.
21. Deyo RA, Gray DT, Kreuter W, Mirza S, Martin BI: United States trends in lumbar fusion surgery for degenerative conditions. *Spine* 2005;30:1441-1445.
22. Kalichman L, Cole R, Kim DH, et al: Spinal stenosis prevalence and association with symptoms: The Framingham Study. *Spine J* 2009;9(7):545-550.
23. Amundsen T, Weber H, Lilleås F, Nordal HJ, Abdelnoor M, Magnaes B: Lumbar spinal stenosis. Clinical and radiologic features. *Spine* 1995;20:1178-1186.
24. Weinstein JN, Tosteson TD, Lurie JD, et al: Surgical versus nonsurgical therapy for lumbar spinal stenosis. *N Engl J Med* 2008;358(8):794-810.
25. Orita S, Yamashita M, Eguchi Y, et al: Pregabalin for refractory radicular leg pain due to lumbar spinal stenosis: A preliminary prospective study. *Pain Res Manag* 2016;2016:10.

   A prospective observational study in 104 patients with LSS and intermittent neurogenic claudication refractory to NSAIDs were treated with pregabalin and demonstrated a tendency toward improved walking distance, although not statistically significant.

26. Ammendolia C, Cote P, Southerst D, et al: Comprehensive nonsurgical treatment versus self-directed care to improve walking ability in lumbar spinal stenosis: A randomized trial. *Arch Phys Med Rehabil* 2018;99(12):2408-2419. [Epub Ahead of Print].

   This was a randomized controlled trial comparing self-directed therapy and structures physical therapy in patients with lumbar spinal stenosis. The structured cohort had improved HRQOL measures and walking distance.

27. Weinstein JN, Tosteson TD, Lurie JD, et al: Surgical versus nonoperative treatment for lumbar spinal stenosis four-year results of the Spine Patient Outcomes Research Trial. *Spine* 2010;35(14):1329-1338.
28. Lurie JD, Tosteson TD, Tosteson A, et al: Long-term outcomes of lumbar spinal stenosis: Eight-year results of the Spine Patient Outcomes Research Trial (SPORT). *Spine* 2015;40(2):63-76.
29. Forsth P, Ólafsson G, Carlsson T, et al: A randomized controlled trial of fusion surgery for lumbar spinal stenosis. *N Eng J Med* 2016;374:1414-1423.

   This is a randomized controlled trial of patients with LSS with or without DS who were randomized to undergo decompression alone or decompression plus fusion. At 2 and 5 years, HRQOL measures and results of a walking test were similar.

30. Yavin D, Casha S, Wiebe S, et al: Lumbar fusion for degenerative disc disease. A systematic review and meta-analysis. *Neurosurgery* 2017;80:701-715.

   A meta-analysis of studies reporting on patients who underwent decompression or decompression plus fusion demonstrated no benefit to fusion in the lumbar spinal stenosis cohort is presented.

31. Chang F, Zhang T, Gao G: Comparison of the minimally invasive and conventional open surgery approach in the treatment of lumbar stenosis: A systematic review and a meta-analysis. *Ann Acad Med Singapore* 2017;46:124-137.

A literature review comparing patients undergoing open versus minimally invasive surgery for LSS demonstrated comparable clinical outcomes, but the minimally invasive group has less blood loss, shorter hospital stay, and less back pain.

32. Ng KKM, Cheung JPY: Is minimally invasive surgery superior to open surgery for treatment of lumbar spinal stenosis? A systematic review. *J Orthop Surg* 2017;25(2):1-11.

A systematic review comparing open versus minimally invasive surgery for LSS concluded that there is no conclusive evidence that MIS approaches reduce revision surgery or demonstrates improved HRQOL scores when compared with open surgery.

33. Jacobsen S, Sonne-Holm S, Rovsing H, Monrad H, Gebuhr P: Degenerative lumbar spondylolisthesis: An epidemiological perspective. The Copenhagen Osteoarthritis Study. *Spine* 2007;32(1):120-125.

34. DeVine JG, Schenk-Kisser JM, Skelly AC: Risk factors for degenerative spondylolisthesis: A systematic review. *Evid Based Spine Care J* 2012;3(2):25-34.

35. Chaput C, Padon D, Rush J, Lenehan E, Rahm M: The significance of increased fluid signal on magnetic resonance imaging in lumbar facets in relationship to degenerative spondylolisthesis. *Spine* 2007;32(17):1883-1887.

36. Matz PG, Meagher RJ, Lamer T, et al: Guideline summary review: An evidence-based clinical guideline for the diagnosis and treatment of degenerative lumbar spondylolisthesis. *Spine J* 2016;16(3):439-448.

This is a summary of evidence-based guidelines published by the North American Spine Society. After review of available evidence, it was concluded that there is a paucity of high-quality evidence to allow for specific nonsurgical recommendations.

37. Abdu WA, Sacks OA, Tosteson ANA, et al: Long-term results of surgery compared with nonoperative treatment for lumbar degenerative spondylolisthesis in the Spine Patient Outcomes Research Trial (SPORT). *Spine (Phila Pa 1976)* 2018;43(23):1619-1630. [Epub Ahead of Print].

This article discusses the 8-year outcomes of SPORT and supports the long-term benefit of surgery over nonsurgical treatment. Level of evidence: I.

38. Herkowitz HN, Kurz LT: Degenerative lumbar spondylolisthesis with spinal stenosis: A prospective study comparing decompression with decompression and intertransverse process arthrodesis. *J Bone Joint Surg Am* 1991;73:802-808.

39. Fischgrund JS, Mackay M, Herkowitz HN, et al: Degenerative lumbar spondylolisthesis with spinal stenosis: A prospective, randomized study comparing decompressive laminectomy and arthrodesis with and without spinal instrumentation. *Spine* 1997;22:2807-2812.

40. Kornblum MB, Fischgrund JS, Herkowitz HN, Abraham DA, Berkower DL, Ditkoff JS: Degenerative lumbar spondylolisthesis with spinal stenosis: A prospective long-term study comparing fusion and pseudarthrosis. *Spine* 2004;29:726-733.

41. Rampersaud YR, Fisher C, Yee A, et al: Health-related quality of life following decompression compared to decompression and fusion for degenerative lumbar spondylolisthesis: A Canadian multicentre study. *Can J Surg* 2014;57(4):E126-E133.

42. Martin BI, Mirza SK, Comstock BA, Gray DT, Kreuter W, Deyo RA: Reoperation rates following lumbar spine surgery and the influence of spinal fusion procedures. *Spine* 2007;32:382-387.

43. Ghogawala Z, Dziura J, Butler W, et al: Laminectomy plus fusion versus laminectomy alone for lumbar spondylolisthesis. *N Engl J Med* 2016;374:1424-1434.

This randomized controlled trial of decompression versus decompression plus fusion for patients with stable grade 1 spondylolisthesis demonstrated improved outcomes in patients who underwent fusion.

44. Vrtovec T, Janssen MMA, Likar B, Castelein RM, Viergever MA, Pernuš F: A review of methods for evaluating the quantitative parameters of sagittal pelvic alignment. *Spine J* 2012;12(5):433-446.

45. Simon J, Longis PM, Passuti N: Correlation between radiographic parameters and functional scores in degenerative lumbar and thoracolumbar scoliosis. *Orthop Traumatol Surg Res* 2017;103(2):285-290.

A single-center retrospective study included 47 patients older than 50 years who had degenerative lumbar scoliosis treated with an instrumented posterolateral fusion and looked at radiographic parameters and functional scores with a mean follow-up of 6.4 years.

46. Bess S, Schwab F, Lafage V, Shaffrey CI, Ames CP: Classifications for adult spinal deformity and use of the Scoliosis Research Society-Schwab Adult Spinal Deformity Classification. *Neurosurg Clin N Am* 2013;24(2):185-193.

47. Schwab F, Ungar B, Blondel B, et al: Scoliosis Research Society-Schwab adult spinal deformity classification: A validation study. *Spine* 2012;37(12):1077-1082.

48. Smith JS, Kilneberg E, Schwab F, et al: Change in classification grade by the SRS-Schwab Adult Spinal Deformity Classification predicts impact on health-related quality of life measures: Prospective analysis of operative and nonoperative treatment. *Spine* 2013;38(19):1663-1671.

49. Braun J, Sieper J: Ankylosing spondylitis. *Lancet* 2007;369(957):1379-1390.

50. Yılmaz O, Tutoğlu A, Garip Y, Ozcan E, Bodur H: Health-related quality of life in Turkish patients with ankylosing spondylitis: Impact of peripheral involvement on quality of life in terms of disease activity, functional status, severity of pain, and social and emotional functioning. *Rheumatol Int* 2013;33(5):1159-1163.

51. Schwab F, Blondel B, Bess S: Radiographical spinopelvic parameters and disability in the setting of adult spinal deformity: A prospective multicenter analysis. *Spine* 2013;38(13):E803-E812.

52. Smith JS, Klineberg E, Lafage V, et al: Prospective multicenter assessment of perioperative and minimum 2-year postoperative complication rates associated with adult spinal deformity surgery. *J Neurosurg Spine* 2016;25(1):1-14.

This prospective multicenter study assesses the rates of complications associated with surgery for ASD with a minimum 2-year follow-up.

Chapter 50

Thoracolumbar Minimally Invasive Surgical Techniques

Don Young Park, MD • Kirkham Wood, MD • Ning Liu, MD

ABSTRACT

Minimally invasive techniques have developed and evolved to become an important aspect of modern spine surgery. From percutaneous pedicle screw placement, kyphoplasty/vertebroplasty, lumbar interbody fusion techniques, spinal deformity, to computer-assisted navigation and robotic surgery, minimally invasive spine surgery has wide-ranging applications with increasing utilization and popularity. This chapter reviews the relevant scientific literature currently available regarding these techniques.

Keywords: computer-assisted navigation; image-guided surgery; kyphoplasty; minimally invasive lumbar fusion; minimally invasive spine surgery; MIS spinal deformity; percutaneous pedicle screw fixation; vertebroplasty

Introduction

Minimally invasive surgery (MIS) techniques are well established in spine surgery and are now widely adopted. Once considered outside the mainstream, MIS techniques are an important part of the surgical armamentarium for spine surgeons today. Whether by consumer-directed or industry-based marketing, minimally invasive spine surgery is now highly sought after by many patients to address their spine pathology because of the commonly held perception that smaller incisions lead to better surgery. Today's patients expect successful surgery to include resolution of pain and symptoms with less postoperative pain, short or no hospital stay, a quick recovery, and rehabilitation that is the least disruptive to their lives.[1] The reality of MIS techniques is that it can be technically difficult with a steep learning curve from the limited surgical exposure. This chapter will review the MIS surgical techniques as applied to the thoracolumbar spine.

A wide spectrum of MIS strategies is used with spine surgery, from mini-open, tubular, expandable, and percutaneous techniques (**Figure 1**). The main strategy is to limit the damage caused by surgical dissection by taking advantage of narrow surgical corridors to accomplish the goals of surgery. Because the surgical exposure is limited, the surgeon must use visual cues from radiographic imaging to successfully perform surgery, thereby increasing the radiation exposure to the surgeon, OR staff, and the patient. This requires a mastery of the three-dimensional anatomy of the spine and being able to translate the radiographic information to the spine to avoid neurological injury and complications. Not only is radiation exposure an issue, but also increased surgical times has been associated with MIS techniques, especially during the learning curve of the procedure. The various MIS techniques used in spine surgery will be reviewed in this chapter.

Percutaneous Pedicle Screw Fixation

Pedicle screw fixation is the mainstay for fixation in the thoracolumbar spine because of the pedicle screw providing biomechanical fixation and stability in all three vertebral columns.[2] The open technique of pedicle screw placement requires full exposure of the bony landmarks, including the transverse process, facet joint, and the pars interarticularis to identify the start point for pedicle screw placement. The open exposure strips the paraspinal musculature off the spine, leading to denervation, devascularization, and ultimately muscle atrophy that may lead to late-onset pain and dysfunction despite a successful fusion.[3,4] In addition,

Dr. Park or an immediate family member serves as a paid consultant to or is an employee of Globus Medical, Nuvasive, and Stryker. Dr. Wood has received royalties from Globus Medical; serves as a paid consultant to or is an employee of Alphatec Spine; and has stock or stock options held in TranS1. Neither Dr. Liu nor any immediate family member has received anything of value from or has stock or stock options held in a commercial company or institution related directly or indirectly to the subject of this chapter.

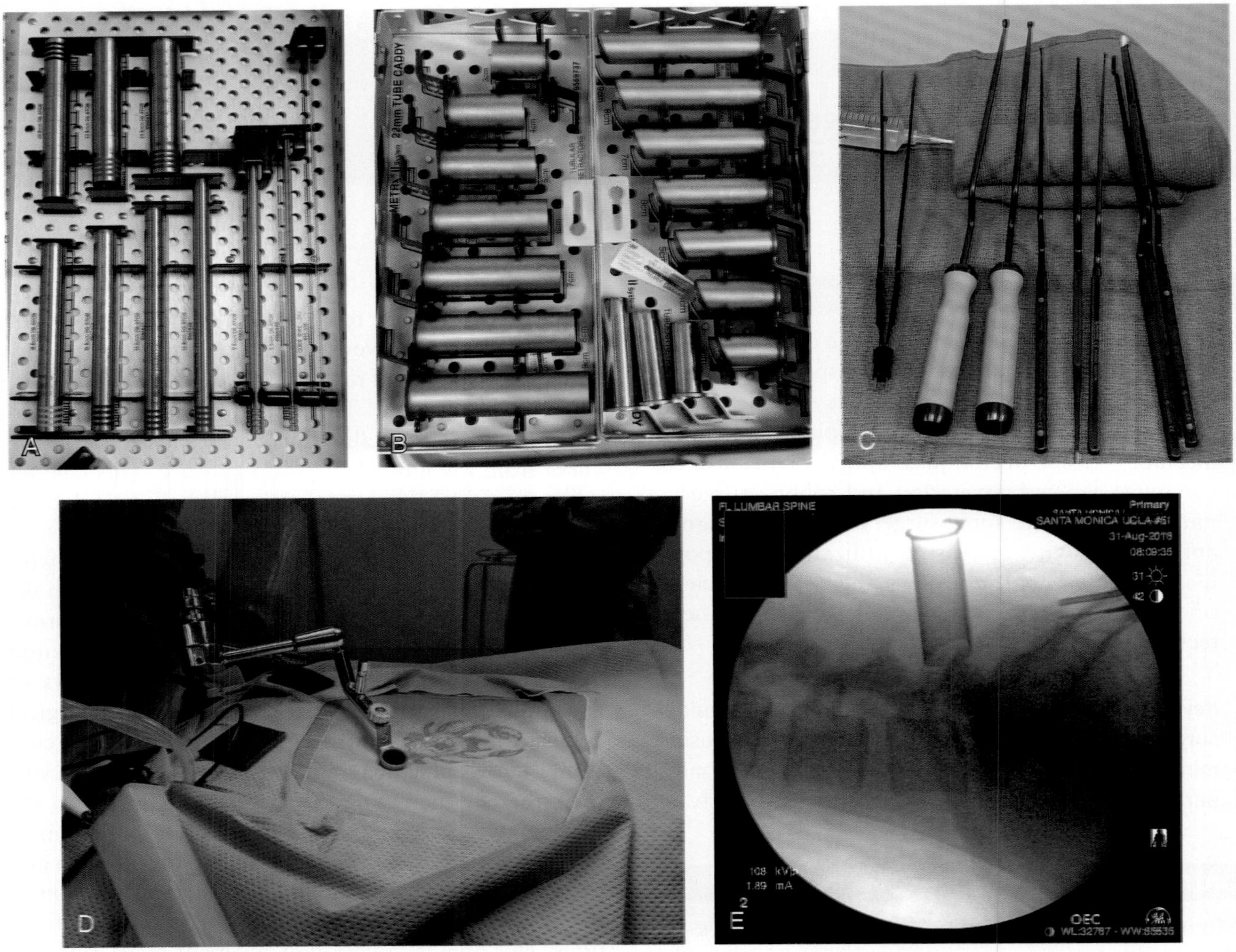

Figure 1 A, Picture of sequential dilators. **B**, Picture of tubular retractors. **C**, Picture of specialized instruments for use with tubular retractors. **D**, Picture of the locking articulating arm attached to the OR table and tubular retractor. **E**, Fluoroscopy image with tubular retractor in place.

prolonged paraspinal muscle retraction greater than 60 minutes can produce muscle necrosis and neuromuscular degeneration, which can lead to increased pain and disability.[5]

Percutaneous techniques in pedicle screw placement use a muscle splitting approach to prevent detachment of the paraspinal muscles off the spine and reduce the muscle injury from retraction. Radiographic guidance with fluoroscopy allows the surgeon to determine the starting point for the pedicle. 1 to 1.5 cm Wiltse type incisions are made on each side for each level and a muscle-splitting approach is used. Cannulated Jamshidi needles are used to create a path through the pedicle and into the vertebral body (**Figure 2**). Guidewires are placed through the cannulated Jamshidi needles, and tubular retractors are placed using the guidewires to retract the paraspinal muscles directly at the site of the pedicle screw insertion. This technique preserves the motor nerve to the multifidus muscle 80% of the time in cadaveric studies, as compared with transection of the nerve 84% of the time with the open technique.[3] The largest study to date evaluating the placement of over 2000 percutaneous pedicle screws demonstrated a pedicle breach rate of 9.4% with the majority of these measuring <2 mm.[6] The percutaneous pedicle screw technique is accurate and versatile and can be used as a strategy for three-column vertebral fixation in many clinical scenarios including degenerative, spinal deformity, trauma, and tumor cases.

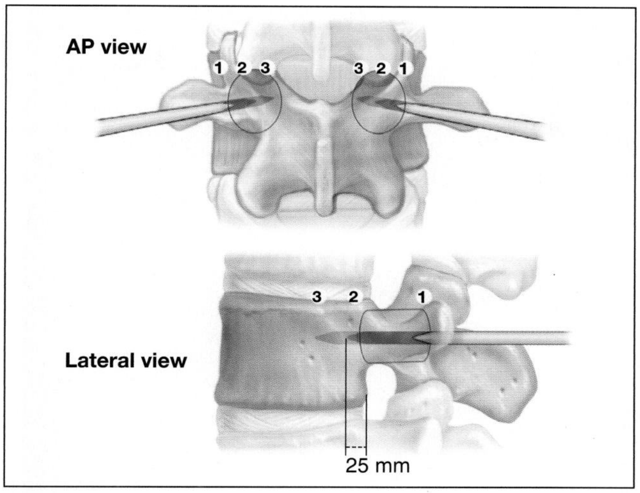

Figure 2 Illustration of the percutaneous pedicle screw technique. Placement of the Jamshidi needle at the 3-o'clock and 9-o'clock positions of the lateral border of the pedicle. The Jamshidi needle is impacted from the lateral border to the midpoint of the pedicle, taking care not to breach the medial border.

Pedicle Screw Fixation in Thoracolumbar Trauma

More than 60% of spine trauma cases are thoracolumbar fractures. In recent years, MIS has been used increasingly and frequently in this setting, especially for cases without neurological deficits. The primary aim of MIS in this setting is to restore segmental stability and spinal alignment while reducing the "approach-related" morbidities associated with open procedures and the long-term sequelae of fusions.

The first long-term (5-year) follow-up study of percutaneous pedicle screw fixation (PPSF) retrospectively compared the outcomes of PPSF (10 patients) and open surgery (11 patients) in thoracolumbar fracture cases.[7] At follow-up, although patient functional scores such as the SF-36 did not significantly differ between groups, nor the loss of correction over time with implant removal, the average blood loss in the MIS group was significantly lower than that in the open group (155.6 vs 194.4 mL). A prospective RCT examined the efficacy of PPSF compared with the paraspinal approach—an open albeit relatively less-invasive procedure—in 61 unstable thoracolumbar burst fracture patients without neurological deficit but with posterior ligamentous complex injury.[8] Again, although the two groups had similar back pain VAS and Oswestry Disability Index (ODI) scores at 3-year follow-up, and much less blood loss (79.0 vs 149.0 mL), PPSF did not correct the local kyphotic angle postoperatively as compared with the open paraspinal approach (0.39° vs 9.25°) and was also associated with a greater average degree of correction loss (3.35° vs 2.33°) at final follow-up. The authors, therefore, suggested using PPSF cautiously with ligamentous disruption, or when a postural reduction of fracture is not achievable during the operation. Another group compared PPSF (11 patients) and open surgery (10 patients) in single-level thoracolumbar burst fractures (**Figure 3**) and found that, although the ultimate degree of kyphosis, as well as postoperative improvement, did not significantly differ between the two techniques, patients treated with PPSF had significantly lower ODI scores than those treated with open surgeries (4 points vs 14 points), both before implant removal and at final follow-up.[9]

What seems certain is that, clinically, PPSF is almost consistently associated with less blood loss, lower infection rates, earlier mobilization, and in many cases, a faster return to work.[10] Patient-reported functional scores and radiographic analysis, however, vary, and overall, do not appear dramatically different between open and MIS approaches. The risk and complications of PPSF appear to be more related to the instrumentation per se—screw misplacement with an incidence between 6.6% and 9.7% in a variety of spinal pathologies treated with MIS— than the traumatic nature of spine fractures.[11,12]

In practice, it is now generally recommended that in thoracolumbar fracture patients without neurological deficits even with mild posterior ligamentous injury, PPSF without fusion can be considered if local instability is determined or nonsurgical treatments are not practically feasible.[11] In patients with significant posterior ligamentous disruption and/or significant deformity, however, a more invasive surgical strategy, either open surgery or PPSF combined with another approach, often with fusion, may be needed. Either way, the fundamental goals of treatment—to reestablish segmental stability and restore spinal alignment—remain the same and the surgical strategy selected is dependent upon the surgeon's experience and preference.

Kyphoplasty and Vertebroplasty

Cement augmentation procedures such as kyphoplasty and vertebroplasty are commonly used to treat painful osteoporotic vertebral compression fractures (VCFs) and metastatic spine lesions. Most osteoporotic VCFs improve over 6 to 8 weeks after injury. However, some patients are afflicted with severe pain and disability that limits early mobilization. In these cases, polymethylmethacrylate (PMMA) cement can be percutaneously introduced into the vertebral body through minimally invasive techniques that are very

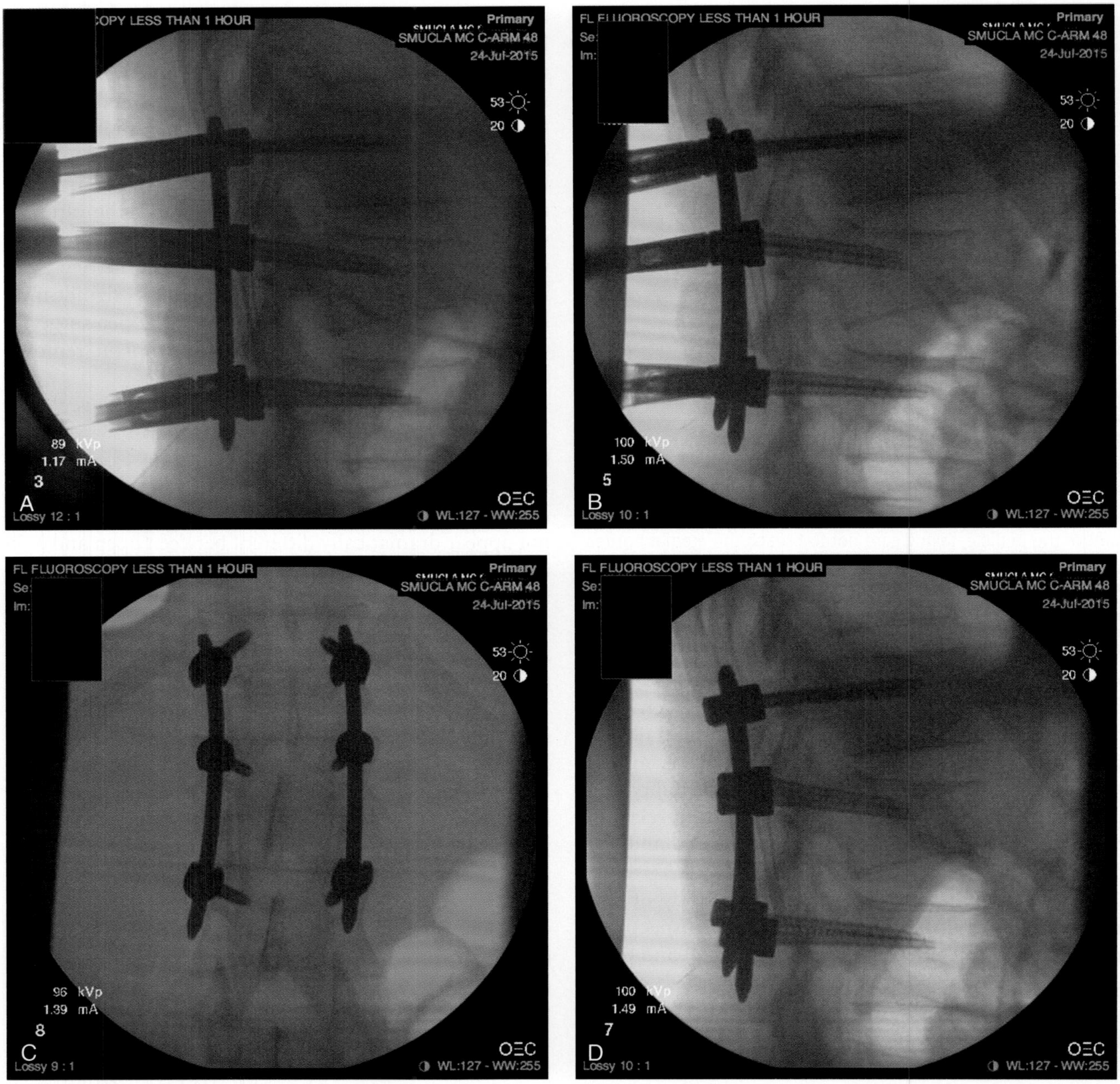

Figure 3 Percutaneous pedicle screw fixation for thoracolumbar trauma. **A**, Lateral fluoroscopy image showing pedicle screw placement before reduction. **B**, Lateral fluoroscopy image showing pedicle screw placement after reduction. **C**, AP fluoroscopy image after final placement of all implants. **D**, Lateral fluoroscopy image after final placement of all implants.

similar to the percutaneous pedicle screw technique.[13] 2 to 3 mm incisions are made using fluoroscopic guidance, and Jamshidi needles are percutaneously impacted into the pedicles and posterior aspect of the vertebral body. Kyphoplasty involves introducing a balloon that is inflated with radiopaque contrast to create a void within the vertebral body and to help reduce the fracture, thereby improving the fracture morphology and alignment. PMMA cement is then injected into the bony void under low pressure. In contrast, vertebroplasty involves injecting PMMA cement into the vertebral body under higher pressure to fill the bony interstices. Complication rates are reported to be less than 1% and most commonly involve cement extravasation and infection.[13] Neurological injury from cement leakage into the spinal canal is rare, as are cement embolism into the lungs. A recent meta-analysis demonstrated no difference in adjacent vertebral fractures with cement augmentation as compared with conservative treatment.[14]

The scientific evidence on vertebroplasty has been mixed and highly controversial, starting with two double-blinded randomized clinical trials by Buchbinder et al and Kallmes et al that were published by the *New England Journal of Medicine* with much publicity.[15,16] These RCTs compared vertebroplasty to sham procedure and demonstrated no difference in pain or disability. These studies included a heterogenous patient population with subacute and chronic VCFs, which biases the results because of the favorable natural history of VCFs. In contrast, RCTs that compared vertebroplasty with standard medical management demonstrated greater pain reduction with vertebroplasty that was sustained through the short term.[17,18] These studies were not blinded, however, leading to questions of a possible placebo effect confounding the results. A recent Cochrane review concluded that the use of vertebroplasty in osteoporotic VCFs was not supported based on the available high to moderate quality evidence with no clinical benefit seen when compared with sham procedure or when performed in the acute period <6 weeks from onset.[19] In addition, sensitivity analyses demonstrated that the trials comparing vertebroplasty with medical management were likely overestimating the actual clinical benefit. The evidence for kyphoplasty is even less robust than vertebroplasty with only one large multicenter RCT demonstrating significant pain reduction and disability with kyphoplasty when compared with medical management that was sustained up to 2 years follow-up.[20] A recent meta-analysis found that both kyphoplasty and vertebroplasty were efficacious in pain relief and functional improvement and kyphoplasty was superior in pain relief in the short term with better improvement in kyphotic angles.[21] Taken together, the scientific evidence demonstrates that cement augmentation procedures are efficacious and safe for a select population of patients with osteoporotic VCFs afflicted with severe pain and disability during the acute period.

Lateral/Oblique Lumbar Interbody Fusion

With the advent of the lateral lumbar interbody fusion (LLIF) technique, spine surgeons have the opportunity to access the anterior column of the spine from T12 to L5, which previously required an anterior approach with a vascular access surgeon.[22,23] A wide array of pathology can be addressed with the LLIF technique, including degenerative spondylolisthesis, trauma, and adult spinal deformity. Limitations of the technique are due to the position and relationship with the iliac crest to the disk space, morphology and location of the iliopsoas musculature, and the position of the femoral nerve and lumbar plexus relative to the disk space, specifically at L4-5. Triggered EMG neuromonitoring can reduce the approach-related morbidity such as femoral nerve and lumbar plexus injury. Specialized curved instruments and equipment can aid in performing the diskectomy and end plate preparation to accomplish successful fusion.

However, the L5-S1 disk space is not accessible with the lateral approach and generally requires an anterior approach because of the anatomic relationship of the iliac vasculature and the iliac crests. In addition, extensive retroperitoneal scarring from prior surgery and transitional anatomy in which anterior psoas and lumbar plexus drift may preclude the LLIF technique to access the disk space safely. Neurological injury to the lumbar plexus and complications related to the psoas dissection can occur, especially at the L4-5 level where the femoral nerve and lumbar plexus is typically adjacent to the midpoint of the lateral disk space. Thigh paresthesias, dysethesias, numbness, and hip flexor weakness can occur up to 23.7% to 30% of cases, which are typically temporary, with up to 90% of cases resolving within 1 year postoperatively.[24-26]

The LLIF technique is a retroperitoneal approach that utilizes minimally invasive techniques to identify and access the disk space of interest. The patient is positioned and secured in the lateral decubitus position with the approach side facing up and the hips and knees flexed to relax tension on the psoas muscle. Once the incision is performed, blunt dissection is carried through the abdominal muscle layers (external, internal oblique, and transversus abdominis), taking care to avoid injury to the iliohypogastric and ilioinguinal nerves. The peritoneum is reflected anteriorly and the psoas muscle is identified. Sequential dilators are then placed through the psoas muscle with EMG guidance to map the location of the lumbar plexus within the psoas (**Figure 4**). The disk space is then identified and targeted with the dilators. K-wires are then placed into the disk space and an expandable retractor is placed over the dilators, exposing the disk space. The diskectomy and disk preparation is performed in standard fashion and an interbody cage with osteobiologic bone graft material is impacted into position. One distinct advantage of the LLIF technique is the ability to span the apophyseal rings from the lateral edges of the disk space, which contain the strongest bone to support the interbody cage. This allows for high fusion rate and the ability to reduce deformity in both the coronal and sagittal planes.[23]

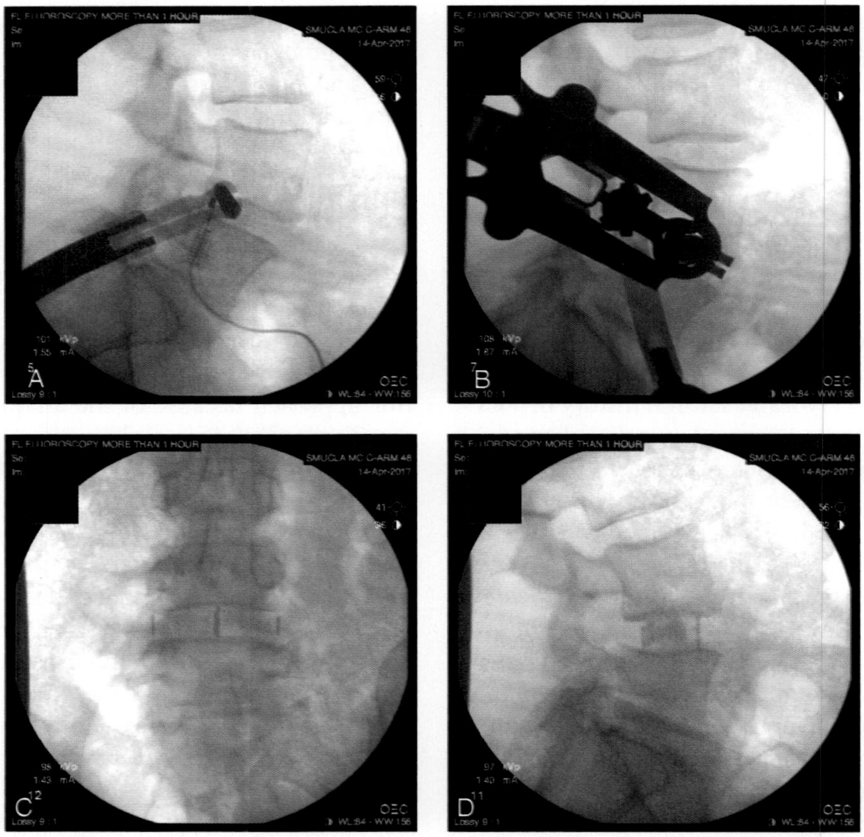

Figure 4 Lateral lumbar interbody fusion technique. **A**, Lateral fluoroscopy image targeting the posterior disk space at L4-5 with the initial dilator. **B**, Lateral fluoroscopy image with the expandable retractor centered at the L4-5 disk space. **C**, AP fluoroscopy image after final placement of the interbody cage. **D**, Lateral fluoroscopy image after final placement of the interbody cage.

The oblique lumbar interbody fusion (OLIF) technique is a modification of the LLIF technique with similar surgical indications (**Figure 5**). Patient positioning and OR setup is similar to LLIF. One striking difference is that triggered EMG guidance is not absolutely necessary as the technique does not depend on dissection within the psoas, reducing the chance for injury to the lumbar plexus. Also, the incision is made anterior to the disk space instead of centered at the lateral midline of the disk space. The retroperitoneal space is entered and the peritoneum reflected anteriorly. The psoas is identified and the target site is the disk space between the great vessels and the psoas. Serial dilators are then placed at the target site and an expandable retractor is placed, retracting the peritoneum and great vessels anteriorly and the psoas posteriorly. The diskectomy and end plate preparation is performed at this point and the interbody cage is introduced, first obliquely into the disk space and then rotating the cage to point direct laterally. Because of the difference in technique, OLIF cages are smaller in dimension than LLIF cages and do not necessarily span the apophyseal rings.[27] Despite this, fusion rates and radiographic and clinical outcomes are similar to ALIF and LLIF.

A significant advantage of the OLIF technique is that the iliac crest is not a limiting factor for access to L4-5 disk space, especially in a deeply seated disk space within the pelvis. The OLIF technique can address pathology at the disk spaces from L1-2 to L5-S1 and is versatile. Also, the technique does not involve dissection within the psoas muscle, reducing the neurological complications and hip flexor weakness associated with LLIF. Despite this, thigh numbness and hip flexor weakness can still occur because the psoas is retracted and compressed transiently as part of the technique. Recent studies demonstrated 16% to 21.4% incidence of thigh numbness and 6.5% to 7.1% incidence of leg weakness that is typically transient and lower than those of LLIF.[27-29] A significant limitation of the technique includes possible vascular injury because the target trajectory to the disk space is between the great vessels and the psoas. This requires that vascular surgery backup be readily available in the event of a

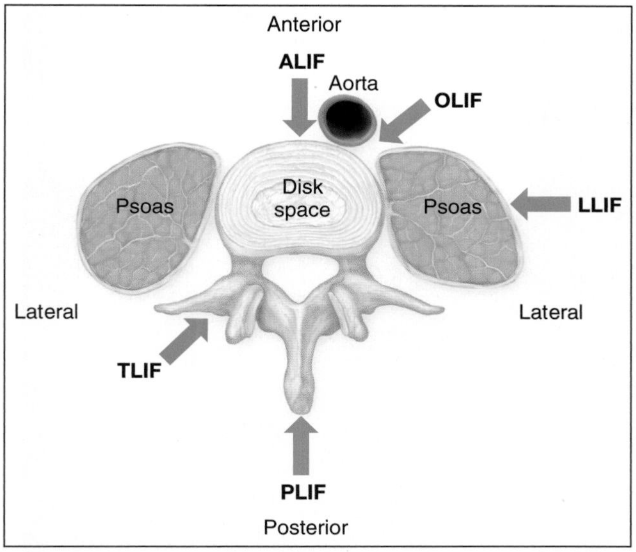

Figure 5 Illustration of the various lumbar interbody approaches.

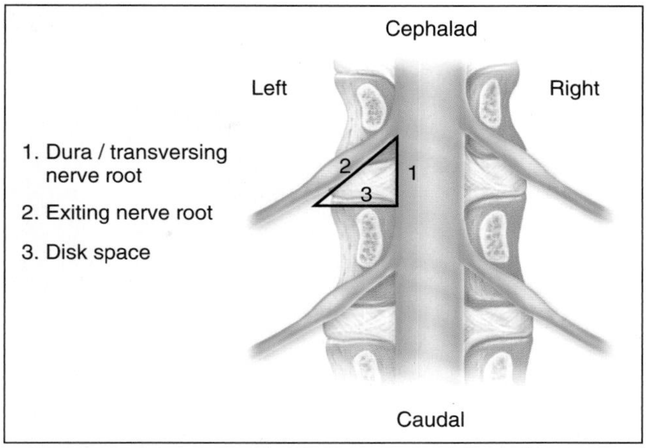

Figure 6 Illustration of Kambin's triangle.

vascular injury, especially with the limited visualization. However, studies have shown that the rates of vascular injury range from 1.1% to 2.8%, making vascular catastrophe a rare occurrence[28,29].

MIS Transforaminal/Posterior Lumbar Interbody Fusion

Transforaminal lumbar interbody fusion (TLIF) is a popular technique to accomplish lumbar fusion because it obviates the need for a vascular approach surgeon or a retroperitoneal approach. TLIF is an all-posterior technique that combines the interbody fusion with pedicle screw placement for stabilization of all three vertebral columns, as well as laminectomy for dorsal decompression. Taking advantage of Kambin's triangle, with the traversing nerve root, exiting nerve root, and disk space comprising the sides of the triangle, the TLIF technique requires less nerve root retraction and less risk of dural tear as compared with the PLIF technique[30] (**Figure 6**).

Small 2 to 3 cm Wiltse type incisions are made 2 to 3 cm lateral to the midline after the level of interest is identified using fluoroscopy. The lumbar dorsal fascia is incised and serial dilators are placed, targeting the facet joint. An expandable retractor is then placed over the dilators and locked into position with an articulating arm attached to the OR table. The facet joint and lamina are exposed and a facetectomy is performed, taking care to avoid violating the pedicles. The pedicles are then skeletonized and a unilateral hemilaminectomy is performed. The contralateral lateral recess and neural foramen can be decompressed by undercutting the undersurface of the spinous process and directing the expandable retractor more medially. At this point, Kambin's triangle is identified and the disk space is exposed. After the diskectomy and end plate preparation is complete, interbody cages of various designs, from oblique cages to "banana cages" that can rotate to the anterior aspect of the disk space, can be filled with bone graft material and impacted into position (**Figure 7**). Pedicle screw fixation can be performed either before or after the TLIF portion of the procedure using minimally invasive techniques.

When comparing the open to the MIS TLIF technique, multiple systematic reviews and meta-analyses demonstrated equivocal results in terms of fusion, VAS, and ODI scores.[31,32] A recent systematic review and meta-analysis by Bevevino et al demonstrated that rates of fusion were similar with the interbody only technique and the interbody fusion combined with posterolateral fusion.[33] In addition, no significant difference in dural tear rates, revision surgery, or surgical complications were found, including surgical site infections, neurologic deficit, or implant malposition. The main differences with MIS versus open TLIF include estimated blood loss (EBL), surgical time, and length of hospitalization. EBL has been shown to be significantly reduced in the MIS TLIF technique in multiple studies, including multiple systematic reviews and meta-analyses.[34,35] Multiple studies demonstrated longer surgical times with the MIS technique as compared with the open technique, which may be due to the learning curve of the MIS technique because surgery can take longer if the surgeon is not familiar with the anatomy within the constrained surgical field.[36] A recent systematic review by Khan et al demonstrated that MIS TLIF was associated with shorter hospital stays as compared with the open technique, which may be related to less muscle

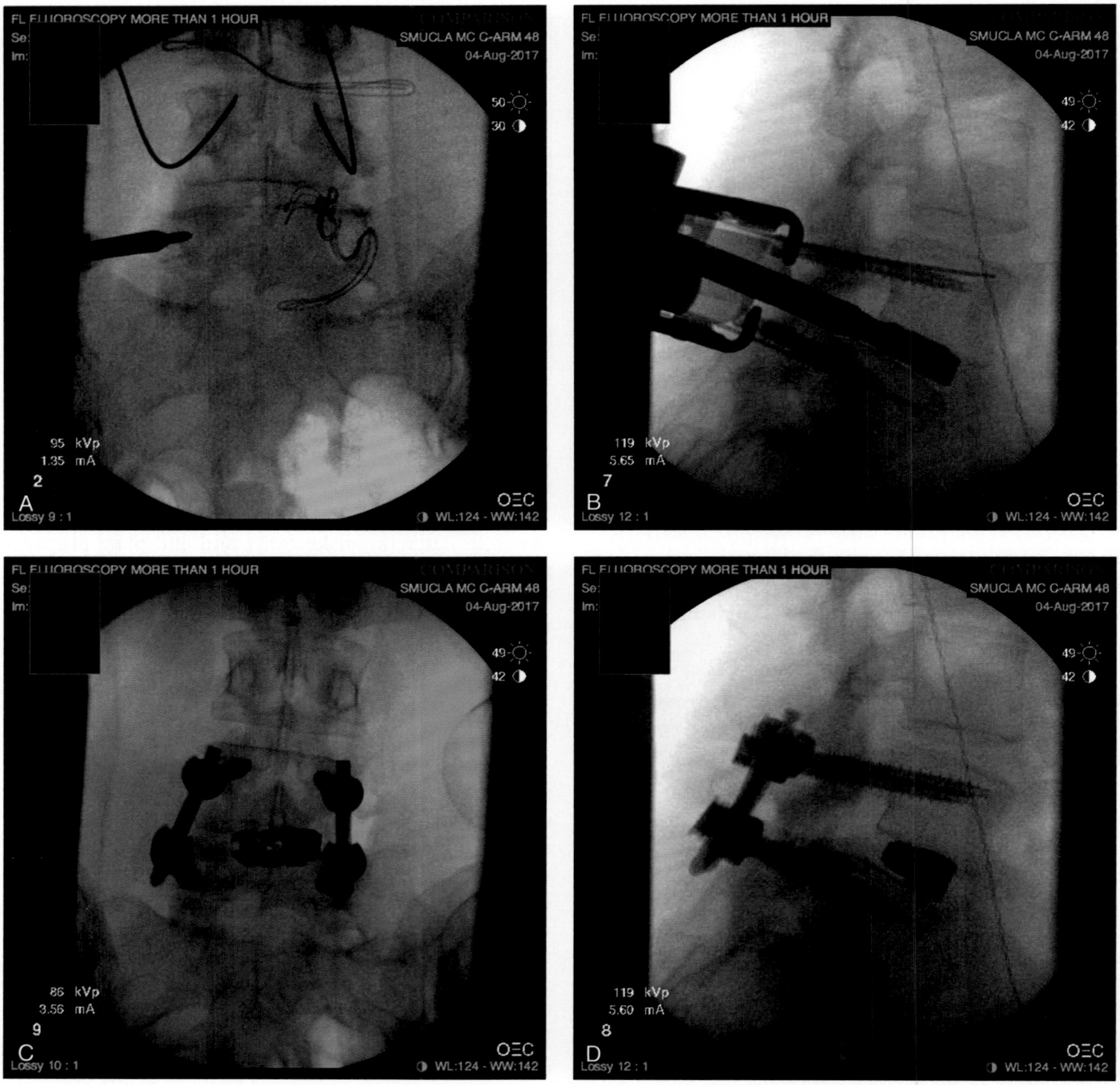

Figure 7 MIS TLIF Technique. **A**, Fluoroscopy image after impacting the Jamshidi needle to the midpoint of the pedicle and the posterior border of the vertebral body. **B**, Lateral fluoroscopy image after placement of expandable TLIF cage. **C**, AP fluoroscopy image after placement of TLIF cage and pedicle screws. **D**, Lateral fluoroscopy image after placement of TLIF cage and pedicle screws.

stripping and surgical dissection, possibly leading to reduced postoperative pain and disability.[37]

Posterior lumbar interbody fusion (PLIF) is also an all-posterior technique similar to TLIF but requires medial retraction of the dura and nerve root to access the posterior disk space after the laminectomy is performed. Because of the retraction required to expose the disk space, the risk for dural tear and nerve root injury from retraction is greater with the PLIF approach as compared with TLIF. Less-invasive, mini-open techniques can be employed by reducing the incision to that required for the laminectomy, typically 3 to 4 cm in length. The literature consists of small retrospective studies regarding MIS versus open techniques for PLIF that are limited by poor study design and short follow-up.[38] Similar to TLIF, MIS PLIF is associated with decreased EBL, shorter hospitalizations, and longer surgical times as compared with open techniques. Longer surgical times may be associated with increased costs with prolonged OR utilization and anesthesia exposure, although Wang et al demonstrated lower overall costs with MIS PLIF after reviewing hospital charges from a national database.[39] Both MIS and open PLIF similarly reduced pain and improved function with no difference between the techniques in clinical outcome or complications with long-term follow-up.[38]

MIS Application of Spinal Deformity

Until recently, the philosophy of MIS was less often applied to treating spinal deformity, especially in the adult patient, likely because of the anatomical complexity, the spine's rigidity, and surgeon preference. Clinical reports in this field are, thus understandably, limited to a few retrospective patient cohorts, with and without controls, and relatively low levels of evidence. Generally speaking, MIS techniques for adult spine deformity (ASD) typically include various combinations of multilevel posterior percutaneous pedicle screw instrumentation, LLIF, and MIS TLIF. ALIF and axial lumbar interbody fusion (AxiaLIF) can also be considered a form of MIS in some institutions. These MIS techniques are often combined as appropriate in actual usage and can also be used together with open techniques such as in a "hybrid" procedure (eg, MIS lateral lumbar interbody fusion combined with open posterior segment fixation).[40]

A multicenter study from the International Spine Study Group compared the surgical outcomes of ASD, defined as a lumbar "Cobb angle greater than 20°," between MIS (42 patients) and an open approach (109 patients).[40] Without inferential statistics, MIS appeared to do well, but did achieve somewhat less deformity correction in lumbar Cobb angle (18.8° vs 22.9°), lordosis (5.6° vs 10.4°), sagittal vertical axis (SVA, 0.3 vs 33.0 mm), and pelvic tilt (PT, 1.1° vs 2.0°) at 1-year follow-up as compared with the open approach, although the first two parameters in the MIS group were smaller preoperatively than those in the open group. Both groups showed improved clinical outcomes including ODI and VAS scores for both back and leg pain that did not significantly differ between groups. Patients in the MIS group did have significantly less estimated blood loss and transfusion rates. The operation time was comparable between groups. MIS was, however, associated with a significantly lower major complication rate (14%) compared with the open approach (45%), although the exact number of specific complications was unclear.

A similar study by the same group based on the same databases compared MIS and open surgery (20 patients of each) at 1-year follow-up through a propensity score matching of patients based on age, preoperative SVA, preoperative Cobb angle, and the number of fused levels, so that the observed outcome difference would be attributed to approach only.[41] It excluded patients with severe thoracic Cobb angles greater than 75°, and the preoperative SVA was 28 and 68 mm in the MIS and open groups. In this study, however, MIS achieved greater lumbar Cobb angle correction (22° vs 14°) and comparable PT correction (3° vs 4°) compared with the open approach, although it still helped little with the SVA correction (2 mm in MIS vs 30 mm in the open group). Still, MIS was associated with less blood loss, albeit in this study, longer surgical time. Clinically, all patients had improved ODI and VAS scores postoperatively except that the MIS patients did not have significant improvement in leg pain, suggesting possibly, some unresolved stenosis. Here the complication rate was less, but not significantly so between the groups (30% in MIS and 63% in the open group).[42]

Overall, it appears that MIS, in selected ASD patients, can achieve adequate coronal realignment and comparable clinical outcomes with those of open approaches with less blood loss. Its utility in correcting sagittal imbalance, however, seems to be limited. As of now, MIS is generally used for patients with baseline SVA <60 mm and PI-LL under 30°.[43] Questions still remain regarding its long-term follow-up results, its utility in adolescent idiopathic scoliosis, and its complications for which future comparative studies may need to be more specific, especially on major complications, so that both surgeons and patients can have a concrete sense of these potential risks. Studies in this field do remain somewhat biased by an emerging specialty disparity, between surgeons trained with open approaches and those who perform MIS. At this time, a consensus seems to be that for surgically eligible ASD patients with moderate deformity mainly in the coronal plane and without severe canal stenosis, especially senior patients or those with significant comorbidities, MIS can be a reasonable and quite useful choice.

Computer-Assisted Navigation and Robotic Spine Surgery

The next evolution of MIS is computer-assisted navigation and robotic spine surgery. Traditional techniques use fluoroscopy as the radiographic means of evaluating

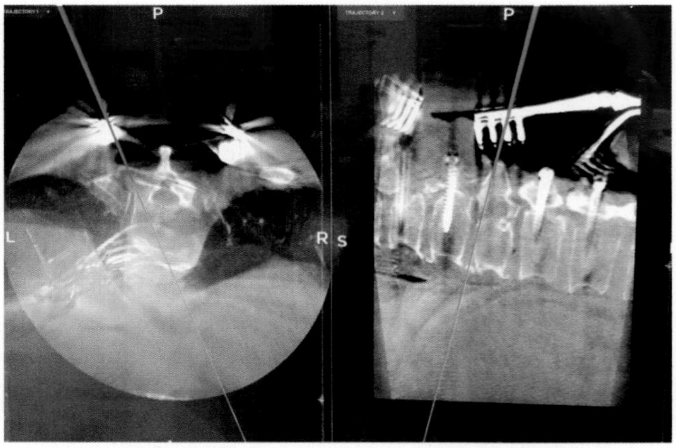

Figure 8 Picture of computer-assisted navigation.

the spinal anatomy intraoperatively. Although effective, this exposes the surgeon, OR staff, and the patient to radiation within the OR. 3D fluoroscopic and CT-based intraoperative platforms are now available to obtain radiographic data while the patient is positioned on the OR table, and computer-assisted navigation programs can use these data to assist the surgeon performing the surgery. A 3D spinal roadmap is created, which provides multiplanar detail as compared with the 2D fluoroscopic images (**Figure 8**). The surgeon and OR staff can exit the OR room during the scan to avoid unnecessary radiation exposure. Anatomic reference clamps are placed on a spinous process or percutaneous pins placed into the iliac crest before the scan to triangulate the spinal anatomic data obtained from the scan to the navigated instruments used during surgery. These navigated instruments are recognized by the stereotactic camera system as the surgeon places spinal instrumentation using either open or MIS techniques. Robotic spine surgery takes the computer-assisted navigation to the next level as the robot itself becomes a navigated instrument and tool. There are several different levels of robotic involvement from full robotic autonomy with preprogrammed and predetermined actions, a telesurgical system such as the Da Vinci robot where the surgeon has complete control of the robot from a remote command station, and co-autonomy with the surgeon and robot simultaneously controlling actions to accomplish the surgical task.[44] Most robotic systems used in spine surgery today use the co-autonomy system in which the robot is used in coordination with the surgeon to accomplish surgery. The robotic arm is positioned based on the trajectory determined by the radiographic data, computer-assisted navigation program, and the surgeon's preoperative plan to place spinal instrumentation.

The existing scientific literature has demonstrated the accuracy and safety of pedicle screw placement with computer-assisted navigation. Two recent large meta-analyses demonstrated significantly higher accuracy with computer-assisted navigation with up to 6% of pedicle breaches as compared with 15% with the freehand technique.[45,46] Not only was computer-assisted navigation accurate but the technique was also safe, as no neurological complications occurred because of screw malposition in the cervical, thoracic, and lumbosacral spine.[46] However, these meta-analyses also did not show a significant difference with neurological injuries, reoperations, or screw revision rates between the various techniques. Not only is computer-assisted navigation accurate and safe, the technique can reduce the radiation exposure to the surgeon and to the patient as the retrospective study by Kraus et al demonstrated with significantly lower radiation experienced by the patient as compared with fluoroscopy-based techniques, even compared with CT-based navigation.[47]

In contrast, the evidence for robotic pedicle screw placement is sparse and lower quality with a recent systematic review concluding that the evidence is inconclusive to recommend robotic technique over the fluoroscopic technique.[48] Interestingly, the largest RCT completed to date demonstrated inferiority of screw placement with 85% accuracy using robotic pedicle screw placement versus 93% using the fluoroscopic technique.[49] This may be due to skiving of the robotic arm and guide from the bone, reducing the accuracy of the start point and trajectory for the pedicle screw. A recent systematic review found that robotic pedicle screw placement was associated with high accuracy up to 99%, low complication rates, but increased surgical time as compared with open nonrobotic techniques.[50] When compared with computer-assisted navigation, the results of robotic spine surgery were similar in terms of accuracy and safety. Given the high cost considerations of the robotic technology, the question remains if robotic spine surgery is necessary and sustainable in today's cost-conscious health care environment.

Summary

Minimally invasive spine surgery is becoming more popular with both surgeons and patients alike. The spine surgeon should be aware of the steep learning curve required to master minimally invasive techniques, which may lead to increased surgical time and radiation exposure. MIS techniques are associated with short-term benefits such as reduced blood loss and shorter hospitalizations. In the long term, there is little difference between MIS and open techniques as long as the goals of surgery are accomplished. Moving forward, the next evolution of MIS techniques will involve computer-assisted navigation and perhaps even robotic spine surgery to improve the accuracy and precision of spine surgery.

Key Study Points

- Percutanenous pedicle screw fixation in thoracolumbar trauma is associated with less blood loss, lower infection rates, earlier mobilization, and faster return to work. Patient-reported functional scores and radiographic results are not significantly different between open and MIS approaches.
- Lateral lumbar interbody fusion is associated with thigh paresthesias, dysethesias, numbness, and hip flexor weakness in up to 30% of cases, with up to 90% resolving within 1 year postoperatively.
- MIS TLIF/PLIF is associated with less blood loss, shorter hospitalization but longer surgical time and radiologic exposure as compared with the open technique.
- MIS adult spinal deformity surgery can achieve coronal correction with comparable clinical outcomes versus open approaches with less blood loss but limited ability to correct sagittal imbalance.
- Computer-assisted navigation is associated with significantly higher accuracy with up to 6% of pedicle breaches versus 15% with the freehand technique.

Annotated References

1. Lykissas MG, Giannoulis D: Minimally invasive spine surgery for degenerative spine disease and deformity correction: A literature review. *Ann Transl Med* 2018;6(6):99.

   The authors performed a literature review of minimally invasive techniques in spine surgery for degenerative spine disease and deformity correction. They describe the clinical outcomes of various minimally invasive techniques from diskectomy, TLIF, LLIF, OLIF, and scoliosis surgery. Level of evidence: II.

2. Verma K, Boniello A, Rihn J: Emerging techniques for posterior fixation of the lumbar spine. *J Am Acad Orthop Surg* 2016;24(6):357-364.

   The authors reviewed the various types of posterior fixation of the lumbar spine and summarized the clinical evidence with each technique. Level of evidence: II.

3. Regev GJ, Lee YP, Taylor WR, Garfin SR, Kim CW: Nerve injury to the posterior rami medial branch during the insertion of pedicle screws: Comparison of mini-open versus percutaneous pedicle screw insertion techniques. *Spine* 2009;34:1239-1242.

4. Kim DY, Lee SH, Chung SK, Lee HY: Comparison of multifidus muscle atrophy and trunk extension muscle strength: Percutaneous versus open pedicle screw fixation. *Spine* 2005;30:123-129.

5. Taylor H, McGregor AH, Medhi-Zadeh S, et al: The impact of self-retaining retractors on the paraspinal muscles during posterior spinal surgery. *Spine* 2002;27(24):2758-2762.

6. Hansen-Algenstaedt N, Chiu CK, Chan CY, Lee CK, Schaefer C, Kwan MK: Accuracy and safety of fluoroscopic guided percutaneous pedicle screws in thoracic and lumbosacral spine: A review of 2000 screws. *Spine* 2015;40(17): E954-E963.

7. Wild MH, Glees M, Plieschnegger C, Wenda K: Five-year follow-up examination after purely minimally invasive posterior stabilization of thoracolumbar fractures: A comparison of minimally invasive percutaneously and conventionally open treated patients. *Arch Orthop Trauma Surg* 2007;127(5):335-343.

8. Jiang XZ, Tian W, Liu B, et al: Comparison of a paraspinal approach with a percutaneous approach in the treatment of thoracolumbar burst fractures with posterior ligamentous complex injury: A prospective randomized controlled trial. *J Int Med Res* 2012;40(4):1343-1356.

9. Kumar A, Aujla R, Lee C: The management of thoracolumbar burst fractures: A prospective study between conservative management, traditional open spinal surgery and minimally interventional spinal surgery. *SpringerPlus* 2015;4(1):204.

10. Gilbert F, Heintel TM, Jakubietz MG, et al: Quantitative MRI comparison of multifidus muscle degeneration in thoracolumbar fractures treated with open and minimally invasive approach. *BMC Muscoskelet Disord* 2018;19(1):75.

    The authors utilized MRI spectroscopy to quantify the fatty degeneration of the multifidus muscle postoperatively. The MIS group did not demonstrate less muscle degeneration as compared to the open group with no difference in clinical outcome at 5.9 years. Level of evidence: IV.

11. Koreckij T, Park DK, Fischgrund J: Minimally invasive spine surgery in the treatment of thoracolumbar and lumbar spine trauma. *Neurosurg Focus* 2014;37(1):E11.

12. Herren C, Reijnen M, Pishnamaz M, et al: Incidence and risk factors for facet joint violation in open versus minimally invasive procedures during pedicle screw placement in patients with trauma. *World neurosurgery* 2018;112:e711-e718.

    The authors conducted a retrospective review of all spine fractures requiring posterior stabilization with 1099 pedicle screws. Facet violation during insertion of the pedicle screws were seen in 39% of screws with less facet violation in the open group. Level of evidence: III.

13. Marcia S, Muto M, Hirsch JA, et al: What is the role of vertebral augmentation for osteoporotic fractures? A review of the recent literature. *Neuroradiology* 2018;60(8):777-783.

    The authors performed a systematic review of the cement augmentation procedures used for treatment of vertebral compression fractures. The authors described the clinical outcomes from the various randomized clinical trials investigating

Spine

vertebroplasty and kyphoplasty. They discussed the limitations of the negative studies pertaining to vertebroplasty, including confounding variables such as sham procedure, and inappropriate inclusion criteria. The overall complication rate was low for these procedures. Level of evidence: II.

14. Zhang H, Xu C, Zhang T, Gao Z, Zhang T: Does percutaneous vertebroplasty or balloon kyphoplasty for osteoporotic vertebral compression fractures increase the incidence of new vertebral fractures? A meta-analysis. *Pain Physician* 2017;20(1):E13-E28.

    The authors performed a meta-analysis examining percutaneous vertebroplasty and balloon kyphoplasty and compared the procedures to conservative treatment. The authors found there was no significant difference in the rates of adjacent vertebral fractures between cement augmentation procedures and conservative treatment. There was also no significant difference in the bone mineral density between the two groups. Level of evidence: II.

15. Buchbinder R, Osborne RH, Ebeling PR, et al: A randomized trial of vertebroplasty for painful osteoporotic vertebral fractures. *N Engl J Med* 2009;361(6):557-568.
16. Kallmes DF, Comstock BA, Heagerty PJ, et al: A randomized trial of vertebroplasty for osteoporotic spinal fractures. *N Engl J Med* 2009;361(6):569-579.
17. Voormolen MH, Mali WP, Lohle PN, et al: Percutaneous vertebroplasty compared with optimal pain medication treatment: Short-term clinical outcome of patients with subacute or chronic painful osteoporotic vertebral compression fractures. The VERTOS study. *AJNR Am J Neuroradiol* 2007;28(3):555-560.
18. Klazen CA, Lohle PN, de Vries J, et al: Vertebroplasty versus conservative treatment in acute osteoporotic vertebral compression fractures (Vertos II): An open-label randomised trial. *Lancet* 2010;376(9746):1085-1092.
19. Buchbinder R, Johnston RV, Rischin KJ, et al: Percutaneous vertebroplasty for osteoporotic vertebral compression fracture. *Cochrane Database Syst Rev* 2015;(4):CD006349.
20. Wardlaw D, Cummings SR, Van Meirhaeghe J, et al: Efficacy and safety of balloon kyphoplasty compared with non-surgical care for vertebral compression fracture (FREE): A randomised controlled trial. *Lancet* 2009;373(9668):1016-1024.
21. Wang H, Sribastav SS, Ye F, et al: Comparison of percutaneous vertebroplasty and balloon kyphoplasty for the treatment of single level vertebral compression fractures: A meta-analysis of the literature. *Pain Physician* 2015;18(3):209-222.
22. Xu DS, Walker CT, Godzik J, Turner JD, Smith W, Uribe JS: Minimally invasive anterior, lateral, and oblique lumbar interbody fusion: A literature review. *Ann Transl Med* 2018;6(6):104.

    The authors reviewed the various minimally invasive lumbar fusion techniques and discussed the differences with the approaches, surgical technique, and clinical outcomes. Level of evidence: III.

23. Teng I, Han J, Phan K, Mobbs R: A meta-analysis comparing ALIF, PLIF, TLIF and LLIF. *J Clin Neurosci* 2017;44:11-17.

    The authors performed a systematic review examining the various lumbar fusion techniques and demonstrated similar fusion rates with ALIF providing superior postoperative disk height and segmental lordosis results. TLIF was associated with better ODI screws, whereas PLIF was associated with the highest blood loss. Complication rates were similar with the various techniques. Level of evidence: II.

24. Rodgers WB, Gerber EJ, Patterson J: Intraoperative and early postoperative complications in extreme lateral interbody fusion: An analysis of 600 cases. *Spine* 2011;36:26-32.
25. Cummock MD, Vanni S, Levi AD, Yu Y, Wang MY: An analysis of postoperative thigh symptoms after minimally invasive transpsoas lumbar interbody fusion. *J Neurosurg Spine* 2011;15:11-18.
26. Knight RQ, Schwaegler P, Hanscom D, Roh J: Direct lateral lumbar interbody fusion for degenerative conditions: Early complication profile. *J Spinal Disord Tech* 2009;22:34-37.
27. Silvestre C, Mac-Thiong JM, Hilmi R, Roussouly P: Complications and morbidities of mini-open anterior retroperitoneal lumbar interbody fusion: Oblique lumbar interbody fusion in 179 patients. *Asian Spine J* 2012;6:89-97.
28. DiGiorgio AM, Edwards CS, Virk MS, Mummaneni PV, Chou D: Stereotactic navigation for the prepsoas oblique lateral lumbar interbody fusion: Technical note and case series. *Neurosurg Focus* 2017;43:E14.

    The authors describe their retrospective small case series of 49 patients who underwent the oblique lumbar interbody fusion using intraoperative computer-assisted navigation and describe their surgical technique and results. There was one surgically related complication with a pre-psoas hematoma and transient hip flexor weakness that resolved spontaneously over time. There were six approach-related complications with thigh dysesthesias and postoperative ileus that also resolved over time. VAS and ODI scores were improved from baseline at 1-year follow-up. Level of evidence: IV.

29. Ohtori S, Mannoji C, Orita S, et al: Mini-open anterior retroperitoneal lumbar interbody fusion: Oblique lateral interbody fusion for degenerated lumbar spinal kyphoscoliosis. *Asian Spine J* 2015;9:565-572.
30. Kambin P, Sampson S: Posterolateral percutaneous suction-excision of herniated lumbar intervertebral discs. Report of interim results. *Clin Orthop Relat Res* 1986;207:37-43.
31. Singh K, Nandyala SV, Marquez-Lara A, et al: A perioperative cost analysis comparing single-level minimally invasive and open transforaminal lumbar interbody fusion. *Spine J* 2014;14(8):1694-1701.
32. Goldstein CL, Macwan K, Sundararajan K, Rampersaud YR: Comparative outcomes of minimally invasive surgery for posterior lumbar fusion: A systematic review. *Clin Orthop Relat Res* 2014;472(6):1727-1737.
33. Bevevino AJ, Kang DG, Lehman RA Jr, Van Blarcum GS, Wagner SC, Gwinn DE: Systematic review and meta-analysis of minimally invasive transforaminal lumbar interbody fusion rates performed without posterolateral fusion. *J Clin Neurosci* 2014;21(10):1686-1690.

34. Wang J, Zhou Y: Perioperative complications related to minimally invasive transforaminal lumbar fusion: Evaluation of 204 operations on lumbar instability at single center. *Spine J* 2014;14(9):2078-2084.

35. Wong AP, Smith ZA, Stadler JA III, et al: Minimally invasive transforaminal lumbar interbody fusion (MI-TLIF): Surgical technique, long-term 4-year prospective outcomes, and complications compared with an open TLIF cohort. *Neurosurg Clin N Am* 2014;25(2):279-304.

36. Phan K, Rao PJ, Kam AC, Mobbs RJ: Minimally invasive versus open transforaminal lumbar interbody fusion for treatment of degenerative lumbar disease: Systematic review and meta-analysis. *Eur Spine J* 2015;24(5):1017-1030.

37. Khan NR, Clark AJ, Lee SL, Venable GT, Rossi NB, Foley KT: Surgical outcomes for minimally invasive vs open transforaminal lumbar interbody fusion: An updated systematic review and metaanalysis. *Neurosurgery* 2015;77(6):847-874.

38. Sidhu GS, Henkelman E, Vaccaro AR, et al: Minimally invasive versus open posterior lumbar interbody fusion: A systematic review. *Clin Orthop Relat Res* 2014;472:1792-1799.

39. Wang MY, Lerner J, Lesko J, McGirt MJ: Acute hospital costs after minimally invasive versus open lumbar interbody fusion: Data from a US national database with 6106 patients. *J Spinal Disord Tech* 2012;25:324-328.

40. Hamilton DK, Kanter AS, Bolinger BD, et al: International Spine Study Group (ISSG). Reoperation rates in minimally invasive, hybrid and open surgical treatment for adult spinal deformity with minimum 2-year follow-up. *Eur Spine J* 2016;25(8):2605-2611.

    The authors examined the MIS versus hybrid versus open technique in the treatment of adult spinal deformity. The MIS group had fewer levels fused as compared to the open group. The most common reason for reoperation for the MIS group was pseudarthrosis. Level of evidence: III.

41. Haque RM, Mundis GM Jr, Ahmed Y, et al: Comparison of radiographic results after minimally invasive, hybrid, and open surgery for adult spinal deformity: A multicenter study of 184 patients. *Neurosurg Focus* 2014;36(5):E13.

42. Tuchman A, Hsieh PC: Comparing minimally invasive, hybrid, and open surgical techniques for adult spinal deformity. *Neurosurg Focus* 2014;36(5):E16.

43. Eastlack RK, Mundis GM Jr, Wang M, et al: Is there a patient profile that characterizes a patient with adult spinal deformity as a candidate for minimally invasive surgery? *Glob Spine J* 2017;7(7):703-708.

    The authors performed a retrospective review comparing MIS versus open techniques in adult spinal deformity and found that MIS patients were older with smaller coronal deformity, sagittal vertical axis less than 6 cm, and baseline pelvic incidence and lumbar lordosis mismatch less than 30°. Level of evidence: III.

Results

44. Overley SC, Cho SK, Mehta AI, Arnold PM: Navigation and robotics in spinal surgery: Where are we now? *Neurosurgery* 2017;80(3S):S86-S99.

    The authors reviewed the literature on computer-assisted navigation and robotics in spine surgery. They discussed the current options available and the similarities and differences with the various technologies. Level of evidence: III.

45. Verma R, Krishan S, Haendlmayer K, Mohsen A: Functional outcome of computer-assisted spinal pedicle screw placement: A systematic review and meta-analysis of 23 studies including 5,992 pedicle screws. *Eur Spine J* 2010;19:370-375.

46. Shin BJ, James AR, Njoku IU, Hartl R: Pedicle screw navigation: A systematic review and meta-analysis of perforation risk for computer-navigated versus freehand insertion. *J Neurosurg Spine* 2012;17:113-122.

47. Kraus MD, Krischak G, Keppler P, Gebhard FT, Schuetz UH: Can computer-assisted surgery reduce the effective dose for spinal fusion and sacroiliac screw insertion? *Clin Orthop Relat Res* 2010;468(9):2419-2429.

48. Marcus HJ, Cundy TP, Nandi D, Yang GZ, Darzi A: Robot-assisted and fluoroscopy-guided pedicle screw placement: A systematic review. *Eur Spine J* 2014;23(2):291-297.

49. Ringel F, Stüer C, Reinke A, et al: Accuracy of robot-assisted placement of lumbar and sacral pedicle screws: A prospective randomized comparison to conventional freehand screw implantation. *Spine* 2012;37(8):E496-E501.

50. Ghasem A, Sharma A, Greif DN, Alam M, Maaieh MA: The arrival of robotics in spine surgery: A review of the literature. *Spine* 2018;43(23):1670-1677.

    The authors performed a systematic review of the use of robotics in spine surgery and demonstrated that pedicle screw placement accuracy and complications are comparable to the freehand technique with longer surgical time, and reduced radiation exposure as the number of robotic cases increased. Inaccuracies were associated with soft-tissue pressure on the robotic arm and skiving of the robotic drill guide on the bony surface. Few high-level studies exist investigating robotic spine surgery, and studies pertaining to cost-effectiveness with the technology are required in the future. Level of evidence: III.

Chapter 51

Spinal Column Infections

Arya Varthi, MD • Comron Saifi, MD • Peter G. Whang, MD, FACS

ABSTRACT

Spinal infections are a common problem that often causes significant morbidity and mortality in affected individuals. When left untreated, spinal infections can cause mechanical instability and possible neurologic compromise. There are a variety of different spinal infections, including osteomyelitis, diskitis, spinal epidural abscess, spinal tuberculosis, and postoperative spinal infections.

Keywords: diskitis; epidural abscess; osteomyelitis; tuberculosis

Osteomyelitis/Diskitis

Epidemiology

Osteomyelitis represents an infection of the osseous spinal column. Osteomyelitis almost always affects the anterior spinal column and rarely involves the posterior elements.[1] Diskitis is an infection of the disk space between vertebral bodies.[1] The intervertebral disk has limited blood supply, with the majority of nutrient delivery occurring via diffusion from the vertebral body.[1] Therefore, for an infection to invade the disk space, it usually originates from the vertebral body.[1]

Osteomyelitis/diskitis are common conditions that can cause significant morbidity and mortality if left untreated. The incidence of osteomyelitis of the spine is 2.2/100,000 people.[2] There are several risk factors for osteomyelitis of the spine, many of which are similar to the risk factors for osteomyelitis of long bones. These include diabetes, smoking, immunocompromise secondary to infections such as HIV or hepatitis C, infections in other parts of the body, previous spine surgery, and skin compromise.[1]

Mylona et al performed a systematic review of 14 studies with a total 1,008 total patients suffering from pyogenic vertebral osteomyelitis (PVO).[3] The authors found that the median age of patients with PVO was 59 years.[3] There was a male predominance (62%) of affected individuals.[3] In terms of medical comorbidities, 24% of the patients had diabetes mellitus and 11% of the patients used intravenous drugs.[3] The lumbar vertebrae were affected in 59% of patients, followed by the thoracic vertebrae in 30% of patients and the cervical vertebrae in 11% of patients[3] (**Figure 1**).

Pathogenesis

The pathogenesis of spinal osteomyelitis/diskitis involves either direct inoculation of the spinal column or hematogenous spread from another organ site.[4] Hematogenous spread is more common than direct inoculation and accounts for the majority of cases of osteomyelitis/diskitis.[1,4] The multiple and redundant sources of vascularity to the spinal column provide a ready avenue for bacterial pathogens to seed vertebrae.[1] Direct inoculation of the spinal column can occur secondary to skin compromise. For example, patients with chronic sacral decubitus ulcers are at risk for vertebral osteomyelitis because of exposure of the bony sacrum to the environment.[5] Direct inoculation of the spinal column can also occur in patients undergoing spinal surgery or spinal procedures (epidural injection, diskography, etc), because

Dr. Saifi or an immediate family member has stock or stock options held in Gilead, Novartis, and Vertera. Dr. Whang or an immediate family member is a member of a speakers' bureau or has made paid presentations on behalf of DePuy, A Johnson & Johnson Company, Medtronic, SI-BONE, and Stryker; serves as a paid consultant to or is an employee of Bio2, Ferring Pharmaceuticals, Histogenics, Life Spine, Medtronic, Orthofix, Inc., Pacira, Paradigm Spine, Relievant, SI BONE, Simplify Medical, and Stryker; serves as an unpaid consultant to DiFusion and SAIL Fusion; has stock or stock options held in DiFusion and SAIL Fusion; and has received research or institutional support from Bioventus, SI BONE, and Spinal Kinetics. Neither Dr. Varthi nor any immediate family member has received anything of value from or has stock or stock options held in a commercial company or institution related directly or indirectly to the subject of this chapter.

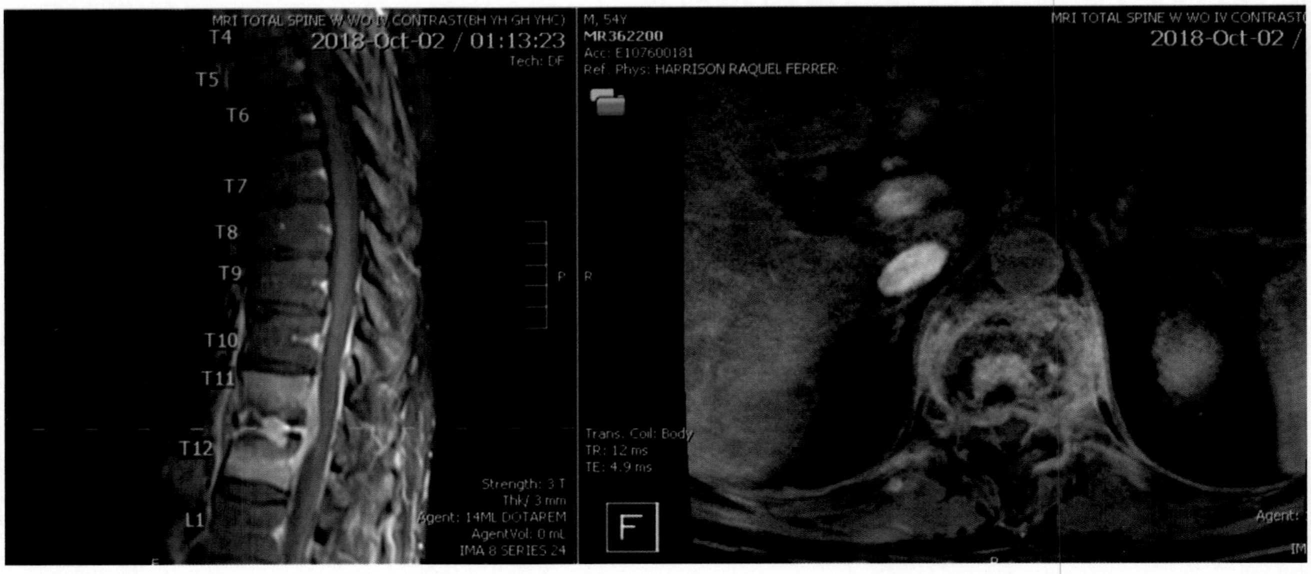

Figure 1 54-year-old male painter with insidious onset of worsening thoracic back pain. After inflammatory markers were noted to be elevated, the patient underwent total spine MRI with and without contrast. This study demonstrates T11 to 12 diskitis/osteomyelitis with ventral epidural phlegmon. The patient was successfully treated with IV antibiotics and bracing treatment.

of iatrogenic contamination of the surgical site.[1] Once a vertebral body is inoculated with a bacterial pathogen, the pathogen may spread to the adjacent disk space via diffusion and cause diskitis.

The most common source of bacterial osteomyelitis/diskitis is *Staphylococcus aureus*. In the previously mentioned systematic review of 1,008 patients with PVO, *S aureus* was the most frequently found organism, with the next most common pathogen being another gram-positive bacterial pathogen, *Streptococcus*.[2] Gram-negative species are also a frequent source of osteomyelitis. Common gram-negative pathogens include *Escherichia coli* and *Klebsiella pneumonia*. These organisms are able to inoculate of the spinal column via hematogenous spread.[6] *Pseudomonas aeruginosa* has been described as a common PVO pathogen in patients with intravenous drug abuse.[7,8]

Park et al compared the outcomes of 313 patients with either MSSA (methicillin-sensitive *Staphylococcus aureus*) or gram-negative hematogenous vertebral osteomyelitis.[9] The authors found that gram-negative bacteria accounted for 20.8% of hematogenous vertebral osteomyelitis cases over the 7-year study period and that clinical outcomes such as in-hospital mortality and recurrence rate were similar between the two groups.[9] Patients with gram-negative organisms had decreased recurrence rates (2.1%) if antibiotics were given for over 8 weeks, compared with antibiotics given for 4 to 6 weeks (40.0%) or 6 to 8 weeks (33.3%).[9]

Diagnosis

Patients with osteomyelitis/diskitis of the spine often have an indolent clinical course in which low-grade back pain increases in severity over several weeks to months.[3] Back pain is the most common presenting report, followed by fever.[10] Although many patients with osteomyelitis/diskitis do not present with neurologic deficit,[3] in the previously described systematic review by Mylona et al, 34% of patients presented with some type of neurologic issue, ranging from radiculopathy to urinary incontinence. As the pyogenic infection spreads, it can cause neurologic compromise secondary to bony retropulsion or extension into the epidural space, causing an epidural abscess. In both of these settings, resultant central or foraminal stenosis can result in neurologic deficits.

Bloodwork can show a normal or elevated white blood cell count.[1] Patients will have an elevated erythrocyte sedimentation rate (ESR) and C-reactive protein (CRP) secondary to the inflammatory response that the body mounts to counter the osteomyelitis/diskitis infection.[1] Blood cultures should be obtained to assess for disseminated infection and identification of microbial pathogen.[1]

Radiographic examination of patients with osteomyelitis of the spine usually demonstrates changes in the architecture of the vertebral body, such as scalloping of end plates and sclerosis of the subchondral bone.[1] Changes in the osteology of the posterior elements of the spine are rarely seen because of the predilection of infectious pathogens for the vertebral body.[1] Radiographic changes in the vertebrae usually take several weeks to develop and may not be seen in a patient with acute vertebral osteomyelitis.[1] In patients with chronic osteomyelitis, loss of bone commonly causes focal kyphosis. Standing full-length scoliosis radiographs can be obtained to assess sagittal spinal alignment in greater detail.[1]

Noncontrast CT scan of the affected part of the spine is commonly performed and can show the above bony morphologic changes in greater detail.[1] Bony retropulsion into the spinal canal, subchondral sclerosis, erosion of the vertebral end plates as well as other bony changes secondary to vertebral osteomyelitis/diskitis are better delineated with CT scan imaging than with MRI.[1] CT-guided bone biopsy can be performed to obtain a sample of the affected vertebral body to allow for guidance of antibiotic therapy.[1]

MRI of the affected area of the spine with and without gadolinium contrast allows for detailed imaging of the soft-tissue structures of the spine and should be obtained in all patients with suspected osteomyelitis of the spine.[1] This imaging modality allows the clinician to assess for local spread of the infection, the development of epidural abscess/diskitis, and the chronicity of the infectious process.[1] On T1-weighted imaging, a patient with vertebral osteomyelitis/diskitis will have hypointense signal at the affected end plate and disk. Meanwhile, T2-weighted imaging will demonstrate hyperintense signal in the vertebral body and disk space.[1] If the infectious process has spread to the spinal canal, MRI will also demonstrate any associated epidural phlegmon or epidural abscess.[1] The addition of gadolinium contrast allows for improved visualization of the infectious process, as the contrast will be taken up at the site of the infection, providing increased visualization of the boundaries of the infection.[1]

Treatment

Isolated vertebral osteomyelitis/diskitis in a patient without neurologic deficit can be treated initially with nonsurgical management. Typical nonsurgical treatment regimens consist of intravenous antibiotics and mobilization of the affected patient. To maximize the efficacy of antibiotics, an organism should be identified to allow for appropriate targeting of antimicrobial therapy. Blood cultures that are obtained before the initiation of antibiotics can help identify an organism. CT-guided bone biopsy is commonly used for obtaining a sample of the affected vertebrae. The efficacy of this treatment modality is controversial. Sehn et al studied 323 patients with possible PVO who underwent image-guided biopsy of the vertebral body. The authors found that among 92 patients who had a high suspicion for infection before the biopsy based upon imaging and clinical data, the biopsy was positive for a bacterial pathogen 30.4% of the time.[11] In patients with intermediate and low prebiopsy probability of infection, the biopsy was positive in 16.1% and 5.0% of cases, respectively.[11]

If a patient with suspected PVO has a negative CT-guided bone biopsy, the next step would commonly be to repeat the biopsy.[12] Gras et al[12] assessed 136 patients with suspected PVO and found that patients who underwent one biopsy only had a pathogen identified 44.1% of the time, whereas patients who underwent an additional biopsy if the first one was negative had a pathogen identified 79.6% of the time. The authors concluded that obtaining a second biopsy if the first biopsy is negative is a reasonable treatment strategy.

Consultation with infectious disease physicians regarding the length and choice of antibiotics should be performed. Typically, intravenous antibiotics are administered for at least 6 weeks with subsequent transition to PO antibiotics.[1] Throughout this time course there should be tracking of WBC, ESR, CRP to monitor the patient's response to the treatment. For non-MRSA gram-positive infections, IV cefazolin is a commonly used antibiotic, whereas IV vancomycin remains the most common antibiotic for MRSA (methicillin-resistant *Staphylococcus aureus*) osteomyelitis.[10]

Bracing treatment is typically performed for patients with osteomyelitis/diskitis as the architectural integrity of the spinal column is compromised from the infectious process, and external bracing treatment is thought to provide additional stability to the spinal column.[1] The specific bracing treatment regimen depends on the level of the vertebral osteomyelitis. For lumbar osteomyelitis, a lumbosacral orthosis is commonly used, whereas for thoracic osteomyelitis a thoracolumbar orthosis or Jewett extension brace can be employed.[1] Bracing treatment has the theoretical benefit of providing external support to the weakened vertebral column although long-term studies have not been performed to demonstrate the added benefit of bracing treatment in patients with vertebral osteomyelitis.

Surgical treatment of vertebral osteomyelitis is commonly performed for a wide spectrum of reasons. Patients who are surgical candidates include those whose infection progresses despite nonsurgical treatment, those who develop associated epidural abscesses/diskitis, those who develop neurologic deficit, and those who develop bony instability of the spinal column or significant kyphotic deformity.[1] The goals of surgical

Spine

treatment of vertebral osteomyelitis are débridement of the infectious pathology, preservation of neurologic function, and stabilization of the spinal column. Secondary goals include the correction of any sagittal or coronal plane deformities caused by the infectious process.[1]

Because vertebral osteomyelitis affects the vertebral body, resection of the infectious process often requires subtotal or total corpectomy with reconstruction of the bony defect with autograft, allograft, or cage placement.[1] This can be accomplished through a variety of anterior, lateral, and posterior surgical approaches depending on the level of pathology.[1] Pedicle screw instrumentation is typically performed to stabilize at least two levels above and below the affected level.[1] If there is a concomitant epidural abscess, a laminectomy can be performed to evacuate the epidural infectious collection.[1]

Dragsted et al performed a retrospective review of 65 patients diagnosed with osteomyelitis/diskitis related to recent spinal surgery.[13] The authors followed up the patients for a median follow-up of 2 years and found that the overall 1-year mortality rate was 6%.[13] Preoperative neurologic impairment was present in 36% of patients and at final follow-up the authors noted that patients with osteomyelitis/diskitis had significantly lower quality of life scores, as measured by EuroQol 5-dimension (EQ-5D) questionnaire and Oswestry Disability Index (ODI) relative to unaffected individuals.[13] Meanwhile, in a retrospective cohort analysis of 1,505 Danish individuals with osteomyelitis/diskitis who were alive 1 year after initial diagnosis and were sex/age matched with unaffected people, Aagaard et al[14] found that osteomyelitis/diskitis patients had a 1.47 mortality rate ratio relative to the affected individuals.

Spinal Epidural Abscess

Epidemiology

Spinal epidural abscess (SEA) is a serious condition with high morbidity and mortality if left untreated.[1] It represents an infection that is inside the spinal canal in the epidural space.[1] The close proximity of the infectious material to the neural elements can lead to devastating complications such as quadriparesis and paraparesis.[1,15] The incidence of SEA is estimated to be 2 to 5/10,000 hospital admissions.[15-17] The most common age for SEA is 50 to 70 years, and males are more frequently affected than females.[16] SEA is uncommon in the pediatric population.[16]

There are several lifestyle and medical risk factors for SEA. Intravenous drug use has been shown in multiple studies to be a significant risk factor for SEA.[15] Additionally, recent trauma and alcohol use have been shown to increase the risk of SEA.[18] Patients who have undergone a recent spinal epidural or facet injection or spine surgery are at risk for SEA secondary to direct bacterial inoculation of the spinal column.[18] Medical comorbidities that cause immunocompromise, such as diabetes and HIV, also place patients at elevated risk for SEA.[18]

S aureus is the most common bacterial pathogen that causes SEA.[18] Both MSSA and MRSA SEA can occur, with MSSA SEA being the most common SEA pathogen in several studies.[18] Less frequent sources of bacterial SEA include coagulase-negative *Staphylococcus* species, *Streptococcus* species and gram-negative bacteria.[18]

In a recent review of 128 patients with SEA, the most common location of SEA was the lumbar spine (54.7%) followed by the thoracic spine (39.1%), and the most common risk factors for SEA were IV drug use (39.1%) and diabetes (21.9%).[19] MSSA was the most frequently isolated bacterial pathogen, followed by MRSA (30%).[19] Arko et al performed a systematic review of SEA patients treated with medical and surgical management.[18] The authors included 12 articles with total of 1,099 patients.[18] Similar to the above study, Arko et al determined that the lumbar spine was the most common location of SEA (48%), males were affected more frequently (62.5%), and the most common pathogen was *S aureus* (63.6%).[18]

Pathogenesis

SEA can occur secondary to direct bacterial inoculation of the spinal column or through hematogenous spread of bacterial pathogens.[1] Direct inoculation occurs through recent spinal surgery, recent spinal injections, and skin defects close to the spinal column.[16] Hematogenous spread occurs when there is a bacterial infection in another part of the body that subsequently spreads via the vascular system to gain access to the spinal column.[16] For example, in IV drug users, bacteria can migrate from the needle insertion site to the spinal column via hematogenous spread.[1] In a review of all SEA cases that occurred over a 10-year time period at a tertiary care hospital, Vakili et al found that hematogenous spread was the most common source of infection with the second most common route of SEA being recent surgery/procedure.[17]

SEA causes neurologic dysfunction secondary to spinal cord ischemia.[15] Ischemia can occur secondary to the mass effect that the infectious collection exerts on the spinal cord or because of bacterial occlusion of local vasculature, which also results in cord ischemia.[15] Commonly, ventral SEA occurs secondary to contiguous spread of bacterial pathogens from osteomyelitis/diskitis, whereas dorsal SEA is more likely to be a de-novo process.[1]

Diagnosis

Signs and Symptoms

Patients with SEA can present in a variety of fashions. Classically, patients with SEA have been thought to experience in a four-stage sequence of increasing disability.[16,20] In the first stage, patients experience focal back pain at the level of the abscess.[16,20] In the second stage, patients develop radicular pain in the distribution of the dermatome that is affected by the SEA.[16,20] In the third stage, patients develop a combination of motor and sensory deficits as well as possible bowel and bladder incontinence.[16,20] In the fourth stage, patients present with paralysis.[16,20] In a recent systematic review of 1,099 patients with SEA, Arko et al found that 66.8% of patients initially presented with back pain, 52% of patients with motor weakness, 40% of patients with sensory abnormalities, 27.1% of patients with bowel/bladder incontinence, and 43.7% of patients with fever.[18]

Labs

Patients with SEA typically have elevated inflammatory markers.[1] All patients should have a white blood cell count, erythrocyte sedimentation rate, and C-reactive protein drawn.[1] In addition, blood cultures should be obtained to assess for systemic spread of infection. Typically, a patient with SEA will have significant elevation of at least one of these markers. C-reactive protein is a marker of acute inflammation and increases/decreases over the shortest time period.[1] However, if these inflammatory markers are not elevated, it does not preclude the diagnosis of SEA.

As previously cited, Patel et al[19] performed a retrospective review of 128 adult patients with SEA who presented to a tertiary care medical center with a mean follow-up of 241 days. Multivariate analysis revealed that diabetes mellitus, CRP > 115, WBC > 12.5, and positive blood cultures predicted failure of medical treatment. The authors concluded that patients treated with medical management should be watched closely and that surgical débridement should be the mainstay of treatment for SEA.

Imaging

In patients with suspected SEA, AP and lateral radiographs of the suspected area of spinal pathology should be obtained to assess for fracture or instability of the spinal segment and to check for bony changes consistent with vertebral osteomyelitis/diskitis.[1] Similarly, CT scan of the affected spinal region can be performed to assess for bony changes consistent with osteomyelitis/diskitis.[1]

The imaging modality of choice for patients with SEA is an MRI with and without gadolinium contrast.[1] On T1-weighted imaging the abscess will have hypointense signal, whereas on T2-weighted imaging, the abscess will have hyperintense signal.[1] Gadolinium contrast is very useful in demonstrating possible rim enhancement of the infectious collection[1] (**Figure 2**).

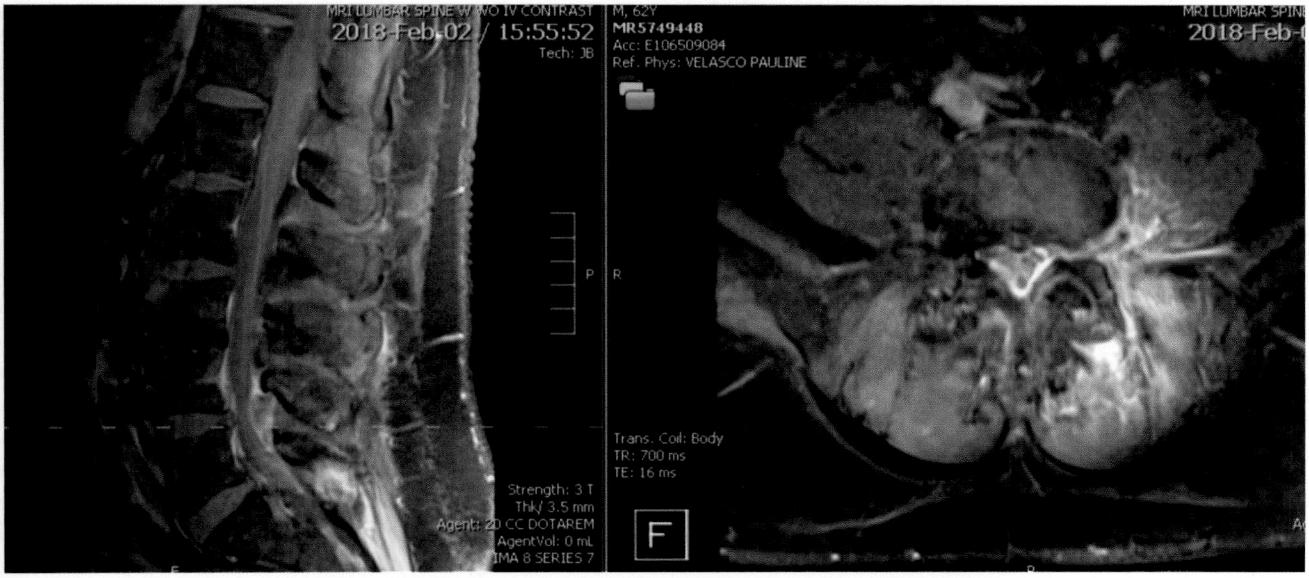

Figure 2 62-year-old man with MSSA bacteremia treated with IV antibiotics. The patient began experiencing significant axial low back pain associated with lower extremity radiculopathy. He was treated with lumbar 3 to 5 laminectomy and evacuation of epidural collection and had significant clinical improvement.

Treatment

Traditionally, surgical irrigation and débridement with evacuation of the infectious collection has been the mainstay of treatment of patients with SEA, because of the fear of neurologic deterioration after conservative management.[1] Surgical intervention allows for removal of the infectious collection from the spinal canal and a laminectomy provides the thecal sac with a larger space to sit in.[1] The potential benefits of this approach are decreased risk of neurologic deficit due to removal of the inflammatory cascade around the thecal sac and decreased mass effect on the thecal sac secondary to the laminectomy and removal of the epidural mass.[1]

However, in recent years conservative management has become a more commonly used treatment option for patients with SEA without neurologic deficit.[1] In these patients, IV antibiotics are given for at least 6 weeks with close monitoring of inflammatory markers, blood cultures, and neurologic status[1] (**Figure 3**). Patients are mobilized throughout this process and can use external bracing treatment for support during this process.[1]

There are mixed outcomes reported for neurologically intact patients treated with IV antibiotics alone. In the previously cited systematic review by Arko et al, the authors included 12 articles with a total of 1,099 patients with a diagnosis of SEA.[18] In this study, patients without neurologic deficits were more likely to be initially treated with medical management rather than surgical management.[18] Overall, surgery was the initial treatment in 59.7% of patients, and conservative management was the initial treatment in 40.3% of patients.[18] The others did not find a difference in the outcomes of patients who were treated with initial conservative or surgical treatment.[18] Meanwhile, in a review of 128 patients with SEA by Patel et al[19], 51 patients were initially treated with antibiotics alone. Of these patients, 21 of 51 (41%) eventually required a surgical intervention because of declining motor function or worsening pain. Patients who were treated with IV antibiotics and immediate surgery had the greatest improvement in motor function as measured by the ASIA motor score.

Surgical intervention for epidural abscess is typically performed for all patients with a neurologic deficit, for patients who have positive blood cultures and systemic illness despite appropriate antibiotic therapy, for patients with significant and ongoing pain despite medical management, and for patients with progressive deformity/fracture at the site of the infection.[1,21] Surgical intervention typically consists of a laminectomy at the site(s) of the infection and irrigation/débridement of the infectious collection.[1] Fusion can be performed if the surgeon feels there is significant instability that would result from bony resection.[1] Chaker et al retrospectively studied 738 patients with SEA who underwent surgical intervention.[22] 608 patients underwent laminectomy alone and 130 patients underwent laminectomy and fusion.[22] The laminectomy/fusion patients had significantly higher rate of return to the operating room (mainly due to recurrent infection) and had higher rates of blood transfusion.[22]

Spinal Tuberculosis

Epidemiology

Tuberculosis (TB) is the second most common cause of infectious mortality worldwide, behind HIV.[23,24] A recent WHO report estimated that there were 10.4 million new cases of tuberculosis worldwide (142 cases per 100,000 people).[23,24] This disease is most common in the developing world, particularly in the continents of Asia and Africa (61% and 26% of new cases in 2015).[23] The disease is frequently seen and treated in the United States because of travel and immigration from these regions to North America. According to CDC data, in 2015 there were 9,557 reported cases of TB in the United States.[25]

There is a synergistic relationship between HIV and TB.[23,24] Patients with HIV have suppressed CD4-related immunity, thereby increasing the ability of TB to penetrate their immune defenses.[23,24] In regions such as Sub-Saharan Africa, 50% of all TB cases were estimated to occur in patients who also had HIV.[23]

Extrapulmonary tuberculosis affects the musculoskeletal system in 10% of cases, with the spinal column being the most common site of osseous involvement.[25] Typically, the spinal column is thought to be involved in 50% of TB cases that spread to the musculoskeletal system.[24,25] The thoracic and lumbar spine are the most commonly infected areas of the spinal column.[24,25]

Pathogenesis

Mycobacterium tuberculosis is an acid-fast bacterium that most commonly seeds the pulmonary system through respiratory droplets from an infected individual.[26] Once the lungs have been seeded, the infection can spread hematogenously to the musculoskeletal system and spinal column.[25] The spinal column has a rich arterial supply, thereby providing the bacteria with an avenue for inoculation.[25] The bacteria typically invade the subchondral bone and cortical bone of the vertebral body, causing lytic destruction of the vertebral body and progressive collapse of the anterior column of the spine[24,25] (**Figure 3**).The disk spaces are usually spared

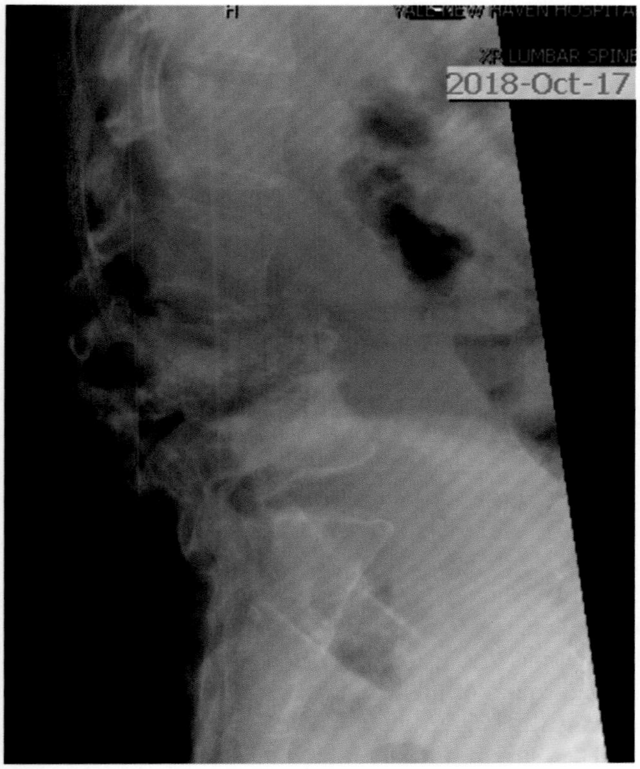

Figure 3 49-year-old male Haitian immigrant with HIV who was transferred to a tertiary care center for management of worsening back pain without neurologic deficits. He was diagnosed with tuberculosis and his radiographs demonstrate changes consistent with tuberculosis of the spinal column. There is preferential destruction of the anterior vertebral body with focal kyphosis and relative sparing of the disk spaces above and below the affected vertebral body.

because of their lack of vascularity.[25] Pott's disease refers to the classic appearance of spinal TB, in which two contiguous vertebral bodies have collapsed into kyphotic alignment, with possible associated soft-tissue infectious granuloma or abscess.[25] The kyphotic deformity seen in patients with spinal TB is commonly called a Gibbus deformity.[25] In spinal TB, the posterior elements are typically spared and patients frequently have involvement of multiple contiguous or noncontiguous vertebral bodies ("skip lesions").[24,25]

Soft-tissue abscesses are frequently seen in association with spinal TB.[24,25] These abscesses can be large in size and spread across multiple levels of the spinal column.[24,25] The abscesses can spread anteriorly under the ALL or posteriorly into the epidural space.[24,25] In the lumbar spine, the soft-tissue spread of TB can cause psoas abscesses.[14,24,25] The soft-tissue abscesses can calcify or cause a large shadow, both of which can be visualized on radiographs of the spine.[24,25]

Neurologic deficits are frequently seen in spinal TB, with studies reporting between 23% and 76% incidence.[24] Neurologic deficits are more frequently seen in the cervical and thoracic spine than the lumbar spine.[24] Neurologic deficits are thought to occur secondary to the combination of focal kyphosis, infectious phlegmon/abscess in the epidural space, and myelopathic cord signal due to focal ischemia.[24,25]

Diagnosis

The diagnosis of pulmonary TB is typically made via sputum analysis for acid-fast bacilli.[26] *M tuberculosis* is a fastidious organism, and laboratory analysis can take up to 6 weeks to demonstrate growth of acid-fast bacilli.[26] The diagnosis of spinal TB should be suspected in any individual with a diagnosis of tuberculosis who develops worsening back pain.[24,25] Similar, to osteomyelitis of the spinal column, the back pain is often insidious in nature and progresses over the course of several months. A kyphotic deformity of the spinal column on physical examination should raise suspicions for spinal TB.[24,25]

Patients can present with motor and/or sensory neurologic deficits, depending on the extent and location of the spinal TB.[24,25] Cervical TB patients can develop quadriplegia and have been noted to suffer from retropharyngeal abscesses.[25] Lumbar TB patients can have restriction of hip flexion secondary to large psoas abscesses rather than true neurologic compromise.[25]

Over the past several years, polymerase chain reaction (PCR) has been used to aid in quicker diagnosis of tuberculosis, through identification of *M tuberculosis* genetic material in a given tissue sample.[24] This test has been shown to have high sensitivity and specificity.[24] In an individual suspected of spinal TB, a biopsy of the suspected vertebrae should be sent for culture for acid-fast bacilli.[24,25] The sample may then be sent for additional PCR analysis to specifically define whether the infection is from *M tuberculosis*.[24,25]

Imaging

Radiographs of the spinal column in a patient with spinal TB will demonstrate kyphotic deformity of the vertebral body with osteolysis of the affected vertebrae, as noted above.[24,25] There is often involvement of multiple vertebrae, and the posterior elements are rarely affected.[24,25] Associated soft-tissue abscesses are frequently calcified or produce shadowing, both of which can be visualized on radiographs of the spinal column.[24,25] CT scan can highlight the above bony and soft-tissue abnormalities in greater detail.[24,25] In addition, CT scan can be used to perform CT-guided bone biopsies of suspected spinal TB and thereby augment in the diagnosis of this condition.[24,25]

MRI with and without gadolinium contrast is the study of choice for the diagnosis of spinal TB.[24,25] MRI demonstrates epidural and paravertebral abscesses, myelopathic cord signal changes, involvement of multiple vertebral bodies, and sparing of the disk space in detail, thus allowing early diagnosis and optimal visualization of spinal TB.[24,25]

Treatment

Pharmacologic therapy is the first-line treatment of spinal TB and can improve both pain and neurologic dysfunction.[24,25] Although there is significant variation with regard to the length and specific medications involved in various treatment regimens, a common cocktail consists of a 6 to 9-month course of rifampin and isoniazid, with the additions of ethambutol and pyrazinamide for a portion of the above treatment course.[24,25] Several studies have demonstrated no additional benefit of surgical intervention in patients with spinal TB who have not yet undergone medical treatment.[24,25] Patients who suffer from paraplegia can experience significant improvement in neurologic function with pharmacologic therapy alone.[24,25]

Currently, surgical treatment is typically reserved for patients who suffer from ongoing neurologic deficits after appropriate medical treatment and patients with severe kyphotic deformity of the spinal column.[24,25] The principles of surgical intervention for spinal TB are removal of the infectious debris and reconstruction/stabilization of the anterior column defect.[24,25] In the thoracic spine this can be accomplished through a transthoracic approach or a posterior approach that allow access to the anterior spinal column, such as costotransversectomy[24] (**Figure 4**). In the lumbar spine, the anterior column is most easily débrided and reconstructed via a retro-peritoneal approach.[24]

Prevention of Postoperative Infections

Prevention of postoperative surgical site infections is critical to good patient outcomes in spine surgery. Recently surgeons, particularly those in pediatric spinal deformity, have come together to release best practice guidelines for infection prevention.[27] The challenge of developing best practice guidelines for infection prevention stems from a lack of strong evidence in the literature. Nevertheless, knowledge of these specific prevention strategies can aid surgeons in minimizing surgical site infections within their own practice.

A recent publication by Vitale et al focused on best practice guidelines for the prevention of surgical site infections in pediatric patients undergoing spine surgery.[27] This study found greater than 90% consensus among pediatric spine surgeons for 13 different infection prevention modalities.[27] This study involved two rounds of voting among the pediatric spine surgeons involved.[27] During the first round, surgeons had a greater than 90% consensus that patient should have chlorhexidine skin wash at home the night before surgery, preoperative urine cultures obtained and treated if positive, preoperative patient education sheets, preoperative nutritional assessment, perioperative intravenous cefazolin, and perioperative intravenous prophylaxis for gram-negative bacilli.[27] Additionally, there was consensus during the first round that operating room access should be limited and there should be adherence to perioperative antimicrobial regimens that should be monitored with regard to agent, time, dosing, redosing, and cessation.[27] During the second round of the loading four additional recommendations were agreed upon including that clipping is preferred to shaving of hair, intrawound vancomycin powder should be used, impervious dressings are preferred postoperatively, and postoperative dressing changes should be minimized before discharge.[27] However, it should be strongly noted that these guidelines are based on a combination of the authors' opinion and evidence; hence the authors state that it is the "unsubstantiated opinion of the authors of the current paper that adherence to recommendations in the best practice guidelines will not only decrease variability in practice but also result in fewer surgical site infections and high-risk children undergoing spinal surgery.[27]"

Patient selection is critical in minimizing the risk of surgical site infections in spine surgery. A study by Ter Gunne et al analysed the incidence of surgical site infection following adult spinal deformity.[28] Some of the factors that predisposed patients to a higher risk of surgical site infection include prior history of the surgical site infection, obesity, diabetes, smoking, and revision surgery.[28] Other factors also included age, urinary incontinence, tumor resection, and 3 or more comorbidities.[28] Although diabetes is a well-known risk factor for postoperative wound infection, the risk of postoperative wound infection is specifically related to the patient's medical management of their diabetes reflected by their glucose control.[28] The hemoglobin A1c, which is a reflection of glucose control over 3 months, has been demonstrated to correlate closely with the risk of postoperative infection.[29] The risk of infection increases

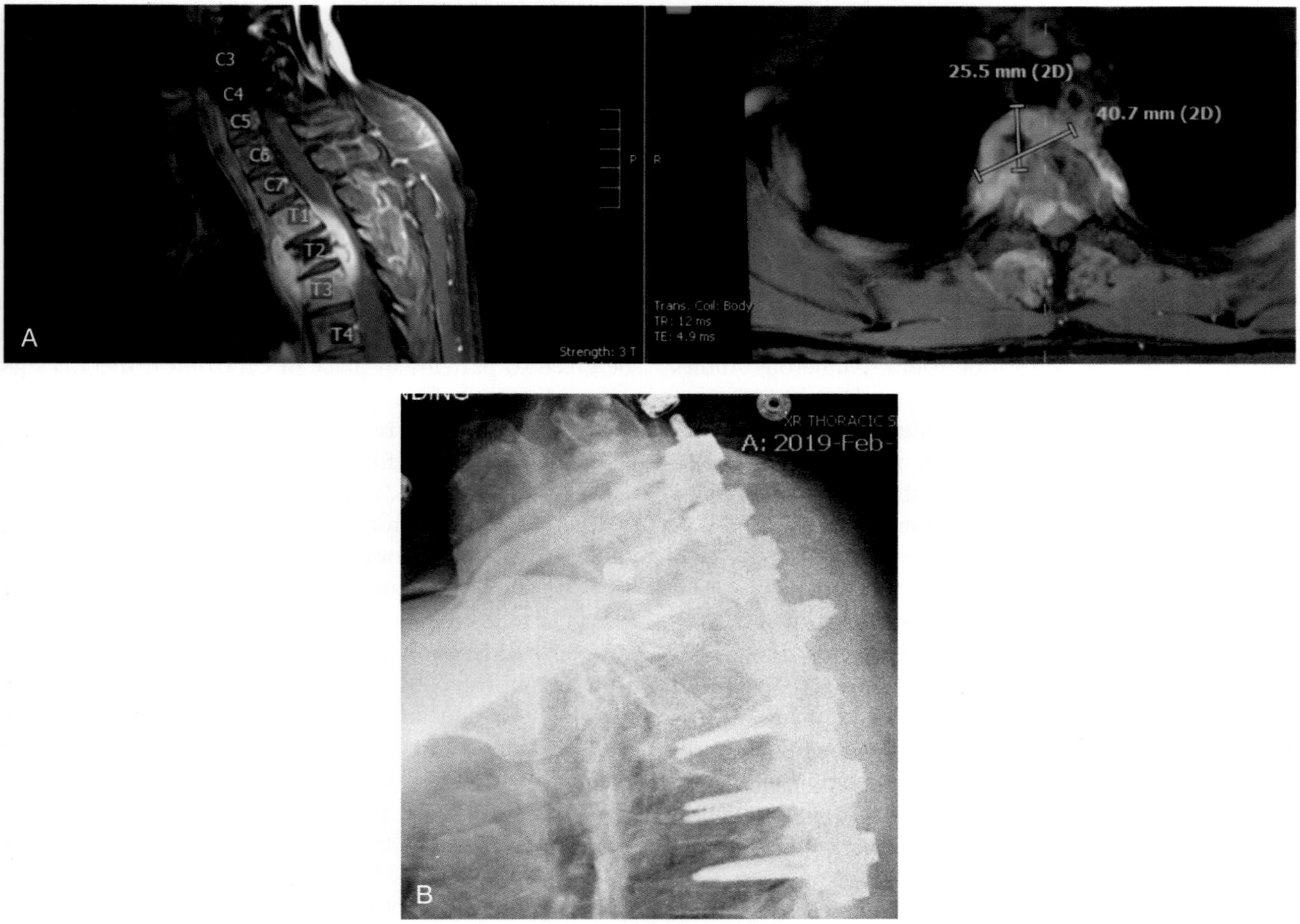

Figure 4 **A**, 30-year-old Indian male with remote exposure to tuberculosis who presented with gait imbalance, urinary retention, and weight loss. He underwent biopsy of the T2 vertebral body, which demonstrated acid-fast bacilli. The T1 postcontrast images demonstrate necrotic lesion within the T2 vertebral body with large soft-tissue component to the infection. There is sparing of the adjacent disk spaces, consistent with tuberculosis. **B**,The patient failed conservative management and underwent C7-T6 posterior spinal fusion, T3 costotransversectomy with application of biomechanical cage. The patient experienced resolution of preoperative symptoms and had an uneventful postoperative course.

proportionally to the patient's A1c value.[29] While there is the debate regarding exact A1c value for surgeons to use to postpone elective surgery, studies have shown that an A1c value greater than 7.5% clearly increases the patient's risk for postoperative infection.[29] A history of previous surgical site infection has been shown in the literature to have an increased odds ratio for postoperative infection of 3.2.[28] Anterior lumbar surgery has a decreased risk of postoperative wound infection compared with posterior surgery with an odds ratio for infection of 0.32.

Several preoperative modalities have been used to minimize surgical site infections in all patients undergoing spine surgery. Antiseptic showers have been suggested as a means to eradicate colonization of the skin flora before surgery. However, this has not been shown to be conclusive in the literature. A Cochrane review that included seven studies demonstrated that there is no consistent effect and no proven effectiveness.[30] Others have studies of aseptic skin clots which had demonstrated a decrease in the rate of positive bacterial culture and surgical site infections; however, there are no randomized controlled trials and the evidence is weak. Skin preparation solutions have been studied through a randomized control trial and may decrease the rate of positive culture results after skin preparation; however, this has not been shown to be conclusively efficacious for the prevention of surgical site infections.

Preoperative MSSA/MRSA screening and eradication has been demonstrated to be effective in adult spine surgery. A recent meta-analysis demonstrated that positive carriers have an increased risk of surgical site infections and that eradication in carriers lowers the rate of surgical site infections. That study recommended preoperative screening and eradication. However, in practice it can be logistically challenging to perform preoperative screening. One of the authors (CS) has all patients treated in the preoperative holding area without prior screening given the low cost of treatment, high prevalence of staph colonization, and high cost associated with screening secondary to the time intensive nature of preoperative screening by ancillary providers.

The surgeon should be cognizant of the potential for contamination in the operating room. Numerous studies have looked at the contamination rate based on various sources in the operating room. Potential sources of contamination include C-arm fluoroscopy, microscope, implants, cadaveric allograft, gowns, and scrubs. A study by Bible et al determined that the contamination rate of sterile gowns in the OR was 6% to 9% in the chest region.[31] Bible et al also studied the contamination rate from microscope use in the operating room. This study demonstrated a 24% contamination rate of the microscope eyepiece and a 44% contamination rate of the microscope drape by overhead structures.[32] A study by Biswas et al[33] found that there was a 56% contamination rate of the top portion of the C-arm and 28% of the upper front portion of the C-arm. A study by Krueger et al[34] demonstrated a 41% contamination rate from unworn scrubs and an 89% contamination rate from scrubs worn post call.

Other intraoperative risk factors for postoperative wound infection include surgical time, estimated blood loss (EBL), and intravenous and intrawound antibiotics. Surgical time has been correlated with increased risk in surgical site infections in spine surgery. The previously discussed study by Ter Gunne et al demonstrated that the odds ratio for a deep postoperative wound infection in patients who had 2 to 5 hours of surgery was 2.4 (*P*-value 0.02) compared with patients who had less than 2 hours of surgery.[28] Patients who had surgeries greater than 5 hours had a 2.85 odds ratio (*P*-value 0.02) of a deep wound infection also compared with patients who had a surgical time of less than 2 hours.[28] Surgical time can be minimized through diligent preoperative planning. Additionally, while surgical times often correlate to EBL, studies have shown that EBL greater than 1 L is an independent risk factor for postoperative wound infection with an odds ratio of 2.2.

One randomized control trial studying wound irrigation with dilute betadine solution demonstrated decreased surgical site infections in spine patients compared with controls.[35] Although close suction drains are commonly used to practice, a Cochrane review of 36 orthopaedic studies demonstrated no difference in surgical site infections with the use of a drain.[36] Antibiotic sutures were shown in one randomized control trial to lower surgical site infections.[37]

IV antibiotics should be administered within 60 minutes of incision and should be redosed appropriately throughout the surgery. Typically a cephalosporin is given preoperatively, unless the patient has an allergy. It is important for the surgeon to communicate with the anesthesia team regarding redosing of antibiotics intraoperatively. For cefazolin, in particular, it should be redosed every 4 hours or once there is approximately 1.5 L of blood loss. Vancomycin or clindamycin can be given to patients in place of cefazolin if there is significant concern for a potential allergic reaction. There is significant debate regarding the use of perioperative vancomycin and gentamicin for MRSA and gram-negative prophylaxis, respectively.

There is also significant debate regarding the efficacy of intrawound vancomycin powder. There are several level III studies supporting the use of intrawound vancomycin to decrease postoperative surgical site infection rates. A study by Sweet et al[38] demonstrated an infection rate in the control group of 2.6% compared with an infection rate in the vancomycin powder group of 0.2% (*P*-value < 0.0001), in patients receiving instrumented fusions. The strength of this study in particular was that it was well powered with 911 patients in the vancomycin powder treatment group and 821 patients in the control group. Of note this study recorded only deep wound infections. A study by Pahys et al[39] of 1,001 patients undergoing posterior cervical spine surgery compared the use of vancomycin in combination with alcohol foam prep and superficial drain placement with a control group, which did not receive any of the three treatments, and found an infection rate of 1.86% in the control group and 0% in the treatment group, despite the treatment group having a significantly higher age and percentage of greater than four-level surgery. However, a randomized control trial comparing the use of standard systemic prophylaxis only to intrawound vancomycin powder in addition to systemic prophylaxis demonstrated a 1.68% infection rate in the control group and a 1.61% infection rate in the treatment group, which was not statistically different.[40] The authors of this study state that the "use of vancomycin powder may not be effective when incidence of infection is low.[40]"

An animal study by Zebala et al[41] used a rabbit spine infection model with and without the use of intrawound vancomycin powder. The group receiving intrawound vancomycin had no bacterial growth, whereas all rabbits that were managed with only prophylactic cefazolin had persistent staph aureus contamination. A study by Rahman et al[42] demonstrated a decreased rate of surgical site infections and patients undergoing adult spinal deformity from 5% to 0.7% with injury wound vancomycin powder. A separate study by Theologis et al[43] also demonstrated a clear decrease in the rate of surgical site infections in patients with adult spinal deformity from 10.9% to 2.6%. This study also determined that the use of intrawound vancomycin powder would result in $244,000 in cost savings per 100 thoracolumbar deformity procedures performed.

More recently attention has been turned to intrawound tobramycin to prevent gram-negative infections given that approximately 30% of all spine surgical site infections are secondary to gram-negative bacteria. Particular patient populations, such as neuromuscular scoliosis patients, have high rates of gram-negative surgical site infections. Most of the literature supporting the use of intrawound tobramycin is based on the orthopaedic trauma literature. A study by Ostermann et al[44] reviewed 1,085 open fractures treated with either IV antibiotics or IV antibiotics with intrawound tobramycin. The control group had an infection rate of 12%, whereas the treatment group receding both IV antibiotics and intrawound tobramycin had an infection rate of only 3.7% (P < 0.001). An animal model study by Laratta et al[45] demonstrated that in a rabbit spine infection model tobramycin powder eliminated *E coli* surgical site contamination. Rabbits in the control group that did not receive intrawound tobramycin had bacterial growth in 39 out of 40 samples, whereas none of the 40 samples from the tobramycin group demonstrated bacterial growth.

Key Study Points

- The optimal study to assess for intraspinal infections is an MRI of the area of interest with and without gadolinium contrast.
- The most common pathogen causing osteomyelitis/diskitis, spinal epidural abscess is *S aureus*.
- Medical treatment, consisting of IV antibiotics and bracing treatment, can be considered for neurologically intact in patients with osteomyelitis/diskitis, spinal epidural abscess. Patients with neurologic deficits are typically treated with surgical intervention and IV antibiotics.
- Tuberculosis infections of the spinal column preferentially affect the anterior column of the spine and spare the disk space (in contrast to diskitis/osteomyelitis). Multiple vertebral bodies can be affected and soft-tissue abscesses are common.
- Multiple studies have shown vancomycin powder decreases the rate of postoperative infections in elective spine surgery.

Annotated References

1. Rothman RH, Simeone FA, Garfin SR: *Rothman-Simeone and Herkowitz's the Spine*. Philadelphia, Elsevier, 2018, 2018.
2. Grammatico L, Baron S, Rusch E, et al: Epidemiology of vertebral osteomyelitis (VO) in France: Analysis of hospital-discharge data 2002-2003. *Epidemiol Infect* 2008;136(5):653.
3. Mylona E, Samarkos M, Kakalou E, Fanourgiakis P, Skoutelis A: Pyogenic vertebral osteomyelitis: A systematic review of clinical characteristics. *Semin Arthritis Rheum* 2009;39(1):10.
4. Sans N, Faruch M, Lapegue F, Ponsot A, Chiavassa H, Railhac JJ: Infections of the spinal column–spondylodiscitis. *Diagn Interv Imaging* 2012;93(6):520.
5. Larson DL, Gilstrap J, Simonelic K, Carrera GF: Is there a simple, definitive, and cost-effective way to diagnose osteomyelitis in the pressure ulcer patient? *Plast Reconstr Surg* 2011;127(2):670.
6. Graham SM, Fishlock A, Millner P, Sandoe J: The management gram-negative bacterial haematogenous vertebral osteomyelitis: A case series of diagnosis, treatment and therapeutic outcomes. *Eur Spine J* 2013;22(8):1845.
7. Wiesseman GJ, Wood VE, Kroll LL, Linda L: Pseudomonas vertebral osteomyelitis in heroin addicts. Report of five cases. *J Bone Joint Surg Am* 1973;55(7):1416.
8. Bryan V, Franks L, Torres H: *Pseudomonas aeruginosa* cervical diskitis with chondro-osteomyelitis in an intravenous drug abuser. *Surg Neurol* 1973;1(3):142.
9. Park KH, Cho OH, Jung M, et al: Clinical characteristics and outcomes of hematogenous vertebral osteomyelitis caused by gram-negative bacteria. *J Infect* 2014;69(1):42.
10. Nickerson EK, Sinha R: Vertebral osteomyelitis in adults: An update. *Br Med Bull* 2016;117(1):121.

    Review of treatment options for vertebral osteomyelitis. Level of evidence: IV.
11. Sehn JK, Gilula LA: Percutaneous needle biopsy in diagnosis and identification of causative organisms in cases of suspected vertebral osteomyelitis. *Eur J Radiol* 2012;81(5):940.
12. Gras G, Buzele R, Parienti JJ, et al: Microbiological diagnosis of vertebral osteomyelitis: Relevance of second percutaneous biopsy following initial negative biopsy and limited yield of post-biopsy blood cultures. *Eur J Clin Microbiol Infect Dis* 2014;33(3):371.
13. Dragsted C, Aagaard T, Ohrt-Nissen S, Gehrchen M, Dahl B: Mortality and health-related quality of life in patients surgically treated for spondylodiscitis. *J Orthop Surg* 2017;25(2):2309499017716068.

    Retrospective review of clinical outcomes in patients undergoing surgery for spondylodiskitis. Level of evidence: III.
14. Aagaard T, Roed C, Dahl B, Obel N: Long-term prognosis and causes of death after spondylodiscitis: A Danish nationwide cohort study. *Infect Dis (Lond)* 2016;48(3):201.

    Danish registry study assessing causes of long-term mortality in patients with spondylodiskitis. Level of evidence: III.

Spine

15. Darouiche RO: Spinal epidural abscess. *N Engl J Med* 2006;355(19):2012.

16. Johnson KG: Spinal epidural abscess. *Crit Care Nurs Clin North Am* 2013;25(3):389.

17. Vakili M, Crum-Cianflone NF: Spinal epidural abscess: A series of 101 cases. *Am J Med* 2017;130(12):1458.

    Retrospective review of outcomes in SEA patients identified through ICD-9 coding. Level of evidence: IV.

18. Arko L, Quach E, Nguyen V, Chang D, Sukul V, Kim BS: Medical and surgical management of spinal epidural abscess: A systematic review. *Neurosurg Focus* 2014;37(2):E4.

19. Patel AR, Alton TB, Bransford RJ, Lee MJ, Bellabarba CB, Chapman JR: Spinal epidural abscesses: Risk factors, medical versus surgical management, a retrospective review of 128 cases. *Spine J* 2014;14(2):326.

20. Heusner AP: Nontuberculous spinal epidural infections. *N Engl J Med* 1948;239(23):845.

21. Shah AA, Ogink PT, Nelson SB, Harris MB, Schwab JH: Nonoperative management of spinal epidural abscess: Development of a predictive algorithm for failure. *J Bone Joint Surg Am* 2018;100(7):546.

    The authors create a predictive algorithm for failure of conservative management of SEA patients based upon retrospective data. Level of evidence: IV.

22. Chaker AN, Bhimani AD, Esfahani DR, et al: Epidural abscess: A propensity analysis of surgical treatment strategies. *Spine* 2018;43(24):E1479-E1485.

    ACS-NSQIP data used to analyze 30-day outcomes in patients with SEA undergoing surgery. Level of evidence: III.

23. Sotgiu G, Sulis G, Matteelli A: Tuberculosis-a world health organization perspective. *Microbiol Spectr* 2017;5(1):1-2.

    Review of current state of tuberculosis treatments and possible future directions. Level of evidence: IV.

24. Dunn RN, Ben Husien M: Spinal tuberculosis. *Bone Joint Lett J* 2018;100-B(4):425.

    Review of the current treatment algorithms for spinal tuberculosis. Level of evidence: IV.

25. Leonard MK, Blumberg HM: Musculoskeletal tuberculosis. *Microbiol Spectr* 2017;5(2):1-2.

    Review of epidemiology and treatment algorithms for musculoskeletal tuberculosis. Level of evidence: IV.

26. Lyon SM, Rossman MD: Pulmonary tuberculosis. *Microbiol Spectr* 2017;5(1):1-2.

    Review of epidemiology and treatment algorithms for pulmonary tuberculosis. Level of evidence: IV

27. Vitale MG, Riedel MD, Glotzbecker MP, et al: Building consensus: Development of a best practice guideline (BPG) for surgical site infection (SSI) prevention in high-risk pediatric spine surgery. *J Pediatr Orthop* 2013;33(5):471.

28. Pull ter Gunne AF, van Laarhoven CJ, Cohen DB: Incidence of surgical site infection following adult spinal deformity surgery: An analysis of patient risk. *Eur Spine J* 2010;19(6):982.

29. Cancienne JM, Werner BC, Chen DQ, Hassanzadeh H, Shimer AL: Perioperative hemoglobin A1c as a predictor of deep infection following single-level lumbar decompression in patients with diabetes. *Spine J* 2017;17(8):1100.

    Retrospective case control study assessing impact of Hb-A1c on rates of deep space infection in single-level lumbar decompression. Level of evidence: III.

30. Webster J, Osborne S: Preoperative bathing or showering with skin antiseptics to prevent surgical site infection. *Cochrane Database Syst Rev* 2015;(2):CD004985.

31. Bible JE, Biswas D, Whang PG, Simpson AK, Grauer JN: Which regions of the operating gown should be considered most sterile? *Clin Orthop Relat Res* 2009;467(3):825.

32. Bible JE, O'Neill KR, Crosby CG, Schoenecker JG, McGirt MJ, Devin CJ: Microscope sterility during spine surgery. *Spine* 2012;37(7):623.

33. Biswas D, Bible JE, Whang PG, Simpson AK, Grauer JN: Sterility of C-arm fluoroscopy during spinal surgery. *Spine* 2008;33(17):1913.

34. Krueger CA, Murray CK, Mende K, Guymon CH, Gerlinger TL: The bacterial contamination of surgical scrubs. *Am J Orthop (Belle Mead NJ)* 2012;41(5):E69.

35. Cheng MT, Chang MC, Wang ST, Yu WK, Liu CL, Chen TH: Efficacy of dilute betadine solution irrigation in the prevention of postoperative infection of spinal surgery. *Spine* 2005;30(15):1689.

36. Parker MJ, Livingstone V, Clifton R, McKee A: Closed suction surgical wound drainage after orthopaedic surgery. *Cochrane Database Syst Rev* 2007;(3):CD001825.

37. Rozzelle CJ, Leonardo J, Li V: Antimicrobial suture wound closure for cerebrospinal fluid shunt surgery: A prospective, double-blinded, randomized controlled trial. *J Neurosurg Pediatr* 2008;2(2):111.

38. Sweet FA, Roh M, Sliva C: Intrawound application of vancomycin for prophylaxis in instrumented thoracolumbar fusions: Efficacy, drug levels, and patient outcomes. *Spine* 2011;36(24):2084.

39. Pahys JM, Pahys JR, Cho SK, et al: Methods to decrease postoperative infections following posterior cervical spine surgery. *J Bone Joint Surg Am* 2013;95(6):549.

40. Tubaki VR, Rajasekaran S, Shetty AP: Effects of using intravenous antibiotic only versus local intrawound vancomycin antibiotic powder application in addition to intravenous antibiotics on postoperative infection in spine surgery in 907 patients. *Spine* 2013;38(25):2149.

41. Zebala LP, Chuntarapas T, Kelly MP, Talcott M, Greco S, Riew KD: Intrawound vancomycin powder eradicates surgical wound contamination: An in vivo rabbit study. *J Bone Joint Surg Am* 2014;96(1):46.

42. Rahman RKK, Lenke LG, Bridwell KH, et al: Intrawound vancomycin powder lowers the acute deep wound infection rate in adult spinal deformity patients: PAPER #36. *Spine* 2011;73.

43. Theologis AA, Demirkiran G, Callahan M, Pekmezci M, Ames C, Deviren V: Local intrawound vancomycin powder decreases the risk of surgical site infections in complex adult deformity reconstruction: A cost analysis. *Spine* 2014;39(22):1875.

44. Ostermann PA, Seligson D, Henry SL: Local antibiotic therapy for severe open fractures. A review of 1085 consecutive cases. *J Bone Joint Surg Br* 1995;77(1):93.

45. Laratta JL, Shillingford JN, Hardy N, et al: Intrawound tobramycin powder eradicates surgical wound contamination: An in vivo rabbit study. *Spine* 2017;42(24):E1393.

   Analysis of efficacy of intrawound tobramycin powder on 20 rabbits that underwent laminectomy and implantation of wire. Level of evidence: IV.

Chapter 52

Concepts in Primary Benign, Primary Malignant, and Metastatic Tumors of the Spine

Arya Nick Shamie, MD • Francis John Hornicek, MD, PhD

Spine

ABSTRACT

Tumors involving the spine comprise various types and subtypes which require meticulous evaluation and diagnosis of the lesion to arrive at the best nonsurgical and/or surgical treatment for the patient. One of the most important steps prior to arriving at the correct diagnosis is to obtain adequate tissue biopsy. Some pathologic conditions have similar clinical presentations and appearances on radiographic and advance study imaging. Therefore, core or open biopsy of the suspicious lesion is critical to arrive at the best treatment for the patient. Some tumors can be treated medically and others require extensive en bloc resections with major reconstruction of the involved anatomic structures. Taking into account the biology of the tumor cells and the overall physiologic status of each individual patient will allow the surgeon and the multidisciplinary team to devise the best plan of care for each patient.

Keywords: chordoma, metastatic spine tumors, primary spine tumors, radiation therapy, surgical treatment of spine tumors

Introduction

Cancers involving the spine are encountered either as primary lesions or more commonly metastatic lesions from a remote location through hematogenous spread. Understanding the disease process is critically important as one devises the proper medical or surgical treatment for the patient. Primary tumors of the spine, although rare, are best treated aggressively with en bloc resection to decrease the risk of local recurrence or distant metastasis. In contrast, metastatic disease needs to be studied to understand the systemic burden on an individual patient before the proper medical or surgical treatment plan is devised.

Background

National Institutes of Health (NIH) and National Cancer Institute estimated that in 2018, more than 1.7 million new cases of cancer will be diagnosed in the United States and over 600,000 people will die from the disease.[1] The most common cancers (listed in descending order according to estimated new cases in 2018) are breast cancer, lung and bronchus cancer, prostate cancer, colon and rectum cancer, melanoma of the skin, bladder cancer, non-Hodgkin lymphoma, kidney and renal pelvis cancer, endometrial cancer, leukemia, pancreatic cancer, thyroid cancer, and liver cancer.

In 2016, there were an estimated 15.5 million cancer survivors in the United States. The number of cancer survivors is expected to rise to 20.3 million by 2026

Dr. Shamie or an immediate family member has received royalties from Seaspine and Stryker; is a member of a speakers' bureau or has made paid presentations on behalf of SI Bone, Stryker, and Vertiflex; serves as a paid consultant to or is an employee of Stryker and Vertiflex; has stock or stock options held in Providence, SI Bone, and Vertiflex; has received research or institutional support from Pfizer; and serves as a board member, owner, officer, or committee member of the American College of Spine Surgery. Dr. Hornicek or an immediate family member serves as a paid consultant to or is an employee of Globus Medical and Stryker; has stock or stock options held in Biome AI, Inc. and Bone Solutions, Inc.; has received research or institutional support from Stryker; has received nonincome support (such as equipment or services), commercially derived honoraria, or other non–research-related funding (such as paid travel) from Biomet; and serves as a board member, owner, officer, or committee member of the American Association of Tissue Banks, FDA, ISOLS, and the Musculoskeletal Tumor Society.

partly due to aging population and improved detection. This increase in overall numbers of people living with cancer will also increase the prevalence of patients with metastatic disease. Approximately, one-third of men and women will be diagnosed with cancer at some point during their lifetimes (based on 2013-2015 data). Estimated national expenditures for cancer care in the United States in 2017 was over $140 billion. In future years, costs are likely to increase as the population ages and cancer prevalence increases. Costs are also likely to increase as more advanced and costly treatments are developed and utilized as standards of care.

In the United States, approximately 1.2 million people are diagnosed with cancer each year, making this disease category the second most common cause of death in the country. Autopsy studies have shown that more than 60% of patients with cancer have evidence of spinal metastasis. Spine tumors can be classified as primary spine tumors, which originate in the spinal elements, or metastatic tumors, which spread from some other location or organ in the body. Further classifications, like all tumors, are made designating a tumor malignant or benign. Metastatic disease substantial enough to cause spinal cord compression occurs in approximately 5% to 14% of patients with metastatic cancer, resulting in approximately 20,000 new instances of tumor-induced myelopathy per year. Approximately half of these patients will lose the ability to ambulate.

Primary benign tumors of the spine, such as hemangioma of bone, are present in up to 10% of the normal population and are often discovered incidentally. Primary malignant spine tumors, by contrast, are exceedingly rare and account for less than 3% of all malignant spine tumors.

Primary Tumors of the Spine

Primary malignant spine tumors are rare and constitute less than 5% of extradural tumors involving the axial skeleton (**Table 1**). Primary tumors of the spine originate mostly from either the bone or cartilage tissue but also from associated tissues like neural structures in or around the spine. The primary lesions that originate from the bony structures are generally extradural in contrast to the intradural nature of most primary tumors arising from neural elements. Intradural tumors may be further subdivided into intramedullary and extramedullary tumors, depending on whether they originate from the spinal cord itself or the nerve roots distal to the spinal cord, respectively. In individuals older than 20 years, majority of primary tumors of the spine are malignant. Proper treatment protocols for these tumors have evolved over the years requiring extensive research and discussions leading to a consensus and leading to well-developed and evidence-based position papers.[2] It is critically important to follow the best practices in treatment for these primary tumors of the spine to minimize local recurrence and provide best quality of life and survival rates for these patients. Typically, a well-planned and more technically challenging en bloc resection is the best approach for these patients with intralesional resection leading to a less favorable outcome for the patient.

Table 1

Anatomic Locations of Most Common Primary Tumors of Spine and Metastases

Vertebral Locations	Benign Tumors	Malignant Tumors
Anterior elements	Eosinophilic granuloma	Chordoma
	Giant cell tumor	Multiple myeloma
	Hemangioma	Metastasis
	Aneurysmal bone cyst	
Posterior elements	Osteoblastoma	
	Osteoid osteoma	
	Osteochondroma	
Adjacent levels	Aneurysmal bone cyst	
	Osteoblastoma	
Multiple noncontiguous levels		Metastasis

Reprinted with permission from Scott DL, Pedlow FX, Hecht AC, Hornicek FJ: Primary benign and malignant extradural spine tumors, in Frymoyer JW, Wiesel SW, eds: *Adult and Pediatric Spine*, ed 3. Philadelphia, PA, Lippincott Williams and Wilkins, 2004, p 192.

Diagnosis and Staging

Patient with tumors involving the spine, typically present with axial pain that is chronic and progressive. They typically report pain that awakens them in the middle of the night and when recumbent, in contrast to degenerative conditions of the spine which are typically activity related. Oftentimes, the delay in diagnosis and severity of the pain results in these patients being placed on narcotic pain medications prior to seeing a surgeon. A minority of patients present with neurologic symptoms or deficits but these symptoms often present later in the disease process as the tumor expands compressing the neural elements.

The evaluation in a patient with a suspected spine tumor should begin with a complete history of symptoms including a familial history followed by observation of the patient's sagittal and coronal balance to assess for signs of reflexive splinting or scoliosis. The posterior spine should be palpated for areas of focal tenderness or masses. Many primary tumors of the spine can be palpable on presentation. The thyroid, breast, and prostate should be palpated for enlargement or irregularities, with the lymph nodes in the neck, axilla, and the groin.

The physical examination should then focus on evaluating the neurologic function with signs of lower or upper motor neuron compression. Patients with upper motor neuron compression may exhibit pathologic reflexes such as the Hoffmann, inverted radial reflex (digit flexion when tapping the brachioradialis tendon) or generalized hyperreflexia. Patients may also walk with a wide-based gait and be unable to perform a tandem heel-to-toe walking.

For patients showing signs of upper motor neuron compression, a thorough cranial nerve evaluation should be performed to check for intracranial involvement.

Radiographs remain the primary imaging tool, but many primary lesions are initially undetected, as, 30% to 50% trabecular bone destruction is required before the lytic lesion appears on traditional radiography. Evaluation of radiographs may also be more challenging with underlying degenerative conditions or metabolic bone diseases. With a higher degree of suspicion, more advance imaging needs to be obtained to evaluate a patient with suspected primary tumor of the spine. CT and MRI are used to evaluate the entirety of the spine. Certain characteristics of various tumors can delineate the specific diagnoses; moth-eaten lesions are typically due to a permeative process in the trabecular bone like multiple myeloma. The intervertebral disks are usually resistant to tumor invasion unless the lesion is producing collagenase and proteinase which is more typically seen in pyogenic processes. CT scan is also an essential tool for staging of malignancies with the typical series of chest, abdomen, and pelvis but can also provide anatomic and bony details not visible on radiographs or MRI. When MRI is not possible, CT myelogram can be used to assess neurologic compression in the spine. MRI's advantage is that it provides detailed imaging in multiple planes of the spine in the absence of ionizing radiation and provides a detailed view of neural elements and can detect small lesions even when they are missed by radiographs or CT scans. Tumor infiltration of the bone marrow decreases the signal on T1-weighted images by displacing the fatty marrow and increases the signal on T2-weighted images due to increase in edema in reactive bone. Technetium bone scan is a low-cost tool for diagnosis of bone metastasis and skip lesions, but it has lower utility in detection of spine tumors when compared with CT and MRI. Recent literature suggests the use of a combination of positron emission tomography (PET) with MRI for earlier detection of disease and for differentiation of tumor versus radiation necrosis.[3] But more investigation is necessary before this positron emission tomography (PET)/MRI or PET/CT modality is standardized and used routinely for evaluation of patients with spine tumors.

When encountering a patient with suspected tumor of the spine, it is critically important to distinguish the suspected disease from other differential diagnoses like trauma and infection and misleading processes like fibrous dysplasia, metabolic bone diseases, and bone islands. Comprehensive evaluation of routine labs, radiographs of involved areas and chest, CT of chest/abdomen/pelvis, and most often a biopsy are necessary to obtain the proper diagnosis. In addition to a complete blood count (CBC) and chemistry panel, serum electrophoresis (multiple myeloma), serum calcium, alkaline phosphatase, and prostate-specific antigen (PSA) (prostate cancer) should be considered.

The anatomic distribution of primary spine tumors based on historical data of Rizzoli institute is 18% in the cervical spine and 41% in each of the thoracic and lumbar spine. Of all 323 tumors reported from 1946 to 1996, 73% of them were benign tumors.[4] Benign tumors are usually discovered in patients younger than 20 years and rarely arise after skeletal maturity. Common forms of benign spine tumors of the spine are osteoid osteoma, osteoblastoma, eosinophilic granuloma (EG), aneurysmal bone cyst (ABC), giant cell tumor (GCT), and hemangioma.

Many of these tumors can be treated with new adjuvant medical treatments like Denosumab for GCT or with stereotactic radiation as these primary tumors are very sensitive to this form of treatment. Radiation, however, raises the risk of malignant degeneration; therefore, surgical resection is preferred in many cases. Denosumab for GCT has been used to initially shrink the tumor size, but ultimately a surgical resection is necessary to decrease the risk of local recurrence or distant metastasis.[5]

Primary Benign Tumor Subtypes

There are distinct types of primary spine tumors that require unique treatment regimen. One type of such class of tumors is osteoid **osteomas and osteoblastoma.** These tumors are characterized by a central nidus of fibrous tissue, lymphocytes osteoid and woven bone with interconnected trabeculae, as well as a background and rim of highly vascularized, fibrous connective tissue. Osteoblastomas are typically larger at 1.5 to 2.0 cm and can have a higher local recurrence rate as compared to osteoid osteomas which can be indolent and even regress without any treatment. These tumors occur in the posterior elements with the smaller lesions best diagnosed by CT scan. NSAIDs are effective in the treatment of pain associated with osteoid osteomas which can be a clue for proper diagnosis of a patient with low back pain of unknown origin. When these benign lesions do not respond to medical treatment, radiofrequency ablation for small lesions and surgical curettage for larger lesions have been shown to be effective in the majority of patients but more research and multidisciplinary collaboration are needed to perhaps change the treatment algorithm in the future.[6]

Osteochondromas

Osteochondromas (osteocartilaginous exostoses) are the most common benign lesions of the long bones and account for 4% of benign spine lesions. These tumors originate from laterally displaced fragments of cartilage from the regions of enchondral bone formation. These tumors can occur randomly or can be associated with an autosomal dominant trait of hereditary multiple osteocartilaginous exostoses (HMOCE). Malignant degeneration can occur in 1% to 15% of these lesions with the higher rates malignancy in patients with multiple lesions. When these lesions occur in the spinal canal, they can cause symptomatic cord compression. These lesions are differentiated on axial CT scans from benign osteosarcomas by their appearance with shared intramedullary canal and the continuity of the bony cortex with the adjacent vertebra. Osteochondromas typically arise from the posterior elements, that is, spinous processes, and can create a palpable and painful mass crossing over to an adjacent level. Surgery is seldom indicated unless the lesions are causing specific symptoms like radiculopathy from tumor extension in the neural foramina or anterior cervical lesions causing dysphagia.

Giant Cell Tumors

Giant cell tumors (GCTs) are characterized by multinucleated giant cells surrounded by richly vascularized networks of spindle-shaped stromal cells. These tumors account for 3% of spine tumors and are more commonly seen in the sacral region and sometimes penetrating the sacroiliac joints. When present in the axial skeleton, it usually arises in the vertebral body or the pedicles. Women between 10 and 40 years of age are more likely to develop these lesions. The GCT lesions in the vertebral body can compress the neural elements in up to 50% of cases. Denosumab shrinkage of the GCT is very successful with a need for reconstructive surgery only if bone lysis is extensive enough to cause spinal instability. Total en bloc resections of more advanced GCT lesions have shown better long-term recurrence-free survival rates as compared to total intralesional resections in recent studies.[7]

Osteosarcomas

Osteosarcomas of the spine account for 3% to 15% of primary spine tumors and have been highly associated (40% prevalence) with survivors of retinoblastoma survivors. Mutations in the tumor-suppressor gene p53 and the Rb gene have been associated.[8] Axial tumors tend to occur in older age groups as compared with appendicular tumors. Clinical presentation is similar to other tumors with pain as the predominant presenting symptom. Radiographically, osteosarcoma of the spine usually appears as mixed lytic and blastic lesions with significant destruction of the surround normal bone. Treatment is usually a combination of wide resection, chemotherapy and radiation with best survival rates seen in patients who receive early surgical resection, although the 5-year survival of these patients is still low at approximately 4% to 17%.

Chondrosarcomas

Chondrosarcomas of the axial skeleton are the second most common primary tumors of the spine. These tumors occur predominantly in men (80%) between the ages of 30 and 70 years. These tumors typically involve the posterior elements resulting in a gradually painful palpable mass. These lesions are typically lytic and with a sclerotic margin. There remains a wide range of chondrosarcoma subtypes with varied responses to different treatments. Surgical resection with adjuvant radiation therapy remains to be the preferred mode of treatment for these locally aggressive tumors. High-dose photon/proton radiation therapy following surgical resection has been shown to improve long-term local control with up to 85% at 8 years for primary tumors.[9]

Chordomas

Chordomas are highly aggressive malignant but low-grade tumors arising from the primitive notochordal origin. Chordomas are the most common primary malignant tumor of the spine in adults. There is a 3:1 male to female ratio, and it usually occurs in patients older than 50 years. Fifty percent of Chordomas occur in the sacrum and coccyx, 35% in the upper cervical-occipital region, and 15% in the mobile segments of the spine; middle-aged men typically have L4, L5 lesions, and elderly men have more incidence of lesions in L3. Histologically, these lesions are characterized by foamy, vacuolated, physaliphorous cells that grow in distinct nodules. These tumors are keratin positive which distinguishes them from the non-keratin-positive chondrosarcomas. Patients present with insidious onset of pain and lumbosacral radiculopathy as the tumor mass engulfs the neural elements emanating from the spine and/or sacrum. Due to their notochordal origin, these lesions show midline bone destruction on CT scans with calcifications in the soft-tissue extensions of these lesions. Sacral lesions can pass across the sacroiliac joint and invade the ilium. Wide en bloc resection of these tumors has been associated with better recurrence-free survival. Various techniques have been described for surgical treatment of Chordomas and meticulous radical en bloc resection of these tumors remains to be the most important factor in assuring the patients the best disease free survival rates.[10]

Surgical Staging

Enneking has been credited for providing the first published oncologic staging system in 1986. Weinstein, Boriani, and Biagini (WBB) modified the Enneking system in 1989 to incorporate tumor location and anatomy in the classification (**Figure 1**). These staging systems are used to identify groups of patients with predictively low or high risk of recurrence, although individual patient's outcome can vary depending on many factors like the cellular behavior of various tumors.

The WBB system for primary spine tumors divides each vertebra into two radial zones like the face of a clock with five layers starting in the outer boundary of the vertebrae all the way to the intradural space (**Figure 1**). The surgical planning and approach is determined by the location of the tumor and the depth of the

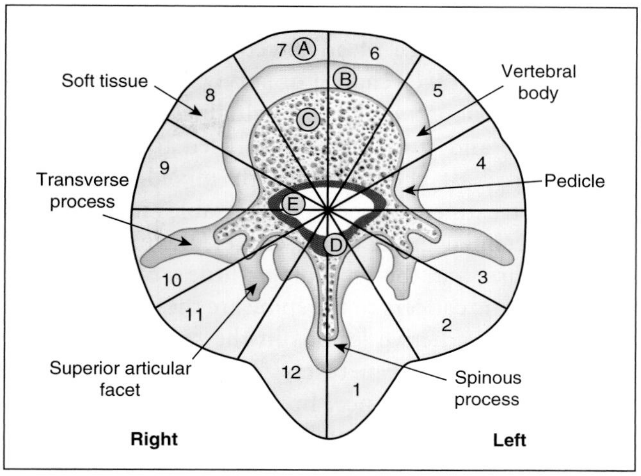

Figure 1 Illustration demonstrating the Weinstein-Boriani-Biagini staging system where the spine is subdivided into 12 equal segments (1–12) and divided in 5 layers (A–E) from superficial to deep. (Adapted from Boriani S, Weinstein JN, Biagini R: Primary bone tumors of the spine: Terminology and surgical staging. *Spine* 1997;22(9):1036-1044.)

involvement. For example, (1) zones 4 to 8 or 5 to 9 with one pedicle free are appropriate for anterior vertebrectomy, (2) zones 3 to 5 or 8 to 11 are appropriate for hemivertebrectomy, and (3) zones 10 to 3 are appropriate for laminectomy or posterior resection alone. The WBB system has been validated for GCTs and chordomas above the sacrum.

Surgical Technique

Surgical techniques for treatment of spine tumors fall under two broad categories of excision or resection. Excision of the tumor usually is subtotal, and some of the tumor tissue is left behind in the tumor bed. In contrast, en bloc resection of the tumor is complete removal of the tumor tissue with the goal of having clear margins. En bloc resection is limited in many occasions due to close proximity of the vital tissues like blood vessels and/or the spinal cord.[10] When en bloc resection of the tumor is not possible, aggressive intralesional resection of maximal amount of tumor that is possible, without compromising safety for the patient, is a good alternative.

Metastatic Tumors of the Spine

The term metastasis was coined in early 1800 by a French gynecologist Joseph Recamier. Since then our understanding of this disease process has improved tremendously; however, there still remains a serious and valid concern by the patients and their physicians when a distant spread of disease is discovered. Metastasis remains to be a sign of advanced disease with poorer outcomes and lower chance of survival for the patient. There are various modalities including radiation, chemotherapy, and surgery that are used to control systemic spread of the cancer with mixed results; the results of treatments depend on variables including the type and cellular grade of the cancer, the extent of systemic disease, and the physiologic fitness of the patient.

Metastatic cancers to the spine are the most common reason for destructive lesions in the spine. Most common carcinomas that metastasize to the spine are those of, in order of prevalence, breast, lung, thyroid, renal, and prostate. Approximately one-quarter of all breast cancer patients will develop metastasis to the spine, followed by 12% to 15% of lung cancer patients; less than 5% of the others listed develop metastasis to the spine. Colon cancer and other gastrointestinal tumors can also spread to the spine through the valveless venous plexus surrounding the intestines connecting it to the epidural vessels, the Batson plexus. Bone is the third most common site of metastasis, with leading locations being the liver and the lung.[11]

Metastatic lesions are most often seen in adults older than 40 years. Most common sites of metastatic lesions are in the spine, due to its size and vascularity, followed by femur and humerus. The thoracic spine is the most common site of metastasis to the spine (**Table 2**).

Pathophysiology

The hematogenous spread of cancer cells, which is the most common route of metastasis, usually occurs in the posterior half of the vertebral body followed by the anterior body and the posterior elements. Cancellous bone, which most of the vertebral bodies is composed of, is highly vascular, making this area of the spine more susceptible to seeding from the hematogenous spread. Furthermore, some tumors like prostate cancer cells have receptors that can attach to adhesion ligands expressed by the bone marrow endothelial cells; interestingly, these ligands are not expressed by hepatic endothelial cells making liver metastasis of prostate cancer less likely.[12]

The bony destruction that occurs with metastatic lesions is caused by tumor cell destruction, osteoclast activation, or cytokine activation. Osteolysis can utilize a mechanism known to be caused by tumor-induced activation of osteoclasts. This osteolysis occurs through a RANK and RANKL osteoprotegerin pathway which is activated in some cancer types like breast cancer. In contrast, some cancer cells like prostate cancer, can stimulate the osteoblasts through various mechanisms including endothelin 1 (ET-1), tumor growth factor-β (TGF-β), and bone morphogenetic protein (BMP) activation.[13] The disks can provide a physical barrier, and therefore, each vertebra acts as a separate compartment initially retarding local spread of the disease.

Table 2

Typical Appearance of Various Metastatic Lesions on Radiographic Studies

Lytic	Blastic	Mixed
Lung	Prostate	Breast
Kidney	Bladder, with prostate	Lung
Thyroid	Bronchial carcinoid	Ovary
Adrenal		Testis
Uterus		Cervix

Evaluation and Diagnosis

Patients with metastatic spine lesions typically present with intractable back pain, escalating over a few days to weeks, or presenting acutely. The pain is present even at night awakening patients and is due to bony destruction, tumorigenic pain, or instability. Patients can also present with metastatic hypercalcemia if the bony destruction is rapid. It has been shown that patients with most discomfort and pain are suffering from spinal instability which should be evaluated carefully for surgical stabilization. The Spinal Instability and Neoplastic Score (SINS) was first published in 2010 and has now been used routinely to indicate patients for surgical stabilization.[14] **Table 3** shows the parameters for scoring a patient on the SINS scale. The total score calculated from the parameters with the following inferred outcomes: 0 to 6 Stable spine, 7 to 12 potentially unstable spine and 13 to 18 unstable spine. A SINS score of 7 to 18 is meant to warrant surgical consideration prior to any radiation treatment is offered to the patient.

Radiographic imaging is the first component of proper diagnosis of a patient with spinal metastasis. The studies should include AP and lateral radiographic views of the involved areas of the spine. Radiographs remain to be the primary and initial imaging technique used and is important in its ability to assess destruction and instability with dynamic radiographs. As radiographs are readily available even in doctors' offices, serial follow-up of radiographs are used to assess lesions' progression or response to treatment. CT scans are used to assess multidimensional bony involvement and are an important tool for preoperative planning and intraoperative navigation. MRI is also an important part of

Table 3

SINS Criteria[5]

SINS Component	Score
Location	
Junctional (occiput-C2, C7-T2, T11-L1, L5-S1)	3
Mobile spine (C3-C6, L2-L4)	2
Semirigid (T3-T10)	1
Rigid (S2-S5)	0
Pain	
Yes	3
Occasional pain but not mechanical	1
Pain-free lesion	0
Bone Lesion	
Lytic	2
Mixed (lytic/blastic)	1
Blastic	0
Radiographic Spinal Alignment	
Subluxation/translation present	4
De novo deformity (kyphosis/scoliosis)	2
Normal alignment	0
Vertebral Body Collapse	
50% collapse	3
50% collapse	2
No collapse with >50% body involved	1
None of the above	0
Posterolateral Involvement of Spinal Elements	
Bilateral	3
Unilateral	1
None of the above	0

SINS = Spinal Instability and Neoplastic Score

Data from Raskin KA, Schwab JH, Mankin HJ, Springfield DS, Hornicek FJ: Giant cell tumor of bone. *J Am Acad Orthop Surg* 2013;21(2):118-126.

the initial evaluation and used to assess the effect of the metastasis on the neural elements. It should be noted that approximately 10% of patients with metastasis have skipped lesions in remote locations of the axial skeleton. Therefore the entire spine needs to be imaged in the initial phases of the evaluation of a patient with metastasis to the spine to be able to assess the overall status of a patient and understand the degree of the progression of the metastatic disease.

Spine tumors must be differentiated from other pathologic conditions such as infections, metabolic bone disorders like osteoporosis, congenital abnormalities, trauma, and pseudotumors like spinal tuberculosis, Paget's disease, and others. Radiographic clues help us diagnose majority of metastatic lesions, but direct biopsy of the lesion remains to be the main tool for our definitive diagnosis. In complex lesions, a core biopsy is more diagnostic than a fine-needle aspiration which could be nondiagnostic in significant percentage of patients.

In the United States, the most prevalent metastatic lesions of the spine are from lung, prostate, breast, thyroid, renal, and gastrointestinal cancers. The cellular biology of each primary cancer dictates the presentation, treatment, and the prognosis of each individual patient.

Management of metastatic spinal disease is controversial, but Patchell's study revealed that patients with evidence of spinal cord compression on imaging studies and physical examination have better results with circumferential spinal decompression compared with radiation alone. This study randomized patients who had evidence of spinal cord compression into several groups receiving either radiation or circumferential surgical decompression followed by postoperative radiation. Patients who were paraplegic for greater than 48 hours with root or cauda equina compression and patients whose tumors were exquisitely sensitive to radiation, such as lymphoma, leukemia, and multiple myeloma, were excluded.

Every patient was given 100 mg of dexamethasone on presentation and then 24 mg every 6 hours until they received either surgery or radiation. Patients who had surgery were compare to radiation alone patients. Patients who underwent surgery were more likely to be ambulatory (84% versus 57%), had shorter hospital stays, and required less narcotics.

Nonsurgical Treatment

Radiation therapy is the preferred treatment for primary tumors such as lymphoma, multiple myeloma, plasmacytoma, and Ewing sarcoma. Unless patients have an indication for early surgical intervention, radiation treatment is traditionally given 30 gray over a 10-day period, and close daily monitoring of patients is required to assess for neurologic deterioration, which may require urgent surgical decompression and reconstruction. Ionizing radiation can cause collateral damage to the surrounding tissues. The organs that are at particular risk are the spinal cord, esophagus, skin, kidney, bowels, heart, lungs, and the great vessels. To avoid injury to the surrounding tissues, stereotactic radiosurgery (SRS) has evolved as the modern technique to deliver high-radiation dose to the tumor cells in a single fraction with high precision.

In cases where the epidural extension of the tumor precludes a safe SRS due to risk of injury to the spinal cord, separation surgery has been recently described to decompress and remove epidural tumor away from the dura so the involved spine can be treated without injury to the spinal cord.[15] Separation surgery can be accomplished either with open decompression or radiofrequency ablation through a percutaneous approach.

Surgical Treatment

Patchell et al are credited for promoting surgery for patients with metastatic lesions that are compressing the spinal cord showing that surgery followed by radiation and/or chemotherapy is superior to nonsurgical management alone for this subgroup of patients.[16] A surgical strategy needs to account for several prognostic factors that has been described by Tomita et al.[17] The three factors include (1) grade of malignancy (slow growth, 1 point; moderate growth, 2 points; rapid growth, 4 points), (2) visceral metastases (no metastasis, 0 points; treatable, 2 points; untreatable, 4 points), and (3) bone metastases (solitary or isolated, 1 point; multiple, 2 points). **Table 4** shows how by adding these points you arrive at a score between 2 and 10 which can guide the surgeon when considering surgery as a treatment for a patient with spinal metastasis. Naturally patients with higher score have a shorter life expectancy, and therefore, more aggressive surgery would be morbid and would not add to the quality of remaining life for these individuals.

The surgical approach to a metastatic lesion is dictated by the location of the tumor in need of resection, anatomic limitations and obstacles, and surgeon's level of comfort with a particular approach. In general, reliance on a fusion mass following these surgeries is unrealistic as the healing potential of these patients is low, especially as radiation therapy and chemotherapy used in the perioperative period will negatively impact the bony union. Surgical stabilization needs to be used with the understanding that healing of the fusion mass will most likely not occur, and the implants along with the implant/bone interface need to bear the weight and forces exerted by the patient for the remainder of their lives.

Surgical Complications

Surgical complications include infection, bleeding, hardware failure, pseudarthrosis, and spinal cord or nerve root injury. Patients who receive perioperative radiation therapy have a potentially two- to threefold greater risk for infection. Highly vascular tumors will increase the risk of significant intraoperative blood loss and should be embolized 24 to 48 hours prior to surgery.

Table 4

Surgical Strategy for Spinal Metastasis

Scoring System			
	Prognostic factors		
Point	Primary Tumor	Visceral Mets.*	Bone Mets.**
1	Slow growth (breast, thyroid, etc.)		Solitary or isolated
2	Moderate growth (kidney, uterus, etc.)	Treatable	Multiple
4	Rapid growth (lung, stomach, etc.)	Untreatable	

Prognostic Score	Treatment Goal	Surgical Strategy
2 3	Long-term local control	Wide or marginal excision
4 5	Middle-term local control	Marginal or intralesional excision
6 7	Short-term palliation	Palliative surgery
8 9 10	Terminal care	Supportive care

* No visceral mets. = 0 point. ** Bone mets. including spinal mets.

Mets. = metastases

Future Direction

There have been some recent discoveries in the field of metabolomics as it pertains to the role of markers in early detection of metastatic disease.[18] With hopes of early detection, the treatments available will be less morbid and more effective in management of the metastasis with better long-term survival of patients. Research in the field of immunotherapy, to train patients own immune systems to attack the cancer cells, has also shown great promise. Nanotechnology uses principles of drug delivery using nanoparticles. This method not only allows for more precise drug targeting, but also greater control of drug release in treating bone cancer, prosthetic joint infections, and osteomyelitis.

Summary

Treatment of spine tumors have evolved over the years, and with better detection, identification on the cellular level, and advancement in medical treatment of cancer, surgical indications are more defined. Surgery remains to be the first line of treatment for more systemically and locally aggressive cancer. With impending neurologic compromise, more urgent need for surgery is recommended but careful identification of the tumor type by direct biopsy decreases the chance of misdiagnosis and performing unnecessary or incorrect surgery.

Key Study Points

- Proper diagnosis of a spine tumor with a biopsy is the critical first step in devising proper treatment for a patient who presents with a spine tumor.
- Primary tumors of the spine are best treated with an en bloc resection to minimize risk of local and distant metastases.
- Proper care for a patient with a spine tumor requires a multidisciplinary team approach with continued follow-up and optimization of the care as the patient's needs can be dynamic and needs to be individualized.

Annotated References

1. NIH/National Cancer Institute. Available at: https://www.cancer.gov/about-cancer/understanding/statistics. Accessed August 2, 2018.
2. Stacchiotti S, Gronchi A, Fossati P, et al: Best practices for the management of local-regional recurrent chordoma: A position paper by the chordoma global consensus group. *Ann Oncol* 2017;28(6):1230-1242.

   This is a position paper discussing the findings of the Chordoma International Group and documents recommendation of this group in proper treatment of patient's with recurrent local chordoma. Level of evidence: IV.
3. Batouli A, Braun J, Singh K, Gholamrezanezhad A, Casagranda BU, Alavi A: Diagnosis of non-osseous spinal metastatic disease: The role of PET/CT and PET/MRI. *J Neuro Oncol* 2018;138(2):221-230.

   In this review, the role of PET/CT and PET/MRI in the diagnostic management of nonosseous metastatic disease of the spinal canal is discussed. It is discussed that recognizing such disease on FDG PET/CT and PET/MRI imaging done routinely in cancer patients can guide treatment strategies and help prevent irreversible neurological damage. Level of evidence: IV.
4. Boriani S, Weinstein JN: Differential diagnosis and surgical treatment of primary benign and malignant neoplasms, in Frymoyer JW, ed: *The Adult Spine*. Philadelphia: Lippincott-Raven, 1997, pp 951-987.
5. Raskin KA, Schwab JH, Mankin HJ, Springfield DS, Hornicek FJ: Giant cell tumor of bone. *J Am Acad Orthop Surg* 2013;21(2):118-126.
6. Charest-Morin R, Boriani S, Fisher CG, et al: Benign tumors of the spine: Has new chemotherapy and interventional radiology changed the treatment paradigm? *Spine* 2016;41(suppl 20):S178-S185.

   Alternative and adjuvant therapy for primary benign bone tumors are discussed in this review paper. The emerging data are reviewed, and benefits of collaboration between the different specialists managing these pathologies are encouraged. Level of evidence: V.
7. Yokogawa N, Murakami H, Demura S, et al: Total spondylectomy for Enneking stage III giant cell tumor of the mobile spine. *Eur Spine J* 2018;27(12):3084-3091.

   This is a retrospective review of 25 consecutive patients with Enneking stage III spinal GCTs undergoing surgery at a single institution who were followed for at least 2 years. Level of evidence: IV.
8. Choy E, Hornicek F, MacConaill L, et al: High-throughput genotyping in osteosarcoma identifies multiple mutations in phosphoinositide-3-kinase and other oncogenes. *Cancer* 2012;118(11):2905-2914.
9. DeLaney TF, Liebsch NJ, Pedlow FX, et al: Long-term results of phase II study of high dose photon/proton radiotherapy in the management of spine chordomas, chondrosarcomas, and other sarcomas. *J Surg Oncol*. 2014;110(2):115-122.
10. Shah AA, Paulino Pereira NR, Pedlow FX, et al: Modified en bloc spondylectomy for tumors of the thoracic and lumbar spine: Surgical technique and outcomes. *J Bone Joint Surg Am* 2017;99(17):1476-1484.

    This manuscript describes a two-stage technique that employs the use of threadwire saws for resection of primary tumors and solitary metastases involving the thoracic or lumbar spine. Level of evidence: IV.

Spine

11. Hecht AC, Scott DL, Cricklow R, Hornicek FJ, Pedlow FX: Matastatic disease, in Frymoyer JW, Wiesel SW, eds: *Adult and Pediatric Spine*, ed 3. Philadelphia, Lippincott Williams and Wilkins, 2004, pp 247-285.
12. Conley-LaComb MK, Saliganan A, Kandagatla P, Chen YQ, Cher ML, Chinni SR: PTEN loss mediated Akt activation promotes prostate tumor growth and metastasis via CXCL12/CXCR4 signaling. *Mol Cancer* 2013;12(1):85.
13. Obenauf AC, Massagué J: Surviving at a distance: Organ specific metastasis. *Trends Cancer* 2015;1(1):76-91.

    This is a review of the metastatic traits that allow cancer cells to colonize distinct organ sites. Organ-specific microenvironments promoting or inhibiting metastatic cancer cells are discussed. Level of evidence: V.
14. Hussain I, Barzilai O, Reiner AS, et al: Patient-reported outcomes after surgical stabilization of spinal tumors: Symptom-based validation of the spinal instability neoplastic score (SINS) and surgery. *Spine J* 2018;18(2):261-267.

    This is a single-institution prospective cohort study of a total of 131 patients who underwent stabilization for metastatic spinal tumor treatment between July 2014 and August 2016. Level of evidence: IV.
15. Laufer I, Iorgulescu JB, Chapman T, et al: Local disease control for spinal metastases following "separation surgery" and adjuvant hypofractionated or high-dose single-fraction stereotactic radiosurgery: Outcome analysis in 186 patients. *J Neurosurg Spine* 2013;18(3):207-214.
16. Patchell RA, Tibbs PA, Regine WF, et al: Direct decompressive surgical resection in the treatment of spinal cord compression caused by metastatic cancer: A randomised trial. *Lancet* 2005;366(9486):643-648.
17. Tomita K, Kawahara N, Kobayashi T, Yoshida A, Murakami H, Akamaru T: Surgical strategy for spinal metastases. *Spine* 2001;26(3):298-306.
18. Dean DC, Shen S, Hornicek FJ, Duan Z: From genomics to metabolomics: Emerging metastatic biomarkers in osteosarcoma. *Cancer Metastasis Rev* 2018;37(4):719-731.

    This is a review focusing on the recently discovered and novel metastatic biomarkers within OS, their molecular and cellular mechanisms, the expansion of humanized OS mouse models amenable to their testing, and the associated clinical trials aimed at managing the metastatic phase of OS. Level of evidence: V.

Section 11
Pediatrics

EDITOR

Amy L. McIntosh, MD

Chapter 53

Pediatric Shoulder, Upper Arm, and Elbow Trauma

Jennifer Nance, DNP • Sarah E. Sibbel, MD

ABSTRACT

Identification and treatment of pediatric upper shoulder, arm, and elbow trauma injuries can be exigent. The ossification patterns of the upper extremity can affect the diagnoses and proposed treatment methods. In addition, pediatric diagnoses such as clavicle, proximal humerus, and medial epicondyle fractures remain controversial for surgical versus nonsurgical treatments. The purpose of this chapter is to propose treatment options for eight different trauma injuries using recent evidence-based studies and American Academy of Orthopaedic Surgeons Clinical Practice Guidelines.

Keywords: clavicle fracture; humerus shaft fracture; lateral condyle fracture; medial epicondyle fracture; pediatric arm trauma; supracondylar humerus fracture

Introduction

Evaluating pediatric upper extremity trauma can be challenging. A thorough history and physical examination are necessary. Neurovascular status of the extremity must be documented accurately. In addition, the physical examination should also include adjacent bones and structures to evaluate for concomitant injuries. Radiographic imaging should always include the joint above and below the area of injury.

It is important to understand the ossification patterns of the upper extremity to accurately identify an injury. Knowledge of the ossification timelines for the pediatric skeleton helps guide the clinician in making appropriate treatment decisions (**Figure 1**). There continues to be controversy regarding indications for surgical versus nonsurgical treatments for pediatric clavicle fractures, proximal humerus fractures and medial epicondyle fractures. The literature is more clear regarding fixation parameters for lateral condyle fractures and supracondylar humerus fractures.

Clinical practice guidelines have been created by the American Academy of Orthopaedic Surgeons (AAOS) to aid in the decision making for pediatric trauma, especially those with vascular compromise.

Dr. Nance or an immediate family member serves as a board member, owner, officer, or committee member of the Pediatric Orthopaedic Society of North America. Neither Dr. Sibbel nor any immediate family member has received anything of value from or has stock or stock options held in a commercial company or institution related directly or indirectly to the subject of this chapter.

Shoulder and Upper Arm Fractures

Sternoclavicular Joint Injuries

The sternoclavicular joint is the connection of the upper extremity to the axial skeleton. The clavicle epiphyses close between the age of 20 and 25 years. Due to this, these injuries present as physeal injuries that mimic dislocations. These dislocations typically only occur with high impact forces. When patients present with pain and swelling near the sternoclavicular joint, a CT scan to assess this area is recommended. Anterior dislocations are typically treated nonsurgically. However, posterior dislocations threaten damage to the brachial plexus, trachea, esophagus, and vascular structures and require more aggressive treatment with reduction and stabilization. A vascular or cardiothoracic surgeon should be available during these procedures because of the potential risk to nearby vascular structures.

One institution recently found that medial third clavicular fractures associated with sternoclavicular dislocations are rare, but should be treated aggressively. Their suggestion is that if there is a displaced medial third clavicle fracture, a CT scan should be obtained to rule out concomitant sternoclavicular joint dislocation.[1]

Clavicle Fractures

Clavicle fractures occur at all ages, including the newborn infant population. Clavicle fractures account for up to 15% of all pediatric fractures.[2] Initial evaluation of clavicle fractures should include radiographs,

Pediatrics

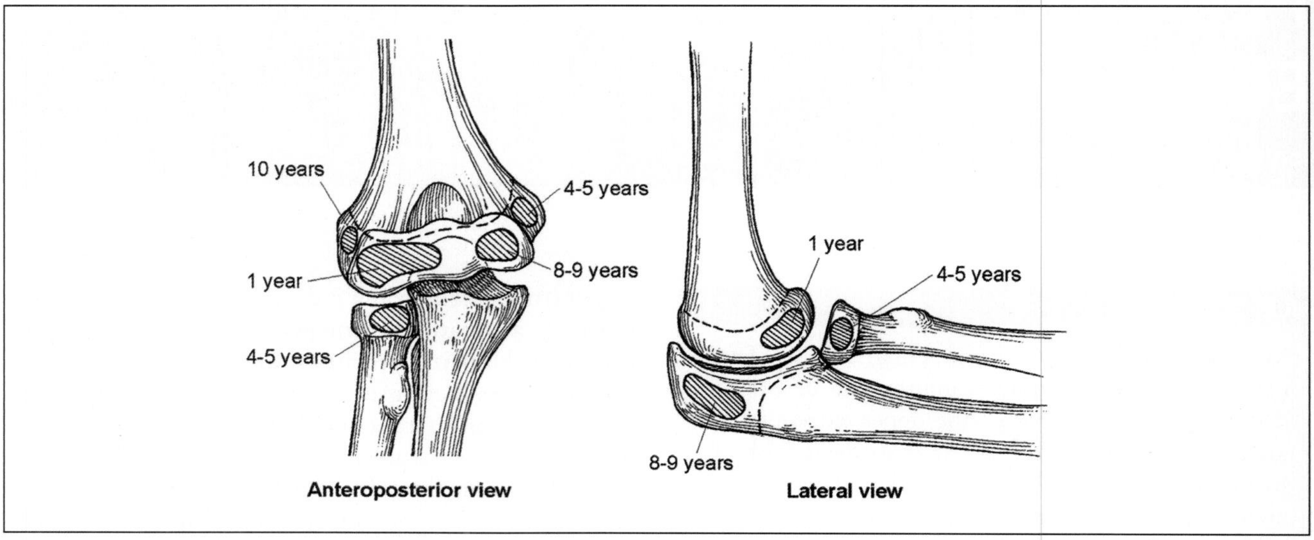

Figure 1 Illustration demonstrating the ages of ossification of the elbow. (Reprinted with permission from Skaggs DL: Elbow fractures in children: diagnosis and management. *J Am Acad Orthop Surg* 5[6]:303-312. https://journals.lww.com/jaaos/Fulltext/1997/11000/Elbow_Fractures_in_Children__Diagnosis_and.2.aspx.)

physical examination, and a complete history. Birth-related clavicle fractures should be assessed for concomitant brachial plexus birth injury. Children will often present with initial pseudoparalysis after this injury, but should be reassessed again several weeks later to rule out the presence of an associated injury to the brachial plexus. Clavicle fractures in this age group can be treated with a swathe, or pinning the sleeve of the affected arm in the desired position of comfort.

The vast majority of clavicle fractures are able to be treated nonsurgically. Indications for surgical treatment include open fractures, severe tenting of the soft tissues, acute vascular injury, or severe shortening of the shoulder girdle (**Figure 2**).

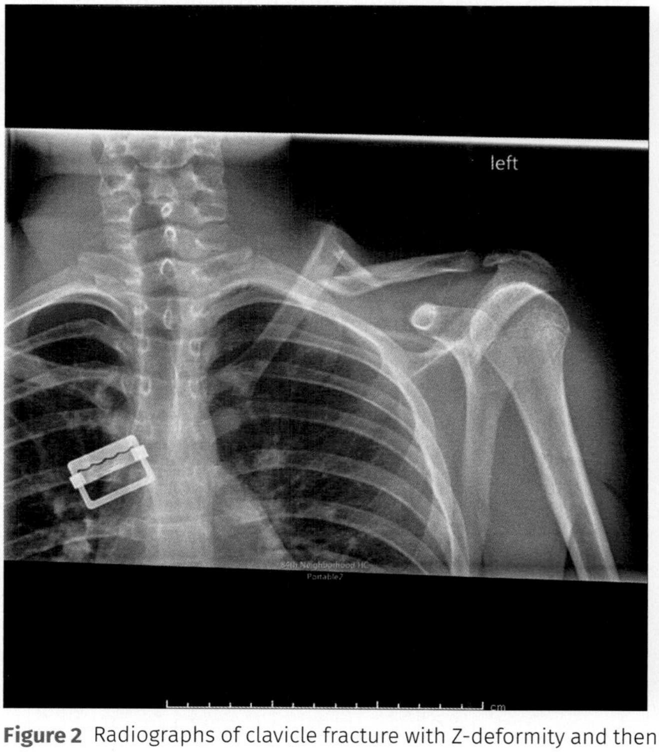

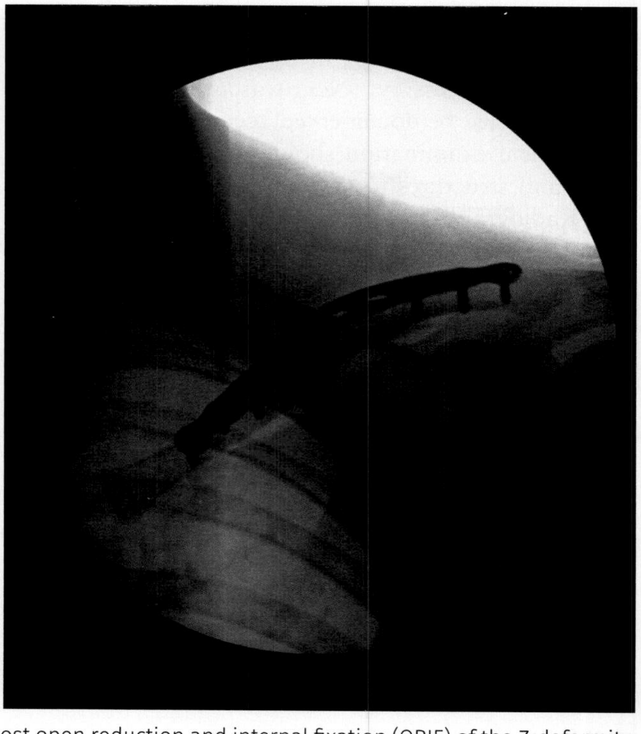

Figure 2 Radiographs of clavicle fracture with Z-deformity and then post open reduction and internal fixation (ORIF) of the Z-deformity.

There has been a recent shift toward surgical intervention in adults with midshaft clavicle fractures and this trend is starting to be seen in the adolescent population.[2] A 2011 study reported on surgical treatment of clavicle fractures with plate fixation in patients 10 to 19 years of age. There was an increase in surgical fixation rates from 12.5% to 21.9% over the course of 4 years. During the study, it was found that functional outcomes were improved and nonunion rates were decreased.[3] Surgical treatment of clavicle fractures in the adolescent population has been found to allow earlier return to activity compared with nonsurgically treated individuals.[4] A two-year functional outcome of surgical versus nonsurgical treatment of completely displaced adolescent midshaft clavicle fractures demonstrated lower complication rates, similar satisfaction, and functional outcomes.[5] Of note, their surgical cohort was older, and demonstrated greater shortening than the nonsurgical group. Surgical versus nonsurgical treatment of adolescent midshaft clavicle fractures remain controversial.

Proximal Humerus Fractures

Proximal humerus fractures in children account for less than 3% of all pediatric fractures.[6] These fractures tend to be treated nonsurgically based on the remodeling potential of the proximal humerus (**Figure 3**). The proximal humeral physis is responsible for 80% of the overall growth of the humerus.[6] In addition to the remodeling capacity, the shoulder arc of motion compensates for malalignment. Proper radiographs of the shoulder should be obtained to ensure that shoulder dislocation is not present

Treatment of proximal humerus fractures is typically nonsurgical. For nondisplaced fractures, the patient may be placed into a sling and swathe. For angulated fractures, a hanging arm cast may placed for three to four weeks and can assist with obtaining improved alignment. For fractures with greater than 30° of angulation and in children older than 10 years, surgical intervention may be considered.[7] Complications associated with surgical fixation of proximal humerus fractures include loss of reduction, pin loosening, and pin tract infections leading to osteomyelitis.[7]

Supracondylar Humerus Fractures

Supracondylar distal humerus fractures are the most common pediatric elbow fracture and account for 16% of all pediatric fractures.[8] A thorough neurovascular examination is critical when evaluating supracondylar humerus fractures.

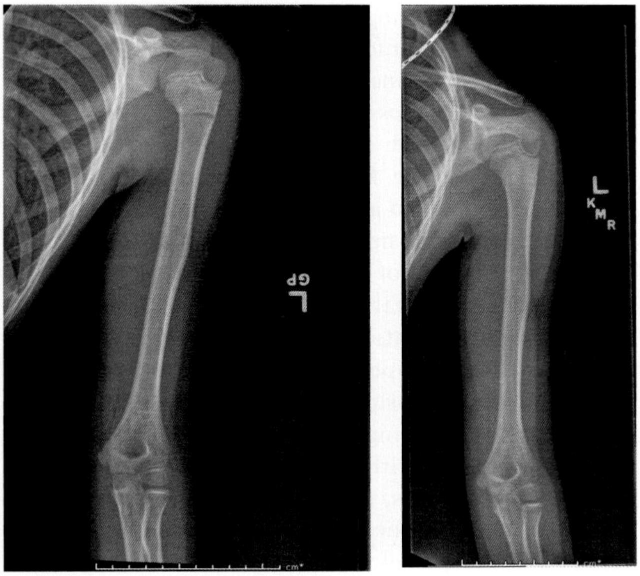

Figure 3 Radiographs of displaced proximal humerus fracture at time of injury and then at 6 weeks post closed treatment of proximal humerus fracture with remodeling present.

The Gartland classification continues to be the most common classification system used to describe these injuries. A type I fracture is nondisplaced. A type II fracture is incomplete and has an intact posterior hinge. A type III fracture is completely displaced. A type IV fracture has complete disruption of both the anterior and posterior periosteum and has multidirectional instability.

Treatment for Gartland type I supracondylar humerus fractures is typically a long arm cast for 3 weeks. There continues to be some controversy regarding nonsurgical versus surgical treatment of type II supracondylar humerus fractures.[9] Nonsurgical treatment of these fractures with closed reduction and casting, increases the risk of cubits varus, malrotation of the elbow, and an altered arc of motion of the elbow.[10] Reduction and Kirschner wire (K-wire) fixation carries a risk of complications such as infection, nerve injury, or pin migration. However, these complications have been found to be rare, and surgical intervention utilizing pin fixation (Gartland type II and II, displaced flexion) continues to be the AAOS recommendation for most patients.[9,10]

Displaced pediatric supracondylar humerus fractures should urgently be reduced in patients with vascular compromise due to risk for permanent injury and muscle and nerve damage. AAOS recommendations support an expert opinion consensus to perform exploration of the antecubital fossa in patients who have absent wrist pulses and underperfusion after reduction and pinning of displaced pediatric supracondylar humerus fractures. Of note, the AAOS recommendations are inconclusive for open exploration of the antecubital fossa in patients with absent wrist pulses but perfused hand after surgical reduction. Surgeons should be flexible in considering options including taking into account patient preference when treating a variety of neurovascular statuses.

Surgical timing of treatment of type III fractures is up to the individual surgeon, as recent studies have reported no correlation between timing of fixation and the need for open reduction. However, it was shown that soft-tissue injury measured by edema, ecchymosis, puckering, and tenting all had a significant association with neurovascular compromise.[11] In many institutions, a pink, well-perfused hand can await surgical treatment until standard daytime hours versus a white pulseless hand which should proceed emergently to the operating room. The combination of diminished pulses, a large amount of edema, ecchymosis, skin puckering, and neurologic deficit should give consideration for more urgent surgical management.

Pin construct is most stable when using larger diameter pins and increasing the number of pins. The addition of a medial pin also increases fracture stability.[11] Acceptable reduction is verified under fluoroscopy and the anterior humeral line should pass through the capitellum (**Figure 4**). There should not be rotation of the condyles of the distal humerus and minimal collapse of the medial or lateral columns to avoid a block to motion or the development of cubitus varus or valgus malalignment.

Medial Epicondyle Fractures

Medial epicondyle fractures are often associated with elbow dislocations, but may also occur in isolation. These fractures account for 20% of all pediatric elbow fractures.[12] It is noteworthy that the medial epicondyle is the attachment point for the ulnar collateral ligament and flexor pronator mass. This is the primary cause for elbow instability in these fractures. Typically, this injury has been treated in a cast for 2 to 4 weeks. However, this treatment is increasingly being replaced by surgical treatment, which allows for stable fixation and early mobilization (**Figure 5**). Surgical indications are controversial, but include the following: fracture displacement greater than 5 mm, ulnar nerve entrapment, elbow instability, or

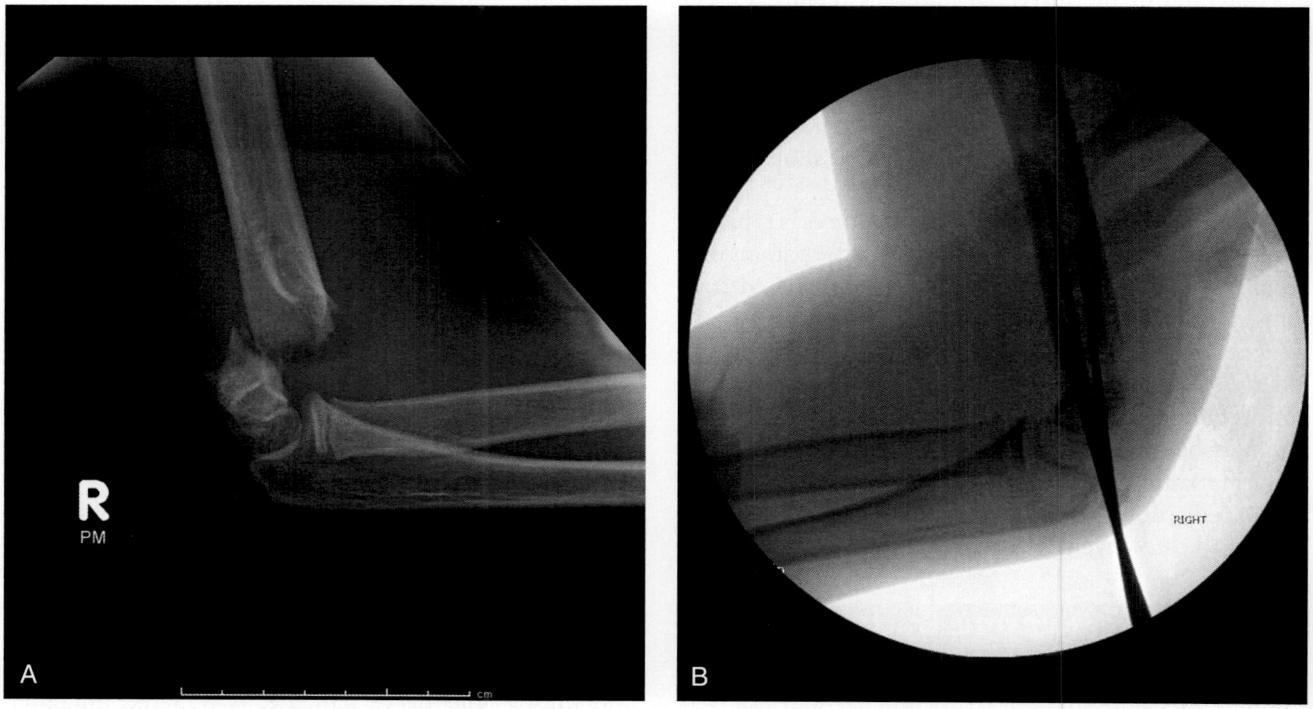

Figure 4 **A,** A preoperative radiograph of a displaced type III supracondylar distal humerus fracture. **B**, An intraoperative radiograph post closed reduction and percutaneous pinning (CRPP).

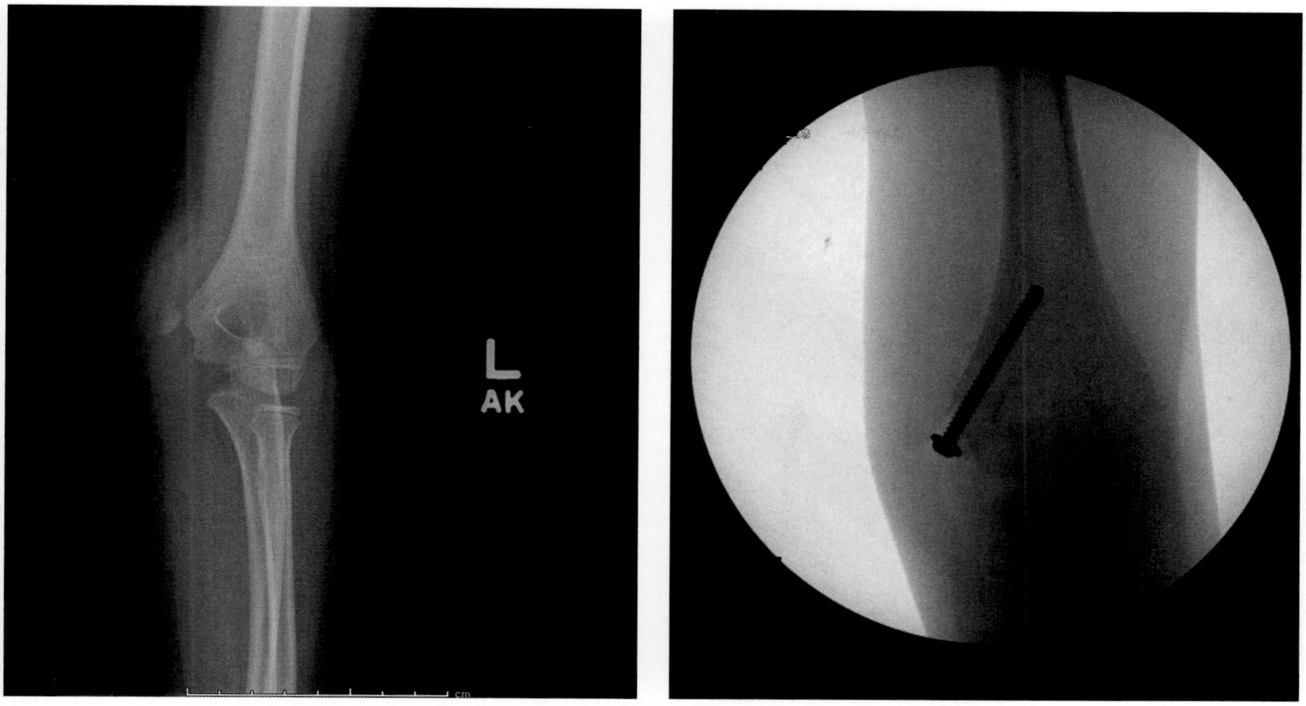

Figure 5 Displaced medial epicondyle fracture initial radiograph and post open reduction and internal fixation (ORIF).

an incarcerated fracture.[12] Some surgeons believe that this fracture in an overhead athlete is a relative indication for surgery, due to concern for elbow instability.[10]

Lateral Condyle Fractures

Lateral condyle fractures are the second most common elbow fracture in children. It can be difficult to assess the amount of true displacement on plain radiographs of the elbow. One recent study demonstrated that the best radiographic view for measurement of the displaced fragment is the internal oblique radiograph.[13] Fractures with less than 2 mm of displacement can often be treated in a long arm cast. It is imperative to monitor these fractures closely for delayed displacement, as this fracture is intra-articular and can lead to joint incongruity if displacement is not identified early. It is suggested to repeat radiographs weekly for the first two weeks to monitor for delayed displacement.[14] A recent German study showed favorable outcomes when initially nondisplaced fractures were reassessed within 5 days of injury to identify late fracture displacement.[15]

Surgical fixation is recommended for those fractures that are displaced more than 2 mm (**Figure 6**). Surgical fixation typically consists of open versus closed reduction and pinning with K-wires, or with screws to stabilize the fracture.[16,17] Lateral condyle fractures are often missed and may present late with nonunion, malunion, valgus deformity, or osteonecrosis of the elbow. Late presenting fractures require open reduction and internal fixation. The surgeon must be careful to protect the blood supply to the lateral condyle fragment, which typically enters the lateral condyle posteriorly.

Radial Neck Fractures

Radial neck fractures make up only 1% of pediatric fractures and less than 10% of fractures involving the elbow in children.[18] Nondisplaced or minimally displaced fractures can be treated in a long arm cast for 2 to 3 weeks. For fractures with more than 50% translation or more than 30° of angulation, intervention is required to improve alignment, as malalignment disrupts the rotational arc of the radius, leading to limited pronosupination. Closed reduction is always attempted

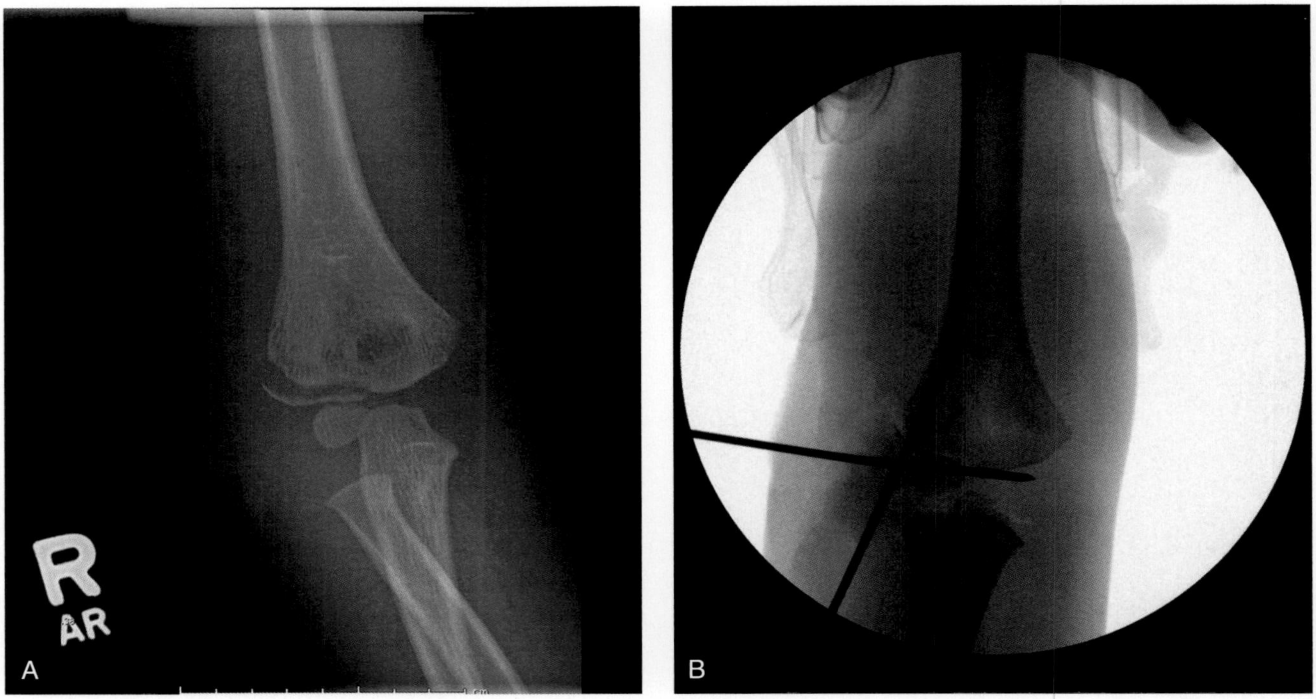

Figure 6 Displaced lateral condyle fracture injury radiographs (**A**) and post open reduction percutaneous pinning (**B**).

first (**Figure 7**). Several maneuvers for closed reduction of these fractures have been described. These include flexing the elbow to 90°, placing direct pressure over the radial head and moving the forearm from a fully supinated position into a pronated position. Another described technique is to place the elbow in full extension, apply distal traction with the forearm supinated, and pull the forearm into varus while applying direct pressure over the radial head. An esmarch bandage may also be used to assist with spontaneous closed reduction of the radial head. The bandage is typically placed from distal to proximal along the forearm and across the elbow.

When closed reduction does not achieve acceptable alignment, then surgical techniques are warranted. These techniques include reduction of the radial head using a percutaneously placed K-wire to act as a lever and elevate to radial neck (**Figure 8**). If reduction is achieved this way, stability of the fracture can be assessed. If the fracture is stable, the patient can be casted in supination; if it is unstable, a K-wire can be placed across the fracture to stabilize it. Should reduction still not be attained, the Metaizeau technique may be used. This technique utilizes an intramedullary device placed in the radial shaft to achieve reduction of the radial head. The device is placed distally and advanced proximally. Once the nail is at the level of the radial neck, it is rotated to move the radial head back into a reduced position. This technique yields excellent results and is minimally invasive with low complication rates.[19]

When these techniques are unsuccessful, open reduction is performed. Care is taken to protect the posterior interosseous nerve during the surgical approach. When performing an open reduction, it is important to avoid excessive stripping of the periosteum to avoid osteonecrosis of the radial head and improve healing. Fixation is placed based upon skeletal maturity, fracture pattern, and surgeon preference. Open reduction is the last step in the treatment pathway, as it has been associated with increased risk of elbow stiffness and poorer clinical outcomes.

Olecranon Fractures

Olecranon fractures account for only 5% of all pediatric elbow fractures. This fracture is often identified in combination with other fractures in the distal humerus or proximal radius.[20] This fracture is also common in children with osteogenesis imperfecta. Most olecranon fractures are nondisplaced or have less than 2 mm of displacement and can be treated in a long arm cast for 4 weeks. For fractures with greater than 2 mm of displacement, surgical treatment is recommended. Fixation options for olecranon fractures include a large-diameter single screw with a washer, a tension band wiring system, K-wire fixation, or plate and screw fixation[21] (**Figure 9**).

The authors utilized a modified Gartland classification system to differentiate type 2 supracondylar fracture of the distal humerus. They found the classification system allows certain type 2 fractures to be treated nonsurgically reducing surgery incidence.

10. Hubbard EW, Riccio AI: Pediatric orthopedic trauma. *Orthop Clin N Am* 2018;49(2):195-210. doi:10.1016/j.ocl.2017.11.008.

Drs. Hubbard and Riccio analyze over 150 references detailing treatment options and outcomes of various pediatric fractures including supracondylar fractures, medial epicondyle fractures, and clavicle fractures. They recommend creating level I evidence studies to simply decision making.

11. Ho CA, Podeszwa DA, Riccio AI, Wimberly RL, Ramo BA: Soft tissue injury severity is associated with neurovascular injury in pediatric supracondylar humerus fractures. *J Pediatr Orthop* 2018;38(9):443. doi:10.1097/BPO.0000000000000855.

The author prospectively collected neurovascular data on surgically treated supracondylar humerus fractures through a standardized note template. Soft-tissue injury identified as swelling, ecchymosis, puckering, and tenting was associated with neurovascular compromise. Level of evidence: II (Therapeutic).

12. Gottschalk HP, Eisner E, Hosalkar HS: Medial epicondyle fractures in the pediatric population. *J Am Acad Orthop Surg* 2012;20(4):223. doi:10.5435/JAAOS-20-04-223.

13. Bland DC, Pennock AT, Upasani VV, Edmonds EW: Measurement reliability in pediatric lateral condyle fractures of the humerus. *J Pediatr Orthop* 2018;38(8):e429. doi:10.1097/BPO.0000000000001200.

This article evaluates intraobserver and interobserver measurements of lateral condyle fracture of the humerus. Agreement was high when using 2 mm as a cutoff on radiographs. The internal oblique projection provided the most reliable measurements. Level of evidence was level two.

14. Knapik DM, Gilmore A, Liu RW: Conservative management of minimally displaced (≤2 mm) fractures of the lateral humeral condyle in pediatric patients: A systematic review. *J Pediatr Orthop* 2017;37(2):e83. doi:10.1097/BPO.0000000000000722.

The authors performed a systemic review of level 1 and 2 studies evaluating conservative treatment of lateral humeral condyle fractures. Pertinent findings included a rate of displacement of 14.9%, and displacement often occurred during the first week of immobilization.

15. Frongia G, Janosi C, Mehrabi A, Schenk J-P, Günther P: Long-term outcome in displaced lateral humeral condyle fractures following internal screw fixation in children. *Acta Orthop Belg* 2016;82(4):889-895.

This study attained excellent clinical outcomes by carefully monitoring lateral condyle fractures for secondary displacement within 5 days of trauma and treating secondary displaced fractures with open reduction and screw fixation.

16. Ganeshalingam R, Donnan A, Evans O, Hoq M, Camp M, Donnan L: Lateral condylar fractures of the humerus in children. *Bone Jt J* 2018;100-B(3):387-395. doi:10.1302/0301-620X.100B3.BJJ-2017-0814.R1.

The authors retrospectively compared screw fixation against K-wire fixation in lateral condylar fractures of the humerus. K-wires trended toward nonunions in their cohort but were associated with reduced costs due to lack of hardware removal.

17. Ormsby NM, Walton RDM, Robinson S, et al: Buried versus unburied Kirschner wires in the management of paediatric lateral condyle elbow fractures: A comparative study from a tertiary centre. *J Pediatr Orthop B* 2016;25(1):69. doi:10.1097/BPB.0000000000000226.

Buried and unburied Kirschner wires were compared in surgically treated lateral condyle elbow fractures. Buried wires were associated with higher rate of skin erosions and infection which resulted in increased complications and treatment costs compared with unburied wires.

18. Gutiérrez-de la Iglesia D, Pérez-López LM, Cabrera-González M, Knörr-Giménez J: Surgical techniques for displaced radial neck fractures: Predictive factors of functional results. *J Pediatr Orthop* 2017;37(3):159. doi:10.1097/BPO.0000000000000617.

This article compared different reduction techniques for Judet grades 3, 4a, and 4b radial neck fractures and associated outcomes. There was no significant association between Mayo Elbow Performance score and reduction technique used. Level of evidence was level three.

19. Guyonnet C, Martins A, Marengo L, et al: Functional outcome of displaced radial head fractures in children treated by elastic stable intramedullary nailing. *J Pediatr Orthop B* 2018;27(4):296. doi:10.1097/BPB.0000000000000502

The authors retrospectively compared functional outcomes in radial head fractures treated by elastic stable intramedullary nailing. They found no association between associated fracture injuries and functional outcomes. QuickDASH outcomes indicated good prognosis.

20. Grimm N, Herman MJ: Pediatric olecranon fractures, in Abzug JM, Herman MJ, Kozin S, eds: *Pediatric Elbow Fractures: A Clinical Guide to Management.* Cham, Springer International Publishing, 2018, 151-167. doi:10.1007/978-3-319-68004-0_11.

This chapter describes evaluation, treatment, and outcomes of olecranon fractures. This includes evaluating for additional fractures, which vary greatly from 14% to 77% of cases, as well as evaluating ossification of the elbow based on age.

21. Persiani P, Ranaldi FM, Graci J, et al: Isolated olecranon fractures in children affected by osteogenesis imperfecta type I treated with single screw or tension band wiring system. *Medicine (Baltimore)* 2017;96(20):e6766. doi:10.1097/MD.0000000000006766.

This article describes the efficacy of a tension band wiring (TBW) system compared with single screw fixation. TBW allowed faster recovery, less complications, and pain when compared with screw fixation. However, early removal of TBW may lead to refracture.

Chapter 54

Pediatric Forearm, Wrist, and Hand Trauma

Mark Dales, MD • Suzanne E. Steinman, MD

ABSTRACT

Fractures of the forearm, wrist, and hand represent the most frequent of skeletal trauma in the pediatric and adolescent age group. Although there has been a trend for surgical stabilization, many of these fractures can be successfully treated nonsurgically with the expectation of an excellent functional result. Early and proper identification of the injury type, the recognition of potential instability, and early recognition of loss of reduction, should it occur, are the key to good results with relatively straight forward management. Late diagnosis or identification of reduction loss is associated with significantly more complex treatment and a more guarded prognosis, but good results can be obtained. Increasing childhood obesity rates have led to an increase in more adult-style fracture patterns and increased need for surgical intervention for a variety of upper extremity fractures.

Keywords: distal radius fracture, forearm fracture, Monteggia, pediatric, phalanx fracture, scaphoid fracture, Seymour

Introduction

Fractures of the forearm, wrist, and hand represent the most common of pediatric fractures.[1] Whereas overall injury rates in children have been declining, upper extremity fracture incidence is increasing.[2] Increased childhood obesity is associated with both causation and a higher incidence of nonsurgical treatment failure in both diaphyseal and distal forearm fractures.[3-5] Somewhat in contrast to fractures about the elbow, many have significant remodeling potential, and many can be successfully managed nonsurgically. As with all pediatric fractures, remodeling potential is variable, with age, location, plane of deformity, and physeal involvement all having to be considered for individual treatment decisions. Although often obvious, more subtle fracture patterns such as traumatic bowing and incomplete fractures must also be looked for, and orthogonal visualization of both the elbow and wrist is mandatory for assessment of all forearm injuries. Missed injury patterns such as the Monteggia fracture, distal radioulnar joint (DRUJ) disruption, subtle physeal injury, and poke-hole open forearm fractures and displaced finger fractures remain too common and can lead to significantly compromised results from delayed appropriate treatment. Preliminary reports from EDs, urgent care clinics, and primary care clinics should be viewed with some skepticism by the orthopedic surgeon, and specific questions or personal evaluation should be pursued.

Neither of the following authors nor any immediate family member has received anything of value from or has stock or stock options held in a commercial company or institution related directly or indirectly to the subject of this chapter: Dr. Dales and Dr. Steinman.

Monteggia Fracture-Dislocation

Dislocation/subluxation of the radiocapitellar joint occurs with fracture or deformity of the ulna with shortening and/or angulation. Therefore, a Monteggia fracture-dislocation should always be considered and assessed radiographically with any identified isolated ulna injury. The majority of Monteggia fractures are Bado type I, with anterior displacement of the radial head. Type III, lateral displacement (which is not always obvious on a lateral view), is the second most commonly reported. Conversely, any identified dislocation or subluxation of the radial head should have a high suspicion of ulnar injury, as an isolated dislocation is rare. This ulnar injury may be quite subtle, but the deformity must be identified and corrected for successful management of the dislocation.

The Monteggia fracture-dislocation typically has an excellent outcome if identified acutely and managed appropriately, but becomes challenging to treat and guarded in prognosis with even modest delay.[2] Occasionally, a dislocated radial head is noted to have a convexity of the articular surface—these are either long-standing traumatic injuries or congenital dislocations and will be irreducible. The radiocapitellar line (RCL) is accurately used on the lateral view, but because of variation in proximal radial ossification is less precise on AP. The lateral humeral line (LHL) has recently been described[6] as a more consistent measure on the AP view, and in particular Bado type III variations, where it will consistently fall lateral to the radial neck with a reduced radiocapitellar joint, and medial in Bado type III injuries (**Figure 1**).

Successful treatment of the Monteggia fracture-dislocation keys on eliminating ulnar deformity and restoring length.[7] This is one situation where near perfect restoration of length and alignment is critical even in a younger patient. Once aligned and out to length, the radiocapitellar joint generally reduces readily in acute situations. Soft-tissue interposition blocking reduction and need for repairing the annular ligament is uncommon. Greenstick and bowing injuries of the ulna, which can be successfully reduced closed and are stable, are amenable to nonsurgical management. For complete fractures of the ulna, surgical stabilization has been recommended. For transverse and short oblique length stable fractures, intramedullary (IM) fixation with either smooth Steinman pin or elastic nail is minimally invasive and advised. Length unstable fractures (fractures with obliquity greater than three times the diameter, those with comminution, and segmental fractures) and

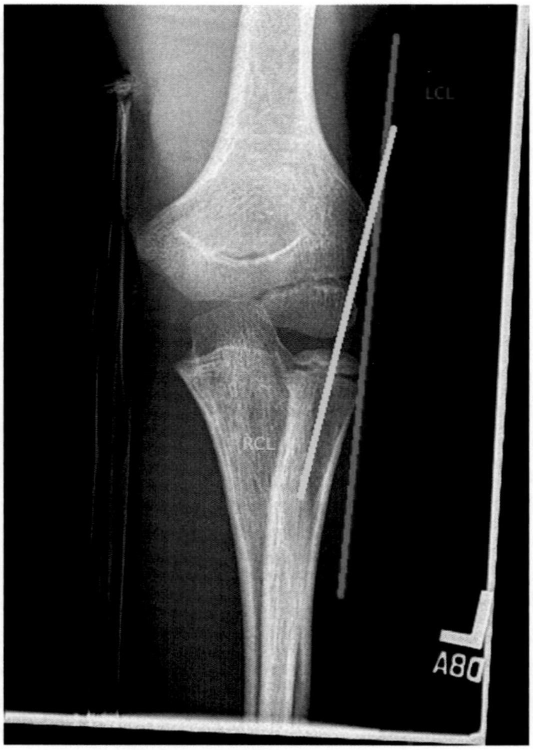

Figure 1 AP radiograph showing lateral humeral line (LCL; red) and radial humeral line (HCL; yellow).

patients nearing skeletal maturity are managed with open reduction and plate fixation. Using this algorithm, a multicenter series showed no treatment failures, whereas roughly 20% treated nonsurgically failed with recurrent radiocapitellar dislocation.[8] However, a more recent series questioned the need for surgical stabilization in all Monteggia fractures with complete ulna fracture and assessed a more conservative approach in 94 isolated, closed, neurovascularly intact Monteggia fractures that underwent initial closed reduction and casting. Eighty-three percent were successfully managed in this way. Of the 16 patients that required surgical intervention, nine were irreducible at presentation. The seven failures were identified in the first 3 weeks of follow-up, and all successfully treated with surgical ulnar restoration.[9] In the relatively uncommon situation where the radiocapitellar joint does not reduce congruently after addressing the ulna, open reduction is indicated, but careful evaluation of whether the ulna is truly aligned and nondeformed should be reassessed.

Close postreduction observation is recommended. The radial head reduction will be most stable in elbow flexion of 90° to 100°, but sometimes swelling and vascular concerns preclude that initially. Radiographs at the first 2 to 3 weeks to confirm maintenance of congruent reduction are appropriate, and a follow-up radiograph 6 to 8 weeks following final cast removal and return to activity may be advisable.

Chronic Monteggia fracture-dislocation, whether initially unrecognized or due to loss of reduction following management (up to 50% and 20%, respectively),[6,10] is often minimally symptomatic initially in terms of pain or functional deficit. Because of this, if unrecognized acutely, eventual diagnosis is often quite delayed. The ulna will have often healed shortened and angulated, and as time goes on the angulation with remodeling becomes much more difficult to correct at the specific initial site of deformity. Pain, cubitus valgus, valgus instability, tardy ulnar nerve palsy, and limited motion have all been reported in longer standing dislocation.[2]

In general, management within 3 years after injury in patients less than 12 years of age has had success, but success in cases of both longer chronicity and older age has been reported. More important may be the degree of secondary deformity of the radial head, with increasingly dysplastic changes of the unarticulated radial head lessening the likelihood of success.[2] Multiple techniques, with and without open reduction of the radiocapitellar joint, and reconstruction of the annular ligament have been described. Open reduction and reconstruction of the annular ligament in a chronically dislocated head without addressing the ulnar deformity is likely to fail. Universal to successful series is osteotomy of the ulna to restore length and allow for stable reduction. A metaphyseal osteotomy with plate osteosynthesis in enough flexion to allow stable reduction is preferred by most recent authors. Eventually, morphologic changes to the radial head with convexity of the articular surface make achieving and maintaining a congruent reduction of the joint less likely, and nonintervention may be the more appropriate choice in a child, especially if relatively asymptomatic.[2]

Radius and Ulna Diaphyseal Fracture

Both bone forearm shaft fractures in the pediatric population are usually the result of FOOSH (fall-on outstretched-hand) type mechanism and can often be successfully managed nonsurgically, especially in those patients younger than 10 years. Particularly, careful assessment of the radiocapitellar joint (Monteggia fracture) and DRUJ (Galeazzi fracture) must be part of the evaluation any time it appears that a single bone is fractured. Both angular and rotational deformities are often present, with the angular deformity being the much more obvious. Greenstick fractures have predictable rotational deformity. With complete fractures the different location of the opposing forearm rotators on the radius makes the exact rotational deformity difficult to anticipate. In the pediatric population with its typically lower energy mechanisms, significant open fractures are less common, but poke-hole grade I fractures are not rare and must be carefully looked for.[11]

Greenstick fractures are usually managed successfully nonsurgically with closed reduction. The key is recognizing that there is a rotational component, so pure attempts to correct angulation alone will be incomplete for both deformities. While angulation is corrected, rotation is also corrected by reversing the rotational mechanism of injury. A simple "rule of thumb" is to rotate the thumb to the apex of the angular deformity. Completion of the fracture is not needed if the rotational deformity is addressed during reduction and can unnecessarily destabilize the fracture.

Limitation of postreduction visits and radiographs may substantially reduce costs and radiation exposure in these stable fractures, as well as lessen the time burden for patient and accompanying adult. A study of 109 greenstick fractures demonstrated a projected 14% decrease in total cost and 40% reduction of radiation if visits were limited to 2 and 6 weeks postreduction only. The highest prevalence of reduction loss was demonstrated by the second-week visit.[12]

Complete fractures in patients younger than 10 years often can be managed nonsurgically with a satisfactory reduction. In general, up to 20° residual angulation can be accepted, but age, BMI, angulation, displacement, location of the fractures, and status of the interosseous space are variables that must be considered in the final acceptance of reduction.[13] Even moderate apex ulnar residual deformity may be cosmetically apparent and looked upon unfavorably by parents, whereas radial angulation or displacement, especially proximal third, may not be as obvious visually, but may affect forearm rotation to a significant degree. Rotational malalignment will not remodel, but 30° to 45° malrotation does not lead to functional deficit in general.[7] Bayonet apposition of less than 1 cm is generally tolerated well as long as angular parameters are acceptable. However, specific activities have different ROM needs, and therefore a reasonable attempt should always be aimed at as near anatomic reduction as possible. For each individual, the balance of accepted residual deformity versus the increased morbidity of more aggressive attempts to improve the reduction must be considered.

Closed reduction is typically accomplished with procedural sedation. Intravenous regional (Bier Block) analgesia is another option. In a comparison of ketamine sedation and Bier block divided between 2,954 patients, mean time in the ED was 31% less in the ED for the IV regional group, with only two failures of adequate analgesia and no major complications.[14]

Following closed reduction of diaphyseal fractures, an above-elbow cast, or double or single plaster sugar-tong splint is appropriate with attention to a good interosseous mold, flat ulnar boarder, and elbow flexion at 90° with a flat posterior arm mold to prevent distal migration. Premade fiberglass splinting material generally does not provide enough moldability for postreduction fracture stability. Multiple casting indices have been described and are predictive in some series. A recent series of 174 diaphyseal fractures had 11% re-reduction, with risk factors for repeat reduction or treatment change being translation of 50% in any plane, age of more than 9 years, and angulation of the radius more than 15° on lateral or ulna of 10° on AP. Cast indices were not found to be different in the re-reduction group.[15] No difference was found in either maintenance of reduction or complications between casts that either had no valve, univalve, or bivalve.[16]

For patients older than 10 years, remodeling capability diminishes progressively, and residual angulation will limit objective rotational range of motion, although functional limitation is less clear.[17] In addition to age, higher energy fractures with greater soft-tissue injury, unstable fractures, irreducible or inadequately reduced fractures, ipsilateral distal humerus or elbow fractures, and re-fracture are considered potential indications for surgical stabilization. In the past decade, surgical management of diaphyseal fractures has been increasingly used despite a majority of clinical studies suggesting initial nonsurgical management may provide satisfactory results.[11,18] Close monitoring over the first 3 weeks is required, and evidence of early loss of reduction should be a consideration for surgical stabilization.

The two most common methods of surgical stabilization in the pediatric and adolescent population are IM fixation and plate and screw osteosynthesis. IM stabilization has the advantage of being generally less invasive, even with reported incidence of 30% to 75% need[11,18] for limited open exposure of the fracture to allow nail passage, but also typically involves a second procedure to remove implants. Elastic nails have become increasingly popular, but a comparison of titanium and stainless steel elastic nails along with smooth Steinman pins found no difference in healing time, complications, or surgical time, but 5 to 30 times less implant cost for the Steinman pins.[19] For the radius, either a dorsal or radial starting point can be used. A systematic review of 22 clinical articles with a total of 1,914 patients revealed a 2.6% rate of EPL rupture with a dorsal start, and a 2.9% incidence (mostly transient) of superficial radial nerve palsy.[20] Single bone fixation can also be successful if the radial bow and interosseous space is subsequently acceptable. A recent systematic review found comparable results for single (either radius or ulna) versus both bone fixation.[4] IM fixation can often be passed across the fracture without opening the fracture if alignment of the narrow canal is close, but more than three attempts may be associated with an increased incidence of compartment syndrome.[11] Open reduction through a limited exposure is recommended in this situation.

Plate and screw fixation has been largely supplanted by IM fixation, but remains a preferred option for some patients, including those nearing skeletal maturity and length unstable patterns. Early unprotected range of motion is possible, but this may not be advantageous in the questionably activity restriction compliant pediatric or adolescent patient, who likewise can be cast protected without significant morbidity. Meta-analysis revealed comparable and overall 90% excellent results, and similar low complication rates up to age 16.[21]

Distal Both-Bone and Distal Radius Fracture

Distal fractures include metaphyseal and physeal injuries. In the pediatric population, intra-articular distal radius fractures are uncommon. Angulation and displacement in the sagittal plane have significant remodeling potential, coronal deformity less so. Guidelines allow for 20° to 30° of angulation in the sagittal plane for patients with significant growth remaining—generally younger than 10 years. Progressively less is acceptable as growth and remodeling potential diminishes. Coronal plane deformity is less capable of remodeling. The majority of these fractures can be managed nonsurgically, either with or without reduction, depending on pattern and remaining growth/remodeling potential.

Torus (buckle) fractures can be managed with a removable splint for 3 to 4 weeks and no follow-up visit or radiograph needed. It is important to evaluate the injury radiographs critically to make sure the injury is not in actuality a complete, but nonangulated, nondisplaced fracture through the far cortex. These can collapse if unrecognized with the torus fracture protocol. A consecutive series of 42 patients treated with this protocol had full return of function, no re-fracture, and 100% parental satisfaction rate. Survey revealed that 67% of parents would have had to take time off work, and 77% of patients time out of school had follow-up been required.[22]

Complete fractures of the distal radius metaphysis may need reduction depending on remodeling potential, which in turn is dependent on age, growth potential, fracture pattern, and concurrent injuries. The majority can be reduced in an acute care setting. Routine use of percutaneous pins for stabilization is not recommended.[23] One hundred percent displaced, bayonet apposed fractures may not require reduction in younger children. In a prospective study of 61 consecutive patients younger than 10 years whose fractures were left unreduced, all healed and remodeling led to satisfactory results in all patients. Wrist range of motion was full and all parents were satisfied with the final result. This protocol was estimated to be between 5 and 9 times less expensive than reduction under sedation/anesthesia.[24] Postreduction immobilization can be successfully accomplished through sugar-tong splint or cast, above or below elbow.[25] The key factors are the reduction and three-point mold.[23] The second metacarpal should be aligned with the axis of the radius to prevent the tendency for radial deviation of the distal fragments. Acceptance of residual angulation or

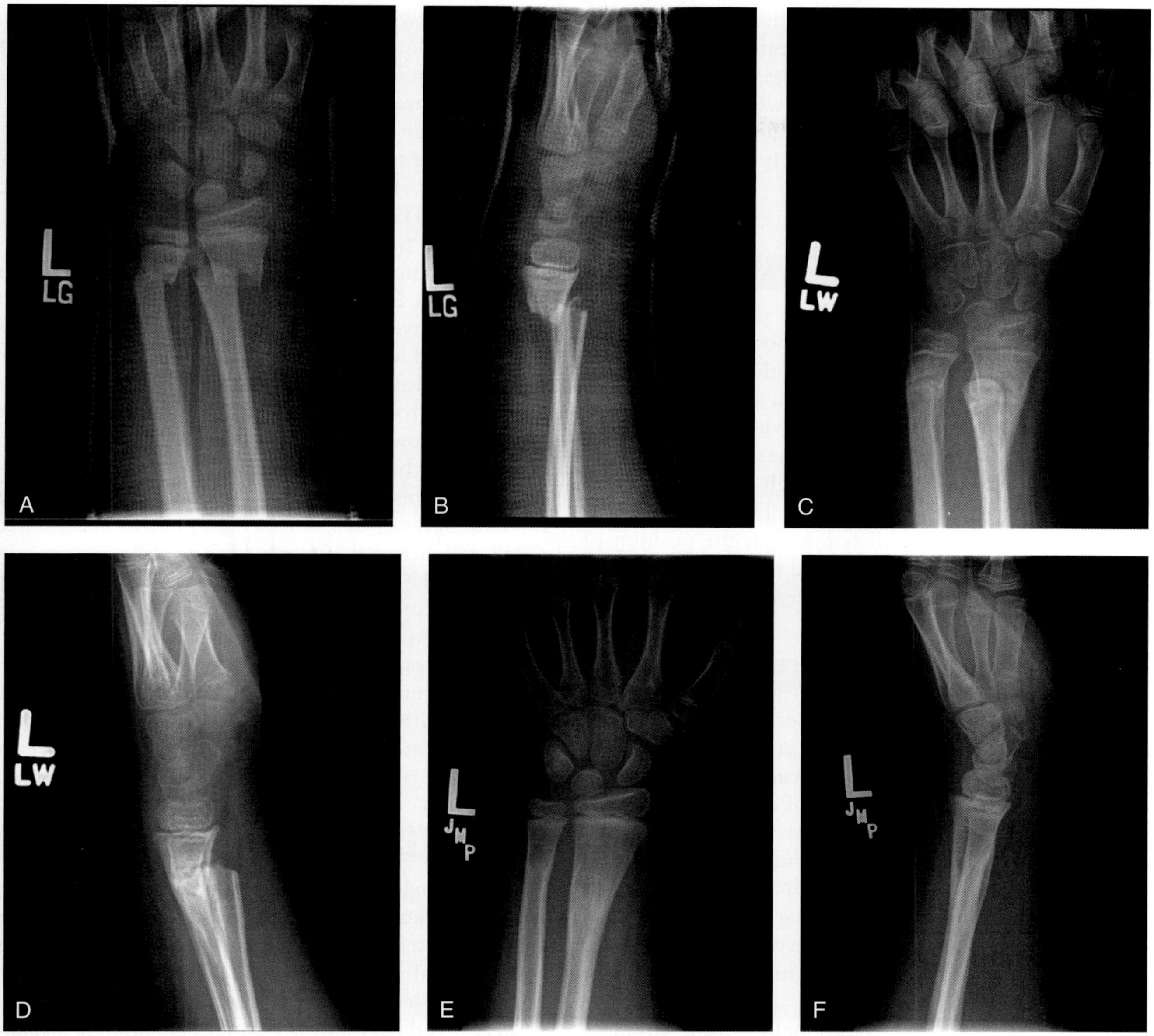

Figure 2 **A and B**, AP and lateral radiographs of distal radius and ulna fractures allowed to stay in bayonet apposition postreduction. **C and D**, AP and lateral radiographs at 6 weeks. **E and F**, AP and lateral radiographs at 9 months demonstrating remodeling.

bayonet apposition with expected satisfactory result through remodeling can sometimes involve a considerable amount of education for the family and at times the primary care providers. Pictures of successful remodeling can be of help (**Figure 2, A** through **D**).

Variability between orthopedic hand surgeons, general orthopedic surgeons, and pediatric orthopedic surgeons in the management of distal radius fractures is known. More recently, a study of classification and treatment recommendation of 100 representative distal radius fractures by nine fellowship trained pediatric orthopaedic surgeons demonstrated only fair agreement of classification, poor agreement on recommended treatment, first follow-up visit and need for radiographs, and no agreement on length of immobilization. Even for buckle fractures, which had 100% diagnostic agreement, there was significant variability in other management areas, despite the presence of published protocols.[26] As distal radius fractures represent 20% to 30% of all childhood fractures,[1] development, validation, and adherence to a clinically reliable and cost-effective algorithm would be of value.

Physeal injury to the distal radius results in growth disturbance in roughly 5%. Repeated attempts and reduction after 10 days may increase the risk. Growth disturbance of the distal ulna following physeal injury may occur up to 50%. Longer term radiographic follow-up of these injuries may identify impending ulnar variance issues.

Galeazzi Fracture

Disruption of the distal radioulnar joint (DRUJ) does occur in the pediatric population, most commonly with isolated fractures of the radius at the middistal third junction. Similar to the Monteggia disruption proximally, the DRUJ generally reduces with anatomic restoration of the radial fracture. Stabilization of the radial fracture may be of benefit, although the advantage of this has not been demonstrated specifically for the pediatric population. Immobilization is in the position of reduction of the joint. As opposed to adults, long-term instability and problems do not seem to be typical.[11]

Scaphoid Fractures

Although relatively uncommon, scaphoid fractures are the most common carpal injury in the pediatric population. They account for approximately 3% of hand and carpal fractures and 0.34% of all fractures in children.[27-29] Traditional thinking was that scaphoid fractures involved the distal pole in children with excellent healing rates but as children participate in higher energy, extreme sports and have increasing BMIs, we are now seeing increased incidence and fracture patterns similar to adults with the majority of fractures occurring at the waist.[30]

Scaphoid fractures traditionally occur from a FOOSH. Pain and swelling can be subtle in the anatomic snuffbox and often these fractures present late. Evaluation for scaphoid fracture includes physical examination, examining for pain in the anatomic snuffbox or over the scaphoid tubercle. PA, lateral, and scaphoid view radiographs should be obtained to evaluate for fracture. If radiographs are equivocal, ultrasonography can be used to diagnose fracture[31] or radiography can be repeated after 2 weeks of immobilization to assess for evidence of healing fracture. Suspected fractures must be immobilized in a thumb spica cast or splint. Nondisplaced, acute fractures are treated in short arm thumb spica casts for 6 to 12 weeks and have a reported union rate of 90%. Surgical intervention is recommended for displaced, chronic, proximal pole or fractures with osteonecrosis. Care must be taken to assess for other associated injuries like distal radius fracture, transscaphoid perilunate dislocations, ulnar styloid fractures, capitate fractures, and bilateral injuries, which can be present in up to 10% of patients.[30]

In a recent study, Bae et al reported on the functional outcomes of children and adolescents with scaphoid fractures.[32] 312 patients aged 8 to 18 years treated for scaphoid fracture over a 15-year period were contacted to complete patient-reported outcome modules including the DASH (Disability of the Arm, Shoulder and Hand) inventory, DASH work and sports modules and Modified Mayo Wrist Score (MMWS) at median of 6.3 years follow-up. They found that chronic fractures and osteonecrosis were independent predictors of worse outcomes. However, 95% of all patients reported functional status better than or equal to the general population per median DASH score. The median MMWS for both surgical and nonsurgical patients represented excellent functional outcome with no difference in outcomes for the two groups. Jauregui et al reported on surgical treatment of pediatric and adolescent scaphoid nonunions via a comprehensive literature review.[33] Eleven studies with 176 surgically treated patients met criteria for inclusion. They found that patients treated surgically with both grafted and nongrafted techniques had union rates greater than 94% with no difference between the groups and excellent functional outcomes.

Hand and Finger Fractures

Hand and finger fractures are extremely common in the pediatric population and are the second most common fracture presenting to emergency departments.[1] There is a bimodal age distribution for these injuries with peaks at 0 to 2 years of age and then 12 to 16 years of age.[34] Toddlers and preschool age children usually sustain their injures while at home and it is usually a crush injury while adolescents most often get injured outside the home with sporting. The most commonly injured locations are the base of the proximal phalanx (67%) of the border rays (little finger 52.2% and thumb 23.5%).[35] The majority of these fractures can be treated with closed reduction, appropriate immobilization, and early motion. Appropriate evaluation of hand and finger fractures includes clinical examination and radiographs. Clinical examination must assess for open injuries and angular and rotational malalignment of the injured ray. Rotational alignment can be confirmed by ensuring that all fingers point to the scaphoid tubercle when the fingers are flexed. Radiographs should include PA, lateral, and oblique views of the injured location.

There are several fractures, however, that do require special attention and some surgical intervention like phalangeal neck and condyle fractures and Seymour fractures.[36-39] Salter-Harris II fractures of the digits are an extremely common hand fracture with the little finger proximal phalanx (know as the extra octave fracture) being the most commonly injured.[35] These injuries usually occur because of a jamming or hyperextension injury to the finger resulting in an abduction deformity. The coronal plane deformity is easy to assess, but extra care must be taken to assess for rotational deformity, which is not as obvious on radiographs. Malrotation does not remodel and this can result in problems with grip formation (**Figure 1**, **A** and **B**).

The classic "jammed" finger with a swollen, painful PIP (proximal interphalangeal) joint is another very common hand injury and the majority of the time it involves a volar plate injury or small nondisplaced avulsion fracture off the volar base of the middle finger epiphysis. These do not require surgical intervention. They should be splinted in approximately 30° of flexion for a week followed by 3 weeks of buddy tape to allow for healing. Prolonged immobilization of these simple injuries can result in significant joint stiffness. Phalangeal neck and condyle fractures, however, have a similar presentation to a simple "jammed" finger and are often missed. These two fractures usually do require surgery, so early diagnosis is essential. Displaced phalangeal neck fractures require reduction and pin fixation which can usually be achieved through a closed fashion.[36] Condyle fractures can often also be treated with closed reduction and pinning. Open procedures increase a risk for osteonecrosis, so all attempts should be made for early diagnosis and treatment of these injuries.[37]

A 2015 article by Boyer et al reviewed displaced proximal phalanx fractures that required surgical treatment[40] and reported complications and outcomes. In a retrospective review, they identified 105 patients treated with closed reduction pin fixation of a displaced proximal phalanx fracture. Average age was 11 years at time of surgery. The majority of fractures involved the physis followed by phalangeal neck and then shaft fractures. They identified a 4.8% complication rate including infection, pin site complication, and malunion. Thirty-six of the 105 patients had postoperative stiffness with 31 requiring therapy. Phalangeal neck fractures had the highest rate of postoperative stiffness. Thirty-one patients available for follow-up at 1 year or greater all reported return of full motion, no pain, and happiness with function and appearance. This was despite 22% (7 of 31) having a measurable coronal plane deformity on radiograph.

Seymour fractures are another special finger fracture in the pediatric population that requires specific attention. They are a Salter-Harris I/II or juxtaphyseal fracture of the distal phalanx with interposed nail bed at the fracture site. These are open fractures but are often missed. Missed Seymour fractures have a high rate of complication including infection and nail or physeal growth disturbance.[38] Radiographs reveal a displaced fracture of the distal phalanx (**Figure 2**), but the key to diagnosis is disruption of the nail plate/cuticle as well (**Figure 3**). This indicates disruption of the nail bed and the likelihood of an open fracture with interposed tissue. Treatment for these fractures involves removal of the nail plate with débridement of the fracture site, extrication of the interposed nail bed, and reduction of the fracture. If the fracture is unstable, it may require

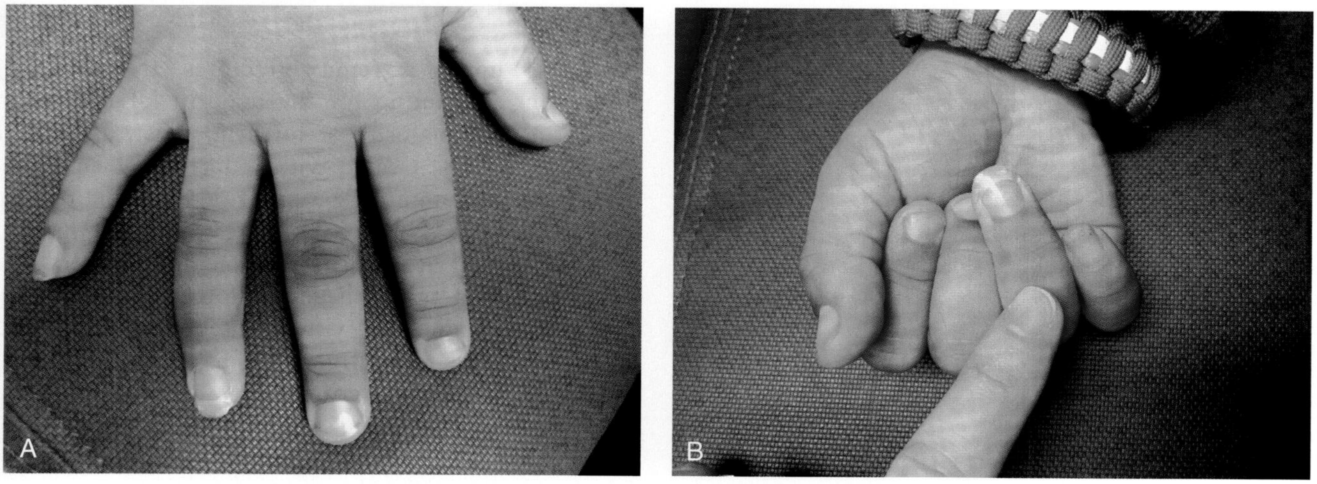

Figure 3 **A and B**, Clinical photographs demonstrating rotational malalignment in a finger fracture.

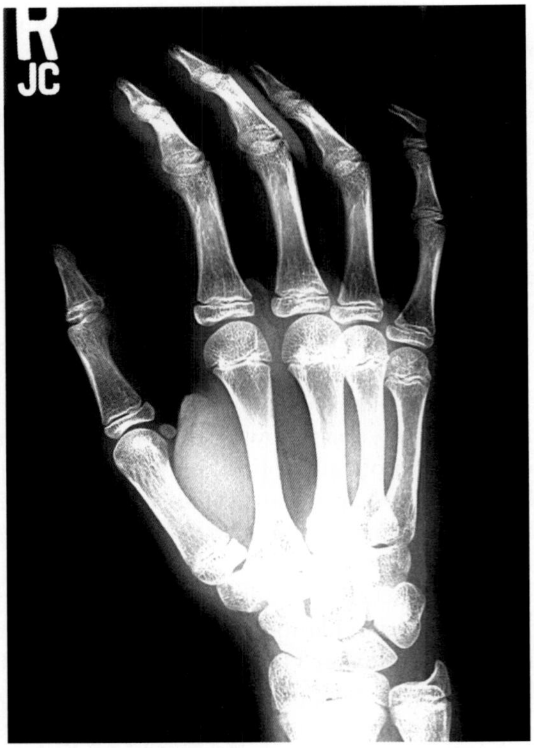

Figure 4 Lateral radiograph of Seymour fracture.

Kirschner wire placement in addition to immobilization in splint/cast. Antibiotics are also a necessity to prevent infection as these are open fractures. Recommended treatment includes a dose of IV antibiotic in the emergency department followed by a 7- to 10-day course of oral antibiotic. A first-generation cephalosporin is the preferred antibiotic.[39] Reyes et al described the high risk of complications in Seymour fractures when treatment was delayed or inadequate.[39] Patients with Seymour fractures were divided into groups depending on the timing and completeness of treatment. "Appropriate" treatment was defined as irrigation and débridement, fracture reduction, and antibiotics versus "partial" treatment defined as any type of incomplete treatment. "Acute" was defined as management within 24 hours of injury and "delayed" treatment greater than 24 hours after injury. Thirty-four patients with 35 Seymour fractures over a 10-year period were identified. Thirty-one percent of patients received acute-appropriate care, 37% acute-partial care, and 31% delayed treatment. They found that delayed and inappropriate care led to increased rates of infection. There were no reports of infection in the acute-appropriate group, a 15% infection rate in the acute-partial group, and a 45% infection rate in the delayed group. This underscores the necessity of identifying and treating these fractures appropriately.

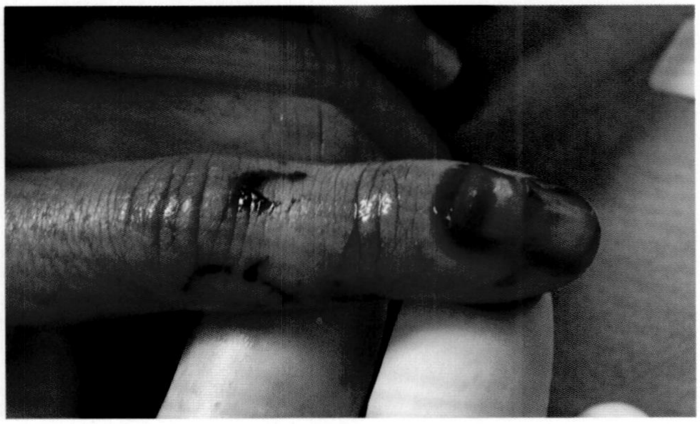

Figure 5 Clinical photograph of Seymour fracture.

Other distal phalanx fractures are also commonly seen in children. Although tuft fractures are the most common injury with a relatively low complication rate, other fracture types can have a high rate of complications like Seymour fractures and bony mallet or Salter-Harris III/IV fractures (**Figures 4** and **5**).[35,38,41] A recent study by Lankachandra et al reviewed complications of all pediatric distal phalanx fractures presenting to their hand clinic over a 1-year period.[42] In their retrospective review of 206 patients with a median of 22 weeks follow-up, they found that complications are common with the most common being infection (22%), stiffness (15%), and nail deformity (13%). The incidence of complication varied based on fracture type with a rate of 62% for Seymour fractures, 50% for SHIII/IV fractures, and 49% for mallet fractures. Combined, these patterns accounted for 26% of the fractures. Overall, one-third of the patients had a documented complication in the medical record.

Summary

Pediatric upper extremity fractures are extremely common, accounting for the majority of injuries in children. The majority of forearm, wrist, and finger fractures can be treated with reduction when necessary and cast immobilization with excellent results. There are several specific fractures, however, that do require special attention and sometimes surgery like Monteggia fractures, displaced forearm fractures in adolescents and those with elevated BMIs, displaced and chronic scaphoid fractures, displaced phalangeal neck and condyle fractures and Seymour fractures. Careful attention to physical examination and radiographs can help identify these specific cases to ensure the best outcome for the patient.

Key Study Points

- Successful management of Monteggia fracture is most likely with early diagnosis (within 3 weeks) and maintenance of ulnar alignment and length. Open reduction of the radiocapitellar joint is rarely needed if the ulna is appropriately addressed.
- Although the trend for both-bone forearm fracture management has increasingly been surgical, clinical research supports nonsurgical management in many cases. Patients older than 10 years with residual angulation after reduction are more likely to fail nonsurgical management. For surgical stabilization, IM fixation is less invasive.
- Obesity may increase likelihood of reduction loss by as much as 50%.
- Buckle fractures of the distal radius are successfully managed with a removable splint and no further visit beyond initial assessment. 100% displaced distal radius fractures in patients less than 10 years of age can be successfully left in bayonet apposition with complete remodeling expected and significant cost savings realized.
- Acute, nondisplaced scaphoid fractures can be treated with cast immobilization with excellent outcomes.
- Seymour fractures that are treated in a delayed fashion with inadequate treatment (lack of complete débridement and/or lack of antibiotics) have a high rate of complication.
- Distal phalanx fractures in children can have a high rate of complication, so appropriate diagnosis and treatment is a necessity.

Annotated References

1. Naranje SM, Erail RA, Warner WC, Sawyer JR, Kelly DM: Epidemiology of pediatric fractures presenting to emergency departments in the United States. *J Pediatr Orthop* 2016;36(4):e45-e48.

   The National Electronic Injury Surveillance System (NEISS) database was searched for all fractures in children between the ages of 0-19 in 2010 to identify the most frequent pediatric fractures per 1,000 population at risk in the United States. The annual occurrence of fractures increases from age 0 to 14 peaking in the 10-14 age range (15.23 per 1,000 children). Fractures of the forearm were most common (17.8% of all fractures) followed by finger and wrist fractures. Finger and hand fractures were most common for age groups 10-14 and 15-19. Overall risk for fracture throughout childhood and adolescence was 180 per 1,000 children or just under 1 in 5. Level of evidence: III.

2. Hubbard J, Chauhan A, Fitzgerald R, Abrams R, Mubarak S, Sangimino M: Missed pediatric Monteggia fractures. *JBJS Rev* 2018;6(6):e2.

   Review article on missed pediatric Monteggia fractures. Reviews diagnosis and treatment options based on an algorithm. Discusses treatment options for missed injuries and outcomes. Level of evidence: II.

3. Manning Ryan L, Teach SJ, Searcy K, et al: The association between weight status and pediatric forearm fractures resulting from ground-level falls. *Pediatr Emerg Care* 2015;31(12):835-838.

4. Kim C, Gentry M, Sala D, et al: Single-bone intramedullary nailing of pediartic both bone forearm fractures. *Bull Hosp Joint Dis* 2017;75(4):227.

   Systematic review article of efficacy of single-bone intramedullary nailing of pediatric both-bone forearm fractures. Medline and Embase were searched identifying 11 articles for review. Studies found that pronation, supination, and radiographic angulation outcomes were comparable in single- and both-bone fixation cohorts. Rates of motion loss and re-angulation were similar across groups. Level of evidence: II.

5. Auer RT, Mazzone P, Robinson L, Nyland J, Chan G: Childhood obesity increases the risk of failure in the treatment of distal forearm fractures. *J Pediatr Orthop* 2016;36(8):e86-e88.

   Retrospective review of 157 consecutive distal radius fractures treated with initial closed reduction and fiberglass casting. Forty-two percent of children were found to be overweight and 29% were obese (BMI > 95%). Twelve percent of normal-sized children required repeat reduction after initial treatment versus 28% of the obese children. Level of evidence: III.

6. Souder CD, Roocroft JH, Edmonds EW: Significance of the lateral humeral line for evaluating radiocapitellar alignment in children. *J Pediatr Orthop* 2017;37(3):e150-e155.

   Radiographs of 37 children were evaluated to determine if the radiocapitellar line (RCL) could be used to evaluate the coronal alignment of the radiocapitellar joint in children as it had previously been only validated on lateral radiographs. They found the RCL intersects the capitellum 30% of the time on lateral imaging and 26% of the time on AP imaging in noninjured elbows. The lateral humeral line (LHL) consistently did fall lateral to the radial neck on normal elbows and medial to the lateral aspect of the radial neck on elbows with Bado III Monteggia fractures. The RCL most commonly intersects the lateral one-third of the ossification center on both radiographs and MRI. Level of evidence: III.

7. Flynn JM, Jones KJ, Garner MR, Goebel J: Eleven years experience in the operative management of pediatric forearm fractures. *J Pediatr Orthop* 2010;30(4):313-319.

8. Ramski DE, Hennrikus WP, Bae DS, et al: Pediatric monteggia fractures: A multicenter examination of treatment strategy and early clinical and radiographic results. *J Pediatr Orthop* 2015;35(2):115-120.

Pediatrics

9. Foran I, Upasani VV, Wallace CD, et al: Acute pediatric Monteggia fractures: A conservative approach to stabilization. *J Pediatr Orthop* 2017;37(6):e335-e341.

Retrospective review of all Monteggia fractures treated at a level 1 trauma center over a 6-year period resulting in 94 patients. At follow-up (mean 18 weeks), there were no cases of residual radiocapitellar joint subluxation or dislocation and all fractures had healed. Majority of patients (87%) were successfully managed in cast. Bado type and ulna angulation greater than 36.5° were only primary predictors requiring surgical stabilization. Level of evidence: IV.

10. Bae DS: Successful strategies for managing Monteggia injuries. *J Pediatr Orthop* 2016;36(suppl 1):S67-S70.

Review article on treatment of Monteggia fractures in acute and late diagnosed settings. Level of evidence: III.

11. Pace JL: Pediatric and adolescent forearm fractures: Current controversies and treatment recommendations. *J Am Acad Orthop Surg* 2016;24(11):780-788.

Review article on pediatric and adolescent forearm fractures. Discusses indications for closed versus open treatment and complications associated with both treatment methods. Level of evidence: III.

12. Ting BL, Kalish LA, Waters PM, Bae DS: Reducing cost and radiation exposure during the treatment of pediatric greenstick fractures of the forearm. *J Pediatr Orthop* 2016;36(8):816-820.

Retrospective review of patients aged 2 to 16 treated with closed reduction and casting of greenstick fractures over a 10-year period. Cost analysis and x-ray exposure were performed. One hundred and nine patients of average age 6.9 were included. On average, patients had 3.6 follow-up visits and 3.5 sets of radiographs. Only one patient required re-reduction. They found if follow-up was limited to two clinic visits and three sets of radiographs, there would be a 14.3% reduction in total cost and 41% decreased radiation exposure. Level of evidence: IV.

13. Okoroafor UC, Cannada LK, McGinty JL: Obesity and failure of nonsurgical management of pediatric both-bone forearm fractures. *J Hand Surg Am* 2017;42(9):711-716.

Retrospective review of pediatric patients older than 2 years treated for radius and ulna shaft fractures with closed reduction and immobilization over a 3-year period. One hundred twenty-nine patients were divided into two groups based on normal-weight children versus overweight and obese children. Fifty-nine percent of patients were normal weight and 20% were overweight and 22% were obese. Eight percent of normal weight children failed cast treatment versus 34% of overweight and obese children. Twenty-nine percent of normal weight children that failed initial cast treatment required surgery versus 56% of overweight and obese children. Level of evidence: II.

14. Chua ISY, Chong SL, Ong GYK: Intravenous regional anaesthesia (Bier's block) for pediatric forearm fractures in a pediatric emergency department-Experience from 2003 to 2014. *Injury* 2017;48(12):2784-2787.

Retrospective cohort study looking at pediatric patients treated with Bier blocks in the emergency department for pediatric forearm fractures. A second subset of patients receiving Bier block versus ketamine sedation were compared. 1781 patients were identified that had Bier blocks with average age of 12. There were two failed blocks. Average length of stay for Bier block patients was significantly shorter than those who had ketamine at 170 versus 238 minutes. Level of evidence: II.

15. Baldwin PC, Han E, Parrino A, Lee MC: Valve or no valve: A prospective randomized controlled trial of casting options for pediatric forearm fractures. *Orthopedics* 2017;40(5):e849-e854.

60 patients with diaphyseal or distal one-third fractures are immobilized in long arm cast following reduction and randomized to no valve, univalve, and bivalve modification. There were no incidents of compartment syndrome or neurovascular complication in any group, and no differences found for reduction loss, cast modification, or need for conversion to surgical stabilization. Minimizing cast splitting may decrease cast saw–related injury. Level of evidence: I.

16. Kutsikovich JI, Hopkins CM, Gannon EW III, et al: Factors that predict instability in pediatric diaphyseal both-bone forearm fractures. *J Pediatr Orthop B* 2018;27(4):304-308.

Retrospective review of pediatric diaphyseal forearm fractures treated with closed reduction casting over a 6-year period. One hundred seventy-four patients were identified. Eleven percentage of patients required a repeat procedure. Risk factors identified for repeat reduction were translation greater than 50% or more in any plane, age more than 9, complete fracture of the radius, and follow-up angulation of the radius more than 15° on lateral radiographs or ulna more than 10° on AP radiographs. Level of evidence: II.

17. Price CT, Scott DS, Kurzer ME, Flynn JC: Malunited forearm fractures in children. *J Pediatr Orthop* 1990;10:705.

18. Eismann EA, Little K, Kunkel ST, Cornwall R: Clinical research fails to support more aggressive management of pediatric upper extremity fractures. *J Bone Joint Surg Am* 2013;95(15):1345-1350.

19. Heare A, Goral D, Belton M, Beebe C, Trizno A, Stoneback J: Intramedullary implant choice and cost in the treatment of pediatric diaphyseal forearm fractures. *J Orthop Trauma* 2017;31(10):e334-e338.

Retrospective review assessing use of titanium elastic nails (TENs), stainless steel elastic nails (SENs), and K-wires for treatment of pediatric diaphyseal forearm fractures with intramedullary fixation. There was no difference between the three groups in time to union, complication rate, or surgical time. There was a significant difference in cost per implant of $639, $172, and $24 for TENs, SENs, and K-wires, respectively. Level of evidence: III.

20. Nørgaard SL, Riber SS, Danielsson FB, Pedersen NW, Viberg B: Surgical approach for elastic stable intramedullary nail in pediatric radius shaft fracture: A systematic review. *J Pediatr Orthop B* 2018;27(4):309-314.

Literature review comparing treatment of children with radial shaft fractures with either dorsal or lateral approach for insertion of an elastic stable intramedullary nail (EISN). PubMed, Cochrane, and EMbase were searched with 2234 articles identified. Twenty-two articles met inclusion criteria for review. Demographics and complications were reviewed. They found the dorsal approach had a 2.6% rate of extensor pollicis longus rupture, whereas the lateral approach had a 2.9% rate of transient superficial radial nerve palsy and 0.3% rate of permanent damage. Level of evidence: II.

21. Baldwin K, Morrison MJ III, Tomlinson LA, Ramirez R, Flynn JM: Both bone forearm fractures in children and adolescents, which fixation strategy is superior – Plates or nails? A systematic review and meta-analysis of observational studies. *J Orthop Trauma* 2014;28(1):e8-e14.

22. Kuba MHM, Izuka BH: One brace: One visit. Treatment of pediatric distal radius buckle fractures with a removable wrist brace and no follow-up visit. *J Pediatr Orthop* 2018;38(6):e338-e342.

    Forty consecutive patients with distal radius buckle fractures were identified to participate in the study. They were treated with a removable wrist brace with a prescribed time to wear the brace. Parents were then contacted by phone at 1 week after brace discontinuation and then at 5-10 months post-injury. Parents reported no complications, no residual pain, and return back to full activity. This protocol saved 67% of parents from missing work and 77% of children from missing work for follow-up appointment. Level of evidence: IV.

23. Bae DS, Howard AW: Distal radius fractures: What is the evidence? *J Pediatr Orthop* 2012;32(suppl 2):S128.

24. Crawford SN, Lee LS, Izuka BH: Closed treatment of overriding distal radial fractures without reduction in children. *J Bone Joint Surg Am* 2012;94:246-252.

25. Acree JS, Schlechter J, Buzin S: Cost analysis and performance in distal pediatric forearm fractures: Is a short-arm cast superior to a sugar-tong splint? *J Pediatr Orthop B* 2017;26(5):424-428.

    Retrospective review of 73 patients aged 5 to 14 treated with closed reduction and then either sugar-tong splint or cast immobilization for distal one-third wrist fracture. There was no statistical difference between maintenance of reduction between the two methods with acceptable alignment in 94% of cases. Cost analysis slightly favored initial placement of short arm cast versus a splint transitioned to cast later. Level of evidence: II.

26. Dua K, Stein MK, O'Hara NN, et al: Variation among pediatric orthopaedic surgeons when diagnosing and treating pediatric and adolescent distal radius fractures. *J Pediatr Orthop* 2019;39(6):306-313.

    Nine pediatric orthopedic surgeons reviewed 100 sets of wrist radiographs and asked to describe fracture type, type of treatment, length of immobilization, and time until next follow-up visit. There was only fair interobserver reliability of diagnosis of fracture type and there was no standardization for type or length of treatment. Level of evidence: II.

27. Mussbichler H: Injuries of the carpal scaphoid in children. *Acta Radiol* 1961;56:361-368.

28. Christodoulou AG, Colton CL: Scaphoid fractures in children. *J Pediatr Orthop* 1986;6:37-39.

29. Kocher MS, Waters PM, Micheli LJ: Upper extremity injuries in the paediatric athlete. *Sports Med* 2000;30:117-135.

30. Gholson JJ, Bae DS, Zurakowski D, Waters PM: Scaphoid fractures in children and adolescents: Contemporary injury patterns and factors influencing time to union. *J Bone Joint Surg Am* 2011;93:1210-1219.

31. Tessaro MO, McGovern TR, Dickman E, Haines LE: Point-of-care ultrasound detection of acute scaphoid fracture. *Pediatr Emerg Care* 2015;31(3):222-224.

32. Bae DS, Gholson JJ, Zurakowski D, Waters PM: Functional outcomes after treatment of scaphoid fractures in children and adolescents. *J Pediatr Orthop* 2016;36(1):13-18.

    Sixty-three of 312 patients treated for scaphoid fractures at a single institution aged 8-18 at time of treatment were contacted to complete patient-reported outcome measures including the DASH inventory and work and sports modules as well as the Modified Mayo Wrist Score (MMWS). At midterm follow-up (6.3 years), all patients had gone on to bony healing. Median DASH score was reported functional status equal to or better than the general population. Chronic fracture presentation and osteonecrosis were predictors of worse outcome. Surgical treatment was not found to influence functional status with an excellent functional outcome per the MMWS for both surgical and nonsurgical patients. Level of evidence: III.

33. Jauregui JJ, Seger EW, Hesham K, Walker SE, Abraham R, Abzug JM: Operative management for pediatric and adolescent scaphoid nonunion: A meta-analysis. *J Pediatr Orthop* 2019;39(2):e130-e133.

    Meta-analysis of 11 studies found to meet the authors criteria of articles reporting on surgical treatment of scaphoid nonunions. This represented 176 surgically treated pediatric/adolescent scaphoid nonunions. Both grafted and non-grafted techniques resulted in high union rates of 94.6% and 94.8%, respectively, and excellent functional outcomes. No difference was found in this study between techniques. Level of evidence: III.

34. Fetter-Zarzeka A, Joseph MM: Hand and fingertip injuries in children. *Pediatr Emerg Care* 2002;18(5):341-345.

35. Vadivelu R, Dias JJ, Burke FD, Stanton J: Hand injuries in children: A prospective study. *J Pediatr Orthop* 2006;26:29-35.

36. Matzon JL, Cornwall R: A stepwise algorithm for surgical treatment of type II displaced pediatric phalangeal neck fractures. *J Hand Surg Am* 2014;39:467-473.

37. Al-Qattan: Nonunion and avascular necrosis following phalangeal neck fractures in children. *J Hand Surg Am* 2010;35:1269-1274.

38. Abzub JM, Kozin SH: Seymour fratures. *J Hand Surg Am* 2013;38:2267-2270.

39. Reyes BA, Ho CA: The high risk of infection with delayed treatment of open Seymour fractures: Salter-Harris I/II or juxta-epiphyseal fractures of the distal phalanx with associated nailbed laceration. *J Pediatr Orthop* 2017;37(4):1-7.

Retrospective review of 34 patients with 35 Seymour fractures. Patients were grouped as treated "appropriately" with irrigation and debridement, fracture reduction and antibiotics versus "partial" defined as any type of incomplete treatment and as "acute" defined as treatment within 24 hours versus "delayed". No infections occurred in the appropriate acutely treated group (0/11) versus 2 in the acute partially treated group (2/11, 15%), versus 5 in the delated treatment group (5/11, 45%).

40. Boyer JS, London DA, Stepan JG, Goldfarb CA: Pediatric proximal phalanx fractures: Outcomes and complications after the surgical treatment of displaced fractures. *J Pediatr Orthop* 2015;35(3):219-223.

41. Bloom JM, Khouri JS, Hammert WC: Current concepts in the evaluation and treatment of mallet finger injury. *Plast Reconstr Surg* 2013;132(4):e560-e566.

42. Lankachandra M, Wells CR, Cheng CJ, Hutchinson RL: Complications of distal phalanx fractures in children. *J Hand Surg Am* 2017;42:574.e1-574.e6.

Retrospective review of patients seen in pediatric hand surgery clinic from 2011 to 2012 with a diagnosis of distal phalanx fracture. Average age of patient was 7.5 years and fracture distribution was tuft (37%), mallet (18%), Salter-Harris I/II (13%), shaft (11%), base (11%), Seymour (6%), Salter-Harris III/IV (2%) and tip amputation (1%). Complications occurred in 31% of patients with highest rates for Salter-Harris IV (100%), Seymour (62%), and mallet fractures (49%). The most common complications were infection (22%), stiffness (15%), and nail deformity (13%). Level of evidence: IV.

Chapter 55

Pediatric Upper Extremity Disorders

Micah Sinclair, MD • Sarah E. Sibbel, MD

ABSTRACT

Classification and understanding of congenital hand and upper extremity disorders has vastly improved since the 1970s. Congenital upper extremity disorders are challenging to treat, and there is a primary focus on achieving optimal function. Recognizing the various types of deformity, identifying potential surgical options, and managing patient expectations may lead to satisfactory results to both the surgeon and patient. It is important to evaluate the risks and benefits of surgery and work on a multidisciplinary team, as well as collaborate with other hand surgeon, to provide the patient with the best potential outcome.

Keywords: congenital hand disorders; dysplasias; malformations; pediatrics; syndactyly

Introduction

Treatment of congenital disorders of the hand and upper extremity requires an understanding of the embryology and developmental anomalies of the pediatric upper extremity. This chapter will include the most frequent congenital disorders that occur in the upper extremity, from the fingertips to the brachial plexus. Each section will feature a brief summary of the disorder and include recent developments in the understanding of the pathophysiology or treatment of each included diagnosis.

Dr. Sibbel or an immediate family member serves as a board member, owner, officer, or committee member of the Pediatric Orthopaedic Society of North America. Neither Dr. Sinclair nor any immediate family member has received anything of value from or has stock or stock options held in a commercial company or institution related directly or indirectly to the subject of this chapter.

Embryology

The upper-limb bud appears in the human embryo 26 days after fertilization and continues until 47 days when the joints of the hand develop. The skeletal elements and connective tissues are derived from a core of mesoderm covered in epithelial cells derived from ectoderm. There are three known signaling centers in the limb that direct development with associated chemical signaling. These are listed in[1-4] **Table 1**. Limb development is complex and specific timing of all of the associated signaling pathways that intersect at multiple points is responsible for the development of the upper extremity. Sonic hedgehog (SHH) protein plays a pivotal role in linking the three axes of growth.

The classification of congenital differences of the upper limb was initially accepted in the 1970s, before the current understanding of molecular and developmental biology and genetics. In 2010, the Oberg-Manske-Tonkin (OMT) classification system was proposed, separating congenital deformities into three groups: malformations, deformations, and dysplasias. This classification system has recently been shown to have excellent intraobserver and intraobserver reliability among pediatric hand surgeons.[5]

Symbrachydactyly

Symbrachydactyly is a congenital hand difference that can present with a variety of morphologic findings including brachydactyly, syndactyly, hand hypoplasia, and the presence of rudimentary nubbins that include elements of nail plate, bone, and cartilage. The central digits are typically absent, with relative sparing of the border digits.[6]

The incidence of symbrachydactyly is approximately 0.6 per 10,000 live births. It occurs primarily in males and is typically unilateral in presentation with the left side being predominantly affected.[7] It is usually not due to a known genetic abnormality, but can be associated with Poland syndrome, in which unilateral hypoplasia or absence of the pectoralis major occurs.[8]

Table 1

Signaling Centers That Direct Development of the Limb

Axis of Growth	Signaling Center	Key Chemical Substrate	Anomaly
Proximodistal—longitudinal growth	Apical ectodermal ridge (AER)	Fibroblast growth factors	Transverse deficiency—phocomelia
Anterioposterior—radial to ulnar	Zone of polarizing activity	Sonic hedgehog	Mirror hand Polydactyly Syndactyly RLD, ULD
Dorsoventral—dorsum to palm	Limb ectoderm	Wnt7	Dorsalization deficiencies—nail-patella syndrome

RLD = radial longitudinal deficiency, ULD = ulnar longitudinal deficiency

The etiology of symbrachydactyly is unknown. A leading hypothesis is the "subclavian artery supply disruption sequence."[9] This hypothesis states that isolated transverse terminal limb deficiencies are associated with interruption of the subclavian artery at the sixth week of embryologic development, leading to a failure of outward limb growth.

The hand affected by symbrachydactyly can present with a variety of findings. The hand or entire limb is shorter and smaller than the uninvolved upper limb with underdeveloped digits: short or webbed digits, digital nubbins, or absent digits. The mesoderm is primarily affected in symbrachydactyly with characteristic preservation of ectodermal elements such as the nail plate and distal phalanges.

The surgical treatment of symbrachydactyly is specific to each patient and focuses on improving hand function if necessary. This includes providing length to the thumb or ulnar sided digits to enhance prehensile function.

Syndactyly and web contractures are released to improve aesthetics, independent digital function, and hand span. Nonvascularized toe phalangeal bone transfers provide additional length and stability for short, hypoplastic digits that have redundant soft tissue present. Distraction osteogenesis lengthening has also been described for the treatment of shortened digits in symbrachydactyly. Microsurgical toe transfers are another option to enhance pinch and prehension in symbrachydactyly.

Radial Longitudinal Deficiency

Radial longitudinal deficiency (RLD) is a spectrum of upper extremity dysplasia and hypoplasia affecting the entire limb. Presentation rests on a spectrum from mild hypoplasia of the thumb, to absence of the radius or proximal humerus. Some forms are spontaneous, but it can be inherited in both autosomal dominant and recessive patterns. RLD is associated with an underlying syndrome 33% to 44% of the time. Associated syndromes include Holt-Oram syndrome, thrombocytopenia absent radius (TAR), Fanconi anemia, and VACTERL association. The hand surgeon may be the first physician to see the child because of the visible upper extremity differences. Appropriate testing must be performed to evaluate for these associated anomalies and syndromes[10] (**Table 2**). The patient and family should also be referred for genetics counseling. Holt-Oram syndrome can have a distinctive or unusual presentation of RLD, which includes atypical radioulnar synostosis, extending distally into the forearm with a reduced radial head and/or first web space syndactyly. If either of these defining features are present, Holt-Oram syndrome should be suspected and a cardiac evaluation and genetic testing should be performed.[11]

Table 2

Recommended Tests for Important Syndromic Associated Conditions in Radial Longitudinal Deficiency Patients

Complete blood count
Echocardiogram
Abdominal ultrasonography
Diepoxybutane testing[a]
Scoliosis radiographs[b]

[a]Patients with café au lait spots and short stature.[10]
[b]Should be performed at an older age.

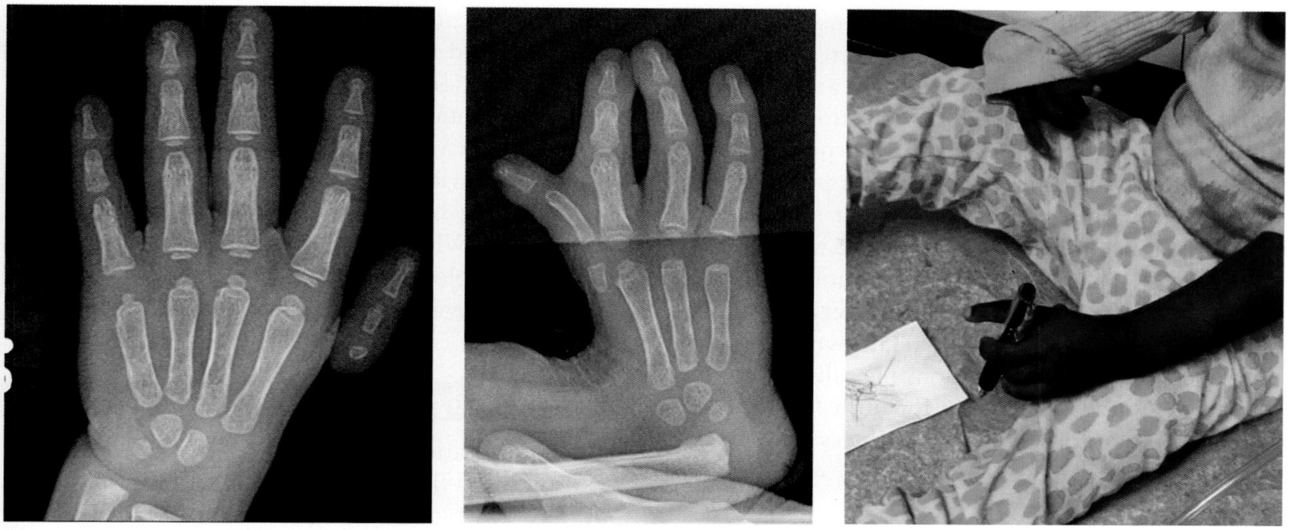

Figure 1 Radiograph images and associated clinical photograph of a child with bilateral thumb hypoplasia. (Courtesy of Micah K. Sinclair, MD.)

Involvement of the forearm in RLD is classified according to the severity of skeletal dysplasia of the radius. The spectrum includes abnormalities of the proximal radius with normal length, to mild shortening of the radius, to complete absence of the radius and severe radial deviation of the hand. In more severe radial shortening, with a radially deviated hand, the initial treatment is stretching and splinting. Soft tissue distraction with an external fixator before centralization is associated with a worse final radial deviation and volar subluxation position compared with centralization alone.[12] Centralization at 1 year of age has been described with overall outcome of further shortening of the ulna due to physeal trauma and recurrence of deformity 36% to 47% of patients.[12] Recently, the release of the radial soft tissue and volar bilobed flap transposition has been shown to be successful at maintenance of wrist motion and avoidance of injury to the ulnar physis, with similar recurrence rates to formal centralization.[13,14] In a study of adults with RLD, grip strength, key pinch, forearm length, and elbow and digital motion were found to be more important to activity than radial angulation of the wrist.[15]

Thumb hypoplasia is included on the spectrum of RLD (**Figure 1**). Treatment is based upon the degree of hypoplasia, with the goal being stable, strong pinch and opposition (**Table 3**). For hypoplastic thumbs, opponensplasty can be performed using abductor digiti minimi with the benefit being increased bulk substituting for absent thenar musculature. Alternatively, the ring finger flexor digitorum superficialis may be used with excellent opposition function.[16] There is no evidence to support one transfer over another; however, one must take into account available anatomy and patient size.

Table 3

Thumb Hypoplasia Classifications and Treatment Options

Type	Findings	Treatment
I	Minor generalized hypoplasia	No treatment
II	Intrinsic thenar muscles hypoplasia	Opponensplasty
	First web space narrowing	First web release
	UCL insufficiency	UCL reconstruction
III	Similar findings as type II plus:	A: Reconstruction
	Extrinsic muscle and tendon abnormalities	B: Pollicization
	Bone deficiency	
	A: Stable TMC joint	
	B: Unstable TMC joint	
IV	*Pouce flottant* or floating thumb	Pollicization
V	Absent thumb	Pollicization

TMC = trapeziometacarpal, UCL = ulnar collateral ligament

Reprinted from Soldado F, Zlotolow DA, Kozin SH: Thumb hypoplasia. *J Hand Surg* 2013;38[7]:1435-1444. Copyright 2013, with permission from Elsevier.

It is critical to differentiate the presence of a stable or unstable carpometacarpal joint when considering reconstruction versus pollicization in a hypoplastic thumb. Thumb ablation and pollicization is recommended for those with an unstable carpometacarpal joint. An important consideration when planning pollicization is the presence of index finger stiffness and patient preference for ulnar sided pinch, which occurs in severe RLD. The benefit of pollicization in this setting is controversial. Although the severity of radial dysplasia has been found to correlate with the quality of function after pollicization, overall satisfaction of the family with pollicization for both function and cosmesis has been shown despite stiffness of the pollicized thumb.[17]

Ulnar Longitudinal Deficiency

Ulnar longitudinal deficiency (ULD) is four times less common than RLD.[7] It is a sporadic condition and is not associated with systemic conditions. It is often associated with other musculoskeletal conditions, including proximal femoral focal deficiency, fibular deficiency, phocomelia, and congenital scoliosis. Unilateral involvement is the most common presentation and the entire limb is involved. There is can be an abnormal or fused elbow. Most patients have missing ulnar digits, up to 70% present with thumb abnormalities and 30% present with syndactyly.

The majority of surgical procedures performed for ULD are for correction of thumb and hand deformity.[18] Wrist and forearm deformities do not typically require surgery.

Radioulnar Synostosis

Congenital radioulnar synostosis (CRUS) is an abnormal connection between the radius and ulna that results from an insult in utero within the second month of gestation. Up to 30% are reported to be associated with syndromes or anomalies, and 60% are bilateral.[19]

Commonly described activity limitations include toileting, hand washing, catching a ball with a baseball glove, and swinging a tennis racket or baseball bat.

Patients present with some degree of fixed forearm rotation. The pronation of the forearm is measured as the angle between the humeral line and the axis of the radial styloid to center of ulnar head. Pain is not a common report.

Most of the patients with CRUS are high functioning and surgery is seldom indicated because of the common presentation of fixed rotation in a functional position. Surgical treatment includes an osteotomy that rotates the fixed forearm position into one that allows bimanual function.

Late presentation of elbow pain in a previously painful elbow can occur in some adolescents, particularly in those with anterior dislocation of their radial head. They may have loss of elbow range of motion and acute locking. When this occurs, excision of radial head to remove the block to motion is found to be successful in restoring previously painful range of motion.[20]

Preaxial Polydactyly

Thumb duplication has a reported incidence of 0.08 to 1.4 in 1,000 live births.[21] The inheritance pattern is sporadic, and typically unilateral in presentation. The etiology is truly a split thumb, rather than a true duplication. The affected thumbs are more slender in appearance compared with the contralateral thumb. The ulnar thumb tends to be the larger and more dominant thumb.

The most common classification is the Wassel classification (**Figure 2**). An easy way to remember this classification is to count the number of abnormal bones, which correlates to the Wassel type. The most common type is a Wassel type IV thumb duplication, which is duplication of both the distal and proximal phalanges of the thumb on a common metacarpal. The pattern of counting abnormal bones yields true for all but the triphalangeal thumb, which is a Wassel type VII. This thumb difference may be associated with genetic syndromes.[22]

Surgical reconstruction typically consists of excision of the less developed digit and reconstruction of the more dominant thumb. The collateral ligaments should be preserved or reconstructed for long-term joint stability.

During reconstruction, a pollex abductus may be encountered. This is an abnormal connection between the extensor pollicis longus and the flexor pollicis longus (FPL), which can lead to angular deformity of the digit.

Postaxial Polydactyly

Postaxial polydactyly, or duplication of a digit on the ulnar border of the hand, is most common in those of African American descent.[23] It is inherited in an autosomal dominant fashion. Postaxial polydactyly in those of Caucasian descent should trigger a more thorough genetic workup, as polydactyly in these individuals may be associated with other system abnormalities.

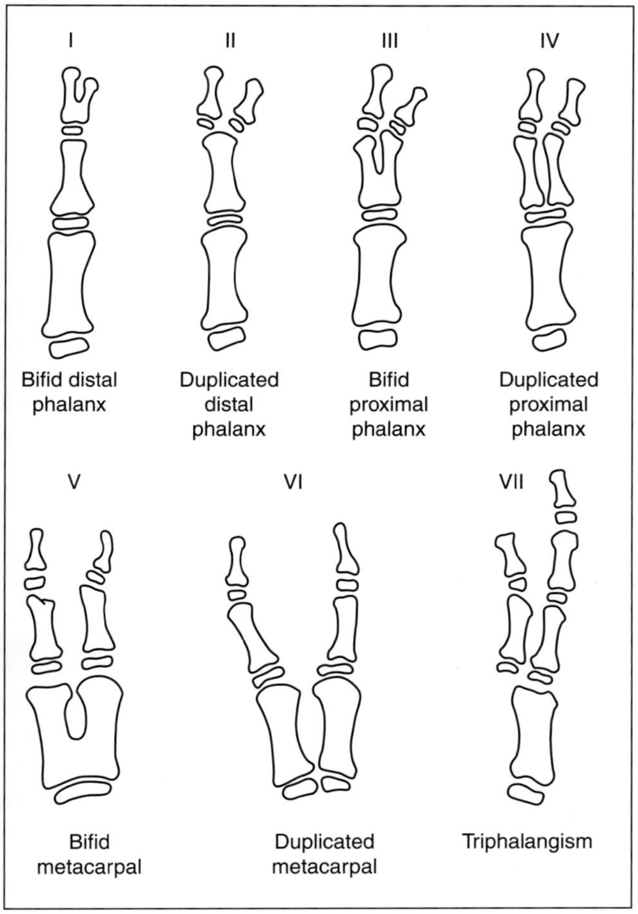

Figure 2 Illustration of Wassel classification for preaxial polydactyly. (Reprinted with permission from Wassel HD: The results of surgery for polydactyly of the thumb. A review. *Clin Orthop Relat Res* 1969;64[22]:175-193. Available at: https://journals.lww.com/clinorthop/Citation/1969/05000/22_The_Results_of_Surgery_for_Polydactyly_of_the.24.aspx.)

Postaxial polydactyly is classified as two types. Type A is a well-formed digit, and type B is a vestigial digit with the appearance of a skin tag. A type A digit should undergo formal surgical reconstruction, should the family elect this. A type B digit has traditionally been ligated with suture or surgical clips as a newborn. This may leave a small bump on the ulnar border of the hand. Formal surgical ablation may be preferred to improve cosmesis and avoid the observation of digit necrosis and autoamputation.

Syndactyly

Syndactyly is a narrowed or fused web space between adjacent digits and is the result of a failure of normal separation of the digits during prenatal development. This separation normally occurs between the fifth and eighth week of gestation. Syndactyly is one of the most common congenital hand differences, with an incidence reported at 1 in 2,500 live births.[24] It affects males more commonly than females.[25,26]

Syndactyly most often presents as an isolated clinical condition and is typically seen as an autosomal dominant inheritance pattern of transmission with variable penetrance.[27] The third web space is most commonly affected, followed by the fourth, second, and first web spaces[28] (**Figure 3**).

The classification of syndactyly is straightforward and based upon anatomic findings. Simple syndactyly involves only the soft tissues, where a complex syndactyly includes bony fusion. When accessory phalanges or abnormal bones between digits are present, this is termed a complex syndactyly. A complete syndactyly occurs when the soft tissue connection extends to the fingertip and is incomplete when the syndactyly ends proximal to the fingertip.

Syndactyly may also be associated with syndromes, including Poland syndrome, acrocephalosyndactyly

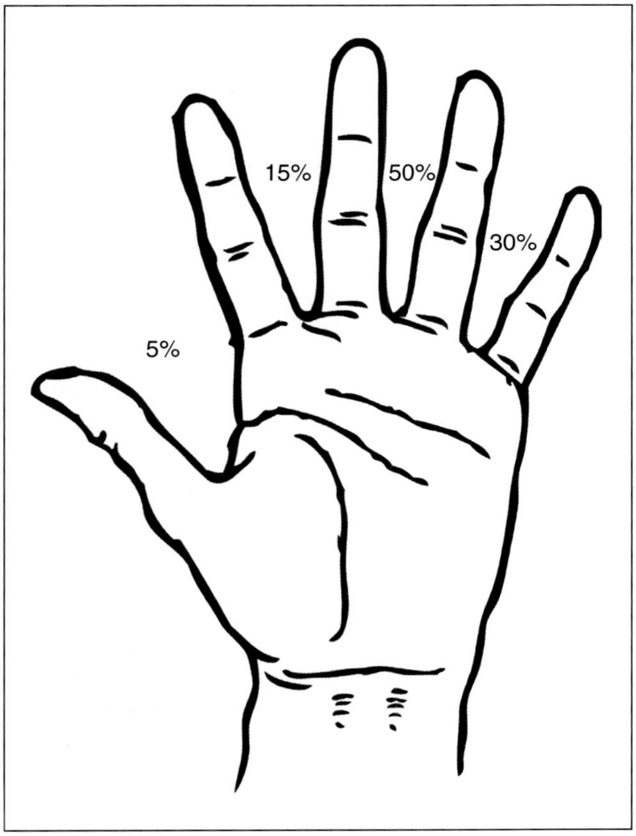

Figure 3 Illustration of syndactyly prevalence of affected web spaces. (Reprinted with permission from Sibbel SE, James MA: Syndactyly and symbrachydactyly, in Weiss A-PC, ed: *Textbook of Hand and Upper Extremity Surgery*. ed 2. Chicago, American Society for Surgery of the Hand, 2019, vol 2, pp 1397-1412.)

(Apert syndrome), amniotic constriction band, and other congenital musculoskeletal abnormalities such as cleft hand, symbrachydactyly, synpolydactyly, or ULD.

Surgical reconstruction is the mainstay of treatment to maximize hand function and appearance. Timing of surgery remains controversial, although most surgeons would agree that surgical intervention should be earlier for border digits as there is a difference in longitudinal growth between thumb and index finger and between ring and small fingers. Separation of these digits around 6 months of age may limit the development of tethering of the digit, which can help diminish the risk of bone or joint deformities and contractures. Separation of the long and ring fingers can be safely accomplished between 12 and 24 months of age with no adverse effect on function or fine motor development.[29-31]

Several techniques are described for syndactyly reconstruction. Interdigitating zigzag flaps are used to avoid longitudinal scar contracture. The web commissure is established using supple dorsal skin flaps, and grafts are avoided in this area to minimize scarring and web creep. Full-thickness skin grafts are typically used to resurface bare areas after complete release and can be easily harvested from the wrist crease or antecubital fossa. Graftless reconstruction techniques have been described as well and rely on the vascularized skin from the dorsum of the hand, which is raised and advanced to reconstitute the web commissure.[32-34] This leaves the skin over the dorsal aspect of the proximal phalanges to cover the skin defects of the separated digits. The resulting donor defect is closed primarily. The distal skin flaps are defatted to decrease digits' circumference and closed.

The complication rate of syndactyly reconstruction is low, reported at 2%, with the most common complication being superficial surgical site infection.[35]

Camptodactyly

Camptodactyly is a nontraumatic flexion deformity of the finger, most commonly affecting the proximal interphalangeal joint. The small finger is most frequently involved.

Presentation of the deformity is bimodal, in young children and adolescents, related to periods of rapid growth. There can also be an association with certain congenital syndromes. In general, in all but the severe forms, the functional deficit is minimal and the concern is more about appearance. Complaints of functional limitations can include difficulty with typing, playing a musical instrument, participating in sporting activities, wearing gloves. Description of the contracture should consider the angle of the contracture and the consideration of whether it is correctible or stiff. Radiographic changes can be seen in 30% of patients. The contracture can lead to a spectrum of bony deformity seen best on lateral radiographs. This includes flattening and loss of the dorsal convex contour of the head of the proximal phalanx and subsequent flattening of the base of the middle phalanx.

Initial treatment of all patients on presentation typically includes stretching and splinting.[36,37] Surgical indications may include severe contracture of greater than 60° with impaired function, unacceptable aesthetics, radiographic changes. When evaluating the patient for surgery, all potential involved soft tissues should be evaluated in a stepwise fashion including the skin, fascia, flexor digitorum superficialis tendon, lumbricals, interosseous muscles, lateral bands, volar plate, collateral ligaments, joint surfaces, central extensor tendon.[37,38]

Kirner Deformity

Kirner deformity is an abnormal volar and radial curvature of the distal phalanx of the small finger (**Figure 4**). There is a female predominance of 2 to 1 and bilateral involvement is common.[39] The etiology is unknown. Surgical correction is rarely necessary as there is no functional deficit.

Metacarpal/Carpal Synostoses

Carpal coalition is an anomalous union of two or more carpal bones. These can be either sporadic and seen in otherwise healthy individuals or in association with syndromes or metabolic disorders.

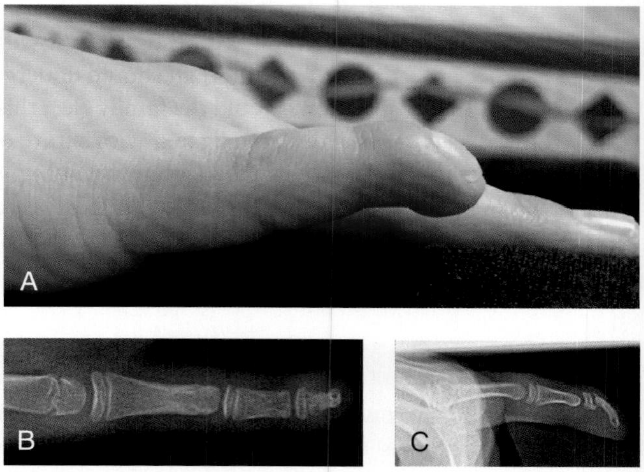

Figure 4 Clinical and radiographic examples of Kirner deformity. (Courtesy of Micah K. Sinclair, MD.)

Isolated coalitions without syndrome involvement most often occur within a carpal row and involve two bones. The most common coalition encountered is between the lunate and triquetrum. There is a 2:1 female to male preponderance and occurrence is most often seen in people of African descent.[40] Most isolated coalitions are asymptomatic.

Syndromic carpal coalitions may be associated with arthrogryposis, diastrophic dwarfism, fetal alcohol syndrome, Holt-Oram syndrome, symphalangism, and Turner syndrome.[40,41]

Metacarpal synostosis is an uncommon bony connection of two or more metacarpals, most commonly the fourth and fifth metacarpal. The synostosis can be either partial or complete and can be isolated or associated with other hand abnormalities including central polydactyly, radial and ulnar deficiencies, cleft hand, symbrachydactyly, clinodactyly, and Apert syndrome.[42] The synostosis can be debilitating if the ulnar digit has an abduction deformity. This deformity affects grip and the ability to hold objects in the palm.

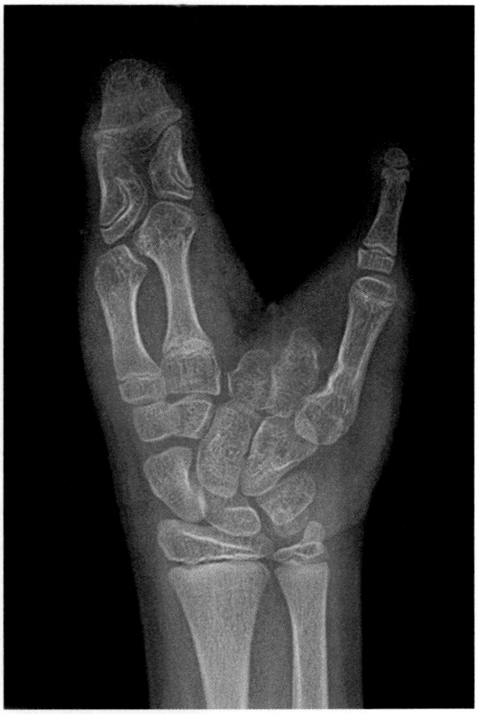

Figure 5 A radiograph of cleft hand. (Courtesy of Micah K. Sinclair, MD.)

Cleft Hand

Cleft hand is a congenital central ray deficiency, with a "V" shaped, central cleft, associated with the absence of one or more rays (**Figure 5**). This anomaly is a longitudinal failure of formation and is isolated to the hand and does not involve the forearm. It can occur sporadically or may be associated with several syndromes and can have associated foot anomalies. Two recent studies of different populations found 25% to 40% of cases are associated with syndromes.[43,44] The embryologic pathway involved is suppression FGF8 which subsequently leads to suppression of FGFF4 expression.[44] Numerous classification systems have been described, and to include all features of the abnormality, two must be considered; most commonly this includes Manske classification considering first web space syndactyly and Ogino classification describing the central deficiency.

Cleft reconstruction must give consideration to both the bony abnormality and soft tissue syndactyly, which can commonly occur in the first web space or the fourth web space. Surgical decision making should include both function and appearance. Multiple surgeries are typically required to complete reconstruction.[45] Surgical outcomes are dependent upon the preoperative deformity. A transverse bone in the cleft was not associated with worse outcomes and surgery was shown to be able to correct the metacarpal and proximal phalangeal divergence angles, maintained at final follow-up.[45] However, preoperative narrowing of the thumb web space and index finger metacarpophalangeal joint abnormality are associated with worse functional outcomes due to pinch limitations.

Amniotic Band Syndrome

Amniotic constriction band (ACB; also called amniotic band syndrome, constriction band syndrome, constriction ring syndrome, amniotic constriction syndrome, Streeter dysplasia) is thought to affect 1:1,200 to 1:15,000 live births.[46-48] The leading theory for how this occurs is that detached strands of amniotic membrane place extrinsic pressure on the fetus, including the limbs, resulting in amputations and the formation of constricting rings. The presentation of amniotic constriction band is variable and may lead to difficulty differentiating it from symbrachydactyly. The identification of bands on multiple limbs or the presence of a fenestrated syndactyly (**Figure 6**) is pathognomonic.

Treatment is variable depending on patient presentation. However, patients with distal ischemia due to a very deep amniotic band acting as a tourniquet should be treated as an emergency. The band is often able to be teased off the digit with surgical forceps. An incision may also be made through the band.

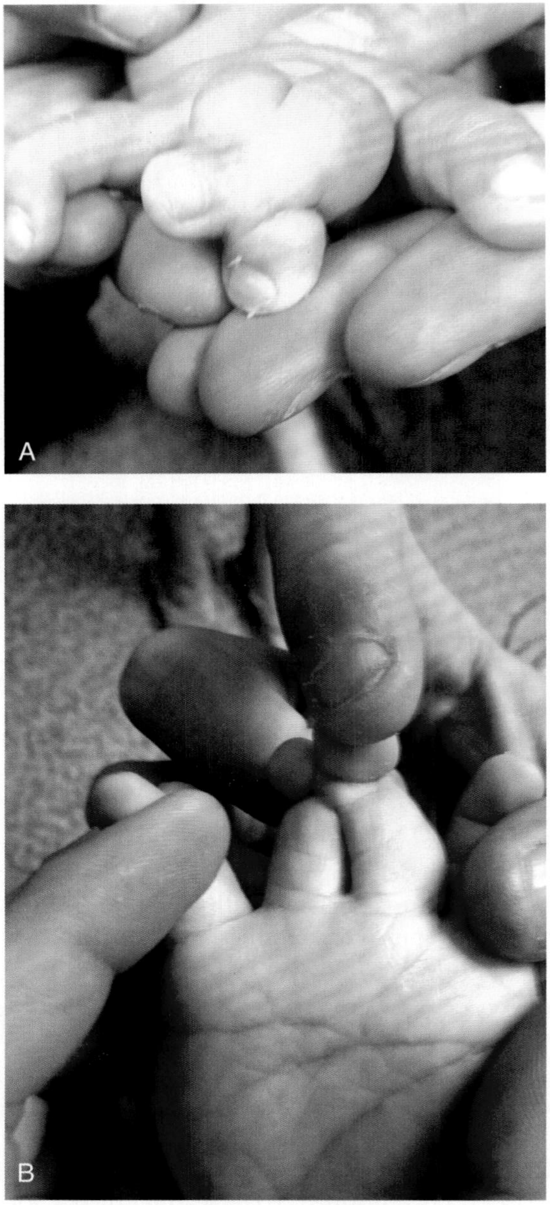

Figure 6 A clinical example of fenestrated syndactyly in amniotic band syndrome. (Reprinted from Williams BR, Van Heest AE: Idiopathic fenestrated complex syndactyly in a unique crisscross fashion. *J Hand Surg* 2016;41[12]:e485-e489. Copyright 2016, with permission from Elsevier.)

Clinodactyly

Clinodactyly is an angular deformity of the finger in the radioulnar plane. The most common occurrence is radial deviation deformity of the small finger due to a bracketed epiphysis causing a trapezoidal shaped middle phalanx. Functionally, the deformity may lead to scissoring and difficulty with gripping. This anomaly can be isolated or associated with a large number of syndromes. An autosomal dominant inheritance pattern has been documented and is often bilateral.

Surgical indications for clinodactyly include angular deformity of >20° and/or unacceptable appearance. The choice of surgical procedure depends upon patient age, pathology, amount of deformity, status of soft tissues, and surgeon's preference. Early physiolysis of the convex side of the bracketed epiphysis and placement of a fat graft requires an adequate amount of growth for correction. It is shown to have greater success in initial deformity >40° and/or age <6 years old. In older children, with little to no growth remaining, an osteotomy is used for correction. A recent study evaluating the results of an opening wedge osteotomy, selected because of its ability to preserve length in an already shortened digit, showed clinical improvement of 32° and radiographic improvement of 29°. The most common complication of clinodactyly correction was stiffness of the DIP joint. This occurred in 3/13 digits, with recurrence of deformity in one of these digits.[49] It was felt to be due to lengthening of the digit and pinning the joint.[50]

Trigger Digit

Trigger Thumb

Trigger thumbs are one of the most common nontraumatic pediatric hand conditions. These most often present in children around age 2 as a flexed thumb interphalangeal joint that cannot be extended. Approximately 25% occur bilaterally, and there is equal incidence between females and males. The etiology remains unknown, although it is thought to be a noninflammatory fibrous proliferation within the FPL tendon. Ultrasonographic studies have recently shown that in locked trigger thumbs, there is an average of 77% enlargement of the FPL tendon than the area under the A1 pulley.[51] If the patient is noted to have triggering and the thumb can be extended, massage and night splinting can be attempted. Resolution has been shown in 30% to 76% of patients in up to 4 years' time. Open surgical release is indicated in locked thumbs that have been present for 3 to 6 months and can be performed with minimal complications. A reported recurrence rate of 4% is due to incomplete release of A1 pulley. Percutaneous release has a recurrence rate up to 35%. In a study of percutaneous followed by open release, an incomplete release was found in 80% of the thumbs and a superficial tendon laceration had occurred.[52] The "squeeze test" can be used to confirm release, which includes maximum wrist extension coupled with compression of FPL muscle belly followed by full wrist flexion and thumb metacarpal flexion. Full flexion and extension with these maneuvers confirms adequate release.[53]

Trigger Finger

Trigger digits are 10 times less common than trigger thumbs. They present at a slightly older age than trigger thumbs, with characteristic triggering rather than presenting in a locked position. They are not present at birth but can have a medical condition associated with triggering, including mucopolysaccharidosis, juvenile rheumatoid arthritis, Ehlers-Danlos syndrome, Down syndrome, central nervous system disorders.

Anatomic anomalies described in trigger fingers have led to a stepwise treatment algorithm. These include proximal decussation of the flexor digitorum superficialis (FDS), aberrant lumbrical muscles, other anomalous relationships between FDS and flexor digitorum profundus (FDP). Splinting has been shown to be twice as successful as observation, with 67% resolution at 10 months after an average of 3 h/d wear. Surgical management requires an extensive Bruner incision, with release of the A1 pulley, removal of one slip of the FDS tendon, and release of the A3 pulley. Splinting is used following surgery for comfort and return to full activity once the incision is healed. Recurrence is the most commonly reported complication; however, the incidence remains low.

Macrodactyly

Macrodactyly is a rare, nonhereditary upper extremity anomaly, characterized by overgrowth within one extremity. It commonly follows a peripheral nerve distribution and involves overgrowth of all tissue types, including skin, subcutaneous tissue, neurovascular bundles, and bone. The involved nerve is also greatly enlarged and infiltrated with fat. Macrodactyly occurs in a male to female ratio of 3:2 and has a 10% syndactyly rate. The radial side of the hand is affected 85% of the time, involving the median nerve or its distal branches. Soft tissue involvement is greater on the volar side of the hand, which was recently quantified radiographically.[54] The enlargement is more pronounced distally and affects multiple digits that are adjacent to one another. Overgrowth syndromes are also described and have a similar presentation. These syndromes include CLOVES syndrome, Proteus syndrome, Klippel-Trenaunay syndrome, Parkes Weber syndrome, Neurofibromatosis type 1.

The extent of involvement and rate of growth can vary widely. The child should be followed regularly in the first few years of life. Compressive neuropathies occur and should be included in the evaluation. Serial radiographs should be obtained to evaluate for angular deformities.

Recently published studies have found the cell signaling pathway affected in these growth disorders is related to PIK3CA cell signaling pathway.[55]

Surgical intervention for macrodactyly is the mainstay of treatment. The patient and their family must understand that there is currently no cure for the condition. Surgical intervention varies based upon the physical examination findings of the extremity. The goal is to maintain function and improve appearance of the extremity. Depending upon involvement of the hand and functional use of the digits, there is a spectrum of procedures that can be performed. These include debulking, epiphysiodesis when the same digit reaches the size of their same-sex parent, corrective osteotomies, phalangectomy, decompression of compressive neuropathies, ablation if the abnormal digit(s). The affected digit is unlikely to be normal in function or appearance and often multiple procedures are required as the child grows. For severe cases, ray resection and/or ablation have been described with satisfaction.[56,57]

Brachial Plexus Birth Injury

The incidence of brachial plexus birth injury (BPBI) is estimated to range from 0.4 to 4 per 1,000 live births.[58-60] The etiology of BPBI is thought to be due to birth trauma, caused by a mechanical traction injury to the nerves of the brachial plexus. Risk factors include large-for-gestational-age infants (macrosomia), multiparous pregnancies, previous deliveries resulting in BPBI, prolonged labor, breech delivery, assisted (vacuum or forceps) and difficult deliveries (shoulder dystocia).[59,60]

The upper trunk of the brachial plexus at C5 and C6 is the most common pattern of injury (Erb's palsy). An extended upper trunk injury will also involve C7. A global injury involves C5-T1. An isolated lower trunk injury (C8-T1), or Klumpke's palsy, is extremely rare. Prognosis is dependent upon the severity of the injury. It is thought that up to >60% of injuries are neurapraxias that will spontaneously recover, but that 10% to 15% of affected individuals will be left with permanent weakness of the limb.[61-63]

Recovery is followed closely in the neonatal period. Functional recovery of elbow flexion by 6 months is the most common benchmark of recovery used by physicians to determine if microsurgical

Pediatrics

reconstruction would be beneficial. Limited recovery of elbow flexion by the age of 6 months suggests neurotmetic nerve injury, which may benefit from postganglionic nerve reconstruction. Most surgeons excise the neuroma and perform cable grafting using autograft of the sural nerve to reconstruct the brachial plexus.

Preganglionic avulsion injuries cannot spontaneously recover, nor can they be directly repaired or reconstructed. Clear physical examination discriminators to evaluate for preganglionic injuries include the presence of a Horner's syndrome (ptosis, miosis, anhidrosis, enophthalmos), phrenic nerve palsy (elevated hemidiaphragm), flail hand, and/or loss of scapular control. These injuries are often treated with nerve transfer surgery using a combination of extraplexus and intra-plexus donors, depending upon injury presentation.

Incomplete neurologic recovery in the shoulder leads to a progressive glenohumeral joint deformity due to persistent muscle imbalance.[64] This is due to the presence of innervated internal rotators and adductors versus the weakened external rotators and abductors.[65-67] The resultant deformity is a progressive internal rotation of the humeral head, placing increased stress along the posterior aspect of the glenoid. These deforming forces cause increased retroversion of the glenoid, as well as flattening and posterior subluxation of the humeral head.[68,69]

Treatment of the shoulder begins in the neonatal period with passive stretching of the glenohumeral joint. Botulinum toxin injections have been used in those cases with persistent contracture.[70] Recurrent contractures and/or glenohumeral dislocations may be indicated for open or arthroscopic glenohumeral joint reduction with or without concomitant tendon transfers. Late presenting patients with limitations in shoulder external rotation may benefit from a humeral rotational osteotomy to move their arc of shoulder internal and external rotation into a more functional space.

Summary

Pediatric congenital disorders can be complex to manage because of variability within a specific diagnosis, patient needs, and families' expectations. A careful history and stepwise examination of the affected extremity is required before providing the patient with a definitive treatment plan. Advances in understanding of the anatomy and/or pathophysiology of these disorders through orthopedic, plastic, and neurosurgery research allows aesthetics to be restored, as well as function and improvement in quality of life. Continuing education, knowledge of new surgical techniques, and collaboration with an interdisciplinary team will equip an orthopedic surgeon to provide optimal care.

Key Study Points

- Treatment of congenital upper extremity disorders requires an understanding of the classification system used to categorize each disorder. This classification system will allow for education of the patient and family as to the anatomic difference and potential treatment options for their deformity.
- Not all deformities require surgery. Each child and their function must be taken into consideration separately, educating the family and often observing the child as they grow before creating a definitive treatment plan.
- Occupational therapy and/or hand therapy are often vital to the function and postoperative recovery of the child's upper extremity who is born with a congenital difference.

Annotated References

1. Yang Y, Kozin SH: Cell signaling regulation of vertebrate limb growth and patterning. *J Bone Joint Surg Am* 2009;91(suppl 4): 76-80. doi:10.2106/JBJS.I.00079.

2. Lyons K, Ezaki M: Molecular regulation of limb growth. *J Bone Joint Surg Am* 2009;91(suppl 4):47-52. doi:10.2106/JBJS.I.00240.

3. Daluiski A, Yi SE, Lyons KM: The molecular control of upper extremity development: Implications for congenital hand anomalies. *J Hand Surg Am* 2001;26(1):8-22. doi:10.1053/jhsu.2001.9419.

4. Oberg KC, Feenstra JM, Manske PR, Tonkin MA: Developmental biology and classification of congenital anomalies of the hand and upper extremity. *J Hand Surg Am* 2010;35(12):2066-2076. doi:10.1016/j.jhsa.2010.09.031.

5. Bae DS, Canizares MF, Miller PE, et al: Intraobserver and interobserver reliability of the Oberg-Manske-Tonkin (OMT) classification: Establishing a registry on congenital upper limb differences. *J Pediatr Orthop* 2018;38(1):69-74. doi:10.1097/BPO.0000000000000732.

6. Goodell PB, Bauer AS, Sierra FJA, James MA: Symbrachydactyly. *Hand* 2016;11(3):262-270. doi:10.1177/1558944715614857.

7. Koskimies E, Lindfors N, Gissler M, Peltonen J, Nietosvaara Y: Congenital upper limb deficiencies and associated malformations in Finland: A population-based study. *J Hand Surg Am* 2011;36(6):1058-1065. doi:10.1016/j.jhsa.2011.03.015.

8. Catena N, Divizia MT, Calevo MG, et al: Hand and upper limb anomalies in Poland syndrome: A new proposal of classification. *J Pediatr Orthop* 2012;32(7):727-731. doi:10.1097/BPO.0b013e318269c898.

9. Bavinck JN, Weaver DD: Subclavian artery supply disruption sequence: Hypothesis of a vascular etiology for Poland, Klippel-Feil, and Möbius anomalies. *Am J Med Genet* 1986;23(4):903-918. doi:10.1002/ajmg.1320230405.

10. Webb ML, Rosen H, Taghinia A, et al: Incidence of Fanconi anemia in children with congenital thumb anomalies referred for diepoxybutane testing. *J Hand Surg Am* 2011;36(6):1052-1057. doi:10.1016/j.jhsa.2011.02.018.

11. Wall LB, Piper SL, Habenicht R, Oishi SN, Ezaki M, Goldfarb CA: Defining features of the upper extremity in Holt-Oram syndrome. *J Hand Surg Am* 2015;40(9):1764-1768. doi:10.1016/j.jhsa.2015.06.102.

12. Manske MC, Wall LB, Steffen JA, Goldfarb CA: The effect of soft tissue distraction on deformity recurrence after centralization for radial longitudinal deficiency. *J Hand Surg Am* 2014;39(5):895-901. doi:10.1016/j.jhsa.2014.01.015.

13. Vuillermin C, Butler L, Ezaki M, Oishi S: Ulna growth patterns after soft tissue release with bilobed flap in radial longitudinal deficiency. *J Pediatr Orthop* 2018;38(4):244-248. doi:10.1097/BPO.0000000000000807.

14. Vuillermin C, Wall L, Mills J, et al: Soft tissue release and bilobed flap for severe radial longitudinal deficiency. *J Hand Surg Am* 2015;40(5):894-899. doi:10.1016/j.jhsa.2015.01.004.

15. Ekblom AG, Dahlin LB, Rosberg H-E, Wiig M, Werner M, Arner M: Hand function in adults with radial longitudinal deficiency. *J Bone Joint Surg Am* 2014;96(14):1178-1184. doi:10.2106/JBJS.M.00815.

16. Vuillermin C, Butler L, Lake A, Ezaki M, Oishi S: Flexor digitorum superficialis opposition transfer for augmenting function in types II and IIIA thumb hypoplasia. *J Hand Surg Am* 2016;41(2):244-249; quiz 250. doi:10.1016/j.jhsa.2015.11.017.

17. de Kraker M, Selles RW, van Vooren J, Stam HJ, Hovius SE: Outcome after pollicization: Comparison of patients with mild and severe longitudinal radial deficiency. *Plast Reconstr Surg* 2013;131(4):544e-551e. doi:10.1097/PRS.0b013e3182818c98.

18. Cole RJ, Manske PR: Classification of ulnar deficiency according to the thumb and first web. *J Hand Surg Am* 1997;22(3):479-488. doi:10.1016/S0363-5023(97)80016-0.

19. Simmons BP, Southmayd WW, Riseborough EJ: Congenital radioulnar synostosis. *J Hand Surg Am* 1983;8(6):829-838.

20. VanHeest AE, Lin TE, Bohn D: Treatment of blocked elbow flexion in congenital radioulnar synostosis with radial head excision: A case series. *J Pediatr Orthop* 2013;33(5):540-543. doi:10.1097/BPO.0b013e318292c187.

21. Abzug JM, Kozin SH, Zlotolow DA, eds: *The Pediatric Upper Extremity*. New York/Heidelberg, Springer, 2015.

22. Wassel HD: The results of surgery for polydactyly of the thumb. A review. *Clin Orthop Relat Res* 1969;64:175-193.

23. Comer GC, Potter M, Ladd AL: Polydactyly of the hand. *J Am Acad Orthop Surg* 2018;26(3):75. doi:10.5435/JAAOS-D-16-00139.

24. Percival NJ, Sykes PJ: Syndactyly: A review of the factors which influence surgical treatment. *J Hand Surg Br* 1989;14(2):196-200.

25. Kozin SH: Syndactyly. *J Am Soc Surg Hand* 2001;1(1):1-13. doi:10.1053/jssh.2001.21778.

26. Eaton CJ, Lister GD: Syndactyly. *Hand Clin* 1990;6(4):555-575.

27. Dao KD, Shin AY, Billings A, Oberg KC, Wood VE: Surgical treatment of congenital syndactyly of the hand. *J Am Acad Orthop Surg* 2004;12(1):39-48.

28. Waters PM, Bae DS: *Syndactyly*, in *Pediatric Hand and Upper Limb Surgery: A Practical Guide*, ed 1. Philadelphia, PA, Lippincott Williams & Wilkins, 2012, pp 12-25.

29. Toledo LC, Ger E: Evaluation of the operative treatment of syndactyly. *J Hand Surg Am* 1979;4(6):556-564.

30. Brown PM: Syndactyly – A review and long term results. *Hand* 1977;9(1):16-27.

31. Kettelkamp DB, Flatt AE: An evaluation of syndactylia repair. *Surg Gynecol Obstet* 1961;113:471-478.

32. Greuse M, Coessens BC: Congenital syndactyly: Defatting facilitates closure without skin graft. *J Hand Surg Am* 2001;26(4):589-594. doi:10.1053/jhsu.2001.26196.

33. Vickers D, Donnelly W: Corrective surgery of syndactyly without the use of skin grafts. *Hand Surg* 1996;01(02):203-209. doi:10.1142/S0218810496000336.

34. Sherif MM: V-Y dorsal metacarpal flap: A new technique for the correction of syndactyly without skin graft. *Plast Reconstr Surg* 1998;101(7):1861-1866.

35. Canizares MF, Feldman L, Miller PE, Waters PM, Bae DS: Complications and cost of syndactyly reconstruction in the United States: Analysis of the Pediatric Health Information System. *Hand* 2017;12(4):327-334. doi:10.1177/1558944716668816.

36. Hori M, Nakamura R, Inoue G, et al: Nonoperative treatment of camptodactyly. *J Hand Surg Am* 1987;12(6):1061-1065.

37. Foucher G, Loréa P, Khouri RK, Medina J, Pivato G: Camptodactyly as a spectrum of congenital deficiencies: A treatment algorithm based on clinical examination. *Plast Reconstr Surg* 2006;117(6):1897-1905. doi:10.1097/01.prs.0000218977.46520.55.

38. Yannascoli SM, Goldfarb CA: Treating congenital proximal interphalangeal joint contracture. *Hand Clin* 2018;34(2):237-249. doi:10.1016/j.hcl.2017.12.013.

39. Satake H, Ogino T, Eto J, Maruyama M, Watanabe T, Takagi M: Radiographic features of Kirner's deformity. *Congenit Anom* 2013;53(2):78-82. doi:10.1111/cga.12010.

40. DeFazio MV, Cousins BJ, Miversuski RA, Cardoso R: Carpal coalition. *Hand* 2013;8(2):157-163. doi:10.1007/s11552-013-9498-5.

41. Gottschalk MB, Danilevich M, Gottschalk HP: Carpal coalitions and metacarpal synostoses: A review. *Hand* 2016;11(3):271-277. doi:10.1177/1558944715614860.

42. Gottschalk HP, Eisner E, Hosalkar HS: Medial epicondyle fractures in the pediatric population. *J Am Acad Orthop Surg* 2012;20(4):223. doi:10.5435/JAAOS-20-04-223.

43. Falcochio DF, Da Costa AC, Durigan CPI, Nascimento VDG, Santili C, Chakkour I: Epidemiological and clinical aspects of cleft hand: Case series from a tertiary public hospital in São Paulo, Brazil. *Hand* 2018. doi:10.1177/1558944718778399.

44. Al-Qattan MM: Central and ulnar cleft hands: A review of concurrent deformities in a series of 47 patients and their pathogenesis. *J Hand Surg Eur Vol* 2014;39(5):510-519. doi:10.1177/1753193413496945.

45. Aleem AW, Wall LB, Manske MC, Calhoun V, Goldfarb CA: The transverse bone in cleft hand: A case cohort analysis of outcome after surgical reconstruction. *J Hand Surg Am* 2014;39(2):226-236. doi:10.1016/j.jhsa.2013.11.002.

46. Moerman P, Fryns JP, Vandenberghe K, Lauweryns JM: Constrictive amniotic bands, amniotic adhesions, and limb-body wall complex: Discrete disruption sequences with pathogenetic overlap. *Am J Med Genet* 1992;42(4):470-479. doi:10.1002/ajmg.1320420412.

47. Foulkes GD, Reinker K: Congenital constriction band syndrome: A seventy-year experience. *J Pediatr Orthop* 1994;14(2):242-248.

48. Seeds JW, Cefalo RC, Herbert WN: Amniotic band syndrome. *Am J Obstet Gynecol* 1982;144(3):243-248.

49. Piper SL, Goldfarb CA, Wall LB: Outcomes of opening wedge osteotomy to correct angular deformity in small finger clinodactyly. *J Hand Surg Am* 2015;40(5):908-913.e1. doi:10.1016/j.jhsa.2015.01.017.

50. Goldfarb CA, Wall LB: Osteotomy for clinodactyly. *J Hand Surg Am* 2015;40(6):1220-1224. doi:10.1016/j.jhsa.2015.03.003.

51. Kim J, Gong HS, Seok HS, Choi YH, Oh S, Baek GH: Quantitative measurements of the cross-sectional configuration of the flexor pollicis longus tendon using ultrasonography in patients with pediatric trigger thumb. *J Hand Surg Am* 2018;43(3):284.e1-284.e7. doi:10.1016/j.jhsa.2017.08.011.

52. Masquijo JJ, Ferreyra A, Lanfranchi L, Torres-Gomez A, Allende V: Percutaneous trigger thumb release in children: Neither effective nor safe. *J Pediatr Orthop* 2014;34(5):534-536. doi:10.1097/BPO.0000000000000119.

53. Wilkerson JA, Strauch RJ: A simple technique for confirmation of complete release in surgical treatment of pediatric trigger thumb. *J Hand Surg Am* 2014;39(11):2348-2349. doi:10.1016/j.jhsa.2014.08.004.

54. Park JW, Kim J, Baek GH: Measurements in plain radiographs of 26 fingers with macrodactyly. *J Hand Surg Eur Vol* 2017;42(8):858-860. doi:10.1177/1753193417690292.

55. Ezaki M, Beckwith T, Oishi SN: Macrodactyly: Decision-making and surgery timing. *J Hand Surg Eur Vol* 2018;44(1):32-42. doi:10.1177/1753193418796441.

56. Waters PM, Gillespie BT: Ray resection for progressive macrodactyly of the hand: Surgical technique and illustrative cases. *J Hand Surg Am* 2016;41(8):e251-e256. doi:10.1016/j.jhsa.2016.05.012.

57. Donohue KW, Zlotolow DA, Kozin SH: Long-finger pollicization for macrodactyly of the thumb and index finger. *J Pediatr Orthop* 2014;34(7):e50-e53. doi:10.1097/BPO.0000000000000232.

58. Foad SL, Mehlman CT, Ying J: The epidemiology of neonatal brachial plexus palsy in the United States. *J Bone Joint Surg Am* 2008;90(6):1258-1264. doi:10.2106/JBJS.G.00853.

59. Hoeksma AF, terSteeg AM, Nelissen RGHH, vanOuwerkerk WJR, Lankhorst GJ, deJong BA: Neurological recovery in obstetric brachial plexus injuries: An historical cohort study. *Dev Med Child Neurol* 2004;46(2):76-83.

60. Waters P: Obstetric brachial plexus injuries: Evaluation and management. *J Am Acad Orthop Surg* 1997;5(4):205-214.

61. Noetzel MJ, Park TS, Robinson S, Kaufman B: Prospective study of recovery following neonatal brachial plexus injury. *J Child Neurol* 2001;16(7):488-492. doi:10.1177/088307380101600705.

62. Pondaag W, Malessy MJA, van Dijk JG, Thomeer RTWM: Natural history of obstetric brachial plexus palsy: A systematic review. *Dev Med Child Neurol* 2004;46(2):138-144.

63. Narakas A, Lamb DW: *Obstetrical brachial plexus injuries*, in *The Paralysed Hand*. Edinburgh, Scotland, Churchill Livingstone, 1987, vol 2, pp 116-135.

64. Kozin SH, Chafetz RS, Barus D, Filipone L: Magnetic resonance imaging and clinical findings before and after tendon transfers about the shoulder in children with residual brachial plexus birth palsy. *J Shoulder Elbow Surg* 2006;15(5):554-561. doi:10.1016/j.jse.2005.11.004.

65. Newman CJ, Morrison L, Lynch B, Hynes D: Outcome of subscapularis muscle release for shoulder contracture secondary to brachial plexus palsy at birth. *J Pediatr Orthop* 2006;26(5):647-651. doi:10.1097/01.bpo.0000233806.72423.30.

66. Waters PM, Monica JT, Earp BE, Zurakowski D, Bae DS: Correlation of radiographic muscle cross-sectional area with glenohumeral deformity in children with brachial plexus birth palsy. *J Bone Joint Surg Am* 2009;91(10):2367-2375. doi:10.2106/JBJS.H.00417.

67. Pöyhiä TH, Nietosvaara YA, Remes VM, Kirjavainen MO, Peltonen JI, Lamminen AE: MRI of rotator cuff muscle atrophy in relation to glenohumeral joint incongruence in brachial plexus birth injury. *Pediatr Radiol* 2005;35(4):402-409. doi:10.1007/s00247-004-1377-3.

68. van Gelein Vitringa VM, van Kooten EO, Mullender MG, van Doorn-Loogman MH, van der Sluijs JA: An MRI study on the relations between muscle atrophy, shoulder function and glenohumeral deformity in shoulders of children with obstetric brachial plexus injury. *J Brachial Plex Peripher Nerve Inj* 2009;4:5. doi:10.1186/1749-7221-4-5.

69. Pearl ML, Edgerton BW: Glenoid deformity secondary to brachial plexus birth palsy. *J Bone Joint Surg Am* 1998;80(5):659-667.

70. Sever JW: Obstetric paralysis: Report of eleven hundred cases. *J Am Med Assoc* 1925;85(24):1862-1865. doi:10.1001/jama.1925.02670240014005.

Chapter 56

Pediatric Pelvis, Hip and Femur Trauma

Elizabeth W. Hubbard, MD

ABSTRACT

Pelvic, hip, and femur fractures in pediatric patients can result from low-energy and sports-related injuries but can also present as a component of significant polytrauma. Although many injuries can be treated nonsurgically, there are specific injuries and fractures which require immediate diagnosis and treatment to minimize patient morbidity and maximize the patient's potential for recovery. This is a review of basic management of these injuries in pediatric patients, with a focus on the most recent literature regarding diagnosis, treatment, and rehabilitation.

Keywords: femoral physeal fracture; pediatric femur fracture; pediatric hip dislocation; pediatric hip fracture; pediatric pelvic fracture

Introduction

Although pelvic, hip, and femur fractures are not the most common pediatric orthopaedic injuries, anatomic features unique to children can complicate management of these injuries and affect a child's subsequent growth and function. Significantly displaced fractures are often associated with high-energy mechanisms and can portend a range of other associated injuries that will affect the patient's resuscitative needs and long-term recovery. This chapter provides an overview of the orthopaedic management of these injuries in pediatric patients and highlights the recent advances published in the literature regarding diagnosis and treatment.

Neither Dr. Hubbard nor any immediate family member has received anything of value from or has stock or stock options held in a commercial company or institution related directly or indirectly to the subject of this chapter.

Pelvic Fractures

Pelvic fractures in children are rare and account for less than 1% of all pediatric fractures.[1] The Torode and Zeig classification has historically been used to describe fracture patterns seen in pediatric patients.[1] This scheme includes four types of fracture patterns. Type I injuries are avulsion injuries of the pelvis, type II are isolated iliac wing fractures, type III are stable pelvic ring fractures, and type IV are unstable ring fractures. However, in 2012, Shore et al revised this classification scheme to differentiate between stable ring fractures involving only either the anterior or posterior portion of the pelvic ring (Torode III-A) and stable ring fractures that involve both the anterior and posterior portions of the ring (Torode III-B; **Figure 1**). Although both Torode III-A and III-B injuries were stable from an orthopaedic perspective, an increased grade from III-A to III-B was associated with an increased need for blood product transfusion, increased volume of blood product required, and a longer ICU stay.[2] Although orthopaedic management of these injuries does not change, this differentiation between patients with stable fractures can help alert the trauma team to those patients who will likely have an increased resuscitative requirement in the immediate postinjury period.

The most common pelvic injury in children is an avulsion fracture of the pelvis (Torode I). These are typically sports-related injuries and have historically been treated nonsurgically. Recently, some authors have recommended considering open reduction and internal fixation for these injuries in adolescent athletes or those with delayed union, with many of these reports focusing on avulsion fractures of the ischial tuberosity and the anterior-superior iliac spine. However, these studies all tend to be small, and limited clinical benefit with surgical fixation has been demonstrated in the literature. A recent retrospective review of 228 patients with pelvic apophyseal fractures showed that 97% were successfully treated nonsurgically.[3] At this time, symptomatic treatment with protected weight bearing and a gradual return to sport continues to be the recommended first-line treatment.[3,4]

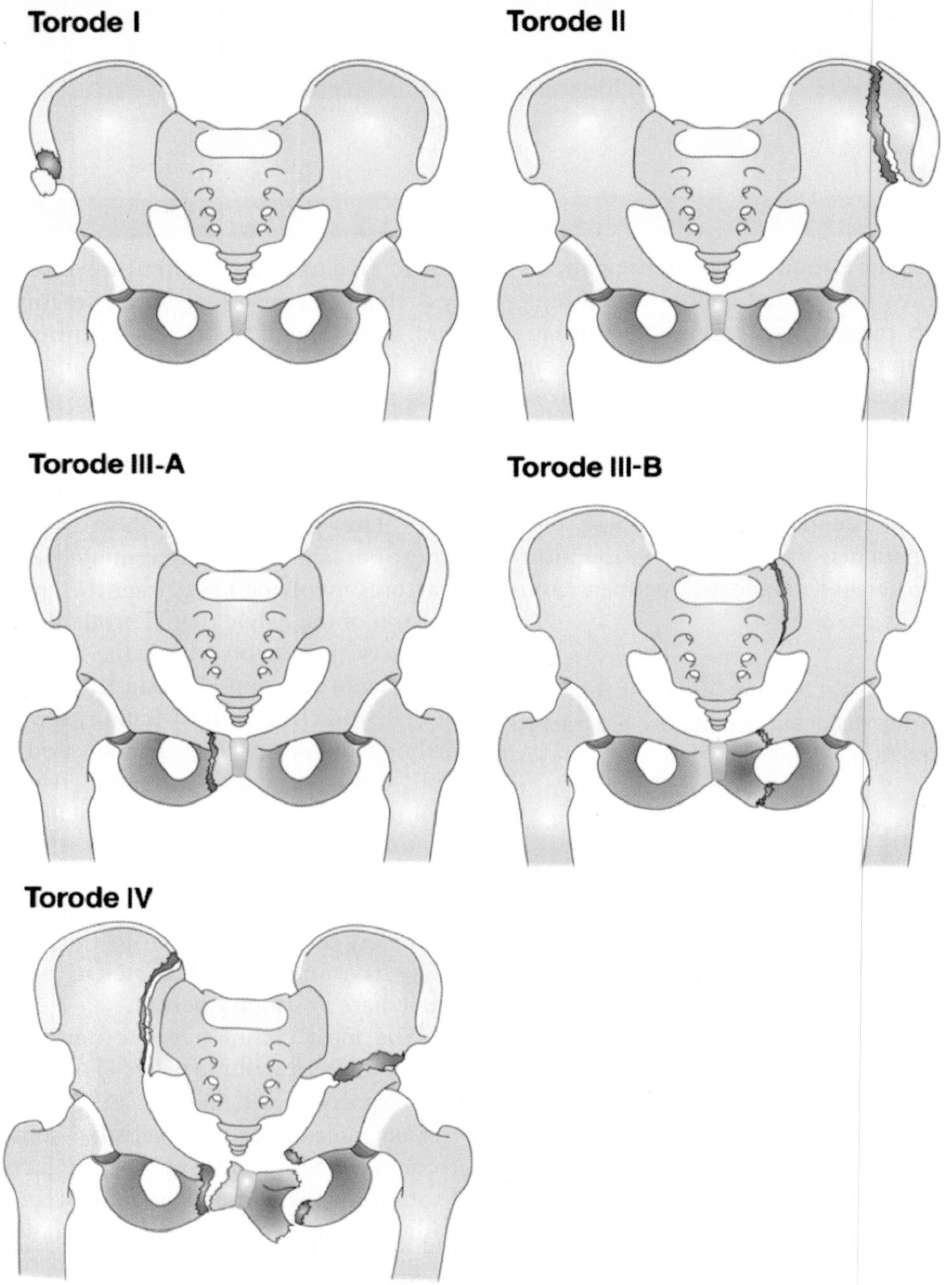

Figure 1 Illustration shows modified Torode-Zieg classification of pelvis fractures. Torode III fractures are stable pelvic ring injuries with type III-A fractures involving *either* the anterior or posterior ring and type III-B fractures involving *both* the anterior and posterior ring. Although all patients with type III fractures have injuries that are clinically stable without fixation, patients with type III-B fractures have significantly greater injury severity scores on presentation and are more likely to require greater resuscitation and longer ICU stays than patients with type III-A injuries. (Reproduced with permission from Shore BJ, Palmer CS, Bevin C, Johnson MB, Torode IP: Pediatric pelvic fracture: A modification of a preexisting classification. *J Pediatr Orthop* 2012;32[2]:162-168. doi:10.1097/BPO.0b013e3182408be6.)

Although uncommon, pelvic ring injuries in children are associated with significant morbidity and mortality. The pediatric pelvis has greater elasticity and thicker periosteum than the adult pelvis.[1] As a result, significant energy is required to generate a true pelvic ring injury. The most common causes in children are motor vehicle collisions (MVC), pediatric versus MVC and fall from height.[5-7] As seen in adults, these patients can have a high rate of associated injuries.[8,9] Hermans et al compared pediatric and adult patients with pediatric pelvic fractures treated over a 10-year period at a level 1 trauma center and found that, although adults tended to have higher injury severity scores and were significantly more likely to require surgical fixation of their fractures, mortality rates were similar between the two groups (8% in adults versus 6% in children).[9] Swaid et al[8] reported a similar mortality rate, citing that this was usually related to nonpelvic injuries including traumatic brain injury, associated organ damage, and blood loss.

Although most pediatric pelvic fractures can be treated nonsurgically, patients with higher energy injuries can have displaced, unstable fractures which require surgical fixation. Immediate stabilization can be achieved with a pelvic binder or an external fixator.[1] Open reduction and internal fixation has been favored to achieve anatomic alignment and stability when needed. However, the increased use of percutaneous screw fixation for adult pelvic fractures has led many surgeons to explore this technique in children as well. Burn et al evaluated pelvic CT scans performed in patients 2 to 16 years of age and reported that 99% had appropriate osseous anatomy that would allow for placement of a S1 ilio-sacral screw and 89% had osseous anatomy which would allow for placement of a trans-sacral-trans-iliac screw at S2.[10] Two small studies have shown that ilio-sacral screws can be placed safely in children as young as 6 years with minimal blood loss and low perioperative complication rates.[11,12]

Patients with residual fracture displacement and pelvic asymmetry greater than 1 cm have reported greater rates of low back and sacroiliac joint pain and worse functional outcome scores than those with less than 1 cm of obliquity.[13] This same study showed that no remodeling occurred after fracture union. In light of these findings, fracture alignment and pelvic obliquity should be corrected intraoperatively as much as possible in those patients who require surgical treatment.[13] Surgical reduction and stabilization should be considered in patients with fracture displacement resulting in pelvic asymmetry greater than 1 cm.

Hip Dislocation and Femoral Neck Fractures

Hip Dislocation

Traumatic hip dislocation in children is a rare but potentially devastating injury. Unlike adults, pediatric patients can sustain hip dislocations after relatively low-energy injuries and spontaneous hip reduction can occur.[1] This is more common in patients younger than 10 years and is likely related to the laxity of the hip capsule and periacetabular structures compared with adults. Older adolescents are more likely to sustain these injuries through higher energy mechanisms and more likely to have ipsilateral acetabular fractures, femoral head fractures, and other associated injuries.[1]

As with adults, roughly 90% of all dislocations are posterior and treatment involves immediate closed versus open reduction. Urgent reduction is essential to minimize the risk of osteonecrosis of the femoral head.[14] Traumatic proximal femoral epiphysiolysis has occurred during both dislocation and reduction attempts.[15-17] It is critical that a reduction be done carefully under general anesthesia to minimize the risk of epiphysiolysis during reduction. The surgeon must also be ready to immediately treat this injury should it occur, given this high associated rate of osteonecrosis if left untreated.[15]

Postreduction imaging is essential as an incongruous reduction is often a sign of entrapped tissue within the hip joint.[18] A recent study comparing MRI with CT studies in children after closed reduction of traumatic hip dislocations demonstrated labral tears, labral entrapment, and entrapped chondral fractures were more easily and frequently detected on MRI, but fractures of the ossified portions of the femoral head and acetabulum were seen on both types of imaging studies.[19] The authors argued that MRI was the preferred imaging modality in this scenario as the results of the MRI would more commonly affect surgical decision making.[19] Labral tears, entrapped capsulolabral tissue, and chondral fractures can effectively be treated with arthroscopic techniques.[18,20] However, more complex fractures of the femoral head and acetabulum may require a surgical hip dislocation to expose the injury and restore alignment.[21]

Femoral Neck Fractures

As with pelvis fractures, femoral neck fractures in children are rare and account for less than 1% of all pediatric fractures. The most commonly used classification scheme is the Delbet classification. Types I-A and I-B are fractures involving the proximal femoral epiphysis, type II are transcervical, type III are basicervical, and

Pediatrics

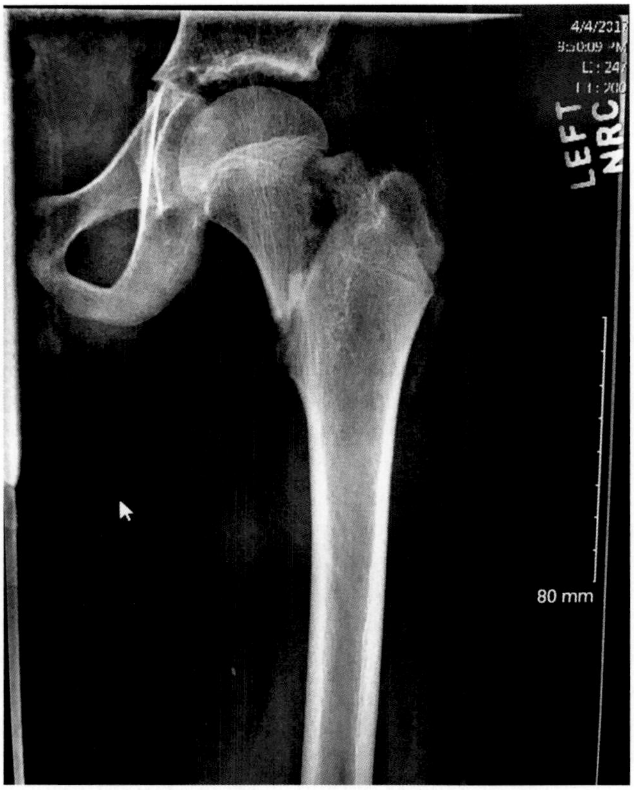

Figure 2 AP view of the left hip of a 10-year-old boy who sustained a closed Delbet II fracture of the left femoral neck while on an all-terrain vehicle. Patient underwent closed reduction and screw fixation within 24 hours of injury and weight bearing was restricted for 6 weeks postoperatively.

type IV fractures are intertrochanteric[1] (**Figure 2**). This classification scheme is both anatomic and prognostic, with fracture type being inversely correlated with osteonecrosis risk. Fracture displacement is directly associated with risk of osteonecrosis. The overall incidence of osteonecrosis after fracture ranges between 20% and 29%, with the highest incidence reported with Delbet I and II fractures. Other complications of femoral neck fractures include nonunion, coxa vara, overgrowth of the femoral neck, and late onset slipped capital femoral epiphysis.[22-24]

Most recent literature has been focused on finding ways to minimize complications, specifically the risk of osteonecrosis after femoral neck fracture. There have been mixed results regarding whether performing an open reduction affects the risk of osteonecrosis. Song and Stone et al both reported significantly improved outcomes among patients who underwent open reduction and internal fixation versus those who were treated with closed reduction and screw or pin fixation.[25,26] However, a systematic review of femoral neck fractures in children showed that, although the likelihood of obtaining an anatomic reduction was greater with open reduction, there was no difference in the reported rates of osteonecrosis, nonunion, or premature physeal closure when compared with patients who were treated with closed reduction and fixation.[27] Urgent or emergent fracture reduction and fixation has been proposed as a method to reduce osteonecrosis risk. However, immediate surgical reduction and stabilization cannot always be achieved. Yeranosian et al[27] specifically analyzed outcomes in children who underwent reduction greater than 24 hours after initial injury. In this scenario, the authors showed that achieving an anatomic reduction had the greatest impact on both clinical outcome and reducing the risk of osteonecrosis.[28]

Stress fractures of the femoral neck have been described in pediatric patients. These can occur as a result of repetitive injury, such as in high-level adolescent athletes. However, compression sided femoral neck fractures in very young patients without known activity or metabolic risk factors have also been described.[29] When a child is diagnosed with a femoral neck stress fracture, the physician should proceed with an endocrine and metabolic workup to rule out underlying factors that may predispose the child to further injury and/or delay union of the fracture. Compression-sided femoral neck fractures can be treated through protected weight bearing, with or without supplemental cast immobilization depending on the patient, and a gradual return to activity.[29] Tension-sided femoral neck fractures are more concerning, and consideration should be given to fracture stabilization with cannulated screws.[30]

Femur Fractures

Subtrochanteric Femur Fractures

This is an uncommon variant of pediatric femur fracture which can be difficult to reduce and treat. As in adults, the muscular attachments of the iliopsoas and abductors can pull the proximal fragment into flexion, abduction, and external rotation. When fractures are minimally displaced or if these muscle forces can be overcome and acceptable alignment can be obtained after closed reduction, spica casting may be the preferred treatment. However, displaced fractures may require open reduction and internal fixation to obtain and maintain anatomic alignment (**Figure 3**). Parikh et al reported that elastic intramedullary nails could be used to treat these injuries, but they reported greater than 20% rate of complications with this technique, including malunion and need for revision surgery with nail reposition or removal before fracture healing.[31] Plate fixation for these fractures has been shown to afford

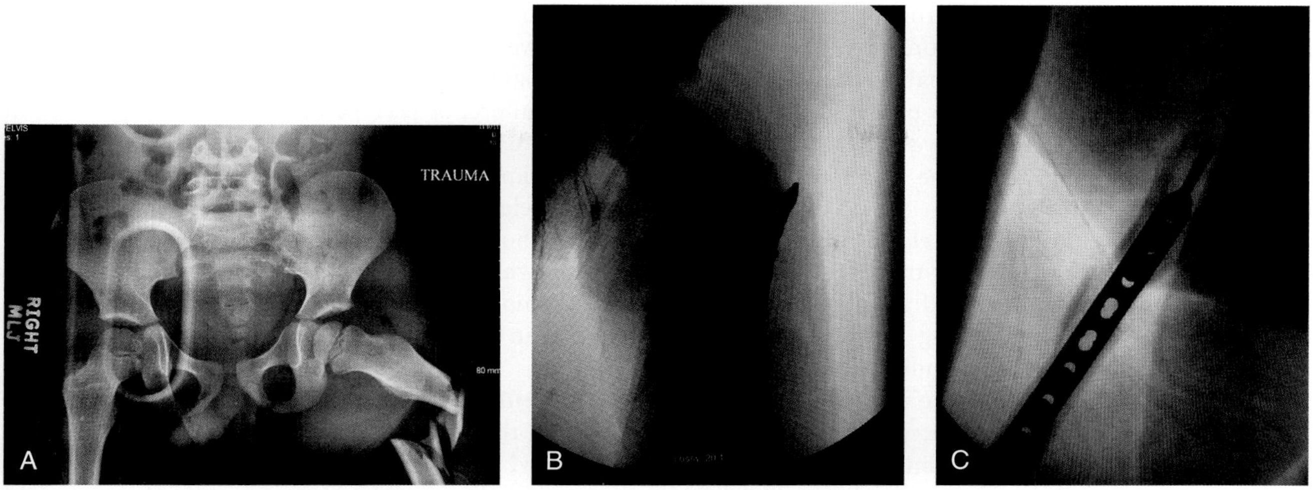

Figure 3 AP view of the pelvis of a 4-year-old boy with a comminuted left subtrochanteric femur fracture who sustained after being ejected from the front passenger seat of a vehicle (**A**). Associated injuries included a comminuted left supracondylar humerus fracture (not shown) and significant traumatic brain injury. Patient was initially stabilized with femoral traction and was taken for open reduction and internal fixation when clinically stable (AP left hip, **B**; lateral left hip, **C**).

equal rate of fracture union, higher patient outcome scores, and lower perioperative complication rates compared with titanium elastic intramedullary nails.[32]

Femoral Shaft Fractures

Although femoral shaft fractures account for only 1% to 2% of all fractures in pediatric patients, they are one of the most common reasons for hospital admissions in this population (**Figure 4**).[1] In 2015, the AAOS released an updated version of the clinical guidelines to treat pediatric femoral shaft fractures to assist physicians who care for this patient population.[33] However, there is limited high-quality literature guiding treatment of these injuries, which is potentially why only 1 of the 14 proposals made by the committee had sufficient supporting evidence to be truly "recommended."[33] Two recent studies have shown that the publication of the original guidelines in 2009 and the updated version in 2015 have had limited impact on the way surgeons at multiple centers are actually treating pediatric patients with femoral shaft fractures.[34,35]

One potential area of controversy is the treatment of children aged 4 to 5. Historically, these children have been treated with closed reduction and spica casting. However, the AAOS clinical guidelines do not provide recommendations for this age group and the increased popularity of elastic intramedullary nails has led some centers to start using this technique in younger patient populations.[33,36] Although these studies reported low rates of complications and faster return to independent ambulation in children treated with elastic intramedullary nails, a recent study of 262 patients showed that school-aged children treated with elastic intramedullary nails had significantly greater perioperative complications compared with those who were treated with spica casting.[37] No differences were seen with regard to

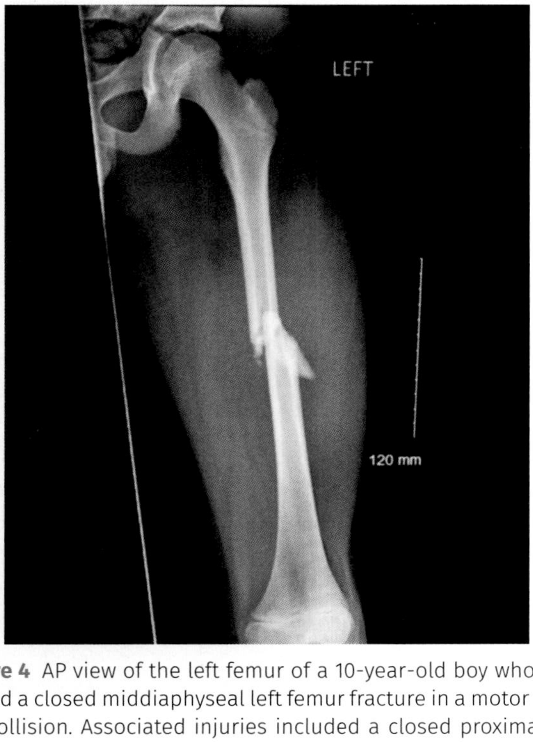

Figure 4 AP view of the left femur of a 10-year-old boy who sustained a closed middiaphyseal left femur fracture in a motor vehicle collision. Associated injuries included a closed proximal 1/3 left tibia fracture. He was treated with retrograde flexible intramedullary nail fixation of the femur fracture and open reduction and internal fixation of the left tibia fracture (not shown).

fracture union, shortening, or coronal or sagittal plane alignment at healing. Furthermore, 89% of children treated with the intramedullary nails required a second surgery versus only 5.1% of the patients treated with spica casting.[37] This difference was largely due to the need for implant removal in the intramedullary nail cohort.

Although the guidelines list elastic intramedullary nails as an implant "option" for treatment of children aged 5 to 11 with femoral shaft fractures, they do not offer recommendations regarding the types of elastic nails available.[33] Most of the studies referenced document results with titanium elastic intramedullary nails and have demonstrated high rates of fracture union and low rates of perioperative complications in length-stable fractures.[38,39] However, multiple studies have published high rates of implant failure, fracture shortening and/or fracture malunion when titanium nails are used to trade length-unstable fractures or fractures in patients who weigh more than 47 kg.[40-42] A direct comparison study between these implants showed that patients treated with the stainless steel elastic intramedullary nails had significantly lower rates of fracture malunion and perioperative complications than those who were treated with titanium nails and that the stainless steel implants cost three to six times less.[43] More recent literature has shown that stainless steel flexible intramedullary nails can be used in length-unstable fractures as well as patients who weigh more than 100 lb without significant increased risk of fracture shortening, implant failure, or perioperative complications, even in clinical situations when only 60% canal fill is achieved with the implant.[44-46] These studies suggest that stainless steel elastic intramedullary nails may be a superior implant choice for femoral shaft fractures, as they have been shown to achieve high rates of fracture union and lower complications in a broader range of clinical situations than their titanium counterparts.

Distal Femur Physeal Fractures

Although this is not the most common area for physeal injury, distal femoral physeal fractures are among the most challenging to manage both in the acute and chronic setting. The reported incidence of distal femoral physeal arrest varies from 40% to 52%, with the greatest incidence seen in displaced fractures[47,48] (**Figure 5**). The close proximity of this physis to the neurovascular bundle in the popliteal fossa means that widely displaced Salter-Harris (SH) I and II fractures can potentially lead to vascular injury and/or compartment syndrome.[1] Therefore, emergent careful reduction and stabilization of widely displaced fractures is critical. Minimally displaced, intra-articular SH III and IV fractures may be difficult to diagnose with routine radiography. In one

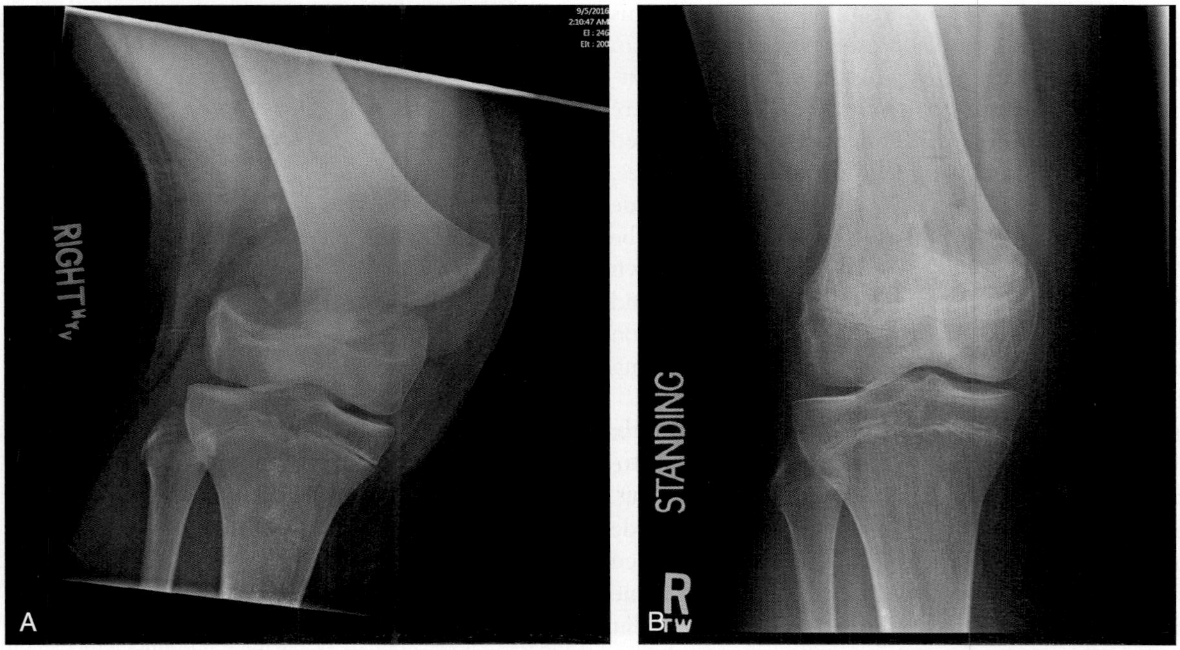

Figure 5 AP view of the right knee of a 13-year-old boy who sustained a closed, displaced Salter-Harris I fracture of the right distal femur after a fall from a bicycle (**A**). He underwent immediate closed reduction and pin fixation (not shown) but demonstrated complete closure of the right distal femoral physis 6 months after injury (**B**). The patient was treated with contralateral distal femoral epiphysiodesis to maintain a 5 mm posttraumatic limb length inequality, right shorter than left.

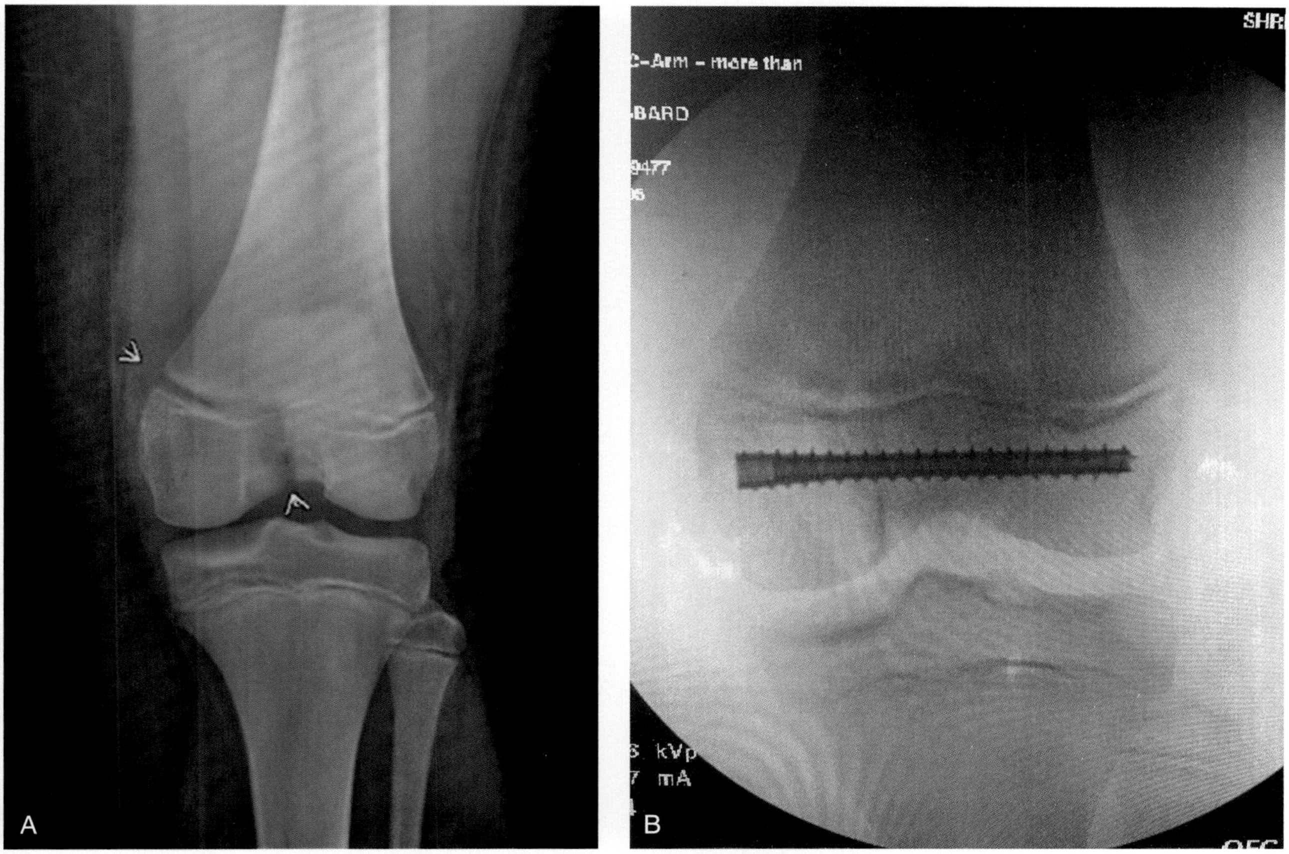

Figure 6 AP view of the left knee of a 14-year-old boy who sustained a left distal femoral Salter-Harris III fracture of the medial condyle when tackled during a football game (**A**). He underwent open reduction and percutaneous placement of an all-epiphyseal screw (**B**).

recent study, almost 40% of patients with SH III and IV fractures of the distal femur were misdiagnosed at the initial evaluation, despite the presence of a knee effusion in the affected extremity.[49] Furthermore, fracture displacement was significantly underestimated on plain radiographs when compared with subsequent CT and MRI scans of these patients.[49] This suggests that advanced imaging should be obtained if there is any concern for an intra-articular fracture to both confirm diagnosis and assist with surgical decision making.

In younger patients with SH I fractures, or SH II fractures with small metaphyseal components, smooth wires are the preferred fixation to cross the physis to minimize further physeal injury[50] (**Figure 5**). Older patients, particularly those who are suspected to be skeletally mature less than 2 years after injury, screws can be used, either partially or fully threaded. For most cases in patients with SH II, III, and IV fractures, all-metaphyseal and/or epiphyseal screw constructs can be used to avoid further physeal damage (**Figure 6**).

Given the high risk of posttraumatic physeal arrest, patients need to be followed up for a minimum of 2 years after injury. Families should be counseled about the risk for angular deformity and/or length discrepancy related to the injury.

Summary

High-energy injuries to the pelvis, hip, and femur can occur in children and require appropriate resuscitation and stabilization. Although many of these injuries can be treated nonsurgically, there are specific fracture patterns that require urgent treatment and the orthopaedic surgeon should be able to recognize these injuries to manage patients appropriately. In addition, because of anatomic characteristics that are unique to the pediatric patient, certain types of pelvic and hip injuries can occur through relatively low-energy mechanisms and a high index of suspicion is required to make the appropriate treatment decisions. Finally, regardless of how the injury is initially managed, these patients often require long-term follow-up to monitor the patient's growth and development.

Key Study Points

- Avulsion injuries are the most common pediatric pelvic fractures. Although recent literature has described surgical indications and techniques for management of these injuries, the current standard of care remains protected weight bearing and a gradual return to activity.
- Pelvic ring fractures can often be treated nonsurgically, but surgical reduction and stabilization should be considered for unstable injuries and fractures that are displaced 1 cm or more.
- Hip dislocation can occur after either high- or low-energy mechanisms in children. Reduction should be done carefully and postreduction imaging should be performed to confirm that the reduction is congruous and to diagnose associated osseous or soft-tissue injuries, which may require treatment.
- Treatment of pediatric femur fracture is determined by the patient's age and size as well as by the fracture pattern.

Annotated References

1. Flynn JM, Skaggs DL, Waters PM: *Rockwood & Wilkins' Fractures in Children*, ed 8. Philadelphia, PA, Wolters Kluwer Health, 2015, pp 921-1027.
2. Shore BJ, Palmer CS, Bevin C, Johnson MB, Torode IP: Pediatric pelvic fracture: A modification of a preexisting classification. *J Pediatr Orthop* 2012;32:162-168.
3. Schuett DJ, Bomar JD, Pennock AT: Pelvic apophyseal avulsion fractures: A retrospective review of 228 cases. *J Pediatr Orthop* 2015;35:617-623.
4. Eberbach H, Hohloch L, Feucht MJ, Konstantinidis L, Sudkamp NP, Zwingmann J: Operative versus conservative treatment of apophyseal avulsion fractures of the pelvis in the adolescents: A systematical review with meta-analysis of clinical outcome and return to sports. *BMC Musculoskelet Disord* 2017;18:162.

   Systematic review of 14 level 4 studies documenting treatment and outcome of patients with avulsion fractures of the pelvis. The studies included 596 patients, 52 of whom underwent surgical intervention. Excellent outcomes were reported in 88% of patients who underwent surgical treatment versus 79% of those treated nonsurgically. However, no standardized method of outcome testing was used and there was no difference in time to full weight bearing or return to sport between the two groups. Level of evidence: IV.
5. Shaath MK, Koury KL, Gibson PD, Adams MR, Sirkin MS, Reilly MC: Associated injuries in skeletally immature children with pelvic fractures. *J Emerg Med* 2016;51:246-251.

   Retrospective review of 60 skeletally immature patients admitted with a pelvic fracture to a single level 1 trauma center between 2001 and 2014. The most common mechanisms included MVC and pedestrian versus MVC. All patients sustained at least one extremity fracture. Only nine patients required reduction of their pelvic injuries (three spica casts; six patients require surgical fixation). Patients who required surgery had higher injury severity scores on presentation, greater resuscitative needs, and longer hospital stays. Level of evidence: IV.
6. Kruppa CG, Sietsema DL, Khoriaty JD, Dudda M, Schildhauer TA, Jones CB: Acetabular fractures in children and adolescents: Comparison of isolated acetabular fractures and acetabular fractures associated with pelvic ring injuries. *J Orthop Trauma* 2018;32:e39-e45.

   Retrospective review of 32 pediatric patients with acetabular fractures seen at a single institution between 2002 and 2011. Twenty-five patients had at least one other pelvic fracture in addition to the acetabular fracture. These patients presented with lower Glasgow coma scores (GCS), higher injury severity scores, and more associated injuries than those patients who sustained isolated acetabular fractures. Level of evidence: IV.
7. Silber JS, Flynn JM, Koffler KM, Dormans JP, Drummond DS: Analysis of the cause, classification, and associated injuries of 166 consecutive pediatric pelvic fractures. *J Pediatr Orthop* 2001;21:446-450.
8. Swaid F, Peleg K, Alfici R, et al: A comparison study of pelvic fractures and associated abdominal injuries between pediatric and adult blunt trauma patients. *J Pediatr Surg* 2017;52:386-389.

   Retrospective review of all patients recorded in the Israeli National Trauma Registry as having sustained a pelvic fracture between 1998 and 2013. Fewer than 1% of all pediatric patients placed on the registry during this time period sustained a pelvic fracture, versus 4.3% of adults ($P < 0.0001$). Mortality rate was similar between the two groups (5.2% in children, 5.4% in adults) with the most common causes of mortality in both groups being traumatic brain injury, severe blood loss, and multiple organ failure. Level of evidence: IV.
9. Hermans E, Cornelisse ST, Biert J, Tan E, Edwards MJR: Paediatric pelvic fractures: How do they differ from adults? *J Child Orthop* 2017;11:49-56.

   Retrospective review of 51 pediatric patients with a pelvic fracture treated at a single institution between 1993 and 2013. Although MVC was a common mechanism for both groups, pediatric patients were more likely to fall from a height and sustained associated injuries over a wider range of body regions, including significant urogenital injury. Mortality rates were similar between the two groups (6% pediatric; 8% adult). Level of evidence: IV.
10. Burn M, Gary JL, Holzman M, et al: Do safe radiographic sacral screw pathways exist in a pediatric patient population and do they change with age? *J Orthop Trauma* 2016;30:41-47.

Retrospective review of all CT scans performed on patients aged 2 to 16 years in a 1 month time period at a single institution. Width and height of screw pathways were recorded for S1 screws, trans-sacral-trans-iliac screws at S1 and trans-sacral-trans-iliac screws at S2. Authors reported that 99% of patients had appropriate anatomy that would allow placement of S1 screws and 89% of patients had anatomy that would allow for safe placement of a trans-sacral-trans-iliac screw at S2. Level of evidence: III.

11. Abdelgawad AA, Davey S, Salmon J, Gurusamy P, Kanlic E: Ilio-sacral (IS) screw fixation for sacral and sacroiliac joint (SIJ) injuries in children. *J Pediatr Orthop* 2016;36:117-121.

    Retrospective review of 11 pediatric patients who underwent percutaneous ilio-sacral screw fixation of sacral fractures and pelvic ring injuries between 2000 and 2012. All screws utilized were either 6.5 mm or 7.3 mm diameter. Nine patients went on to fracture union without complication, one patient required revision fixation with anterior symphysis stabilization, and one patient developed postoperative weakness and paresthesias in distribution of the L5-S1 nerve root. Average follow-up was 15.1 months (range 1 to 75 months). Level of evidence: IV.

12. Scolaro JA, Firoozabadi R, Routt MLC: Treatment of pediatric and adolescent pelvic ring injuries with percutaneous screw placement. *J Pediatr Orthop* 2018;38:133-137.

    Retrospective review of 67 patients who underwent percutaneous screw fixation of pelvic ring injuries at a single center between 2005 and 2012. Almost 50% of patients in this cohort underwent both posterior and anterior pelvic fixation and average follow-up was 8 months (range 1 to 81 months). There were no reported intraoperative or immediate postoperative complications. One patient was noted to have screw backout 4.5 months postoperatively and underwent implant removal and one patient underwent a single-level posterior spinal fusion for persistent radicular back pain after injury. Level of evidence: IV.

13. Smith W, Shurnas P, Morgan S, et al: Clinical outcomes of unstable pelvic fractures in skeletally immature patients. *J Bone Joint Surg Am* 2005;87:2423-2431.

14. Mehlman CT, Hubbard GW, Crawford AH, Roy DR, Wall EJ: Traumatic hip dislocation in children. Long-term followup of 42 patients. *Clin Orthop Relat Res* 2000;(376):68-79.

15. Kennon JC, Bohsali KI, Ogden JA, Ogden J 3rd, Ganey TM: Adolescent hip dislocation combined with proximal femoral physeal fractures and epiphysiolysis. *J Pediatr Orthop* 2016;36:253-261.

    Retrospective review of 12 patients who sustained associated hip dislocation and proximal femoral physeal injury. Eleven patients were injured during high level athletic competition, most commonly football, soccer, field hockey, and ice hockey. No patient had preceding hip, groin, or thigh pain suggestive of a developing slipped capital femoral epiphysis. Nine of the 12 patients developed partial or complete avascular necrosis of the ipsilateral femoral head, with radiographic changes seen between 7 and 15 months after surgery. Level of evidence: IV.

16. Van Nortwick S, Beck N, Li M: Adolescent hip fracture-dislocation: Transphyseal fracture with posterior dislocation of the proximal femoral epiphysis: A case report. *JBJS Case Connect* 2016;6:e62.

    Case report of a 13-year-old boy who sustained a Delbet 1B femoral neck fracture when he was tackled during a football game. The patient underwent a surgical hip dislocation, open reduction and internal fixation of the fracture within 9 hours of injury. Two years postoperatively, the patient has no pain, no radiographic evidence of avascular necrosis, and has returned to full athletic activity. Level of evidence: V.

17. Shaath MK, Shah H, Adams MR, Sirkin MS, Reilly MC: Management and outcome of transepiphyseal femoral neck fracture-dislocation with a transverse posterior wall acetabular fracture: A case report. *JBJS Case Connect* 2018;8:e64.

    Case report of a 10-year-old girl involved in a pedestrian versus MVC. She sustained a right hip dislocation, Delbet 1B femoral neck fracture and posterior acetabular wall fracture, in addition to a pubic symphysis separation, right inferior ramus fracture, and left sacroiliac joint disruption. She underwent open reduction and internal fixation of all fractures 28 hours after injury. She was followed up for 13 years and developed coxa breva as well as mild difference in hip range of motion but has returned to all activity without pain or functional limitation. Level of evidence: V.

18. Blanchard C, Kushare I, Boyles A, Mundy A, Beebe AC, Klingele KE: Traumatic, posterior pediatric hip dislocations with associated posterior labrum osteochondral avulsion: Recognizing the acetabular "fleck" sign. *J Pediatr Orthop* 2016;36:602-607.

    Retrospective review of 10 patients who underwent surgical treatment after sustaining closed posterior hip dislocations. All patients had a small posterior wall fragment displaced 2 to 3 mm after hip reduction noted on pelvic radiography. All patients had documented complete posterior labral detachment noted intraoperatively. The authors warn that this posterior fleck sign can represent significant posterior labral injury in patients with known or suspected hip dislocation or subluxation. Level of evidence: IV.

19. Thanacharoenpanich S, Bixby S, Breen MA, Kim YJ: MRI is better than CT scan for detection of structural pathologies after traumatic posterior hip dislocations in children and adolescents. *J Pediatr Orthop* 2018. doi:10.1097/BPO.0000000000001127.

    Retrospective review of 27 patients who underwent postreduction MRI after sustaining traumatic hip dislocations. Sixteen patients also underwent postreduction CT. Although all fractures seen on CT were also noted on MRI, magnetic resonance images showed soft-tissue injuries and chondral injury not demonstrated on CT. Twelve patients underwent surgery and authors cite MRI findings as being an important adjunct to surgical decision making. Level of evidence: IV.

20. Morris AC, Yu JC, Gilbert SR: Arthroscopic treatment of traumatic hip dislocations in children and adolescents: A preliminary study. *J Pediatr Orthop* 2017;37:435-439.

Retrospective review of seven patients who underwent hip arthroscopy after closed reduction of traumatic hip dislocations. All patients had a preoperative CT scan, which noted intra-articular osteochondral fragments after reduction. At the time of surgery, posterior labral injury, ligamentum teres tears, and chondral fractures not seen on CT were also noted. Labral repair, osteochondral fracture fixation, and loose body removal were all performed arthroscopically and no intraoperative or immediate perioperative complications were noted. Average follow-up was 10 months (range 6 to 52 months). Level of evidence: IV.

21. Novais EN, Heare TC, Hill MK, Mayer SW: Surgical hip dislocation for the treatment of intra-articular injuries and hip instability following traumatic posterior dislocation in children and adolescents. *J Pediatr Orthop* 2016;36:673-679.

    Retrospective review of eight patients who underwent surgical hip dislocation for surgical treatment of associated injuries after traumatic hip dislocation. Patients underwent surgical treatment of labral injuries as well as femoral head and acetabular fractures. Patients were followed up for an average of 27 months (range 13 to 67 months) and none of the patients developed avascular necrosis of the femoral head. At final follow-up, five patients were actively participating in organized sports and all but one patient reported having no residual hip pain. Level of evidence: IV.

22. Eberl R, Singer G, Ferlic P, Weinberg AM, Hoellwarth ME: Post-traumatic coxa vara in children following screw fixation of the femoral neck. *Acta Orthop* 2010;81:442-445.

23. Kuo FC, Kuo SJ, Ko JY: Overgrowth of the femoral neck after hip fractures in children. *J Orthop Surg Res* 2016; 11:50.

    Retrospective review of 30 pediatric patients treated for femoral neck fractures at a single institution. All patients with Delbet I, II, and III femoral neck fractures were treated with either closed or open reduction and screw fixation. At follow-up, 37% of patients developed AVN and 40% developed clinically asymptomatic femoral neck overgrowth. Patients who developed overgrowth tended to be younger at time of injury, did not develop AVN, and had better functional outcomes compared to the nonovergrowth patients. Level of evidence: IV.

24. Li H, Zhao L, Huang L, Kuo KN: Delayed slipped capital femoral epiphysis after treatment of femoral neck fracture in children. *Clin Orthop Relat Res* 2015;473:2712-2717.

25. Song KS: Displaced fracture of the femoral neck in children: Open versus closed reduction. *J Bone Joint Surg Br* 2010;92:1148-1151.

26. Stone JD, Hill MK, Pan Z, Novais EN: Open reduction of pediatric femoral neck fractures reduces osteonecrosis risk. *Orthopedics* 2015;38:e983-e990.

27. Yeranosian M, Horneff JG, Baldwin K, Hosalkar HS: Factors affecting the outcome of fractures of the femoral neck in children and adolescents: A systematic review. *Bone Joint J* 2013;95-B:135-142.

28. Ju L, Jiang B, Lou Y, Zheng P: Delayed treatment of femoral neck fractures in 58 children: Open reduction internal fixation versus closed reduction internal fixation. *J Pediatr Orthop B* 2016;25:459-465.

    Retrospective review of 58 patients who underwent closed or open reduction and internal fixation of femoral neck fractures more than 24 hours after initial injury. Reduction quality was judged on postreduction radiographs of the affected side. Anatomic reduction was achieved in 89% of patients who underwent open reduction versus only 33.3% of patients treated closed. The AVN rate was 18.9% overall, with a significantly fewer cases of AVN seen in those who underwent open reduction. When surgical treatment of femoral neck fractures cannot be performed within 24 hours of injury, these authors recommend open reduction as a means to achieve more anatomic alignment, reduced risk of AVN, and improved overall functional outcome. Level of evidence: IV.

29. Boyle MJ, Hogue GD, Heyworth BE, Ackerman K, Quinn B, Yen YM: Femoral neck stress fractures in children younger than 10 years of age. *J Pediatr Orthop* 2017;37:e96-e99.

    Case series of six patients who developed compression-sided femoral neck stress fractures. All patients were younger than 10 years and achieved resolution of pain and radiographic fracture union with nonsurgical treatment. Two patients required spica cast immobilization after failure to abide by weight-bearing restrictions. Level of evidence: IV.

30. Lehman RA Jr, Shah SA: Tension-sided femoral neck stress fracture in a skeletally immature patient. A case report. *J Bone Joint Surg Am* 2004;86-A:1292-1295.

31. Parikh SN, Nathan ST, Priola MJ, Eismann EA: Elastic nailing for pediatric subtrochanteric and supracondylar femur fractures. *Clin Orthop Relat Res* 2014;472:2735-2744.

32. Li Y, Heyworth BE, Glotzbecker M, et al: Comparison of titanium elastic nail and plate fixation of pediatric subtrochanteric femur fractures. *J Pediatr Orthop* 2013;33:232-238.

33. AAOS: *Treatment of Pediatric Diaphyseal Femur Fractures: Evidence-Based Clinical Practice Guideline*. Rosemont, IL, AAOS, 2015. Available at: https://www.aaos.org/research/guidelines/PDFF_Reissue.pdf. Accessed July 7, 2017.

34. Oetgen ME, Blatz AM, Matthews A: Impact of clinical practice guideline on the treatment of pediatric femoral fractures in a pediatric hospital. *J Bone Joint Surg Am* 2015 ;97:1641-1646.

35. Roaten JD, Kelly DM, Yellin JL, et al: Pediatric femoral shaft fractures: A multicenter review of the AAOS clinical practice guidelines before and after 2009. *J Pediatr Orthop* 2017;39:394-399.

    This is a retrospective review of all pediatric femoral shaft fractures treated at four trauma centers from 2004 through 2013. The study found a significant increase in both the use of rigid intramedullary nails in patients younger than 11 years with femoral shaft fractures as well as an increased rate of surgical treatment of femoral shaft fractures in children younger than 5 years. Both findings contradict the general guidelines of femoral shaft fractures in pediatric patients as documented in the clinical practice guidelines. Authors also found significant variability in treatment practices between the four centers involved in the study. These results suggest that the current guidelines are either not being used for treatment decisions for patients or are not reflective of current practice patterns.

36. Heffernan MJ, Gordon JE, Sabatini CS, et al: Treatment of femur fractures in young children: A multicenter comparison of flexible intramedullary nails to spica casting in young children aged 2 to 6 years. *J Pediatr Orthop* 2015;35:126-129.

37. Ramo BA, Martus JE, Tareen N, Hooe BS, Snoddy MC, Jo CH: Intramedullary nailing compared with spica casts for isolated femoral fractures in four and five-year-old children. *J Bone Joint Surg Am* 2016;98:267-275.

    Retrospective review of 262 patients treated for isolated femoral diaphyseal fractures at a single institution between 2000 and 2012. Patients were 4 to 5 years of age and 158 were treated with spica casting, while 104 underwent open reduction and placement of flexible intramedullary nails (IMNs). The IMN group was statistically older, heavier and injuries were sustained through higher energy mechanisms. No statistically significant differences were seen in fracture shortening or alignment after fracture union. The overall complication rate was higher in the IMN group. These patients also required more clinic visits and 89% underwent reoperation for implant repositioning and/or removal. IMN did not obviate the need for spica casting in 13% of patients. Level of evidence: III.

38. Shemshaki HR, Mousavi H, Salehi G, Eshaghi MA: Titanium elastic nailing versus hip spica cast in treatment of femoral-shaft fractures in children. *J Orthop Traumatol* 2011;12:45-48.

39. Garner MR, Bhat SB, Khujanazarov I, Flynn JM, Spiegel D: Fixation of length-stable femoral shaft fractures in heavier children: Flexible nails vs rigid locked nails. *J Pediatr Orthop* 2011;31:11-16.

40. Moroz LA, Launay F, Kocher MS, et al: Titanium elastic nailing of fractures of the femur in children. Predictors of complications and poor outcome. *J Bone Joint Surg Br* 2006;88:1361-1366.

41. Lascombes P, Haumont T, Journeau P: Use and abuse of flexible intramedullary nailing in children and adolescents. *J Pediatr Orthop* 2006;26:827-834.

42. Sink EL, Gralla J, Repine M: Complications of pediatric femur fractures treated with titanium elastic nails: A comparison of fracture types. *J Pediatr Orthop* 2005;25:577-580.

43. Wall EJ, Jain V, Vora V, Mehlman CT, Crawford AH: Complications of titanium and stainless steel elastic nail fixation of pediatric femoral fractures. *J Bone Joint Surg Am* 2008;90:1305-1313.

44. Ellis HB, Ho CA, Podeszwa DA, Wilson PL: A comparison of locked versus nonlocked Enders rods for length unstable pediatric femoral shaft fractures. *J Pediatr Orthop* 2011;31:825-833.

45. Shaha J, Cage JM, Black S, Wimberly RL, Shaha SH, Riccio AI: Flexible intramedullary nails for femur fractures in pediatric patients heavier than 100 pounds. *J Pediatr Orthop* 2018;38(2):88-93.

    Retrospective review of 261 patients treated at a single center with stainless steel flexible intramedullary nails for femoral diaphyseal fractures. Twenty-four patients weighed greater than 100 lb at the time of surgery (average weight was 121.8 lb). Compared with patients who weighed less than 100 lb, no significant difference was seen in fracture shortening, malunion, or implant failure. Level of evidence: III.

46. Shaha JS, Cage JM, Black SR, Wimberly RL, Shaha SH, Riccio AI: Redefining optimal nail to medullary canal diameter ratio in stainless steel flexible intramedullary nailing of pediatric femur fractures. *J Pediatr Orthop* 2017;37:e398-e402.

    Retrospective review of 261 patients treated at a single center with stainless steel flexible intramedullary nails for femoral diaphyseal fractures. Postoperative radiographs were used to determine the medullary canal diameter, and a nail diameter to medullary canal diameter ratio was calculated for each patient. Almost 60% of patients were treated with implants that achieved less than 80% canal fill (average canal fill 68.4%). In contrast to patients with ≥80% canal fill, there was no significant difference in fracture shortening, malunion, or implant failure in patients with less than 80% implant canal fill. Level of evidence: III.

47. Basener CJ, Mehlman CT, DiPasquale TG: Growth disturbance after distal femoral growth plate fractures in children: A meta-analysis. *J Orthop Trauma* 2009;23:663-667.

48. Arkader A, Warner WC Jr, Horn BD, Shaw RN, Wells L: Predicting the outcome of physeal fractures of the distal femur. *J Pediatr Orthop* 2007;27:703-708.

49. Pennock AT, Ellis HB, Willimon SC, et al: Intra-articular physeal fractures of the distal femur: A frequently missed diagnosis in adolescent athletes. *Orthop J Sports Med* 2017;5. doi:10.1177/2325967117731567.

    Case series of 49 patients treated for intra-articular physeal fractures of the distal femur between 2006 and 2016. This is a multicenter study involving three institutions. The majority of fractures were SH III fractures involving the distal femur medial condyle and the diagnosis was missed on presentation in 39% of patients. CT and/or MRI demonstrated greater fracture displacement than radiography (6 mm versus 3 mm). Authors recommend having a high index of suspicion for fracture when treating skeletally immature athletes with acute knee injuries and recommend obtaining advanced imaging to help both with diagnosis and surgical planning. Level of evidence: IV.

50. Wall EJ, May MM: Growth plate fractures of the distal femur. *J Pediatr Orthop* 2012;32(suppl 1):S40-S46.

Chapter 57

Pediatric Hip Disorders

Daniel Augusto Maranho, MD, MSc, PhD • Eduardo Novais, MD

ABSTRACT

Pediatric hip disorders involve a spectrum of anatomical and functional abnormalities that are associated with instability, joint incongruence, and femoroacetabular impingement (FAI). Developmental dysplasia of the hip (DDH) is characterized by acetabular dysplasia with or without hip instability or proximal femur abnormalities. Early diagnosis in newborns is recommended through active investigation using clinical examination and ultrasonographic imaging. The main risk factors to consider when evaluating a newborn with suspected DDH includes female sex, breech presentation, and family history. Treatment is based on concentric reduction of the femoral head into the acetabulum which can be achieved by bracing treatment (ie, Pavlik harness, abduction splints), closed or open reduction, and spica casting. The Pavlik method is the main treatment in newborns. Legg-Calvé-Perthes disease is characterized by the idiopathic osteonecrosis of the capital femoral epiphysis. The disease is an important cause of limping and decreased range of motion (mainly abduction) in children from 4 to 8 years of age. The diagnosis is often confirmed with radiographs. Recently, magnetic resonance imaging has been proposed as adjunct to diagnosis and prognosis. Observation is typically recommended for treatment of children younger than 4 years. Surgical or nonsurgical containment principle is usually recommended for hips with increased risk of capital epiphysis collapse (persistent pain, necrosis greater than 50% of the epiphysis, extensive involvement of the lateral pillar, extrusion, subluxation, and patients older than 8 years). Prognosis depends on the morphology of the healed femoral head and its relationship with the acetabulum. Slipped capital femoral epiphysis is characterized by the displacement of the femoral capital epiphysis in relation to the femoral neck, affecting mostly adolescents. Delayed diagnosis may aggravate the prognosis. Treatment includes prevention of slip progression with stabilization of the epiphysis, and in some instances, correction of the proximal femoral deformity. The FAI syndrome is a dynamic mechanical conflict between the proximal femur and the acetabular rim that is associated with hip pain. *Cam*-type FAI morphology is thought to arise during the adolescence, especially in young athletes. *Pincer* morphology is usually associated with local or global acetabular overcoverage or acetabular retroversion. Surgical treatment of FAI is controversial and requires full understanding of the hip morphology and the extent of the intra- and extra-articular pathology.

Keywords: developmental dysplasia of the hip; femoroacetabular impingement; Legg-Calvé-Perthes disease; slipped capital femoral epiphysis

Neither of the following authors nor any immediate family member has received anything of value from or has stock or stock options held in a commercial company or institution related directly or indirectly to the subject of this chapter: Dr. Maranho and Dr. Novais.

Introduction

Pediatric hip disorders involve a spectrum of anatomical and functional abnormalities affecting the normal development of acetabulum and capital femoral epiphysis, from the prenatal to late adolescent stages. The disease recognition and diagnosis are essential to ensure a prompt diagnosis and effective treatment, avoiding the progression of the disease and maximizing long-term function of the hip. The therapeutic time window is often relatively short for diseases like developmental dysplasia of the hip, Legg-Calvé-Perthes disease, and slipped capital femoral epiphysis (SCFE).

Developmental Dysplasia of the Hip

Definition, Etiology, and Epidemiology

Developmental dysplasia of the hip (DDH) is a condition characterized by a developmental anomalous anatomical relationship between the femoral head and the acetabulum. A spectrum of abnormalities may be present including joint instability, ligamentous laxity, acetabular dysplasia, excessive femoral anteversion, hip subluxation, and complete dislocation. The normal development of the acetabulum depends on the concentric centralization of the femoral head into the acetabular cavity, with the presence of articular motion. Minimal femoral head displacement from the center of the acetabular cavity may predispose to abnormal acetabular development and further instability. Family history, ethnicity, ligamentous laxity, intrauterine positioning, and postnatal positioning are considered risk factors. Possibly, there are intrinsic genetic but also extrinsic factors that classify the etiology as multifactorial.

The natural history of DDH presents via three evolutional courses. First, the instability may spontaneously resolve during the first few weeks of life, resulting in a stable normal hip. Second, the instability and acetabular dysplasia may progress, and the hip may eventually subluxate or even completely dislocate. Third, a subclinical instability may be present without obvious signs or symptoms, and acetabular dysplasia may persist beyond the childhood if not diagnosed correctly. It is unclear whether the acetabular dysplasia diagnosed during the adolescence or later is a residual deformity of DDH in the childhood, or a distinct acetabular growth abnormality with later presentation, because late dysplasia is more likely to be bilateral.[1]

Clinical and Imaging Diagnosis

In newborns, DDH may be a silent disease with subtle or even no abnormalities in the physical examination. Newborns with DDH have no pain, no evident deformity, and no limitation of the hip motion. Therefore, DDH in newborns can only be diagnosed if adequately examined and imaged. Dislocated or subluxated hips may be identified with the Ortolani maneuver, where a palpable clunk is perceived when the hip in 90° of flexion, is abducted and the greater trochanter is pushed upward by the examiner's fingers. A positive Ortolani sign means that the dislocated hip is able to be reduced. On the contrary, the provocative Barlow maneuver may be performed to test the hip stability. With the hip in 90° of flexion, the examiner adducts the hip applying axial posterior force through the knee and lateral force using the thumb through the lesser trochanter. The Barlow maneuver means that a reduced hip can be dislocated or subluxated with stress. This examination should be done gently. Nevertheless, hip instability maneuvers may become spontaneously negative within 2 to 4 weeks of life. Although the specificity of these tests are high, sensitivity may be as low as 60%,[2] and Barlow and Ortolani maneuvers may fail to predict further surgical treatment in almost two-thirds of hips.[3] Dislocated hips may also shorten the limb length, allowing for discrepancy and positive Galeazzi sign.

Patients aged 3 to 6 months with dislocated hips present asymmetry in cutaneous creases of the thigh, gluteal, or inguinal region. An important clinical sign is limitation of hip abduction, that usually becomes evident after age 3 months. In walking patients, an obvious limping with abductor insufficiency is present, or the patient toe walks on the side of the dislocated hip.

Ultrasonographic imaging is recommended for breech presentation, family history, and any instability suspicion (Ortolani or Barlow signs, persistent hip click). Universal ultrasonographic screening is performed in some countries, but it may increase the rate of false-positive cases and overtreatment. Hip ultrasonography is the benchmark imaging method to search for DDH in patients until 4 to 6 months, when the secondary ossification center of the capital femoral epiphysis is still absent. Anatomical landmarks are important to determine the hip morphology. The Graf method[4] is accepted worldwide and considers the acetabular inclination angle (alpha) and the femoral head coverage determined by the chondrolabral angle (beta) (**Figure 1**). In normal hips, the alpha angle is greater than 60° and the beta angle is smaller than 55°. DDH is classified according to several Graf's grades. The dynamic Harcke method is helpful to evaluate hip stability. The percentage of femoral head coverage (**Figure 1**) is also a helpful measurement and values greater than 50% are considered normal.[5] The pubofemoral distance (**Figure 1**) has been suggested to be comparable to the Graf method for DDH diagnosis.[6] Whereas Graf angles assessment may vary between observers, the pubofemoral distance has good reliability even with inexperienced examiners.[6] Cutoff values are 6.0 mm with the hip in flexion and adduction,[7] 4.9 mm in flexion, and 4.6 mm in neutral position.[6] The pubofemoral distance has significative correlation with the percentage of coverage of femoral head, and both decrease with DDH treatment in patients younger than 6 months.[8]

Ultrasonography should be performed in the first or second week of life for newborns with clinical instability, determined by positive Barlow or Ortolani signs. The early accurate diagnosis allows for prompt treatment onset and optimal outcomes. Notably, ultrasound at diagnosis has been shown to have prognosis importance as more severe hips have been found to respond worse to treatment.[9,10] For patients with clinically reduced, stable hips but with risk factors, ultrasonography should

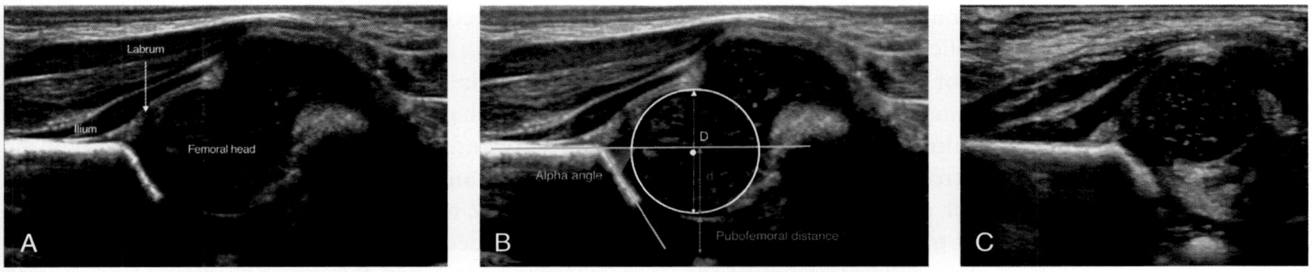

Figure 1 Ultrasonographic imaging of the hip in a newborn showing: (**A**) the main anatomical landmarks for developmental dysplasia of the hip screening including the ilium and osseous roof of the acetabulum, the labrum, and the femoral head; (**B**) the alpha angle, the percentage of femoral head coverage, and the pubofemoral distance; and (**C**) the subluxation with the instability maneuver.

be postponed to 6 weeks of life, avoiding false positives of dysplastic morphological aspect due to physiological immaturity of the hip.[11]

In patients younger than 6 months, radiographs may have the disadvantage to depict only the ossifying proximal femur and acetabulum, but not the cartilaginous components (**Figure 2**). Therefore, the radiographic assessment is based on indirect measurements rather than the morphology of the acetabulum and femoral head coverage. The Tönnis classification considers the position of the ossification nucleus of the femoral capital epiphysis in relation to the Hilgenreiner and Perkin lines. As the ossification is not present in young patients, the International Hip Dysplasia Institute suggested the use of the superior midpoint of the metaphysis (**Figure 2**), and the inferolateral quadrant is divided into two through a 45° line.[12]

Treatment and Prognosis

The principles of treatment are to provide stable reduction of the femoral head concentrically into the acetabular cavity. The biology potential of the growing acetabulum in young children usually promotes significant remodeling of the acetabulum when the femoral head is reduced.[13] Therefore, outcomes are expected to be better with earlier diagnostic and treatment onset.

In newborns, the most popular treatment is the closed reduction using the Ortolani maneuver, determining the Ramsey safe arc, and stabilization using the Pavlik method. The Pavlik harness allows for hip stability by dynamic flexion while abduction is achieved with gravity. The flexion abduction positioning maintains a concentric hip reduction, and its use during the initial child development is associated with adequate acetabular remodeling in almost 90% of cases. Forced

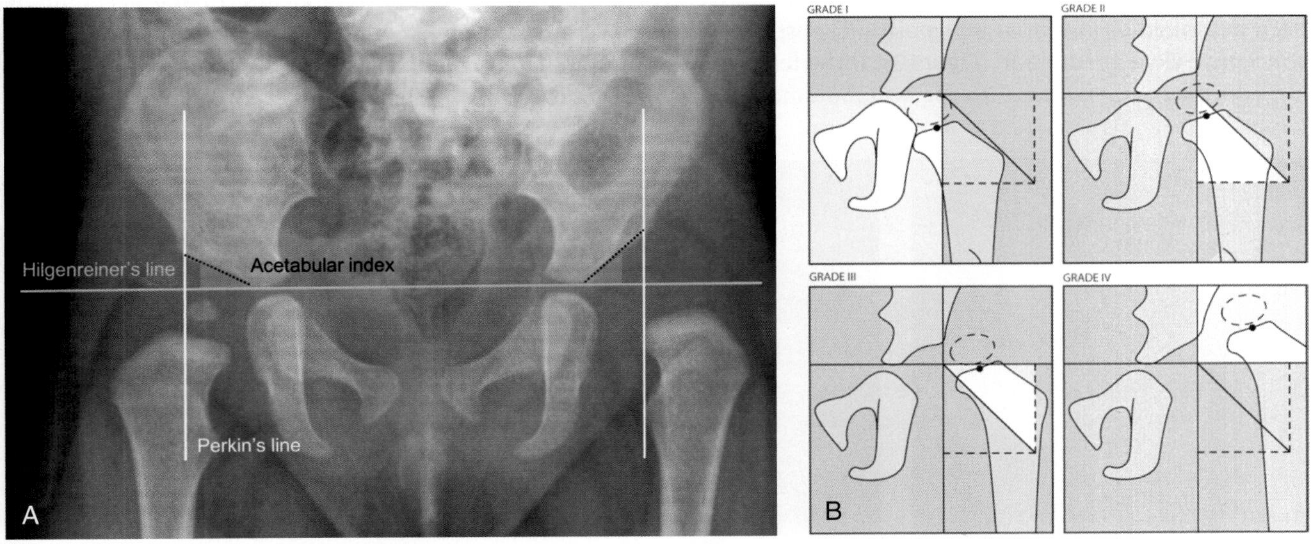

Figure 2 **A**, AP pelvic radiograph of a 6-month-old girl with developmental dysplasia of the left hip and complete dislocation. The Hilgenreiner line, Perkin line, and acetabular index are important tools to assess hip dysplasia in children. **B**, The Tönnis classification modified by the International Hip Dysplasia Institute, in which the superior midpoint of the metaphysis is used and the inferolateral quadrant is divided into two through a 45° line.

flexion abduction positioning must be avoided because of the increased risk of complication such as femoral nerve palsy and osteonecrosis of the femoral head. The Pavlik harness is usually recommended for full-time use, with serial clinical visits and ultrasonographic control. The length of treatment is controversial, but in general, the harness should be used for minimum of 8 weeks, although we favor 12 weeks of treatment for dislocated hips at initial presentation. As a general recommendation, treatment should be discontinued if the hip is not reduced on ultrasound by 3 or 4 weeks of use, although it may be tried up to 6 weeks. Independent factors associated with failure of the Pavlik harness include male sex, age older than 4 months, and severe dislocation (Graf type IV).[9]

In patients older than 6 months up to the walking age, acetabular dysplasia in reduced hips can be treated with an abduction rigid brace, to improve the acetabular index. In dislocated hips older than 6 months, the decision making benefits from an arthrogram study to confirm if a concentric reduction can be achieved by closed treatment, and whether the femoral head can be reduced under the acetabular labrum. Additionally, it is crucial to assess the hip range of motion, stability, and the safe zone of Ramsey, where the minimal range of flexion and adduction are determined for the limit in which the hip becomes unstable. If necessary, the adductors lengthening can be performed to provide greater abduction and lower pressure on the capital epiphysis. The iliopsoas tendon, the hypertrophic ligamentum teres, the transverse acetabular ligament, the fibrofatty pulvinar, and a hypertrophic inverted labrum are structures that have been described as potential interposition, obstructing a concentric closed reduction (**Figure 3**). If the femur does not concentrically reduce into the acetabulum, an open reduction is recommended to treat the interposed blocking structures. After concentric reduction is achieved, the child is placed in a spica cast for about 6 weeks. Often a cast change with repeated arthrogram to assess the stability and improvement of the relationship of the femoral head and acetabulum is performed at 6 weeks. After about 12 weeks in a spica cast, an abduction brace is recommended until normalization of radiographic acetabular parameters for age. Advanced imaging with MRI or CT scan may be useful to assess the concentric reduction after surgery.

Open reduction can be performed through anterior or anteromedial approach. Recent systematic review of the literature has shown similar proportion of osteonecrosis of the femoral head between patients treated with closed versus open reduction and those treated with open anterior versus anteromedial approach.[14] The anteromedial approach is preferably recommended during the first year of life and in bilateral hip dislocations which can be operated on simultaneously. However, it does not allow for a complete capsulorrhaphy or supra-acetabular osteotomy to be performed. The anterior approach allows for capsulorrhaphy; however, in patients with bilateral dislocation, the procedure typically is staged. After walking age, femoral shortening osteotomy with or without anteversion correction is often performed to alleviate the tension of the hip reduction, which may potentially decrease the risk of osteonecrosis. Pelvic osteotomy is also performed often during the same surgical setting in patients after 18 months of age to augment the stability of the reduction and improve the remodeling of the acetabulum. Several osteotomies of the pelvis, including the Salter innominate, Pemberton, and Dega osteotomy, have been described. The specific technique of osteotomy

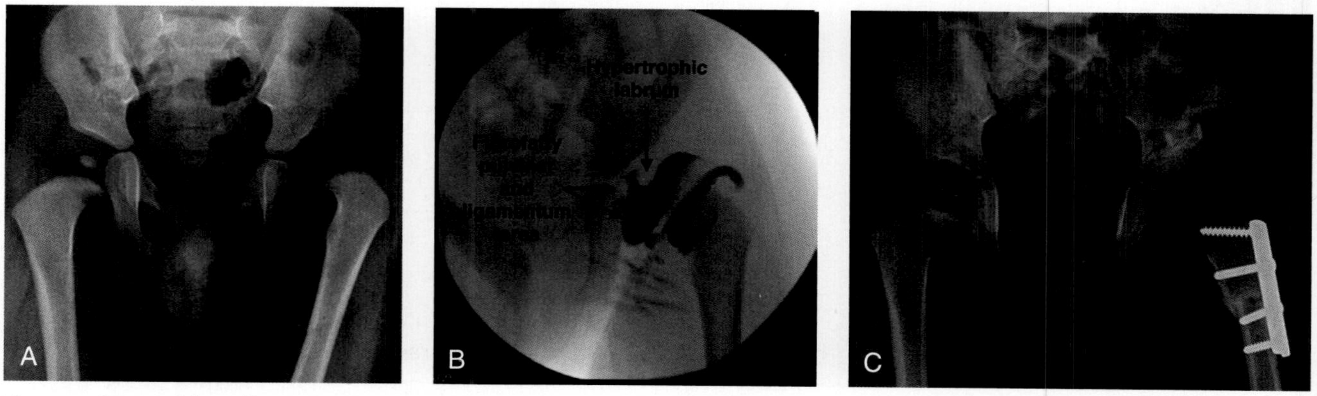

Figure 3 **A**, AP pelvic radiograph of a 1.5-year-old boy with developmental dysplasia of the left hip and complete dislocation. **B**, The hip was unreducible and the arthrogram showed as obstructing structures the hypertrophied labrum and fibrofatty pulvinar. **C**, An open reduction was required, along with femoral derotational and pelvic Pemberton osteotomies. The hip was stable after 6 weeks of surgery and casting.

may be less important than the attention to the position of the acetabular fragment. DDH typically leads to anterolateral acetabular insufficiency; therefore, the osteotomy should be planned to improve the femoral head coverage anteriorly and laterally. The Salter osteotomy is a rotational complete osteotomy with fulcrum in the pubic symphysis, whereas the Pemberton and Dega incomplete osteotomies have the main fulcrum at the triradiate cartilage. Attention to the correction is mandatory and overcorrection should be avoided because it may lead to femoroacetabular impingement (FAI) during skeletal maturity age.

Complications of any treatment include redislocations, residual acetabular dysplasia, and osteonecrosis of the femoral head. The younger the patient at treatment onset, the lower the risk of complications. Older patients (>4 months), bilateral dislocation, severe dysplasia (Graf IV), fixed complete dislocation are important risk factors for Pavlik harness failure.[9,10] Osteonecrosis has been described but is rare with Pavlik method. Transient femoral nerve palsy is a potential complication of the Pavlik harness that has been reported in up to 3% of patients. Early recognition is key to successful treatment. Once diagnosed, the harness should be discontinued, and the hip should be left untreated for minimum of 2 weeks when the function of the femoral nerve should return. Abduction bracing treatment is an alternative to the harness once function is restored.

Osteonecrosis of the femoral head is the most severe complication associated with treatment of DDH. Current investigations are studying the ability of intra- and postoperative assessment of femoral head with MRI to identify epiphyseal hypoperfusion after closed reduction.[15] One important modifiable factor that has been associated with osteonecrosis is the degree of hip abduction in spica casting, which should be limited to a maximum of 60° and the so-called “frog-leg” position in cast should be avoided. If the hip cannot be maintained reduced with less than 60° of abduction, open reduction should be performed.

Patients with DDH must be followed up at least up to skeletal maturity. Those with excellent outcomes may be expected to achieve normal acetabular morphology and no instability. Nevertheless, there is a potential for residual acetabular dysplasia which can be identified at any point in time during growth. Up to 10% of patients treated with Pavlik harness have been reported to present with residual acetabular dysplasia at 6 and 12 months.[10] At this age, abduction bracing treatment is recommended as there is current evidence that bracing treatment between 6 and 12 months allows for better correction of the acetabular index when compared with observation. Remodeling of residual dysplasia is higher during the first 4 years of life, and minimal improvement in acetabular morphology is typically observed after 4 years. Patients with persistent severe acetabular dysplasia and subluxation may be considered for surgical treatment with pelvic osteotomy. Residual acetabular dysplasia at skeletal maturity may present with instability, abductor fatigue, and pain. In teenagers and young adults, the hip should be carefully assessed with radiographs and MRI to investigate for the presence of associated intra-articular abnormality including chondral damage and labral tear. Surgical treatment of acetabular dysplasia in symptomatic adolescents and young adults is recommended. Current evidence of low complication rate and the good long-term results of the Bernese periacetabular osteotomy (PAO) are encouraging. The surgery involves an incomplete osteotomy of the ischium, a complete osteotomy of the superior pubic ramus, and a supra-acetabular iliac osteotomy with a split osteotomy of the posterior column.

Legg-Calvé-Perthes Disease

Definition, Etiology, and Epidemiology

Legg-Calvé-Perthes disease (LCPD) is an idiopathic osteonecrosis of the capital femoral epiphysis in skeletally immature patients. The cause of LCPD remains controversial and unknown. Currently, LCPD is thought to be a multifactorial disease process that is a consequence of unclear genetic factors influenced by environmental conditions. Genetical factors associated with LCPD include mutation in the type II collagen gene (COL2A1). Thrombophilia has been described in association with LCPD, including protein-C, protein-S deficiency, and a high prevalence of factor V Leiden mutation. Recent studies have suggested that there is a high inflammatory response in the synovial fluid of patients with LCPD.[16] Environmental factors include exposure to smoking and hyperactivity with potential exposure to increased load to the femoral head and period (lacking)[17] It is well accepted that disruption of the blood supply to the femoral head is the keystone pathologic event that triggers the ischemic injury and osteonecrosis. A recent hypothesis considered the mechanical resistance of the epiphysis as a potential etiology. The intraepiphyseal vessels would be subject of occlusion in the setting of delayed ossification or reduced cartilage stiffness.[18] Following the ischemic injury, pathologic changes involve the articular cartilage including osteochondral disruption; the epiphyseal bone including fracture of the trabeculae; epiphyseal plate, and metaphysis leading to the formation of cysts in the early phases of the disease[19] (**Figure 4**).

Clinical and Imaging Diagnosis

LCPD is one of the most important causes of hip pain and limping in childhood, especially between 4 and 8 years. Pain is referred in the groin area, thigh, or knee. Limping is often the first sign of disease even in the absence of pain. Subsequent and progressive reduction in hip motion is usually found, particularly abduction and internal rotation. The early symptoms including limp and slight pain may be differentiated from transient hip synovitis and juvenile arthritis. LCPD is most commonly a unilateral disease, and bilateral synchronous epiphyseal deformity resembling LCPD should be differentiated from systemic skeletal dysplasia including multiple epiphyseal dysplasia, spondyloepiphyseal dysplasia, and other systemic or endocrine disorders. Another differential diagnosis to consider is Meyer's dysplasia which is more commonly bilateral and characterized by mild involvement of the epiphysis with delayed ossification or granular fragmentation. Adolescents with healed LCPD deformity may present with symptoms related to FAI or hip instability associated with potential intra-articular pathology including chondral damage, labral tear, and loose bodies.

Children presenting with a limp with or without associated pain should be promptly evaluated with an anteroposterior (AP) pelvic radiograph and a frog-leg lateral radiograph. Usually, the first radiographic abnormality is a decrease in the height of the epiphyseal ossification nucleus, followed by sclerosis. Each stage of disease has some particular radiographic findings. MRI is helpful to detect the extent of necrosis, and chondral and labral abnormalities.[20]

Classifications

Classifying LCPD is important to help staging the disease, plan for treatment, and assess the prognosis. The Waldenström classification is the most commonly used classification for staging the disease. Recently, the Waldenström classification has been slightly modified and reported to have excellent intra- and interobserver reliability[21] (**Figure 5**). The classification includes four stages from early sclerosis to complete healing of the epiphysis.

The extent of epiphyseal involvement can be assessed by different classification schemes (**Figure 6**). Necrosis is the basis for the Salter and Thompson classification, especially considering the subchondral fracture in lateral radiographic view (necrosis of less than 50% of the epiphysis, or more than 50%). The Herring classification is the most commonly used, and it is based on the height of the lateral pillar defined as the lateral one-fourth of the epiphysis on an AP radiograph. Lateral pillar-A hips have no involvement of the lateral pillar; pillar-B hips have a lucency in the lateral pillar and slight loss of height not exceeding 50% of the original height. Those considered B/C borderline hips have a very narrow lateral pillar (2 to 3 mm wide) with more than 50% of the original height but with very little ossification or

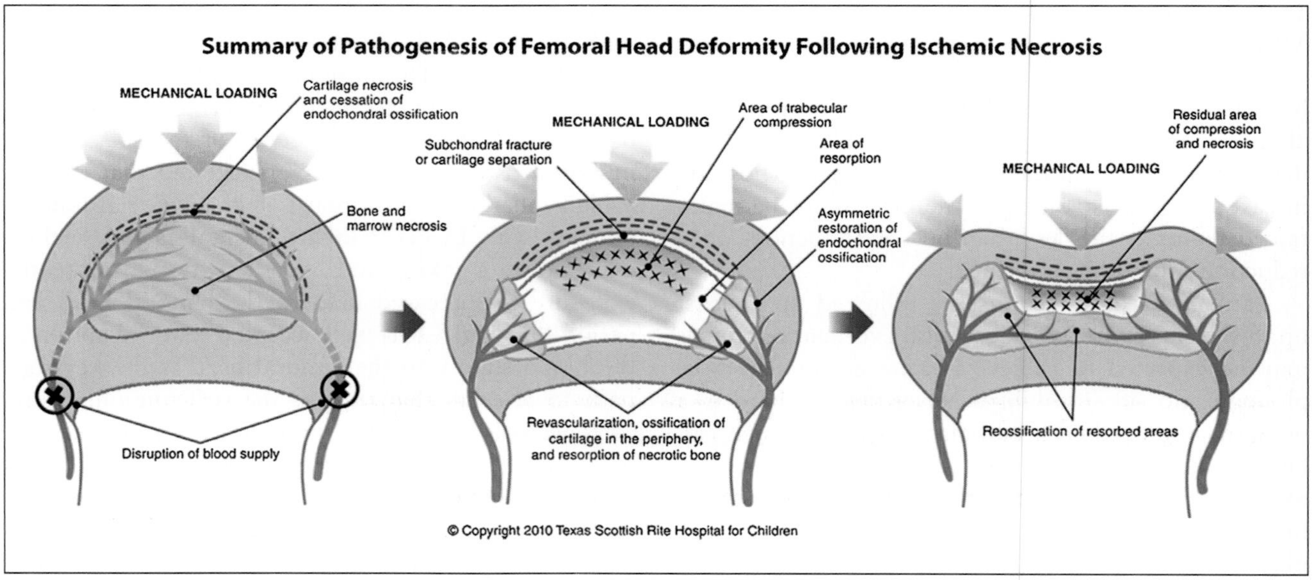

Figure 4 Illustration of a hypothesis on the pathogenesis of Legg-Calvé-Perthes disease. (©2010, Texas Scottish Rite Hospital for Children, Dallas, Texas, All Rights Reserved.)

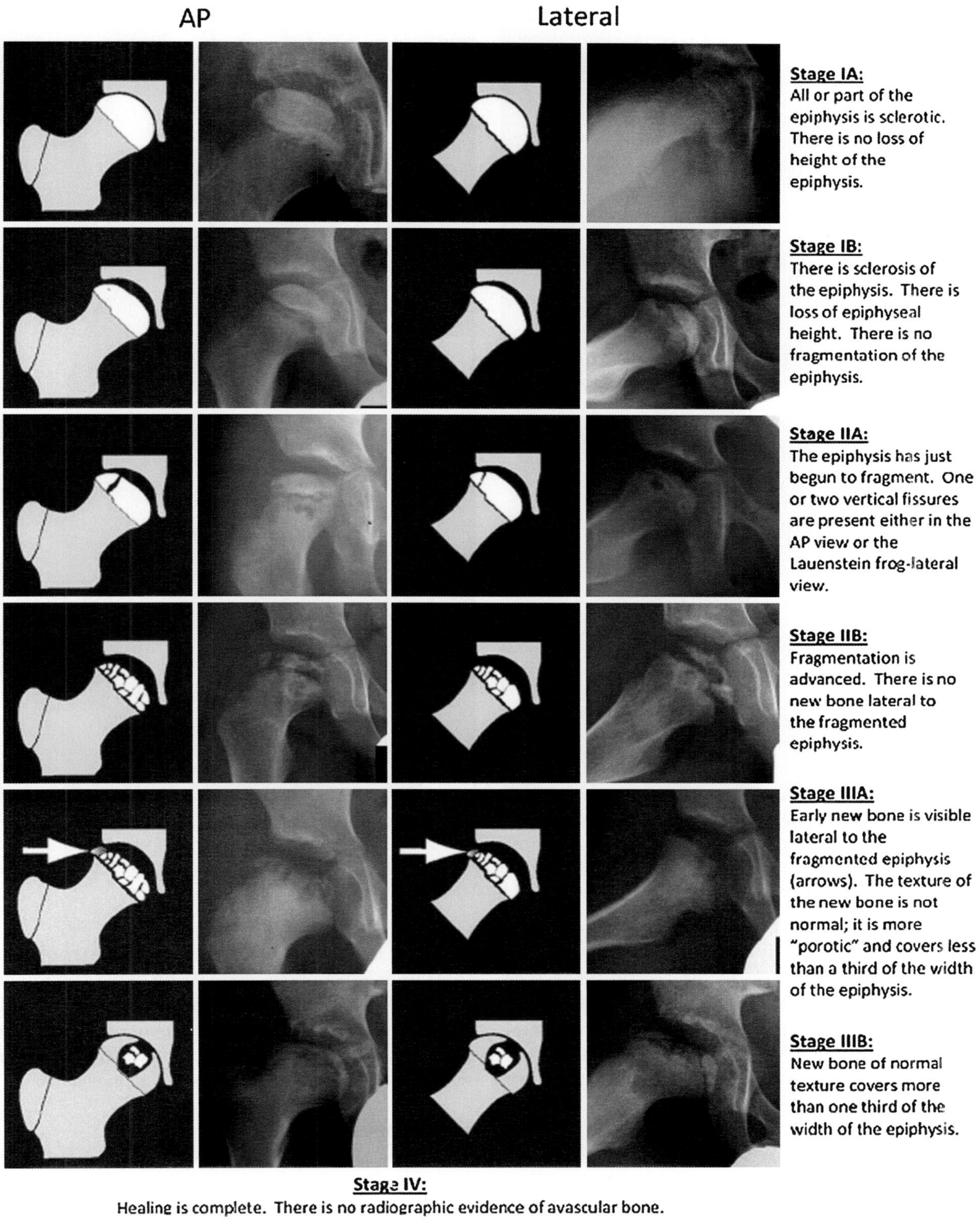
AP
Lateral
Stage IA:
All or part of the epiphysis is sclerotic. There is no loss of height of the epiphysis.
Stage IB:
There is sclerosis of the epiphysis. There is loss of epiphyseal height. There is no fragmentation of the epiphysis.
Stage IIA:
The epiphysis has just begun to fragment. One or two vertical fissures are present either in the AP view or the Lauenstein frog-lateral view.
Stage IIB:
Fragmentation is advanced. There is no new bone lateral to the fragmented epiphysis.
Stage IIIA:
Early new bone is visible lateral to the fragmented epiphysis (arrows). The texture of the new bone is not normal; it is more "porotic" and covers less than a third of the width of the epiphysis.
Stage IIIB:
New bone of normal texture covers more than one third of the width of the epiphysis.
Stage IV:
Healing is complete. There is no radiographic evidence of avascular bone.

Figure 5 AP and frog-leg lateral radiographs of the right hip, and representative illustrations of each stage of the modified Waldenström classification system for Legg-Calvé-Perthes disease. Classification of Legg-Calvé-Perthes disease. (Reprinted with permission from Hyman JE, Trupia EP, Wright ML, et al: Interobserver and intraobserver reliability of the modified Waldenstrom classification system for staging of Legg-Calve-Perthes disease. *J Bone Joint Surg Am* 2015;97(8):643-650. doi:10.2106/JBJS.N.00887.)

Pediatrics

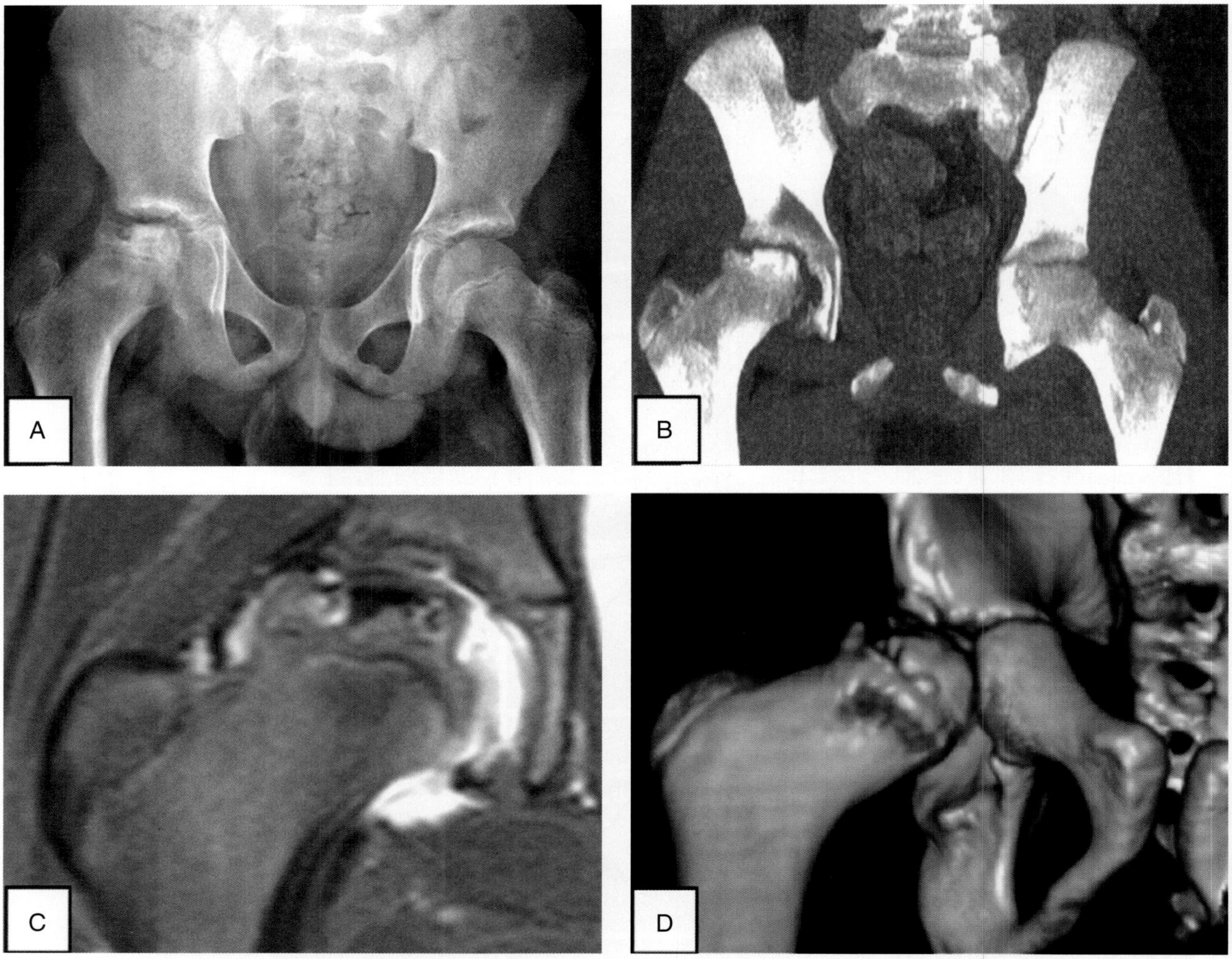

Figure 6 AP pelvic radiograph (**A**), CT scan (**B**), magnetic resonance image (**C**), and 3D reconstruction (**D**) of the right hip of an 8-year-old boy with Legg-Calvé-Perthes disease. There is a central necrosis with less than 50% of head involvement (Salter-Thompson A) and about 50% of lateral pillar involvement (Herring B). However, the child is older, there is lateral subluxation, and the lateral pillar is extruded, exposing the necrotic area to increased loading, risk of collapse, and worse prognosis.

a lateral pillar with exactly 50% of the original height that is depressed in relation to the central pillar. The most involved pillar-C hips have more than 50% loss of epiphyseal height. Although widely used, the lateral pillar classification does not have excellent reliability.[22] The percentage of epiphyseal extrusion is an important factor to be considered beyond the extent of involvement the femoral head. Hips with more than 20% of epiphyseal extrusion are at higher risk for worse prognosis. The long-term prognosis of LCPD is usually determined by the sphericity of the femoral head once the disease has completely healed. The most commonly used system to assess the residual deformity after LCPD is the Stulberg et al classification, which basically classifies the hip as normal (class I); spherical femoral head that may be large in diameter (coxa magna) or with a short neck (coxa brevis, class II); an ovoid femoral head that still has congruency with the acetabulum (class III); a slightly flat femoral head with maintained congruency with the acetabulum (class IV); and a flat femoral head with a round acetabulum (class V, incongruent).

Treatment and Prognosis

Treatment of LCPD is highly controversial but specific patient and disease-related factors should be considered in the decision-making process. Those include the patient's age, range of motion, and percentage of femoral head involvement and stage of disease. Classic treatment of LCPT is based on the principle of containment. By definition, the femoral head should be concentrically reduced into the acetabulum to allow for appropriate spherical development of the femoral head while the acetabulum remodels around it. Because containment is based on the ability of the femoral head and acetabulum to develop concentrically, treatment should start as early as possible. The objective is to concentrically reduce and maintain the femoral head into the acetabular cavity to provide protective effect against collapse, and allow for spherical remodeling of the capital epiphysis according to the acetabular coverage. The containment principle is valid only for the plastic stages (necrosis and fragmentation), but not for reossification and healed stages because there is insufficient remodeling potential in late stages. Containment can be achieved through abduction casting or bracing treatment, or surgeries including femoral and acetabular osteotomies. Adductor tenotomy may be performed in association with any treatment, depending on the tension or contracture of the hip adductors.

Patients who are younger than 4 years, and those with small involvement of the femoral head necrosis less than 50% (Salter-Thompson I), mild involvement of the lateral pillar (Herring A), no femoral head extrusion, and no subluxation can be treated symptomatically with preservation of motion by physical therapy or a home-based exercise program for abduction preservation. In addition, relative rest avoiding impact activities is encouraged. Notably, surgical treatment has been suggested to not improve outcomes in patients younger than 8 years at onset of LCPD with lateral pillar A and B groups.[23]

Older patients, particularly over 6 years, may benefit from surgical treatment for containment which can be achieved by soft-tissue release with extensive casting/bracing treatment program, femoral varus osteotomy or pelvic osteotomy.[24] The definition of age as a surrogate for surgical treatment remains controversial. In lateral pillar-B or lateral pillar-B/C patients older than 8 years, surgical treatment (femoral or pelvic osteotomy) demonstrated improvement in outcomes in one study, while lateral pillar-C had poor outcomes independently of patients' age or surgical versus nonsurgical treatment.[23] Another study noted that in children older than 6 years and more than 50% of femoral head necrosis, proximal femoral varus osteotomy provided better outcomes than nonsurgical treatment, but no difference was found in patients younger than 6 years.[25]

One of the keystones of containment principle for the management of LCPD is that hip abduction should be preserved. A hip that is concentrically reduced would have a wide range of abduction (at least 30°). Gradual loss of abduction should be seen as a risk factor for worse prognosis and is associated with extrusion of the femoral head. Femoral head extrusion can be quantified by measuring the index of extrusion as the percentage of the femoral head that is lateral to the vertical Perkin line divided by the femoral head diameter. Subluxation can be seen as a discontinuity in the arch of Shenton, and these are important radiographic markers for disease progression. Hip abduction should be preserved to avoid severe deformity of the femoral head and acetabulum called hinged abduction. In this phenomenon, the femoral head moves farther from the acetabular fossa while the hip is abducted, and an abnormal contact between the extrusion portion of the femoral epiphysis against the acetabular rim promotes a peripheral fulcrum during motion. In the early stages of limited abduction, an arthrogram should be performed with the patient under anesthesia, and if the femoral head can be reduced completely under the acetabular labrum, then release of the adductor tendons and immobilization in a Petrie cast followed by brace can be attempted as an alternative to rescue the hip and gain mobility. Definitive treatment of hinged abduction can follow by continuation of bracing treatment (**Figure 7**) or femoral or pelvic osteotomies. Valgus femur osteotomy is the classic surgical indication in the setting of hinged abduction. However, the classic valgus osteotomy does not allow for assessment of potential intra-articular deformities, neither it allows for correction of the potential instability associated with hinged abduction. Pelvic osteotomies to achieve containment in LCPD include the Salter osteotomy and the triple osteotomy, which are redirectional osteotomies, and the shelf osteoplasty and Chiari osteotomy that increase extra-capsular coverage of the femoral head. Another alternative for the treatment of severe hip deformity with hinged abduction is the principle of arthrodiastasis with external fixator and reduction of the femoral head into the acetabulum. However, the long-term outcomes of arthrodiastasis for the treatment of LCPD remain unclear.

Treatment of residual healed deformity of Perthes disease in adolescent and young adults includes the application of the surgical hip dislocation technique with dissection of the free retinacular flap containing the nutrient vessels to the femoral head with relative lengthening of the femoral neck[26] with or without an associated PAO to improve the stability of the hip. A contemporary technique of femoral head reduction osteotomy can be performed during the surgical hip dislocation approach with promising early results.[27] However, the technique is difficult and currently only available in tertiary specialized hip centers.

Patients with spherical congruency (Stulberg I and II) have usually good prognosis. The proportion of poor outcomes in aspherical congruency may be as high as 60% to 70% in long term. Incongruent hips usually

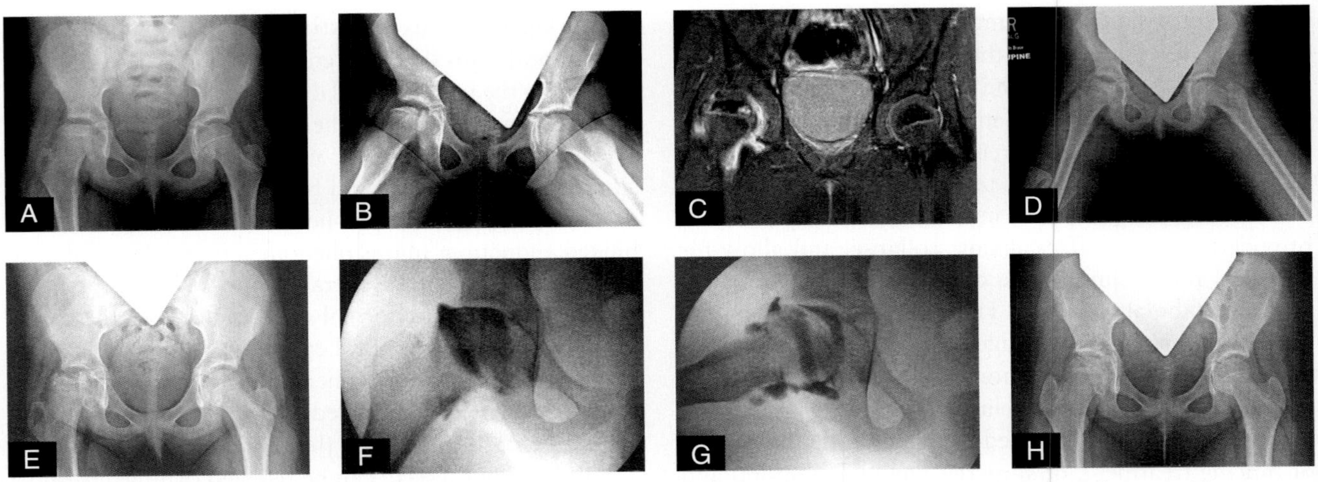

Figure 7 Anteroposterior (**A**) and frog-leg (**B**) radiographs from a 8-year-old girl with right Legg-Calvé-Perthes disease, with an extensive necrotic area. Coronal magnetic resonance imaging of the hip (**C**) confirmed a necrosis proportion greater than 50%. The patient was initially treated with an abduction orthosis, as shown by the AP pelvis radiograph (**D**). After 6 months of follow-up, the femoral head collapsed, developing lateral superior extrusion and subluxation (**E**, AP radiograph), raising a concern for the presence of the hinged abduction phenomenon. An AP arthrogram confirmed the hinged abduction, in which the femoral head moved eccentrically with peripheral fulcrum and farther from the acetabular fossa (medial contrast pooling with hip abduction). However, the labrum was still covering the lateral pillar and the head was reduced under the acetabular labrum in AP and lateral radiographs (**F**, **G**). A Petrie cast was applied for 6 weeks than a removable abduction cast was used for hygiene and physical therapy for more 6 weeks. A night-time bracing was used for one extra year. At 11 years, the hip was near spherical, congruent and concentric in the AP radiographs (**H**).

present with early failure (third decade of life). The optimal treatment for LCPD would be the early prevention of femoral head collapse, and future research will be essential to determine new methods to enhance the long-term hip survivorship in LCPD.

Slipped Capital Femoral Epiphysis

Definition, Etiology, and Epidemiology

Slipped capital femoral epiphysis (SCFE) is defined by the rotational deformity of the capital femoral epiphysis in relation to the metaphysis, at the level of the capital epiphyseal plate in skeletally immature patients. It has been proposed that the capital femoral epiphyseal plate is susceptible to mechanical failure in the presence of systemic endocrine or osteometabolic disorders. Along with the onset of cam deformity in the FAI syndrome, SCFE is one of the most common causes of acquired deformities in the adolescent hip. The incidence has been reported around 10 cases per 100.000 habitants, and it is more prevalent in Polynesians and African Americans. The disease onset is around 12 years and it is more common in boys (2:1.4), but in girls the onset is usually 2 years earlier. The increasing rate of obesity may be changing the epidemiology of SCFE, with the onset at younger ages and higher prevalence of bilaterality. SCFE may be bilateral at initial presentation in 9% to 23% of cases, and in initial unilateral SCFE, a subsequent contralateral SCFE may occur in 18% to 41% of patients.

The etiology of SCFE remains not completely understood, although novel hypothesis have been recently reported. The most acceptable concept involves proximal femur overloading, biochemical abnormalities of the capital epiphyseal plate, and morphologic variations of the femur and acetabulum during a period of rapid skeletal growth. The presence of one or more of these factors may generate instability at the level of the epiphyseal plate and predispose the epiphysis to slip. Endocrine disorders (growth hormone therapy or abnormalities, hypothyroidism, etc) and osteometabolic disorders (renal insufficiency, osteodystrophy, etc) are thought to disturb the physiological mechanical resistance of the capital epiphyseal plate. However, the most common systemic abnormality in patients with SCFE is obesity. It is possible that obesity affects the resistance of the capital epiphyseal plate by three mechanisms: (1) biochemical abnormalities associated with endocrine and metabolic disorders, (2) morphologic inclination of the femoral epiphysis,[28] and (3) mechanical overloading. Leptin level elevation has been suggested to be associated with SCFE regardless the presence of obesity.[29]

Acetabular retroversion is one of the anatomical factors that may cause shear stress across the epiphyseal plate in SCFE. A recent CT study[30] suggested that the acetabulum has reduced version and a higher proportion of the crossover sign is found in patients with SCFE.[31] Femoral morphology may play a role in SCFE pathogenesis. Shear stress may be aggravated by femoral retroversion, posterior epiphyseal inclination, and decreased head-neck offset,[32] but an increased epiphyseal cupping or extension may be protective against physeal instability.[33] The surface anatomy of the epiphyseal plate has been focus of recent advanced studies. The physeal surface of the epiphysis has two distinct anatomical landmarks that may play an important role in the epiphysis stability (**Figure 8**). The epiphyseal tubercle is a bone prominence located at the superoposterior surface of the epiphysis and insinuates into a metaphyseal socket.[34-37] Peripherally, there is a circumferential expansion of the epiphysis around the metaphysis nominated as epiphyseal extension or cupping.[36,37] The epiphyseal tubercle has been suggested to be a primary stabilizer of the epiphysis, particularly when the epiphyseal plate is damage.[38] A rotational theory has been proposed for the pathogenesis of SCFE, in which the epiphysis would rotate over the metaphysis with the epiphyseal tubercle acting as a fulcrum.[34,39] In chronic SCFE, a progressive external rotation of the metaphysis would occur around the epiphyseal tubercle. Furthermore, a bone remodeling process at the metaphyseal socket would raise in response to tubercle shearing stress and micromotion.[40] Radiographic lucency around the tubercle has been described as an early sign of SCFE.[40] It has been proposed that the epiphyseal tubercle could protect the superior-posterior vessels against traumatic damage and osteonecrosis in SCFE. In acute slips, a sudden and complete dislodgment of the epiphysis would occur, predisposing the vessels to disruptions.[36]

Clinical and Imaging Diagnosis

SCFE has basically four distinct presentations. The most common is the onset of hip, thigh, or knee pain with limping. Pain may be referred at the knee in up to one-quarter of patients because of proximity of obturator nerve, being a cause of diagnosis delay. The natural history is the progression of pain and external rotation deformity along several weeks or months, characterizing the chronic SCFE. Patients walk with an antalgic limp and external rotation progression angle of the knee and foot. In supine, there are varying degrees of loss of internal rotation and flexion because of synovitis and mechanical conflict of the anteriorly displaced metaphysis against the acetabular rim. The attempting to flex the hip beyond the limit will be associated with abduction and external rotation (Drehman sign). A subset of SCFE patients presents with a complete sudden dissociation of the epiphysis from the metaphysis, characterizing an

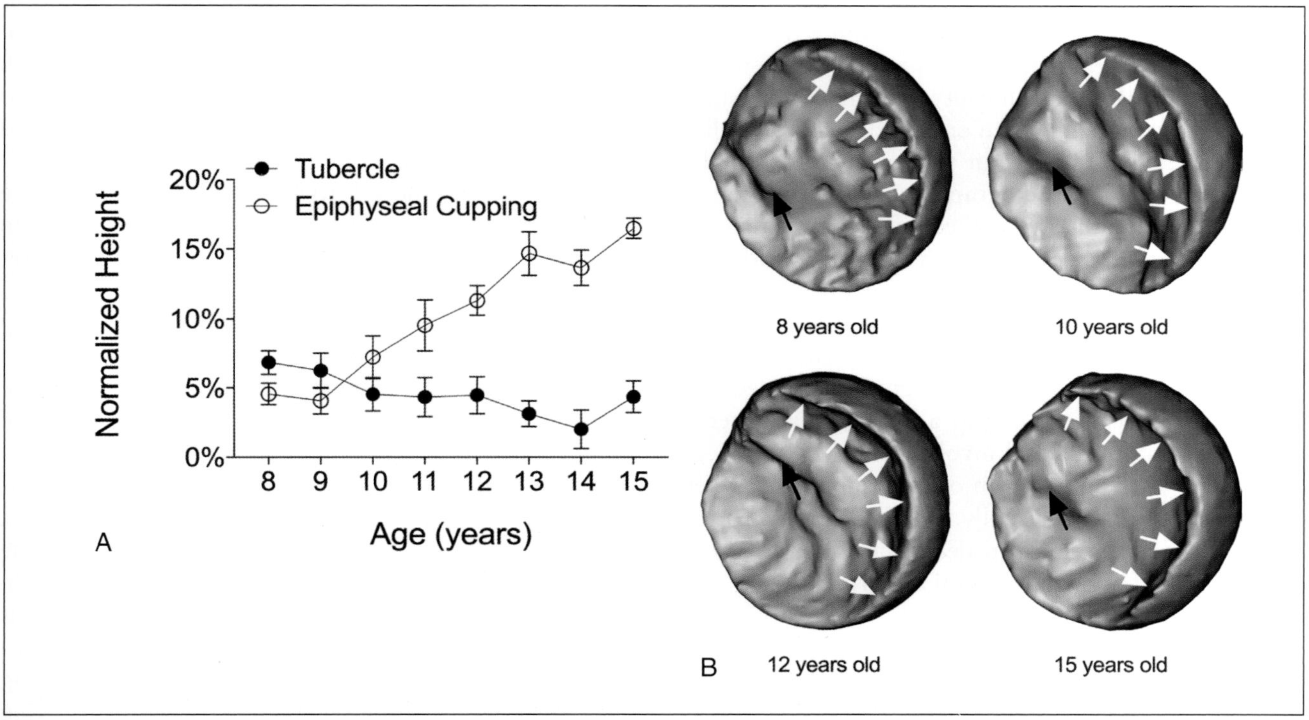

Figure 8 **A**, Graph representing the normal growth of the physeal surface anatomy of capital femoral epiphysis from 8 to 15 years. **B**, 3D-CT reconstructions at ages 8, 10, 12, and 15 years. The epiphyseal tubercle (black arrow) is a bone prominence located at the postero-superior quadrant of the epiphysis, and the epiphyseal cupping is the peripheral bone extension of the epiphysis into the metaphysis (white arrow). In comparison with the epiphysis diameter, the epiphyseal tubercle size decreases with the skeletal growth, whereas the epiphyseal cupping increases. (Reprinted from Novais EN, Maranho DA, Kim YJ, Kiapour A: Age- and sex-specific morphologic variations of capital femoral epiphysis growth in children and adolescents without hip disorders. *Orthop J Sports Med* 2018;6[6]:2325967118781579.)

acute SCFE. A third form of presentation is the presence of hip pain with no epiphyseal displacement on radiographs, defining a preslip stage. Fourth, if the disease process remains entirely asymptomatic with no significant progression, a subclinical slip may occur and heals without timely diagnosis. A comprehensive knowledge of kinds of disease manifestation is important, because chronic and acute SCFE differ in clinical presentation, diagnosis, treatment, complications and prognosis.

SCFE is clinically classified according to acuity and stability. Chronic slips are those with more than 3 weeks of symptoms, whereas acute slips have less than 3 weeks of pain. The slip can also be acute on chronic, when the length of symptoms is greater than 3 weeks, but there is a significant and acute intensification on pain. Stable SCFE is defined by the ability of walking even with assistive devices, whereas in unstable SCFE, patients are not able to ambulate.

AP and Lauenstein pelvic radiographs are essential for the diagnosis of stable SCFE, whereas only the AP is recommended for acute unstable slips. Subtle slips are more evident in lateral views. The eccentricity of the epiphysis is usually assessed by the Klein line and the angle of slip. Physeal widening with adjacent bone irregularities is important for the early diagnosis. Slip severity is classified according to Southwick that originally considers the difference between the affected and contralateral epiphyseal-diaphyseal slip angles. CT scan is helpful to evaluate the deformity and the healing status of the epiphyseal plate (open or closed) in chronic slips.

The presence of hip pain with no evident epiphyseal eccentricity on radiographs suggesting a preslip status will demand more detailed imaging investigation. Careful observation of physeal asymmetry (widening) is mandatory. More recently, the peritubercle lucency sign has been described.[40] A radiolucency around the epiphyseal tubercle on radiographs may correspond to a scenery of micromotion, that might be observed even before symptoms according to a longitudinal observation study of contralateral involvement. MRI is recommended for the confirmation of a preslip status, where juxtaphyseal edema is usually observed at the metaphysis. MRI is also helpful to determine the presence of osteonecrosis and chondrolabral abnormalities.

Treatment and Prognosis

Treatment of SCFE is basically surgical. In stable SCFE, the index procedure must prevent the progression of SCFE by means of epiphyseal stabilization. The most preferred method of epiphyseal stabilization is epiphysiodesis; however, recent studies suggested that fixation techniques without promoting epiphysiodesis may allow for a residual physeal growth and remodeling.[41,42] Percutaneous in situ pinning (**Figure 9**) remains the standard of care for stable SCFE given the low rate of complications with the procedure. For stable slips, a single cannulated screw inserted nearly orthogonal into the center of the epiphysis is recommended. Greater the slip angle, more anterior must be the entry point; however, the screw should not be inserted medial to the intertrochanteric line to avoid screw impingement against the acetabular rim. The main criticism against the in situ pinning is the residual deformity. Mild SCFE deformities may lead to a cam-inclusion FAI type, whereas more severe deformities may cause a cam-type impaction that alters the range of motion and lead to chondrolabral damage (**Figure 9**).

Recent evidence suggests that SCFE deformities related to FAI may lead to chondral damage that could ultimately result in hip osteoarthritis.[43] Correction of SCFE deformity is typically recommended for patients with symptoms of FAI after in situ fixation although few authors recommend acute correction of deformity in patients with severe SCFE. Several techniques have been described to improve the femoral deformity associated with a stable SCFE and are classified according to the level of correction. Capital realignment performed at the level of the epiphyseal plate through a surgical hip dislocation approach allows for optimal realignment. However, several studies have reported a high proportion of complications including hip instability with dislocation[44,45] and osteonecrosis of the femoral head following capital realignment.[46] Osteotomies performed distal to the subcapital level, including the base of neck, intertrochanteric and subtrochanteric osteotomies, have traditionally been thought to have less complications in comparison with the capital realigment. However, careful planning is necessary to avoid creating a major deformity of the proximal femur that would make a total hip replacement surgery more difficult in the future.

Unstable SCFE presents with an increased rate of complications and osteonecrosis. Beyond the risk of epiphyseal blood supply disruption, the acute epiphyseal displacement may be associated with severe hemarthrosis that may tamponade the epiphyseal perfusion, although there is controversial evidence about the effect of capsular decompression on the rate of osteonecrosis.[47] The treatment of unstable SCFE remains controversial. The most popular method is the so-called inadvertent reduction and percutaneous pinning associated with capsular decompression.[48] Measuring the epiphyseal perfusion intraoperatively has been described as an adjunct to the treatment of unstable SCFE.[49] Open reduction through an anterior or anterolateral approach (Parsch et al technique) may have the

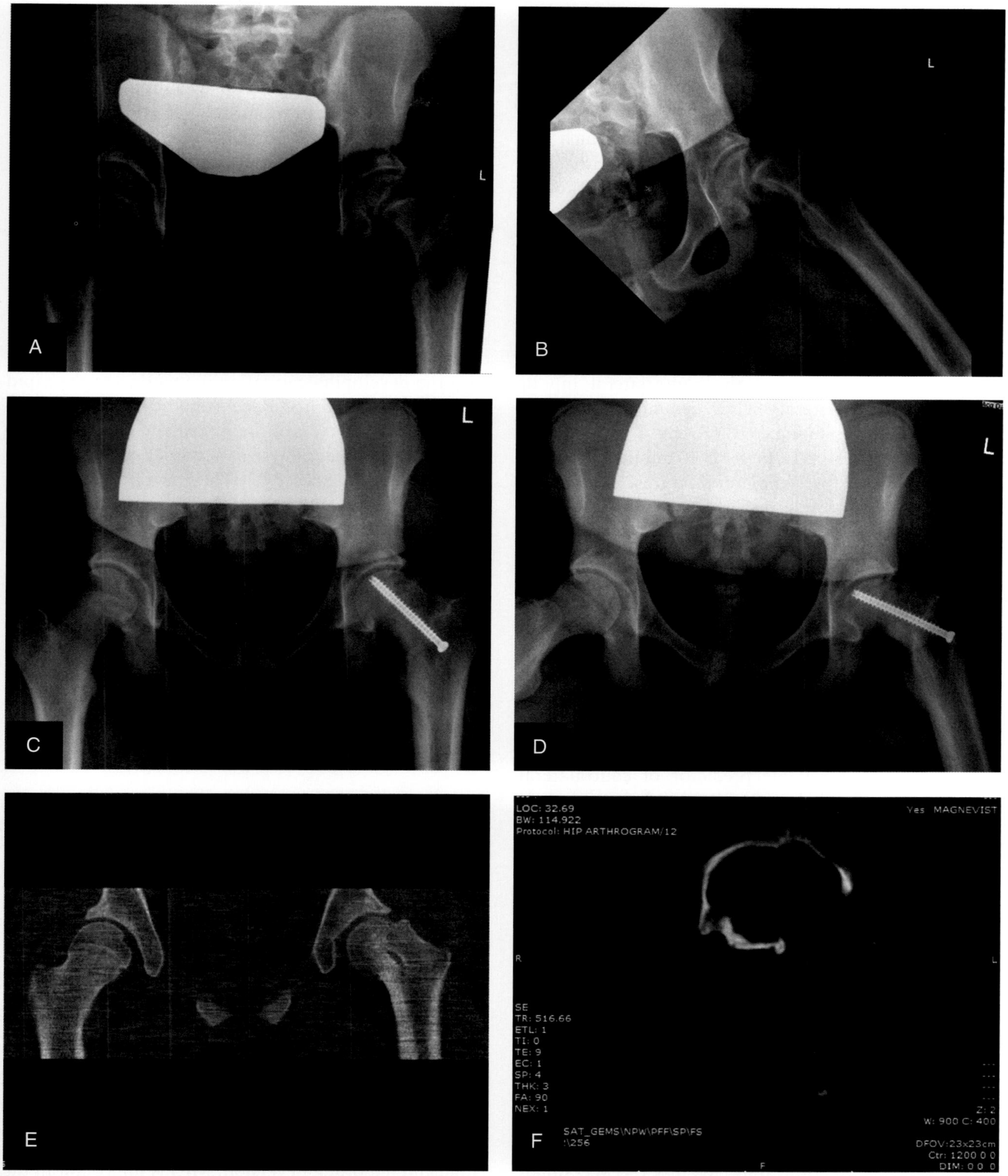

Figure 9 AP (**A**) and lateral (**B**) radiographs of the hip of a 12-year-old girl with a history of 4 months of left hip pain due to slipped capital femoral epiphysis. In situ epiphysiodesis was performed (**C** and **D**); however, there was persistent metaphyseal deformity leading to pain and limited range of motion. After screw removal, a CT scan (**E**) and a magnetic resonance image (**F**) were obtained, showing the cam deformity and chondrolabral abnormalities (**F**).

advantage to control the epiphyseal reduction by digital pressure, avoiding hypercorrection or abrupt maneuvers. The rate of osteonecrosis after open reduction was reported as low as 5% according to Parsch et al. The modified Dunn procedure is the capital realignment using the surgical hip dislocation approach which has the advantage of controlling the reduction with preservation of the periosteal retinacular flap. Although the initial series of this procedure reported low rates of osteonecrosis, recent studies in North America have reported a rate of osteonecrosis around 25%.[50,51] The capital epiphysis perfusion has been suggested to be reduced in unstable SCFE, and surgical treatment with modified Dunn procedure may have the potential to improve the perfusion.[52]

Prophylactic fixation of the contralateral hip in patients with unilateral SCFE remains controversial. Prophylactic pinning may prevent a further contralateral slip; however, there is a minimal risk for osteonecrosis and peri-implant fractures, aside from the potential for growth disturbance of the proximal femur. Systemic endocrine, metabolic, and genetic diseases (autism, Down syndrome) are relative indications for contralateral prophylactic pinning, given the increased likelihood of bilateral disease. Reduced skeletal maturity assessed by the modified Oxford scale and the status of the triradiate cartilage is a helpful tool to predict the likelihood of contralateral slip. The morphology of the femur may also predispose the capital epiphysis to slip, particularly the epiphyseal inclination. Posterior sloping angle greater than 14° has been suggested to be a reliable predictor of contralateral disease.[53] Peritubercle lucency sign has been suggested to be useful in the follow-up period of patients with unilateral SCFE.[40] These criteria should be considered in combination with the family education and decision for prophylactic contralateral pinning or closed surveillance. Moreover, the final morphology of the contralateral femur in unilateral SCFE resembles a sliplike deformity.[54]

Femoroacetabular Impingement

Definition, Etiology, and Epidemiology

Femoroacetabular impingement (FAI) is the dynamic mechanical conflict between the proximal femur and acetabulum. Intra-articular FAI occurs when the femoral head-neck junction abuts against the acetabular rim. Extra-articular FAI occurs because of relatively distant conflicts between the lesser trochanter and the ischium (ischiofemoral impingement), between the greater trochanter and the supra-acetabular region, or between the femoral neck and the anterior-inferior iliac spine (subspine impingement). Intra-articular is the most common form and arises from anatomical variations of the femur or acetabulum. The term "pincer" designates morphologic variations of the acetabulum causing focal or global overcoverage such as acetabular retroversion and coxa profunda. Femoral head-neck deformities are known as cam-type FAI. The origin of cam deformities is controversial and has been focus of investigations. Cam deformity can be secondary to pediatric hip diseases including SCFE and LCPD. However, idiopathic cam deformity has been suggested to be the most common acquired hip deformity in adolescents. Moreover, the etiology of both SCFE and cam deformities may have association with the developing capital epiphysis during the rapid growth in adolescents. Recent studies suggested that the cam deformity is more prevalent in adolescents who practice impact physical activities such as basketball, hockey, and soccer.[55,56] There is a hypothesis that the intense physical activity during adolescence may cause mechanical overloading across the epiphyseal plate, leading to an increase in the epiphyseal extension.[56] This increased cupping phenomenon would make the head-neck junction broader, flattening the physiological convexity, or even creating a convex cam morphology (**Figure 10**). On the contrary, in SCFE the mechanical overloading would lead to epiphyseal displacement because of different baseline factors such as biochemical physeal abnormalities, obesity, posterior inclination of the epiphysis, among others.

Clinical and Imaging Diagnosis

FAI is a common cause of hip pain in young adults, but symptoms may initiate in adolescence. Classic clinical presentation involves anterior or anterolateral hip pain with positive FAI test (pain with passive flexion, adduction, and internal rotation maneuver). An AP pelvic radiograph and a lateral radiograph of the femur are recommended. The most sensitive and specific view is the Dunn 45° lateral which allows for inspection of the anterosuperior aspect of the femoral head-neck junction, which is the most common location of cam deformity. CT may be helpful to quantify the severity of deformity and to localize specifically areas of potential impingement as well as to measure the acetabular coverage and femoral anteversion. MRI is important in the evaluation of chondral or labral pathology associated with FAI and can be performed with intra-articular contrast or without contrast if high-level 3-Tesla protocol is used.

45. Upasani VV, Birke O, Klingele KE, Millis MB, International SSG: Iatrogenic hip instability is a devastating complication after the modified Dunn procedure for severe slipped capital femoral epiphysis. *Clin Orthop Relat Res* 2017;475:1229-1235.

This multicentric retrospective study described postoperative hip instability in 4% of 406 patients (17) who underwent modified Dunn procedure for the treatment of SCFE. Instability was identified as persistent hip pain or radiographically as subluxation or dislocation. Fourteen of 17 patients developed femoral head osteonecrosis and 3 of 17 patients underwent THA during this short-term follow-up. Although uncommon, instability following the modified Dunn procedure is a devastating complication, and factors associated with surgical techniques and primary acetabular insufficiency must be considered. Level of evidence: IV (Therapeutic study).

46. Sikora-Klak J, Bomar JD, Paik CN, Wenger DR, Upasani V: Comparison of surgical outcomes between a triplane proximal femoral osteotomy and the modified Dunn procedure for stable, moderate to severe slipped capital femoral epiphysis. *J Pediatr Orthop* 2019;39(7):339-346.

This retrospective study compared two cohort of patients with stable SCFE who underwent interthrocanteric triplanar osteotomy (Imhäuser, 12 patients) or capital realignment (modified Dunn procedure, 14 patients). The triplanar osteotomy group had no osteonecrosis, whereas four cases (29%) were observed in the modified Dunn group. Radiographic outcomes and the overall complication rate were similar between groups, except for decreased neck-shaft angle in the osteotomy group. The authors pointed out the challenging treatment of severe SCFE with a high rate of complications; however, the occurrence of 29% of osteonecrosis following the Dunn procedure was a critical concern against the technique. Level of evidence: III (Retrospective comparative study).

47. Ibrahim T, Mahmoud S, Riaz M, Hegazy A, Little DG: Hip decompression of unstable slipped capital femoral epiphysis: A systematic review and meta-analysis. *J Child Orthop* 2015;9:113-120.

48. Thawrani DP, Feldman DS, Sala DA: Current practice in the management of slipped capital femoral epiphysis. *J Pediatr Orthop* 2016;36:e27-e37.

This study used a questionnaire for the orthopaedic surgeons, members of POSNA, and reported that the most preferred method to treat SCFE is still in situ fixation, but treatment varies according to each center and surgeon practice. Level of evidence: V (Therapeutic study).

49. Schrader T, Jones CR, Kaufman AM, Herzog MM: Intraoperative monitoring of epiphyseal perfusion in slipped capital femoral epiphysis. *J Bone Joint Surg Am* 2016;98:1030-1040.

A description of percutaneous method of monitoring the femoral head perfusion during surgical treatment. Level of evidence: IV (Therapeutic).

50. Sankar WN, Vanderhave KL, Matheney T, Herrera-Soto JA, Karlen JW: The modified Dunn procedure for unstable slipped capital femoral epiphysis: A multicenter perspective. *J Bone Joint Surg Am* 2013;95:585-591.

51. Novais EN, Maranho DA, Heare T, Sink E, Carry PM, O'Donnel C: The modified Dunn procedure provides superior short-term outcomes in the treatment of the unstable slipped capital femoral epiphysis as compared to the inadvertent closed reduction and percutaneous pinning: A comparative clinical study. *Int Orthop* 2019;43(3):669-675.

Two cohorts of patients with unstable SCFE treated with the modified Dunn procedure or inadvertent reduction plus percutaneous pinning were retrospectively evaluated with clinical and radiographic criteria. Although the proportion of osteonecrosis (26% vs 28%, respectively) and unplanned reoperations (26% vs 33%) were similar between both groups, the modified Dunn procedure was associated with improved clinical and radiographic outcomes. Level of evidence: III (Therapeutic study).

52. Jackson JB III, Frick SL, Brighton BK, Broadwell SR, Wang EA, Casey VF: Restoration of blood flow to the proximal femoral epiphysis in unstable slipped capital femoral epiphysis by modified Dunn procedure: A preliminary angiographic and intracranial pressure monitoring study. *J Pediatr Orthop* 2018;38:94-99.

The perfusion of the capital femoral epiphysis was evaluated with an intracranial pressure monitor and selective angiography during the modified Dunn procedure, in nine patients who experienced an unstable SCFE. The authors observed that most patients (two-thirds, 6/9) had no epiphyseal perfusion preoperatively, but the blood flow was restored postoperatively in four of these patients. Two of these nine patients developed osteonecrosis, being one with no epiphyseal perfusion, and one with perfusion after reduction according to the pressure monitor. The modified Dunn procedure was associated with restoration of perfusion in five of nine patients, but the presence of blood flow was not a guarantee against osteonecrosis. Level of evidence: I (Therapeutic and prognostic).

53. Phillips PM, Phadnis J, Willoughby R, Hunt L: Posterior sloping angle as a predictor of contralateral slip in slipped capital femoral epiphysis. *J Bone Joint Surg Am* 2013;95:146-150.

54. Hesper T, Bixby SD, Maranho DA, Miller P, Kim YJ, Novais EN: Morphologic features of the contralateral femur in patients with unilateral slipped capital femoral epiphysis resembles mild slip deformity: A matched cohort study. *Clin Orthop Relat Res* 2018;476:890-899.

The morphology of the contralateral femur in unilateral SCFE (39 patients) was assessed with CT scan reformatting imaging, comparing with matched controls. The contralateral femur had decreased concavity of the head-neck junction assessed by a higher alpha angle and reduced head-neck offset compared with age- and sex-matched control subjects. A lower epiphyseal extension and a more posteriorly tilted epiphysis were observed; therefore the reduced concavity resembles a mild slip deformity rather than an idiopathic cam morphologic feature. Level of evidence: III (Prognostic).

55. Wyles CC, Norambuena GA, Howe BM, et al: Cam deformities and limited hip range of motion are associated with early osteoarthritic changes in adolescent athletes: A prospective matched cohort study. *Am J Sports Med* 2017;45:3036-3043.

This prospective cohort study included 13 young athletes (12 to 18 years) with limited hip internal rotation (<10°), and 13 individuals matched by sex and age with normal internal rotation (>10°). Clinical examination, radiographs, and MRI were performed at the study enrollment and after 5 years. The cohort with limited hip motion had increased proportion of MRI chondrolabral abnormalities and greater alpha angle, compared with controls. After 5 years, the cohort with limited hip motion presented greater proportion of degenerative changes at MRI and radiographs, suggesting the presence of early osteoarthritis. Level of evidence: II (Cohort study, prognosis).

56. Palmer A, Fernquest S, Gimpel M, et al: Physical activity during adolescence and the development of cam morphology: A cross-sectional cohort study of 210 individuals. *Br J Sports Med* 2018;52:601-610.

    A cross-sectional study of young football players between 9 and 18 years, who underwent hip MRI. The alpha angle and epiphyseal extension increased between 12 and 14 years, but soft-tissue hypertrophy, evident at age 10 years, preceded the osseous cam morphology. Cam morphology was greater at 1 o'clock, in males, and in individuals with regular sport activities. Level of evidence: III (Diagnostic study).

57. Griffin DR, Dickenson EJ, Wall PDH, et al: Hip arthroscopy versus best conservative care for the treatment of femoroacetabular impingement syndrome (UK FASHIoN): A multicentre randomised controlled trial. *Lancet* 2018;391:2225-2235.

    A prospective multicenter randomized controlled clinical trial was performed to evaluate outcomes of conservative versus surgical treatment of FAI. 177 participants underwent hip arthroscopy and 171 underwent specific hip physical therapy. Hip arthroscopy and personalized hip therapy both improved hip-related quality of life in FAI syndrome; however, hip arthroscopy led to a greater improvement. Level of evidence: I (Therapeutic, randomized trial).

58. Fairley J, Wang Y, Teichtahl AJ, et al: Management options for femoroacetabular impingement: A systematic review of symptom and structural outcomes. *Osteoarthr Cartil* 2016;24:1682-1696.

    A systematic review about effects of surgical and nonsurgical treatment of FAI on clinical and radiographic outcomes. Surgery has been suggested to improve symptoms and alpha angle. Until 2016, no study compared surgical versus non-surgical treatment of FAI, raising a concern on the lack of evidence in FAI literature. Level of evidence: III (Therapeutic study).

59. Beaule PE, Speirs AD, Anwander H, et al: Surgical correction of cam deformity in association with femoroacetabular impingement and its impact on the degenerative process within the hip joint. *J Bone Joint Surg Am* 2017;99:1373-1381.

    The study evaluated patients with FAI who underwent surgical treatment for the cam morphology. At 2 years of follow-up, they showed significant improvement in clinical function scores, but also in the cartilage aspect in MRI. The authors suggested that this is the first evidence suggesting that the treatment of FAI improves the overall health of the hip joint. Level of evidence: IV (Therapeutic).

Chapter 58

Pediatric Knee, Leg, Foot, and Ankle Trauma

Megan Johnson, MD

ABSTRACT

Children and adolescents are vulnerable to lower extremity trauma due to an imbalance between limb length and limb mass during growth. Due to the unique anatomy of children, many lower extremity injuries involve the epiphyseal plate, which increases the risk of long-term sequelae, including limb-length discrepancy and angular deformity from premature physeal arrest. It is the presence of an open physis, however, that allows for the tremendous remodeling potential of bone in children. Therefore, in many cases, excellent results can still be achieved in fractures that are not reduced back to an anatomic position. Periarticular fractures in the lower extremity are also common in children and adolescents. As in adults, special attention must be paid to restoring the articular surface back to an anatomic position. Children with lower extremity fractures are at risk for developing acute compartment syndrome and present differently than adults. Care must be taken when placing children and adolescents with high-risk injuries into circumferential dressings, and these patients should be admitted for elevation and careful monitoring.

Keywords: compartment syndrome; growth arrest; physeal injury; Salter-Harris; tibia fracture; triplane fracture

Introduction

Children are particularly vulnerable to injury of the lower extremity due to rapidly changing limb length, mass, and moments of inertia as they change in age. Limb length increases 1.4 times from age 6 to 14 years, but limb mass increases by 3 times, leading to musculoskeletal imbalance.[1,2] This puts strain on tendons, musculotendinous junctions, and apophyses. This in combination with the presence of open physes puts children and adolescents at risk for bony injury in the lower body.[1]

The Salter-Harris (SH) classification is the most commonly used classification system to describe periarticular fractures in children. SH I and II fractures have a better prognosis than III and IVs, which often require open reduction to restore anatomical alignment of the joint surface. Additionally, periarticular fractures involving the epiphyseal plate can cause premature physeal arrest, leading to limb-length discrepancy and angular deformity.

Neither Dr. Johnson nor any immediate family member has received anything of value from or has stock or stock options held in a commercial company or institution related directly or indirectly to the subject of this chapter.

Patellar Fracture/Patellar Sleeve

Patellar fractures in children are uncommon. Less than 2% occur in skeletally immature patients and over half of those in children with open physes are patellar sleeve fractures.[3-5] A sleeve fracture is a traumatic avulsion of the inferior or superior pole in which a small osseous fragment gets pulled off along with a sleeve of periosteum and cartilage. Most cases of patellar sleeve fractures involve the inferior pole of the patella.[3]

Patients report the sudden onset of pain after explosive acceleration during activity. Physical examination of the knee may reveal an effusion, pain over the inferior or superior pole of the patella, a palpable gap, or extension lag with straight leg raise.[3,4] Patellar sleeve fractures may be hard to diagnose on plain radiographs as the only finding may be a small fragment of bone adjacent to the proximal or inferior pole of the patella. In fractures that are largely cartilaginous, the only findings may be a joint effusion and patella alta or baja.[3,6]

MRI is useful for diagnosing a sleeve fracture when the diagnosis is not clear on plain radiographs.[7] MRI can also help assess the true extent of the injury by evaluating the size of the chondral fragment, injury to the articular surface of the patella, extent of periosteal avulsion, and the size of the fracture fragment.[3,8]

Surgical treatment of patellar sleeve fractures is recommended. Fixation can be achieved by a tension band construct with either suture or wire, transosseous sutures, or suture anchor fixation.

Pediatrics

Proximal Tibia Physeal Fractures

Fractures of the proximal tibia physis are uncommon and represent <1% of all physeal fractures.[9] These fractures are classified by the Salter-Harris system, with type II being the most common.[9] The metaphyseal fragment can be displaced posteriorly or anteriorly depending on the mechanism of injury (posterior with extension and anterior with flexion).[9] As with a knee dislocation, there is a risk for injury to the popliteus neurovascular structures due to their proximity to the proximal tibia physis. Therefore, a thorough examination should be done, including assessment of the neurologic and vascular status of the limb, as well as evaluation for compartment syndrome. While plain radiographs are usually adequate for diagnosis, CT can help assess the amount of articular surface displacement in SH III and IV fractures, while MRI may be helpful for diagnosis of ligamentous injuries.[9] Nondisplaced fractures and SH I and II fractures that can be closed reduced can be successfully managed with a long leg cast for 4 to 6 weeks. If adequate reduction is unable to be obtained, then open reduction and internal fixation (ORIF) is necessary. There may be interposed periosteum, tendon, or ligament in the fracture site. Internal fixation can be done with percutaneously placed Kirschner wires (K-wires) or Steinman pins either in an antero- or retrograde fashion. When there is a large metaphyseal fragment, partially threaded cannulated screw fixation can be used.[9]

SH III or IV fractures that are nondisplaced can be treated nonsurgically in a long leg cast; however, screw fixation should be considered to prevent late displacement in the cast.[9] Displaced SH III or IV fractures require open reduction to obtain anatomic alignment at the joint surface. Internal fixation is achieved by partially threaded cannulated screws placed in the epiphysis and or metaphysis parallel to the joint surface depending on the fracture pattern.[9]

The incidence of growth arrest after proximal tibial physeal injuries is 25%.[9,10] Patients with these types of fractures should be followed until skeletal maturity to assess for this complication.

Tibial Tubercle Fractures

The proximal tibia physis closes between ages 13 and 15 years in girls and 15 to 17 years in boys. Tibial tubercle fractures are most common in adolescent boys, between the ages of 12 and 17 years. They are caused by a rapid eccentric contraction of the quadriceps and occur most frequent with jumping sports, especially basketball.[1,11] Osgood-Schlatter disease is present in 23% of patients with tibial tubercle fractures.[11]

The most common classification system used for tibial tubercle fractures is the Ogden modification of the Watson-Jones classification. Type I is an avulsion of the distal portion of the tubercle—type IA fractures are non- or minimally displaced and type IB are displaced. Type IIA involves the entire secondary ossification center and is hinged upward at the level of the proximal tibial physis and type IIB fractures are comminuted. A type IIIA fracture has extension through the proximal tibia epiphysis and into the knee joint and IIIB are both intraarticular and comminuted.[1,9] Type III fractures are the most common.[11] Associated injuries include patellar or quadriceps tendon avulsions, meniscal tears, and compartment syndrome.[11]

Nondisplaced fractures can be placed into either a long leg cast or cylinder cast with the knee extended for 4 to 6 weeks. Displaced fractures require ORIF with partially threaded cannulated screws that are placed in the metaphysis parallel to the physis (**Figure 1**). For fractures that extend into the joint, a screw can be placed within the epiphysis, parallel to the physis, from anterior to posterior. Complications occur in 28% of patients. The most common complication is painful hardware requiring removal (56%), prominence of the tubercle (18%), refracture (6%), wound infection (3%), recurvatum (4%), and limb-length discrepancy (5%).[11] All instances of recurvatum occurred in patients <13 years of age at the time of the injury.[11] This complication is due to premature physeal arrest of the anterior proximal tibia physis. Outcomes of tibia tubercle fractures are generally good, with an overall union rate close to 100%.[11] One quarter of patients with this injury have

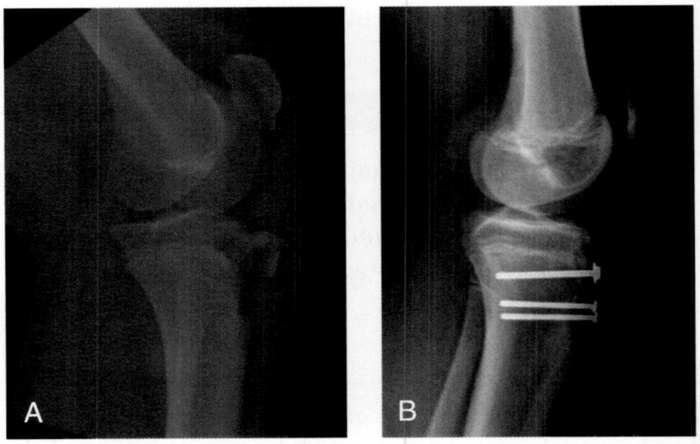

Figure 1 **A**, Lateral radiograph of a displaced tibial tubercle fracture in a 13-year-old male. **B**, Lateral radiograph 12 months after open reduction and internal fixation (ORIF) with three partially threaded cannulated screws.

a significant quadriceps extension strength deficit after surgical management;[12] however, 94% of patients are able to return to preinjury levels of activity and 98% achieve full knee range of motion.[11]

Patients with tibial tubercle fractures should be monitored closely for compartment syndrome as the anterior tibial recurrent artery, which lies near the tubercle, can be torn at the time of fracture.[1] The anterior compartment can be prophylactically released at the time of ORIF.[9]

Floating Knee

A tibial shaft fracture with an ipsilateral femur fracture ("floating knee") is an uncommon injury in children. It is usually the result of a high-energy mechanism. The most commonly used classification system is the Letts-Vincent system for pediatric floating knees. In this classification, type A fractures are both closed and both diaphyseal, type B fractures are both closed, with one diaphyseal and one metaphyseal fracture, type C are both closed, with one diaphyseal and one epiphyseal fracture, type D is one open fracture, and type E are both open fractures.[13,14]

The majority of open floating knee fractures occur in the tibia, and 75% of the femur and tibia fractures are diaphyseal.[13] There are many treatment combinations available for these fractures. In one series of 97 patients, over half were treated nonsurgically with casting and/or traction.[13] Stable internal fixation of both the tibia and femur fractures, however, allows for earlier range of motion and weight bearing and may improve outcomes in children.[15,16] Younger patients are more likely to be treated nonsurgically than adolescent children. Complications from floating knee injuries include limb-length discrepancy (33%), mostly due to overgrowth of the injured side, malunion (20%), secondary surgery (13%), infection (9%), nonunion (7%), and premature physeal closure (3%).[13]

Tibial Shaft Fracture

Tibial shaft fractures represent 15% of all pediatric long bone fractures[17] and occur due to a variety of mechanisms, including minor trauma, sporting activities, and high-energy mechanisms, such as motor vehicle accidents.[15,18] In 30% of children, there is also a fibular shaft fracture, and these fractures are usually the result of a higher energy mechanism.[15,19,20] When both the tibia and fibula are fractured, there is valgus angulation of the distal fragment due to the pull of the anterior and lateral muscle groups. In the other 70% of fractures where the fibula is intact, there can be varus angulation due to the pull of the posterior compartment muscles. These fractures usually occur in younger children due to a twisting injury.[15,20,21]

Most tibial shaft fractures in children can be treated successfully with cast immobilization in a long leg cast for the first 4 to 6 weeks, followed by a short leg cast/walking boot with progressive weight bearing for an additional 4 to 6 weeks.[15,18] Displaced fractures should undergo closed reduction with conscious sedation or general anesthesia. A long leg cast should be applied with three-point molding to counteract deforming forces (especially varus) and maintain fracture reduction. Plantarflexion of 15° to 20° is helpful to prevent a recurvatum deformity. Flexion of 30° to 45° at the knee provides rotational control of the fracture and can help prevent weight bearing.[22] The amount of knee flexion introduced at the time of casting, however, may not be significant for fracture healing. There was no significant difference in time to union or alignment between a group of adolescents with low-energy tibial shaft fractures treated with long leg casts in 60° of flexion of the knee versus long leg casts with 10° of knee flexion with permission to weightbear as tolerated.[23,24] In younger children (<8 years), up to 10° of varus/valgus angulation, 10° of procurvatum/recurvatum, and translation up to one full cortical shaft width are acceptable. In older children and adolescents, ≤5° of varus/valgus angulation, ≤5° of procurvatum/recurvatum, 1 cm of shortening, and 50% translation are acceptable.[15,25] Fractures should be followed weekly for the first 2 to 3 weeks to ensure that loss of reduction does not occur. Cast-wedging or repeat reduction can be used for fractures that start to displace in the cast after the initial reduction. In a large series of adolescents with tibia fractures, 21% of patients required a cast change or wedging in clinic for loss of reduction. Immobilization for 3 months or longer was required in 60% of fractures.[23,26]

Fractures that lose reduction after an initial attempt at nonsurgical treatment, irreducible or unstable fractures, fractures with ipsilateral femur fractures (floating knees), fractures in obese children that are difficult to cast, open fractures, and fractures in the polytrauma setting may require surgical treatment.[18] Up to 40% of patients may ultimately require surgical fixation due to loss of reduction. Predictors of failure for fractures treated with closed reduction and casting are initial fracture displacement >20% and the presence of a fibula fracture.[27] Despite the increased risk of failure with nonsurgical management for tibial shaft fractures with intact fibulas, surgical treatment of these fractures with flexible intramedullary nails yields similar outcomes with a significantly shorter time of immobilization (6.6 versus 10.3 weeks for closed reduction and casting).[23,28]

Pediatrics

For children with an open proximal tibia physis, flexible intramedullary titanium nails can be used for fracture fixation (**Figure 2**). This technique avoids injury to the anterior proximal tibia physis, which can lead to limb-length discrepancy and recurvatum. This type of fixation works best for length stable fractures, but can also be used in fractures with comminution, or significant obliquity. In the latter case, a supplemental cast is helpful to maintain alignment.[15] In younger children with unstable fracture patterns, closed reduction with percutaneous pin fixation can be performed. Open reduction and plate fixation of tibia shaft fractures is rarely utilized in children; however, it can be useful in unstable fracture patterns or in certain open fractures[15] (**Figure 2**). Advantages of ORIF with plate and screws include more anatomic reductions, lower rates of subsequent surgeries, and decreased time to weight bearing; however, there is an increased incidence of wound-related complications and longer operating room times with this type of fixation.[29]

In adolescent children who are within a year of the end of growth, or in whom the proximal tibia physis has already closed, a rigid, locked, intramedullary nail can be used for fracture fixation. The use of a suprapatellar nailing technique has become popular in adult orthopaedic trauma and can be utilized in adolescents as well (**Figure 2**).

Open tibia fractures in children are treated in the same manner as adults. Antibiotics should be started as soon as possible after presentation, followed by irrigation and débridement. Early stabilization of open tibial shaft fractures has been shown to protect the soft tissues and decrease the risk of infection.[18,30] Flexible intramedullary nails are the implant of choice in most open fractures; however, external fixation is a good option for fractures with significant comminution, segmental bone loss, severe soft-tissue injury, or gross contamination. Wound closure/coverage following fixation should not be delayed.[15] As in adults, the soft-tissue injury can be managed by primary closure, vacuum-assisted closure, skin grafting, and flap coverage.[18]

The rate of delayed union or nonunion in children with tibial shaft fractures is 25%.[15,31] The risk is higher in older children/adolescents and those with open fractures. Malunion of tibial shaft fractures is better tolerated in younger children. Below the age of 8 years, remodeling of 10° of angulation either in the coronal or sagittal plane can be expected.[32] Most remodeling is achieved in the first 2 years after fracture.[18] Malrotation

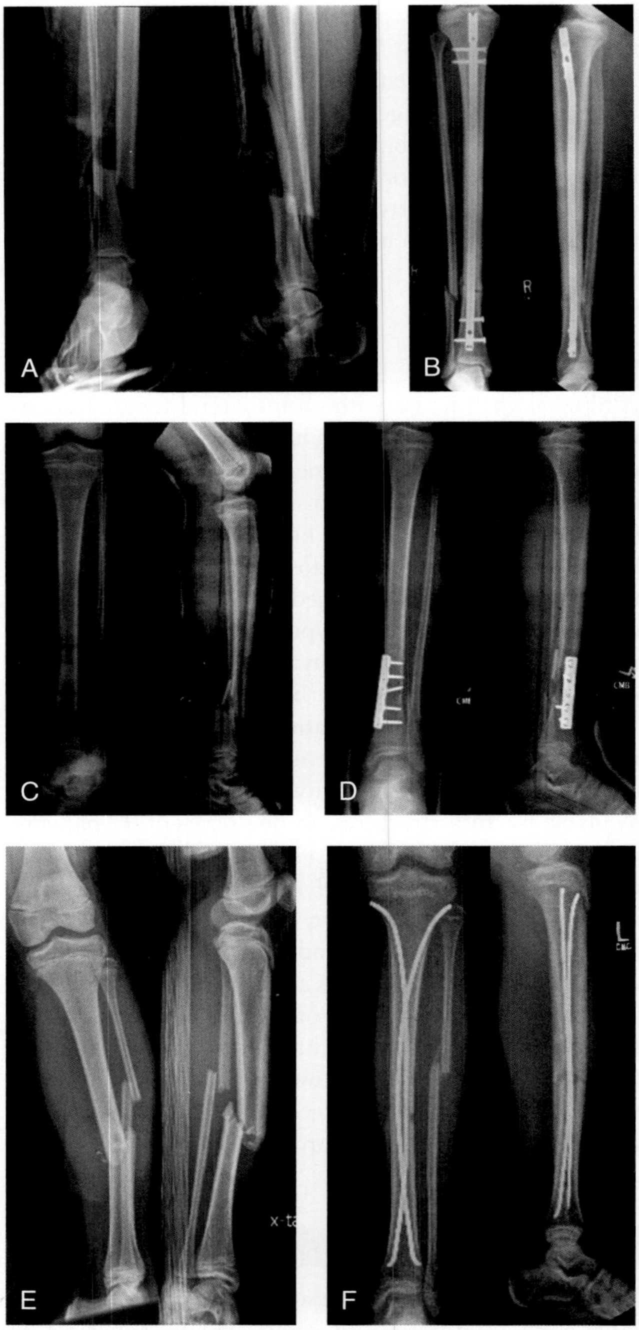

Figure 2 **A**, AP and lateral radiographs of a 16-year-old male with a distal third tibial shaft fracture. **B**, Follow-up radiographs 12 weeks after intramedullary nail (IMN). **C**, AP and lateral radiographs of a 10-year-old female with a grade II open tibial shaft fracture. **D**, Initial post-op radiographs after open reduction and internal fixation (ORIF) with plate and screws. **E**, AP and lateral radiographs of a 9-year-old female with a poke hole open tibial shaft fracture. **F**, AP and lateral radiographs taken 8 weeks after fixation with intramedullary flexible nails.

of the fracture does not remodel over time. Rotational malalignment of >10° may lead to functional and cosmetic problems requiring correction through a derotational osteotomy.[15]

Compartment Syndrome

Pediatric acute compartment syndrome (PACS) is rare. The pathophysiology is a rise in interstitial pressures within a closed fascial compartment resulting in microvascular compromise. Decreased perfusion causes tissue ischemia leading to nerve injury and muscle death.[17] PACS is most commonly caused by trauma; however, nontraumatic etiologies occur as well, often resulting in delayed recognition and treatment. Traumatic PACS occurs more commonly in the lower leg (60%) than in the forearm (27%).[33] Tibial shaft fractures account for >40% of all PACS cases[15,17,34] and can be seen with minimally displaced fractures of the proximal tibia, closed shaft fractures that require reduction and casting, fractures treated with flexible intramedullary nails, and with open fractures.[18] The overall incidence of PACS after tibial shaft fractures is 11.6% with a fivefold higher risk for patients >14 years involved in a high-speed motor vehicle accident.[35] There is also an increased incident of PACS in patients >50 kg, comminuted fractures, and in cases with a preoperative neurologic deficit.[36]

Unlike adults who present with the five P's (pain, paresthesias, paralysis, pallor, and pulselessness), PACS presents with the three A's: (increasing) analgesia, anxiety, and agitation (Herman et al). Increased use of pain medication is the earliest and most sensitive indicator of PACS than neurovascular changes or uncontrolled pain.[34]

Measurement of compartment pressures can provide objective data when the clinical picture is not clear; however, this is challenging in the pediatric population. Compartment pressures >30 mm Hg or a delta *P* value <20 mm Hg when compared with the diastolic blood pressure have been suggested as thresholds for the diagnosis of ACS. This may not be accurate in children, as children have been shown to have higher normal resting compartment pressures in the leg than adults and can tolerate higher pressures after injury with lower pressure gradients.[17,37] For example, children seem to be able to tolerate compartment pressures of >30 mm Hg and perfusion gradients <30 mm Hg without developing PACS.[37,38]

For injuries with a high risk for developing PACS or those that present with significant swelling, circumferential dressings should be avoided. Splints can be applied initially and converted to casts after swelling has decreased. If a cast is applied in the acute setting, it should be at least univalved or bivalved depending on the clinical situation. Bivalving the cast and cast padding by 0.5 cm reduces compartment pressures by 47% in the anterior compartment and 33% in deep posterior compartment.[39] Patients at high risk for PACS should be admitted for elevation of the extremity and serial examinations.

When concern for PACS arises, any circumferential dressings should be removed. Casts that are not bivalved initially should be bivalved down to the cast padding. The anterior half of the cast can be removed if needed. The limb should be elevated to the level of the heart to reduce the arteriorvenous gradient, and supplemental oxygen can be given to optimize tissue perfusion.[38]

Tissue ischemia begins within 4 hours after elevated compartment pressures and irreversible tissue necrosis occurs after 8 hours.[17] Therefore, early recognition and treatment is crucial to achieving good outcomes in PACS. Lower extremity compartment releases are performed in the same manner as in adults, with a medial and lateral calf incision. The anterior and lateral compartments are released from the lateral incision, and the medial incision is used to release the superficial and deep posterior compartments. A vacuum-assisted wound closure system is then applied to the wounds with plans to return to the operating room every 48 to 72 hours for delayed closure.[17,18] An average of three serial washouts is needed for simple wound closure.[40] Wounds that cannot be primarily closed require more complex closure, such as split-thickness skin grafting. The outcome of PACS is generally favorable, with 85% of children achieving full functional recovery. The most common complication is range of motion deficit, which occurs in 10% of cases.[33]

Toddler's Fracture

Toddler's fractures occur in children aged 9 months to 6 years. The injury mechanism is usually a twisting of the foot which leads to a nondisplaced oblique fracture of the distal third of the tibial shaft.[41] The fracture may not be noticed by the caregiver and usually presents as a limp or refusal to bear weight. Physical examination findings include local tenderness over the fracture site, as well as pain elicited by external rotation of the foot. In 39% of children, radiographs are normal at the time of presentation, with the fracture only becoming evident as periosteal reaction along the diaphysis of the tibia develops with healing.[42] Unlike tibial shaft fractures in older children, toddler's fractures do not require manipulation, as they are nondisplaced. These fractures can be successfully treated with either a walking boot or short leg weight-bearing cast for 3 to 4 weeks (Herman et al). Advantages of a walking boot over a short leg cast include earlier return to weight bearing and a lower risk of skin breakdown.[41,42]

Distal Tibia Physeal Fracture

Ankle injuries are the second most common injury in adolescents, with hand and wrist injuries being the most common.[43] A thorough knowledge of the ligamentous attachments around the ankle is essential to evaluating and treating distal tibia physeal fractures. The deltoid ligament stabilizes the medial ankle while the lateral ligamentous complex (posterior talofibular ligament, calcaneofibular ligament, anterior talofibular ligament) stabilizes the lateral side. Distal ligamentous attachments include the posterior and anterior tibiofibular ligament, and they attach to the epiphysis of the tibia and fibula. Because these ligamentous structures are stronger than the physis, physeal and bony injuries are more common than ligamentous injury in the growing child and adolescent.[43] The distal tibia contributes 40% of the overall growth of the tibia with 3 to 4 mm of growth per year.[44]

Patients with distal tibia physeal fractures typically present after a twisting injury to the ankle. It is necessary to distinguish an ankle fracture from an ankle sprain. Fractures usually present with inability to bear weight, bony tenderness, swelling, and/or deformity.[44] Tenderness located over the ligaments distal to the malleoli may indicate a sprain, rather than a fracture. Ankle radiographs with three views are used to evaluate for fractures in children with an ankle injury. The Low Risk Ankle Rule, similar to the Ottawa Rules for adults, has been developed for children to determine when a radiograph is needed to evaluate ankle injuries and has been shown to reduce the number of radiographs used in the emergency department.[44,45]

The Salter-Harris classification is the most widely used system for distal tibia physeal fractures. SH II fractures are the most common type of fracture (40%), followed by SH type III (25%), SH type IV (25%), SH Type I (3% to 15%), and SH type V (<1%).[44,46,47] Growth arrest is most common after type III and IV fractures. Type V fractures are often missed because of the lack of a visible fracture line; however, these fractures also have a high risk of growth arrest due to the crush injury that occurs at the physis.[43]

Nondisplaced SH type I and IIs can be managed with a cast for 4 to 6 weeks. Both fractures occur through the physis in the zone of hypertrophy, with type II fractures exiting through the metaphysis, creating a Thurston-Holland fragment. Displaced type I and II fractures should be reduced to decrease the risk of growth disturbance. Displacement of ≥3 mm at the physis has been found to be a risk factor for premature physeal arrest.[43,48] Reduction attempts should be limited to one or two and should be done with sufficient anesthesia. Repetitive attempts at reduction can cause further damage to the physis. When closed reduction fails, it may be due to the presence of periosteum or tendon within the fracture site. Open reduction must then be performed to achieve anatomic alignment at the physis, decreasing the risk of physeal arrest. Fractures that are stable once the interposed tissue is removed and reduction is performed can be treated without internal fixation; however, any instability requires internal fixation to prevent later displacement. If the Thurston-Holland fragment is large enough, cannulated screws can be inserted through this fragment, parallel to the physis. In younger children, or older children with a smaller fragment, K-wires can also be used.[43]

Type III fractures are common and typically occur at the medial malleolus or through the anterolateral physis (Tillaux fracture). Fractures with <2 mm gap or step-off at the articular surface can be treated in a cast. When displacement >2 mm is present at the joint surface, an attempt at closed reduction should be made. The patient is placed into a long leg cast following reduction. A postreduction CT scan can be performed to determine the amount of residual articular displacement. If >2 mm of displacement remains, ORIF should be performed to restore anatomic alignment of the joint surface.[49] After reduction under direction visualization, 1 to 2 partially threaded cannulated screws are placed parallel to the physis and joint line within the epiphysis.[43] Due to the theoretical risk of increased contact forces and articular pressures when metal implants are placed within the epiphysis close to the joint surface, fixation with bioabsorable screws has been advocated.[44,50,51] In younger children, fixation across the physis should be avoided; however, if necessary for fracture fixation, smooth pins should be used to minimize damage to the open physis.[44]

Type IV fractures are also common and are seen with triplane fractures and also in the medial malleolus (**Figure 3**). The same principles apply as with type III fractures.[43] If there is displacement at the physis, reduction is recommended to decrease the risk of physeal bar formation. If the metaphyseal fragment is large enough, a partially threaded cannulated screw can be placed in the metaphysis parallel to the physis.[52]

Premature physeal closure occurs in up to 38% of SH III and IV fractures.[53] The risk is much lower for SH I and II fractures; however, the risk is increased if there is >3 mm of widening at the physis after final reduction and may be as high as 43%.[48,54] Children with physeal fractures should be followed for at least 2 years after their injury or until growth stops to evaluate for the development of a growth arrest. Park-Harris growth arrest lines can be seen in the metaphysis parallel to the physis once normal growth resumes. Park-Harris growth arrest lines that are incomplete or track to the physis are indicative

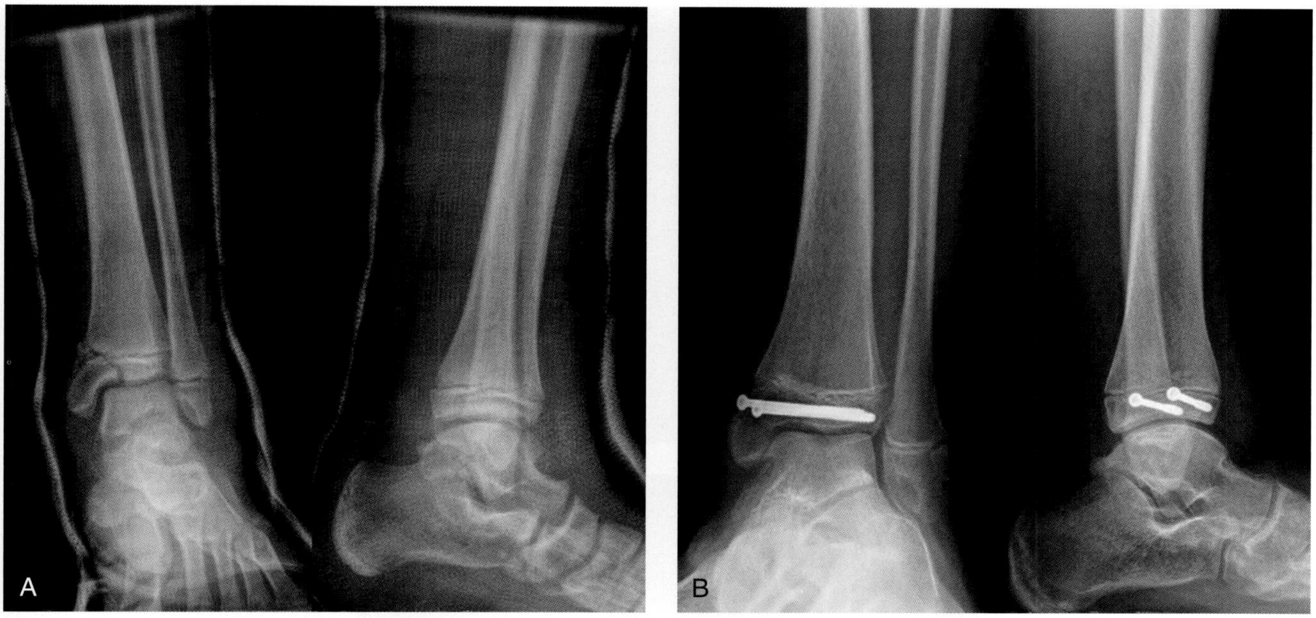

Figure 3 **A**, AP and lateral radiographs of a Salter-Harris (SH) IV medial malleolus fracture after attempted reduction. **B**, AP and lateral radiographs 12 months after open reduction and internal fixation (ORIF) with screws.

of physeal bar formation. Partial growth arrests can lead to angular deformity of the limb while complete growth arrests that involve the whole physis can lead to a limb-length discrepancy.[43] Physeal arrest can be evaluated using CT or MRI. In 65% of cases, bar formation occurs in the anteromedial portion of the physis.[53,55] Treatment of partial physeal arrest is determined by the age of the child, the amount of growth remaining, and the size of the physeal bar. For a child who has a year or less of growth remaining, the recommended treatment is to complete the arrest with a distal tibia epiphysiodesis in combination with an ipsilateral distal fibula epiphysiodesis. When there is more than a year of growth remaining, treatment of partial physeal arrest includes resection of the physeal bar when <50% of the physis is involved, epiphysiodesis for bars that are more than 50% of the physis, and osteotomy if angular deformity is present[53] (**Figure 4**).

Complex regional pain syndrome (CRPS) is rare, but happens most frequently after foot and ankle injuries in children and adolescents.[53] It is seen more

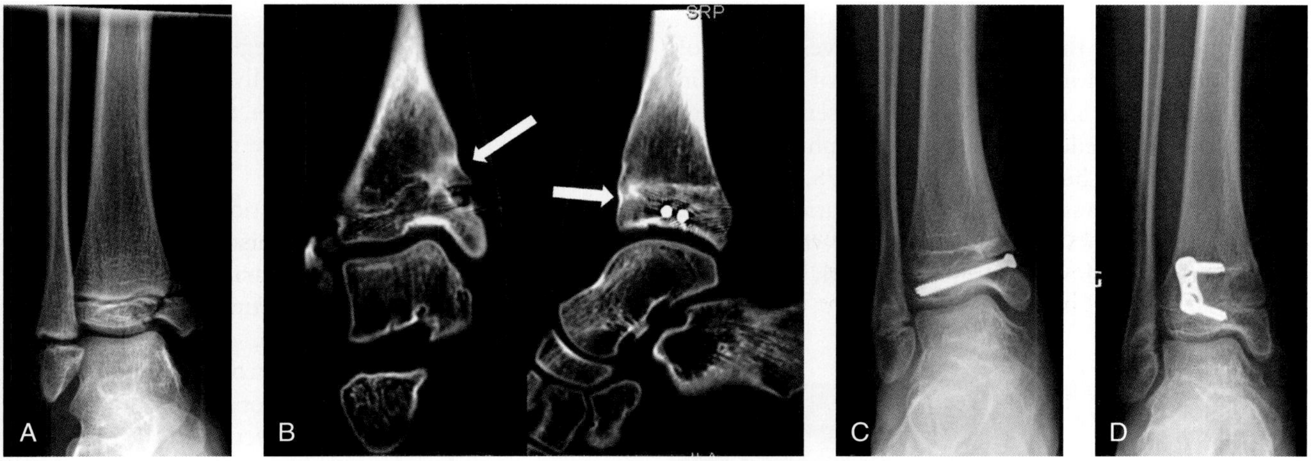

Figure 4 **A**, Injury AP radiograph showing a Salter-Harris (SH) IV medial malleolus fracture in a 9-year-old female. **B** and **C**, CT scan and AP radiograph taken 18 months post open reduction and internal fixation (ORIF) showing an anteromedial physeal bar (arrows) causing varus angulation and distal fibular overgrowth. **D**, AP radiograph taken 1 year after bar resection, guided growth of the lateral distal tibia epiphysis, and epiphysiodesis of the distal fibula.

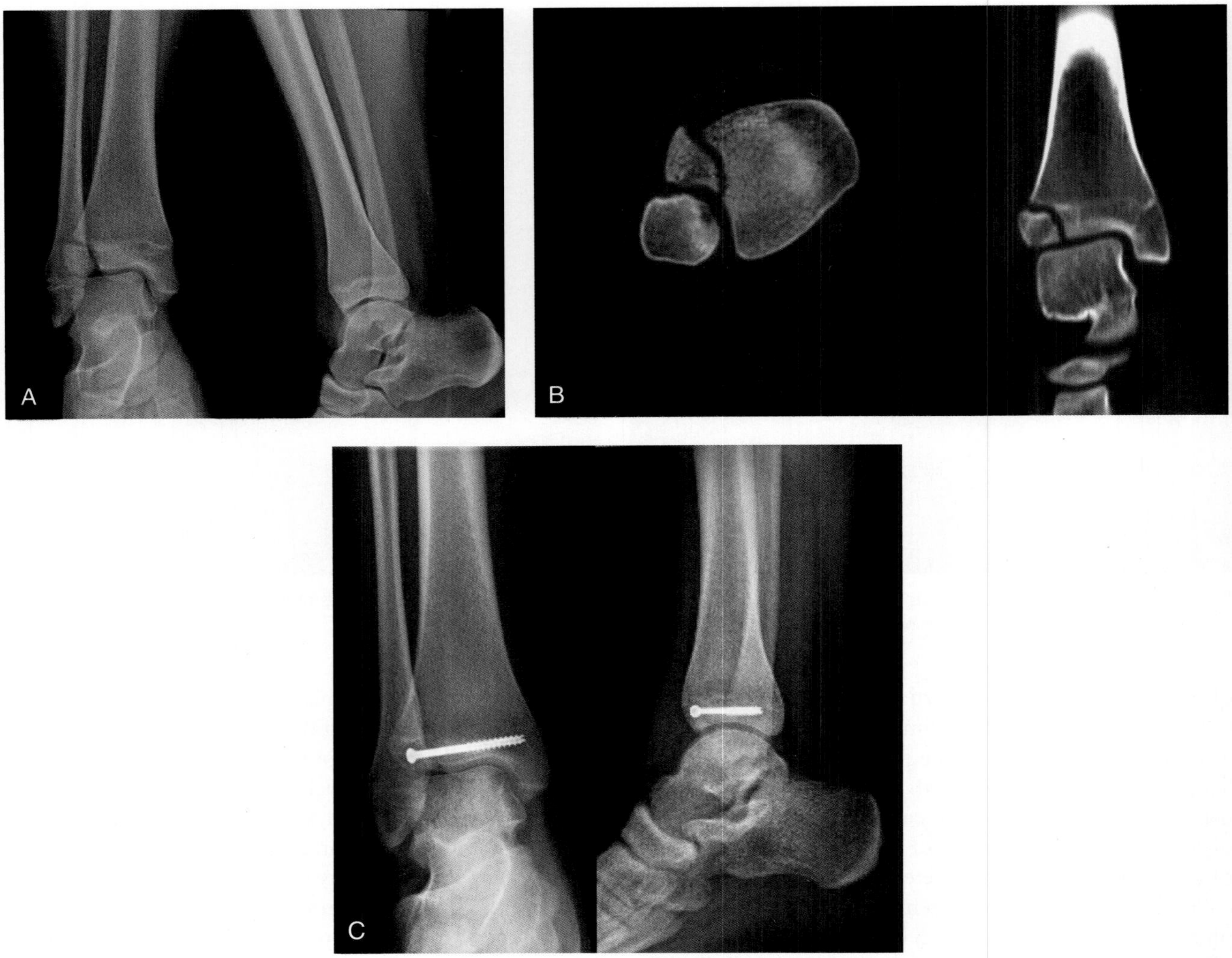

Figure 5 **A**, AP and lateral radiographs showing displaced Tillaux fracture. **B**, CT scan showing displacement of the fracture fragment at the articular margin. **C**, AP and lateral radiographs taken 12 months after open reduction and internal fixation (ORIF).

commonly in girls than boys, with an average age of 12.5 years.[56] Symptoms include pain out of proportion to the initial injury and a combination of sensory, vasomotor, sweating, edema, motor, or trophic changes. Gabapentin can be helpful in cases of CRPS, along with physical therapy, massage, and desensitization therapy. Children with CRPS generally have a better prognosis than adults, although it can recur with subsequent injury.[53]

Ankle Fractures (Tillaux, Triplane, Supination External Rotation)

The distal tibia physis accounts for a large portion of tibia growth. Prior to the closure of the distal tibia physis at age 14 years in girls and 16 years in boys, there is a transitional period in which specific types of fractures can occur. The physis begins to close centrally, then medially, and finally, laterally. This process takes 18 months to complete. Therefore, the unfused portions of the physis are most vulnerable to injury during this transitional period.[43]

The Dias-Tachdjian classification of pediatric ankle fractures is based on the mechanism of injury and also takes into account the Salter-Harris classification system. The four types are supination-inversion, pronation/eversion-external rotation, supination-plantar flexion, and supination-external rotation with the first term being the position of the foot at the time of injury and the second indicating the direction of the force. The two transitional fracture types, Tillaux and triplane, have since been added to this system.[43]

Tillaux fractures are SH III fractures that involve the anterolateral portion of the distal tibia in adolescents.[43] The mechanism of injury is an avulsion of the anterolateral portion of the epiphysis (which is the last portion of the physis to close) by the anterior tibiofibular ligament when an external rotation force is applied to the ankle. The fracture exits horizontally through the physis and vertically through the epiphysis causing an intra-articular fracture.[43] The fracture line is best visualized on a mortise view of the ankle; however, the true amount of displacement is difficult to judge on plain radiographs. CT is helpful in cases where the amount of displacement is in question and can also aid in surgical planning.[43] Nondisplaced Tillaux fractures can be managed nonsurgically in a cast. Reduction using plantarflexion and internal rotation can be attempted for displaced fractures.[43,57] For those fractures with ≥2 mm of displacement at the articular surface, ORIF with either one or two partially threaded screws or, in younger children, K-wires are recommended[43] (**Figure 5**).

Triplane fractures are SH IV injuries in which the fracture line is in the sagittal plane through the epiphysis, axial through the physis, and coronal in the metaphysis. The mechanism of injury is external rotation of a supinated foot.[43,58] In addition to plain radiographs, CT is useful to assess the intra-articular portion of the fracture and also for surgical planning. Treatment algorithm is similar to other distal tibia physeal fractures. Nondisplaced triplane fractures can be treated with cast immobilization. An attempt at closed reduction with axial traction and internal rotation of the foot can be performed. Fractures with residual displacement of >2 mm at the articular surface or >3 mm at the physis require ORIF to restore the anatomic alignment of the articular surface and the epiphyseal plate.[59] When open reduction is necessary, it can be achieved through an anteromedial or anterolateral approach depending

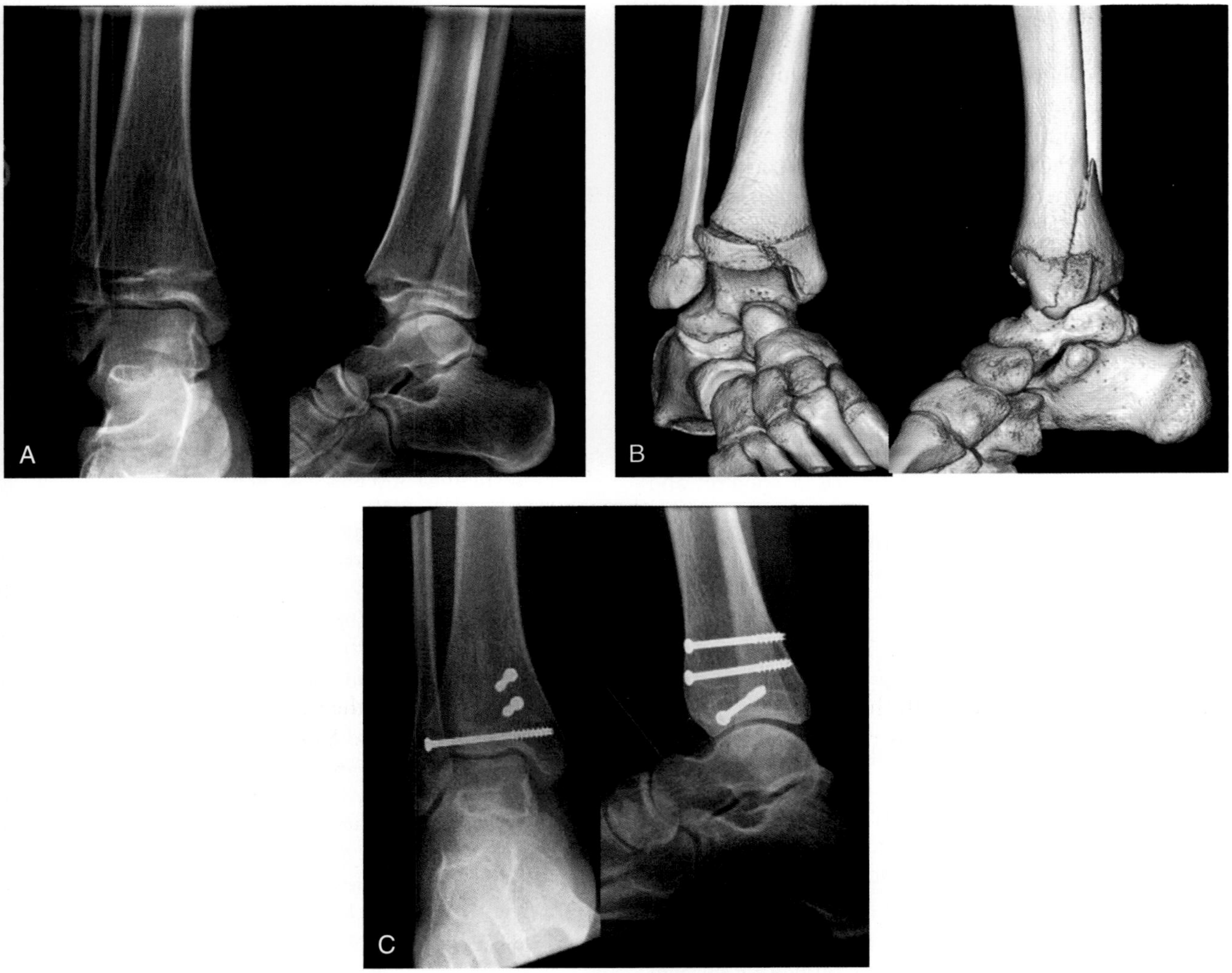

Figure 6 **A**, Radiographs showing triplane fracture with sagittally oriented Salter-Harris (SH) III fracture on the AP view and coronally oriented SH II fracture on the lateral. **B**, 3D CT images showing the three fracture planes. **C**, Postoperative AP and lateral radiographs taken 8 months after open reduction and internal fixation (ORIF).

on the fracture pattern. Fixation is generally achieved with one transepiphyseal cannulated screw and one to two metaphyseal partially threaded cannulated screws placed from anterior to posterior depending on the size of the metaphyseal fragment[43] (**Figure 6**). K-wires can be used in younger patients.

Problems from early physeal closure are less common with transitional fractures because these patients are usually older and closer to the end of growth. Children with >2 years of growth remaining at the time of the injury should be followed until growth ceases.[43]

Summary

Fractures of the lower extremity are very common in children and adolescents and can occur due to a variety of mechanisms, from minor trauma, to sporting activities, to high-energy mechanisms like motor vehicle accidents. Many of these injuries involve the epiphyseal plate and have an increased risk of long-term sequelae such as limb-length discrepancy and angular deformity caused by premature physeal arrest. Children with lower extremity fractures are also at increased risk of developing acute compartment syndrome. Therefore, special attention must be paid when putting children with acute lower extremity injuries into circumferential dressings, such as casts and splints. With appropriate treatment, however, children and adolescents with fractures of the lower extremity can achieve excellent results.

Key Study Points

- The physis is particularly vulnerable to injury and leads to unique patterns of injury in children and adolescents. Injury to the growing physis puts children at risk for long-term sequelae including limb-length discrepancy and angular deformity due to premature physeal arrest.
- Surgical treatment of tibial shaft fractures yields similar results to nonsurgical management, with a shorter period of immobilization and better fracture alignment at final follow-up.
- Compartment syndrome in children and adolescents presents with increasing analgesia, anxiety, and agitation. Children have higher resting compartment pressures and can tolerate higher pressures after injury with lower pressure gradients.
- The risk of premature physeal arrest is greatest after SH III and IV fractures of the lower extremities, with an overall rate of 38%. The rate of premature physeal arrest of the proximal tibia is 25%.

Annotated References

1. Frank JB, Jarit GJ, Bravman JT, Rosen JE: Lower extremity injuries in the skeletally immature athlete. *J Am Acad Orthop Surg* 2007;15(6):356-366.
2. Hawkins D, Metheny J: Overuse injuries in youth sports: Biomechanical considerations. *Med Sci Sports Exerc* 2001;33(10):1701-1707.
3. Gettys FK, Morgan RJ, Fleischli JE: Superior pole sleeve fracture of the patella: A case report and review of the literature. *Am J Sports Med* 2010;38(11):2331-2336.
4. Hunt DM, Somashekar N: A review of sleeve fractures of the patella in children. *Knee* 2005;12(1):3-7.
5. Bostrom A: Fracture of the patella. A study of 422 patellar fractures. *Acta Orthop Scand Suppl* 1972;143:1-80.
6. Khanna G, El-Khoury GY: Sleeve fracture at the superior pole of the patella. *Pediatr Radiol* 2007;37(7):720-723.
7. Zionts LE: Fractures around the knee in children. *J Am Acad Orthop Surg* 2002;10(5):345-355.
8. Bates DG, Hresko MT, Jaramillo D: Patellar sleeve fracture: Demonstration with MR imaging. *Radiology* 1994;193(3):825-827.
9. Mayer S, Albright JC, Stoneback JW: Pediatric knee dislocations and physeal fractures about the knee. *J Am Acad Orthop Surg* 2015;23(9):571-580.
10. Gautier E, Ziran BH, Egger B, Slongo T, Jakob RP: Growth disturbances after injuries of the proximal tibial epiphysis. *Arch Orthop Trauma Surg* 1998;118(1-2):37-41.
11. Pretell-Mazzini J, Kelly DM, Sawyer JR, et al: Outcomes and complications of tibial tubercle fractures in pediatric patients: A systematic review of the literature. *J Pediatr Orthop* 2016;36(5):440-446.

    This systematic review was performed to evaluate tibial tubercle fractures in children. Type III fractures were the most common. The overall incidence of anterior compartment syndrome was low, 3.57%. Results after treatment were excellent, nearly all patients returning to preinjury activity level and obtaining normal ROM of the injured knee. Level of evidence: V.
12. Riccio AI, Tulchin-Francis K, Hogue GD, et al: Functional outcomes following operative treatment of tibial tubercle fractures. *J Pediatr Orthop* 2019;39(2):e108-e113.

    The authors of this study looked at 42 patients with tibial tubercle fractures treated with ORIF. Twenty-six percent of patients were found to have a deficit in quadriceps extension strength compared to the uninjured side. Level of evidence: III.
13. Anari JB, Neuwirth AL, Horn BD, Baldwin KD: Ipsilateral femur and tibia fractures in pediatric patients: A systematic review. *World J Orthop* 2017;8(8):638-643.

    In this systematic review, the authors found that >50% of patients with floating knee injuries were treated nonsurgically. Nonsurgical treatment was favored in younger children. Twenty-five percent of floating knee injuries involve at least one open fracture and 75% involve the diaphysis. Level of evidence: V.

14. Letts M, Vincent N, Gouw G: The "floating knee" in children. *J Bone Joint Surg Br* 1986;68(3):442-446.

15. Mashru RP, Herman MJ, Pizzutillo PD: Tibial shaft fractures in children and adolescents. *J Am Acad Orthop Surg* 2005;13(5):345-352.

16. Yue JJ, Churchill RS, Cooperman DR, Yasko AW, Wilber JH, Thompson GH: The floating knee in the pediatric patient. Nonoperative versus operative stabilization. *Clin Orthop Relat Res* 2000;(376):124-136.

17. Livingston KS, Glotzbecker MP, Shore BJ: Pediatric acute compartment syndrome. *J Am Acad Orthop Surg* 2017;25(5):358-364.

    Review of the literature highlighting the different presentation of children with acute compartment syndrome (three A's) versus adults. Different in resting compartment pressures between children and adults also noted. Overall, outcomes after fasciotomy in children tend to be excellent, as long as the diagnosis is not delayed. Level of evidence: V.

18. Herman MJ, Martinek MA, Abzug JM: Complications of tibial eminence and diaphyseal fractures in children: Prevention and treatment. *J Am Acad Orthop Surg* 2014;22(11): 730-741.

19. Shannak AO: Tibial fractures in children: Follow-up study. *J Pediatr Orthop* 1988;8(3):306-310.

20. Yang JP, Letts RM: Isolated fractures of the tibia with intact fibula in children: A review of 95 patients. *J Pediatr Orthop* 1997;17(3):347-351.

21. Teitz CC, Carter DR, Frankel VH: Problems associated with tibial fractures with intact fibulae. *J Bone Joint Surg Am* 1980;62(5):770-776.

22. Ho CA: Tibia shaft fractures in adolescents: How and when can they be managed successfully with cast treatment? *J Pediatr Orthop* 2016;36 suppl 1:S15-S18.

    The author of this review noted an increase in popularity of surgical treatment of pediatric tibial shaft fractures with no evidence to support surgical management over closed reduction and casting. Level of evidence: V.

23. Rickert KD, Hosseinzadeh P, Edmonds EW: What's new in pediatric orthopaedic trauma: The lower extremity. *J Pediatr Orthop* 2018;38(8):e434-e439.

    In this systematic review, the authors noted that fractures with larger displaced and those with associated fibula fractures were more likely to require delayed stabilization due to loss of reduction after initial treatment with closed reduction and casting. Level of evidence: IV.

24. Silva M, Eagan MJ, Wong MA, Dichter DH, Ebramzadeh E, Zionts LE: A comparison of two approaches for the closed treatment of low-energy tibial fractures in children. *J Bone Joint Surg Am* 2012;94(20):1853-1860.

25. Gordon JE, O'Donnell JC: Tibia fractures: What should be fixed? *J Pediatr Orthop* 2012;32 suppl 1:S52-S61.

26. Ho CA, Dammann G, Podeszwa DA, Levy J: Tibial shaft fractures in adolescents: Analysis of cast treatment successes and failures. *J Pediatr Orthop B* 2015;24(2):114-117.

27. Kinney MC, Nagle D, Bastrom T, Linn MS, Schwartz AK, Pennock AT: Operative versus conservative management of displaced tibial shaft fracture in adolescents. *J Pediatr Orthop* 2016;36(7):661-666.

    The authors of this retrospective review of 74 patients noted fracture displacement of >20% and the presence of a fibula fracture to be predictors of failure of closed reduction and casting for pediatric tibial shaft fractures. Patients treated surgically had better alignment at final follow up, but longer hospital stays and a higher incidence of anterior knee pain. Level of evidence: III.

28. Canavese F, Botnari A, Andreacchio A, et al: Displaced tibial shaft fractures with intact fibula in children: Nonoperative management versus operative treatment with elastic stable intramedullary nailing. *J Pediatr Orthop* 2016;36(7):667-672.

    This retrospective case series on 80 children with displaced tibial shaft fractures with intact fibulae noted equal outcomes in patients treated with intramedullary elastic nailing versus closed reduction and casting. Level of evidence: III.

29. Pennock AT, Bastrom TP, Upasani VV: Elastic intramedullary nailing versus open reduction internal fixation of pediatric tibial shaft fractures. *J Pediatr Orthop* 2017;37(7): e403-e408.

    In this retrospective review, the authors evaluated 70 patients with tibial shaft fractures treated with either elastic intramedullary nailing or ORIF with plate/screws. They patients in the ORIF group to have shorter cast duration, better alignment at final follow-up, and lower rates of subsequent surgery, but longer operating room times and higher rates of wound complications. Level of evidence: III.

30. Pandya NK, Edmonds EW: Immediate intramedullary flexible nailing of open pediatric tibial shaft fractures. *J Pediatr Orthop* 2012;32(8):770-776.

31. Hope PG, Cole WG: Open fractures of the tibia in children. *J Bone Joint Surg Br* 1992;74(4):546-553.

32. King J, Diefendorf D, Apthorp J, Negrete VF, Carlson M: Analysis of 429 fractures in 189 battered children. *J Pediatr Orthop* 1988;8(5):585-589.

33. Lin JS, Balch Samora J: Pediatric acute compartment syndrome: A systematic review and meta-analysis. *J Pediatr Orthop B* 2019.

    In this systematic review, the authors noted pediatric acute compartment syndrome to be most common in the lower leg. Eighty-five percent of patients achieved full recovery with the most common deficit being range of motion. Level of evidence: IV.

34. Bae DS, Kadiyala RK, Waters PM: Acute compartment syndrome in children: Contemporary diagnosis, treatment, and outcome. *J Pediatr Orthop* 2001;21(5):680-688.

35. Shore BJ, Glotzbecker MP, Zurakowski D, Gelbard E, Hedequist DJ, Matheney TH: Acute compartment syndrome in children and teenagers with tibial shaft fractures: Incidence and multivariable risk factors. *J Orthop Trauma* 2013;27(11):616-621.

36. Pandya NK, Edmonds EW, Mubarak SJ: The incidence of compartment syndrome after flexible nailing of pediatric tibial shaft fractures. *J Child Orthop* 2011;5(6):439-447.

37. Bussell HR, Aufdenblatten CA, Subotic U, et al: Compartment pressures in children with normal and fractured lower extremities. *Eur J Trauma Emerg Surg* 2019;45(3):493-497.

    The authors of this prospective study evaluated compartment pressures in children up to the age of 16 years with lower extremity fractures requiring reduction. They noted that children have higher normal compartment pressures than adults and are able to tolerate higher absolute compartment pressures than adults before clinically significant acute compartment syndrome occurs. Level of evidence: IV.

38. Mars M, Hadley GP: Raised compartmental pressure in children: A basis for management. *Injury* 1998;29(3):183-185.

39. Weiner G, Styf J, Nakhostine M, Gershuni DH: Effect of ankle position and a plaster cast on intramuscular pressure in the human leg. *J Bone Joint Surg Am* 1994;76(10):1476-1481.

40. Livingston K, Glotzbecker M, Miller PE, Hresko MT, Hedequist D, Shore BJ: Pediatric nonfracture acute compartment syndrome: A review of 39 cases. *J Pediatr Orthop* 2016;36(7):685-690.

    In this retrospective review of 37 children, the authors noted that there was a delay in diagnosis of acute compartment syndrome in nonfractures cases with a high rate of myonecrosis. Only 54% made a full recovery. Level of evidence: IV.

41. Schuh AM, Whitlock KB, Klein EJ: Management of toddler's fractures in the pediatric emergency department. *Pediatr Emerg Care* 2016;32(7):452-454.

    The authors of this retrospective cohort study of 75 patients with toddler's fractures noted that children who were treated in a splint or cast had a longer duration of immobilization, higher rate of follow-up in orthopaedic clinic and a greater number of repeat radiographs than those treated with a CAM walker boot or nothing. They also noted a 17.3% rate of skin breakdown in children placed in splints or casts. Level of evidence: III.

42. Bauer JM, Lovejoy SA: Toddler's fractures: Time to weight-bear with regard to immobilization type and radiographic monitoring. *J Pediatr Orthop* 2019;39(6):314-317.

    In this retrospective review of 192 patients with toddler's fractures, the authors found that children treated in a boot returned to walking sooner. 98% of all patients were walking by 4 weeks. Level of evidence: III.

43. Wuerz TH, Gurd DP: Pediatric physeal ankle fracture. *J Am Acad Orthop Surg* 2013;21(4):234-244.

44. Su AW, Larson AN: Pediatric ankle fractures: Concepts and treatment principles. *Foot Ankle Clin* 2015;20(4):705-719.

45. Boutis K, von Keyserlingk C, Willan A, et al: Cost consequence analysis of implementing the low risk ankle rule in emergency departments. *Ann Emerg Med* 2015;66(5):455-463 e454.

46. Spiegel PG, Cooperman DR, Laros GS: Epiphyseal fractures of the distal ends of the tibia and fibula. A retrospective study of two hundred and thirty-seven cases in children. *J Bone Joint Surg Am* 1978;60(8):1046-1050.

47. Leary JT, Handling M, Talerico M, Yong L, Bowe JA: Physeal fractures of the distal tibia: Predictive factors of premature physeal closure and growth arrest. *J Pediatr Orthop* 2009;29(4):356-361.

48. Barmada A, Gaynor T, Mubarak SJ: Premature physeal closure following distal tibia physeal fractures: A new radiographic predictor. *J Pediatr Orthop* 2003;23(6):733-739.

49. Kling TF Jr, Bright RW, Hensinger RN: Distal tibial physeal fractures in children that may require open reduction. *J Bone Joint Surg Am* 1984;66(5):647-657.

50. Podeszwa DA, Wilson PL, Holland AR, Copley LA: Comparison of bioabsorbable versus metallic implant fixation for physeal and epiphyseal fractures of the distal tibia. *J Pediatr Orthop* 2008;28(8):859-863.

51. Charlton M, Costello R, Mooney JF III, Podeszwa DA: Ankle joint biomechanics following transepiphyseal screw fixation of the distal tibia. *J Pediatr Orthop* 2005;25(5):635-640.

52. Kay RM, Matthys GA: Pediatric ankle fractures: Evaluation and treatment. *J Am Acad Orthop Surg* 2001;9(4):268-278.

53. Denning JR: Complications of pediatric foot and ankle fractures. *Orthop Clin North Am* 2017;48(1):59-70.

    In this review, the author discusses a variety of complications associated with foot and ankle fractures in children, highlighting the special risk of limb-length discrepancy or angular deformity that can occur as a result of premature physeal arrest. Level of evidence V.

54. Russo F, Moor MA, Mubarak SJ, Pennock AT: Salter-harris II fractures of the distal tibia: Does surgical management reduce the risk of premature physeal closure? *J Pediatr Orthop* 2013;33(5):524-529.

55. Ecklund K, Jaramillo D: Patterns of premature physeal arrest: MR imaging of 111 children. *AJR Am J Roentgenol* 2002;178(4):967-972.

56. Wilder RT, Berde CB, Wolohan M, Vieyra MA, Masek BJ, Micheli LJ: Reflex sympathetic dystrophy in children. Clinical characteristics and follow-up of seventy patients. *J Bone Joint Surg Am* 1992;74(6):910-919.

57. Manderson EL, Ollivierre CO: Closed anatomic reduction of a juvenile tillaux fracture by dorsiflexion of the ankle. A case report. *Clin Orthop Relat Res* 1992;(276):262-266.

58. Feldman DS, Otsuka NY, Hedden DM: Extra-articular triplane fracture of the distal tibial epiphysis. *J Pediatr Orthop* 1995;15(4):479-481.

59. Schnetzler KA, Hoernschemeyer D: The pediatric triplane ankle fracture. *J Am Acad Orthop Surg* 2007;15(12):738-747.

Chapter 59

Pediatric Lower Extremity and Foot Disorders

Daniel (Dan) J. Miller, MD • Andrew G. Georgiadis, MD • Aaron J. Huser, DO • Jennifer C. Laine, MD

ABSTRACT

Lower extremity anomalies in children are a common reason for referral to an orthopaedic surgeon. These conditions may be congenital, developmental, or acquired in nature. A thoughtful diagnostic approach including elements from the patient's medical history, family history, and a carefully performed physical examination is diagnostic in most cases. Radiographs may help in equivocal cases and provide additional quantifiable measures that help direct treatment.

Differentiating between age-appropriate variations and pathologic conditions requires a thoughtful understanding of normal skeletal growth and development. Observation and familial reassurance is indicated in benign variations known to have a favorable natural history. Numerous treatment options exist for pathologic conditions expected to adversely affect patient health–related quality of life. Several of these modalities take advantage of physeal growth and/or the remarkable plasticity of the pediatric musculoskeletal system to achieve deformity correction.

Keywords: foot deformity; limb deficiency; limb deformity; rotational alignment

Dr. Miller or an immediate family member serves as a board member, owner, officer, or committee member of the Pediatric Orthopaedic Society of North America. Dr. Georgiadis or an immediate family member serves as a board member, owner, officer, or committee member of the Pediatric Orthopaedic Society of North America. Dr. Laine or an immediate family member serves as a board member, owner, officer, or committee member of the Pediatric Orthopaedic Society of North America. Neither Dr. Huser nor any immediate family member has received anything of value from or has stock or stock options held in a commercial company or institution related directly or indirectly to the subject of this chapter.

Introduction

Lower extremity anomalies represent a diverse set of conditions, ranging from normal physiologic variations to severe limb deficiencies. These may occur in isolation or be part of a multisegmental condition. Understanding and appreciating normal musculoskeletal growth and gait maturation is essential to proper diagnosis. A thoughtful evaluation and a patient-centered approach are critical to optimizing health-related quality of life while minimizing the cost, burden, and morbidity of treatment.

Rotational Variations

The rotational alignment of long bones influences lower extremity appearance, arc of motion, and foot progression angle. Torsional abnormalities resulting in deviations of foot progression (eg, "in-toeing" or "out-toeing") are a frequent source of caregiver anxiety and reason for referral.

The rotational orientation of a child's lower extremities changes considerably from birth to age 10. As such, determining normal versus pathologic abnormalities in torsion is contingent upon the child's age at the time of evaluation.

Femoral version refers to the angle of the femoral neck relative to the transcondylar axis of the distal femur. Femoral version can be inferred clinically by assessing hip range of motion with the patient prone and the pelvis level. A hip arc of motion skewed toward internal rotation relative to external rotation suggests a greater degree of anteversion. Femoral anteversion averages approximately 40° at birth and typically decreases to an average of 10° to 15° by 8 to 10 years of age.[1]

Tibial torsion is defined as the rotational relationship between the proximal and distal articular axes of the tibia around its longitudinal axis. Tibial torsion is typically quantified on physical examination by measuring a patient's thigh-foot angle while prone with the knee flexed 90°. Using this technique, tibial torsion averages approximately 5° internal at birth, changing to approximately 10° external by 8 years of age.[2]

Pediatrics

Evaluation of a perceived rotational abnormality in a child should begin with a thorough history and physical. It is important to elucidate the perceived influence of the rotational abnormality on the patient's functional status with respect to pain, balance, and function. Functional difficulties such as frequent tripping should be understood with knowledge of a typical evolution of gait. A gradual deterioration in gait over time should alert the provider as to the possibility of an underlying neuromuscular condition.

Physical examination of a perceived rotational abnormality should include evaluation of the patient's rotational profile as described by Staheli.[2] This includes measuring the patient's internal rotation of the hip, external rotation of the hip, thigh-foot angle, heel-bisector angle, and foot progression angle. The foot progression angle is the summation of the torsional contributions from the lower extremity segments (eg, femur, tibia, and foot). As such, a neutral foot progression angle does not exclude the presence of abnormalities in multiple segments. The combination of external tibial torsion with excessive femoral anteversion places increased stress at the patellofemoral joint and has been termed miserable malalignment syndrome.

Radiographs are not typically required for assessment of torsional profile and do little to change management. A CT scan is the most accurate means of quantifying torsion in children, but this exposes the child to significant, often unnecessary, radiation exposure.

Because the vast majority of rotational abnormalities in young children improve with growth, reassurance and observation are the mainstays of treatment. Abnormalities in torsional profile, such as increased femoral anteversion or tibial torsion, have not been associated with long-term problems such as osteoarthritis of the knee or hip.[3] Nonsurgical treatment of benign childhood torsional abnormalities (eg, physical therapy or orthoses) has not been shown to be effective and may be associated with adverse psychologic effects.[4] Surgical treatment of torsional abnormalities in otherwise healthy children should only be considered for severe abnormalities that are causing functional and/or cosmetic problems deemed unacceptable to patients and their families in children beyond 10 years of age. Surgical treatment of tibial torsion generally consists of a supramalleolar osteotomy, whereas surgical treatment of femoral rotational abnormalities can be considered through a variety of approaches.

Coronal Plane Variations of the Knee

Coronal plane variations of the knee are common. As with rotational variations, an understanding of the typical changes in lower extremity appearance with growth is critical to differentiating normal variations from pathologic conditions.

Newborns are born with mild genu varum (~10° to 15° of varus). This typically decreases to neutral tibial-femoral alignment by 18 to 24 months of age and progresses to genu valgum thereafter. Knee valgus reaches a maximum at around 3 years of age (10° to 15° of valgus), after which knee valgus generally decreases to adult norms (~7° to 8°) by age 6.[5] Developmental changes in coronal plane knee alignment are uncommon in late childhood or adolescence in the absence of physeal disturbance.

Evaluation of coronal plane abnormalities of the knee begins with a detailed history and physical. History should focus on the perceived change in alignment with growth, motor development, nutrition, and queries regarding potential prior insults to the physis (eg, trauma or infection). As with rotational abnormalities, the provider should try and assess how the knee alignment may be influencing the patient's status with respect to pain and function.

Physical examination should determine the location and acuteness of deformity. The patient's growth and stature should be scrutinized for any evidence of skeletal dysplasia. It is important to assess for the presence of concomitant rotational abnormalities and/or ligamentous laxity, both statically and during gait.

When pathologic coronal plane variations are suspected, radiographic evaluation should include full-length lower extremity radiographs with the patient standing (if possible). Imaging should be obtained with the patella facing forward to minimize distortion caused by torsional abnormalities. Radiographs allow the provider to evaluate for physeal disturbances and allow one to characterize the degree of limb length discrepancy, mechanical axis deviation, and location or locations of deformity.

Genu Valgum

Pathologic genu valgum may be idiopathic in nature or may be secondary to metabolic disorders, skeletal dysplasias, or injury to the lateral femoral and/or tibial physes. A medial metaphyseal proximal tibia fracture may also result in posttraumatic genu valgum (eg, Cozen phenomenon).[6] This phenomenon is important to recognize because it typically resolves spontaneously over time without treatment.

Idiopathic genu valgum is variably defined as greater than two standard deviations above age-matched controls. These deformities are commonly associated with laxity of the medial soft-tissue structures of the knee and hypoplasia of the lateral femoral condyle.

Nonsurgical modalities such as orthoses or physical therapy have not been demonstrated to change the natural history of genu valgum. Typical indications for surgical intervention in pathologic genu valgum include a clinically unacceptable deformity and/or lateral deviation of the mechanical axis to the outer 25% of the tibial plateau (or greater) in children older than 10 years. Surgical intervention can also be considered for patients <10 years of age with >20° of valgus.[7]

Surgical options for pathologic genu valgum includes medial hemiepiphysiodesis (temporary or permanent) or acute osteotomy. Goals of surgical treatment for pathologic genu valgum include restoration of a normal mechanical-axis and joint orientation while minimizing complications. Guided growth is dependent upon sufficient growth potential of the lateral-sided physes to correct deformity with time. As such, it is not a reliable option for patients who are at (or near) skeletal maturity, or in patients with pathologic lateral physes.

Genu Varum

As with genu valgum, distinguishing between normal variants and pathologic cases of genu varum is crucial. As described above, persistence of genu varum beyond age 2 is abnormal and warrants further evaluation.[5] Physiologic genu varum is associated with early walking, internal tibial torsion, and a positive family history. Physiologic genu varum demonstrates a broad, sweeping deformity, whereas pathologic forms are typified by an acute, focal apex of deformity. On imaging, physiologic genu varum tends to demonstrate gradual bowing in the distal femur and proximal tibia without physeal abnormalities. Physiologic genu varum frequently resolves spontaneously with growth and has a favorable natural history. As such, observation and reassurance is recommended.[8]

Numerous causes of pathologic genu varum exist in the pediatric population including metabolic bone diseases, skeletal dysplasias, and physeal growth disturbances. Pathologic idiopathic tibia vara (aka Blount disease) is characterized by an abrupt varus deformity at the proximal tibia. Although defined primarily on the basis of coronal plane deformity, Blount disease is frequently associated with internal rotation and flexion deformities as well. The specific etiology of Blount disease is unknown, but it is thought to be related to deceleration or arrest of growth in the posteromedial proximal tibia physis. Left untreated, Blount disease is associated with progressive coronal deformity, leg length discrepancy (in unilateral cases), gait abnormality, and premature arthritis.[9]

Blount disease is classified based on the age of onset with two forms predominating, the infantile type (typified by onset before age 5) and the adolescent form (onset after age 10). A third, juvenile, type has been described for patients aged 4 to 10 at diagnosis with intermediate findings.

Infantile Blount disease is bilateral in approximately 50% of cases. Imaging findings of infantile Blount disease include physeal changes and medial metaphyseal beaking (**Figure 1**). Infantile Blount disease may be associated with a valgus deformity of the distal femur. Distinguishing between physiologic genu varum and infantile Blount disease can be challenging. The metaphyseal-diaphyseal angle, described by Levine and Drennan,[10] provides prognostic value in equivocal cases. This angle is defined as the angle between the proximal tibial metaphysis and a line perpendicular to the long axis of the tibial diaphysis (**Figure 2**). A metaphyseal-diaphyseal angle ≤9° is associated with a 95% chance of spontaneous resolution, whereas angles ≥16° are with a 95% chance of pathologic and progressive tibia vara.[11] Infantile Blount disease is classified according to the Langenskiöld classification.[12]

Orthotic management aimed at unloading the medial tibial physis is considered for the young patient with mild, early, Blount disease (eg, age ≤3 years, Langenskiöld stage I or II), though the evidence for this is poor. For older children, or for advanced and/or progressive cases, surgical intervention is recommended. Surgical options include growth modulation or proximal tibial and fibular osteotomy. Hemiplateau elevation or physeal bar resection may be considered in severe cases. In infantile cases, the surgeon typically aims to overcorrect the deformity into valgus to prevent deformity recurrence.

Adolescent Blount disease is typically less severe than infantile forms and is more often unilateral. Adolescent Blount disease may be associated with varus deformities of the distal femur and/or valgus deformities of the distal tibia.[9] Recognition and concomitant treatment of these deformities is important to successful outcomes. Adolescent Blount disease is strongly associated with obesity. Because of the limited growth potential and

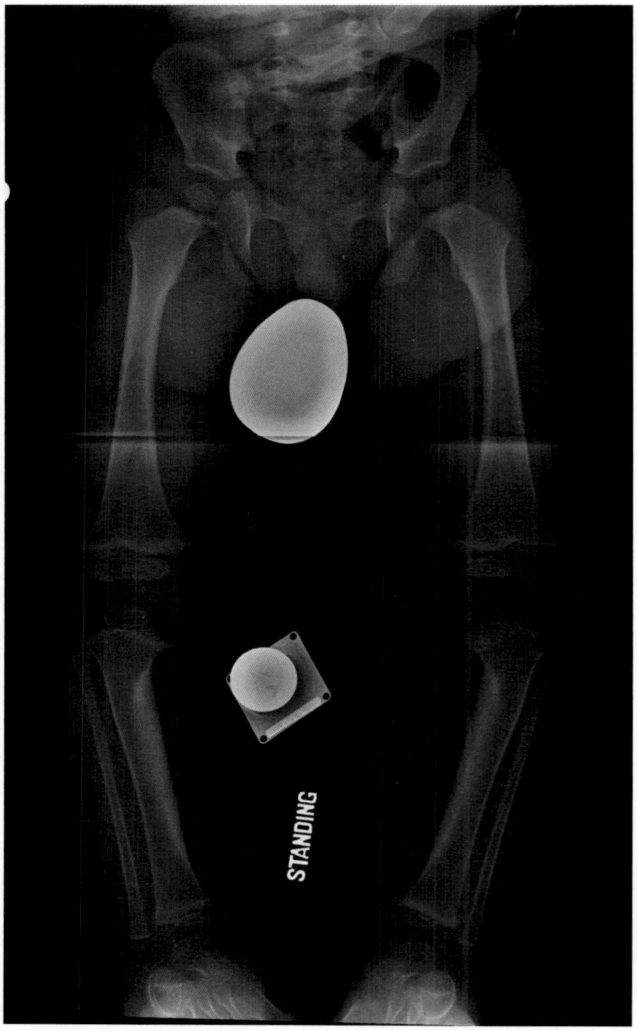

Figure 1 AP standing lower extremity radiograph of a patient with bilateral infantile Blount disease. Note the abrupt varus deformity at the proximal tibiae with associated physeal changes and medial metaphyseal beaking.

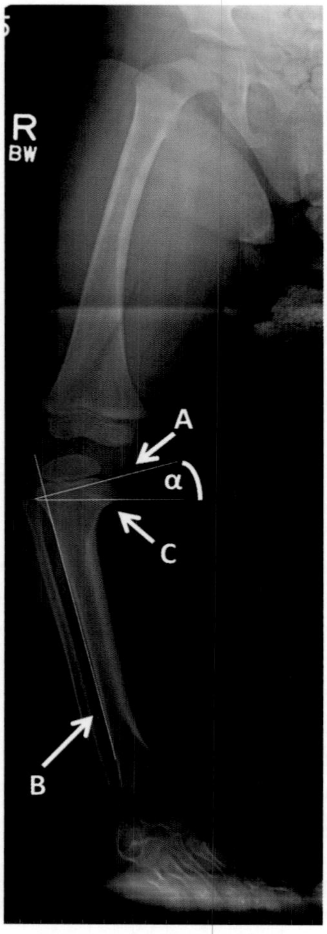

Figure 2 Standing PA radiograph of the right lower extremity with an illustration of the metaphyseal-diaphyseal angle of Levine and Drennan. This represents the angle subtended by a line perpendicular (A) to the longitudinal axis of the tibia (B) and a line connecting the medial and lateral metaphyseal beaks (C). In this patient, the metaphyseal-diaphyseal angle measured 17°, suggesting a high chance of deformity progression.

frequent association of obesity, nonsurgical management has no role in adolescent Blount care. Surgical options include growth modulation or a proximal tibial osteotomy with either acute or gradual correction.

Congenital Limb Deficiencies

Congenital lower limb deficiencies are rare, with an estimated incidence of 2 in 10,000.[13] Management of these complex and rare conditions benefits from a multidisciplinary approach. The primary goal of management is achieving a durable, functional lower extremity for the child while minimizing the morbidity of treatment.

Congenital Femoral Deficiency

Congenital femoral deficiency (CFD) includes the diagnoses of proximal femoral focal deficiency and congenitally short femur. CFD represents a wide spectrum of pathology ranging from a mild limb length discrepancy to severe limb shortening with an absent femoral head and/or acetabulum. CFD is associated with numerous anomalies including acetabular dysplasia, delayed ossification or pseudarthrosis of the femoral neck (**Figure 3**), femoral retroversion, coxa vara, hip flexion deformity, multidirectional knee instability, distal femoral lateral condyle hypoplasia, fibular hemimelia, dynamic ankle instability, shortened soft-tissues, and ray deficiency.[14]

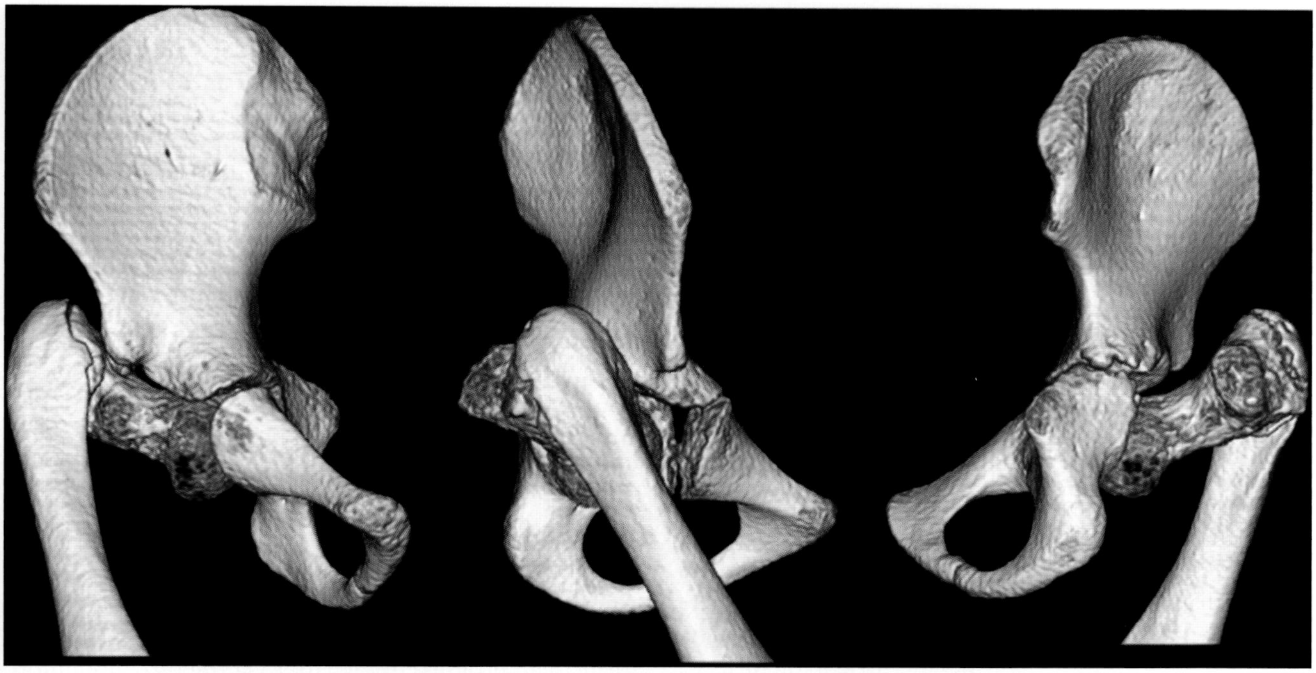

Figure 3 A CT-based three-dimensional reconstruction of a hip in a patient with congenital femoral deficiency. Note the pseudarthrosis of the femoral neck and coxa vara.

Management options of CFD and its associated deformities are broad and should be individualized to a patient's anatomy, functional status, and goals of care. Treatment may be as simple as supportive care for limb length difference or may include orthoses, corrective osteotomies of the femur, soft-tissue reconstructions, hemiepiphysiodesis, contralateral epiphysiodesis, limb lengthening, rotationplasty and/or amputation. Limb lengthening is considered if the projected limb length discrepancy is ≤20 cm at maturity in the presence of a stable and functional hip and foot. In general, proximal femoral abnormalities and/or acetabular dysplasia should be corrected before initiating lengthening. For patients with discrepancies predicted to be ≥20 cm, a foot-ablating amputation or rotationplasty is an alternative surgical option.[15]

Fibular Hemimelia

Fibular hemimelia (FH), also known as congenital fibular deficiency, is the most common long bone deficiency. Although the name fibular hemimelia is used to describe the hypoplastic or aplastic fibula, this condition is associated with numerous other conditions of functional import including limb length discrepancy, knee instability, genu valgum, tarsal coalitions, ankle instability, absent rays of the foot, CFD, and upper extremity anomalies.[16,17] FH is also associated with anterior or anteromedial bowing of the tibia (**Figure 4**) thought secondary to a tethering effect of the fibular anlage.[16,17]

As with CFD, numerous treatment options exist for FH and these should be tailored to the patient and the family's goals of care. Treatment of FH is driven primarily based on the expected degree of limb length inequality at maturity, the stability of the foot and

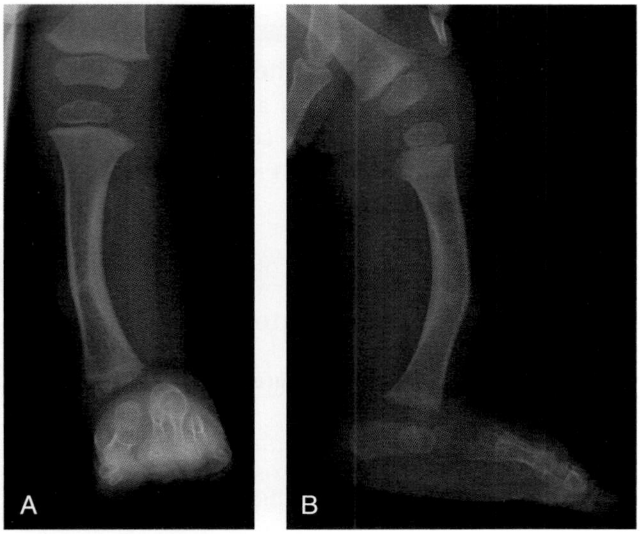

Figure 4 AP (**A**) and lateral (**B**) radiographs of a patient with fibular hemimelia and associated anteromedial bowing of the tibia.

ankle, and the functional ability of the upper extremities.[16] Patients with mild limb length inequalities may be managed with epiphysiodesis with limb lengthening available for patients with more substantial inequalities. Amputation (Boyd or Syme type) and prosthetic reconstruction are considered in cases of a poorly functioning foot and ankle that is not amenable to reconstruction. Limb salvage and foot reconstruction should be strongly considered if upper extremity function is compromised in order for the foot to substitute for upper extremity prehension in these cases.[16]

Tibial Hemimelia

Tibial hemimelia (TH) is the rarest of the three congenital lower limb deficiencies. TH has been found to have both autosomal dominant and autosomal recessive inheritance patterns.[18] TH has a variety of presentations ranging from mild shortening of the tibia to complete absence of the tibia. Aside from the tibial deficiency, associated deformities may include absent quadriceps muscle, absent patella, knee flexion deformity, knee instability, ankle instability, talipes equinovarus, duplication of fibula, and duplication or deficiency of the tarsals, metatarsals, and/or phalanges.[19,20]

Treatment of TH and its associated deformities may include tibial lengthening, transfer of the fibula to the distal or proximal tibia, ankle arthrodesis, patelloplasty, soft-tissue lengthening, contralateral epiphysiodesis, ipsilateral fibular epiphysiodesis, ipsilateral tibial epiphysiodesis, Syme amputation, below-knee amputation, or through-knee amputation.[19,20]

Tibial Bowing

Posteromedial Bowing of the Tibia

Posteromedial tibial bowing is a congenital deformity which has traditionally been considered self-limited. Bowing commonly presents in combination with an ipsilateral calcaneovalgus foot, itself exaggerating the appearance of apex posteromedial deformity. Treatment is initially expectant, with most foot and tibial deformity resolving in the first year of life.[21] Continued surveillance should continue until skeletal maturity to fully assess residual deformity and limb length discrepancy (**Table 1**).

If deformity has not corrected by age 4, it is unlikely to undergo remodeling thereafter. Angular deformity of the tibia or foot can be treated with guided growth of the distal tibia, oblique plane osteotomy, or multifocal osteotomy.[22] If length discrepancy exists, a lengthening procedure may be incorporated into the angular correction. Recent series suggest that a significant proportion of congenital posteromedial tibial bowing may not remodel with expectant management as previously reported.[23]

Anterolateral Bowing and Congenital Pseudarthrosis of the Tibia

Anterolateral bowing of the tibia exists on a continuum with congenital pseudarthrosis of the tibia (CPT). The former can progress to the latter via fracture, nonunion, and pseudarthrosis. There is a strong association with neurofibromatosis type 1 with CPT (50% of cases).

Prefracture management can include bracing treatment, guided growth, or prophylactic allogeneic grafting bypassing the prefracture segment. Surgical management of fractured or pseudarthrosed tibiae can include intramedullary fixation, external fixation, or a combination.[24] Four-in-one osteosynthesis (a single union of two tibial and two fibular segments) has been proposed with reportedly high union rates.[25] There is not clear evidence for the role of recombinant human bone morphogenetic proteins as adjuncts[26] or which surgical or patient factors truly affect the outcome of surgical CPT treatment.[27] Union can be achieved with similar outcomes whether surgery is undertaken before or after age 3.[28] The maintenance of fibular length is now understood to affect functional outcome of treatment, particularly of the foot and ankle.[29]

Table 1

Tibial Bowing and Associated Features

	Features	Associations
Posteromedial bowing	Often self-limited, may result in limb length discrepancy.	Calcaneovalgus foot
Anterolateral bowing	High risk for fracture and pseudarthrosis; bone is often pathologic	Neurofibromatosis type I (50%) Fibrous dysplasia (15%)
Anteromedial bowing	Often associated with fibular hemimelia/deficiency	Ipsilateral femoral deformity (PFFD, coxa vara)

Foot Conditions

Congenital Vertical Talus

Congenital vertical talus (CVT) is a rare, congenital rigid flatfoot deformity often described as a rocker-bottom foot. It is characterized by dorsolateral dislocation of the navicular on the talus, ankle equinus, hindfoot valgus, and forefoot dorsiflexion and abduction. The incidence of CVT is approximately 1 per 10,000 live births. Approximately 50% of cases are associated with underlying neuromuscular or genetic conditions or syndromes.[30] Frequent associations include myelomeningocele, distal arthrogryposis, and chromosomal abnormalities. Because of these common associations, a thorough physical examination is essential. If an underlying cause is suspected, MRI of the spine, neurology referral and/or genetics referral should be considered.

CVT should be differentiated from a number of other conditions, including the calcaneovalgus foot and oblique talus. Often, clinical examination alone can differentiate CVT from calcaneovalgus, based on the presence or absence of rigid hindfoot equinus, respectively. Plain radiographs (AP and three lateral views: neutral, dorsiflexion, and plantar flexion) can be used to aid in the diagnosis of CVT and to differentiate it from oblique talus. On a plantar flexion lateral radiograph, the talonavicular joint reduces with an oblique talus and remains dislocated in CVT (**Figure 5**). Owing to the cartilaginous nature of the newborn midfoot, it can be difficult to visualize the pathologic anatomy. The talocalcaneal angle, the tibiocalcaneal angle, and the lateral talar axis–first metatarsal base angle can be useful radiographic measurements. Dynamic ultrasonography can also be used to assist in diagnosis.[31]

Without treatment, the foot deformity persists or worsens and can lead to significant pain, gait dysfunction, and difficulty with shoe wear. Similar to the treatment of clubfoot, the standard approach to CVT treatment has transitioned from extensive surgical release to a more minimally invasive treatment course. This technique, often called the Dobbs method, consists of serial manipulations and casting, pinning the talonavicular joint, and percutaneous Achilles tenotomy.[32] Once the postsurgical cast has been removed, the child is then transitioned to a brace/orthoses. The Dobbs method has been shown to be superior compared with extensive surgical release with respect to pain and foot flexibility.[33] This is now the recommended first-line treatment in both idiopathic and teratologic cases.[34]

Clubfoot

Clubfoot, or talipes equinovarus (TEV), is a complex congenital limb deformity characterized by cavus, forefoot adductus, hindfoot varus, and equinus, as well as calf atrophy and shortness of the foot (**Figure 6**). The diagnosis is typically made at birth on physical examination, though the features of the foot position can be observed on prenatal ultrasonography. Incidence is estimated at approximately 1 per 1,000 live births, affecting males twice as commonly as females.[35] Approximately 50% of cases are bilateral. TEV is most commonly

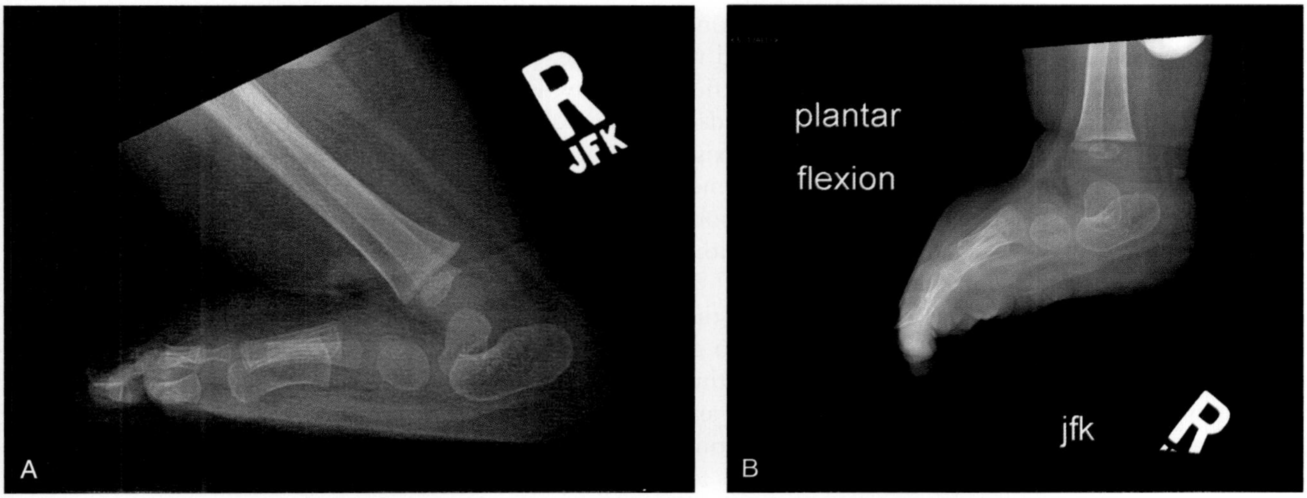

Figure 5 Dorsiflexion (**A**) and plantar flexion (**B**) lateral radiographs of an infant with congenital vertical talus. Note that the hindfoot remains in equinus despite ankle dorsiflexion (**A**) and that the talus remains vertical and the talonavicular joint remains dislocated despite plantar flexion (**B**).

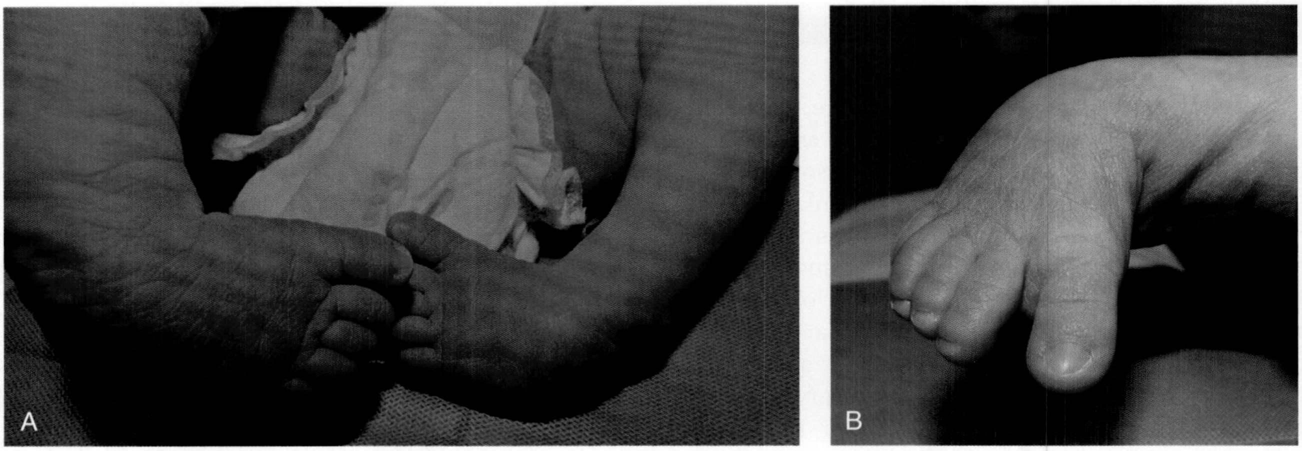

Figure 6 Clinical photographs show bilateral idiopathic clubfoot in a newborn. **A**, The adductus and varus can be appreciated. **B**, Looking at the right foot from the medial aspect, the equinus, cavus, and medial crease are more apparent.

isolated and idiopathic, but can also be associated with genetic or neuromuscular disorders. The exact etiology of TEV is unknown and is likely multifactorial, involving both environmental and genetic factors.

Without treatment, TEV can lead to significant foot dysfunction, pain, and morbidity. The most common treatment for both idiopathic and teratologic TEV is the Ponseti method. This consists of weekly manipulations and serial long leg casting, followed by percutaneous Achilles tenotomy in most patients. Randomized, controlled, blinded study has shown that infants who are given either an oral sucrose solution or milk during manipulation and casting have a decreased pain response.[36] Traditional recommendations have been to start treatment as early as possible in the newborn period. Recent study has challenged this thinking. Patients initiating treatment at ≤26 weeks showed no significant difference as a function of age at presentation for treatment with respect to number of casts needed, skin problems, or early relapse.[37] Controversy exists whether the Achilles tenotomy should be performed in the outpatient clinic setting or the operating room, though the outpatient setting has been associated with a lower complication rate and decreased cost.[38]

After the deformity is corrected through casting +/− Achilles tenotomy, patients are transitioned to an abduction foot orthosis. The orthosis is worn full-time for three months and then part-time, often at night and during naps. The appropriate duration of part-time wear is controversial, with typical recommendations for brace-wear falling between 2 and 4 years.[39]

Success rates for achieving initial correction using the Ponseti method are high, but relapse is common within the first 5 years, with reported rates ranging from 26% to 48%.[40] Early relapse, especially before the age of 2 years, has been associated with poor brace compliance.[41] Actual brace use, as recorded by temperature sensors, has been shown to be lower than prescribed brace use and parent-reported use, and mean brace-wear was lower in patients who experienced early relapse.[42]

Early relapse is often addressed with manipulation and casting, with or without repeat tenotomy, followed by bracing treatment. Anterior tibial tendon transfer (ATTT) to the third cuneiform is a frequently used procedure in patients 2.5 years or older to address dynamic supination, often with preoperative casting.[40] Nearly 30% of TEV patients undergo ATTT.[43] Additional procedures used to address relapse include posterior release, plantar fascial lengthening, and midfoot osteotomy. Extensive posteromedial release and correction using circular external fixation are reserved for severe deformities that have not corrected with less-invasive means. The Ponseti method has been shown to be superior at long-term follow-up in comparison with extensive release with respect to range of motion, strength, pain and arthritis.[44]

Tarsal Coalition

Tarsal coalition represents an abnormal fusion between two bones of the hindfoot or midfoot. The embryologic precursor is considered to be a failure of mesenchymal cell segmentation, and symptomatic coalitions can be fibrous or osseous.

Coalitions can occur between any two adjacent bones, but most commonly affected are the talocalcaneal

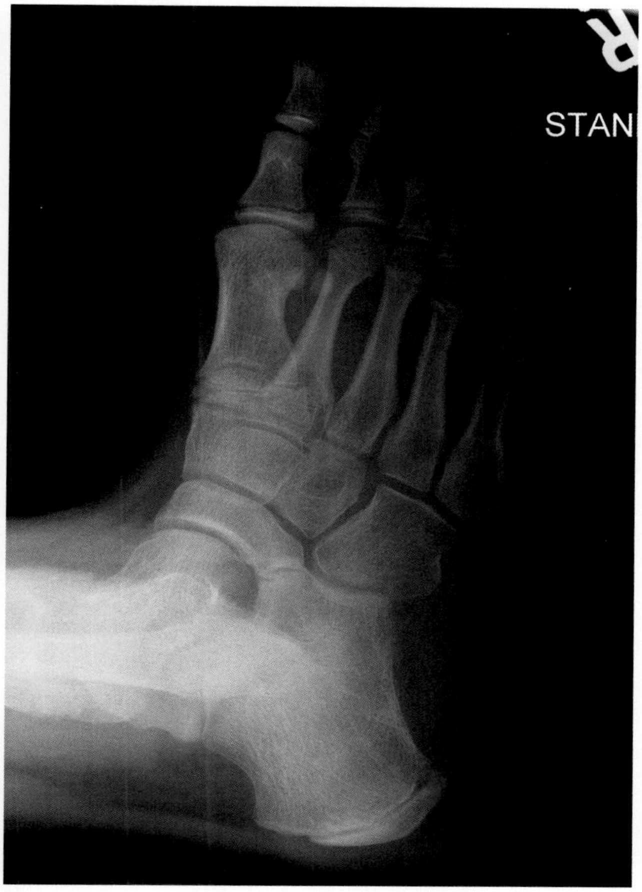

Figure 7 Oblique radiograph of a right foot with a calcaneonavicular coalition.

(TCC) and the calcaneonavicular articulations (CNC, **Figure 7**). Clinical presentation is characteristically that of a painful adolescent flatfoot with decreased or absent subtalar motion and/or recurrent ankle sprains. Both CNCs and TCCs can be identified by surface palpation in some cases. Radiographic identification of a CNC is best achieved on an oblique plain radiographic projection of the foot, and a TCC coalition can be viewed on the lateral projection in 50% of cases. If surgical resection is planned, many authors advocate for cross-sectional imaging for planning by MRI or three-dimensional CT.

Initial management of tarsal coalition may consist of activity modification, nonsteroidal anti-inflammatories, orthotic use, and/or a period of immobilization. If nonsurgical management fails, coalition resection and interposition of a non-osteoinductive material is the recommended treatment. Open approaches are traditional, although limited endoscopic results have been reported in TCC with comparable outcomes.[45] Interposition material can be local muscle, autogenous fat, or bone wax. A recent study demonstrated a higher rate of coalition reossification and worse functional outcomes with muscle interposition compared with bone wax or fat.[46] Arthrodesis is considered for advanced coalitions that fail attempts at resection.

Cavovarus Foot

A cavovarus foot represents a multisegmental deformity characterized by a plantarflexed first ray, elevated medial longitudinal arch, and hindfoot varus. Clinical assessment should include a focused history and physical examination evaluating for an underlying neurogenic or intraspinal etiology to the cavovarus, particularly if findings are unilateral and/or rapidly progressive. Hereditary motor and sensory neuropathies (eg, Charcot-Marie-Tooth disease) are classically associated with progressive deformities.

On physical examination, plantar callosities under the first and fifth metatarsal heads are common, as is plantar intrinsic wasting. The medial longitudinal arch is elevated when viewed from the side, and the heel is inverted on standing when viewed from behind. Viewed from anterior, a peek-a-boo heel can signify hindfoot varus. Multiple clinical methods have been described to assess the flexibility of the hindfoot, including the Coleman block test, oblique block test, and the prone Price and Mubarak tests.[47] If lateral foot elevation and first ray plantar flexion (achieved by all examination maneuvers) succeeds in everting the hindfoot, it connotes that the hindfoot deformity is driven by the plantarflexed first ray (aka forefoot driven hindfoot varus). As such, the hindfoot deformity should correct with treatment of the midfoot/forefoot plantar flexion.

Radiographic assessment is with AP and lateral weight-bearing foot radiographs. Quantitative segmental foot alignment has been described with normative values published for all major radiographic measures.[48] Among the many metrics, hindfoot varus can be assessed using the AP-talocalcaneal angle and midfoot cavus by the lateral talar–first metatarsal angle. Foot supination can be quantified by metatarsal overlap.

Initial management includes an orthotic that recesses the first ray and elevates the entire lateral foot, and is reserved for deformities with flexible hindfoot varus. Surgical treatment can include osteotomies of the areas of fixed deformity (forefoot, midfoot, or hindfoot), and tendon transfers in neurogenic etiologies.[49]

Summary

Evaluation of pediatric lower extremity anomalies requires a careful approach and a thorough understanding of musculoskeletal growth and development. Observation and reassurance are indicated in conditions known to have a favorable natural history. Treatment, in the form of manipulation, bracing treatment, and/or surgery can have a substantial effect on patient quality of life for anomalies known to have deleterious effects on comfort and/or function.

Key Study Points

- Rotational variations of the lower extremity are typically managed with observation and reassurance, whereas nonphysiologic significant lower limb coronal angular deformities are treated with growth modulation or osteotomy.
- Congenital limb deficiencies are complex, multistructural deformities that benefit from a comprehensive approach aimed at achieving a stable, functional limb.
- Congenital vertical talus and clubfoot are congenital foot deformities best managed with early serial casting and minimally invasive procedures. Long-term orthosis use is critical to preventing deformity recurrence.

Annotated References

1. Lincoln TL, Suen PW: Common rotational variations in children. *J Am Acad Orthop Surg* 2003;11(5):312-320.
2. Staheli LT: Rotational problems in children. *Instr Course Lect* 1994;43:199-209.
3. Weinberg DS, Park PJ, Morris WZ, Liu RW: Femoral version and tibial torsion are not associated with hip or knee arthritis in a large osteological collection. *J Pediatr Orthop* 2017;37(2):e120-e128.

   The authors examined 1158 cadaveric tibiae and femora from a large osteological collection. Femoral version and tibial torsion were measured for each specimen. The amount of degenerative joint disease of the hip and knee for each specimen was graded and correlated with torsional measures. Neither tibial torsion nor femoral version was a predictor of hip or knee arthritis on regression analysis. Level of evidence: not applicable.
4. Driano AN, Staheli L, Staheli LT: Psychosocial development and corrective shoewear use in childhood. *J Pediatr Orthop* 1998;18(3):346-349.
5. Salenius P, Vankka E: The development of the tibiofemoral angle in children. *J Bone Joint Surg Am* 1975;57(2):259-261.
6. Jackson DW, Cozen L: Genu valgum as a complication of proximal tibial metaphyseal fractures in children. *J Bone Joint Surg Am* 1971;53(8):1571-1578.
7. White GR, Mencio GA: Genu valgum in children: Diagnostic and therapeutic alternatives. *J Am Acad Orthop Surg* 1995;3(5):275-283.
8. Brooks WC, Gross RH: Genu varum in children: Diagnosis and treatment. *J Am Acad Orthop Surg* 1995;3(6):326-335.
9. Birch JG: Blount disease. *J Am Acad Orthop Surg* 2013;21(7):408-418.
10. Levine AM, Drennan JC: Physiological bowing and tibia vara. The metaphyseal-diaphyseal angle in the measurement of bowleg deformities. *J Bone Joint Surg Am* 1982;64(8):1158-1163.
11. Feldman MD, Schoenecker PL: Use of the metaphyseal-diaphyseal angle in the evaluation of bowed legs. *J Bone Joint Surg Am* 1993;75(11):1602-1609.
12. Langenskioeld A, Riska EB: Tibia vara (osteochondrosis deformans tibiae): A survey of seventy-one cases. *J Bone Joint Surg Am* 1964;46:1405-1420.
13. Syvanen J, Nietosvaara Y, Ritvanen A, Koskimies E, Kauko T, Helenius I: High risk for major nonlimb anomalies associated with lower-limb deficiency: A population-based study. *J Bone Joint Surg Am* 2014;96(22):1898-1904.
14. Lange DR, Schoenecker PL, Baker CL: Proximal femoral focal deficiency: Treatment and classification in forty-two cases. *Clin Orthop Relat Res* 1978;(135):15-25.
15. Westberry DE, Davids JR: Proximal focal femoral deficiency (PFFD): Management options and controversies. *Hip Int* 2009;19 suppl 6:S18-S25.
16. Birch JG, Lincoln TL, Mack PW, Birch CM: Congenital fibular deficiency: A review of thirty years' experience at one institution and a proposed classification system based on clinical deformity. *J Bone Joint Surg Am* 2011;93(12):1144-1151.
17. Hamdy RC, Makhdom AM, Saran N, Birch J: Congenital fibular deficiency. *J Am Acad Orthop Surg* 2014;22(4):246-255.
18. Richieri-Costa A, Ferrareto I, Masiero D, da Silva CR: Tibial hemimelia: Report on 37 new cases, clinical and genetic considerations. *Am J Med Genet* 1987;27(4):867-884.
19. Paley D: Tibial hemimelia: New classification and reconstructive options. *J Child Orthop* 2016;10(6):529-555.

    This is a recent review article that discusses the etiology, presentation, and treatment options for tibial hemimelia. The author proposes a new classification to guide management and surgical reconstruction of these challenging cases. Level of evidence: V.
20. Schoenecker PL, Capelli AM, Millar EA, et al: Congenital longitudinal deficiency of the tibia. *J Bone Joint Surg Am* 1989;71(2):278-287.

21. Shah HH, Doddabasappa SN, Joseph B: Congenital posteromedial bowing of the tibia: A retrospective analysis of growth abnormalities in the leg. *J Pediatr Orthop B* 2009;18(3):120-128.

22. Napiontek M, Shadi M: Congenital posteromedial bowing of the tibia and fibula: Treatment option by multilevel osteotomy. *J Pediatr Orthop B* 2014;23(2):130-134.

23. Wright J, Hill RA, Eastwood DM, Hashemi-Nejad A, Calder P, Tennant S: Posteromedial bowing of the tibia: A benign condition or a case for limb reconstruction? *J Child Orthop* 2018;12(2):187-196.

This study is a retrospective review of 38 patients who presented with posteromedial bowing of the tibia. At a mean follow-up of 78 months, 20/38 patients (53%) were indicated for surgery for limb length discrepancy and/or residual tibial deformity. The authors noted that spontaneous deformity correction of the tibia was greatest in the first year of life but limited after 4 years. Level of evidence: IV.

24. O'Donnell C, Foster J, Mooney R, Beebe C, Donaldson N, Heare T: Congenital pseudarthrosis of the tibia. *JBJS Rev* 2017;5(4):e3.

This is a recent review article that discusses the history, pathophysiology, presentation, and management options of congenital pseudarthrosis of the tibia. Level of evidence: V.

25. Choi IH, Lee SJ, Moon HJ, et al: "4-in-1 osteosynthesis" for atrophic-type congenital pseudarthrosis of the tibia. *J Pediatr Orthop* 2011;31(6):697-704.

26. Richards BS, Anderson TD: rhBMP-2 and intramedullary fixation in congenital pseudarthrosis of the tibia. *J Pediatr Orthop* 2018;38(4):230-238.

This study is a single-center, retrospective review of 21 patients with CPT treated with intramedullary fixation, autogenous bone grafting, and topical rhBMP-2. Mean follow-up was 7.2 years. Bony union was achieved following the index surgery in 16/21 of patients (76%) at an average of 6.6 months postoperatively. Of the five patients who did not achieve osseous healing after the index surgery, three eventually underwent amputation. Level of evidence: IV.

27. Shah H, Joseph B, Nair BVS, et al: What factors influence union and refracture of congenital pseudarthrosis of the tibia? A multicenter long-term study. *J Pediatr Orthop* 2018;38(6):e332-e337.

This study is a multicenter, retrospective review of 119 patients with CPT treated surgically and followed to skeletal maturity. Primary osseous healing occurred in 102/119 of children (86%); however, by skeletal maturity, only 82/119 (69%) remained soundly united. Failure of primary union was associated with BMP use (OR 3.9, $P = 0.042$). A combination of the Ilizarov technique and intramedullary nailing was associated with unsound union at maturity (OR 6.2, $P = 0.026$). Level of evidence: IV.

28. Liu Y, Mei H, Zhu G, et al: Congenital pseudarthrosis of the tibia in children: Should we defer surgery until 3 years old? *J Pediatr Orthop B* 2018;27(1):17-25.

This single-center, case-control study evaluated clinical and biomechanical outcomes of 24 patients with CPT treated with an Ilizarov technique. Mean score of the American Orthopaedic Foot & Ankle Society (AOFAS) ankle-hindfoot scale was 89.9 and the mean score of the Oxford Ankle Foot Questionnaire (OAFQ) was 42.8. When compared with healthy control subjects, patients with CPT demonstrated abnormal biomechanics including slower walking speeds, diminished ankle push-off power, and delayed time to heel-rise. Level of evidence: III.

29. Seo SG, Lee DY, Kim YS, Yoo WJ, Cho TJ, Choi IH: Foot and ankle function at maturity after ilizarov treatment for atrophic-type congenital pseudarthrosis of the tibia: A comprehensive outcome comparison with normal controls. *J Bone Joint Surg Am* 2016;98(6):490-498.

This study is a single-center, retrospective review of 42 patients with CPT. The authors sought to determine if age at the time of treatment was associated with outcome. They divided the cohort into two groups based on their age at the time of index surgery, group A (<3 years) and group B (>3 years). There was no significant difference in primary bone union between patients in group A and group B (97% vs 92%, $P > 0.05$). Limb length discrepancy was less frequent in group A compared with group B (41% vs 77%, $P = 0.033$). The authors conclude that there is no advantage to deferring surgical intervention in patients with established CPT. Level of evidence: III.

30. Jacobsen ST, Crawford AH: Congenital vertical talus. *J Pediatr Orthop* 1983;3(3):306-310.

31. Supakul N, Loder RT, Karmazyn B: Dynamic US study in the evaluation of infants with vertical or oblique talus deformities. *Pediatr Radiol* 2013;43(3):376-380.

32. Dobbs MB, Purcell DB, Nunley R, Morcuende JA: Early results of a new method of treatment for idiopathic congenital vertical talus. *J Bone Joint Surg Am* 2006;88(6):1192-1200.

33. Yang JS, Dobbs MB: Treatment of congenital vertical talus: Comparison of minimally invasive and extensive soft-tissue release procedures at minimum five-year follow-up. *J Bone Joint Surg Am* 2015;97(16):1354-1365.

34. Chan Y, Selvaratnam V, Garg N: A comparison of the Dobbs method for correction of idiopathic and teratological congenital vertical talus. *J Child Orthop* 2016;10(2):93-99.

The authors performed a retrospective comparison of idiopathic and teratological cases of CVT treated with the Dobbs method. Clinical and radiographic outcomes of 10 children (18 feet) were reviewed at a mean follow-up of 53 months. Sixty-seven percent of feet were successfully corrected and had significant radiographic improvement at final follow-up compared with initial radiographs. There was a higher recurrence rate in the teratological group, though this was not statistically significant. Level of evidence: IV.

35. Wynne-Davies R: Genetic and environmental factors in the etiology of talipes equinovarus. *Clin Orthop Relat Res* 1972;84:9-13.

36. Milbrandt T, Kryscio R, Muchow R, Walker J, Talwalkar V, Iwinski H Jr: Oral sucrose for pain relief during clubfoot casting: A double-blinded randomized controlled trial. *J Pediatr Orthop* 2018;38(8):430-435.

This is a randomized double-blinded controlled trial of 33 patients with idiopathic TEV. Each of the 131 casting events was randomized to giving a bottle with: sucrose solution, water, or milk. The sucrose solution and milk were associated with a decreased pain response during casting. The sucrose solution had a more lasting effect in the post–casting period. Level of evidence: I.

37. Zionts LE, Sangiorgio SN, Cooper SD, Ebramzadeh E: Does clubfoot treatment need to begin as soon as possible? *J Pediatr Orthop* 2016;36(6):558-564.

This is a prospective study of 176 patients with idiopathic TEV with a minimum of 1 year follow-up. Age at presentation for treatment was correlated with the early treatment course. All patients began treatment by 26 weeks, with a median age of 4 weeks. An increased rate of cast slippage was noted in younger patients. No other difference in early treatment was noted based on age. Level of evidence: II.

38. Hedrick B, Gettys FK, Richards S, Muchow RD, Jo CH, Abbott MD: Percutaneous heel cord release for clubfoot: A retrospective, multicentre cost analysis. *J Child Orthop* 2018;12(3):273-278.

This is a retrospective chart review of 382 patients who underwent percutaneous Achilles tenotomy for idiopathic TEV either in the outpatient clinic setting or in the operating room. The clinical setting was associated with significantly lower cost, and there were no complications in the outpatient clinic group. Level of evidence: III.

39. Hosseinzadeh P, Kiebzak GM, Dolan L, Zionts LE, Morcuende J: Management of clubfoot relapses with the Ponseti method: Results of a survey of the POSNA members. *J Pediatr Orthop* 2017;25(3):195-203.

This study reports the results of a survey on TEV relapse management sent to the members of the Pediatric Orthopedic Society of North America (POSNA). Ninety-eight percent of respondents reported using the Ponseti method, but there were wide variations in the recommendations for duration of bracing and management of relapse. Level of evidence: not applicable.

40. Hosseinzadeh P, Kelly DM, Zionts LE: Management of the relapsed clubfoot following treatment using the Ponseti method. *J Am Acad Orthop Surg* 2017;25(3):195-203.

This is a recent review article highlighting the causes, clinical presentation, and treatment options for TEV relapse. Level of evidence: V.

41. Mahan ST, Spencer SA, May CJ, Prete VI, Kasser JR: Clubfoot relapse: Does presentation differ based on age at initial relapse? *J Child Orthop* 2017;11(5):367-372.

This study is a retrospective review of 70 patients with TEV recurrence. Over half (56%) of patients had initial relapse before the age of 2 years. In this early relapse group, the brace adherence was 28% compared with 74% adherence in the group with relapse after age 2 years. Level of evidence: IV.

42. Sangiorgio SN, Ho NC, Morgan RD, Ebramzadeh E, Zionts LE: The objective measurement of brace-use adherence in the treatment of idiopathic clubfoot. *J Bone Joint Surg Am* 2016;98(19):1598-1605.

Brace compliance was evaluated using wireless temperature sensors in 48 patients over a 3-month period. Actual brace use was significantly lower than recommended brace use and parent-reported brace use. Duration of brace use per day was significantly lower in the patients who relapsed during the study period compared with those patients who did not relapse. Level of evidence: III.

43. Zionts LE, Jew MH, Bauer KL, Ebramzadeh E, Sangiorgio SN: How many patients who have a clubfoot treated using the Ponseti method are likely to undergo a tendon transfer? *J Pediatr Orthop* 2018;38(7):382-387.

This is a prospective case series of 137 patients with idiopathic TEV who underwent the Ponseti method of treatment with minimum age at final follow-up of 2.5 years. Nearly 25% underwent ATTT. Based on survivorship analysis, there is a 29% probability of undergoing ATT by age 6 years. The most significant factor associated with need for ATTT was parent-reported nonadherence to bracing protocol. Level of evidence: III.

44. Smith PA, Kuo KN, Graf AN, et al: Long-term results of comprehensive clubfoot release versus the Ponseti method: Which is better? *Clin Orthop Relat Res* 2014;472(4):1281-1290.

45. Knorr J, Soldado F, Menendez ME, Domenech P, Sanchez M, Sales de Gauzy J: Arthroscopic talocalcaneal coalition resection in children. *Arthroscopy* 2015;31(12):2417-2423.

46. Masquijo J, Allende V, Torres-Gomez A, Dobbs MB: Fat graft and bone wax interposition provides better functional outcomes and lower reossification rates than extensor digitorum brevis after calcaneonavicular coalition resection. *J Pediatr Orthop* 2017;37(7):e427-e431.

This is a multicenter case-control study that sought to compare the efficacy of three interposition materials (fat graft, bone wax, or local extensor digitorum brevis muscle) at preventing reossifcation following calcaneonavicular coalition resection. It included 48 patients and 56 feet. Coalition reossification was significantly more common with interposition of local muscle (6/15, 40%) compared with fat (1/23, 4%) or bone wax (1/18, 6%), P =0.004). Interposition of local muscle was associated with inferior American Orthopaedic Foot and Ankle Society (AOFAS) functional scores as well. Level of evidence: III.

47. Georgiadis AG, Spiegel DA, Baldwin KD: The cavovarus foot in hereditary motor and sensory neuropathies. *JBJS Rev* 2015;3(12):e4.

48. Davids JR, Gibson TW, Pugh LI: Quantitative segmental analysis of weight-bearing radiographs of the foot and ankle for children: Normal alignment. *J Pediatr Orthop* 2005;25(6):769-776.

49. Mubarak SJ, Van Valin SE: Osteotomies of the foot for cavus deformities in children. *J Pediatr Orthop* 2009;29(3):294-299.

Chapter 60

Pediatric Athletic Injuries

Allison E. Crepeau, MD • Jennifer M. Weiss, MD

ABSTRACT

Pediatric athletic injuries are on the rise because of a number of factors including early sports specialization and year-round play. Some of these injuries are overuse-type injuries, such as Little Leaguer's shoulder, Little Leaguer's elbow, and osteochondritis dissecans of the knee and ankle. Many of the injuries are acute and can include anterior shoulder instability, medial epicondyle fractures, anterior cruciate ligament tears, meniscus tears. Some injuries, such as discoid meniscus and patellar instability, may have both congenital and acute components.

Keywords: ankle; elbow; hip; knee; shoulder; sports injuries

Introduction

Sports-related injuries in youth athletes have become increasingly more common. The increase has been attributed to early sports specialization and year-round play. There has been a rise in both acute and overuse injuries in this population, and procedures previously reserved for college or professional athletes are now commonly performed in youth athletes.

Little Leaguer's Shoulder

Little Leaguer's shoulder (LLS) is an overuse injury that occurs in skeletally immature overhead athletes and causes epiphysiolysis of the proximal humeral physis. It primarily affects male baseball players aged 12 to 14 years who pitch, but it can also be seen in catchers, tennis players, and female pitchers playing in baseball leagues. The incidence of LLS has increased significantly over the last 14 years.[1]

It is caused by increased stress at the proximal humeral physis due to repetitive forces seen during throwing. Risk factors for physeal stress at the proximal humerus even in asymptomatic Little Leaguers include year-round play and single-sport specialization.[2]

Symptoms include shoulder or upper arm pain with throwing, shoulder weakness, and occasionally mechanical symptoms or pain at rest. Physical examination often reveals tenderness over the proximal humeral physis, limited range of motion (ROM; specifically GIRD—glenohumeral internal rotation deficit), and possibly weakness. 13% of patients diagnosed with LLS also have concomitant elbow pain.[1]

Imaging should include standard plain radiographs of the shoulder with an external rotation AP view to assess for changes to the proximal humeral physis (**Figure 1**). Comparison radiographs of the contralateral shoulder can help with diagnosis. Classic findings include widening of the physis, adjacent sclerosis, or metaphyseal fragmentation. MRI will show similar edema at the proximal humeral physis but is often not needed for diagnosis.

The mainstay of treatment includes rest from throwing until symptoms resolve. Additionally, physical therapy can be used to address any ROM and strength deficits. Therapy is useful in patients with GIRD to work on stretching the posterior capsule. In persistent or recurrent situations, players may be advised to consider position changes. Ultimately, this is a self-limiting condition that will resolve as the physis closes. Prevention of LLS can involve preseason ROM assessments as well as in season adherence to pitch count and rest day recommendations.

Anterior Shoulder Instability

Anterior traumatic shoulder dislocation is a common injury among adolescent athletes and represents the vast majority of shoulder dislocations in this age group. It occurs most frequently in contact and collision sports,

Dr. Crepeau or an immediate family member serves as a board member, owner, officer, or committee member of the Pediatric Orthopaedic Society of North America. Dr. Weiss or an immediate family member serves as a board member, owner, officer, or committee member of the American Academy of Orthopaedic Surgeons and the Pediatric Orthopaedic Society of North America.

Pediatrics

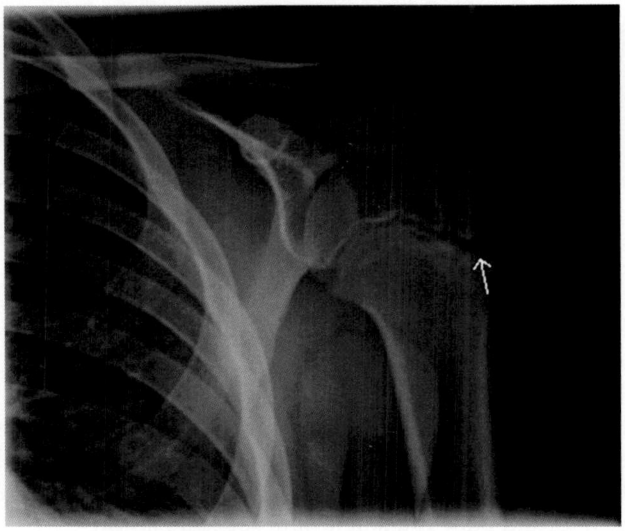

Figure 1 Radiograph showing Little Leaguer's shoulder. AP radiograph of a 12-year-old male pitcher with shoulder pain showing widening of the lateral proximal humerus epiphysis (arrow).

with football being the most common sport.[3,4] The mechanism is often a fall or blow to an outstretched, abducted arm. Incidence and rate of recurrence increase in athletes older than 14 years.[5]

Presentation includes pain, limited ROM, and deformity at the shoulder. Plain radiographs including an axillary view should be obtained, including postreduction radiographs (**Figure 2**). These radiographs are useful for assessing direction of dislocation and bony injury involving the glenoid or humeral head (Hill-Sachs lesion). When pain limits the ability to obtain an axillary view, scapular y view is a good alternative. Initial treatment should include closed reduction and immobilization of the shoulder in a sling.

There is ongoing debate surrounding the treatment of first-time shoulder dislocations as the rate of recurrence in the adolescent age group is reported up to 92%. MRI can be used to assess for tears of the labrum, rotator cuff, and biceps, as well as evaluate for Hill-Sachs lesions and glenoid bone loss. MRI aids in surgical planning and should be obtained only if the patient and surgeon are considering surgery. In a study comparing surgical versus nonsurgical treatment for anterior shoulder dislocation, the recurrence rates were 13.1% versus 70.3%, respectively. Most were not sports related.[4]

When there is no significant bone loss, surgical options include arthroscopic labral repair with or without capsular imbrication and open Bankart repair. In one study, there was no difference between arthroscopic and open Bankart repair in pediatric patients as far as outcomes or redislocation rates. Redislocation rate was 21%.[3] When bone loss is established by CT scan (or MRI scan), open procedures with bone augmentation such as the Latarjet should be considered.[6]

Risk factors for recurrent instability include age ≥14, male sex, and glenoid bone loss.[5] One study found that 48.2% of adolescent patients with recurrent instability

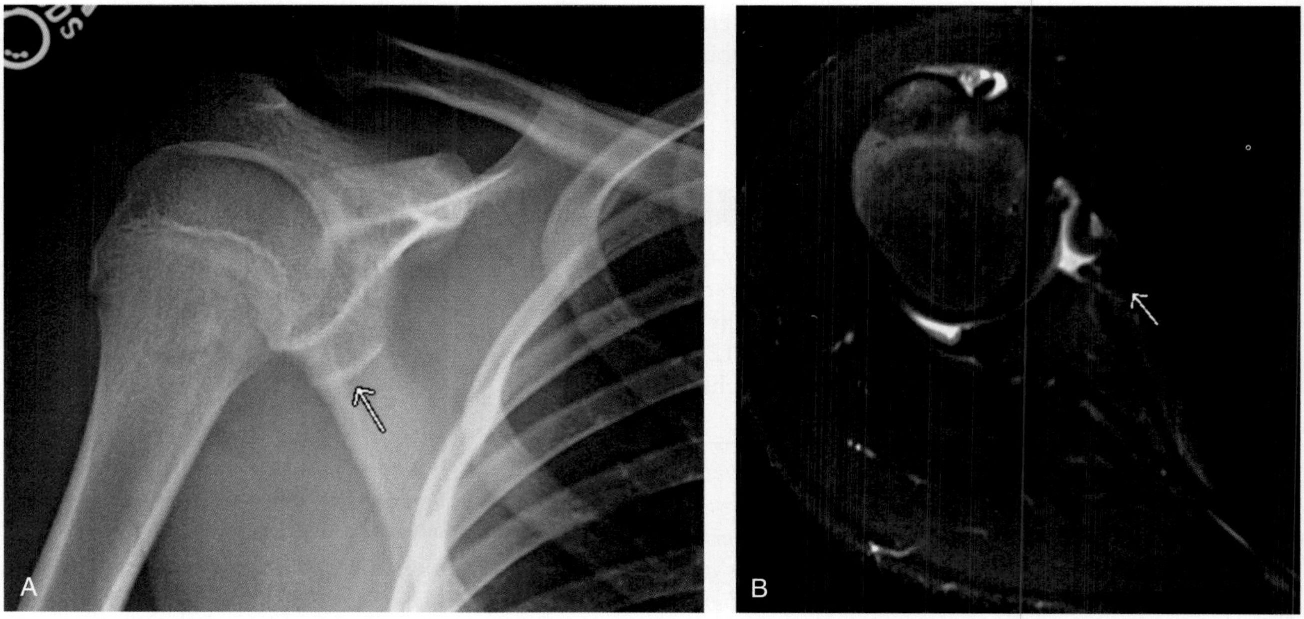

Figure 2 Imaging of a 12-year-old boy following an anterior shoulder dislocation. **A**, AP radiograph of the shoulder showing glenoid fracture (arrow). **B**, Axial T2 MRI showing a displaced bony Bankart lesion (arrow).

had glenoid bone loss, with 27% of them having critical bone loss.[7] Contact athletes younger than 16 years had a significantly higher rate of redislocation than those aged 16 and older after arthroscopic Bankart repair.[8] Factors associated with recurrence after arthroscopic Bankart repair in patients younger than 30 years included more preoperative dislocations, off-track Hill-Sachs, and increased time to surgery.[9]

Little Leaguer's Elbow (Medial Epicondyle Apophysitis)

Little Leaguer's elbow is an overuse injury in which there is stress at the medial epicondyle apophysis due to valgus overload. It is caused by repetitive throwing, primarily pitching, in the youth baseball player. The maximal valgus moment on the elbow occurs during the late cocking through early acceleration phase. It has become more prevalent as athletes specialize at younger ages and play baseball year-round. The true incidence is unknown as many athletes do not seek treatment. However, a 2015 survey of healthy youth baseball players found that 74% and 80% of them had at least some pain during or after throwing, respectively.[10] MRI studies in symptomatic youth athletes often show edema at the distal humerus or medial epicondyle apophysis.[11] Preseason MRI abnormalities in youth baseball players were associated with year-round play, private coaching, loss of shoulder internal rotation.[12] Postseason MRI evaluation of dominant elbows revealed abnormalities in 46% of Little League players. Additionally, players lost an average of 11.2° of internal rotation of the shoulder during the season.[13]

Little Leaguer's elbow presents primarily as medial elbow pain in the throwing athlete, loss of velocity, tenderness over the medial epicondyle, and pain with valgus stress. Shoulder ROM should be assessed when plain radiographs of the elbow can potentially show widening of the apophysis or fragmentation of the medial epicondyle. Comparison views can be useful in diagnosis.

Treatment of Little Leaguer's elbow is similar to that of LLS in that it involves complete rest from throwing activities until symptoms resolve and then a gradual return to throwing program. Physical therapy can also be useful to address any strength or ROM deficits. Pitching analysis to assess for proper pitching mechanics can also help to prevent elbow injuries in the long term. The risk of pitching through pain includes medial epicondyle fracture and ulnar collateral ligament (UCL) injury.

Risk factors for developing elbow pain during a season include recent increase in height, shoulder or elbow pain during the previous season, team training 4 days or more per week, self-training 7 days per week, and being in the starting lineup.[14,15]

Other risk factors for shoulder and elbow pain in the youth baseball player include age, height, higher velocity pitches, playing for multiple teams, and arm fatigue.[16,17] A study looking at pitch types found that fastballs produced the greatest torque across the elbow while curveballs required the greatest arm speed. Increased torque across the elbow was found in higher velocity, higher BMI, and decreased arm slot, but pitchers who started throwing curveballs at an older age had lower torque in the elbow while pitching.[18]

USA Baseball has published guidelines (MLB Pitch Smart) for youth pitchers that include recommendations by age on pitch count, pitch type, and days of rest.[19] There are additional recommendations that players rest from baseball for 3 months a year, avoid playing on multiple teams in the same season, and avoid throwing curveballs and sliders. Some affected athletes may be advised to hold off on pitching until they are more mature.

Medial Epicondyle Avulsion Fractures

The medial epicondyle is the attachment site for the flexor-pronator mass as well as the UCL. Ossification of the medial epicondyle typically begins between the ages of 5 to 7 and fuses between the ages of 15 to 18, earlier in females than males. Medial epicondyle avulsion fractures represent up to 20% of pediatric elbow fractures and are most common between the ages of 9 and 15, with a peak age of 11 to 12.

Medial epicondyle fractures often present with a pop and sudden pain at the medial elbow, accompanied by swelling and ecchymosis. When these fractures occur in pitchers, there is often a prodromal period of medial elbow pain consistent with Little Leaguer's elbow (or medial epicondyle apophysitis). Up to 60% of the time, there may be a concurrent elbow dislocation, sometimes with spontaneous reduction. The medial epicondyle may become incarcerated in the joint in up to 15% of dislocations.

Controversies exist regarding the accuracy of measuring fracture displacement and the indications for surgical management. Diagnosis is made with plain radiographs (**Figure 3**). CT imaging provides more accurate measurement of actual displacement; however, concerns about radiation exposure and cost have led to a continued search for improved measurement

Pediatrics

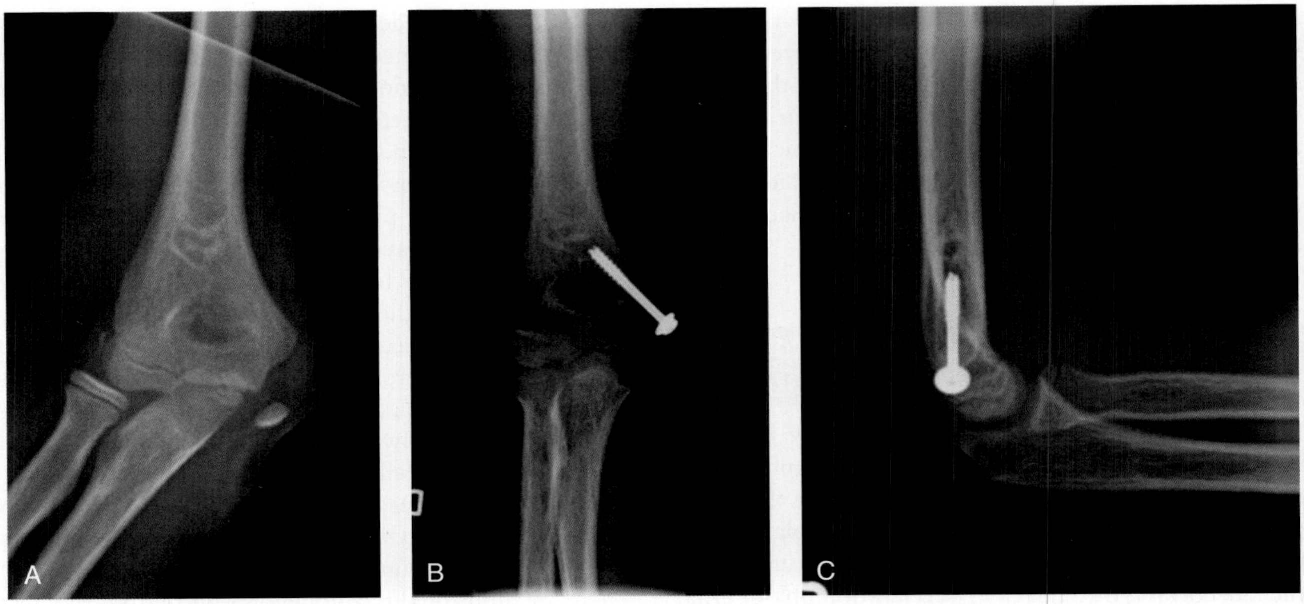

Figure 3 Radiographs showing elbow dislocation with medial epicondyle fracture. **A**, AP radiograph of injury radiograph showing 13-year-old boy with an elbow fracture/dislocation. **B**, AP radiograph showing fixation of the medial epicondyle fracture. **C**, Lateral radiograph showing fixation of the medial epicondyle fracture.

techniques using plain radiographs. The 45-degree internal oblique view and the distal humerus axial view have been shown to improve reliability of the measurement of fracture displacement when added to standard AP and lateral views.[20,21]

Nonsurgical management has been the mainstay of treatment for medial epicondyle fractures, despite the high rate of bony nonunion.[22,23] Because of the attachment of the UCL, there is concern about valgus stability of the elbow in the setting of a nonunion or malunion. Nonsurgical treatment is typically a long arm cast for 3 to 4 weeks followed by ROM exercises. Absolute indications for surgical treatment are open fractures or incarceration of the fragment in the joint, whereas relative indications include valgus elbow instability, ulnar nerve entrapment, significant fracture displacement, and overhead or upper extremity weight-bearing athlete. Surgical techniques include screw, screw/washer, K-wire, and suture anchor fixation. Fragment excision and soft-tissue reattachment has been shown to have poor outcomes. Addition of a washer may increase likelihood of hardware symptoms and need for removal.[24] Chronic nonunion may occur after nonsurgical management, and in this case delayed surgical open reduction with internal fixation has been shown to lead to acceptable results.[25] A recent study showed no difference in return to sports, functional limitations, ROM, or pain between moderately displaced medial epicondyle fractures treated surgically or nonsurgically in upper extremity athletes.[26]

Hip Avulsion Fractures

Pelvic apophyseal avulsion fractures occur in a narrow range of adolescent years. They can involve the anterior superior iliac spine or ASIS (avulsion of sartorius), anterior inferior iliac spine or AIIS (avulsion of the rectus femoris), ischial tuberosity (avulsion of the hamstrings), iliac crest (avulsion of the tensor fascia lata), or the lesser trochanter (avulsion of the psoas tendon). 76% occur in males, most of whom are participating in sports, with an average age of 14.4 years.[27,28] Running/sprinting and kicking are the most common activities associated with this injury. In one study, AIIS fractures were the most common (49%), followed by ASIS (30%), ischial tuberosity (11%), and iliac crest (10%).

Presentation generally involves a pop and subsequent pain and swelling during an activity. Some patients may report a prodromal period of pain before the fracture. Imaging can include standard AP and frog lateral radiographs (**Figure 4**). ASIS and AIIS fractures may also be visualized with a false profile view.

Treatment of pelvic avulsion fractures is primarily nonsurgical, usually with 4 to 6 weeks of protected weight-bearing, or until normal gait can be restored, followed by physical therapy to increase flexibility. Fractures with initial displacement >20 mm are more likely to go on to a nonunion and therefore this may be an indication for surgical fixation.[27] A meta-analysis found that for fractures displaced >15 mm, surgical

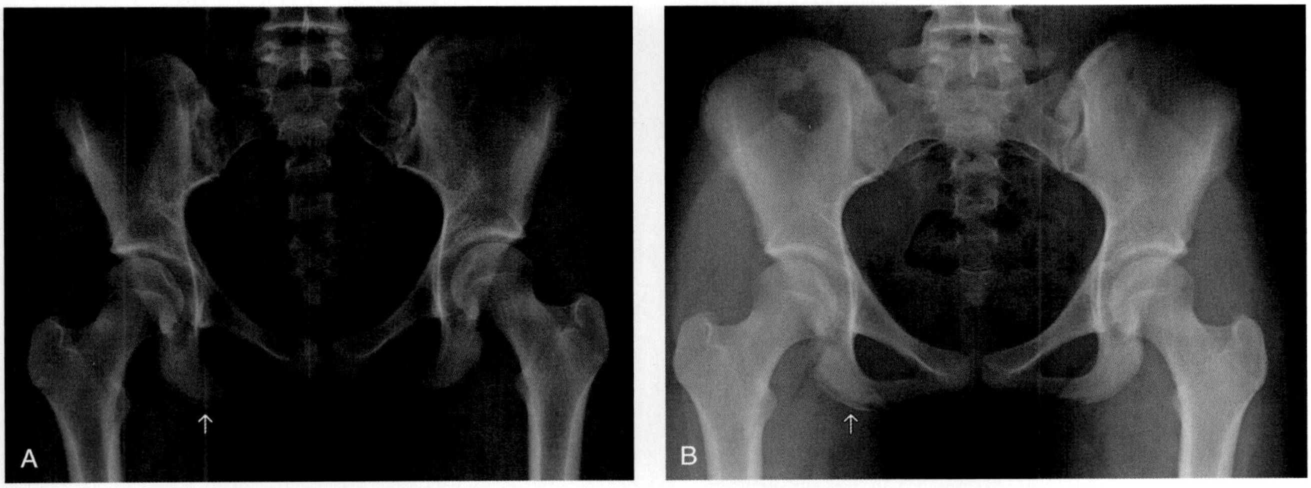

Figure 4 Radiographs of a 14-year-old girl who was injured while doing a splint in dance class. **A**, AP radiograph at the time of injury showing a subtle ischial avulsion fracture (arrow) missed on the original read. **B**, AP radiograph 10 weeks post injury showing healing at the fracture site (arrow).

treatment resulted in 84% excellent results versus only 50% in nonsurgical treatment.[28] However, the complication rate is higher for surgically treated fractures. Painful nonunion or sciatic nerve irritation (ischial tuberosity) may be indications for surgical treatment. Patients with AIIS fractures were the most likely to have hip pain >3 months out from surgery. This fracture type can cause extra-articular subspine hip impingement. Because of this, more research regarding the best initial treatment is needed.

Anterior Cruciate Ligament Injury

The incidence of anterior cruciate ligament (ACL) injury and ACL reconstruction among pediatric and adolescent athletes has been increasing over the last 20 years.[29] Adolescents aged 13 to 17 who are competing in sports are at the highest risk for ACL injury. Female athletes in this age group are more likely to injure their ACL than males. Patients with an acute ACL tear will often report a plant, pivot, or contact injury, sometimes with a "pop," and subsequent pain, swelling, and inability to continue their activity. The mechanism is often a valgus load on an extended knee and may be a contact or noncontact injury. Physical examination shows effusion, limited ROM, and a positive Lachman and pivot shift, though these examination findings are often difficult to appreciate because of guarding. Radiographs of the knee can show a joint effusion and occasionally a Segond fracture of the proximal lateral tibia. MRI is the study of choice to confirm diagnosis of ACL tear and evaluate for concomitant injuries to the meniscus, cartilage, and other ligaments (**Figure 5**). Bone age radiographs and long leg alignment radiographs may aid in preoperative planning for skeletally immature patients.

One factor leading to the increasing rate of ACL reconstruction in this population is the development of techniques to safely perform this surgery in skeletally immature patients. Previously, it was often recommended to postpone surgical intervention until skeletal maturity. However, studies have shown a significant rate of meniscal and cartilage injury in patients treated nonsurgically. Nonsurgical treatment still has a role in certain patients, such as those who are skeletally immature, have partial tears, or have low physical demand. Risks of proceeding with activities with an ACL-deficient knee should be discussed. Partial ACL tears can have good results in patients younger than 14 years with no instability and less than 50% of the ligament ruptured.[30]

ACL repair has historically been unsuccessful, though there are successful indications for femoral-sided avulsion repair and new work being done on the additional of a biologic matrix. The current mainstay of treatment involves reconstruction of the ACL (ACLR). Surgical technique/graft choice depends on skeletal maturity and surgeon/patient preference.[31] In patients with more than 2 years of growth remaining, reconstruction should avoid the physis. Options include extraphyseal or all-epiphyseal. With <2 years of growth remaining, a surgeon can use the previously mentioned techniques or an all soft-tissue transphyseal reconstruction. Skeletally mature patients have options of

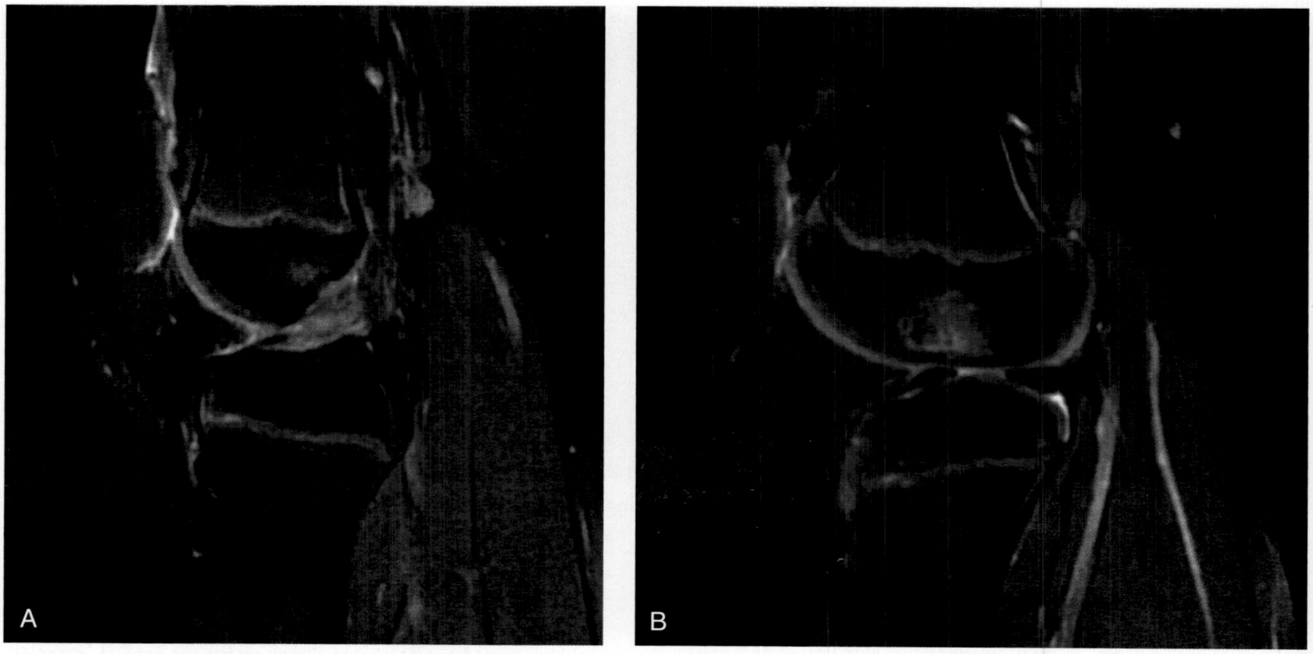

Figure 5 Imaging of an 11-year-old boy injured while playing football. **A**, Sagittal MRI showing a complete tear of the ACL. **B**, Sagittal MRI showing classic bone bruising of the lateral femoral condyle associated with ACL injury.

hamstring tendon, bone–patellar tendon–bone, quadriceps tendon (with or without a bone block) autograft or allograft.

Complications of ACLR include retear, meniscal injury, arthrofibrosis, flexion or extension deficits, graft harvest site morbidity, and contralateral ACL rupture. Although uncommon, skeletally immature patients who undergo ACLR are at risk for growth arrest and should be monitored closely.[32,33] The overall incidence of ACL reinjury (ipsilateral or contralateral) in young patients within 2 years of ACLR is reported around 30%, substantially higher than is reported in the adult population.[34,35] Graft rerupture has been reported at varying rates from 6 to 30%. Patient age has been found to be a significant risk factor for re-rupture.[36] Longer time to return to sport can be protective.[34] Graft choice can also be correlated to re-rupture rate, with some studies showing hamstring grafts failing more often than BPTB.[36] Smaller graft size has also been found to increase risk of re-tear, though hybrid grafts (autograft supplemented with allograft) have an even higher rate of failure.[37] The use of allograft in the adolescent age group has been shown to have an increased rate of re-rupture.

Overall, the rate of return to sport after ACLR in the pediatric population is high, but the reinjury rate is also high. Neuromuscular re-education, ACL prevention training, and delayed return to sport should be encouraged.

Tibial Spine Fractures

Tibial spine (tibial eminence) fractures occur when the osteochondral attachment of the ACL fails. Although they were historically considered the pediatric version of an ACL tear, it is now known that a tibial spine fracture can coexist with an ACL injury 19.4% of the time.[38] All patients had type II or type III fractures and 20% went on to require later ACL reconstructions.

Tibial spine fractures occur most commonly in males aged 8 to 14 years. The overall average age of injury is 11 years, though females have a lower average age of 9.6 years.[39] The Myers and McKeever classification is useful both for description and treatment guidance.[40] Type I fractures are non- or minimally displaced. Type II fractures are displaced anteriorly but have an intact posterior hinge (**Figure 6**). Type III fractures are completely displaced and/or comminuted (**Figure 7**). Zaricznyj later added a type IV to describe displaced fractures that also had a rotational component.[41]

Patients with tibial spine avulsion fractures present with acute knee pain and a joint hemarthrosis. Often the diagnosis can be made on standard AP and lateral radiographs, particularly if the fracture is displaced. CT imaging can give a more accurate measure of displacement, whereas MRI can reveal concomitant injuries to the ACL, meniscus, and cartilage. Another study showed that 59% of displaced tibial spine fractures had associated injuries

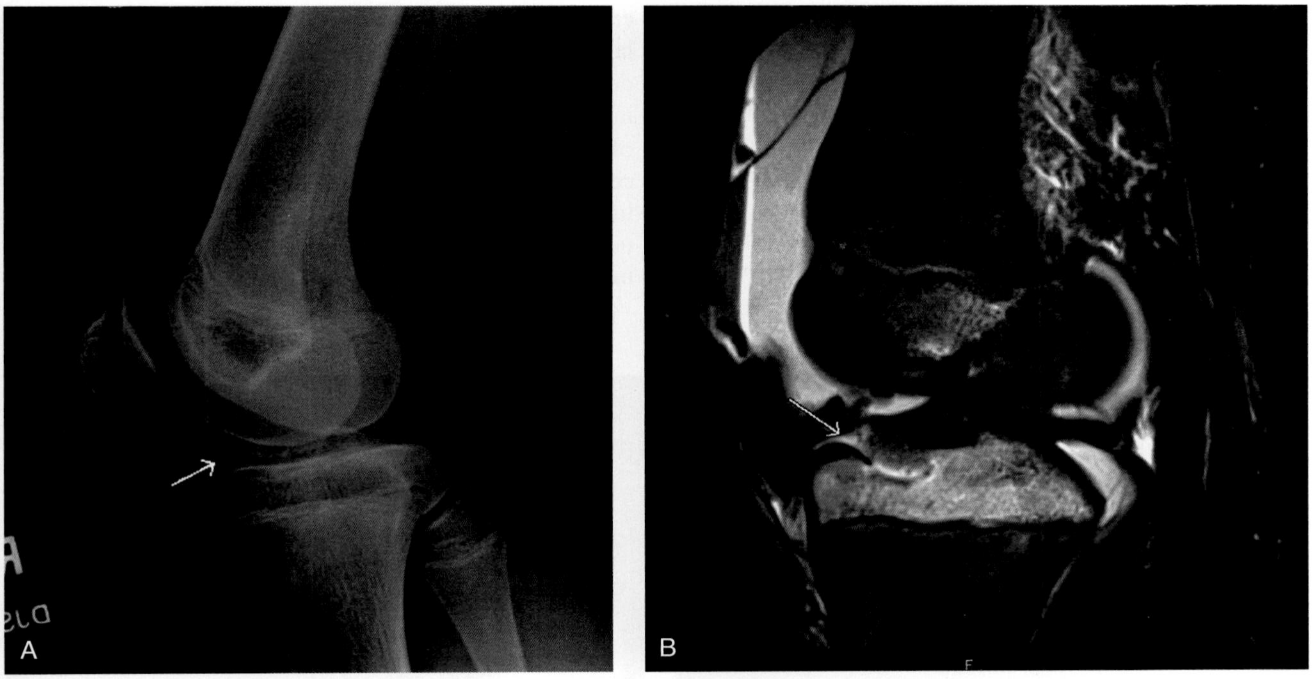

Figure 6 Imaging of a 14-year-old boy with a type II tibial spine fracture. **A**, Lateral radiograph shows a hinged fracture fragment (arrow) and large effusion. **B**, Sagittal T2 MRI shows a hinged fracture fragment (arrow) and large hemarthrosis.

with meniscal or intra-meniscal ligament entrapment being the most common, followed by meniscal tear.[42] The incidence of entrapment may be underestimated by MRI.[43]

Nonsurgical management with closed reduction and cast immobilization can be used in type I and some type II fractures. Surgical management is indicated for significantly displaced or irreducible fracture, as well as fractures with concomitant injuries or meniscal entrapment. Surgical options include arthroscopic or open fixation of the fracture using various techniques such as screw or suture fixation. Screw fixation has been shown to have a higher revision surgery rate for hardware removal.

The most common complication following treatment for a tibial spine fracture is arthrofibrosis. Early surgical intervention and early mobilization can decrease arthrofibrosis. Delayed ACL rupture is also a concern as one recent study has shown that 19% of patients required later ACL reconstruction.[44]

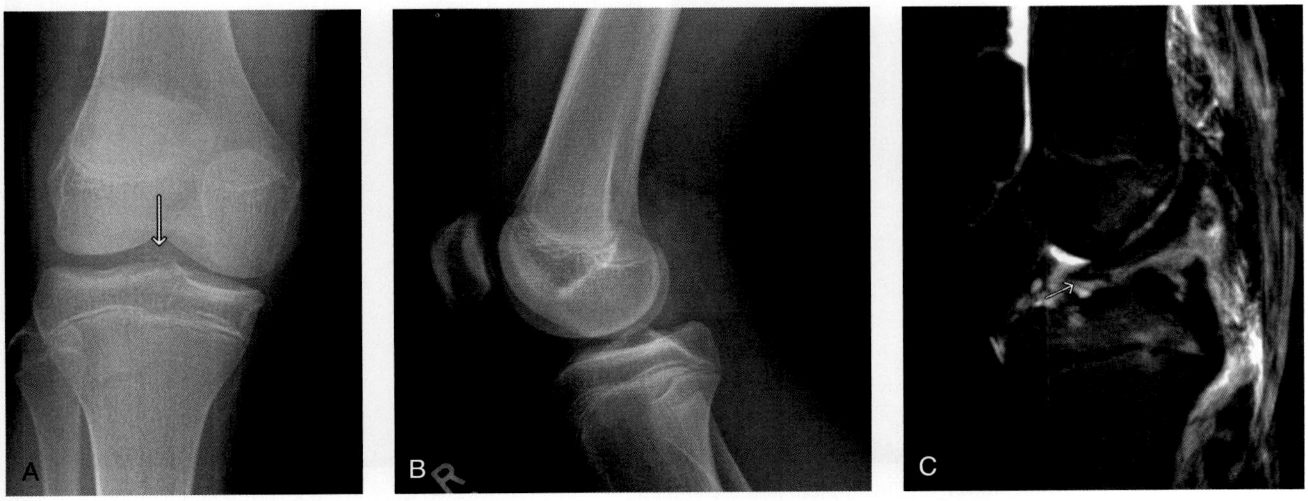

Figure 7 Imaging of a 16-year-old boy with a type III tibial spine fracture. **A**, AP radiograph shows a small fleck of bone in the notch (arrow). **B**, Lateral radiograph shows a large effusion. **C**, Sagittal T2 MRI shows the avulsed ACL with small bony fragment (arrow).

Meniscus Tear

Meniscus tears are common knee injuries that often require treatment in the pediatric and adolescent population. In young children, the cause is often a discoid lateral meniscus. Discoid lateral meniscus (DLM) is a congenital anomaly affecting the size and shape of the lateral meniscus (**Figure 8**). Abnormal thickness, motion, meniscocapsular attachments, and histopathology all contribute to the development of symptomatic discoid lateral meniscus and tears. There is an increased incidence of DLM in the Asian population. One study looking at the incidence of DLM showed that up to 75% of isolated lateral meniscus tears were found to be discoid in nature at the time of arthroscopy, particularly in the younger age group, whereas teens >14 years were more likely to have traumatic tears in normal shaped menisci.[45] The mechanism is often a twisting injury to

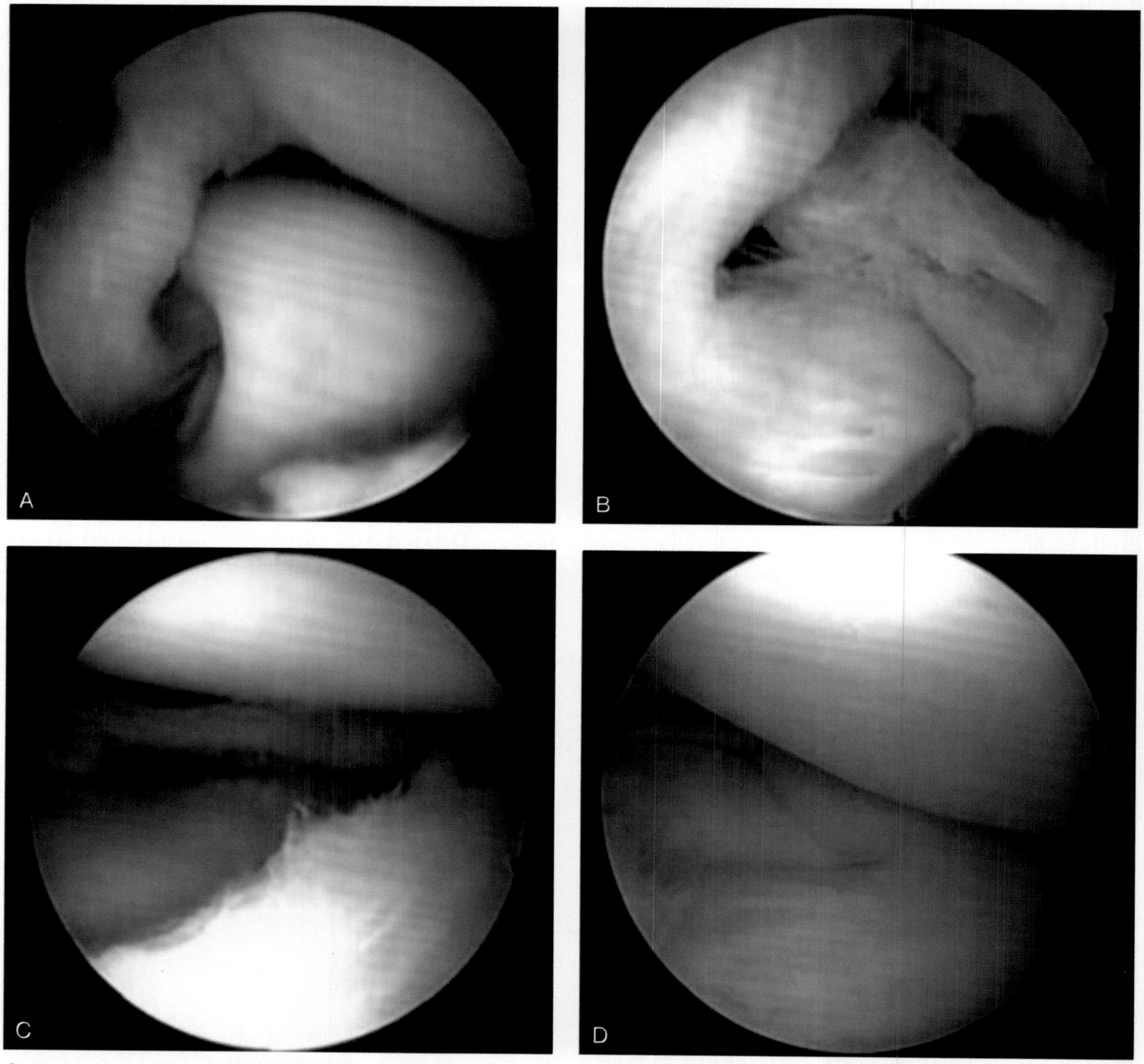

Figure 8 Arthroscopy images showing an incomplete and a complete discoid meniscus. **A**, 10-year-old girl with an incomplete discoid lateral meniscus. **B**, 12-year-old boy with a complete discoid meniscus. **C**, During saucerization, the complete discoid meniscus shows degeneration and a horizontal cleavage tear. **D**, Final image of the complete discoid after saucerization and repair.

the knee, commonly occurring during sports. The most common tear patterns in young patients are complex, vertical, bucket-handle, radial, horizontal, oblique, and root, and the lateral meniscus is most often affected.[46]

Symptoms of meniscal injury include knee swelling, pain particularly with twisting or cutting, and locking/mechanical symptoms. Patients with symptomatic discoid lateral meniscus may present with swelling (though often not), locking, limited ROM, lateral joint line popping or clunking, and tenderness. Patients with acute meniscal tears may exhibit the following on physical examination: effusion, joint line tenderness, extension deficit, and a positive McMurray's test. Radiographs of the knee may reveal squaring of the lateral condyle (discoid) or knee effusion. MRI is often used for diagnosis of meniscus injuries. Meniscus tears are also associated with ACL tears (up to 50% of the time), tibial spine fractures, and chondral injuries.

Treatment of the asymptomatic discoid can be observational, though any signs of mechanical instability should be addressed. Discoid lateral meniscus is typically treated with arthroscopy and partial meniscectomy (saucerization of the meniscus) as well as repair of any peripheral instability. In cases of catastrophic tears, it is sometimes not possible to preserve the meniscus. Surgical treatment of acute meniscal tears also includes partial or total meniscectomy and repair and depends on the tear pattern, age of patient, chronicity of tear, and zone of injury. Repair techniques include inside-out, outside-in, all-inside, and side to side and a wide variety of instruments and products are available.

There are limited data on the outcomes of isolated meniscus tears in the pediatric population, with a majority of the available literature focusing on discoid lateral meniscus. A recent study of partial meniscectomy in patients with discoid lateral meniscus showed improved clinical outcomes but also significant rates of degeneration of the remaining meniscus (52%) as well as arthritic changes in the lateral compartment (68%) with long-term follow-up.[47] Revision surgery rate in the setting of discoid lateral meniscus is reported between 10 and 30%.[47,48] In general, all attempts should be made for repair in young patients, as the long-term results of meniscectomy are poor.[49] Good clinical outcomes have been found in arthroscopic meniscal repair in the pediatric population with reported success rates of 80% to 90%.[49,50] Revision surgery may be required in about 13% of patients, often for acute retear of the meniscus, and can include repair or meniscectomy.[51]

Patellofemoral Instability

Lateral patellar dislocation is a common knee injury in the pediatric population with the incidence peaking between the ages of 10 and 17.[52] Most injuries occur during athletic activities. Patients may present with pain, effusion, limited ROM, and a history of spontaneous or assisted patella reduction. Physical examination in the recurrent dislocator should include an assessment of limb alignment (specifically genu valgum, femoral anteversion, external tibial torsion, and Q angle) as well as patellar tracking (lateral tilt, J-sign, crepitus, and lateral excursion).

Initial imaging typically includes standard radiographs to assess for fracture, loose bodies, effusion, and trochlear dysplasia. MRI can be used to confirm diagnosis, evaluate chondral injury, assess concomitant injuries, and aid in preoperative planning. Measurements of patella alta, trochlear dysplasia, sulcus angle, tibial tubercle–trochlear groove distance (TT-TG) can aid in decision making for surgery. Preoperative planning may also include long leg alignment radiographs to assess for genu valgum.

Risk factors for patellofemoral instability include trochlear dysplasia, previous patella dislocation, ligamentous laxity, patella alta, and skeletal immaturity. Risk factors for recurrent patellofemoral instability include trochlear dysplasia, patella alta (Caton-Deschamps index >1.45), skeletal immaturity, and history of contralateral patellar dislocation.[53,54]

First-time patella dislocations are generally treated with rest, immobilization/bracing treatment, and physical therapy unless there is a significant chondral or osteochondral fracture. Indications for surgical stabilization can include recurrent subluxation or dislocation, continued pain, mechanical symptoms, or inability to return to sports.

There are many surgical options to treat patellar instability, and procedure selection depends primarily on skeletal maturity and the anatomic abnormalities of each individual patient. Proximal realignment procedures can include VMO (vastus medialis obliquus) advancement with medial retinacular plication. Medial patellofemoral ligament repair has been shown to be a viable option in the adolescents.[55] Medial patellofemoral ligament reconstruction (MPFLR) has become a mainstay of treatment in the setting of both MPFL tears and ligamentous laxity. A recent study showed no difference in return to activity, pain, or failure rate when comparing autograft with allograft MPFL reconstruction in adolescents.[56] A pedicled quadriceps tendon graft can also be used with the advantage of hardware-free patella fixation. Lateral release or lateral retinacular lengthening can be added to correct significant patella tilt. Tibial tubercle transfer is often advocated for patients who have a TT-TG distance ≥20 mm, though MRI may underestimate this distance. This procedure can also be used to distalize the tubercle to correct patella alta. Genu valgum can be corrected with hemiepiphysiodesis in the skeletally immature patient or osteotomy in the mature patient. Trochleoplasty is also an option to address trochlear dysplasia and, while it has typically been reserved for skeletally mature patients, a recent study showed no growth disturbance following the procedure in skeletally immature patients with less than 2 years of growth remaining.[57]

Skeletal immaturity can pose some challenges in the surgical management of patellofemoral instability. Medial patellofemoral ligament reconstruction can be modified to avoid the physis by either placing the tunnel distal to the physis or by using soft-tissue fixation.[58] Tibial tubercle transfer is not recommended in the setting of an open physis. Multiple nonanatomic distal realignment procedures have been described for this situation, such as the modified Roux-Goldthwait and Galeazzi procedures.

Osteochondritis Dissecans of the Knee

Osteochondritis dissecans is a focal, idiopathic compromise of the subchondral bone which can lead to collapse and damage to the overlying cartilage. In a large demographic and epidemiologic study, males had 79% of OCD lesions of the knee and the 12- to 19-year-old group had 2.6 times as many OCD lesions than the 6- to 12-year-old group. No patients under the age of 6 were found to have OCD lesions. African Americans had an increased rate of OCD.[59] The medial condyle is most commonly affected, but OCD lesions can be found in the lateral condyle, trochlea, and patella.

Although some OCD lesions in young patients are found incidentally, most present with a vague history of knee pain, often activity related. In unstable lesions, patients may present with intermittent swelling, pain, and mechanical symptoms such as catching and locking. Physical examination may show an effusion, quadriceps atrophy, and deep tenderness to palpation over the affected condyle. Diagnosis can be made with standard radiographs, which should include AP, lateral, tunnel/notch, and sunrise/Merchant views (**Figure 9**). MRI is useful for determining stability of OCD lesions. In the setting of a lateral condyle OCD lesion, long leg alignment radiographs can assess for genu valgum, which may affect healing.

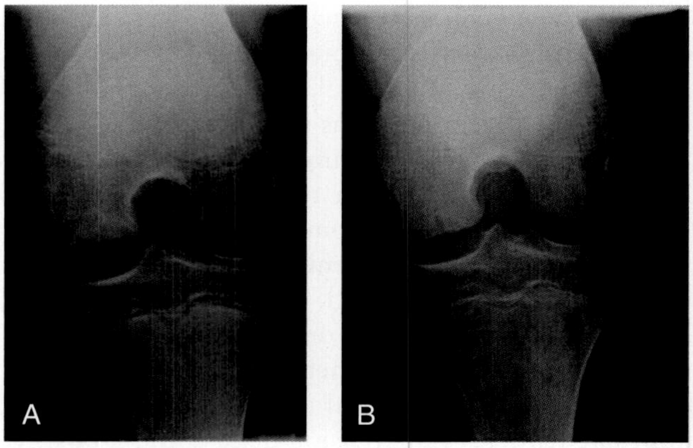

Figure 9 Radiographic images of a 12-year-old boy with a symptomatic medial femoral condyle OCD lesion. **A**, Tunnel radiograph at age 12. **B**, Tunnel radiograph at age 14 showing healing of the OCD lesion following arthroscopic drilling and fixation.

Stable OCD lesions can be treated nonsurgically with observation, activity modification, immobilization, and bracing treatment. In skeletally immature patients, one study evaluating healing (based on imaging) with activity modification only found that at 6 months, 26% of lesion had progressed toward healing, while at 12 months, it was 49% of lesions.[60] In assessing for stability, age has been found to be predictive of the integrity of the overlying cartilage. In one study, patients >13 years had a low probability of disrupted cartilage (3%), whereas those >17 years had disrupted cartilage 100% of the time.[61] A study looking at progression to surgery found the rate in OCD of the knee to be 33.5%, with a significantly higher odds ratio in older patients.[62]

Surgical treatment is indicated for unstable lesions and persistently symptomatic stable lesions and may be considered in patients nearing or at skeletal maturity, large lesions, or lateral condyle lesions. Surgical options include a variety of arthroscopic and open procedures. For stable lesions, antegrade and retrograde drilling have been found to promote healing. If the fragment is unstable, fixation with absorbable and nonabsorbable implants is recommended if the overlying cartilage is in good condition. This is often augmented with drilling, curettage, and bone grafting as needed. For unsalvageable lesions, fragment excision can be followed by microfracture, orthobiologic products, autologous chondrocyte implantation, osteochondral autograft transfer (OATS), or osteochondral allograft (OCA).

There are limited outcomes studies comparing surgical treatment for OCD of the knee. In a study looking at fixation of OCD lesions and skeletal maturity, there

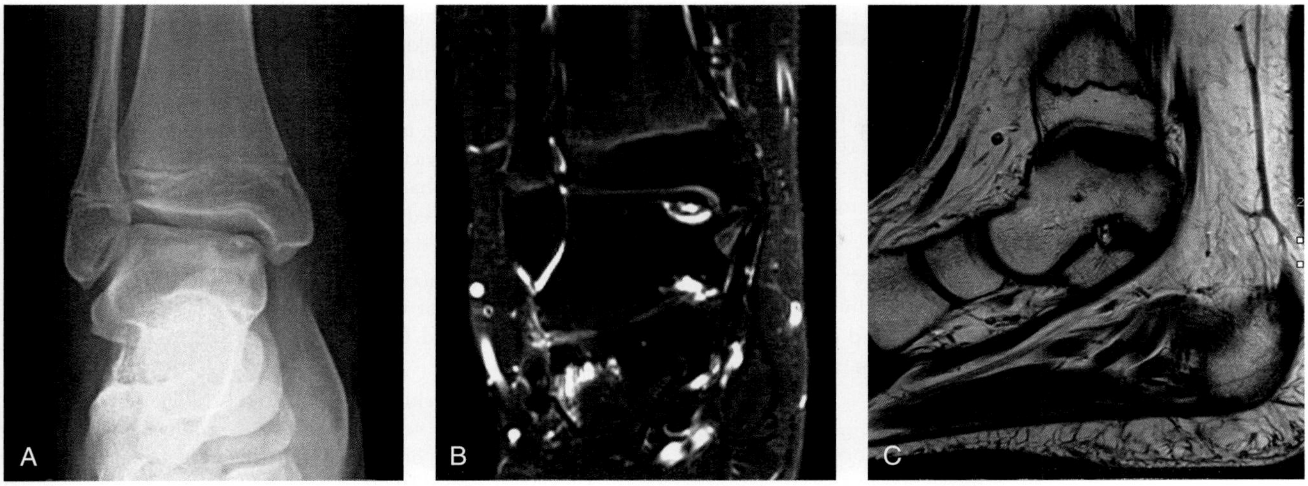

Figure 10 Radiographic images of an 11-year-old boy with an OCD lesion of the talus. **A**, AP radiograph showing the medial talus OCD lesion. **B**, Coronal T2 MRI of the OCD showing significant fluid signal behind the lesion. **C**, Sagittal T1 MRI showing the large OCD.

was no difference in healing rates between mature and immature patients. Overall failure rate was 24%, with lateral condyle lesions being a risk factor for failure.[63]

A long-term study looked at the rate of arthritis and arthroplasty after OCD. At 30 years, the incidence of arthritis and arthroplasty in patients with fragment excision was 70% and 51%, respectively, versus 50% and 11% in the fragment preservation group, and zero in the chondral grafting group.[64]

Osteochondritis Dissecans of the Talus

Osteochondritis dissecans of the talus (OCDT) represents around 25% of all juvenile OCD lesions.[62] It occurs most commonly in females (up to 75%) and in the teen age group (average age 14 years).[65,66] The most common location of the lesion is the medial talus (about 70%), followed by lateral talus. Central talus lesions occur but are rare. Risk factors for OCDT include non-Hispanic whites and extreme obesity.[66,67]

Patients with OCDT may present with a history of vague ankle pain, stiffness, swelling, and mechanical symptoms. There may also be a history of recurrent ankle injuries or instability. Symptoms are typically worsened with weight-bearing and impact activities. Initial imaging should include AP, lateral, and mortise views of the ankle. If there is clinical suspicion but no visible lesion, MRI can be used to further evaluate. MRI is also helpful for assessing the size and stability of OCDT lesions (**Figure 10**). The Berndt and Hardy classification is more commonly used.

Nonsurgical management is indicated for skeletally immature patients with stable or partially stable lesion. This includes immobilization in a boot or cast, protected weight-bearing, and activity modification. Around 30% of OCD lesions of the talus will require surgery with older age being a risk factor.[62] Surgical indications include symptomatic stable lesions that fail 6 months of nonsurgical treatment and symptomatic unstable lesions. Surgical interventions depend on the size and stability of the OCD lesion and can be arthroscopic or open depending on the location of the lesion. An anterior arthrotomy can be used for some anterior-based lesions, whereas posteromedial or posterolateral arthrotomy with the ankle in full dorsiflexion can allow access to more posterior lesions. This can be particularly useful in skeletally immature patients for whom a medial malleolar osteotomy is not an option. Surgical options include drilling (antegrade or retrograde), fixation, or excision/microfracture. There are also limited data on the use of autologous chondrocyte implantation, bone marrow–derived cell implantation, osteochondral allograft or autograft.[68] Even with surgical treatment, the rate of lesions progressing to full radiographic healing is low (16%), though they may still have good clinical results.[65]

Overall revision surgery rate was 26% in one study and most commonly followed lesions that either did not change or worsened radiographically after initial procedure. Female sex and increased BMI were risk factors for worse outcomes.[65]

Key Study Points

- Shoulder and elbow pain are common in the overhead throwing young athlete. Families, coaches, and athletes should be counseled on the risk of early sports specialization and year-round play, as well as pitch count and pitch type recommendations for their age groups.
- Anterior shoulder instability has a high rate of recurrence in the adolescent population. Surgical procedures should be selected based on age, sport, and glenoid bone loss to decrease postoperative recurrence rates.
- Surgical management of ACL tears can be accomplished safely at all stages of skeletal maturity using a variety of techniques. There is significant risk of further meniscal or cartilage injury in the young patient with an ACL-deficient knee. Reinjury rate following ACLR in the adolescent patient is 30% in the first 2 years.
- Discoid lateral meniscus is the most common cause of isolated lateral meniscus pathology in patients aged 13 years or younger. Teens 14 years or older are more likely to have traumatic tears of normal menisci, often occurring with a twisting injury to the knee during sports.
- Treatment of patellar instability in the young athlete may be accomplished with a variety of surgical techniques to correct underlying anatomic issues, such as ligamentous laxity, genu valgum, patella alta, lateralization of the tibial tubercle, and trochlear dysplasia. Medial patellofemoral ligament reconstruction (MPFLR) has become the mainstay of treatment.

References

1. Heyworth BE, Kramer DE, Martin DJ, Micheli LJ, Kocher MS, Bae DS: Trends in the presentation, management, and outcomes of Little League shoulder. *Am J Sports Med* 2016;44(6):1431-1438.

   Ninety-five patients with Little League shoulder were analyzed with respect to demographics and risk factors. From 1999 to 2013, the number of cases increased. The most common patients were male pitchers, but the condition was found in catchers, tennis players, and two girls. Age ranged from 8 to 16, with average age of 13.1. Average length of symptoms was 2.6 months. Only 7% had recurrent episode. Level of evidence: IV.

2. Pennock AT, Dwek J, Levy E, et al: Shoulder MRI abnormalities in asymptomatic Little League baseball players. *Orthop J Sports Med* 2018;6(2):2325967118756825.

   MRI was performed on 23 asymptomatic Little League baseball players' shoulders bilaterally. Throwing arm abnormality was 8.5 times more likely than nondominant shoulder. More than half of the players had MRI findings, including edema, physeal widening, labral tear, partial thickness rotator cuff tear, acromioclavicular joint abnormality, subacromial bursitis, and cystic change of the greater tuberosity. Single-sport players who played baseball year-round were most likely to have abnormalities. Level of evidence: III.

3. Shymon SJ, Roocroft J, Edmonds EW: Traumatic anterior instability of the pediatric shoulder: A comparison of arthroscopic and open bankart repairs. *J Pediatr Orthop* 2015;35(1):1-6.

4. Gigis I, Heikenfeld R, Kapinas A, Listringhaus R, Godolias G: Arthroscopic versus conservative treatment of first anterior dislocation of the shoulder in adolescents. *J Pediatr Orthop* 2014;34(4):421-425.

5. Leroux T, Ogilvie-Harris D, Veillette C, et al: The epidemiology of primary anterior shoulder dislocations in patients aged 10 to 16 years. *Am J Sports Med* 2015;43(9):2111-2117.

6. Baverel L, Colle PE, Saffarini M, Anthony Odri G, Barth J: Open Latarjet procedures produce better outcomes in competitive athletes compared with recreational athletes: A clinical comparative study of 106 athletes aged under 30 years. *Am J Sports Med* 2018;46(6):1408-1415.

   106 patients underwent open Latarjet procedure for shoulder instability. Only three recurrences of dislocation were noted, two in competitive athletes and one in a recreational athlete. Level of evidence: III.

7. Ellis HB Jr, Seiter M, Wise K, Wilson P: Glenoid bone loss in traumatic glenohumeral instability in the adolescent population. *J Pediatr Orthop* 2017;37(1):30-35.

   Bone loss after shoulder instability was measured retrospectively in 114 shoulders. Almost half of the patients (48%) sustained bone loss. Bone loss was not appreciated on plain radiographs 45% of the time. Male sex, older age, taller stature, sports injuries, and the presence of apprehension on physical examination were risk factors for bone loss. Level of evidence: II.

8. Torrance E, Clarke CJ, Monga P, Funk L, Walton MJ: Recurrence after arthroscopic labral repair for traumatic anterior instability in adolescent rugby and contact athletes. *Am J Sports Med* 2018;46(12):2969-2974.

   Adolescent rugby players were studied post arthroscopic stabilization for shoulder instability. Players younger than 16 years were 2.2 times as likely to sustain recurrent instability events than patients older than 16 years. 51% of the rugby players sustained recurrent shoulder dislocation after surgical stabilization. Level of evidence: IV.

9. Lee SH, Lim KH, Kim JW: Risk factors for recurrence of anterior-inferior instability of the shoulder after arthroscopic bankart repair in patients younger than 30 years. *Arthroscopy* 2018;34(9):2530-2536.

   Patients younger than 30 years are less likely to sustain recurrent dislocation of the shoulder when surgery is performed within 6 months of their dislocation. Level of evidence: III.

10. Makhni EC, Morrow ZS, Luchetti TJ, et al: Arm pain in youth baseball players: A survey of healthy players. *Am J Sports Med* 2015;43(1):41-46.

11. Wei AS, Khana S, Limpisvasti O, Crues J, Podesta L, Yocum LA: Clinical and magnetic resonance imaging findings associated with Little League elbow. *J Pediatr Orthop* 2010;30(7):715-719.

12. Pennock AT, Pytiak A, Stearns P, et al: Preseason assessment of radiographic abnormalities in elbows of Little League baseball players. *J Bone Joint Surg Am* 2016;98(9):761-767.

    MRI was performed in 26 asymptomatic Little League players between ages 10 and 13. Abnormalities were more common in year-round players, players with internal rotation deficit, and those who had private coaches. Level of evidence: III.

13. Pytiak AV, Stearns P, Bastrom TP, et al: Are the current Little League pitching guidelines adequate? A single-season prospective MRI study. *Orthop J Sports Med* 2017;5(5):2325967117704851.

    Prospective study of 26 Little League players with pre- and postseason MRI and physical exam. Despite compliance with pitching guidelines, 48% of players had abnormal MRI findings. There was a significant loss of shoulder internal rotation. Year-round play was associated with changes on MRI. Level of evidence: II.

14. Yukutake T, Nagai K, Yamada M, Aoyama T: Risk factors for elbow pain in Little League baseball players: A cross-sectional study focusing on developmental factors. *J Sports Med Phys Fitness* 2015;55(9):962-968.

15. Yukutake T, Kuwata M, Yamada M, Aoyama T: A preseason checklist for predicting elbow injury in Little League baseball players. *Orthop J Sports Med* 2015;3(1):2325967114566788.

16. Greenberg EM, Lawrence JTR, Fernandez-Fernandez A, et al: Physical and functional differences in youth baseball players with and without throwing-related pain. *Orthop J Sports Med* 2017;5(11):2325967117737731.

    A group of 84 youth baseball players were divided into those with and without throwing-related pain. Those with pain were taller, were heavier, played more baseball per year, and had a greater loss of internal rotation and asymmetric humeral retrotorsion. Level of evidence: III.

17. Norton R, Honstad C, Joshi R, Silvis M, Chinchilli V, Dhawan A: Risk factors for elbow and shoulder injuries in adolescent baseball players: A systematic review. *Am J Sports Med* 2019;47(4):982-990.

    A meta-analysis of throwing injuries in adolescent baseball throwers examined 19 independent risk factors for elbow and shoulder injuries. Risk factors for throwing injuries included age, height, playing for multiple teams, pitch velocity, and arm fatigue. Pitch number (per game) was a risk factor for shoulder injuries only. Level of evidence: III.

18. Okoroha KR, Lizzio VA, Meta F, Ahmad CS, Moutzouros V, Makhni EC: Predictors of elbow torque among youth and adolescent baseball pitchers. *Am J Sports Med* 2018;46(9):2148-2153.

    To analyze torque on adolescent pitchers' elbows, sensors were placed on 20 pitchers' elbows. Eight fastballs, 8 curveballs, and 8 changeups were analyzed. The greatest torque was found with fastballs and the greatest arm speed was found with curveballs. Older age and larger size were protective against elbow torque. Level of evidence: III.

19. USA Baseball Pitch Smart. https://www.mlb.com/pitch-smart/pitching-guidelines. Accessed December 12, 2018.

20. Gottschalk HP, Bastrom TP, Edmonds EW: Reliability of internal oblique elbow radiographs for measuring displacement of medial epicondyle humerus fractures: A cadaveric study. *J Pediatr Orthop* 2013;33(1):26-31.

21. Souder CD, Farnsworth CL, McNeil NP, Bomar JD, Edmonds EW: The distal humerus axial view: Assessment of displacement in medial epicondyle fractures. *J Pediatr Orthop* 2015;35(5):449-454.

22. Knapik DM, Fausett CL, Gilmore A, Liu RW: Outcomes of nonoperative pediatric medial humeral epicondyle fractures with and without associated elbow dislocation. *J Pediatr Orthop* 2017;37(4):e224-e228.

    A systematic review of the literature reporting on papers looking at the outcome of nonsurgical treatment of medial epicondyle fractures. Bony nonunion occurred in 69% of fracture dislocations and 49% of isolated fractures. Range of motion deficits were more likely in the setting of a dislocation, though clinical outcomes in all patients were good. Level of evidence: II.

23. Stepanovich M, Bastrom TP, Munch J III, Roocroft JH, Edmonds EW, Pennock AT: Does operative fixation affect outcomes of displaced medial epicondyle fractures? *J Child Orthop* 2016;10(5):413-419.

    12 patients treated surgically (6) and nonsurgically (6) for medial epicondyle fractures were examined at an average of 3 years postinjury. There was a high rate of osseus nonunions (5) and malunions (1) noted in the nonsurgical group versus none in the surgical group. Both had high patient satisfaction and elbow function scores. Level of evidence: III.

24. Pace GI, Hennrikus WL: Fixation of displaced medial epicondyle fractures in adolescents. *J Pediatr Orthop* 2017;37(2):e80-e82.

    A series of 17 elbows treated with fixation of a medial epicondyle fracture in the setting of a fracture/dislocation were evaluated. Those treated with a screw and washer were compared with those treated with screw only. The presence of a washer increased risk of hardware prominence and request for removal. No fragmentation was seen in the screw-only group. Level of evidence: IV.

25. Shukla SK, Cohen MS: Symptomatic medial epicondyle nonunion: Treatment by open reduction and fixation with a tension band construct. *J Shoulder Elbow Surg* 2011;20(3):455-460.

26. Axibal DP, Carry P, Skelton A, Mayer SW: No difference in return to sport and other outcomes between operative and nonoperative treatment of medial epicondyle fractures in pediatric upper-extremity athletes. *Clin J Sport Med* 2018.

Pediatrics

Retrospective chart review and phone interviews compared patients with medial epicondyle fractures, 24 treated without surgery and 14 with surgery. Outcomes were not different in terms of return to play or complication rate among those with moderately displaced fractures. Level of evidence: III.

27. Schuett DJ, Bomar JD, Pennock AT: Pelvic apophyseal avulsion fractures: A retrospective review of 228 cases. *J Pediatr Orthop* 2015;35(6):617-623.

28. Eberbach H, Hohloch L, Feucht MJ, Konstantinidis L, Südkamp NP, Zwingmann J: Operative versus conservative treatment of apophyseal avulsion fractures of the pelvis in the adolescents: A systematical review with meta-analysis of clinical outcome and return to sports. *BMC Musculoskelet Disord* 2017;18(1):162.

    Meta-analysis of 596 patients (14 studies) comparing return to sports and preinjury activity level after pelvic avulsion fracture was performed. In fragments displaced more than 1.5 cm return to preinjury level of sport was slightly higher in patients who had higher demand in their sports. Level of evidence: III.

29. Tepolt FA, Feldman L, Kocher MS: Trends in pediatric ACL reconstruction from the PHIS database. *J Pediatr Orthop* 2018;38(9):e490-e494.

    Data from the Pediatric Health Information Services database were analyzed for patients younger than 18 years who underwent ACL reconstruction between 2004 and 2014. The rate of ACL reconstruction was compared with the number of orthopaedic surgeries performed on this population. Over this time period, there was a 2.8-fold increase in the number of ACL reconstructions relative to the total increase in orthopaedic surgeries. Level of evidence: IV.

30. Kocher MS, Micheli LJ, Zurakowski D, Luke A: Partial tears of the anterior cruciate ligament in children and adolescents. *Am J Sports Med* 2002;30(5):697-703.

31. Popkin CA, Wright ML, Pennock AT, et al: Trends in management and complications of anterior cruciate ligament injuries in pediatric patients: A survey of the PRiSM Society. *J Pediatr Orthop* 2018;38(2):e61-e65.

    A survey of 71 orthopaedic members of the Pediatric Research in Sports Medicine Society was performed to look at treatment trends of the young and very young athlete undergoing ACL reconstruction. Level of evidence: V.

32. Shifflett GD, Green DW, Widmann RF, Marx RG: Growth arrest following ACL reconstruction with hamstring autograft in skeletally immature patients: A review of 4 cases. *J Pediatr Orthop* 2016;36(4):355-361.

    A case report of four patients who underwent transphyseal ACL reconstruction with hamstring autograft and developed growth disturbances, three of which required further surgery to address the deformity. Level of evidence: IV.

33. Cruz AI Jr, Fabricant PD, McGraw M, Rozell JC, Ganley TJ, Wells L: All-epiphyseal ACL reconstruction in children: Review of safety and early complications. *J Pediatr Orthop* 2017;37(3):204-209.

    Retrospective review of 103 patients who underwent all-epiphyseal ACL reconstruction. Overall complication rate was 16.5% and included rerupture, subsequent meniscus tear, growth disturbance, and arthrofibrosis. Level of evidence: IV.

34. Dekker TJ, Godin JA, Dale KM, Garrett WE, Taylor DC, Riboh JC: Return to sport after pediatric anterior cruciate ligament reconstruction and its effect on subsequent anterior cruciate ligament injury. *J Bone Joint Surg Am* 2017;99(11):897-904.

    A continuous cohort of 112 patients <18 years old who underwent isolated primary ACL reconstruction with autograft were followed up for a minimum of 2 years. 91% of patients returned to sport. 32% of patients sustained either an ipsilateral re-rupture or a contralateral ACL tear, with time to return to sport being predictive of a second injury. Level of evidence: IV.

35. Paterno MV, Rauh MJ, Schmitt LC, Ford KR, Hewett TE: Incidence of second ACL injuries 2 years after primary ACL reconstruction and return to sport. *Am J Sports Med* 2014;42(7):1567-1573.

36. Ho B, Edmonds EW, Chambers HG, Bastrom TP, Pennock AT: Risk factors for early ACL reconstruction failure in pediatric and adolescent patients: A review of 561 cases. *J Pediatr Orthop* 2018;38(7):388-392.

    Retrospective review of 561 ACL reconstructions in pediatric and adolescent patients. Overall graft failure rate was 9.6%, with soft-tissue grafts almost twice as likely to fail as patellar tendon grafts. Level of evidence: IV.

37. Pennock AT, Ho B, Parvanta K, et al: Does allograft augmentation of small-diameter hamstring autograft ACL grafts reduce the incidence of graft retear? *Am J Sports Med* 2017;45(2):334-338.

    Retrospective review of primary ACL reconstructions with hamstring autograft comparing 20 patients with small graft size (<7 mm) and 20 patients with small graft size augmented with allograft who were followed up for a minimum of 2 years. There was a significantly higher rate of graft failure in the allograft augmented group, 30% versus 1%, most within 1 year of surgery. Level of evidence: III.

38. Mayo MH, Mitchell JJ, Axibal DP, et al: Anterior cruciate ligament injury at the time of anterior tibial spine fracture in young patients: An observational cohort study. *J Pediatr Orthop* 2019;39(9):e668-e673.

    ACL injury was found to occur with tibial spine fracture in 25 out of 129 patients studied. Older male patients were more likely to sustain concomitant injuries. MRI was not sufficient to detect ACL injury; most were found at the time of surgery. Level of evidence: III.

39. Axibal DP, Mitchell JJ, Mayo MH, et al: Epidemiology of anterior tibial spine fractures in young patients: A retrospective cohort study of 122 cases. *J Pediatr Orthop* 2019;39(2):e87-e90.

    Retrospective review of 122 tibial spine fractures found the average age at injury to be 11 years. 21% were type I, 44% were type II, and 34% were type III. Organized sports was the most common mechanism, 36%, then bicycle accidents. 69% males. Males were older (11.6 vs 9.8). Organized sport more common in males; outdoor sports (skiing, snowboarding, skateboarding) more common in females. Level of evidence: IV.

40. Meyers MH, McKeever MF: Fracture of the intercondylar eminence of the tibia. *J Bone Joint Surg Am* 1959;41-A(2):209-220.

41. Zaricznyj B: Avulsion fracture of the tibial eminence: Treatment by open reduction and pinning. *J Bone Joint Surg Am* 1977;59(8):1111-1114.

42. Mitchell JJ, Sjostrom R, Mansour AA, et al: Incidence of meniscal injury and chondral pathology in anterior tibial spine fractures of children. *J Pediatr Orthop* 2015;35(2):130-135.

43. Rhodes JT, Cannamela PC, Cruz AI, et al: Incidence of meniscal entrapment and associated knee injuries in tibial spine avulsions. *J Pediatr Orthop* 2018;38(2):e38-e42.

    Meniscal entrapment was found in 39.9% of the 163 patients enrolled in a multicenter study of tibial spine avulsions. Concomitant injuries are common in patients who sustain tibial spine avulsion fractures. These include meniscal, chondral, and ligamentous injuries. Level of evidence: IV.

44. Mitchell JJ, Mayo MH, Axibal DP, et al: Delayed anterior cruciate ligament reconstruction in young patients with previous anterior tibial spine fractures. *Am J Sports Med* 2016;44(8):2047-2056.

    Retrospective review of 101 pediatric patients with tibial spine fractures followed up for a minimum of 2 years. 19% of patients underwent a subsequent delayed ACL reconstruction. The risk of progression to ACL reconstruction increased with age at the time of injury for the tibial spine fracture. Level of evidence: IV.

45. Ellis HB Jr, Wise K, LaMont L, Copley L, Wilson P: Prevalence of discoid meniscus during arthroscopy for isolated lateral mensicus pathology in the pediatric popluation. *J Pediatr Orthop* 2017;37:285-292.

    Retrospective review of 261 arthroscopic procedures for isolated lateral meniscus pathology found that 75% of the menisci were discoid in nature. 97% of patients younger than 13 years with lateral meniscus pathology had discoid meniscus and 66% had no reported injury. This rate dropped in the 14 to 16 age group to 59%. MRI criteria were unreliable for diagnosing discoid after the age of 13. Level of evidence: III.

46. Shieh A, Bastrom T, Roocroft J, Edmonds EW, Pennock AT: Meniscus tear patterns in relation to skeletal immaturity: Children versus adolescents. *Am J Sports Med* 2013;41(12):2779-2783.

47. Lee CR, Bin SI, Kim JM, Lee BS, Kim NK: Arthroscopic partial meniscectomy in young patients with symptomatic discoid lateral meniscus: An average 10-year follow-up study. *Arch Orthop Trauma Surg* 2018;138(3):369-376.

    Retrospective review of 73 knees in 66 patients who underwent partial lateral meniscectomy for discoid lateral meniscus age ≤40. There was a mean 10-year follow-up. Reoperation rate was 32.9%. Radiographs showed progression of lateral compartment arthritis in 68.5% of knees and MRI showed degeneration of the residual meniscus in 52.9% of knees.

48. Carter CW, Hoellwarth J, Weiss JM: Clinical outcomes as a function of meniscal stability in the discoid meniscus: A preliminary report. *J Pediatr Orthop* 2012;32(1):9-14.

49. Mosich GM, Lieu V, Ebramzadeh E, Beck JJ: Operative treatment of isolated meniscus injuries in adolescent patients: A meta-analysis and review. *Sports Health* 2018;10(4):311-316.

    Systematic review and meta-analysis of nine studies on isolated meniscus tears in adolescents found a recent increase in meniscus repair versus meniscectomy, possibly because of poor long-term results with meniscectomy. Retear rate for repair was 37%. Level of evidence: IV.

50. Vanderhave KL, Moravek JE, Sekiya JK, Wojtys EM: Meniscus tears in the young athlete: Results of arthroscopic repair. *J Pediatr Orthop* 2011;31(5):496-500.

51. Shieh AK, Edmonds EW, Pennock AT: Revision meniscal surgery in children and adolescents: Risk factors and mechanisms for failure and subsequent management. *Am J Sports Med* 2016;44(4):838-843.

    Retrospective review of arthroscopic surgery performed on 324 menisci in a pediatric population. At a mean of 40 months follow-up, the revision procedure rate was 13%. Primary repairs had the highest failure rate of 18%, followed by discoid saucerization (15%) and partial meniscectomy (7%). Patients with open physes and bucket-handle meniscus tear had the highest retear rate of 46%. Level of evidence: III.

52. Fithian DC, Paxton EW, Stone ML, et al: Epidemiology and natural history of acute patellar dislocation. *Am J Sports Med* 2004;32(5):1114-1121. [PubMed].

53. Jaquith BP, Parikh SN: Predictors of recurrent patellar instability in children and adolescents after first-time dislocation. *J Pediatr Orthop* 2017;37(7):484-490.

    Retrospective review of all patients at a single institution who presented with first-time patellar dislocation. Of those treated nonsurgically, the most significant risk factors for recurrent dislocation included trochlear dysplasia, skeletal immaturity, patella alta, and history of contralateral patellar dislocation. A predictive model for recurrence risk was created. Level of evidence: IV.

54. Sanders TL, Pareek A, Hewett TE, Stuart MJ, Dahm DL, Krych AJ: High rate of recurrent patellar dislocation in skeletally immature patients: A long-term population-based study. *Knee Surg Sports Traumatol Arthrosc* 2018;26(4):1037-1043.

55. Bryant J, Pandya N: Medial patellofemoral ligament repair restores stability in pediatric patients when compared to reconstruction. *Knee* 2018;25(4):602-608.

    Primary MPFL repair was compared with historical control of MPFL reconstruction with allograft. Sixteen repairs were compared with 22 historical reconstructions. Results were similar in this study. There were three complications in reconstruction group and none in the repair group. Level of evidence: III.

56. Kumar N, Bastrom TP, Dennis MM, Pennock AT, Edmonds EW: Adolescent medial patellofemoral ligament reconstruction: A comparison of the use of autograft versus allograft hamstring. *Orthop J Sports Med* 2018;6(5):2325967118774272.

Retrospective chart review compared patients who underwent MPFL reconstruction using autograft versus allograft reconstruction. Allograft was used in 36 patients, and autograft in 23. The outcomes were similar, without any statistically significant difference. The authors concluded that allograft is as effective and safe as autograft in this population for MPFL reconstruction. Level of evidence: III.

57. Nelitz M, Dreyhaupt J, Williams SRM: No growth disturbance after trochleoplasty for recurrent patellar dislocation in adolescents with open growth plates. *Am J Sports Med* 2018;46(13):3209-3216.

    18 consecutive patients with trochlear dysplasia and less than 2 years of growth remaining underwent trochleoplasty. At 2-year follow-up, no clinical or radiographic growth disturbances were found. No redislocations occurred. Level of evidence: IV.

58. Nelitz M, Dreyhaupt J, Williams SRM: Anatomic reconstruction of the medial patellofemoral ligament in children and adolescents using a pedicled quadriceps tendon graft shows favourable results at a minimum of 2-year follow-up. *Knee Surg Sports Traumatol Arthrosc* 2018;26(4):1210-1215.

    The authors describe a technique that respects the physis for MPFL reconstruction, with quadriceps pedicle, no hardware in the patella, and physeal sparing in the femur. No recurrent instability was reported with 2.6-year follow up. Study design was prospective. Level of evidence: III.

59. Kessler JI, Nikizad H, Shea KG, Jacobs JC Jr, Bebchuk JD, Weiss JM: The demographics and epidemiology of osteochondritis dissecans of the knee in children and adolescents *Am J Sports Med* 2014;42(2):320-326.

60. Krause M, Hapfelmeier A, Möller M, Amling M, Bohndorf K, Meenen NM: Healing predictors of stable juvenile osteochondritis dissecans knee lesions after 6 and 12 months of nonoperative treatment. *Am J Sports Med* 2013;41(10):2384-2391.

61. Siegall E, Faust JR, Herzog MM, Marshall KW, Willimon SC, Busch MT: Age predicts disruption of the articular surface of the femoral condyles in knee OCD: Can we reduce usage of arthroscopy and MRI? *J Pediatr Orthop* 2018;38(3):176-180.

    Retrospective review of 119 patients treated for OCD of the femoral condyle was performed. Age was found to be a statistically significant predictor of cartilage status when patients were 13 or younger or 17 or older. The authors point out that age is an independent predictor and may be a factor in decreasing need for MRI studies in some patients. Level of evidence: IV.

62. Weiss JM, Nikizad H, Shea KG, et al: The incidence of surgery in osteochondritis dissecans in children and adolescents. *Orthop J Sports Med* 2016;4(3):2325967116635515.

    Retrospective review of 334 OCD lesions in 317 patients was reported. Progression to surgery was 35%; it did not differ significantly between sexes with OCD of any joint. In OCD of the knee, elbow, and ankle, progression to surgery strongly correlated with patient age at the time of diagnosis. Level of evidence: IV.

63. Wu IT, Custers RJH, Desai VS, et al: Internal fixation of unstable osteochondritis dissecans: Do open growth plates improve healing rate? *Am J Sports Med* 2018;46(10):2394-2401.

    Multicenter retrospective study of 87 patients with fixation of OCD of the knee found that rate of healing did not correlate with open physes or age. Lateral femoral condyle lesions were found to be a risk factor for healing failure. Level of evidence: III.

64. Sanders TL, Pareek A, Obey MR, et al: High rate of osteoarthritis after osteochondritis dissecans fragment excision compared with surgical restoration at a mean 16-year follow-up. *Am J Sports Med* 2017;45(8):1799-1805.

    Retrospective review of 221 patients treated to OCD of the knee with mean follow-up of over 15 years is reported. Fragment of excision correlated with higher rate of arthritis than fragment preservation or defect grafting. Other risk factors for arthritis were BMI greater than 25 kg/m^2 and older age at diagnosis. Level of evidence: III.

65. Kramer DE, Glotzbecker MP, Shore BJ, et al: Results of surgical management of osteochondritis dissecans of the ankle in the pediatric and adolescent population. *J Pediatr Orthop* 2015;35(7):725-733.

66. Kessler JI, Weiss JM, Nikizad H, et al: Osteochondritis dissecans of the ankle in children and adolescents: Demographics and epidemiology. *Am J Sports Med* 2014;42(9):2165-2171.

67. Kessler JI, Jacobs JC Jr, Cannamela PC, Shea KG, Weiss JM: Childhood obesity is associated with osteochondritis dissecans of the knee, ankle, and elbow in children and adolescents. *J Pediatr Orthop* 2018;38(5):e296-e299.

    Review of 269 patients with OCD was performed. Extreme obesity correlated especially with OCD Of the elbow and ankle. Moderate obesity correlated with increased risk of knee OCD. Patients with OCD had higher average BMI compared to patients without OCD. Level of Evidence IV.

68. Pagliazzi G, Baldassarri M, Perazzo L, Vannini F, Castagnini F, Buda R: Tissue bioengineering in the treatment of osteochondritis dissecans of the talus in children with open physis: Preliminary results. *J Pediatr Orthop* 2018;38(7):375-381.

    Seven patients with open physes with OCD of the talus were treated with arthroscopic bone marrow aspirate concentrate (BMAC) transplantation. Follow-up showed that 43% fully healed their OCD lesions, and all were satisfied with the procedure. Level of evidence: IV.

Chapter 61

Pediatric Spine Disorders and Trauma

A. Noelle Larson, MD • Lindsay M. Andras, MD

ABSTRACT

Spinal deformity is frequently encountered in children. Adolescent idiopathic scoliosis is the most common form of scoliosis, but scoliosis can also present in younger children and in children with congenital vertebral anomalies or associated syndromes. Treatment includes observation, bracing, and surgery. Specialized techniques may be needed in immature children to preserve growth, particularly in children younger than 10 years. Spondylolysis is most commonly seen in ambulatory athletic patients. Although pars repair or fusion surgery may be indicated on occasion, most patients respond to conservative management. High-grade spondylolisthesis may necessitate surgical treatment due to concern for progression and neurologic deterioration. Finally, trauma can result in vertebral fracture and, in rare cases, spinal cord injury. An understanding of pediatric spinal deformities is essential to provide appropriate care, treatment, and referral.

Keywords: congenital scoliosis; pars defect; spine deformity; spondylolisthesis; spondylolysis

Dr. Larson or an immediate family member serves as a paid consultant to or is an employee of Medtronic and serves as a board member, owner, officer, or committee member of the Pediatric Orthopaedic Society of North America and the Scoliosis Research Society. Dr. Andras or an immediate family member is a member of a speakers' bureau or has made paid presentations on behalf of Biomet, Medtronic, and Nuvasive; serves as a paid consultant to or is an employee of Biomet, Medtronic, Nuvasive and Zimmer; has stock or stock options held in Eli Lilly; and serves as a board member, owner, officer, or committee member of the Pediatric Orthopaedic Society of North America and the Scoliosis Research Society.

Introduction

Adolescent idiopathic scoliosis is the most common spine condition found in children. However, familiarity with other traumatic and nontraumatic causes of spinal deformity is essential for prompt diagnosis, treatment, and referral. Early-onset scoliosis can be life threatening, as can scoliosis associated with neuromuscular conditions. This section will summarize recent developments in the treatment of scoliosis, kyphosis, and spine deformities associated with trauma.

Early-Onset Scoliosis

Early-onset scoliosis (EOS) is defined as a spinal curvature in the coronal plane of greater than 10° with onset under 10 years of age. Children with EOS are at risk for impaired pulmonary function from their spinal deformity due to constraints on the thorax during a critical time of lung development.[1] The natural history of untreated EOS is associated with significant morbidity and potential for cardiopulmonary compromise, including respiratory failure and cor pulmonale.

A Swedish study evaluating children treated between 1927 and 1937 compared expected population death rates and demonstrated more than double the mortality rate by the age of 40 years in patients with EOS compared with that of the general population.[2] Early spinal fusion was once routine in children with severe progressive EOS, which addressed the scoliosis, but limited spine and thoracic growth resulting in poor pulmonary outcomes.[3] Currently, the objective of EOS treatment is to maximize growth of the spine and thorax by controlling the spinal deformity, with the goal of promoting normal lung development and pulmonary function. This population is also challenging due to the diverse and often medically complex nature of these patients. The etiology of the spinal deformity may be idiopathic, associated with underlying systemic syndromes, secondary to a neuromuscular condition, or caused by a structural congenital spinal

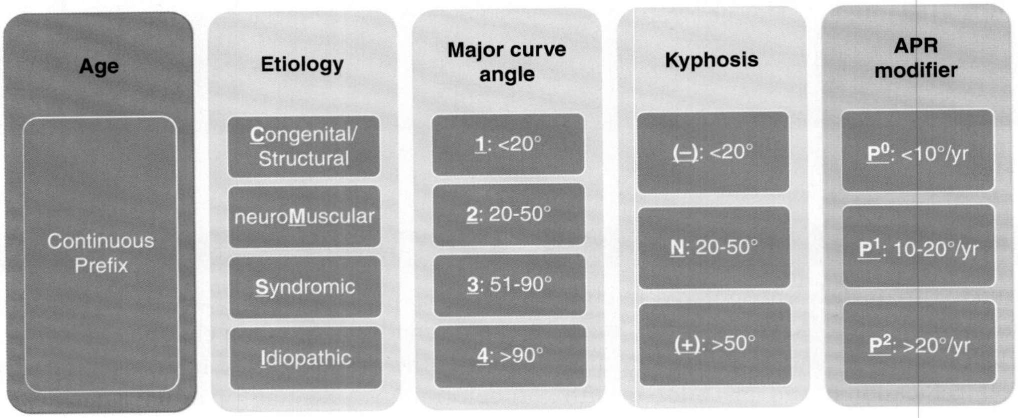

Figure 1 Early-onset scoliosis (EOS) classification system by Vitale et al takes into account etiology, curve magnitude, kyphosis, and rate of progression.

deformity. This heterogeneous group of patients may require a variety of treatments. Vitale et al have developed the C-EOS classification system to aid in studying these patients and optimizing their management[4] (see **Figure 1**).

Infantile Idiopathic Scoliosis

Unlike adolescent idiopathic scoliosis, infantile idiopathic scoliosis (IIS) is more common in boys (1:1 male to female ratio), is most often a left thoracic curve, and improves spontaneously in the majority of cases. While 74% to 92% of early-onset idiopathic scoliosis in children younger than 2 years spontaneously resolves, some of these curves do not improve and are in fact progressive. Mehta identified predictors of progression including: Cobb angle >20°; rib vertebral angle difference >20°; and rib phase 2 (rib head overlaps the vertebral body). In cases that do not have these risk factors for progression, patients can be observed and reassessed in 6 months.

In cases with these predictors of progression or those who have already demonstrated clinical or radiographic progression, the initial assessment is confirming that the scoliosis is in fact idiopathic. An MRI of the entire spine is warranted to evaluate for any intraspinal anomalies such as a tethered cord, syrinx, or Chiari malformation that may be associated with the scoliosis. Intraspinal anomalies have been shown to be present in 13% to 22% of patients with presumed idiopathic infantile scoliosis.[5,6] Both Pahys and Dobbs et al reported that a neurosurgical intervention was indicated in 70% of the cases in which these anomalies were identified. Consequently, managing the concomitant intraspinal pathology is of utmost importance, as it may prevent potential neurologic problems in addition to halting progression or even improving curve magnitude.

In IIS cases that are progressing or have risk factors for progression, bracing treatment is sometimes considered, but its efficacy in EOS continues to be a source of debate and compliance with brace wear is often challenging in this age group. Currently, casting is typically the first line in treatment. Mehta et al have demonstrated that casting may not only slow progression, but in some cases may also lead to curve resolution, especially when initiated in younger children with smaller curves (mean Cobb angle 32°, mean age 19 months).[7] This type of casting is also known as EDF casting for the elongation, derotation, and flexion maneuver that is performed. The positive outcomes seen in Mehta's series have driven a resurgence of enthusiasm for casting. Alternative techniques include placing the cast with the child suspended instead of in traction, casts that do not go over the shoulder, or even those placed without anesthesia are being trialed in an effort to optimize conservative management.[8-10] While many cases of IIS may be successfully managed conservatively, some curves continue to progress despite this, prompting consideration of surgical management with growing spine instrumentation (see **Figure 2**).

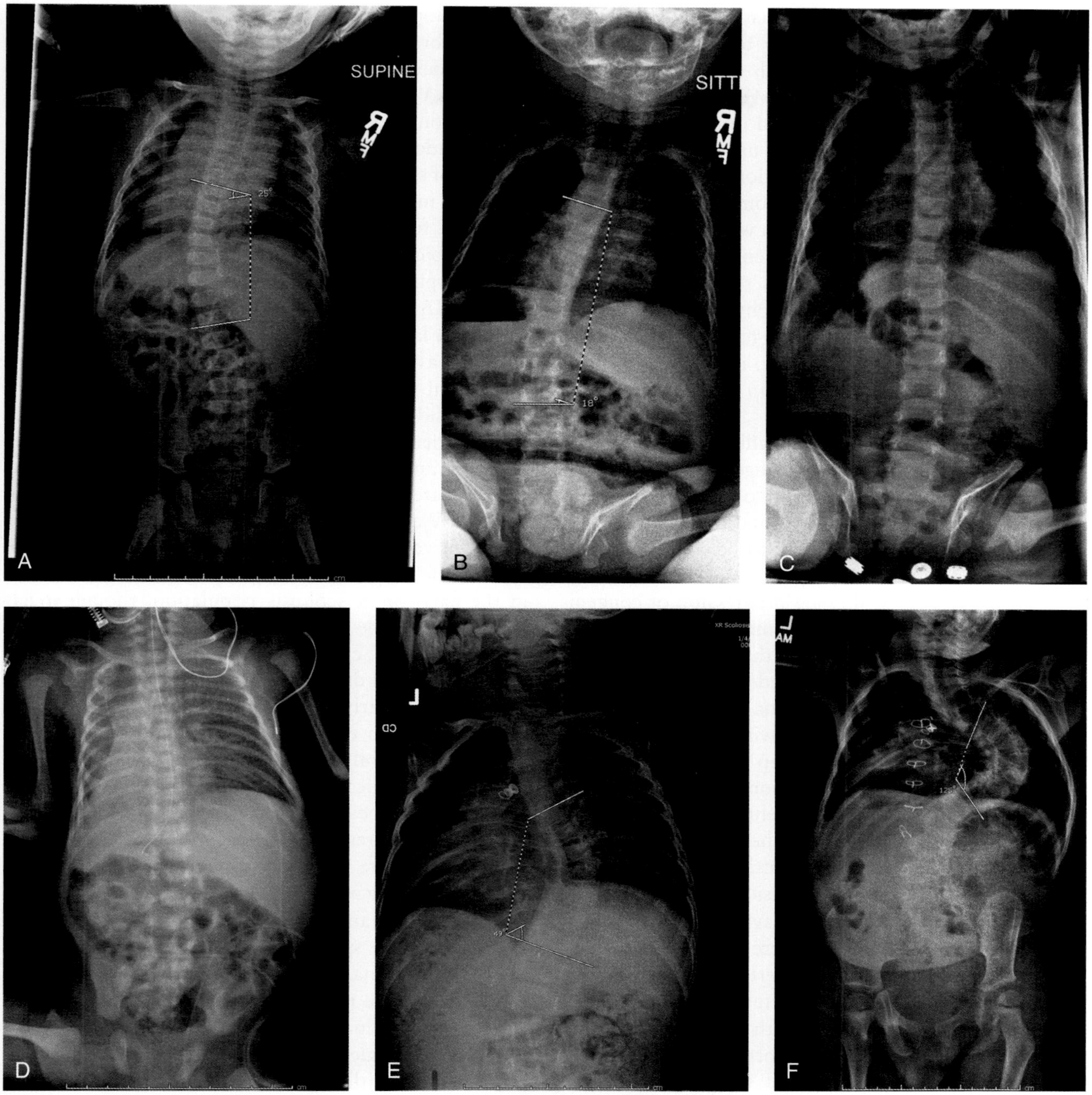

Figure 2 **A** through **C**, Radiographs show a patient with IIS and complete resolution of the curve with observation alone. **D** through **F** Shows a patient with a similar curve magnitude on presentation but characteristics predictive of progression. The patient's curve progressed and surgery for growing rod placement has been scheduled.

Congenital Scoliosis

Congenital scoliosis consists of a variety of vertebral anomalies that can be broadly categorized as either defects of vertebral formation or defects of segmentation. These two types of defects may occur separately or in combination, which can be particularly problematic. A unilateral failure of segmentation (bar) opposite a contralateral hemivertebrae is known to progress rapidly. Of note, a true hemivertebrae consists of half the vertebral body, a hemilamina and a single pedicle, but there are many variations of this that may be encountered. Additionally these deformities are often associated with rib deformities that may also impact the child's pulmonary function.

An important aspect of evaluating the child with congenital scoliosis is evaluating for other concomitant anomalies. For patients with significant or progressive congenital scoliosis, an MRI is recommended due to the high rate of associated intraspinal anomalies, which have a prevalence of up to 37% in some series.[11] An additional consideration is the evaluation of the genitourinary system, as anomalies will be found in approximately 20% of children with congenital scoliosis.[12] While many MRI protocols will also image the genitourinary system, this is traditionally evaluated with a renal ultrasonography. Similarly, these patients with congenital scoliosis have around a 25% incidence of cardiac anomalies, so if the child has not had a formal cardiac evaluation an echocardiogram is warranted.

Although bracing treatment will not alter the natural history of the anomalous congenital deformity, it may be of benefit to address the longer, flexible compensatory curves that often surround these deformities. Casting was historically thought to be contraindicated in cases of congenital EOS; however, several series have now shown success in slowing progression of congenital curves and delaying instrumentation.[13,14] For young children with congenital scoliosis that progresses despite casting or whose rib deformity and/or pulmonary status prevent them from being a casting candidate, growing spine instrumentation with growing rods or VEPTR implants is typically the next step in management. Of note, the initial VEPTR description advocated for thoracoplasty in addition to placement of rib anchors, but due to concerns about creating chest wall stiffness and rigidity, most surgeons reserve cutting the ribs for cases in which there are multiple rib fusions.

One notable exception to avoiding early spinal fusion is congenital scoliosis where the spine deformity is limited to a small number of vertebrae. For example, in the case of an isolated hemivertebra causing progressive scoliosis, an early fusion (with or without excision of the hemivertebrae) can often correct the scoliosis in a single surgery between the ages of 3 and 6 years, with a fusion of only two to four vertebrae.

Neuromuscular/Syndromic Scoliosis

Neuromuscular and syndromic scoliosis comprises a diverse group of conditions, many of which have their own unique considerations. While treatment with bracing treatment or casting is generally the initial management in these cases, there are some diagnoses where this is either ineffective or contraindicated. For example, in patients with spinal muscular atrophy (SMA), scoliosis will develop in over 90% of patients. In these SMA patients, bracing treatment has been unable to prevent scoliosis development and can lead to respiratory complications.[15] Although a soft TLSO is sometimes used for positional support in these flaccid curves, the treatment to address the SMA scoliosis is typically surgical. In cases of slow progression and stable pulmonary function, this may be delayed until the child is old enough for spinal fusion, though many of these children experience rapid progression and undergo treatment with growing spine instrumentation. A notable consideration in the SMA population is skipping fusion levels or performing a laminectomy in the lumbar spine as the only currently available treatment for this condition requires intrathecal drug delivery which can be more difficult with a solid fusion.

In patients with cerebral palsy, scoliosis commonly develops and is more frequently observed in patients with greater functional involvement, with 30% of GMFCS V cerebral palsy patients having a moderate to severe curve by the age of 10 years.[15] There are limited data on the impact of bracing treatment on these curves in the early-onset scoliosis population, though it has been shown to be ineffective in preventing progression in the adolescent cerebral palsy population.[16] Although there are limited data on casting for patients with cerebral palsy for early-onset scoliosis, these patients have been included in other studies of neuromuscular EOS patients in general and casting is often used in attempt to postpone surgical management though this would not be expected to be curative.[14,17] In patients with continued, severe progression, growing rods have been shown to be an effective treatment though the deep infection rate is reportedly as high as 30%.[18] A frequent question in both the EOS and adolescent neuromuscular patients with progressive spinal deformity is whether the benefits of surgical management exceed the risks given the frequently severe medical comorbidities. Though each case must be evaluated individually in this respect, most series favor surgical intervention despite a high complication rate with a preference for early fusion when patient size permits.[7,19,20]

Growing Spine Instrumentation

In many EOS cases, management with observation, bracing treatment or casting is sufficient to either prevent the need for instrumentation or postpone surgical intervention until an age where a definitive fusion can be performed. Nevertheless, when the scoliosis progresses aggressively despite these conservative measures or the child is not a candidate for bracing treatment or casting due to concomitant medical comorbidities, earlier intervention may be necessary. Fusion of the very young child with a spinal deformity was once standard but has fallen out of favor as this approach resulted in small lung volumes and subsequent restrictive lung disease.[3] The last decade has witnessed the development of several "growth-friendly" alternatives. The objectives of these implants are to maximize growth of the spine and facilitate development of the thorax and lungs while controlling curve progression. Nevertheless, use of these modern implants should be delayed for as long as possible as early instrumentation is fraught with both a high complication rate and a decrease in the amount of growth or expansion over time.[21,22] These "growth-friendly" implants can be classified into three distinct subtypes including distraction-based, guided growth, and compression-based strategies.[23] Of note, due to the relatively rare nature of these curves, the majority of studies of "growth-friendly" instrumentation are comprised of series of patients with not only IIS but a diverse group of patients with early onset scoliosis.

Of the "growth-friendly" techniques, distraction-based strategies are the most commonly used including traditional growing rods, vertical expandable prosthetic titanium rib (VEPTR) device, and magnetically lengthening growing rods. Traditional growing rods consist of a proximal and distal anchor with either a screw or hook attached to the spine. These anchors are then connected by either a single rod, or preferably dual rods, with expandable segments in the middle. This segment between the anchors is intentionally not fused to allow for growth and expansion and is surgically lengthened at approximately 6 month intervals. In a series of 24 patients by Akbarnia et al. with a mean of 4-year follow-up, there was an improvement of coronal plane scoliosis curve from 82° to 36° and an average of 1.2 cm growth in T1-S1 length per year.[24] An additional series found that patients who were lengthened at ≤6 month intervals had significantly higher annual T1-S1 growth rate of 1.8 cm/yr compared with 1.0 cm/yr in patients lengthened less frequently, leading many to believe that distraction may in fact promote growth of the spine.[25] An alternative to the traditional growing rod is the vertical expandable prosthetic titanium rib (VEPTR) device developed by Robert Campbell who furthered our understanding of the chest wall deformity and resultant thoracic insufficiency syndrome that many of these children endure. VEPTRs consist of rib anchors and were initially described for the primary purpose of chest expansion. However, as the thorax and spinal development are closely linked, they have also demonstrated the ability to control the coronal curve while promoting spinal growth.[26,27]

Another option is a hybrid construct, combining both the traditional concept of growing rods and VEPTR using rib anchors as the proximal attachment for a growing rod construct. This allows the theoretical advantage of avoiding any fusion of the spine at the proximal anchor site. Additionally the flexibility of the ribs as upper anchors may reduce the rigidity of the construct and help protect against rod fractures. While all of these options initially require surgical lengthenings through the growth period, a magnetically lengthening option has now obtained FDA approval. While the overall construct is similar to prior growing rods, this allows the implants to be lengthened in an office setting. The initial studies of magnetically lengthening growing rods (MCGR) appear promising with regard to achieving similar curve correction and increases in spine length with far fewer surgical procedures.[28] For example, a case-control study comparing 12 matched MCGR and traditional growing rod patients demonstrated no significant difference in spine length gains, though 57 fewer surgical procedures were performed in the MCGR group.[29] While implant complications continue to occur with MCGR, avoiding the need for routine surgical lengthening will likely have both physical and psychosocial benefits for this patient population (**Figure 3**).

Although distraction-based techniques remain the most popular option for "growth-friendly" instrumentation, there are also guided growth and compression-based alternatives. Guided growth techniques aim to straighten the spine with instrumentation that allows the vertebrae to continue to grow along the path of the implants. Authors have described the Shilla technique in which there is an apical fusion and sliding screws at either end placed with minimal dissection in the hopes of avoiding spontaneous fusion.[30] The major theoretical advantage of growth guidance techniques over growing rods is that children avoid multiple surgical lengthenings though there is some evidence that less spinal growth and less correction of scoliosis is seen with Shilla compared with growing rods.[31]

Another alternative approach is compression-based implants which aim to correct the scoliosis by stopping the growth of the convex side of the scoliosis without fusion and allowing growth of the concave side of the curve. This is performed via an anterior approach typically thoracoscopically in which staples, tethers, or other devices are placed across the vertebral epiphyseal plate on the convex side of the scoliosis. Although several case series on compression-based implants have demonstrated improvement in curve magnitude in scoliosis patients, due to the risk of overcorrection, these techniques are generally

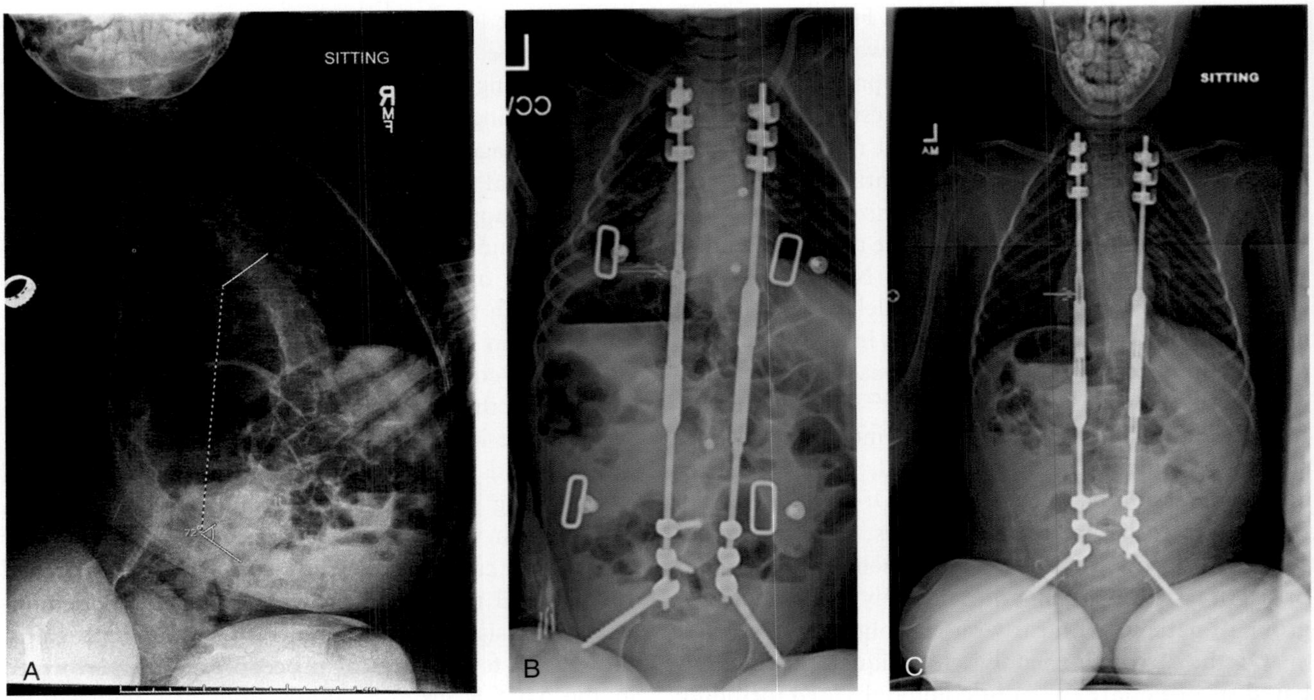

Figure 3 **A** through **C**, Preoperative, postoperative, and most recent radiographs of a patient with early-onset scoliosis associated with spinal muscular atrophy (SMA) who underwent magnetically lengthening growing rods (MCGR) which allows for lengthening in the clinic setting as shown (red arrows showing device distraction).

reserved for patients with more limited growth potential, such as those aged 9 years or above.[32] Prospective studies are underway to study efficacy and complications. Data on thoracoscopic anterior spinal instrumentation have shown minimal effect on pulmonary function, but there are concerns regarding the pulmonary impact of one or more transthoracic surgeries if performed through an open approach. Open anterior surgery should be avoided as serial measures of lung function in older children with scoliosis treated with anterior open spine surgery have shown greater loss of pulmonary function postoperatively than with posterior spinal instrumentation.[33]

Adolescent Idiopathic Scoliosis

Adolescent idiopathic scoliosis (AIS) is the most common type of scoliosis in children. Mild curvatures are present in up to 1 in 20 children. Moderate scoliosis is found in up to one in 300 children and one in 3,000 children require surgical management for severe curves over 45° to 50° due to concern of ongoing progression in adulthood. Treatment options include observation, bracing treatment, and surgery. The etiology is unknown, but genetic and structural factors are actively being explored. Up to 30% of patients with AIS have been shown to have lower bone mineral density than population controls, which is associated with increased risk of curve progression and corrects with calcium and vitamin D treatment.[34]

Nonsurgical Management of Adolescent Idiopathic Scoliosis

Bracing treatment in a corrective TLSO for curves between 20° and 40° is recommended for children with growth remaining either Risser 2 or less or Sanders Stage 5 or less. The greatest risk for curve progression is at peak growth velocity or Sanders Stage 3. The simplified Tanner-Whitehouse (Sanders digital maturity stage classification, **Table 1, Figure 4**) has been found to be highly predictive of peak growth velocity with good inter-and intraobserver reliability and is preferred over Risser staging.[35-38] At peak growth velocity, all digital physes are capped (Sanders Stage 3) and children are 90% of final adult height. At Sanders Stage 4, children are 96% of their final adult height (**Figure 5**).

Increased hours of brace wear and correction in brace are predictive of a successful brace outcome.[39] Standing radiographs should be obtained in brace to ensure at least 25% to 50% curve correction in brace. The BrAIST study was a prospective randomized controlled study which was stopped early by the data safety monitoring board due to the efficacy of bracing treatment, which found it unethical to withhold full-time bracing treatment from enrolled patients in the control

Table 1

Key Findings of the Simplified Tanner-Whitehouse III Skeletal Maturity Assessment

Stage	Key Features	Greulich and Pyle Reference	Related Maturity Signs
1. Juvenile slow	Digital epiphyses are not covered.	Female 8 yr + 10 mo Male 12 yr + 6 mo (note fifth middle phalanx)	Tanner stage 1
2. Preadolescent slow	All digital epiphyses are covered.	Female 10 yr Male 13 yr	Tanner stage 2. starting growth spurt
3. Adolescent rapid—early	The preponderance of digits are capped. The second through fifth metacarpal epiphyses are wider than their metaphyses.	Female 11 and 12 yr Male 13 yr + 6 mo and 14 yr	Peak height velocity, Risser stage 0, open pelvic triradiate cartilage
4. Adolescent rapid—late	Any of distal phalangeal physes are clearly beginning to close (see detailed description in the text).	Female 13 yr (digits 2,3, and 4), male 15 yr (digits 4 and 5)	Girls typically in Tanner stage 3, Risser stage 0, open triradiate cartilage
5. Adolescent steady—early	All distal phalangeal physes are closed. Others are open.	Female 13 yr + 6 mo Male 15 yr + 6 mo	Risser stage 0, triradiate cartilage closed, menarche only occasionally starts earlier than this
6. Adolescent steady—late	Middle or proximal phalangeal physes are closing.	Female 14 yr Male 16 yr (late)	Risser sign positive (stage 1 or more)
7. Early mature	Only distal radial physis is open. Metacarpal physeal scars may be present	Female 15 yr Male 17 yr	Risser stage 4
8. Mature	Distal radial physis is completely closed.	Female 17 yr Male 19 yr	Risser stage 5

Reprinted with permission from Sanders JO, Khoury JG, Finegold DN: Predicting scoliosis progression from skeletal maturity: A simplified classification during adolescence. *J Bone Joint Surg Am* 2008;90[3]:540-553. doi: 10.2106/JBJS.G.00004.

group. Treatment failure (progression to curve 50° or greater) was 28% with bracing treatment versus 52% without bracing treatment, with a mean of 12 hours of daily brace wear.

Latest studies show bracing treatment with a TLSO does not adversely affect patient quality of life, although historic studies showed permanent decrease in body image from Milwaukee brace treatment. Counseling using a brace monitor may increase daily hours of brace wear by a mean of 3 hours.[40] Interest in Rigo Cheneau bracing treatment is high, but currently there is no comprehensive data showing superiority of these braces over a standard TLSO or Boston brace. Minsk et al showed lower rates of surgery in the Rigo Cheneau group at 0% (0 out of 13 patients) versus 32% (32 out of 95 patients) in a retrospective group of patients with a mean of 16 to 17 hours of daily brace wear; however, there may be selection bias in these cohorts.[41] Further interest exists in the role of scoliosis-specific exercises. Limited short-term preliminary data show potentially less curve progression and improved health-related quality of life scores in those who participate in scoliosis-specific exercises.[42] Similarly, data regarding the role and efficacy of night-time hypercorrection bracing treatment are forthcoming.

In a retrospective series of patients undergoing brace treatment, Thompson et al reported higher rates of braced patients progressing to surgery for thoracic (34% or 44 out of 129 patients) compared with lumbar curves (15% out six of 69 patients) with a mean of 12 to 13 hours of daily brace wear.[43] Karol et al reported that 63% of Risser 0, open triradiate patients treated with bracing treatment went on to surgical management (29 out of 46 patients). Of the patients with Risser 0 who wore their brace more than 18 hours per day, 35% (7 out of 20) went on to surgery.[40] Thus, for very skeletally immature patients, even full-time brace wear does not guarantee avoidance of surgery. Clinical tools are emerging which will provide more accurate risk assessment for families and surgeons as they consider the role of bracing treatment.

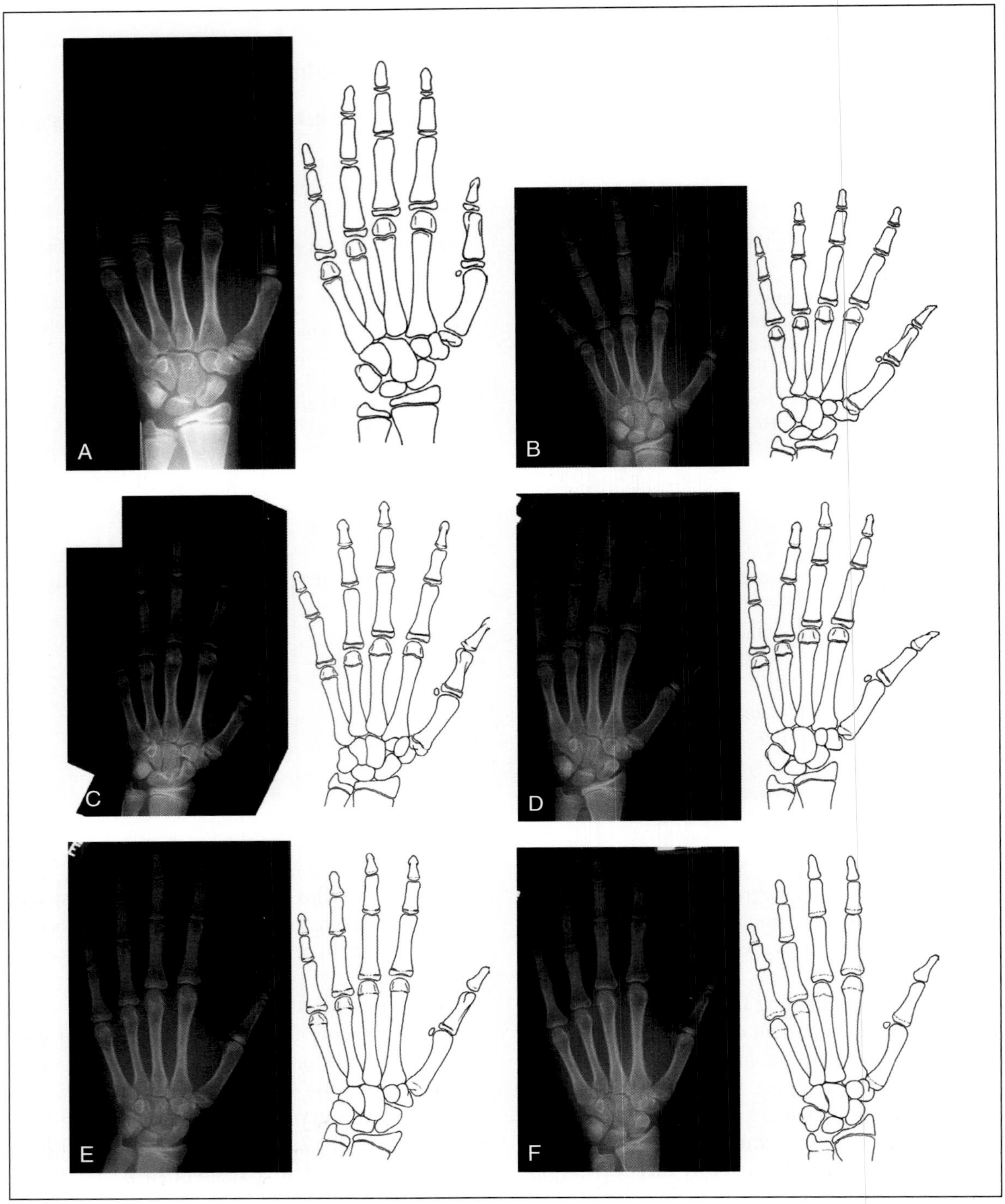

Figure 4 The simplified Tanner-Whitehouse staging or the Sanders digital maturity stage classification is highly predictive of growth remaining. **A**, In stage 2, all digital epiphyses are covered, or the epiphyses are as wide as the metaphyses. **B**, In stage 3, most of the epiphyses are capping the metaphysis, or curling around the edge of the metaphysis. **C**, In stage 4, the distal phalangeal physes are starting to close and the digital physes are fully capped. **D**, In stage 5, the distal phalangeal physes are completely closed, with no black cartilaginous material remaining. **E**, In stage 6, the proximal or middle phalangeal physes are closing. **F**, In stage 7, all digital physes are closed and spinal growth is essentially complete.

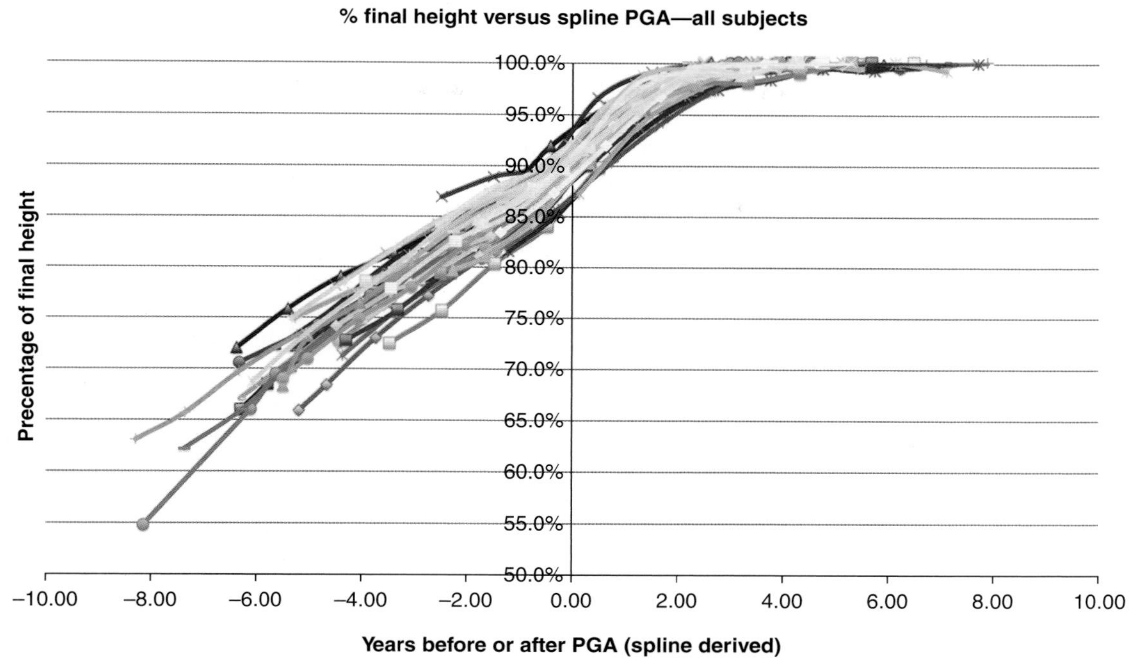

Figure 5 Graph of data from the Brush Foundation Study performed between 1931 and 1942, including 4,483 children followed with radiographs and measurements over time. Although peak growth age (PGA; age at peak growth velocity) widely varies, children uniformly undergo an adolescent growth spurt at their peak growth age with a rapid linear growth rate. Ninety percent of adult height corresponds to Sanders hand bone age of 3 years and peak growth velocity, which subsequently levels off with 2 years. Reprinted from Sanders JO, Qui X, Lu X, et al: The uniform pattern of growth and skeletal maturation during the human adolescent growth spurt. Scientific Reports 2017;7[1]. doi:10.1038/s41598-017-16996-w. (CC BY 4.0).

Surgical Management and Perioperative Considerations

Surgical treatment is indicated for patients with progressive curves with a Cobb angle of more than 45° to 50° due to concerns of lifelong curve progression.[44] The treatment of AIS can be a financial burden both on families and on the healthcare system. Out of all pediatric conditions requiring inpatient treatment, AIS ranks as the 48th most common reason for hospitalization in US children, and scoliosis fusion surgery ranks as the 5th most expensive pediatric inpatient procedure.[45] The US nationwide inpatient hospital charge estimates for AIS surgery exceeded $1.1 billion in 2012.[46] Accelerated discharge pathways may help reduce length of stay and hospital charges.[47] Utilization of fewer pedicle screws or constructs with lower implant density may also result in cost savings, as intraoperative costs under the control of the surgeon contribute more to total costs of surgery than room and board.[48]

Improving patient safety and reducing complications is an ongoing priority for pediatric spine surgery. Reported 2-year return to OR for AIS patients treated with all pedicle screw constructs is 3.5%,[49] and at 5-years, reported at 7.5% to 9.9% return to OR.[50] Neurologic deficit following AIS surgery is reported at 0.2% to 0.8%.[51] Use of Ponte osteotomies for routine AIS surgery has been shown to increase the incidence of neurologic monitoring alerts.[52] Compliance with perioperative antibiotic administration guidelines including use of a first-generation cephalosporin within 1 hour of incision and continued for 24 hours afterward was associated with a lower rate of surgical site infections for pediatric spine surgery.[53] If acute infection does occur, the majority can be cleared without implant removal; however, infection may be more difficult to eradicate in patients who have stainless steel instrumentation.[54]

CT-guided navigation can be used to reduce the rate of pedicle screw malposition down to 3% for scoliosis patients, although the significance of screw malposition is not well-agreed upon in the literature.[55,56] For centers using intraoperative CT-guided navigation, a pediatric setting (such as 80 kV, 20 mA, 80 mA) should be used to reduce patient radiation exposure.[57,58] At 25-year follow-up, Simony et al found a 4.8 relative risk of developing cancer for scoliosis patients compared with the normal Danish population.[59] These patients received a mean of 16 radiographs at 0.8 to 1.4 mSv per radiograph or around 16 mSv total exposure (for reference, annual background radiation is 3 mSv). Dermal discoloration may occur at neuromonitoring needle electrode sites in up to 16% of patients, although permanent discoloration/burns are uncommon (1 in 200 or 0.5%).[60] Lateral femoral cutaneous nerve palsy occurs in 25% of patients undergoing surgery for AIS, is associated with longer surgical times, and reliably resolves postoperatively.[61] Thus, as there is increased focus on perioperative complications and cost of care, presumably rates of adverse events and quality of care will improve.

Outcomes of Adolescent Idiopathic Scoliosis Treatment

Fusion surgery is recommended to prevent curve progression in adulthood and to improve pain and cosmesis. Long-term outcome studies, however, are limited,[44] and it is difficult to link health-related quality of life or mortality with curve magnitude in the context of the modern world.[2] At a mean of 25 years, Simony et al. found 3° curve progression in the Harrington rod group (n = 93) and 5.5° progression in the braced group (n = 66).[62] Three of the surgical patients had additional surgery due to distal adding on (3%). There was no difference in health-related quality of life with the exception of better satisfaction scores in the surgical group.[63] Jeans et al. found reduced VO2 max reduction in 23 patients at two years following spinal fusion surgery; however, all AIS patients were within accepted limits before and after surgery.[64] Thus, further efforts are needed to refine the indications for fusion surgery for AIS to predict which patients will progress in adulthood and require prophylactic fusion surgery in childhood. Nonfusion techniques such as anterior vertebral body tethering are emerging technologies for AIS treatment; however, there is no long-term data showing improved outcomes, motion, or safety for these approaches. Prospective trials are underway.

Kyphosis

Although less common than severe scoliosis, severe kyphosis can result in deformity, back pain, and in rare cases neurologic compromise. Kyphosis is defined as curvature of the spine in the sagittal plane. Normal thoracic kyphosis in adults is 40° to 60°, and 20° to 40° in children. Thoracic kyphosis over 70° to 80° may warrant surgical intervention depending on patient symptoms and deformity. Congenital kyphosis occurs in fetal life with malformation of the vertebrae, classically with wedging or a hemivertebrae. Due to the high incidence of concomitant renal, spinal cord, and cardiac abnormalities, patients with newly diagnosed congenital scoliosis or kyphosis should undergo renal and cardiac ultrasonography, ultrasonography of the spinal cord if under 2 months of age, or more typically MRI of the entire spine. Congenital kyphosis can be rapidly progressive and can result in spinal stenosis and myelopathy. Patients with congenital spine deformity should have routine monitoring with both PA and lateral spine radiographs. The deformity most typically occurs at the thoracolumbar junction. Surgical management of congenital kyphosis is among the highest risk of all pediatric spinal deformity surgery, with a 1.3% risk of neurologic deficit.[51] Patients should be screened for associated syndromic diagnoses, such as mucopolysaccharidoses.

In general, surgical management of pediatric kyphosis is high risk, with a reported 14.7% rate of complications. Scheuermann kyphosis is an idiopathic curvature of the spine associated with 5° of wedging at three adjacent vertebra (Sorenson criteria). Scheuermann kyphosis is frequently associated with Schmorl nodes, or end plate irregularities (**Figure 6**). The role for bracing treatment in Scheuermann kyphosis is unclear and has not been shown to be of long-term benefit to prevent deformity progression. Scheuermann kyphosis surgery is associated with higher rates of complications compared with AIS surgery, including a 0.7% rate of neurologic injury.[51] Patients undergoing surgery for Scheuermann kyphosis more frequently have pain over the prominence, are older in age, and have larger magnitude T2-T12 kyphosis than those treated nonsurgically.[65] Although historically anterior disk releases were performed for kyphosis treatment, posterior fusion alone with Ponte osteotomies has become the treatment of choice[66] (**Figure 7**). Routine preoperative MRI to assess for disk herniation and intrathecal abnormalities should be considered.[67,68] Severe kyphosis may limit aerobic capacity.[69]

Spondylolysis/Spondylolisthesis

Spondylolysis is a defect in the pars interarticularis, with a prevalence of 6% to as high as 25% in some populations.[70] In children, these defects are most commonly of the isthmic (associated with a lesion of the pars interarticularis) or dysplastic type (in which facet joints allow anterior translation). In isthmic spondylolisthesis, the defect occurs at L5 in 87% of the patients, at L4 in 10%, and at L3 in 3%.[71]

By far the most common cause of back pain in adolescents, spondylolysis accounts for up to 47% of cases in some series.[72] Approximately 80% of cases are bilateral, whereas 20% of cases are unilateral. An associated slippage of a vertebra in relation to the adjacent vertebra is termed a "spondylolisthesis." The Meyerding grading

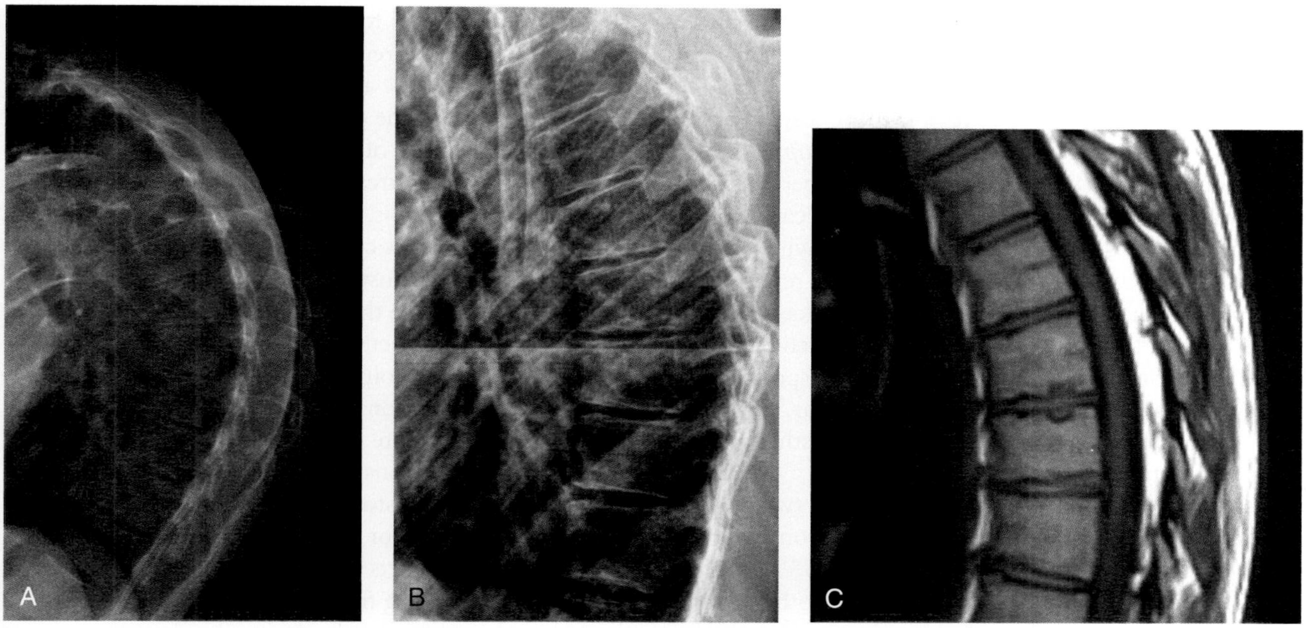

Figure 6 Scheuermann kyphosis is defined by three adjacent vertebral bodies with at least 5° of wedging (**A**). Schmorl nodes as well as end plate irregularities are frequently present and can be seen on radiograph (**B**) or MRI (**C**). In contrast to adolescent postural kyphosis, a benign condition, Scheuermann patients have a rigid spine deformity most evident on forward bend (**D**).

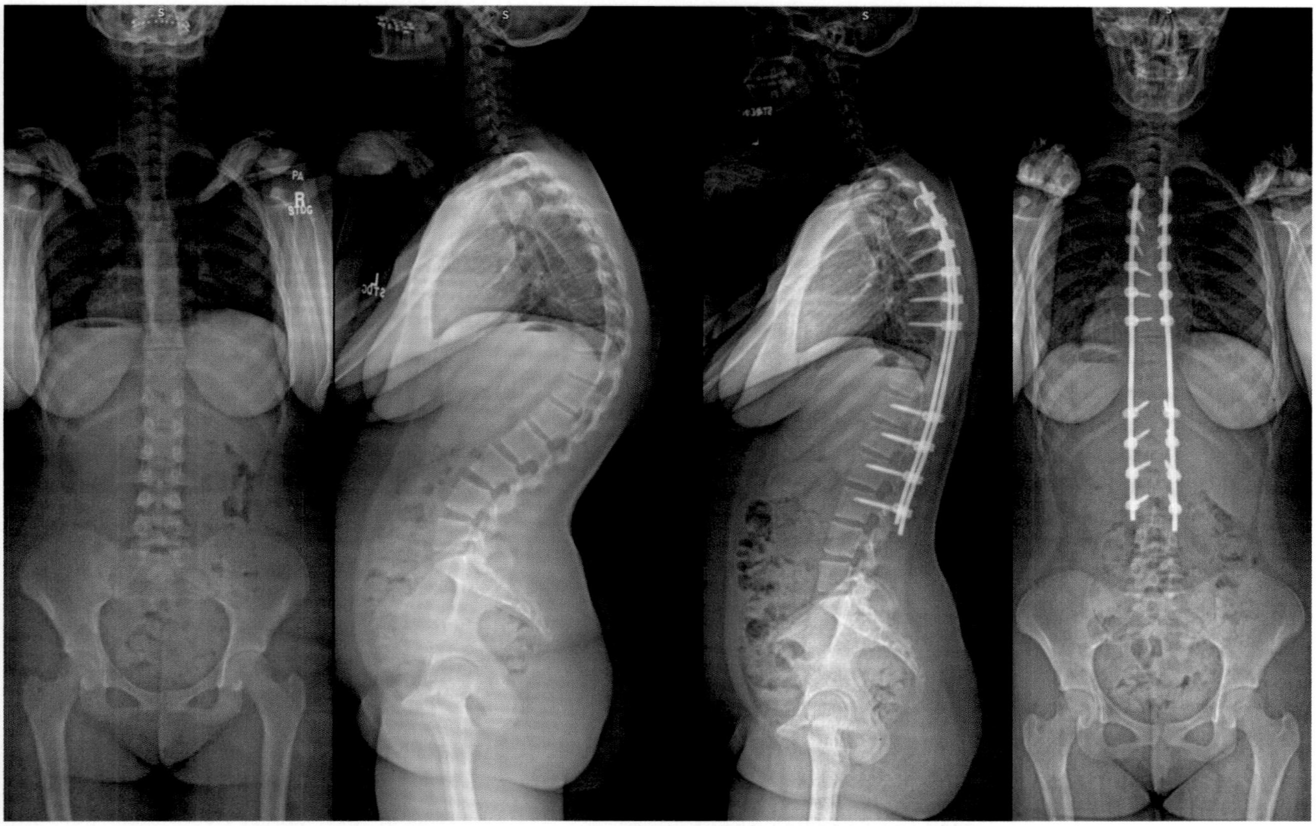

Figure 7 Preoperative and postoperative imaging for a 14-year-old female who underwent posterior spinal fusion with Ponte osteotomies for treatment of Scheuermann kyphosis.

system is used to classify cases of spondylolisthesis by the degree of displacement in relation to the adjacent vertebra, where 1% to 24% = 1, 25% to 49% = 2, 50% to 74% = 3, and 75% to 100% = 4. If the displacement exceeds 100% this is referred to as *spondyloptosis*.

Spondylolysis is associated with hyperextension sports (gymnastics, volleyball, football) but can be seen with almost any sport, or even in children who are not athletes. The history is typically of activity-related low back pain, with radiating pain in the buttocks or legs in some cases. Physical examination often demonstrates lumbar hyperlordosis, though in high-grade spondylolisthesis flattening of the lumbar spine may occur.[73] Patients with symptomatic spondylolysis/spondylolisthesis have pain with standing spine hyperextension, especially during single-leg stance or with concomitant twisting.

The optimal imaging protocol remains controversial with more than half of spondylolysis lesions (53%) missed on plain films alone in some series. MRI is another option for imaging of spondylolysis, but the reported sensitivity ranges from 25% to 86%.[74] A CT scan is more sensitive than either MRI or plain radiographs in detecting spondylolytic lesions and also may assess the acuity which can aid in treatment planning, but to limit the radiation one should only image the area of clinical concern, typically L4 to S1.[75,76] Oblique radiographs should be avoided, as a four-view lumbar spine series carries as much radiation as a limited lumbar spine CT.

Nonsurgical Management

In most cases of spondylolysis, symptoms resolve with conservative treatment consisting primarily of activity modification and bracing treatment. For acute cases, ideally an osseous union is achieved and rest and bracing treatment are typically continued for 3 months to facilitate this. Sakai et al found 94% healing with conservative treatment in the early stage and 80% in the healing stage.[77] Other series have shown that an estimated 75% to 100% of acute unilateral lesions and 50% of acute bilateral lesions heal, whereas essentially no chronic defects heal.[73] Nevertheless, by an average of 5 to 6 months approximately 90% of athletes have returned to their prior level of sports participation.[78] This suggests that in many cases a fibrous union is sufficient for symptomatic improvement because the rates of returning to sport exceed the rate of achieving bony union.[73] There is significant variability in the type of brace and wear hours recommended with the Boston thoracolumbar sacral orthosis, antilordotic braces, and braces with a thigh cuff all being used. In chronic spondylolysis cases, the bone is not expected to heal and conservative treatment is based on symptoms. Often an SI belt or other low-profile brace may prevent hyperextension and alleviate discomfort. This can even be used for participation in athletic activities, allowing a rapid return in some cases.

While conservative management is successful in the majority of cases, if the patient has unresolved pain after more than 6 months of conservative treatment, intolerance of conservative treatment, a greater than 50% slip of the spondylolisthesis, or severe neurologic symptoms, surgical intervention is considered. Several techniques for direct repair and for fusion of the involved segment have been described. While this remains controversial, there is agreement that a direct repair should not be performed in cases with spondylolisthesis or associated disk disease at adjacent levels. Consequently, an MRI scan should be obtained to evaluate the intervertebral disk prior to a repair. Fusion may consist of a posterior only approach, with or without a transforaminal lumbar interbody fusion, or a combined posterior and anterior fusion. Fortunately, rates of return to sports participation after surgical treatment are high, ranging from 80% to 100%[79] (**Figure 8**).

Although posterior only approaches have been more traditionally performed, a high rate of implant failure and late complications have been observed for posterior fusion alone for high grade spondylolisthesis. This may in fact be a greater concern than earlier studies suggest as a recent report from four pediatric centers saw a 30% rate of implant failure with mean 5 year follow up, which may be higher than other series due to the longer follow up as the mean time to revision surgery was over 2 years.[80] Consequently, many surgeons are moving toward a combined anterior and posterior fusion, to try to expeditiously develop a solid fusion, although an anterior approach holds the risk of retrograde ejaculation in males. Another controversial area is the degree to which a reduction of the spondylolisthesis should be performed. The increased neurologic risks of reduction must be weighed against the risks of implant failure, slip progression, and pseudarthrosis associated with in situ fusion.[81,82]

Trauma

C-Spine

Care of the pediatric C-spine injury can be challenging due to unique aspects of anatomy that may cause both normal findings to be perceived as injuries or conversely true injuries to be overlooked.

Pseudosubluxation

From birth to 8 years of age, lateral radiographs show a progressively increasing facet angle. At younger ages the more horizontal orientation of the facets allows for motion through flexion and extension and contributes to the appearance of pseudosubluxation often seen at C2-C3 and

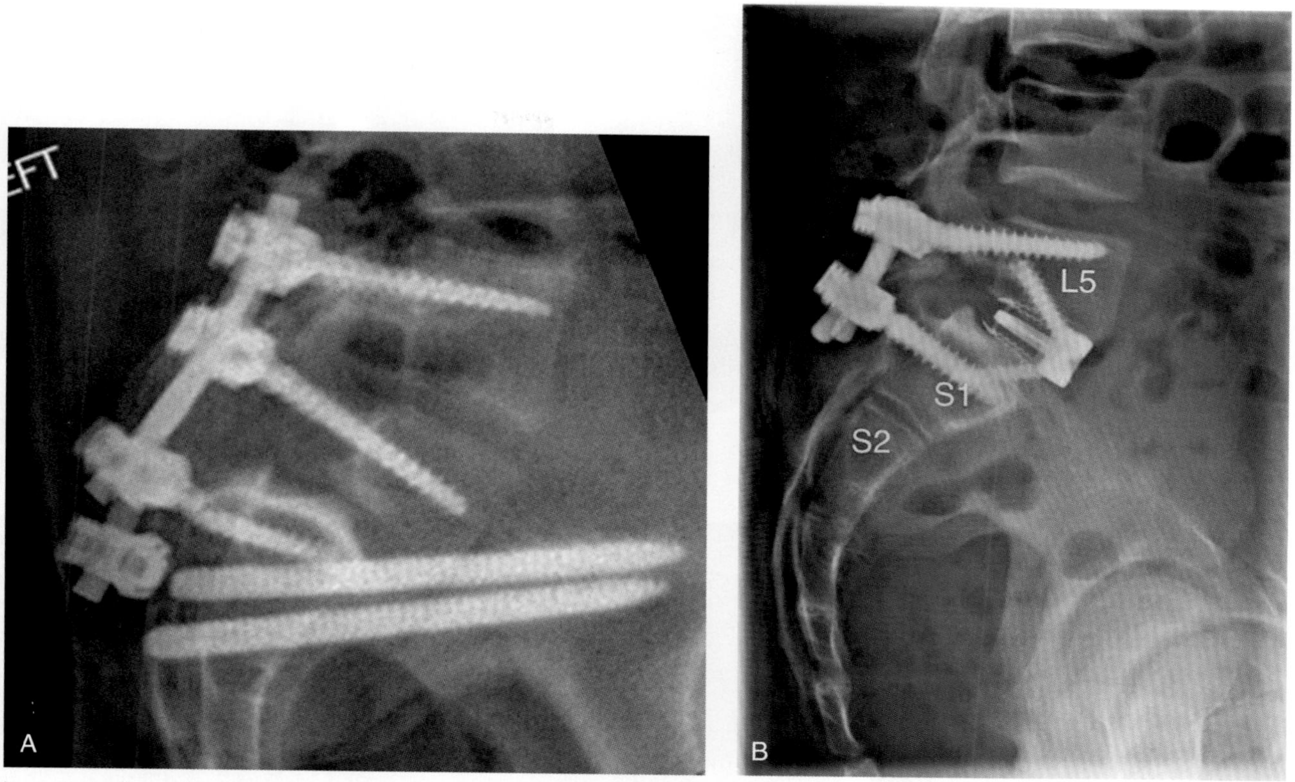

Figure 8 Radiographs show that although the majority of patients with spondylolysis/spondylolisthesis that undergo surgical management do return to sports and can continue to be highly competitive athletes, implant failures are not uncommon for treatment of high-grade spondylolisthesis (**A**), prompting some surgeons to opt for a combined anterior and posterior fusion (**B**).

C3-C4. Pseudosubluxation can be differentiated from true subluxation on plain radiographs by the maintenance of a straight line drawn along the spinolaminar line (the anterior edge of the posterior neural arch), known as Swischuk line. However, care should be taken as while pseudosubluxation is a normal finding and does not require treatment, injuries can also occur at this level (**Figure 9**).

Rotatory Atlantoaxial Subluxation

Rotatory atlantoaxial subluxation, which occurs when the lateral mass of the atlas locks behind the ipsilateral lateral mass of the axis, is a common cause of acute torticollis. This may be due to trauma (often minor), Grisel or Sandifer syndrome, or associated with conditions causing laxity such as Down syndrome or Marfan syndrome. Patients typically present with a "cock robin" torticollis, and clinically, there is difficulty rotating the head passively to the affected side. This can be differentiated from congenital muscular torticollis by history and also by the fact that the sternocleidomastoid will be soft on the side to which the head is tilted and may feel taut on the contralateral side because it is lengthened.

A dynamic CT scan can confirm the diagnosis and avoid an ambiguous test result due to positioning. To minimize radiation, this should be limited to the upper cervical spine (occiput to C3). Treatment depends on the time to presentation, as with time the subluxation becomes more difficult to reduce and may also result in subsequent instability and recurrence if a reduction is obtained.[83] For patients presenting within a week of onset, typically a soft collar and muscle relaxants will be sufficient to achieve and maintain a reduction though this should be monitored closely. Beyond that traction followed by a CT scan to confirm the reduction and a noninvasive halo for 4 to 6 weeks is used.[84] It was once thought that late presentation (>4 weeks) of rotatory atlantoaxial instability frequently resulted in irreducible or recurrent subluxation and fusion was frequently needed. Two recent series have challenged this assertion reporting a 73% to 100% success rate with mean presentations greater than 10 weeks.[85,86]

Atlantoaxial Instability

As opposed to adults, for whom a normal ADI is less than 3 mm, in young children the ADI may be up to 4.5 mm without signifying injury. Children who have an ADI of 5 mm or more on plain radiographs may have atlantoaxial instability either acutely due to trauma or chronic due to conditions of ligamentous

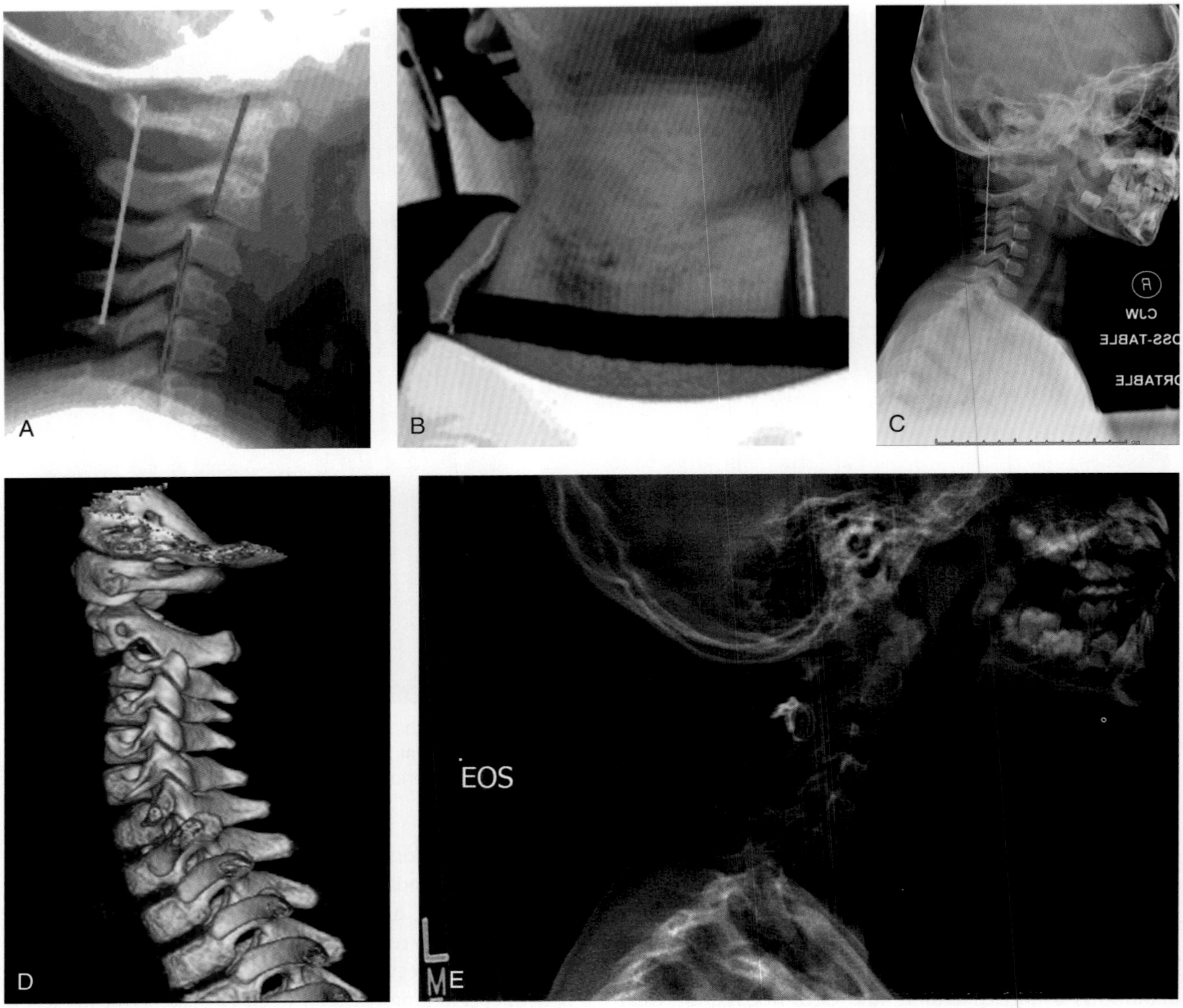

Figure 9 Radiographs show an example of pseudosubluxation (red line) on a patient who sustained minor trauma. Note how Swischuk line (green) is maintained (**A**). Conversely in this patient involved in a high-speed motor vehicle collision with a seat belt sign (**B**), the disruption of Swischuk line (green) is noted (**C**) in conjunction with jumped facets confirmed with CT scan (**D**). Final post-op image (**E**).

laxity, most commonly Down syndrome. MRI can be used to further evaluate this condition. In traumatic cases where the transverse ligament is injured, posterior spinal fusion of C1 and C2 is indicated to protect the spinal cord.

More commonly the physician is faced with management of chronic atlantoaxial instability in patients with Down syndrome. The estimated incidence of asymptomatic atlantoaxial instability in Down syndrome is up to 22%, while only 2% to 3% of persons with Down syndrome have symptomatic atlantoaxial instability.[87] In these patients the history is of critical importance as the literature currently does not include any reports of children with Down syndrome without preceding neurologic symptoms who have had a traumatic injury resulting in a neurologic decline. The revised American Academy of Pediatrics 2011 guidelines mark a shift away from routine radiographic screening and emphasize the need for a physical examination and parental counseling to monitor for development of any symptoms on a biannual basis.[88]

Although many techniques for atlantoaxial fusion have been described, fusion rates in the setting of atlantoaxial instability in persons with Down syndrome have historically been poor and range from

40% to 80% prompting some authors to recommend including the occiput and routine use of halo immobilization.[89] Additionally, Segal et al[90] have reported a 100% complication rate and an 18% mortality rate. Due to this high complication rate, caution is warranted with surgical intervention and typically reserved for patients who are symptomatic or have an ADI of >10 mm.

Dens Fractures

Odontoid fractures account for 10% of all cervical spine injuries in children and the majority of pediatric cervical spine fractures.[91] Between 3 and 6 years of age, fusion of the dens to the neural arches and anterior body occurs. This can be mistaken for a fracture at the base of the odontoid, or conversely, a fracture may be assumed to be the synchondrosis and overlooked. Assessment for swelling in the retropharyngeal space can be helpful in this differentiation. If a clinical suspicion is present and the diagnosis is unclear, an MRI may be obtained for further evaluation. Most of these injuries can be treated by stabilization in a halo vest. The alignment of the fracture is generally improved with the head positioned in slight extension. The amount of acceptable angulation and the potential for remodeling varies with age and remains controversial, although one report of patients younger than 3 years with angulation of greater than 30° showed that remodeling led to a normal structure with no associated sequelae.[92]

Thoracolumbar Fractures

While many of the thoracolumbar fractures seen in children are similar to those seen in adults, there are some unique injuries that may be seen, particularly in the adolescent population.

Apophyseal Ring Fractures

The vertebral ring apophysis develops at the age of 6 years and fuses to the vertebral body at the age of 17 years. Trauma to the apophyseal ring can lead to a fracture of the vertebral epiphyseal plate, resulting in an apophyseal ring fracture. This not only causes pain similar to that of the adult disk herniation but may also appear to be a disk herniation on MRI because the thin bony component of the apophysis is not appreciated. CT scan allows one to differentiate these similar clinical entities. It is an important distinction to make as while disk herniations may often resorb somewhat over time, the osseous component typically causes persistent pain and failure of conservative treatment. Consequently, the mainstay of treatment is surgical excision of the protruding fragment. A recent report by Higashino et al[93] demonstrated favorable long-term outcomes in patients with these injuries (**Figure 10**).

Chance Fractures

Chance fractures are due to a flexion-distraction mechanism with failure of both the anterior elements in flexion and the posterior elements in distraction. It is important to distinguish these from the more common compression fractures that do not have failure of the posterior elements in distraction. Some Chance fractures may be purely osseous in nature and thus potentially treated conservatively. However, many have a ligamentous component and are associated with significant instability. Arkader et al demonstrated superior results in Chance fractures managed surgically (84% good results in the surgical group compared with 45% in the conservative group). In their review, patients in the surgical group had more kyphosis initially (22°) as compared with the nonsurgical group (11.4°) but had less posttreatment kyphotic deformity (3.5° for surgical group; 20° for nonsurgical group).[94]

Sacral Facet Fractures

Sacral facet fractures are a rare injury but an important diagnosis to recognize. Presentation is typically a young athlete who has localized back pain with extension. This diagnosis may be easily missed on plain radiographs, bone scans, and MRI, which are frequently negative in these cases.[95,96] CT is the imaging modality of choice in these cases. Ideally, these are identified early, in which case, pain relief and return to activities is the expected outcome after removal of the intra-articular fracture fragments by a minimally invasive muscle-sparing approach.[96] In cases where the diagnosis is delayed, the issue may be complicated by additional cartilage damage to the facet joint.

Summary

Spinal deformity is frequently seen in children. Pattern recognition and knowledge of indications for imaging and surgery are needed for appropriate treatment. Early-onset scoliosis remains a potentially life-threatening disorder with patients who have specialized needs and frequent concomitant conditions. Adolescent idiopathic scoliosis is the most common cause of pediatric spinal deformity and responds to treatment with bracing treatment or surgery. Treatment of pediatric cervical spine imaging and interpretation of imaging is challenging and requires familiarity with common disease presentations.

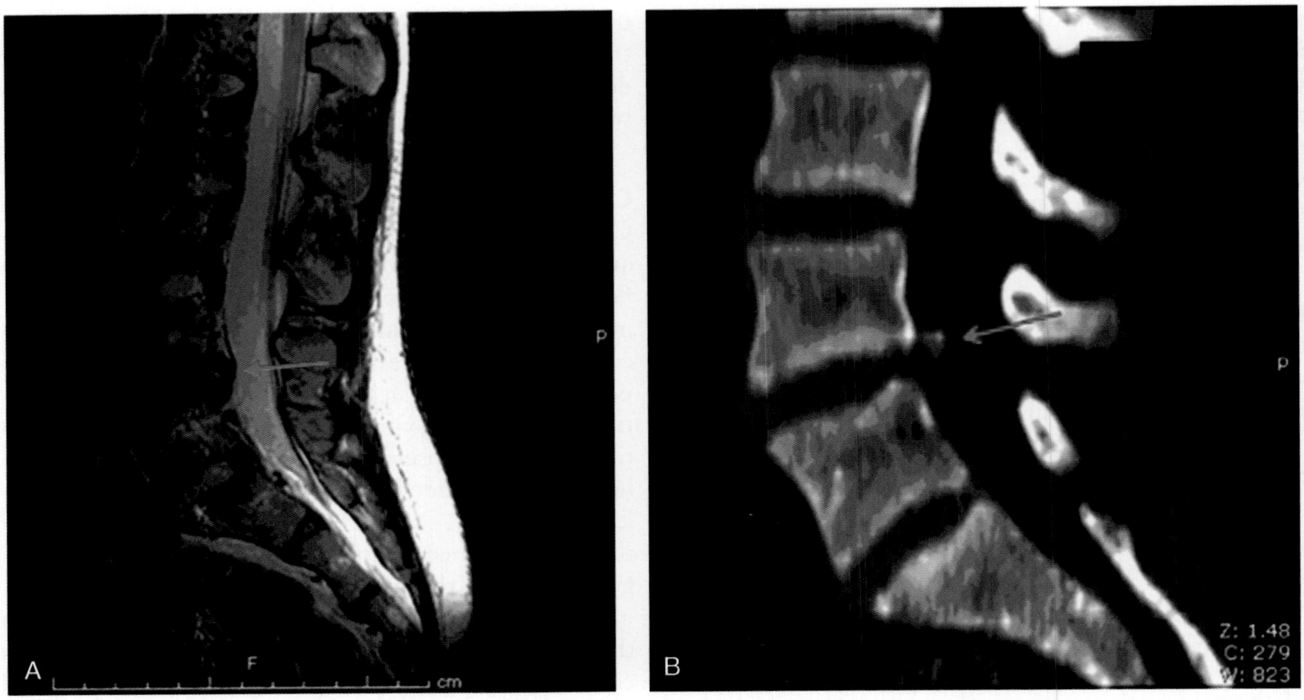

Figure 10 MRI showing what appears to be a disk herniation (**A**), though CT scan shows this to in fact be an apophyseal end plate fracture (red arrow) (**B**). The patient underwent removal via a limited approach and returned to full sports and activities at 2 weeks.

Key Study Points

- Patients with congenital scoliosis have vertebral abnormalities, such as a hemivertebra, and require screening with spinal MRI, renal and cardiac ultrasonography to detect associated spinal cord and organ abnormalities.
- Bracing treatment with a TLSO has been shown to be effective for reducing the rate of surgery for patients with AIS curves between 20° and 40° who are Risser 2 or less with a 12 hours mean daily brace wear.
- Hand bone age is the new standard for maturity in patients undergoing bracing treatment and surgery as it provides information regarding skeletal maturation prior to peak growth velocity.
- MRI or limited CT is the benchmark for workup of spondylolysis, which typically responds to nonsurgical measures, while single photon emission CT (SPECT) and oblique radiographs should be avoided to limit radiation exposure.
- Rotatory atlantoaxial subluxation can occur in children without history of trauma, and early treatment with NSAIDs and traction may obviate the need for halo treatment, which may be required with late presentation, although fusion is rarely indicated.

Annotated References

1. Herring MJ, Putney LF, Wyatt G, Finkbeiner WE, Hyde DM: Growth of alveoli during postnatal development in humans based on stereological estimation. *Am J Physiol Lung Cell Mol Physiol* 2014;307(4):L338-L344.
2. Pehrsson K, Larsson S, Oden A, Nachemson A: Long-term follow-up of patients with untreated scoliosis. A study of mortality, causes of death, and symptoms. *Spine* 1992; 17(9):1091-1096.
3. Karol LA, Johnston C, Mladenov K, Schochet P, Walters P, Browne RH: Pulmonary function following early thoracic fusion in non-neuromuscular scoliosis. *J Bone Joint Surg Am Vol* 2008;90(6):1272-1281.
4. Williams BA, Matsumoto H, McCalla DJ, et al: Development and initial validation of the Classification of Early-Onset Scoliosis (C-EOS). *J Bone Joint Surg Am Vol* 2014;96(16):1359-1367.
5. Pahys JM, Samdani AF, Betz RR: Intraspinal anomalies in infantile idiopathic scoliosis: Prevalence and role of magnetic resonance imaging. *Spine* 2009;34(12):E434-E438.
6. Dobbs MB, Lenke LG, Szymanski DA, et al: Prevalence of neural axis abnormalities in patients with infantile idiopathic scoliosis. *J Bone Joint Surg Am Vol* 2002;84-A(12):2230-2234.
7. Jain A, Sullivan BT, Shah SA, et al: Caregiver perceptions and health-related quality-of-life changes in cerebral palsy patients after spinal arthrodesis. *Spine* 2018;43(15):1052-1056.

Caregivers report improvement in health related quality of life after spinal fusion surgery in patients with GMFCS level IV and V. Level of evidence: III.

8. Kawakami N, Koumoto I, Dogaki Y, et al: Clinical impact of corrective cast treatment for early onset scoliosis: Is it a worthwhile treatment option to suppress scoliosis progression before surgical intervention? *J Pediatr Orthop* 2018;38(10):e556-e561.

   Addition of casting to brace treatment alone for early onset scoliosis resulted in reduced curve progression. Level of evidence: III.

9. Hassanzadeh H, Nandyala SV, Puvanesarajah V, Manning BT, Jain A, Hammerberg KW: Serial Mehta cast utilization in infantile idiopathic scoliosis: Evaluation of radiographic predictors. *J Pediatr Orthop* 2017;37(6):387-391.

   Serial Mehta casting resulted in improved Cobb angle in 45 patients with infantile idiopathic scoliosis. Level of evidence: IV.

10. Dede O, Sturm PF: A brief history and review of modern casting techniques in early onset scoliosis. *J Child Orthop* 2016;10(5):405-411.

    Technique of Mehta casting is described in detail including a brief literature review. Level of evidence: V.

11. Suh SW, Sarwark JF, Vora A, Huang BK: Evaluating congenital spine deformities for intraspinal anomalies with magnetic resonance imaging. *J Pediatr Orthop* 2001;21(4):525-531.

12. MacEwen GD, Winter RB, Hardy JH: Evaluation of kidney anomalies in congenital scoliosis. *J Bone Joint Surg Am Vol* 1972;54(7):1451-1454.

13. Cao J, Zhang XJ, Sun N, et al: The therapeutic characteristics of serial casting on congenital scoliosis: A comparison with non-congenital cases from a single-center experience. *J Orthop Surg Res* 2017;12(1):56.

    Cobb angle decreased in a series of 8 patients with congenital scoliosis treated with casting. Level of evidence III.

14. Fletcher ND, McClung A, Rathjen KE, Denning JR, Browne R, Johnston CE III: Serial casting as a delay tactic in the treatment of moderate-to-severe early-onset scoliosis. *J Pediatr Orthop* 2012;32(7):664-671.

15. Mesfin A, Sponseller PD, Leet AI: Spinal muscular atrophy: Manifestations and management. *J Am Acad Orthop Surg* 2012;20(6):393-401.

16. Miller A, Temple T, Miller F: Impact of orthoses on the rate of scoliosis progression in children with cerebral palsy. *J Pediatr Orthop* 1996;16(3):332-335.

17. Waldron SR, Poe-Kochert C, Son-Hing JP, Thompson GH: Early onset scoliosis: The value of serial Risser casts. *J Pediatr Orthop* 2013;33(8):775-780.

18. McElroy MJ, Sponseller PD, Dattilo JR, et al: Growing rods for the treatment of scoliosis in children with cerebral palsy: A critical assessment. *Spine* 2012;37(24):E1504-E1510.

19. Miyanji F, Nasto LA, Sponseller PD, et al: Assessing the risk-benefit ratio of scoliosis surgery in cerebral palsy: Surgery is worth it. *J Bone Joint Surg Am Vol* 2018;100(7):556-563.

    Reported health-related quality of life (CP-CHILD) improved for 69 patients with GMFSC level IV and V cerebral palsy treated with spinal fusion surgery. Level of evidence: IV.

20. Sewell MD, Malagelada F, Wallace C, et al: A preliminary study to assess whether spinal fusion for scoliosis improves carer-assessed quality of life for children with GMFCS level IV or V cerebral palsy. *J Pediatr Orthop* 2016;36(3):299-304.

    Over a 2-year period, reported health-related quality of life (CP-CHILD) improved for 18 patients with GMFSC level IV and V cerebral palsy treated with spinal fusion surgery and declined in 15 patients treated with observation. Level of evidence: III.

21. Bess S, Akbarnia BA, Thompson GH, et al: Complications of growing-rod treatment for early-onset scoliosis: Analysis of one hundred and forty patients. *J Bone Joint Surg Am Vol* 2010;92(15):2533-2543.

22. Sankar WN, Skaggs DL, Yazici M, et al: Lengthening of dual growing rods and the law of diminishing returns. *Spine* 2011;36(10):806-809.

23. Skaggs DL, Akbarnia BA, Flynn JM, et al: A classification of growth friendly spine implants. *J Pediatr Orthop* 2014;34(3):260-274.

24. Akbarnia BA, Marks DS, Boachie-Adjei O, Thompson AG, Asher MA: Dual growing rod technique for the treatment of progressive early-onset scoliosis: A multicenter study. *Spine* 2005;30(17 suppl):S46-S57.

25. Akbarnia BA, Breakwell LM, Marks DS, et al: Dual growing rod technique followed for three to eleven years until final fusion: The effect of frequency of lengthening. *Spine* 2008;33(9):984-990.

26. Schulz JF, Smith J, Cahill PJ, Fine A, Samdani AF: The role of the vertical expandable titanium rib in the treatment of infantile idiopathic scoliosis: Early results from a single institution. *J Pediatr Orthop* 2010;30(7):659-663.

27. Hasler CC, Mehrkens A, Hefti F: Efficacy and safety of VEPTR instrumentation for progressive spine deformities in young children without rib fusions. *Eur Spine J* 2010;19(3):400-408.

28. Akbarnia BA, Cheung K, Noordeen H, et al: Next generation of growth-sparing techniques: Preliminary clinical results of a magnetically controlled growing rod in 14 patients with early-onset scoliosis. *Spine* 2013;38(8):665-670.

29. Akbarnia BA, Pawelek JB, Cheung KM, et al: Traditional growing rods versus magnetically controlled growing rods for the surgical treatment of early-onset scoliosis: A case-matched 2-year study. *Spine Deform* 2014;2(6):493-497.

30. Wilkinson JT, Songy CE, Bumpass DB, McCullough FL, McCarthy RE: Curve modulation and apex migration using Shilla growth guidance rods for early-onset scoliosis at 5-year follow-up. *J Pediatr Orthop* 2017. doi:10.1097/BPO.0000000000000983. [Epub ahead of print] PubMed PMID:28375968.

    This paper reports on 21 patients with minimum 5-year follow-up treated with the Shilla technique with a mean of 45 mm spinal growth. Level of evidence: IV.

31. Andras LM, Joiner ER, McCarthy RE, et al: Growing rods versus Shilla growth guidance: Better Cobb angle correction and T1-S1 length increase but more surgeries. *Spine Deform* 2015;3(3):246-252.

32. Crawford CH III, Lenke LG: Growth modulation by means of anterior tethering resulting in progressive correction of juvenile idiopathic scoliosis: A case report. *J Bone Joint Surg Am Vol* 2010;92(1):202-209.

33. Lonner BS, Auerbach JD, Estreicher MB, et al: Pulmonary function changes after various anterior approaches in the treatment of adolescent idiopathic scoliosis. *J Spinal Disord Tech* 2009;22(8):551-558.

34. Yip BH, Yu FW, Wang Z, et al: Prognostic value of bone mineral density on curve progression: A longitudinal cohort study of 513 girls with adolescent idiopathic scoliosis. *Sci Rep* 2016;6:39220.

Scoliosis patients who were osteopenic at the time of presentation were at higher risk of curve progression necessitating surgical management, even when correction for menarchal status, age, and initial Cobb angle. Level of evidence: II.

35. Sitoula P, Verma K, Holmes L Jr, et al: Prediction of curve progression in idiopathic scoliosis: Validation of the Sanders skeletal maturity staging system. *Spine* 2015;40(13):1006-1013.

36. Vira S, Husain Q, Jalai C, et al: The interobserver and intraobserver reliability of the Sanders classification versus the Risser stage. *J Pediatr Orthop* 2017;37(4):e246-e249.

Sanders classification has moderate reliability for physicians and good reliability among spine surgeons, and was noted to have greater reliability than the Risser score. Level of evidence: III.

37. Sanders JO, Khoury JG, Kishan S, et al: Predicting scoliosis progression from skeletal maturity: A simplified classification during adolescence. *J Bone Joint Surg Am Vol* 2008;90(3):540-553.

38. Minkara A, Bainton N, Tanaka M, et al: High risk of mismatch between Sanders and Risser staging in adolescent idiopathic scoliosis: Are we guiding treatment using the wrong classification? *J Pediatr Orthop* 2018. doi: 10.1097/BPO.0000000000001135.

There is significant mismatch between Risser sign and Sanders stage, particularly in males and those of Hispanic ethnicity. Level of evidence: III.

39. Weinstein SL, Dolan LA, Wright JG, Dobbs MB: Effects of bracing in adolescents with idiopathic scoliosis. *N Engl J Med* 2013;369(16):1512-1521.

40. Karol LA, Virostek D, Felton K, Jo C, Butler L: The effect of the Risser stage on bracing outcome in adolescent idiopathic scoliosis. *J Bone Joint Surg Am Vol* 2016;98(15):1253-1259.

70% of Risser 0, open triradiate cartilage patients went on to require surgery despite brace wear. Level of evidence: II.

41. Minsk MK, Venuti KD, Daumit GL, Sponseller PD: Effectiveness of the Rigo Cheneau versus Boston-style orthoses for adolescent idiopathic scoliosis: A retrospective study. *Scoliosis Spinal Disord* 2017;12:7

In a retrospective comparative study, 13 patients who wore a Rigo Cheneau orthosis did not progress to surgery, whereas 32 out of 95 patients with a standard TLSO progressed to surgery; however, 2 patients in the Rigo Cheneau orthosis had a curve over 45 degrees and 36 patients in the TLSO group. Level of evidence: III.

42. Kwan KYH, Cheng ACS, Koh HY, Chiu AYY, Cheung KMC. Effectiveness of Schroth exercises during bracing in adolescent idiopathic scoliosis: Results from a preliminary study-SOSORT award 2017 winner. *Scoliosis Spinal Disord* 2017;12:32.

24 patients were treated with bracing and 24 patients with bracing and Schroth PT with a mean 18 month follow-up. Level of evidence: III.

43. Thompson RM, Hubbard EW, Jo CH, Virostek D, Karol LA: Brace success is related to curve type in patients with adolescent idiopathic scoliosis. *J Bone Joint Surg Am Vol* 2017;99(11):923-928.

In a retrospective review of 168 patients treated with bracing, there was a higher rate of curve progression in thoracic compared to lumbar curves. Level of evidence: III.

44. Weinstein SL, Ponseti IV: Curve progression in idiopathic scoliosis. *J Bone Joint Surg Am Vol* 1983;65(4):447-455.

45. Keren R, Luan X, Localio R, et al: Prioritization of comparative effectiveness research topics in hospital pediatrics. *Arch Pediatr Adolesc Med* 2012;166(12):1155-1164.

46. Vigneswaran HT, Grabel ZJ, Eberson CP, Palumbo MA, Daniels AH: Surgical treatment of adolescent idiopathic scoliosis in the United States from 1997 to 2012: An analysis of 20,346 patients. *J Neurosurg Pediatr* 2015;16(3):322-328.

47. Sanders AE, Andras LM, Sousa T, Kissinger C, Cucchiaro G, Skaggs DL: Accelerated discharge protocol for posterior spinal fusion patients with adolescent idiopathic scoliosis decreases hospital postoperative charges 22. *Spine* 2017;42(2):92-97.

An accelerated discharge pathway resulted in a modest saving of $5280 in postoperative charges. Level of evidence: IV.

48. Raudenbush BL, Gurd DP, Goodwin RC, Kuivila TE, Ballock RT: Cost analysis of adolescent idiopathic scoliosis surgery: Early discharge decreases hospital costs much less than intraoperative variables under the control of the surgeon. *J Spine Surg* 2017;3(1):50-57.

An accelerated discharge pathway resulted in decreased length of stay and cost neutrality, but reducing implants and bone graft expenses had a greater effect on reduced costs (9% drop). Level of evidence: III.

49. Samdani AF, Belin EJ, Bennett JT, et al: Unplanned return to the operating room in patients with adolescent idiopathic scoliosis: Are we doing better with pedicle screws? *Spine* 2013;38(21):1842-1847.

50. Ramo BA, Richards BS: Repeat surgical interventions following "definitive" instrumentation and fusion for idiopathic scoliosis: Five-year update on a previously published cohort. *Spine* 2012;37(14):1211-1217.

51. Burton DC, Carlson BB, Place HM, et al: Results of the Scoliosis Research Society Morbidity and Mortality Database 2009-2012: A report from the Morbidity and Mortality Committee. *Spine Deform* 2016;4(5):338-343.

The SRS M&M database reports an overall rate of neurologic deficits from 0.44% to 0.79% following spine deformity surgery. Level of evidence: IV.

52. Buckland AJ, Moon JY, Betz RR, et al: Ponte osteotomies increase the risk of neuromonitoring alerts in adolescent idiopathic scoliosis correction surgery. *Spine* 2019;44(3):E175-E180.

For 2210 patients including 1611 undergoing Ponte osteotomies, curve magnitude and Ponte osteotomies are independent risk factors for intraoperative neuromonitoring alerts. Level of evidence: III.

53. Vandenberg C, Niswander C, Carry P, et al: Compliance with a comprehensive antibiotic protocol improves infection incidence in pediatric spine surgery. *J Pediatr Orthop* 2018;38(5):287-292.

    Overall level of compliance with standardized perioperative antibiotics dosing was only 85%, and lack of compliance was associated with a higher rate of infection. Level of evidence: III.

54. Glotzbecker MP, Gomez JA, Miller PE, et al: Management of spinal implants in acute pediatric surgical site infections: A multicenter study. *Spine Deform* 2016;4(4): 277-282.

    24% of patients who sustained a postoperative spinal infection had recurrent chronic infection requiring further treatment. Level of evidence: III.

55. Oba H, Ebata S, Takahashi J, et al: Pedicle perforation while inserting screws using O-arm navigation during surgery for adolescent idiopathic scoliosis: Risk factors and effect of insertion order. *Spine* 2018;43(24):E1463-E1468.

    This series reports on the use of navigation for 23 consecutive patients with adolescent idiopathic scoliosis. Level of evidence: IV.

56. Luo TD, Polly DW Jr, Ledonio CG, Wetjen NM, Larson AN: Accuracy of pedicle screw placement in children 10 years or younger using navigation and intraoperative CT. *Clin Spine Surg* 2016;29(3):E135-E138.

    This series reports on the use of navigation for 16 consecutive patients age 10 or younger. Level of evidence: IV.

57. Su AW, Luo TD, McIntosh AL, et al: Switching to a pediatric dose O-arm protocol in spine surgery significantly reduced patient radiation exposure. *J Pediatr Orthop* 2016;36(6):621-626.

    Use of an 80 kV, 20 mA, 80 mAs setting on intraoperative CT navigation reduced the radiation dose to the patient by nearly 80% compared to the manufacturer settings. Level of evidence: III.

58. Sarwahi V, Payares M, Wendolowski S, et al: Low-dose radiation 3D intraoperative imaging: How low can we go? An O-arm, CT scan, cadaveric study. *Spine* 2017;42(22):E1311 -E1317.

    In this study of 8 cadavers, imaging resulted in accurate pedicle screw placement on all O-arm settings. Medial breeches were most frequently misclassified. Level of evidence: N/A.

59. Simony A, Hansen EJ, Christensen SB, Carreon LY, Andersen MO: Incidence of cancer in adolescent idiopathic scoliosis patients treated 25 years previously. *Eur Spine J* 2016;25(10):3366-3370.

    At 25 year follow-up, 209 adolescent idiopathic scoliosis patients monitored with radiographs in childhood had a 4.3% cancer risk which is 5 times higher than the age-matched Danish population. Level of evidence: III.

60. Sanders A, Andras L, Lehman A, Bridges N, Skaggs DL: Dermal discolorations and burns at neuromonitoring electrodes in pediatric spine surgery. *Spine* 2017;42(1): 20-24.

    One in 201 scoliosis patients had a dermal burn following neuromonitoring. Level of evidence: III.

61. Sanders AE, Andras LM, Choi PD, Tolo VT, Skaggs DL: Lateral femoral cutaneous nerve palsy after spinal fusion for adolescent idiopathic scoliosis (AIS). *Spine* 2016;41(19): E1164-E1167.

    14 out of 55 patients had a lateral femoral cutaneous nerve palsy following spine surgery which subsequently resolved. Level of evidence: III.

62. Simony A, Christensen SB, Carreon LY, Andersen MO: Radiological outcomes in adolescent idiopathic scoliosis patients more than 22 years after treatment. *Spine Deform* 2015;3(5):436-439.

    Prospective VO2 max testing correlated best with activity level in AIS patients following spinal fusion surgery. Level of evidence: III.

63. Simony A, Hansen EJ, Carreon LY, Christensen SB, Andersen MO: Health-related quality-of-life in adolescent idiopathic scoliosis patients 25 years after treatment. *Scoliosis* 2015;10:22.

64. Jeans KA, Lovejoy JF, Karol LA, McClung AM: How is pulmonary function and exercise tolerance affected in patients with AIS who have undergone spinal fusion? *Spine Deform* 2017;5(6):416-423.

65. Polly DW Jr, Ledonio CG, Diamond B, et al: What are the indications for spinal fusion surgery in Scheuermann kyphosis? *J Pediatr Orthop* 2019;39(5):217-221. doi:10.1097/BPO.0000000000000931.

    Patients undergoing surgery for Scheuermann kyphosis are older, have increased sagittal plane deformity, and more pain over the prominence compared to those opting for nonoperative management. Level of evidence: III.

66. Riouallon G, Morin C, Charles YP, et al: Posterior-only versus combined anterior/posterior fusion in Scheuermann disease: A large retrospective study. *Eur Spine J* 2018;27(9):2322-2330.

    Multicenter review of 67 Scheuermann kyphosis patients treated with posterior fusion alone compared with 64 patients treated with anterior/posterior fusion showed no difference in functional results, complications, and radiologic correction between the two groups at mean 4.2 year follow-up. Level of evidence: III.

67. Lonner BS, Toombs CS, Mechlin M, et al: MRI screening in operative Scheuermann kyphosis: Is it necessary? *Spine Deform* 2017;5(2):124-133.

    Retrospective review of MRI for 86 patients with Scheuermann kyphosis showed that 4.7% of cases had a neurologic abnormality which changed the surgical plan. Level of evidence: IV.

68. Cho W, Lenke LG, Bridwell KH, et al: The prevalence of abnormal preoperative neurological examination in Scheuermann kyphosis: Correlation with X-ray, magnetic resonance imaging, and surgical outcome. *Spine* 2014;39(21):1771-1776.

Pediatrics

69. Lorente A, Barrios C, Lorente R, Tamariz R, Burgos J: Severe hyperkyphosis reduces the aerobic capacity and maximal exercise tolerance in patients with Scheuermann disease. *Spine J* 2019;19(2):330-338.

Maximal oxygen consumption (VO2 max testing) was carried out in 41 patients with Scheuermann kyphosis and 20 healthy controls matched in age. Patients with curvature over 75° had lower VO2 max and significant respiratory inefficiency. Level of evidence: II.

70. Frederickson BE Baker D, McHollick WJ, et al: The natural history of spondylolisthesis and spondylolysis. *J Bone Joint Surg Am Vol* 1984;66:669-707.

71. Eisenstein S: Spondylolysis. A skeletal investigation of two population groups. *J Bone Joint Surg Br* 1978;60-B(4):488-494.

72. Micheli LJ, Wood R: Back pain in young athletes. Significant differences from adults in causes and patterns. *Arch Pediatr Adolesc Med* 1995;149(1):15-18. [Epub 1995/01/01].

73. Hu SS, Tribus CB, Diab M, Ghanayem AJ: Spondylolisthesis and spondylolysis. *J Bone Joint Surg Am Vol* 2008;90(3): 656-671. [Epub 2008/03/11].

74. Campbell RS, Grainger AJ, Hide IG, Papastefanou S, Greenough CG: Juvenile spondylolysis: A comparative analysis of CT, SPECT and MRI. *Skelet Radiol* 2005;34(2):63-73. [Epub 2005/01/26].

75. Anderson K, Sarwark JF, Conway JJ, Logue ES, Schafer MF: Quantitative assessment with SPECT imaging of stress injuries of the pars interarticularis and response to bracing. *J Pediatr Orthop* 2000;20(1):28-33. [Epub 2000/01/21].

76. Sairyo K, Sakai T, Yasui N: Conservative treatment of lumbar spondylolysis in childhood and adolescence: The radiological signs which predict healing. *J Bone Joint Surg Br* 2009;91(2):206-209. [Epub 2009/02/05].

77. Sakai T, Tezuka F, Yamashita K, et al: Conservative treatment for bony healing in pediatric lumbar spondylolysis. *Spine* 2017;42(12):E716-E720.

Sixty consecutive patients diagnosed with lumbar spondylolysis were prospectively followed. Patients who presented early in the disease course had more rapid and reliable healing when treated with rest, avoidance of sports, and use of a TLSO. Level of evidence: II.

78. Iwamoto J, Sato Y, Takeda T, Matsumoto H: Return to sports activity by athletes after treatment of spondylolysis. *World J Orthop* 2010;1(1):26-30. [Epub 2010/11/18].

79. Debnath UK, Freeman BJ, Gregory P, de la Harpe D, Kerslake RW, Webb JK: Clinical outcome and return to sport after the surgical treatment of spondylolysis in young athletes. *J Bone Joint Surg Br* 2003;85(2):244-249. [Epub 2003/04/08].

80. Nielsen E, Andras L, Michael N, et al: 46% reoperation rate in adolescents with spondylolisthesis. *Spine Deform* 2018.

All posterior approach for treatment of high grade spondylolisthesis resulted in a high rate of revision surgery. Level of evidence: IV.

81. Molinari RW, Bridwell KH, Lenke LG, Ungacta FF, Riew KD: Complications in the surgical treatment of pediatric high-grade, isthmic dysplastic spondylolisthesis. A comparison of three surgical approaches. *Spine* 1999;24(16): 1701-1711. [Epub 1999/09/03].

82. Newton PO, Johnston CE II. Analysis and treatment of poor outcomes following in situ arthrodesis in adolescent spondylolisthesis. *J Pediatr Orthop* 1997;17(6):754-761. [Epub 1998/05/20].

83. Phillips WA, Hensinger RN: The management of rotatory atlanto-axial subluxation in children. *J Bone Joint Surg Am Vol* 1989;71(5):664-668. [Epub 1989/06/01].

84. Skaggs DL, Lerman LD, Albrektson J, Lerman M, Stewart DG, Tolo VT: Use of a noninvasive halo in children. *Spine* 2008;33(15):1650-1654. [Epub 2008/07/03].

85. Glotzbecker MP, Wasser AM, Hresko MT, Karlin LI, Emans JB, Hedequist DJ: Efficacy of nonfusion treatment for subacute and chronic atlanto-axial rotatory fixation in children. *J Pediatr Orthop* 2014;34(5):490-495. [Epub 2013/11/28].

86. Chechik O, Wientroub S, Danino B, Lebel DE, Ovadia D: Successful conservative treatment for neglected rotatory atlantoaxial dislocation. *J Pediatr Orthop* 2013;33(4): 389-392. [Epub 2013/05/09].

87. Pueschel SM, Herndon JH, Gelch MM, Senft KE, Scola FH, Goldberg MJ: Symptomatic atlantoaxial subluxation in persons with Down syndrome. *J Pediatr Orthop* 1984;4(6):682-688. [Epub 1984/11/01].

88. Bull MJ: Health supervision for children with Down syndrome. *Pediatrics* 2011;128(2):393-406. [Epub 2011/07/27].

89. Menezes AH, Ryken TC: Craniovertebral abnormalities in Down's syndrome. *Pediatr Neurosurg* 1992;18(1):24-33. [Epub 1992/01/01].

90. Segal LS, Drummond DS, Zanotti RM, Ecker ML, Mubarak SJ: Complications of posterior arthrodesis of the cervical spine in patients who have Down syndrome. *J Bone Joint Surg Am Vol* 1991;73(10):1547-1554. [Epub 1991/12/01].

91. Apple JS, Kirks DR, Merten DF, Martinez S: Cervical spine fractures and dislocations in children. *Pediatr Radiol* 1987;17(1):45-49. [Epub 1987/01/01].

92. Tokunaga S, Ishii Y, Aizawa T, Koizumi Y, Kawai J, Kokubun S: Remodeling capacity of malunited odontoid process fractures in kyphotic angulation in infancy: An observation up to maturity in three patients. *Spine* 2011;36(23):E1515-E1518. [Epub 2011/01/22].

93. Higashino K, Sairyo K, Katoh S, Takao S, Kosaka H, Yasui N: Long-term outcomes of lumbar posterior apophyseal endplate lesions in children and adolescents. *J Bone Joint Surg Am Vol* 2012;94(11):e74. [Epub 2012/05/29].

94. Arkader A, Warner WC Jr, Tolo VT, Sponseller PD, Skaggs DL: Pediatric chance fractures: A multicenter perspective. *J Pediatr Orthop* 2011;31(7):741-744.

95. McCormack RG, Athwal G: Isolated fracture of the vertebral articular facet in a gymnast. A spondylolysis mimic. *Am J Sports Med* 1999;27(1):104-106. [Epub 1999/02/06].

96. Skaggs DL, Avramis I, Myung K, Weiss J: Sacral facet fractures in elite athletes. *Spine* 2012;37(8):E514-E517. [Epub 2011/10/06].

Chapter 62

Pediatric Skeletal Dysplasias, Connective Tissue Disorders, and Other Genetic Conditions

Klane K. White, MD, MSc • Samantha A. Spencer, MD • Craig M. Birch, MD

Pediatrics

ABSTRACT

Genetic disorders affecting the musculoskeletal system are commonly encountered by the pediatric orthopaedic surgeon. Syndromes of orthopaedic importance can result from disorders of growth or function of bone, cartilage, or muscle while the skeletal dysplasias specifically are genetic disorders of the epiphyseal plate. The orthopaedic surgeon must be aware of the clinical and radiographic manifestations of these disorders to appropriately diagnose and treat patients so affected. An update on the specifics of the more common forms is presented.

Keywords: connective tissue disorders; genetics; orthopaedic syndromes; skeletal dysplasia

Introduction

Genetic mutations and chromosomal abnormalities can result in an array of cytokine, enzyme, and structural malfunctions of the tissues in which they are expressed. The physis, specifically, responds to multiple systemic (endocrine) and local (paracrine) regulatory factors, which can be affected by both intrinsic and extrinsic (environmental) factors. Dysregulation of these processes through either mutations in germ line DNA or post fertilization can manifest a skeletal deformity at any point in this process, either through upregulation or downregulation of cellular activity.

Dr. White or an immediate family member is a member of a speakers' bureau or has made paid presentations on behalf of Biomarin; serves as a paid consultant to or is an employee of Biomarin; has received research or institutional support from Biomarin and Ultragenyx; has received nonincome support (such as equipment or services), commercially derived honoraria, or other non–research-related funding (such as paid travel) from Genzyme; and serves as a board member, owner, officer, or committee member of the Pediatric Orthopaedic Society of North America. Neither of the following authors nor any immediate family member has received anything of value from or has stock or stock options held in a commercial company or institution related directly or indirectly to the subject of this chapter: Dr. Birch and Dr. Spencer.

Marfan Syndrome

Marfan syndrome results from a mutation in the gene encoding for the fibrillin protein.[1] Fibrillin is an extracellular glycoprotein essential in the formation of the elastic fibers found in connective tissues. An increased availability of growth factors also is also responsible for changes in the mechanical properties of the soft tissues, most importantly the aortic root and the ocular lens.

The revised Ghent nosology (2010) emphasizes the importance of family history, aortic root aneurysm, and ectopia lentis as the cardinal diagnostic features of Marfan syndrome[2] (**Table 1**). Other musculoskeletal findings are a part of this systemic score, including laxity of the wrist and thumb, chest deformity, pes planovalgus, protrusio acetabuli, scoliosis, and loss of elbow extension.[3] In patients with Marfan syndrome, scoliosis is often diagnosed first, and consequently, it is important for the orthopaedic surgeon to recognize the underlying condition for diagnostic referral and appropriate management of potentially life-threatening cardiovascular abnormities. Scoliosis in Marfan syndrome is treated in a manner similar to idiopathic scoliosis, although bracing treatment appears to be less effective, with a reported success rate of only 17% in patients with mild to moderate curves.[4] Management of scoliosis in these patients, however, differs from idiopathic scoliosis in several important ways. First, the incidence of dural ectasia is higher in these patients, and appropriate imaging (CT and MRI) is recommended for all patients indicated for surgical intervention. Associated small pedicles in the lumbar spine, particularly on the concave side, make pedicle screw fixation more challenging[5] (**Figure 1**). Second, the complication rate in scoliosis surgery is higher for

Table 1

Revised Ghent Criteria—2010

Absence of Family History
Aortic diameter ≥ +2 Z-score, ectopia lentis
Aortic diameter ≥ +2 Z-score, FBN1 mutation
Aortic diameter ≥ +2 Z-score, systemic score ≥ 7
Ectopia lentis, FBN1 mutation, known aortic dilatation
Family History (as defined above)
Ectopia lentis
Systemic score ≥ 7
Aortic diameter ≥ +2 Z-score, > 20 years old
Aortic diameter ≥ +3 Z-score, < 20 years old
Systemic Scores
Wrist and thumb sign—3 (wrist or thumb sign—1)
Pectus carinatum deformity—2 (pectus excavatum or chest asymmetry—1)
Hindfoot deformity—2 (plain pes planus—1)
Pneumothorax—2
Dural ectasia—2
Protrusio acetabuli—2
Reduced US/LS and increased arm/height and no severe scoliosis—1
Scoliosis or thoracolumbar kyphosis—1
Reduced elbow extension—1
Facial features (3/5)—1 (dolichocephaly, enophthalmos, downslanting palpebral fissures, malar hypoplasia, retrognathia)
Skin striae—1
Myopia >3 diopters—1
Mitral valve prolapse (all types)—1

patients with Marfan syndrome when compared with those with idiopathic scoliosis. Infection, implant failure, pseudarthrosis, or coronal and sagittal curve decompensation are reported to occur in 10% to 20% of patients, while overcorrection can cause cardiovascular complications.[6] Traction should be used with caution, as subluxation of vertebrae can occur and worsen, especially in the presence of associated kyphosis.[7,8] Infection is often associated with a dural tear (increased risk due to dural ectasia). Perioperative death from valvular insufficiency has been reported.

Osteogenesis Imperfecta

Osteogenesis imperfecta (OI) occurs in about 1 in 20,000 children and is most commonly the result of a mutation in the genes that code for type I collagen (*COL1A1* and *COL1A2*) or the genes that encode for processing of these strands.[9] Defects in type I collagen can be quantitative (type I) or qualitative (types II-IV) in nature. A substitution of glycine by another amino acid, leading to structural abnormalities, prevents proper triple helix formation of the collagen molecule and subsequent qualitative deficiency of the bone matrix.[10] Meanwhile, mutations that result in a premature stop codon lead to abnormal messenger RNA production and, therefore, less collagen production. There is an increased number of osteoblasts and osteoclasts, which are biologically hypermetabolic. Bone in patients affected by OI shows a decreased number of trabeculae and decreased cortical thickness. Despite an increase in the frequency of

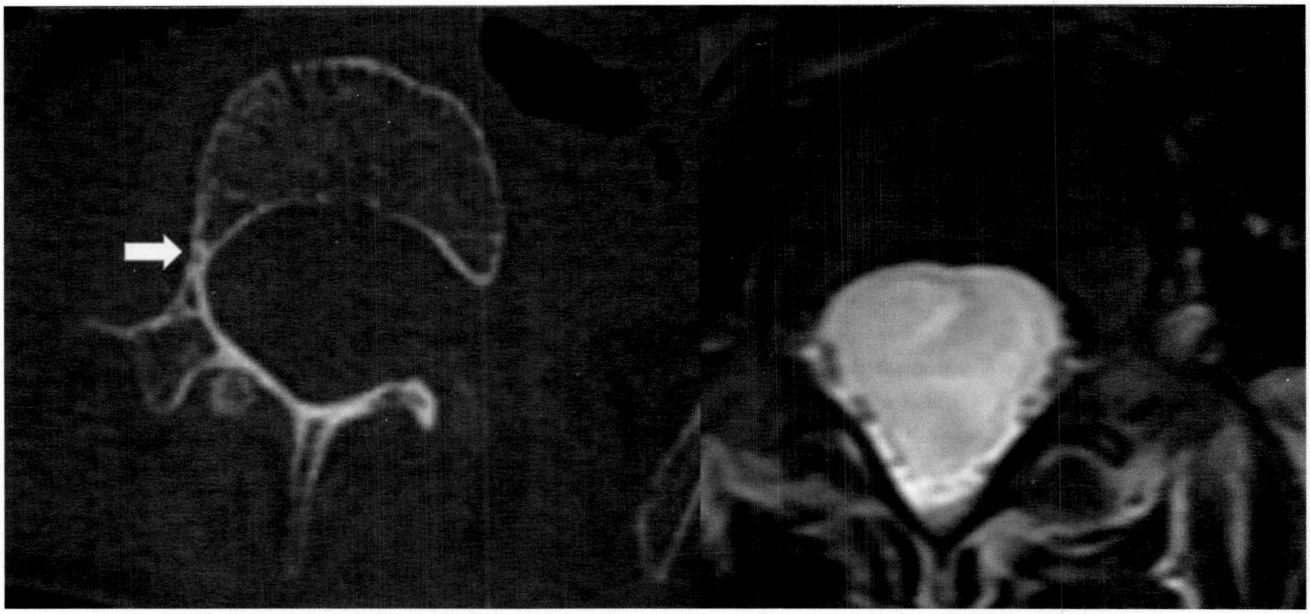

Figure 1 Axial views of CT scan and MRI of lumbar spine in a patient with Marfan syndrome. Surgeons should be aware of the anatomy in these patients in which the pedicles (arrow) are quite narrow and dural ectasia is common.

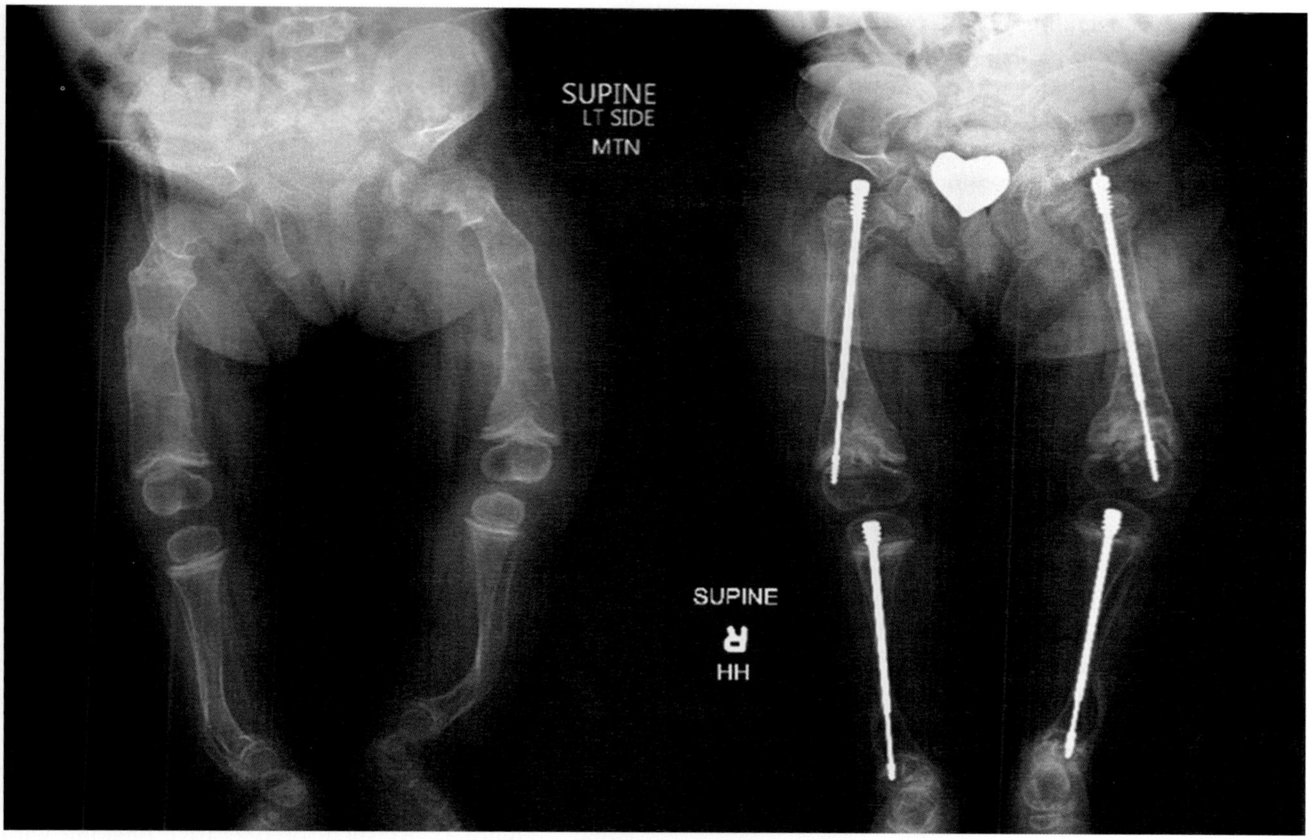

Figure 2 MRI showing multiple fractures in the lower extremities in patients with osteogenesis imperfecta. Placement of telescoping rods can be challenging in these small patients, but very beneficial to their long-term quality of life.

fractures in patients with OI during childhood, bone healing occurs at a normal rate, but with abnormal bone.

Nonsurgical management of fractures consists of a short course of splinting to minimize the effects of disuse osteoporosis and to prevent cyclic fracturing. Realignment osteotomies with intramedullary fixation (commonly with telescoping rods) are the standard treatment in children with bone deformities that interfere with function.[11] Age at realignment is dictated by the size of the patient and, in the author's experience, can be performed as early as 18 months of age, but in more severely affected individuals may have to wait until four to five years of age. Intramedullary fixation, particularly of the tibiae, with telescoping rods may still be challenging, even at this age (**Figure 2**).

Pharmacologic treatment with diphosphonates is commonly used in the care for children with OI sustaining two or more long bone fractures per year.[12] Cyclical treatment with intravenous pamidronate results in improved bone mineral density, reduction in fracture incidence, reduction in pain, and improved remodeling of vertebral body compression fractures. Data supporting the use of other forms of diphosphonates (zoledronate) exist in the treatment of low bone mineral density in children and in children with OI, but pamidronate remains the standard in diphosphonate therapy. Because animal data suggest that impaired bone healing may occur in the presence of diphosphonate therapy, elective osteotomies should be timed accordingly (infusions should be delayed approximately three months after surgical intervention).[13]

Fassier-Duval telescoping rods (FD rods) have become the mainstay for orthopaedic treatment of upper and lower extremity deformities in OI.[11] Treatment of multiple long bones (eg, femurs and tibiae) in one setting, with reasonable blood loss is possible. Short- and medium-term (4-5 years) outcomes are good, with regard to reducing fracture recurrence and improving mobility. Complications include refracture, pseudarthrosis, rod migration, and failure to elongate. Revision surgery rates for lower extremities are approximately 50% by four years and about 35% at three years for upper extremities.

Spinal manifestations in OI include scoliosis, kyphosis, craniocervical junction abnormalities (ie, basilar invagination), and spondylolysis and spondylolisthesis.[14] The prevalence of scoliosis in OI ranges from

39% to 80%, depending on the type of OI.[15] Scoliosis is rarely observed in patients younger than 6 years but can progress rapidly after it is diagnosed.[16]

Craniocervical junction abnormalities are seen in 37% of patients with OI, including basilar invagination (13%), basilar impression (15%), and platybasia (29%).[17] Skull base abnormalities are correlated with the severity of disease and older age.[18] Advanced imaging including CT and MRI are recommended to best understand the complex anatomy that can be quite difficult to discern on plain radiography. Treatment of basilar invagination may be by odontoid resection, foramen magnum decompression, or both, and may require occipitocervical fusion.[19]

Spinal fusion has been recommended for deformities as small as 35° to halt curve progression, but the patient's age and truncal height need to be taken into account to avoid thoracic insufficiency. While reports indicate that children with severe OI may benefit from fusion when curves are 35°, delay of treatment to 50° is unlikely to significantly compromise pulmonary function or increase difficulty in deformity correction.[20] Recent evaluation of contemporary instrumentation and correction techniques has shown improved outcomes. The authors of a 2014 study[21] reviewed a series of 10 patients with OI who underwent posterior spinal fusion for the treatment of scoliosis. These authors recommend surgical stabilization at 40°. All of their patients underwent preoperative pamidronate therapy, and seven had cement-augmented pedicle screw instrumentation at the proximal and distal foundations. These authors emphasize the difficulty of exposure of the thoracic spine due to rib overgrowth and thoracic lordosis. Utilizing rib and Ponte osteotomies, they report an average correction of 48% with no loss of correction at follow-up, no neurologic deficits, and no implant failures. They also noted improved quality of life scores, pain, and sitting tolerance in these patients. While not supported by the literature, the author now utilizes polyester sublaminar bands to reduce pullout stresses on pedicle screws and a rigid postoperative thoracolumbosacral orthosis for three months postoperatively to help reduce stresses on the spinal instrumentation.

Neurofibromatosis

Neurofibromatosis (NF) is the most common single-gene disorder in humans. This disorder has several forms, of which NF type 1 (NF1) is the most relevant to orthopaedic surgeons. These children appear normal at birth, showing disease progression with age. Diagnosis is made based on the presence of at least two of the seven cardinal clinical findings (**Table 2**).

Table 2

Cardinal Clinical Findings for the Diagnosis of Neurofibromatosis

- Six or more café-au-lait spots (larger than 5 mm in diameter in a child or 15 mm in an adult)
- Two neurofibromas or a single plexiform neurofibroma
- Freckling in the axilla or inguinal region
- An optic glioma
- Two or more Lisch nodules (hamartoma of the iris)
- A distinctive osseous lesion such as vertebral scalloping or cortical thinning
- A first-degree relative with neurofibromatosis type 1

Common orthopaedic manifestations of NF include scoliosis, limb overgrowth, and pseudarthrosis of long bones. Scoliosis in NF is categorized as idiopathic or dystrophic.[22,23] Dystrophic curves are generally single thoracic curves that are kyphotic and typically involve a short (sharp) segment. These curves typically present early and are aggressively progressive. Brace treatment is largely ineffective in dystrophic curves. Surgical intervention can be complicated by the presence of severe dural ectasia and rib head dislocation into the spinal canal[24] (**Figure 3**). As such, preoperative imaging with CT and MRI is mandatory for patients with dystrophic curves. The risk of paraplegia is increased in patients with dystrophic curves, particularly those with severe

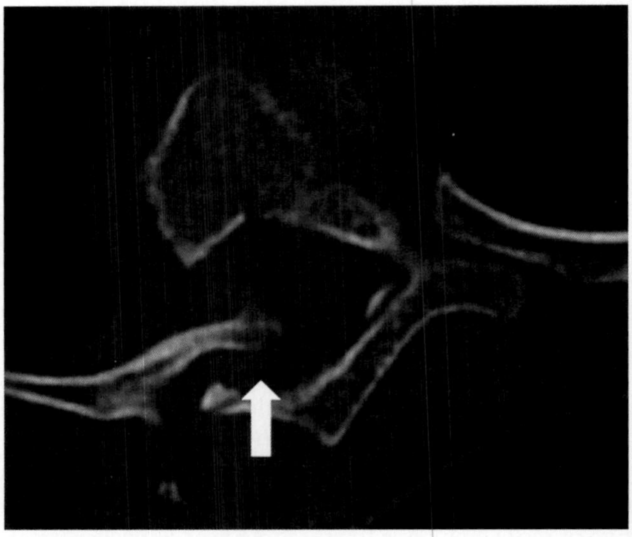

Figure 3 Dystrophic scoliosis in neurofibromatosis type 1 can often present with rib head intrusion of the spinal canal. Preoperative CT scan and MRI are strongly recommended to evaluate for unusual anatomy including rib head intrusion (arrow), dural ectasia, neuraxial neurofibromas, and dystrophic pedicles.

kyphosis. Nondystrophic curves are managed using standard techniques applicable to idiopathic scoliosis. Excision of rib heads invading the spinal canal is controversial, with some authors suggesting that rib head resection is unnecessary.[25] Early-onset scoliosis (EOS) in NF, typically dystrophic in nature, is amenable to growth friendly spine treatments, without concern for additional complications as compared with other etiologies for EOS.

Congenital pseudarthrosis of the long bones, most commonly the tibia (tibial dysplasia), is common in NF. Tibial dysplasia presents with a characteristic anterolateral bow that is usually obvious in infancy. The dysplastic site is composed of a hamartoma of undifferentiated mesenchymal cells.[26] Early management of tibial dysplasia should be directed at preventing fracture with a clamshell orthosis. Surgical intervention in not warranted until a fracture is established, as osteotomy may lead to true pseudarthrosis. Although many approaches have been proposed, common elements leading to successful treatment include aggressive débridement of the hamartoma and adequate stabilization of the tibia and fibula. Intramedullary fixation, free vascularized bone graft, and Ilizarov bone transport have been described.[27-30] Studies utilizing bone morphogenetic protein (BMP) at the pseudarthrosis site suggest that this modality may help in achieving union.[31] The results of BMP use have demonstrated variable success. Concerns about the use of bone morphogenetic protein in patients with an inherited premalignant condition still exist.[32]

Ehlers-Danlos Syndrome

Ehlers-Danlos syndrome (EDS) is a group of clinically and genetically heterogeneous, heritable connective tissue disorders characterized by joint hypermobility, skin hyperextensibility, and tissue fragility. The most recent nosology recognizes 13 subtypes, with variations in tissue types involved, including the skin, ligaments, joints, eyes, intestines, and cardiovascular structures.[33] Ninety percent of EDS is represented by two of these subtypes: classic EDS (cEDS) and hypermobile EDS (hEDS). cEDS is an autosomal dominant disorder, most commonly (>90%) associated with mutations in COL5A1 or COL5A2, but can also be associated with COL1A1 and COL1A2 mutations when clinical criteria are met. hEDS is also transmitted in an autosomal dominant fashion, but no reliable or appreciable genetic underpinning has yet been identified.

Diagnosis of EDS relies on unique major and minor criteria for each subtype. Generalized joint laxity is a hallmark of both of these EDS subtypes. Generalized joint laxity with regard to EDS has been defined as a Beighton score of ≥6 for prepubertal children and adolescents, ≥5 for pubertal men and women up to the age of 50 years, and ≥4 for those >50 years of age for hEDS (**Table 3**). Lower Beighton scores may be found in patients with molecular confirmation of cEDS.

Other orthopaedic manifestations of hEDS include chronic musculoskeletal pain, recurrent joint dislocations, or frank instability in the absence of trauma.[34] There are no described pathognomonic radiographic findings associated with EDS. Physical therapy focusing on core muscle strength or stabilization of specific joints may be successful. Recognition that EDS patients have loose joints and tight muscles is requisite to rehabilitation success. According to a 2017 study, exercise programs that emphasize "range of motion" or repetitive, forceful actions can often make symptoms worse.[34]

Higher complication rates after surgery are commonly associated with EDS.[35] The literature, however,

Table 3

Beighton Score

Palm and forearm resting on a flat surface with the elbow flexed at 90°, the metacarpal-phalangeal joint of the fifth finger can be hyperextended more than 90°	1point each hand
With arms outstretched forward, hand pronated, the thumb can be passively moved to touch the ipsilateral forearm	1point each hand
With the arms outstretched to the side and hand supine, the elbow extends more than 10°	1 point each elbow
While standing with knees locked in extension, the knee extends more than 10°	1 point each knee
With knees locked straight and feet together, the patient places the total palm of both hands flat on the floor	1 point
Total possible score	**9 points**

lacks detailed analysis or explanation of why surgery does not go well.[36] Avoidance of surgical complications depends largely on appropriate and strict indications. Surgery is an option for a select number of specific conditions in EDS, including the spine, shoulders, elbow, and hands as well as hips and lower extremities. The rate of failure of surgical intervention is higher in EDS, particularly for conditions where ligaments are repaired. Wound healing is generally good, but may result in widened scars.

Achondroplasia

Achondroplasia is the most common cause of disproportionate dwarfism, with a prevalence of 1 in 15,000 live births, and is an autosomal dominant disorder caused by a gain of function mutation in the transmembrane portion of the developmental receptor gene *FGFR3*.[37,38] Mutations in the gene coding for fibroblast growth factor receptor-3 (*FGFR-3*) result in upregulation of *FGFR-3* receptor tyrosine kinase activity and consequently impaired differentiation of physeal cartilage and diminished growth of the proliferative and hypertrophic zones.

The mutations for hypochondroplasia and thanatophoric dysplasia reside in different locations within the *FGFR-3* gene than in achondroplasia, resulting in the differing phenotypes.[39,40] Thanatophoric dysplasia is the more severe phenotype and is almost always fatal before two years of age. It is characterized by severe rhizomelic shortening, platyspondyly, a protuberant abdomen, and a small thoracic cavity that is responsible for cardiorespiratory failure. Other FGFR-3 disorders that result in skeletal dysplasia include SADDAN (severe achondroplasia with developmental delay and acanthosis nigricans) and Crouzon syndrome with acanthosis nigricans.[40,41]

An increased mortality rate has been observed in infants with achondroplasia, approaching 7%.[42] The increased incidence of sudden death observed in this population has been at least partially attributed to central sleep apnea resulting from spinal cord compression at the foramen magnum.[43,44] Routine surveillance in infants with achondroplasia is critical and consists of a combination of history and physical examination and polysomnography. Neuraxial imaging (MRI) should be performed only if indicated by abnormal findings with any of the above.[45]

Thoracolumbar kyphosis is found in up to 95% of infants with achondroplasia, and often worsens prior to achieving independent ambulation.[46] The deformity at this age is typically supple and it is thought to be preventable through sitting modifications and bracing.[47,48] Persistence of kyphosis beyond childhood can lead to myelopathy, paraparesis and rarely paraplegia.[49] Deformity correction by a combined anterior and posterior approach, or through an all-posterior approach with osteotomy, both allow for correction of most deformities and avoid lengthening of the spinal cord.[50,51] Surgery is recommended when thoracolumbar kyphosis exceeded 60° with more than 10° of progression per year.

Spinal stenosis is essentially universal in achondroplasia, but not typically symptomatic until the third or fourth decade of life. Symptoms can present as early as adolescence, particularly in the presence of residual thoracolumbar kyphosis.[52] Symptoms include leg weakness and pain with walking, and are often relieved by flexion of the lumbrosacral spine achieved by squatting, sitting, bending forward at the waist, or lying down. Treatment of symptomatic disease in the skeletally immature patient is recommended, as neglect may result in permanent neurological dysfunction. Preoperative MRI may be helpful, but is often difficult to interpret due to multilevel stenosis.

Current treatment recommendations for stenosis are for laminectomy from one to two levels above the most cranial segment of compression, as determined by imaging extending caudally to the first sacral level. Inadequate decompression results in a high rate of recurrence. In the skeletally immature, fusion of the decompressed levels is necessary to avoid postlaminectomy kyphosis. If a kyphotic deformity is present, then concomitant deformity correction with oinsrumented fusion is recommended.

The lower extremity malalignment found in achondroplasia is genu varum with associated internal tibial torsion, typically with ligamentous laxity at the knees (accentuated by slight knee flexion). With few exceptions the genu varum in achondroplasia is asymptomatic and rarely leads to precocious arthritis.[53] Genu varum in achondroplasia rarely requires treatment; however, osteotomy may be required for reduced function caused by lateral leg or foot pain (which must be differentiated from pain of spinal origin). When symptomatic at younger ages, guided growth techniques may be considered.[21] It is suggested that surgeons consider addressing both the distal femoral and proximal tibial and fibular physes. Complete deformity correction by guided growth may take up to three years or may not be attained at all. Discoid meniscus appears to be more common in achondroplasia and may require arthroscopic débridement when symptomatic.[54]

In the upper extremities, flexion contractures of the elbows and subluxation of the radial heads are present. Humeral lengthening is indicated for children lacking the ability to independently engage in personal hygiene because of rhizomelic shortening. Nonorthopaedic manifestations of achondroplasia include difficulty with weight control, sleep apnea, recurrent otitis media, and hydrocephalus. These patients have normal intelligence, and life expectancy is not significantly diminished.

Medical therapies are currently under investigation. Use of C-natriuretic peptide (CNP) analogues, which inhibit the tyrosine kinase-mediated MAPK pathway in both short acting and long acting forms are being evaluated. Soluble FGFR-3 is also being investigated as a therapy. Soluble protein acts as a decoy receptor and prevents FGF from binding to mutant FGFR3, thus reducing the upregulation of FGFR-3 seen in schondroplasia. None of these therapies is FDA approved, nor has efficacy been established.

Pseudoachondroplasia

Pseudoachondroplasia (1 in 20,000 births) bears many phenotypic similarities to achondroplasia, but is a quite different disorder. Pseudoachondroplasia is transmitted in an autosomal dominant fashion and results from a defect in the cartilage oligomeric matrix protein (COMP), an important mediator of chondrocyte-extracellular matrix interactions, and a potent suppressor of apoptosis.[55] Mutant COMP is retained in the rough endoplasmic reticulum resulting in premature intracellular assembly of extracellular matrix ("endoplasmic reticulum stress") and physeal chondrocyte apoptosis.

This disruption results in radiographically evident delays in epiphyseal ossification.[56] Pseudoachondroplasia is typified by normal facial features, rhizomelic short stature, ligamentous laxity, windswept knees, and severe osteoarthritis.[56] Children with pseudoachondroplasia have a normal appearance at birth. Clinical changes are often not apparent until the age of 3 years, although radiographic changes are certainly present earlier.

The pathognomonic radiographic finding in pseudoachondroplasia is a tongue-like anterior projection of the vertebral bodies best seen on the lateral spine view. This occurs as a result of delayed ossification of the vertebral endplates (**Figure 4**). Although this finding is pathognomonic, it is seen in early in life and gradually normalizes with age, making early investigation important in the radiographic diagnosis.

Scoliosis is common in this condition.[49] A high prevalence of C1-C2 instability is of primary importance in pseudoachondroplasia.[57,58] As is the case with other skeletal dysplasias, routine radiographic examination is warranted and occipitocervical fusion is indicated when radiographic evidence of instability or myelopathy is present.

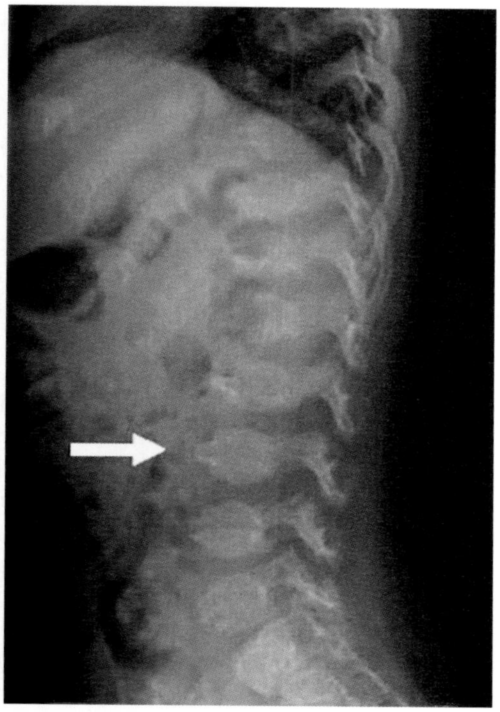

Figure 4 Lateral view of the lumbar spine depicts classical, pathgnomonic vertebral finding for pseudoachondroplasia. Superior and inferior endplates lack ossification at anterior aspect, resulting in a squared anterior projection mid body (arrow).

Lower extremity deformities can manifest as either varus or valgus malalignment of the knees. Often these deformities occur concomitantly in contralateral limbs (ie, windswept deformity). Maintenance of deformity correction in the skeletally immature patients can be exceedingly difficult, often requiring multiple revision surgeries.[21] Given the propensity for precocious arthritis in this group, correction of malalignment is believed to be important in the preservation of long-term function. Like type II collagen disorders, guided growth can be effective at younger ages, but ultimately osteotomies at skeletal maturity to achieve appropriate alignment are necessary.

Diastrophic Dysplasia

Diastrophic dysplasia (DTD) is an autosomal recessive, short-limbed dwarfism associated with multiple severe and, at times, life-threatening spinal deformities.[59,60] Clinically, these patients present with multiple joint contractures, severe clubfeet, patellar dislocation, and joint instability; the presence of the classic hitchhiker's thumb

Pediatrics

and cauliflower ears are pathognomonic for the condition.[61] Normal intelligence is associated with DTD.

This disorder is the result of a sulfate transporter protein defect, resulting from mutations in the *SLC26A2* gene (solute carrier family 26, member 2; formerly DTDST), which on histopathology results in a paucity of sulfated proteoglycans in cartilage matrix.[62] While the exact prevalence of diastrophic dysplasia is not known, it is estimated that DTD affects about 1 in 500,000 newborns in the United States. Variability in phenotypic expression may result in less severe forms of the disorder, with the most mild form manifesting as "autosomal recessive multiple epiphyseal dysplasia."[63]

Epiphyseal dysplasia and painful degenerative arthrosis of the hip is common in young adults. The spine frequently develops excessive lumbar lordosis, thoracolumbar kyphosis, and scoliosis.[64] The knee may be unstable in childhood, and flexion contractures develop with progressive valgus deformity and lateral subluxation or dislocation of the patella. The description of "clubfoot," generally used for the foot deformity in DTD, is often a misnomer.[65] Three-dimensional analysis of "clubfeet" in diastrophic dysplasia demonstrates that clubfeet in this disorder are very different than idiopathic clubfeet.[66] Hindfoot valgus and metatarsus adductus, more consistent with a skewfoot-type deformity, is the most common presentation. Equinovarus adductus, metatarsus adductus, or isolated equinus also occur.

Casting for clubfeet may result in limited correction. Equinus deformity tends to be recalcitrant and persists. Even with attempted correction of clubfoot deformities, many adults with DTD are unable to place their heels on the ground. Typically, the adult with classic DTD stands on his toes with knee and hip flexion deformities and marked lumbar lordosis with limited ambulatory ability.[67]

In the rare absence of flexion deformities of the knees and hips, dorsiflexion osteotomy of the distal tibia may be indicated to create a plantigrade foot. Treatment of lateral patellar subluxation has been recommended by some authors.[67,68] Bayhan et al recommend early treatment of patellar subluxation to slow flexion deformity of the knee and consequently improve and extend ambulatory status in children with DTD.

Cervical kyphosis tends to resolve in most children with DTD (**Figure 5**). Kyphosis exceeding 60°, typically associated with severely hypoplastic vertebrae, tends not to resolve and usually progresses. Bracing treatment has been recommended in young children for cervical kyphosis with good results, but this likely represents the benign natural history of the condition for most individuals. Severe complications can be expected from progressive kyphosis, with multiple reports of quadriplegia and cardiopulmonary failure existing in the literature.[69]

Scoliosis is the hallmark deformity of diastrophic dysplasia, being reported in 37% **to** 88% of affected individuals.[59,63,70,71] The most common curve pattern is a thoracic scoliosis with hyperkyphosis. Treating surgeons should be aware of the high incidence (up to 75%) of spina bifida occulta within the cervical spine when planning their surgical approach, with good preoperative imaging including CT angiography and MRI.[74]

Spine deformities often present prior to the age of 5 years, and are prone to severe progression, become extremely rigid, and adversely affect pulmonary function. Individuals with diastrophic dysplasia generally do not develop trunk height after the age of 10 years, and as such early intervention (curves >50°) regardless of age has been recommended.[75] Severe complications can be expected with surgical treatment, however, with

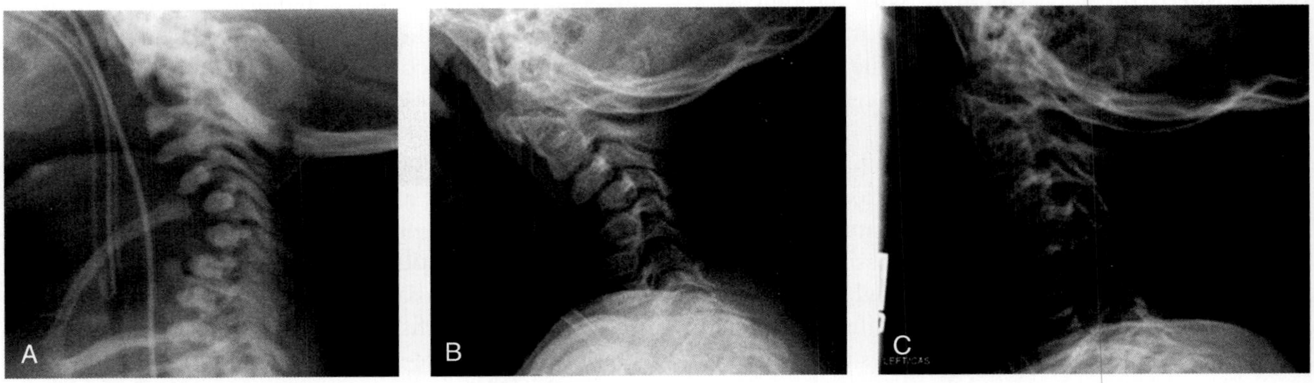

Figure 5 Cervical kyphosis is common in young children with diastrophic dysplasia, but tends to resolve as demonstrated here (**A**) at age 2 years, (**B**) age 5 years, and (**C**) age 9 years. Bracing has been recommended with good results, but likely represents the benign natural history of this condition.

multiple reports of quadriplegia and cardiopulmonary failure. In younger children, growth-friendly instrumentation has been successfully implemented.[72] Because of the kyphosis, spine to rib constructs that bypass the kyphotic segment of the spine are useful. With increased age and rigidity, posterior fusion and instrumentation with posterior osteotomies may be required.

Camptomelic Dysplasia

Camptomelic dysplasia results from mutations in the *SOX9* gene, which is critical to the ossification of long bone cartilage anlagen during fetal development.[73] No reliable data exist regarding the prevalence of camptomelic dysplasia, but estimates are in the range of 1:40,000 to 1:80,000 live births. Diaphyseal bowing of the long bones, primarily the tibia and femur, are the hallmarks of camptomelic dysplasia, while absence of thoracic pedicles on plain radiograph is diagnostic (**Figure 6**). Plagiocephaly, cleft palate, micrognathia, renal and cardiac defects, and sex reversal (phenotypic females with an XY karyotype) are common in this disorder.[74] Defective tracheal cartilage and restricted chest size often result in respiratory failure and death during the neonatal period.

Cervical kyphosis, spondylolisthesis, hydromyelia, or diastematomyelia may be present, and neurologic complications and pseudarthrosis are common after spine treatment.[75] As in diastrophic dysplasia, early deformity treatment with growth friendly devices is recommended. Because of the extremely hypoplastic vertebrae and radiographically absent pedicles, spine-to-rib constructs are favored by the author in this patient group.

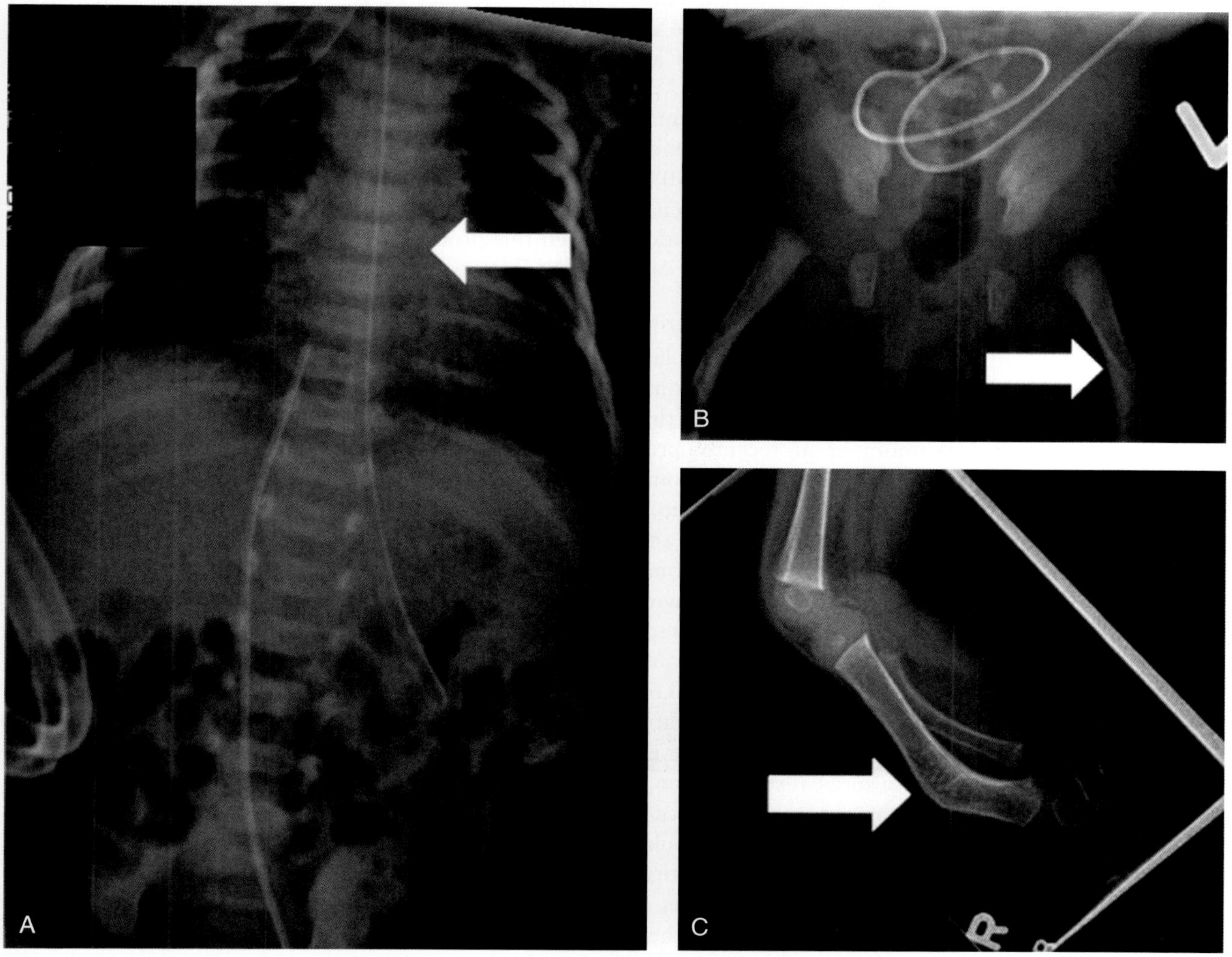

Figure 6 Camptomelic dysplasia is typified by (**A**) an absence of thoracic pedicles (arrow) and diaphyseal bowing of the (**B**) femurs and (**C**) tibias (arrows). Acamptomelic camptomelic dysplasia presents with the absence of pedicles on spine radiographs seen in (**A**), but lacks the bowing of the long bones.

Cleidocranial Dysplasia

The gene mutation in cleidocranial dysplasia is in runt-related transcription factor 2 (*RUNX2*), which is transferred in an autosomal dominant fashion. RUNX2 is an osteoblast-specific transcription factor that regulates osteoblast differentiation.[76] Failure of development of membranous bones is manifested as a deficiency of the clavicles and pelvis as well as delayed closure of the cranial fontanels. As a result, the shoulders appear narrow and sloping and can be brought close together in front of the body. Mild short stature, coxa vara or valga, a high palate, and abnormal permanent tooth development also are present, with lumbar spondylolysis occurring in 24% of patients.[77] Scoliosis requiring treatment has been reported in small case series, as has treatment of hip deformities.[78-82]

Trisomy 21 (Down Syndrome)

Down syndrome is the most common chromosomal abnormality in humans with an occurrence of approximately 1 in 800 to 1,000 live births with an increased incidence with increased maternal age.[83,84] Nonorthopaedic manifestations include developmental delay including both gross motor and cognitive impairment. Congenital heart disease is present in about 50% of patients, most commonly septal defects. Duodenal atresia is associated with Down syndrome, as is endocrinopathy, specifically hypothyroidism. Leukemia can occur about 1% of the time.

Of the patients with Down syndrome, 10% to 30% have an increased atlantodens interval (ADI) on lateral radiographs.[85-87] Only 1% of the Down syndrome population has neurologic findings associated with this instability however.[88] Nakamura et al recently proposed a new radiographic measure in Down syndrome called the C1/C4 space available for cord (SAC) ratio.[89] Neutral lateral cervical spine radiographs are taken and the SAC at the level of C1 and C4 are measured. Normal controls had an average of 1.29 (±0.14), patients with Down syndrome not requiring surgery had an average of 1.15 (±0.13), and patients with Down syndrome who underwent posterior fusion had an average of 0.63 (±0.1). The authors concluded that C1/C4 SAC ratio <0.8 was associated with increased likelihood for developing myelopathy and therefore surgical stabilization.

Patients with Down syndrome have a significant risk of scoliosis with 10% of the ambulatory population being affected and rates as high as 50% in institutionalized patients.[90,91] Most recently, Abousamra et al reviewed all cases of scoliosis and trisomy 21 at their institution with a prevalence of 21% of patients over the age of 8. Most patients have an idiopathic curve pattern, most commonly a double major curve.[92,94] Bracing treatment as a nonsurgical treatment option remains controversial in Down syndrome.[91,93,96] Surgical treatment with posterior spinal fusion has been reported to have higher rates of complications when compared with the general population.[94]

Congenital dislocation of the hips is rare in the Down syndrome infant; however, acetabular dysplasia develops in childhood and can be progressive past skeletal maturity.[95-97] Twenty-eight percent of adults with trisomy 21 have radiographic evidence of hip pathology which is associated with a significant reduction in ambulatory ability.[100] The combination of established generalized ligamentous laxity and unique pelvic anatomy and acetabular morphology contribute to instability with potential for recurrent and habitual dislocations. Traditionally, surgical intervention was met with significant complication and high recurrent instability[98-100] (**Figure 7**). Recurrent subluxation, infection, and periprosthetic fracture remain major complications in this population.[101] Reportedly, outcomes have improved with better understanding of the pathoanatomy.[101] The mainstay of surgical treatment in the skeletally immature patient with recurrent hip subluxation is varus osteotomy with derotation when anatomically indicated.[102] Improved outcomes have been reported when this procedure is performed between the ages of 5 and 7 years. Previously, procedures failed to address the acetabular retroversion present in trisomy 21 hip instability.[103] Other study authors reported their experience with anteverting acetabular osteotomy resulting in significantly improved outcomes.[107,109]

Lower extremity alignment in Down syndrome is overwhelmingly genu valgum with many patients having asymptomatic patellar instability and recurrent dislocations that require no intervention.[104] In the patient with symptomatic patellar instability, the authors recommend nonsurgical intervention initially. Specific modalities include patellar stabilizing orthoses and physical therapy. Multiple methods of surgical management have been reported with varying levels of success.[105-107] The most important factor for success remains surgical intervention that addresses all aspects of the deformity of the individual.

Mucopolysaccharidoses

The mucopolysaccharidoses (MPS) are a family of lysosomal storage disorders resulting from single gene defects in the enzymes responsible for the normal degradation of glycosaminoglycans (GAG).[108] The MPS disorders are autosomal recessive disorders (with MPS II being X-linked recessive), with a combined incidence of 1 in 25,000 live births[109] (**Table 4**). Each MPS

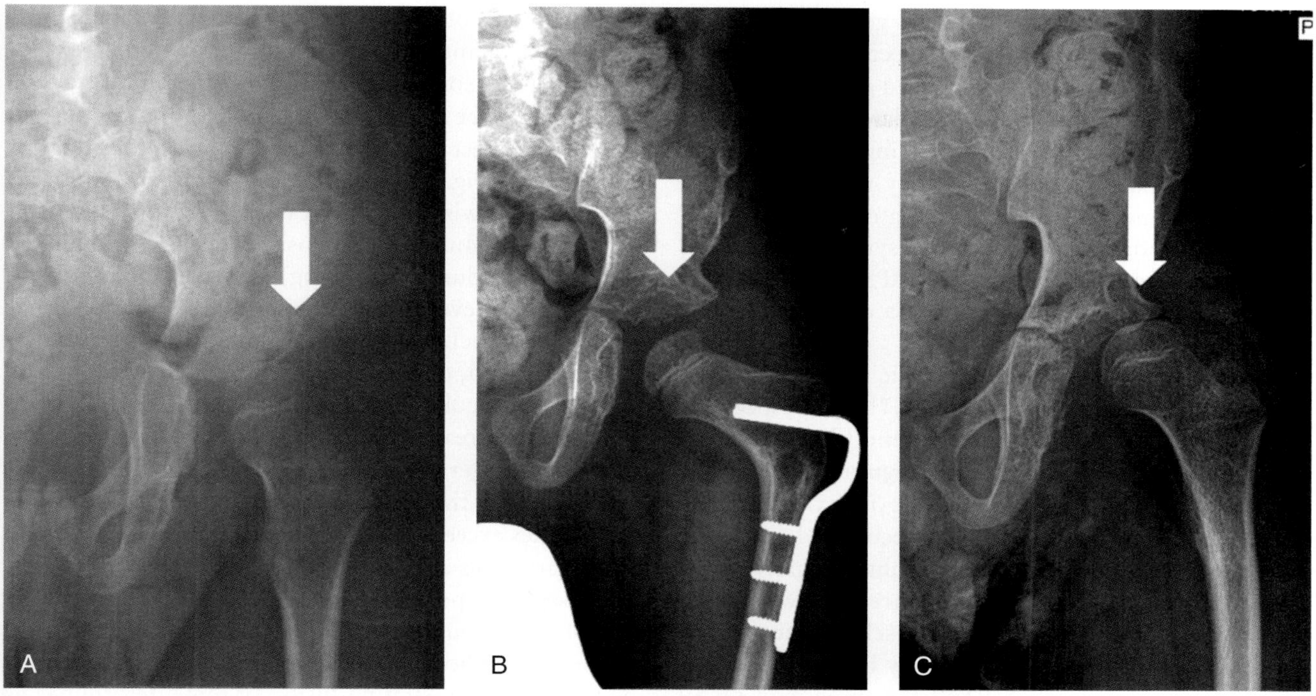

Figure 7 On AP view of the hip, progressive subluxation of the hip (arrow) associated with voluntary dislocation in a boy with Down syndrome (**A**). Recurrent subluxation (**C**) is common even after open reduction, capsulorrhaphy, femoral varus osteotomy, and acetabuloplasty (**B**).

Table 4

The Mucopolysaccharidoses

Designation	Syndrome	Enzyme Defect	Substance Stored	Inheritance Pattern
MPS IH	Hurler	α-l-Iduronidase	HS, DS	Autosomal recessive
MPS 1HS	Hurler/Scheie			
MPS1S	Scheie			
MPS II	Hunter	Iduronidase-2-sulfatase	HS, DS	X-linked recessive
MPS IIIA	Sanfilippo A	Heparin-sulfatase (sulfamidase)	HS	Autosomal recessive
MPS IIIB	Sanfilippo B	α-N-acetylglucosamidase	HS	Autosomal recessive
MPS IIIC	Sanfilippo C	Acetyl-CoA: α-glucosaminide-N-acetyltransferase	HS	Autosomal recessive
MPS IIID	Sanfilippo D	Glucosamine-6-sulfatase	HS	Autosomal recessive
MPS IVA	Morquio A	N-acetyl galactosamine-6-sulfate sulfatase	KS, CS	Autosomal recessive
MPS IVB	Morquio B	β-d-Galactosidase	KS, CS	Autosomal recessive
MPS VI	Maroteaux-Lamy	Arylsulfatase B, N-acetylgalactosamine-4-sulfatase	HS, DS	Autosomal recessive
MPS VII	Sly	β-d-Glucuronidase	CS, HS, DS	Autosomal recessive
MPS VIII	No eponym	Glucosamine-6-sulfatase	CS, HS	Autosomal recessive

CS = chondroitin sulfate, DS = dermatan sulfate, HS = heparan sulfate, KS = keratan sulfate, MPS = mucopolysaccharidosis disorder is associated with a single gene defect and a corresponding enzyme function defect. Common musculoskeletal findings in MPS include a gibbus deformity of the spine, hip dysplasia, or bilateral Perthes-like disease of the hips.[110-112] Later findings include lower extremity malalignment, particularly valgus deformity of the knees and ankles and wasting of the hand musculature secondary to carpal tunnel syndrome. There is some element of joint stiffness in MPS disorders, with the exception of MPS IV, which is characterized by excessive joint laxity.

The constellation of radiographic findings in MPS is known as "dysostosis multiplex."[113] Platyspondyly with anterior "beaking" in the vertebral bodies should always arouse suspicion of MPS (**Figure 8**). Wide iliac wings with inferior tapering of the ilium, acetabular dysplasia, and coxa valga are also seen. Madelung type deformity of the distal radius and ulnar negative variance are common. The metacarpals are short with proximal pointing in older children. The sella turcica can be J-shaped, and the ribs are universally broad (ribs wider than intercostal spaces). MRI of the spine may reveal stenosis at the occipital-cervical junction, the subaxial cervical spine, or the cervicothoracic level.

Surgical indications for cervical spinal stenosis and atlantoaxial instability are not established, but signs and symptoms of myelopathy, significant instability, and cord signal change on MRI are minimum indicators for treatment.[114] Isolated stenosis at the occipital-cervical junction can be treated by decompression alone, but is probably best combined with fusion in MPS IV due to associated ligamentous laxity.[115] When instability is present otherwise, decompression with fusion is recommended. Multilevel stenosis is seen in attenuated MPS I (from dural thickening) and in MPS IV and VI (due to multilevel disk prominence).[116,117] Options for these cases include multilevel laminectomy, with or without fusion, or laminoplasty.

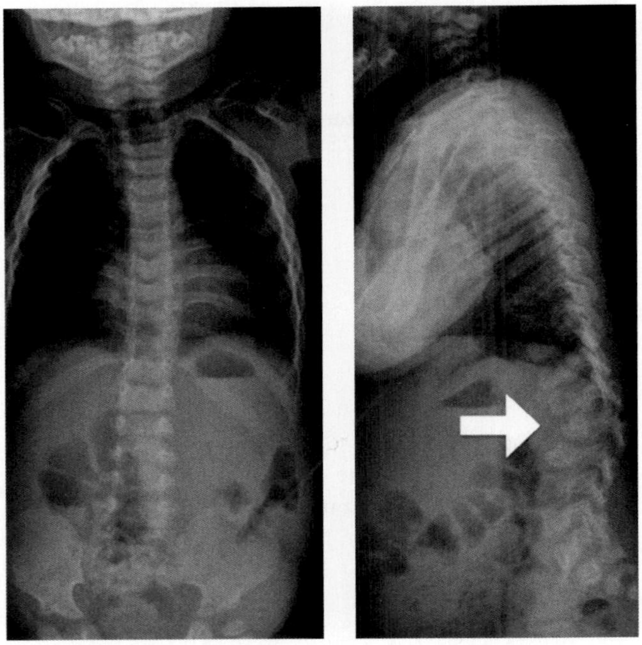

Figure 8 Thoracolumbar kyphosis, seen on lateral radiograph of the spine, with L1 or L2 hypoplasia and "beaking" (arrow) is often a presenting feature of mucopolysaccharidoses (MPS), as in this two-year-old with MPS VI. This finding should always trigger diagnostic testing for MPS.

For thoracolumbar kyphoses, treatment can be much less aggressive allowing continued growth of the spine in younger children, as these deformities are typically caudal to the conus medularis. Practically speaking deformities exceeding 70° should be stabilized, as should those rare cases associated with myelopathy.[120] Isolated short segment posterior fusion without deformity correction is discouraged, as failure rates increase significantly.[118] Kyphotic deformities may be accompanied by scoliosis, necessitating fusion of these deformities as well. The role of delay tactics, such as bracing treatment and casting are not defined in MPS, nor is the role of "growth-friendly" spinal instrumentation, but could certainly be entertained in appropriate circumstances.

Surgical treatment for hip dysplasia and subluxation may be considered to prevent progressive subluxation.[119] Literature suggests that excellent radiographic outcomes can be achieved with surgical reconstruction of the hip.[120] Long-term outcomes, however, suggest that patients treated surgically may not fare better than those not treated surgically with regard to eventual development of radiographic arthrosis.[121] The San Diego (Dega) innominate osteotomy with a femoral varus osteotomy is preferable. Patients with MPS IV are prone to resubluxation, so augmentation with an acetabular shelf procedure has also been recommended. Total hip arthroplasty is advocated in adults who have pain-limiting disease that is beyond traditional reconstructive capabilities.

Genu valgum is responsive to guided growth techniques, but recurrence is common.[126] Osteotomy of the proximal tibia or distal femur may be required in patients with limited growth potential. Total knee arthroplasty has been reported for severe degenerative arthritis. Significant lateral release and allograft augmentation may be required.[122]

Nerve recovery from carpal tunnel syndrome is more likely with early intervention, so aggressive surgical treatment is recommended.[123] Even early signs of nerve conduction deficiency warrant open carpal tunnel release, including excision of hypertrophic tenosynovium, concomitant A1 pulley releases and resection of thickened tendon slips for associated trigger digits.[124]

Multiple Epiphyseal Dysplasia

The multiple epiphyseal dysplasias (MED) represent a heterogeneous group of genetic disorders with a commonality of clinical manifestations, which include mild short stature (often presenting in late childhood), genu valgum, and precocious arthritis, most pronounced in the hips and knees. The five autosomal dominant forms of MED appear to result from five different genes (*COMP*, *COL9A1*, *COL9A2*, *COL9A3*, and *MATN3*).[55] Radiographically, there is a commonality of underdevelopment or delayed ossification of the epiphyses (**Figure 9**) or the presence of osteochondritis dissecans-like lesions. When multiple sites of osteochondritis dissecans are present and associated with a Robin Sequence, the mutations in common with Stickler syndrome (*COL9A1*, *COL9A2*, *COL9A3*) should be considered. The recessive form of MED has been attributed to mutations in the *SLC26A2* gene. Radiographically, this form of MED is typified by a double-layer patella on lateral views. These patients have milder characteristics of those seen in diastrophic dysplasia. Unlike the autosomal dominant forms, up to 50% of affected individuals with the recessive form have an abnormal finding at birth (such as clubfoot, cleft palate, or clinodactyly).

Orthopaedic management of these patients is mostly supportive and revolves around management of lower extremity malalignment and precocious arthritis. Like other skeletal dysplasias, guided growth works well in these patients at younger ages, but due to growth restraints, may have limited benefits in later childhood, and time to correction may be prolonged. Similarly, early joint arthroplasty can be extremely effective a reliving pain and improving quality of life.

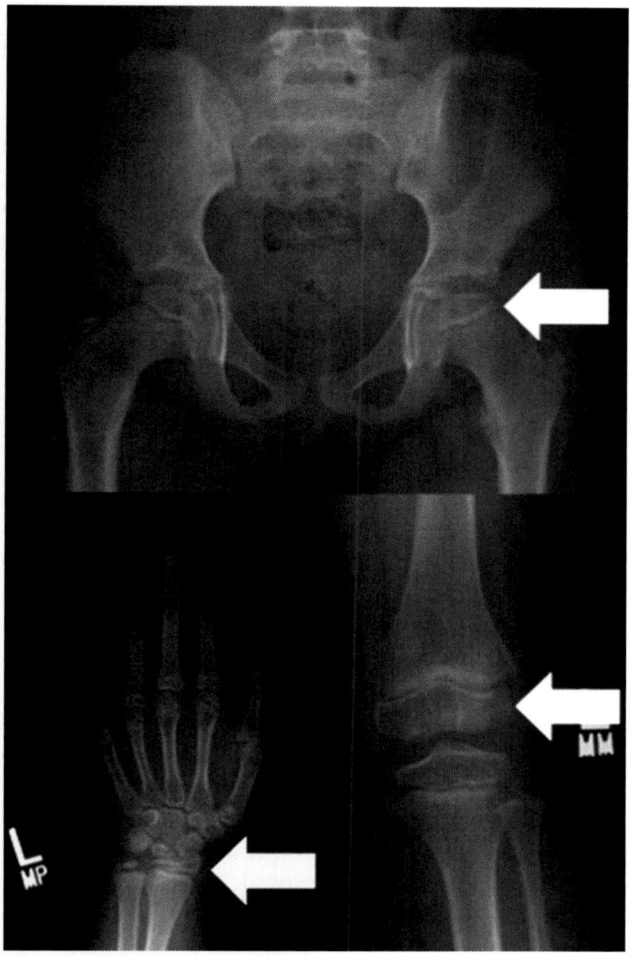

Figure 9 Multiple epiphyseal dysplasia is most commonly associated with underdevelopment of the epiphyses (arrows) throughout the extremities (shown here on AP pelvis, AP hand, and AP knee radiographs), without involvement of the spine. Other findings include osteochondritis dissecans like lesions, or in the case of the autosomal recessive form, a double layer patella on lateral radiograph of the knee.

X-Linked Hypophosphatemic Rickets

X-linked hypophosphatemic rickets (XLH) is characterized by renal phosphate loss associated with a normal to low vitamin D serum concentration and is the most common form of heritable rickets.[125] As the name implies XLH is inherited in an X-linked manner, and its incidence is estimated at 1 in 20,000 live births. XLH is caused by mutations in the phosphate-regulating endopeptidase homolog, X-linked (PHEX) gene.[126] Mutations in PHEX lead to an increase in the activity of fibroblast growth factor 23 (FGF23). FGF23 is a bone-derived hormone that regulates phosphate metabolism. FGF23 reduces serum phosphate by suppressing proximal tubular phosphate reabsorption and intestinal phosphate absorption.[127] The upregulation of FGF23 in XLH leads to the phosphate-wasting characteristic of the disorder. The aberration in phosphate availability to the skeleton contributes to a decrease in the mineralization of the long bones and teeth in patients with XLH.

The phenotypic spectrum of XLH ranges from isolated hypophosphatemia to severe lower extremity bowing.[128] XLH frequently manifests in the first 2 years of life with progressive varus deformity; however, it may not manifest until adulthood, as previously unevaluated short stature. In adults, enthesopathy (calcification of the tendons, ligaments, and joint capsules) associated with joint pain and impaired mobility. Persons with XLH are prone to spontaneous dental abscesses and sensorineural hearing loss.

The rachitic skeletal changes of nutritional rickets and XLH are clinically indistinguishable. In children the metaphyses may be widened, frayed, or cupped, typically with greater involvement at the knees than the wrists when compared with nutritional rickets. In severe cases, rachitic rosary (beading of the ribs) results from poor skeletal mineralization and overgrowth of the costochondral joint cartilage. Looser zone or pseudofractures that may or may not be symptomatic are commonly seen and have been reported to occur at any age.

Clinical findings in XLH include short stature, lower extremity deformity (both varus and valgus), and, in adults, enthesopathy and tendon/ligament calcification. Adults with XLH have a significantly reduced final height of −1.9 standard deviations from reference standards, with disproportionate short legs. In adults enthesopathy can cause joint pain and impair mobility. Enthesopathy of vertebral ligaments has been reported, including case reports of spinal cord compression and paraplegia following calcification of the ligamenta flavum.[129]

Conventional therapy for XLH consists of phosphate supplementation in multiple daily doses and active vitamin D analogues (calcitriol, 1,25 HO-Vitamin D). In a recent trial, inhibition of FGF-23 activity with a recombinant human IgG1 monoclonal antibody was associated with an increase in renal tubular phosphate reabsorption and radiographic improvements in the severity of rickets.[130] The improvement in radiographic changes was most profound in those with most severe scores at baseline. These improvements were associated with concurrent improvements in growth, physical activity, and a reduction in pain.

Both varus and valgus deformities of the lower extremities are found in XLH, with the classic deformity at skeletal maturity consisting of an anterolateral bow of the femur with distal femoral valgus and proximal tibia vara (**Figure 10**). With prompt treatment at a young age (younger than3 years), medical management often suffices in the management of lower extremity deformity. Historically, deformity correction was accomplished via osteotomies, with a high rate of recurrence when performed in growing children.[131,132] Because of these outcomes, surgery has been reserved for children with progressive bony deformities that result in significant gait disturbance, activity limitation, and pain. Optimization of medical management is encouraged

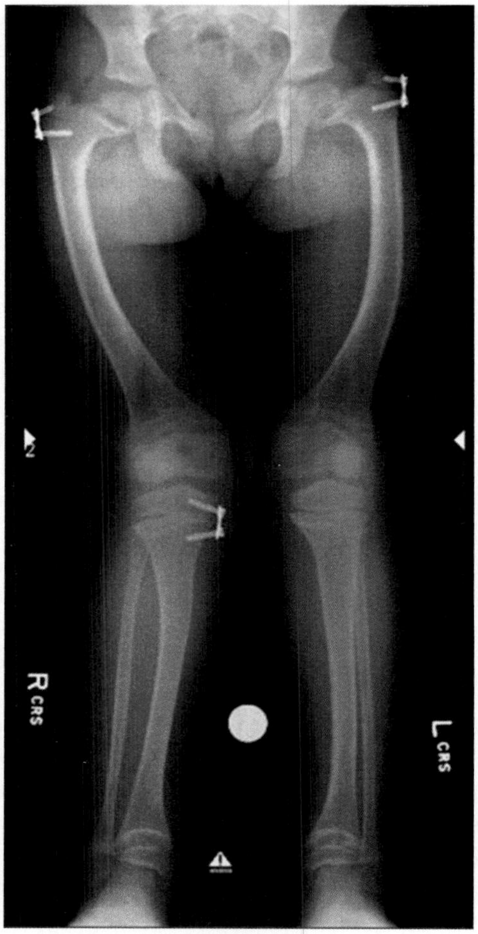

Figure 10 An AP standing alignment film of the lower extremities shows coxa vara, varus and/or valgus deformities of the knees and metaphyseal cupping, all of which are typical findings in X-linked hypophosphatemic rickets. The femora often have a distal anterolateral bow with compensatory valgus at the metaphysis.

prior to engaging in surgical management. Healing rates with distraction osteogenesis have been correlated with serum phosphate levels, with the recommendation that lengthenings not be undertaken when serum phosphate levels are <2.5 mg/dL.[133] At minimum, normalization of parathyroid hormone and alkaline phosphatase are recommended prior to surgical intervention, as normal serum phosphate levels may be difficult to maintain.[134] Guided growth can be quite effective in younger children. Periarticular deformities correct at a rate of 0.3° and 0.7° per month for the mMPTA and mLDFA, respectively, with improvement of femoral and tibial diaphyseal bowing also occurring.[134] Outcomes with valgus deformities seem to be better than varus deformities where one must be vigilant for recurrence of deformity.

Summary

Genetic conditions with orthopaedic manifestations are a common part of pediatric orthopaedic practice. The orthopaedic surgeons' unique training makes their involvement critical to the diagnosis and management of theses individually rare disorders. Although surgical management is paramount for many of these disorders, there is a quickly evolving landscape with regard to medical therapies that are changing the way the orthopaedic surgeon approaches and treats individuals included in this group of patients.

Key Study Points

- Many genetic disorders manifest with musculoskeletal deformities. Most of these disorders are uncommon or rare. Familiarity with the conditions most associated with orthopaedic manifestations is provided.
- Presentation of musculoskeletal disease in genetically mediated conditions varies widely among these conditions, as does the natural history.
- Surgery is often indicated for genetically mediated musculoskeletal conditions. Surgical indications vary by condition, and recommendations are made for the conditions reviewed.

Annotated References

1. Pearson GD, Devereux R, Loeys B, et al: Report of the national heart, lung, and blood institute and national Marfan foundation working group on research in Marfan syndrome and related disorders. *Circulation* 2008;118(7):785-791.
2. Loeys BL, Dietz HC, Braverman AC, et al: The revised ghent nosology for the Marfan syndrome. *J Med Genet* 2010;47(7):476-485.
3. De Maio F: Orthopaedic aspects of Marfan syndrome: The experience of a referral center for diagnosis of rare diseases. *Adv Orthop* 2016;2016:8275391.
4. Sponseller PD, Bhimani M, Solacoff D, Dormans JP: Results of brace treatment of scoliosis in Marfan syndrome. *Spine* 2000;25(18):2350-2354.
5. Qiao J, Zhu F, Xu L, et al: Accuracy of pedicle screw placement in patients with Marfan syndrome. *BMC Musculoskelet Disord* 2017;18(1):123.

   A study concerning safety and accuracy of pedicle screw placement in Marfan syndrome. CT scanning was performed to analyze accuracy of pedicle screw placement. Placement of pedicle screw in Marfan syndrome is accurate and safe. Special attention should be paid when screws were placed at the lumber spine and the concave side of spine deformity to avoid the higher rate of complications. Level of evidence: III.
6. Skaggs DL, Bushman G, Grunander T, Wong PC, Sankar WN, Tolo VT: Shortening of growing-rod spinal instrumentation reverses cardiac failure in child with Marfan syndrome and scoliosis: A case report. *J Bone Joint Surg Am* 2008;90(12):2745-2750.
7. Yang S, Andras LM, Redding GJ, Skaggs DL: Early-onset scoliosis: A review of history, current treatment, and future directions. *Pediatrics* 2016;137(1). doi:10.1542/peds.2015-0709.
8. DeMaio F, Fichera A, De Luna V, Mancini F, Caterini R: Orthopaedic aspects of Marfan syndrome: The experience of a referral center for diagnosis of rare diseases. *Adv Orthop* 2016;2006:8275391.

   The aim of this study was to report the most frequent musculoskeletal alterations observed in 146 patients affected by Marfan syndrome. Musculoskeletal anomalies were observed in all patients with Marfan syndrome: severe flatfoot in 21.2%, hindfoot deformity 36.9%, scoliosis or thoracolumbar kyphosis in 15%, and acetabular protrusio was found on radiographs in 18.4%. Level of evidence: IV.
9. Sillence DO, Senn A, Danks DM: Genetic heterogeneity in osteogenesis imperfecta. *J Med Genet* 1979;16(2):101-116.
10. Rauch F, Glorieux FH: Osteogenesis imperfecta. *Lancet* 2004;363(9418):1377-1385.
11. Azzam KA, Rush ET, Burke BR, Nabower AM, Esposito PW: Mid-term results of femoral and tibial osteotomies and Fassier-Duval Nailing in children with osteogenesis imperfecta. *J Pediatr Orthop* 2018;38(6):331-336.

    Retrospective chart review identified 58 children with OI who had realignment osteotomies with Fassier-Duval (FD) intramedullary nailing of the lower extremity. Fifty-eight patients had 179 lower extremity FD intramedullary rods placed. Revisions were required in 53% of patients, which occurred at a mean time of 52 months after initial rodding surgery. Diphosphonate infusion was not postponed after surgical procedures. Patients had improvement in mobility status at the latest follow-up. Level of evidence: IV.
12. Glorieux FH: Bisphosphonate therapy for severe osteogenesis imperfecta. *J Pediatr Endocrinol Metab* 2000;13 suppl 2:989-992.
13. Meganck JA, Begun DL, McElderry JD, et al: Fracture healing with alendronate treatment in the Brtl/+ mouse model of osteogenesis imperfecta. *Bone* 2013;56(1):204-212.
14. Wallace MJ, Kruse RW, Shah SA: The spine in patients with osteogenesis imperfecta. *J Am Acad Orthop Surg* 2017;25(2):100-109.

    Review article on the treatment of spinal deformities in patients with osteogenesis imperfecta. Level of evidence: V.
15. Widmann RF, Bitan FD, Laplaza FJ, Burke SW, DiMaio MF, Schneider R: Spinal deformity, pulmonary compromise, and quality of life in osteogenesis imperfecta. *Spine* 1999;24(16):1673-1678.

16. Benson DR, Newman DC: The spine and surgical treatment in osteogenesis imperfecta. *Clin Orthop Relat Res* 1981;(159):147-153.
17. Arponen H, Makitie O, Haukka J, et al: Prevalence and natural course of craniocervical junction anomalies during growth in patients with osteogenesis imperfecta. *J Bone Miner Res* 2012;27(5):1142-1149.
18. Cheung MS, Arponen H, Roughley P, et al: Cranial base abnormalities in osteogenesis imperfecta: Phenotypic and genotypic determinants. *J Bone Miner Res* 2011;26(2):405-413.
19. Klekamp J: Treatment of basilar invagination. *Eur Spine J* 2014;23(8):1656-1665.
20. Kocher MS, Shapiro F: Osteogenesis imperfecta. *J Am Acad Orthop Surg* 1998;6(4):225-236.
21. Yilmaz G, Oto M, Thabet AM, et al: Correction of lower extremity angular deformities in skeletal dysplasia with hemiepiphysiodesis: A preliminary report. *J Pediatr Orthop* 2014;34(3):336-345.
22. Crawford AH: Neurofibromatosis in children. *Acta Orthop Scand Suppl* 1986;218:1-60.
23. Akbarnia BA, Gabriel KR, Beckman E, Chalk D: Prevalence of scoliosis in neurofibromatosis. *Spine* 1992;17(8 suppl):S244-S248.
24. Funasaki H, Winter RB, Lonstein JB, Denis F: Pathophysiology of spinal deformities in neurofibromatosis. An analysis of seventy-one patients who had curves associated with dystrophic changes. *J Bone Joint Surg Am* 1994;76(5):692-700.
25. Ton J, Stein-Wexler R, Yen P, Gupta M: Rib head protrusion into the central canal in type 1 neurofibromatosis. *Pediatr Radiol* 2010;40(12):1902-1909.
26. Cho TJ, Seo JB, Lee HR, Yoo WJ, Chung CY, Choi IH: Biologic characteristics of fibrous hamartoma from congenital pseudarthrosis of the tibia associated with neurofibromatosis type 1. *J Bone Joint Surg Am* 2008;90(12):2735-2744.
27. Grill F, Bollini G, Dungl P, et al: Treatment approaches for congenital pseudarthrosis of tibia: Results of the EPOS multicenter study. european paediatric orthopaedic society (EPOS). *J Pediatr Orthop B* 2000;9(2):75-89.
28. Dobbs MB, Rich MM, Gordon JE, Szymanski DA, Schoenecker PL: Use of an intramedullary rod for treatment of congenital pseudarthrosis of the tibia. A long-term follow-up study. *J Bone Joint Surg Am* 2004;86-A(6):1186-1197.
29. Romanus B, Bollini G, Dungl P, et al: Free vascular fibular transfer in congenital pseudoarthrosis of the tibia: Results of the EPOS multicenter study. European Paediatric Orthopaedic Society (EPOS). *J Pediatr Orthop B* 2000;9(2):90-93.
30. Paley D, Catagni M, Argnani F, Prevot J, Bell D, Armstrong P: Treatment of congenital pseudoarthrosis of the tibia using the Ilizarov technique. *Clin Orthop Relat Res* 1992;280:81-93.
31. Richards BS, Oetgen ME, Johnston CE: The use of rhBMP-2 for the treatment of congenital pseudarthrosis of the tibia: A case series. *J Bone Joint Surg Am* 2010;92(1):177-185.
32. Senta H, Park H, Bergeron E, et al: Cell responses to bone morphogenetic proteins and peptides derived from them: Biomedical applications and limitations. *Cytokine Growth Factor Rev* 2009;20(3):213-222.
33. Malfait F, Francomano C, Byers P, et al: The 2017 international classification of the Ehlers-Danlos syndromes. *Am J Med Genet C Semin Med Genet* 2017;175(1):8-26.

    A revised classification of Ehler-Danlos syndrome is presented. The definite diagnosis of all EDS subtypes, except for the hypermobile type, relies on molecular confirmation with identification of a causative genetic variant. The clinical criteria for hypermobile EDS are revised in order to allow for a better distinction from other joint hypermobility disorders. Level of evidence: V.
34. Ericson WB Jr, Wolman R: Orthopaedic management of the Ehlers-Danlos syndromes. *Am J Med Genet C Semin Med Genet* 2017;175(1):188-194.

    Review article on orthopaedic surgical treatment of Ehlers-Danlos syndrome patients. Conclusions are that specific joint stabilization and nerve decompression procedures can provide symptomatic relief when conservative measures fail. Level of evidence: V.
35. Freeman RK, Swegle J, Sise MJ: The surgical complications of Ehlers-Danlos syndrome. *Am Surg* 1996;62(10):869-873.
36. Weinberg J, Doering C, McFarland EG: Joint surgery in Ehlers-Danlos patients: Results of a survey. *Am J Orthop (Belle Mead NJ)* 1999;28(7):406-409.
37. Horton WA, Hall JG, Hecht JT: Achondroplasia. *Lancet* 2007;370(9582):162-172.
38. Oberklaid F, Danks DM, Jensen F, Stace L, Rosshandler S: Achondroplasia and hypochondroplasia. comments on frequency, mutation rate, and radiological features in skull and spine. *J Med Genet* 1979;16(2):140-146.
39. Heuertz S, Le Merrer M, Zabel B, et al: Novel FGFR3 mutations creating cysteine residues in the extracellular domain of the receptor cause achondroplasia or severe forms of hypochondroplasia. *Eur J Hum Genet* 2006;14(12):1240-1247.
40. Bellus GA, Bamshad MJ, Przylepa KA, et al: Severe achondroplasia with developmental delay and acanthosis nigricans (SADDAN): Phenotypic analysis of a new skeletal dysplasia caused by a Lys650Met mutation in fibroblast growth factor receptor 3. *Am J Med Genet* 1999;85(1):53-65.
41. Passos-Bueno MR, Serti Eacute AE, Jehee FS, Fanganiello R, Yeh E: Genetics of craniosynostosis: Genes, syndromes, mutations and genotype-phenotype correlations. *Front Oral Biol* 2008;12:107-143.
42. Simmons K, Hashmi SS, Scheuerle A, Canfield M, Hecht JT: Mortality in babies with achondroplasia: Revisited. *Birth Defects Res A Clin Mol Teratol* 2014;100(4):247-249.
43. Stokes DC, Phillips JA, Leonard CO, et al: Respiratory complications of achondroplasia. *J Pediatr* 1983;102(4):534-541.
44. Pauli RM, Horton VK, Glinski LP, Reiser CA: Prospective assessment of risks for cervicomedullary-junction compression in infants with achondroplasia. *Am J Hum Genet* 1995;56(3):732-744.

45. White KK, Bompadre V, Goldberg MJ, et al: Best practices in the evaluation and treatment of foramen magnum stenosis in achondroplasia during infancy. *Am J Med Genet* 2016;170A(1):42-51.

Best-practice guidelines for management of foramen magnum stenosis in infants with achondroplasia, based on Delphi consensus panel. Level of evidence: V.

46. Kopits SE: Thoracolumbar kyphosis and lumbosacral hyperlordosisin achondroplastic children. *Basic Life Sci* 1988;48:241–255.

47. Siebens AA, Hungerford DS, Kirby NA: Achondroplasia: Effectiveness of an orthosis in reducing deformity of the spine. *Arch Phys Med Rehabil* 1987;68:384–388.

48. Lonstein JE: Treatment of kyphosis and lumbar stenosis in achondroplasia. *Basic Life Sci* 1998;48:283–292.

49. Tolo VT: Surgical treatment of kyphosis in achondroplasia. *Basic Life Sci* 1988;48:257–259.

50. Bradford DS, Tribus CB: Vertebral column resection for the treatment of rigid coronal decompensation. *Spine (Phila Pa 1976)* 1997;22(14):1590–1599.

51. Suk SI, Kim JH, Kim WJ, Lee SM, Chung ER, Nah KH: Posterior vertebral column resection for severe spinal deformities. *Spine (Phila Pa 1976)* 2002;27(21):2374–2382.

52. Ponsetti IV: Skeletal growth in achondroplasia. *J Bone Joint Surg Am* 1970;52A:701–716.

53. Tang J, Su N, Zhou S, et al: Fibroblast growth factor receptor 3 inhibits osteoarthritis progression in the knee joints of adult mice. Arthritis Rheumatol 2016;68(10):2432-2443.

54. Hoernschemeyer DG, Atanda A Jr, Dean-Davis E, Gupta SK: Discoid meniscus associated with achondroplasia. Orthopedics 2016;39(3):e498-e503.

A case series of four patients with achondroplasia with symptoms of knee pain and discoid lateral meniscus. The authors propose that symptomatic discoid lateral meniscus should be added to the differential diagnosis for lower-extremity pain in the achondroplasia population. Level of evidence: IV.

55. Jackson GC, Mittaz-Crettol L, Taylor JA, et al: Pseudoachondroplasia and multiple epiphyseal dysplasia: A 7-year comprehensive analysis of the known disease genes identify novel and recurrent mutations and provides an accurate assessment of their relative contribution. Hum Mutat 2012;33(1):144-157.

56. Posey KL, Alcorn JL, Hecht JT: Pseudoachondroplasia/COMP - translating from the bench to the bedside. *Matrix Biol* 2014;37:167-173.

57. Svensson O, Aaro S: Cervical instability in skeletal dysplasia. Report of 6 surgically fused cases. *Acta Orthop Scand* 1988;59(1):66-70.

58. Shetty GM, Song HR, Lee SH, Kim TY: Bilateral valgus-extension osteotomy of hip using hybrid external fixator in spondyloepiphyseal dysplasia: Early results of a salvage procedure. *J Pediatr Orthop B* 2008;17(1):21-25.

59. Bethem D, Winter RB, Lutter L: Disorders of the spine in diastrophic dwarfism. *J Bone Joint Surg Am* 1980;62(4):529-536.

60. Poussa M, Merikanto J, Ryoppy S, Marttinen E, Kaitila I: The spine in diastrophic dysplasia. *Spine* 1991;16(8):881-887.

61. Horton WA, Rimoin DL, Lachman RS, et al: The phenotypic variability of diastrophic dysplasia. *J Pediatr* 1978;93(4):609-613.

62. Superti-Furga A: Defects in sulfate metabolism and skeletal dysplasias, in Scriver CR, Beaudet AL, Sly WS, Valle D, Vogelstein B, Childs B, eds: *The Metabolic and Molecular Bases of Inherited Disease*. 2001, p 5189.

63. Makitie O, Savarirayan R, Bonafe L, et al: Autosomal recessive multiple epiphyseal dysplasia with homozygosity for C653S in the DTDST gene: Double-layer patella as a reliable sign. *Am J Med Genet* 2003;122A(3):187-192.

64. Remes V, Poussa M, Lonnqvist T, et al: Walking ability in patients with diastrophic dysplasia: A clinical, electroneurophysiological, treadmill, and MRI analysis. *J Pediatr Orthop* 2004;24(5):546-551.

65. Ryoppy S, Poussa M, Merikanto J, Marttinen E, Kaitila I: Foot deformities in diastrophic dysplasia. an analysis of 102 patients. *J Bone Joint Surg Br* 1992;74(3):441-444.

66. Weiner DS, Jonah D, Kopits S: The 3-dimensional configuration of the typical foot and ankle in diastrophic dysplasia. *J Pediatr Orthop* 2008;28(1):60-67.

67. Bayhan IA, Er MS, Nishnianidze T, et al: Gait pattern and lower extremity alignment in children with diastrophic dysplasia. *J Pediatr Orthop* 2016;36(7):709-714.

A retrospective review of clinical data and radiographs on patients with diastrophic dysplasia who had gait analysis before lower extremity skeletal surgery. Gait analysis showed limited lower extremity function of the children with diastrophic dysplasia. Those with patella dislocation had increased crouch gait, suggesting that surgery may be indicated. Level of evidence: IV.

68. Langenskiold A, Ritsila V: Congenital dislocation of the patella and its operative treatment. *J Pediatr Orthop* 1992;12(3):315-323.

69. Jalanko T, Remes V, Peltonen J, Poussa M, Helenius I: Treatment of spinal deformities in patients with diastrophic dysplasia: A long-term, population based, retrospective outcome study. *Spine* 2009;34(20):2151-2157.

70. Herring JA: The spinal disorders in diastrophic dwarfism. *J Bone Joint Surg Am* 1978;60(2):177-182.

71. Matsuyama Y, Winter RB, Lonstein JE: The spine in diastrophic dysplasia. The surgical arthrodesis of thoracic and lumbar deformities in 21 patients. *Spine* 1999;24(22):2325-2331.

72. White KK, Bompadre V, Shah SA, et al: Early-onset spinal deformity in skeletal dysplasias: A multicenter study of growth-friendly systems. *Spine Deform* 2018;6(4):478-482.

A retrospective, multicenter study of 23 patients with skeletal dysplasia and early onset scoliosis. Patients with skeletal dysplasia were found to start with shorter spine lengths, but gains in spine length were comparable to other forms of EOS. Pulmonary complications were more common in the SKD group. Level of evidence: III.

73. Meyer J, Sudbeck P, Held M, et al: Mutational analysis of the SOX9 gene in campomelic dysplasia and autosomal sex reversal: Lack of genotype/phenotype correlations. *Hum Mol Genet* 1997;6(1):91-98.

74. Mansour S, Offiah AC, McDowall S, Sim P, Tolmie J, Hall C: The phenotype of survivors of campomelic dysplasia. *J Med Genet* 2002;39(8):597-602.

75. Thomas S, Winter RB, Lonstein JE: The treatment of progressive kyphoscoliosis in camptomelic dysplasia. *Spine* 1997;22(12):1330-1337.

76. Jaruga A, Hordyjewska E, Kandzierski G, Tylzanowski P: Cleidocranial dysplasia and RUNX2-clinical phenotype-genotype correlation. *Clin Genet* 2016;90(5):393-402.

A review article on cleidocranial dysostosis, with focus on RUNX2 function, mutations and their phenotypic consequences in patients.

77. Cooper SC, Flaitz CM, Johnston DA, Lee B, Hecht JT: A natural history of cleidocranial dysplasia. *Am J Med Genet* 2001;104(1):1-6.

78. Balioglu MB, Kargin D, Albayrak A, Atici Y: The treatment of cleidocranial dysostosis (scheuthauer-marie-sainton syndrome), a rare form of skeletal dysplasia, accompanied by spinal deformities: A review of the literature and two case reports. *Case Rep Orthop* 2018;2018:4635761.

Report of two cases and review of the literature of patients with cleidocranial dysostosis and spinal deformity. Level of evidence: IV.

79. Trigui M, Pannier S, Finidori G, Padovani JP, Glorion C: Coxa vara in chondrodysplasia: Prognosis study of 35 hips in 19 children. *J Pediatr Orthop* 2008;28(6):599-606.

80. Stelling FH: The hip in heritable conditions of connective tissue. *Clin Orthop Relat Res* 1973;(90):33-49.

81. Aktas S, Wheeler D, Sussman MD: The "chef's hat" appearance of the femoral head in cleidocranial dysplasia. *J Bone Joint Surg Br* 2000;82(3):404-408.

82. Richie MF, Johnston CE II: Management of developmental coxa vara in cleidocranial dysostosis. *Orthopedics* 1989;12(7):1001-1004.

83. Gath A: Parental reactions to loss and disappointment: The diagnosis of down's syndrome. *Dev Med Child Neurol* 1985;27(3):392-400.

84. Collins VR, Muggli EE, Riley M, Palma S, Halliday JL: Is down syndrome a disappearing birth defect? *J Pediatr* 2008;152(1):20-24.e1.

85. MacLachlan RA, Fidler KE, Yeh H, Hodgetts PG, Pharand G, Chau M: Cervical spine abnormalities in institutionalized adults with down's syndrome. *J Intellect Disabil Res* 1993;37(pt 3):277-285.

86. Pueschel SM, Scola FH, Tupper TB, Pezzullo JC: Skeletal anomalies of the upper cervical spine in children with down syndrome. *J Pediatr Orthop* 1990;10(5):607-611.

87. Grobovschek M, Strohecker J: Congenital atlanto-axial subluxation in down's syndrome. *Neuroradiology* 1985;27(2):186.

88. Nakamura N, Inaba Y, Aota Y, et al: New radiological parameters for the assessment of atlantoaxial instability in children with down syndrome: The normal values and the risk of spinal cord injury. *Bone Joint Lett J* 2016;98-B(12):1704-1710.

A total of 272 children with Down syndrome were compared to controls. ADI and SAC in those with Down syndrome requiring surgery and those with Down syndrome not requiring surgery were 9.8 mm (sd 2.8) and 4.3 mm (sd 1.0), respectively. Level of evidence: III.

89. Nakamura N, Inaba Y, Oba M, et al: Novel 2 radiographical measurements for atlantoaxial instability in children with Down syndrome. *Spine* 2014;39:E1566–E1574.

90. Diamond LS, Lynne D, Sigman B: Orthopedic disorders in patients with down's syndrome. *Orthop Clin North Am* 1981;12(1):57-71.

91. Krompinger JA, Renshaw TS: *Scoliosis in Down's Syndrome.* Milwaukee, WI: Scoliosis Research Society; 1983.

92. Abousamra O, Duque Orozco MDP, Er MS, Rogers KJ, Sees JP, Miller F: Scoliosis in down's syndrome. *J Pediatr Orthop B* 2017;26(4):383-387.

93. Milbrandt TA, Johnston CE II: Down syndrome and scoliosis: A review of a 50-year experience at one institution. *Spine* 2005;30(18):2051-2055.

94. Lerman JA, Emans JB, Hall JE, Karlin LI: Spinal arthrodesis for scoliosis in down syndrome. *J Pediatr Orthop* 2003;23(2):159-161.

95. Hresko MT, McCarthy JC, Goldberg MJ: Hip disease in adults with down syndrome. *J Bone Joint Surg Br* 1993;75(4):604-607.

96. Roberts GM, Starey N, Harper P, Nuki G: Radiology of the pelvis and hips in adults with down's syndrome. *Clin Radiol* 1980;31(4):475-478.

97. Shaw ED, Beals RK: The hip joint in down's syndrome. A study of its structure and associated disease. *Clin Orthop Relat Res* 1992;(278):101-107.

98. Aprin H, Zink WP, Hall JE: Management of dislocation of the hip in down syndrome. *J Pediatr Orthop* 1985;5(4):428-431.

99. Bennet GC, Rang M, Roye DP, Aprin H: Dislocation of the hip in trisomy 21. *J Bone Joint Surg Br* 1982;64(3):289-294.

100. Gore DR: Recurrent dislocation of the hip in a child with down's syndrome. A case report. *J Bone Joint Surg Am* 1981;63(5):823-825.

101. Kelley SP, Wedge JH: Management of hip instability in trisomy 21. *J Pediatr Orthop* 2013;33 suppl 1:S33-S38.

102. Knight DM, Alves C, Wedge JH: Femoral varus derotation osteotomy for the treatment of habitual subluxation and dislocation of the pediatric hip in trisomy 21: A 10-year experience. *J Pediatr Orthop* 2011;31(6):638-643.

103. Sankar WN, Millis MB, Kim YJ: Instability of the hip in patients with down syndrome: Improved results with complete redirectional acetabular osteotomy. *J Bone Joint Surg Am* 2011;93(20):1924-1933.

104. Dugdale TW, Renshaw TS: Instability of the patellofemoral joint in down syndrome. *J Bone Joint Surg Am* 1986;68(3):405-413.

105. Bettuzzi C, Lampasi M, Magnani M, Donzelli O: Surgical treatment of patellar dislocation in children with down syndrome: A 3- to 11-year follow-up study. *Knee Surg Sports Traumatol Arthrosc* 2009;17(4):334-340.

106. Joo SY, Park KB, Kim BR, Park HW, Kim HW: The 'four-in-one' procedure for habitual dislocation of the patella in children: Early results in patients with severe generalised ligamentous laxity and aplasis of the trochlear groove. *J Bone Joint Surg Br* 2007;89(12):1645-1649.

107. Kocon H, Kabacyj M, Zgoda M: The results of the operative treatment of patellar instability in children with down's syndrome. *J Pediatr Orthop B* 2012;21(5):407-410.

108. Neufeld E, Muenzer J: The mucopolysaccharidoses, in Scrivers CF, Beaudet AL, Sly WS, Valle D, eds: *The Metabolic and Molecular Bases of Inherited Diseases.* 2001, p 3421.

109. Baehner F, Schmiedeskamp C, Krummenauer F, et al: Cumulative incidence rates of the mucopolysaccharidoses in Germany. *J Inherit Metab Dis* 2005;28(6):1011-1017.

110. Tandon V, Williamson JB, Cowie RA, Wraith JE: Spinal problems in mucopolysaccharidosis I (hurler syndrome). *J Bone Joint Surg Br* 1996;78(6):938-944.

111. Belmont PJ Jr, Polly DW Jr: Early diagnosis of hurler's syndrome with the aid of the identification of the characteristic gibbus deformity. *Mil Med* 1998;163(10):711-714.

112. Mendelsohn NJ, Wood T, Olson RA, et al: Spondyloepiphyseal dysplasias and bilateral legg-calve-perthes disease: Diagnostic considerations for mucopolysaccharidoses. *JIMD Rep* 2013;11:125-132.

113. Lachman R, Martin KW, Castro S, Basto MA, Adams A, Teles EL: Radiologic and neuroradiologic findings in the mucopolysaccharidoses. *J Pediatr Rehabil Med* 2010;3(2):109-118.

114. Solanki GA, Martin KW, Theroux MC, et al: Spinal involvement in mucopolysaccharidosis IVA (morquio-brailsford or morquio A syndrome): Presentation, diagnosis and management. *J Inherit Metab Dis* 2013;36(2):339-355.

115. Kachur E, Del Maestro R: Mucopolysaccharidoses and spinal cord compression: Case report and review of the literature with implications of bone marrow transplantation. *Neurosurgery* 2000;47(1):223-228; discussion 228-9.

116. Mut M, Cila A, Varli K, Akalan N: Multilevel myelopathy in maroteaux-lamy syndrome and review of the literature. *Clin Neurol Neurosurg* 2005;107(3):230-235.

117. Baratela WA, Bober MB, Thacker MM, et al: Cervicothoracic myelopathy in children with morquio syndrome a: A report of 4 cases. *J Pediatr Orthop* 2014;34(2):223-228.

118. Bekmez S, Demirkiran HG, Dede O, Ismayilov V, Yazici M: Surgical management of progressive thoracolumbar kyphosis in mucopolysaccharidosis: Is a posterior-only approach safe and effective? *J Pediatr Orthop* 2018;38(7):354-359.

Case series of patients with MPS treated for thoracolumbar kyphosis by posterior only approach. Of the six patients, two were revisions for previously failed posterior only surgery and two more required subsequent revision. The authors concluded that posterior only techniques are safe and effective. Level of evidence: IV.

119. Langereis EJ, Borgo A, Crushell E, et al: Treatment of hip dysplasia in patients with mucopolysaccharidosis type I after hematopoietic stem cell transplantation: Results of an international consensus procedure. *Orphanet J Rare Dis* 2013;8:155.

120. Dhawale AA, Thacker MM, Belthur MV, Rogers K, Bober MB, Mackenzie WG: The lower extremity in morquio syndrome. *J Pediatr Orthop* 2012;32(5):534-540.

121. Thawrani DP, Walker K, Polgreen LE, Tolar J, Orchard PJ: Hip dysplasia in patients with hurler syndrome (mucopolysaccharidosis type 1H). *J Pediatr Orthop* 2013;33(6):635-643.

122. de Waal Malefijt MC, van Kampen A, van Gemund JJ: Total knee arthroplasty in patients with inherited dwarfism–a report of five knee replacements in two patients with morquio's disease type A and one with spondylo-epiphyseal dysplasia. *Arch Orthop Trauma Surg* 2000;120(3-4):179-182.

123. Yuen A, Dowling G, Johnstone B, Kornberg A, Coombs C: Carpal tunnel syndrome in children with mucopolysaccaridoses. *J Child Neurol* 2007;22(3):260-263.

124. Van Heest AE, House J, Krivit W, Walker K: Surgical treatment of carpal tunnel syndrome and trigger digits in children with mucopolysaccharide storage disorders. *J Hand Surg Am* 1998;23(2):236-243.

125. Carpenter TO: New perspectives on the biology and treatment of X-linked hypophosphatemic rickets. *Pediatr Clin North Am* 1997;44(2):443-466.

126. A gene (PEX) with homologies to endopeptidases is mutated in patients with X-linked hypophosphatemic rickets. the HYP consortium. *Nat Genet* 1995;11(2):130-136. doi:10.1038/ng1095-130.

127. Kinoshita Y, Fukumoto S: X-linked hypophosphatemia and FGF23-related hypophosphatemic diseases: Prospect for new treatment. *Endocr Rev* 2018;39(3):274-291.

Review on the phosphate metabolism and the pathogenesis and treatment of FGF23-related hypophosphatemic diseases. Level of evidence: V.

128. Capelli S, Donghi V, Maruca K, et al: Clinical and molecular heterogeneity in a large series of patients with hypophosphatemic rickets. *Bone* 2015;79:143-149.

129. Vera CL, Cure JK, Naso WB, et al: Paraplegia due to ossification of ligamenta flava in X-linked hypophosphatemia. A case report. *Spine* 1997;22:710-715.

130. Burosumab therapy in children with X-linked hypophosphatemia. *N Engl J Med* 2018;378(21):1987-1998. doi:10.1056/NEJMoa1714641.

131. Sharkey MS, Grunseich K, Carpenter TO: Contemporary medical and surgical management of X-linked hypophosphatemic rickets. *J Am Acad Orthop Surg* 2015;23:433-442

132. Gizard A, Rothenbuhler A, Pejin Z, et al: Outcomes of orthopedic surgery in a cohort of 49 patients with X-linked hypophosphatemic rickets (XLHR). *Endocr Connect* 2017;6:566-573.

Retrospective assessment of surgical limb correction in XLH. Surgery before puberty and poor metabolic control are associated with a higher risk of recurrence of limb deformity. Level of evidence: IV.

133. Choi IH, Kim JK, Chung CY, et al: Deformity correction of knee and leg lengthening by Ilizarov method in hypophosphatemic rickets: Outcomes and significance of serum phosphate level. *J Pediatr Orthop* 2002;22(5):626-631.

134. Horn A, Wright J, Bockenhauer D, Van't Hoff W, Eastwood DM: The orthopaedic management of lower limb deformity in hypophosphataemic rickets. *J Child Orthop* 2017;11:298-305.

Chapter 63

Neuromuscular Disorders in Children

Caroline Tougas, MD, FRCSC • Rachel M. Thompson, MD

Pediatrics

ABSTRACT

Cerebral palsy, myelomeningocele, muscular dystrophy, spinal muscular atrophy, hereditary sensory motor neuropathy, and Friedreich ataxia are the most common neuromuscular conditions treated by orthopaedic surgeons. While their etiologies vary, they share commonalities in terms of musculoskeletal manifestations. These neuromuscular conditions present with limb deformities and scoliosis resulting from weakness and/or muscular imbalance. Available medical and surgical treatment for each condition differs, but the treatment goals are consistent—increase comfort, ease care, and promote mobility, whether wheelchair-dependant or ambulatory. Treating orthopaedic surgeons must be cognizant of new medical and genetic treatments available for some of these diagnoses and be familiar with modern surgical techniques, risk stratification, and novel patient-reported outcomes to guide appropriate care in this unique patient population.

Keywords: cerebral palsy; Charcot-Marie-Tooth; Duchenne muscular dystrophy; Friedreich ataxia; hereditary sensory motor neuropathy; myelomeningocele; spina bifida; spina muscular atrophy

Introduction

Neuromuscular conditions encompass a broad range of diseases, including those whose primary pathology originates in the brain and those in which the pathologic process begins at the muscle fiber. While their etiology, natural history, and treatments vary, they share commonalities in terms of musculoskeletal manifestations. In all of the included diseases, muscular weakness or imbalance is present, which may result in diminished function, contracture, deformity, gait disturbance, and, in many cases, scoliosis, all of which present challenges to the treating orthopaedic surgeon. There is currently no cure for any of the included conditions, but advances in medical management, genetic treatment, and surgical care have increased life expectancy. As such, the orthopaedic manifestations of these disease processes are no longer confined to the pediatric population, and both pediatric and adult providers should be familiar with these diseases and the most up-to-date treatments available to improve quality of life and function for this patient population.

Neither of the following authors nor any immediate family member has received anything of value from or has stock or stock options held in a commercial company or institution related directly or indirectly to the subject of this chapter: Dr. Tougas and Dr. Thompson.

Cerebral Palsy

Background

Cerebral palsy (CP) is a descriptive term for a group of disorders affecting motor function as a result of nonprogressive disturbances that occur in the developing brain. It is the leading cause of childhood disability worldwide, affecting nearly 3 in every 1,000 live births. Individuals affected by CP have varying degrees of physical disability, which may be accompanied by seizure disorders, as well as cognitive, speech, behavioral, and/or feeding impairment. The management of children and adults with CP requires a multidisciplinary approach, which necessarily includes orthopaedic surgery.

While there are many classification schemes, the most commonly utilized and most useful is the Gross Motor Function Classification Scale (GMFCS), which categorizes patients by functional level from I-V.[1] In broad terms, GMFCS I-III are independently ambulatory and GMFCS IV-V primarily utilize wheelchairs for mobility. Treatment for patients classified as GMFCS I-III—both surgical and medical—are aimed to improve gait efficiency and mobility while treatments for patients classified as GMFCS IV-V are aimed to improve comfort, sitting balance, and assisted care. Orthopaedic-related care for individuals with CP include physical and occupational therapy, bracing treatment, tone management, and orthopaedic surgery.

Tone Management

The majority of individuals with CP have spasticity, at least in part. Spasticity and increased tone can cause discomfort, decreased range of motion, difficulty with brace wear, and diminished mobility and should be addressed if it is functionally limiting. Tone may be managed by locally acting agents, botulinum toxin A, or globally by oral medications, most commonly baclofen, or surgery, intrathecal baclofen therapy or selective dorsal rhizotomy. In certain patients, both local and global management are warranted.

Botulinum toxin A selectively blocks the release of acetylcholine at the neuromuscular junction, allowing for muscle relaxation. It has been widely used off-label for pediatric and adult spasticity management for many years, but the FDA approved its use in lower extremity spasticity in children in 2016 and in adults in 2017. It is short acting and cannot prevent surgery, nor is it more effective than other treatment modalities—therapy, casting, or surgery. However, it can provide temporary control and delay surgical intervention in very young children.

Oral baclofen is most commonly a first-line treatment for global spasticity control. It works as an inhibitory neurotransmitter, blocking synaptic reflexes at the spinal cord. Taken orally, it can be sedating and may lead to tolerance in many patients. While it is frequently prescribed, a recent systematic review of six randomized controlled trials comparing oral baclofen to placebo or antispasmodics found poor evidence to support or refute the efficacy of this medication in terms of tone management or improving motor function in children and adolescents.[2]

A common alternative to oral baclofen is intrathecal baclofen therapy (ITB). ITB utilizes a surgically implanted battery-powered pump to deliver baclofen directly to the thecal space (**Figure 1**), bypassing the blood-brain barrier and significantly decreasing its systemic adverse effect profile. This therapy can safely be utilized in ambulatory and nonambulatory patients. Its efficacy in nonambulatory children was demonstrated recently. In midterm follow-up, researchers in Austria demonstrated significant sustained improvement in spasticity as measured by the modified Ashworth scale as well as improvements in quality of life, as measured by CPCHILD, a validated patient and/or parent-reported outcomes measure.[3] However, these authors did report a nearly 30% complication rate with a 14% unexpected return-to-OR rate. Nonetheless, ITB remains a valuable treatment option for global spasticity control.

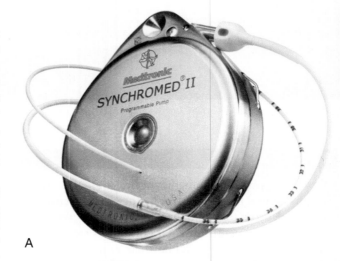

A

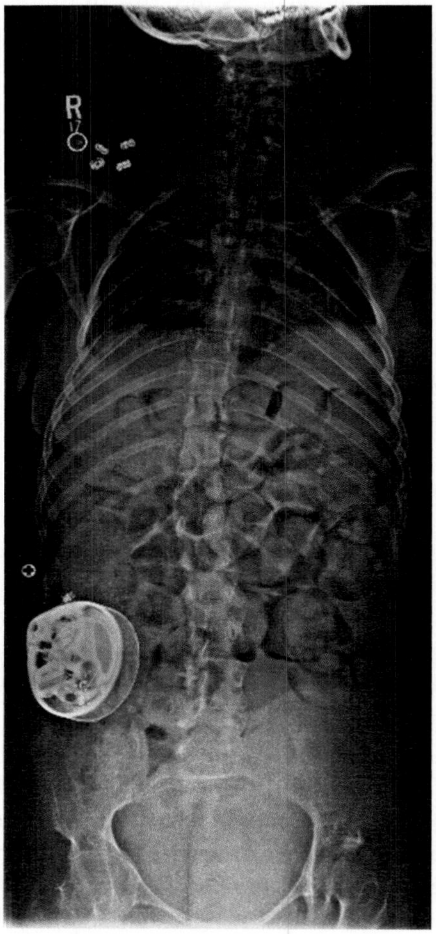

B

Figure 1 **A**, Clinical image of a baclofen pump, including the medication reservoir/battery, which is placed deep to the external oblique musculature, with associated intrathecal tubing, which is tunneled along the flank and into the intrathecal space; **B**, Radiographic image—PA scoliosis radiograph—of patient after implantation of baclofen pump for function-limiting spasticity.

Selective dorsal rhizotomy (SDR) is an alternative surgical option in which a neurosurgeon selectively cuts dorsal nerve rootlets between L1 and S1, preventing sensory feedback from muscle spindles and effectively diminishing spinal reflexes. It has historically been indicated for ambulatory patients (GMFCS II-III), but it is becoming more popular in nonambulatory patients for comfort and ease of care, even in the setting of previous ITB therapy.[4] However, the long-term outcomes of SDR are mixed. In a case-control study of adults with CP comparing those treated with SDR and those who did not have SDR, researchers found no difference in pain intensity, pain interference, or fatigue utilizing PROMIS (Patient-Reported Outcomes Measurement Information System) patient-reported quality of life measures, yet they noted a decrease in need for assistance and a lower perceived decline in functionality in the SDR group without any decrease in orthopaedic intervention.[5] As such, similar to ITB, SDR is a viable treatment for global spasticity in appropriately selected patients.

Spine Surgery

The risk of developing scoliosis in this population is closely correlated to functional status. Patients who are nonambulatory have a significant risk of developing scoliosis; and those that are ambulatory have no increased risk compared with the general population.[6] Typically, wheelchair modifications are made for relatively small (<50°) flexible curves, and surgery is reserved for curves measuring >50°, with the goal of halting progression, preserving seating balance, and supporting pulmonary and GI function. Surgical management typically consists of posterior spinal fusion with pedicle screws and sacral-alar iliac fixation in nonambulators. A recently published five-year outcome study revealed excellent initial correction and maintenance of scoliosis and pelvic obliquity correction without neurologic compromise or pseudarthrosis utilizing this surgical technique.[7] Despite acceptable outcomes in terms of deformity correction, a recent review of the literature reported an associated complication rate of 38.1% with essentially equivocal findings in terms of quality of life/health outcomes following surgical intervention.[8]

However, a multicenter prospective registry study demonstrated consistent improvement in CPCHILD scores following spinal fusion in 199 included individuals.[9] These authors stratified this cohort of GMFCS V patients by number of associated comorbidities (presence of a gastrostomy tube, tracheostomy, seizure disorder, nonverbal status) and found that risk of complication was directly correlated to each patient's comorbidity burden. Those with no confounding comorbidities had a major complication rate of 12%, and those with three or more had a rate of 49%. Of note, baseline CPCHILD scores directly correlated with number of comorbidities, but there was no difference in the absolute improvement in scores from pre- to post-operative assessment between groups.

Hip Surveillance and Surgery

The risk for hip dysplasia/dislocation directly correlates with GMFCS level. Hip dislocation may lead to pain, functional impairment affecting the ability to sit, stand, or walk, and impaired quality of life. Along those lines, a prospective cohort study including 38 children with CP reported a negative correlation between migration percentage (MP) (radiographic measure which denotes the percentage of the femoral head lateral to the lateral aspect of the acetabulum relative to the entire width of the femoral head) and CPCHILD scores.[10] Further, a recent population-based cohort study found a reported incidence of hip pain in 72% of adults with MP >30%.[11]

Population-based hip surveillance and access to appropriate surgical management of hips-at-risk can significantly reduce or eliminate the incidence of painful, debilitating dislocations and need for unpredictable salvage surgery.[12] Regular surveillance allows for early intervention. Typically, soft-tissue surgery is recommended for migration percentage between 30% and 40% with associated adductor contracture, which includes adductor and iliopsoas lengthening. Osseous reconstructive surgery is recommended for migration percentages between 40% and 50% or more, which includes femoral varus derotational osteotomy with or without associated pelvic osteotomy. With correct indications, CPCHILD scores improve following surgery such that there is an increase in overall score by 0.2 points per additional 1% MP correction achieved, regardless of surgical procedure performed.[10]

These surgeries are not without risks, with one retrospective case-control series reporting a 65% complication rate following bony hip surgery, with 26% of patients experiencing multiple complications.[13] Of these complications, only 15% required return-to-OR and an additional 2% were life-threatening (Clavien-Dindo III-IV), with no reported perioperative deaths.

Salvage surgery is indicated for those who present late with painful, debilitating hip dislocations. There are multiple options described in the literature, all of which have high complication rates. A recent systematic review of 28 studies reporting on salvage procedure outcomes revealed similar pain reduction following femoral head resection (FHR), valgus-producing osteotomy

Pediatrics

(VO), total hip arthroplasty (THA), and shoulder prosthetic interposition (SPI) (90.4%, 88.4%, 93.8%, and 90.9%, respectively), all of which performed better than arthrodesis, with a reported pain reduction of 56.3%.[14] Further, complication rates were similar between FHR, VO, THA, and SPI (24%, 33.3%, 35.3%, and 28.6%, respectively), and all were significantly lower than that of arthrodesis (106.3%). These authors did not advocate for a specific salvage procedure, but they did conclude that hip arthrodesis should be avoided in this population. In choosing a salvage procedure, the surgeon and family must weigh the risks and benefits of each option's specific complication profile.

Knee Surgery

In ambulatory patients, hamstring spasticity and eventual contracture can lead to excessive knee flexion during stance, which increases pressure at the patellofemoral joint and increases the energy required for walking. First-line treatments include botulinum toxin A injections, stretching, and ground-reaction force ankle-foot orthoses. Surgical hamstring lengthening is typically recommended for worsening flexion without fixed contracture. Fixed contractures of small magnitude (<10°) in growing children may be addressed with guided growth[15] or posterior knee capsulotomy, but larger contractures should be addressed with distal femoral extension osteotomy (DFEO) with or without patellar tendon advancement (PTA) (**Figure 2**). PTA has previously been shown to decrease midstance knee flexion at short- and midterm follow-up. Recently, a long-term follow-up study compared gait analysis and patient-reported outcomes in patients who underwent DFEO and PTA to those whose crouched gait was treated by other methods and found that those who underwent DFEO with PTA had improved stance phase extension and decreased knee flexion contractures, but there was no associated improvement in activity, participation, or knee pain.[16]

Some patients present with swing phase dysfunction secondary to rectus femoris spasticity. Historically, rectus femoris transfer has been recommended. However, a retrospective matched cohort study reported no difference in stride length, speed, peak knee flexion in swing, time to peak knee flexion, or Gait Deviation Index when comparing patients who underwent transfer with those who underwent lengthening at 1 year out.[17] Simple lengthening is a viable alternative to transfer and should be considered.

Foot and Ankle Surgery

Foot and ankle deformities are common in patients with CP. The goal in treatment is maintaining a plantigrade, painless foot that provides a stable base in stance. Common procedures include gastrocnemius recession and, less commonly, Achilles lengthening. However, Achilles lengthening should be reserved primarily for children with hemiplegic involvement and severe contractures as there is a risk of overlengthening and subsequent crouching inherent in isolated Achilles tendon lengthening. Furthermore, tibialis anterior tendon shortening should be considered in combination with Achilles tendon lengthening for severe equinus to ensure proper ankle dorsiflexion power after correction of equinus. A long-term study (mean 5.8-year follow-up) of 23 patients following this procedure (with and without concomitant lower extremity procedures) found significant, durable improvements in stance phase and swing phase dorsiflexion without need for postoperative bracing treatment.[18]

Pes planovalgus and pes equinovalgus are common in patients with spastic diplegia, while equinovarus deformities are more common in patients with hemiplegic involvement. In all cases, management begins with bracing treatment. Surgical management is reserved for patients with unbraceable deformities or in patients who are brace-intolerant. Equinovarus is treated surgically through a combination of muscular rebalancing and corrective osteotomy as needed. In addition to soft-tissue balancing and appropriate midfoot osteotomies, calcaneal lengthening is a common procedure for moderate planovalgus deformity, but a recent retrospective review of 20 patients (30 limbs) identified two preoperative radiographic markers closely correlated with radiographic undercorrection following calcaneal lengthening,[19] suggesting that patients with an AP talonavicular angle >24° and a calcaneal pitch < −5° may require subtalar fusion. Alternatively, naviculectomy with midfoot arthrodesis may be a viable alternative in severe cases. A recently published series of 44 feet reported 81% excellent or good outcomes based on pain, radiographic union, and alignment of the forefoot and hindfoot at a mean of 5 years.[20]

Single-Event Multilevel Surgery

Single-event multilevel surgery (SEMLS), sometimes termed multilevel surgery (MLS), first described in 1985, has become the norm in the surgical management of ambulatory children with cerebral palsy, with multiple authors reporting durable improvements in gait profile postoperatively. A review of 231 patients with long-term MLS postoperative gait analysis and clinical examination (mean 9.1 years) revealed an average improvement in gait profile scores (GPS) of 5° (minimally clinically important difference: 1.6°) at short-term (1 year) follow-up, which was well maintained at an average of

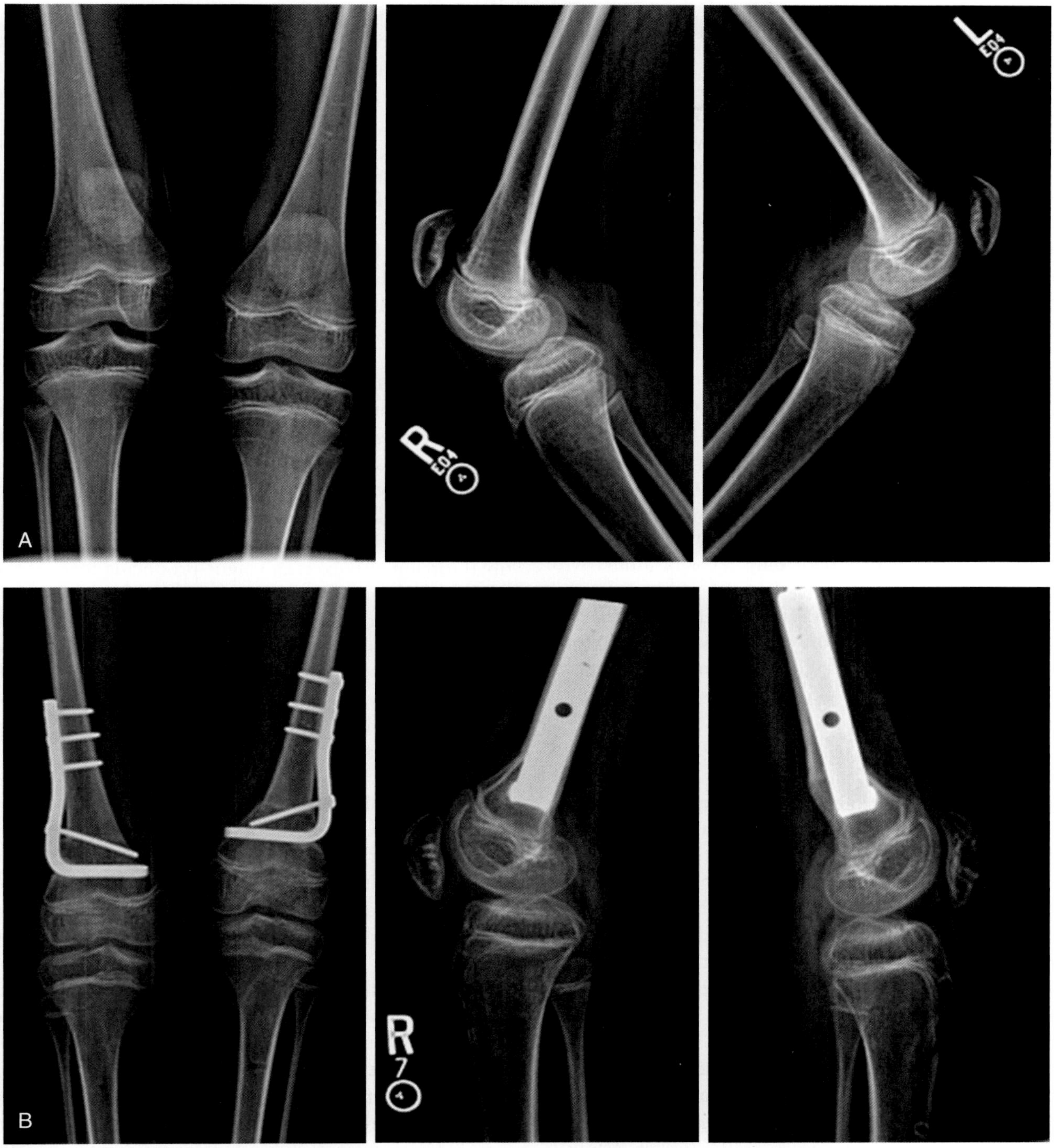

Figure 2 **A**, AP and lateral radiographs of a 13-year-old male with spastic diplegia and bilateral significant knee flexion contractures, resulting in crouched gait, with associated patella alta; **B**, postoperative radiographs of the same patient after bilateral distal femoral extension osteotomies and patellar distalization with soft-tissue procedure only.

9 years.[21] In total, 76.6% of children maintained their GPS improvements. Of note, 39% required subsequent surgery other than removal of hardware, all of which were less invasive than the index procedure. This is in line with the series published by Rutz et al in 2013.[22] In this patient population, the need for subsequent surgery following SEML/MLS surgery is not unexpected, and patients/parents should be counseled accordingly.

Pediatrics

Myelomeningocele

Background

Myelomeningocele (MMC) is the most common and severe form of spina bifida characterized by a failure of closure of the neural tube in utero with extrusion of the underlying neural structures and resultant dysfunction. Open fetal repair is a new option in select patients with MMC and is associated with improved neurologic outcomes compared with postnatal repair.[23] Subsequent care for these patients requires a multidisciplinary approach as they have bladder, bowel, motor, and sensory dysfunction below the level of the neurologic lesion. Specific orthopaedic manifestations of MMC depend on neurologic level of involvement but include spinal deformity, hip dysplasia, joint contracture, limb deformity, and skin breakdown. Unfortunately, the natural history is consistent with an expected decline in functional status. Utilizing cross-sectional data from the National Spina Bifida Patient Registry, one study[24] reported a 60% rate of community ambulation at age 7 years, which decreased to only 35% in adults with MMC.

Of note, gradual deformity is a known sequela of flaccid paralysis, but rapidly progressive deformity may be associated with tethered cord syndrome, syringomyelia, or hydrocephalus, and should be evaluated by a neurosurgeon.

Spinal Deformity

Spinal deformity, including scoliosis, kyphosis, and lordosis, is common and can be associated with seating imbalance, pressure sores, and respiratory compromise. A recent systematic review reported a pooled prevalence rate of 53%, which was directly correlated to neurologic level of involvement, suggesting the importance of frequent monitoring and early intervention for patients with higher levels of involvement.[25] Surgical complication rates as high as 53% were also reported, which includes an infection risk of 33.3%.[26]

Common spine surgeries include tethered cord release, spinal fusion, and guided-growth procedures. Tethered cord release may result in stabilization or even improvement in milder curves (<50°), lower lesions,[25] and in patients older than 10 years.[27] Young children with moderate mobile deformities may be safely and effectively treated with dual growing rod constructs, allowing continued thoracic growth and pulmonary development.[28] Posterior spinal fusion and instrumentation may be utilized in moderate deformities in older children, while fixed severe kyphotic deformities may require kyphectomy and combined AP fusion.[25]

Hip Deformity

Hip status correlates with neurologic level and the resultant imbalanced muscular forces acting across the hip joint. The primary goal of treatment is maintenance of functional range of motion for seating, hygiene, and, in some patients, ambulation. Surgery to reduce a subluxated or dislocated hip is often unnecessary and unsuccessful. Rather, efforts should be made to maintain motion with contracture release and tendon transfer as needed. It remains unclear whether independently ambulatory children with low sacral lesions and a unilateral dislocation benefit from surgical reduction to restore gait symmetry.

Knee Deformity

Knee deformities can be functionally limiting. Knee flexion contractures are common in patients with higher level lesions and are treated with surgical release if functionally limiting. In most ambulatory patients, abductor weakness results in lateral trunk sway, which produces an external valgus force at the knee. External tibial torsion also exerts a valgus-producing force at the knee, and the combination can produce a fixed deformity and arthrosis. Forearm crutches can be utilized to decrease the effects of abductor weakness, and tibial derotational osteotomies can correct lever arm disease. Less frequently, extension contractures occur and can be treated by manipulation and serial casting, reserving modified V-Y-plasty for resistant cases.

Foot and Ankle Deformity

Foot and ankle deformities may be congenital or acquired. Level of neurologic involvement is not predictive of deformity. Congenital deformities include clubfoot and vertical talus. Acquired deformities range from calcaneovalgus to cavovarus. The goal in treating any foot deformity is to provide a supple, plantigrade foot that will fit into an orthosis without skin breakdown. Specific treatment depends on the deformity and the patient's functional status but may include tenotomy, guided growth, and/or osteotomy. Arthrodesis should be avoided in this patient population as insensate feet are susceptible to skin breakdown and ulceration.

MMC-associated clubfeet deformities are typically severe and difficult to manage. A retrospective review[29] of the outcomes following modified Ponseti technique in 17 MMC-associated clubfeet demonstrated an initial correction in *all* children following an average of seven casts and Achilles tenotomy with a relapse rate of 53%. Of those who recurred, 44% required extensive surgical release. A similar study of 48 clubfeet treated with the modified Ponseti method and an open Achilles tenotomy reported a 10% failure rate along with a 15% incidence of residual deformity limiting shoe wear following successful casting.[30] Taken together, these studies demonstrate the effectiveness of the modified Ponseti method as a first-line treatment for complex clubfoot.

Duchenne Muscular Dystrophy

Background

Duchenne muscular dystrophy (DMD) is the most common inherited pediatric muscle disorder. The genetic pathology results in an absence of dystrophin, which leads to progressive muscle atrophy and weakness (**Table 1**). Without this important component of the basement membrane, myofiber content is released into the extracellular matrix, causing inflammation, fibrosis, and eventual dysfunction of the myofibers. Progressive degeneration of skeletal and cardiac muscles leads to weakness, loss of ambulation, musculoskeletal deformities, respiratory insufficiency, cardiac disease, and eventual death.

In 2018, a comprehensive review[31,32] was published on the requisite assessments and available interventions for appropriate care in DMD. It describes multidisciplinary management goals for each stage of DMD including diagnosis, early ambulatory, late ambulatory, early nonambulatory, and late nonambulatory. Musculoskeletal management goals throughout these phases include the preservation of mobility, minimization of joint contracture, maintenance of a straight spine, and promotion of bone health.

Ambulatory Phase

The orthopaedic surgeon may be the first point of contact for patients with DMD, who are typically referred for impaired walking in early childhood. It is important to counsel these patients and their families regarding the role of stretching in the prevention of joint contracture. As weakness increases and contractures progress, there is a progressive loss of ambulation in late childhood. Nighttime orthoses are indicated for passive dorsiflexion <10°.[32] Use of knee-ankle-foot orthoses (KAFOs) with locked knee joints may preserve walking, and certain contractures may need to be released surgically to permit brace fit. However, tendon lengthening may increase weakness and hasten loss of ambulation and should be undertaken cautiously.[33]

Disuse osteopenia and steroid-induced osteoporosis are common. Extremity fractures can lead to premature and permanent loss of ambulation. Prompt and aggressive surgical management of fractures can delay this decline by permitting early range of motion and weight bearing (**Figure 3**). Due to preexisting cardiac and respiratory muscle dysfunction, fat emboli syndrome (FES) after fractures are often unrecognized and can result in major complications, including death.[34]

Nonambulatory Phase

Patients with DMD are often wheelchair dependent before adolescence. After becoming nonambulatory, contractures progress rapidly. Supported standing devices can be used if contractures are not too severe to prevent positioning or tolerance. Contractures of the foot, ankle, and upper extremities can impede shoe wear and activities of daily living (ADLs) and

Pediatrics

Table 1

Inheritable Neuromuscular Conditions

	Prevalence	Inheritance	Gene	Protein Involved	Location of Pathology	Nonorthopaedic Manifestations
DMD	1/4,000	X-linked	DMD—Xp21	Dystrophin	Muscle	Cardiomyopathy, respiratory insufficiency
SMA	1/11,000	AR	SMN 1—5q	Survival Motor Neuron 1 (SMN1)	Anterior Motor Neurons	Dysarthria, dysphagia, respiratory compromise
FDRA	1/30,000	AR	FXN—9q	Frataxin	Cerebellum	Cardiomyopathy, glucose metabolism dysfunction, dysarthria, dysphagia
CMT[a]	1/2,500	AD*	PMP22	Peripheral Myelin Protein 22	Peripheral Nerves	

CMT = Charcot-Marie-Tooth; DMD = Duchenne muscular dystrophy; FDRA = Friedreich ataxia; SMA = spinal muscular atrophy

[a]Type 1a, most common form.

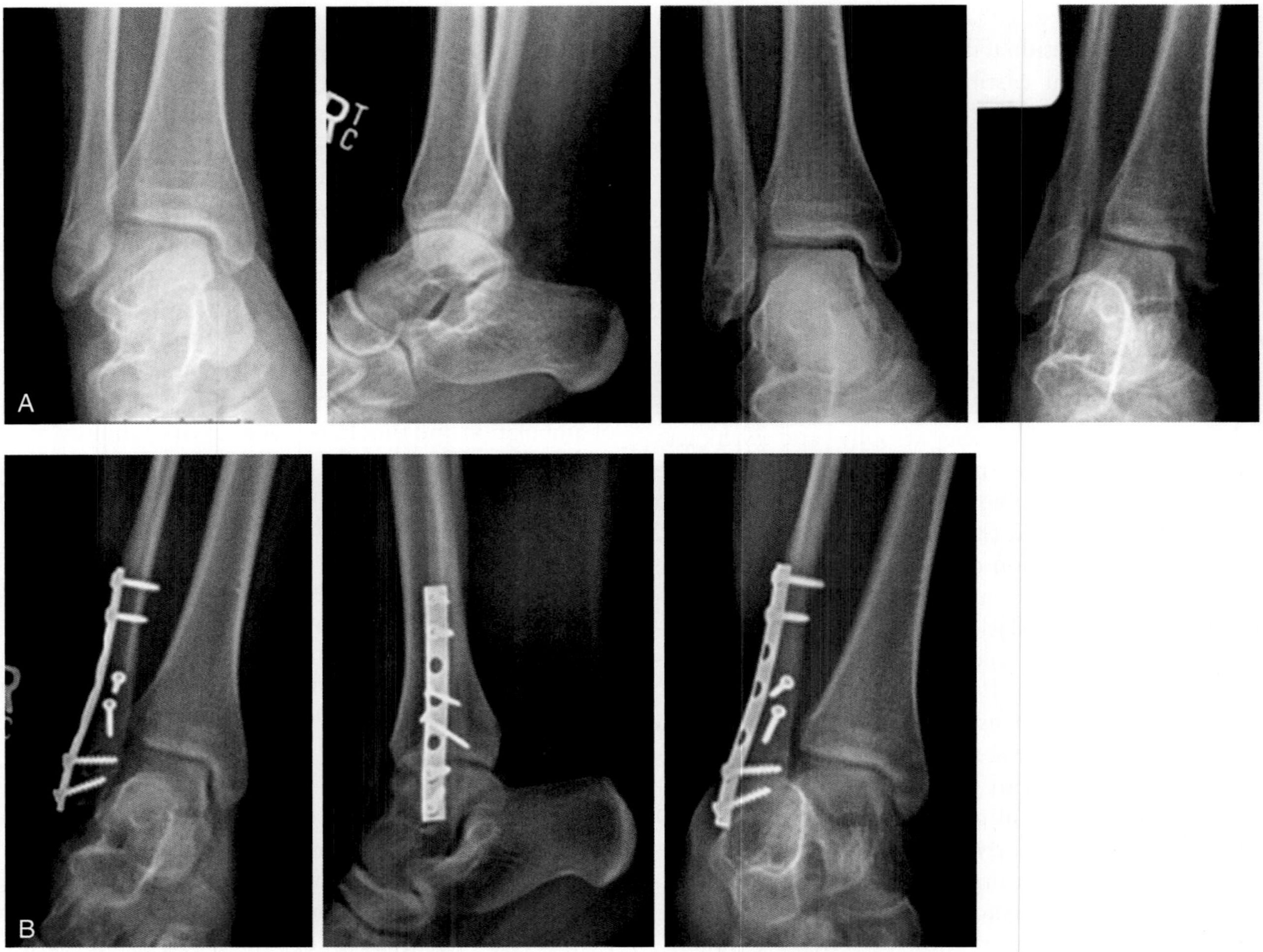

Figure 3 **A**, AP, lateral, mortise, and gravity external rotation stress radiographs of the ankle of a 15-year-old ambulatory male with muscular dystrophy who presented 3 days after a fall out of a car with these radiographs; **B**, AP, lateral, and mortise views of the ankle 3 months following open reduction and internal fixation, allowing for early weight bearing and resultant maintenance of ambulatory status 6 months postoperatively.

necessitate surgical releases if painful, position limiting, or compromising to the skin. Scoliotic curves progress rapidly in the nonambulatory phases and should be monitored closely. Wheelchair modifications must be made for trunk support, and surgery is generally recommended for curves measuring >30°, given the inherent risk of progression. Surgical correction of scoliosis has been shown to improve quality of life, reduce pain, improve sitting balance, and enhance function.[35] Preoperative assessment by a cardiologist and pulmonologist is required. It is further important to recruit an anesthesiologist familiar with DMD as there is a risk of fatal rhabdomyolysis and hyperkalemia if exposed to inhalational anesthetics or succinylcholine.[32]

A 2017 single-center review of 30 years' experience treating scoliosis in patients with DMD reported a trend toward delaying treatment and operating in older, heavier patients with larger curves with all-pedicle screw constructs as compared with those who were historically treated with Luque rod constructs.[36] Despite these differences, all patients had improvement in their spinal deformity and high complication rates. The reported benefits on cardiopulmonary function was not significant in this study; however, a 2017 review of 29 patients demonstrated a decrease in the rate of pulmonary decline after scoliosis correction (7.80% per year preoperatively to 4.26% per year postoperatively, $P < 0.001$).[37]

Corticosteroids

There is currently no cure for DMD, but the mainstay of medical management is corticosteroid therapy. It should be initiated prior to functional deterioration and continue after loss of ambulation.[31] In 2018, a multicenter prospective cohort study of 440 patients reported a reduced risk of losing clinically meaningful mobility and upper extremity function as well as a reduced risk of death in patients on glucocorticoid therapy.[38] This study supports previously published work, including a 2016 systematic review reporting similar reductions in death rates and need for scoliosis surgery, improved strength and pulmonary function, delayed cardiomyopathy, and prolonged independent ambulation. However, steroid treatment is not without consequence, and reported complications include cataracts, weight gain, short stature, hirsutism, delayed puberty, Cushingoid appearance, and osteoporosis.[32,39]

Spinal Muscular Atrophy

Background

Spinal muscular atrophy (SMA) is an autosomal recessive disease (**Table 1**). Affecting roughly 1 in 11,000,[40] it is the second most common inherited neuromuscular disorder in children. Degeneration of the anterior motor neurons results from a mutation in the SMN1 gene, which codes for the survival motor neuron (SMN) protein. The number of remaining functional SMN proteins produced from the near-identical SMN2 gene determines disease severity. SMA is classified into four types (I-IV) reflecting age of onset, life expectancy, and functional status.

SMA is characterized by proximal weakness, hypotonia, and hyporeflexia predominantly in the lower extremities. Cranial nerves V-XII can also be involved, affecting speech, feeding, and breathing. In its most severe form, SMA causes respiratory insufficiency resulting in death during the first decade of life. There is no cure for SMA; however, a major milestone in the treatment of SMA was the development of nusinersen (Spinraza), an antisense oligonucleotide drug, recently approved by the FDA and the Agency for Medicines in Europe. Nusinersen is administered intrathecally and alters the SMN2 gene to produce more functional SMN protein. The drug has shown promising results in motor function in patients with the most severe form of SMA.[41]

SMA standard of care recommendations[41,42] were recently published, establishing consensus statements where data were lacking. Orthopaedic recommendations were based on the functional status of the child: nonsitters, sitters, and walkers. Orthopaedic manifestations of SMA include joint contracture, hip dysplasia, pathologic fractures, and scoliosis.

Limb Involvement

Hip flexion, abduction and external rotation contractures, knee flexion contractures, and ankle equinus contractures are common. Contracture should be addressed surgically if painful or functionally limiting.

Hip dysplasia is common in SMA and may cause intermittent—mostly asymptomatic—hip instability. Older studies recommended against surgical reconstruction due to high redislocation rates. However, these studies did not utilize modern techniques, and new consensus recommendations[42] suggest hip reconstruction for symptomatic dysplasia.

Scoliosis

Scoliosis occurs in 60% to 90% of patients with SMA.[41] It is often rapidly progressive and significantly impacts respiratory function secondary to associated rib deformity and resultant thoracic insufficiency. Surgical indications are based on curve progression, skeletal maturity, and overall health status. Dependent-sitters are rarely candidates for surgery due to their poor functional and respiratory status. These patients may benefit from custom-molded lightweight orthoses to improve sitting balance; however, there is no evidence to suggest that bracing treatment reduces the rate of progression and improves pulmonary function or gastric emptying. For independent sitters, bracing treatment may provide truncal support for curves between 20° and 50°. In this cohort, surgery is recommended for curves >50° and those with significant progression. Surgery should be delayed until 4 years of age, at which point growth-sparing instrumentation should be utilized up to 10 to 12 years of age to achieve sufficient trunk height.[42] Surgical intervention has been associated with a decreased rate of pulmonary decline, although the frequency of chest infections is unaffected. With the advent of nusinersen, surgical techniques must consider the need for long-term intrathecal access for medication administration.

Hereditary Peripheral Neuropathies

Background

The most common type of hereditary peripheral neuropathy is Charcot-Marie-Tooth (CMT) disease. Despite there being over 75 associated genes (**Table 1**), a classic clinical presentation exists consisting of distal sensory loss, distal lower followed by upper extremity amyotrophy, loss of deep tendon reflexes, and gait disturbances. Orthopaedic manifestations common to all genetic permutations of this disease include hand and foot deformity, ankle instability, hip dysplasia, and scoliosis.[43]

Foot Deformity

Foot and ankle deformities are common and may present as the first clinical manifestation of disease. A 2018 review found a 71% incidence of foot deformities, of which 30% required surgery.[44] The most common deformity is pes cavus (63%) followed by hammer toes (26%) and pes planus (8%). The goal of surgery is to achieve a plantigrade balanced foot, and the surgical plan must be individualized according to type, severity, and flexibility of the deformity. Current surgical procedures can be divided into (1) soft-tissue procedures to rebalance the involved muscles, (2) osteotomies to correct fixed deformity, and (3) fusion as salvage of uncorrectable deformity.

The same study surveyed 16 surgeons experienced in treating CMT foot deformities and found high variability in preferred treatment. The most common procedures cited were calcaneal osteotomy, peroneal tendon transfer, first metatarsal osteotomy, and plantar fascia release. The median number of procedures per surgery was five at a median age of 15 years. One-third required repeat surgery.[44]

Scoliosis

Scoliosis occurs in 15% of patients with CMT, 70% of which are progressive and 30% eventually require surgery.[45] Bracing treatment is rarely effective in halting curve progression or preventing surgery. Surgical treatment is similar to that for adolescent idiopathic scoliosis, with similar complication rates. Intraoperative neurologic monitoring is difficult due to their demyelinating polyneuropathy. Increased latencies may require adjustments in neuromonitoring settings.

Hip Deformity

In a 2017 French review, hip dysplasia reportedly affected approximately 6% of patients with CMT, especially in those with CMT1, presenting as early as 8 years of age with ambulatory pain.[46] It is associated with more severe deformity than idiopathic dysplasia (DDH). The pathogenesis may result from selective hip abductor and extensor weakness causing progressive subluxation. Presentation may be delayed due to decreased sensation, and in the absence of treatment, early secondary arthritis may develop. Once symptoms develop, surgery is the only appropriate treatment option. As such, all children with CMT should be screened with a pelvic radiograph to allow for early treatment. Although associated with worse radiographic parameters than DDH, treatment follows the same algorithm with periacetabular osteotomies (PAO) offered to symptomatic skeletally mature patients. A 2016 review comparing 27 patients with CMT who underwent PAO to 54 matched patients with DDH demonstrated similar outcomes and radiographic correction, albeit with a higher complication rate in the CMT population, likely due to severity of disease.[47]

Friedreich Ataxia

Background

Friedreich ataxia (FRDA) is an autosomal recessive spinocerebellar disorder affecting 1/30,000 people.[48] It is caused by a mutation of the FXN gene that codes for frataxin, a protein involved in mitochondrial iron metabolism (**Table 1**). Dysfunction of frataxin results in the accumulation of iron within the mitochondria and subsequent nerve and muscle dysfunction.

FRDA typically presents as slowly progressive ataxia, weakness, and areflexia beginning in adolescence. Other clinical features include dysarthria or dysphagia, hand clumsiness, upgoing plantar responses, and peripheral sensory neuropathy. Nonorthopaedic manifestations include cardiomyopathy and glucose metabolism dysfunction. Individuals with this disorder are typically wheelchair dependent in adulthood and die from heart failure by the age of 50 years. Currently, there is no cure, and no treatment has been shown to modify the natural history. Current and emerging therapies involve reducing mitochondrial iron accumulation, decreasing oxidative and inflammatory stress, enhancing mitochondrial function, and modulating frataxin production.[49]

Scoliosis

Scoliosis occurs in almost all patients with FRDA with a variable pattern of deformity, not all of which are progressive. Bracing treatment is ineffective at preventing surgery but can be utilized in younger patients to delay surgical intervention.[50] When surgery is indicated, a preoperative cardiopulmonary assessment is required, as the presence of cardiomyopathy and respiratory compromise determine life expectancy and surgical risks, which should be weighed against surgical benefits—halting progression, restoring balance, and improving function.

Summary

Currently, neuromuscular conditions with orthopaedic manifestations are incurable, but appropriate orthopaedic intervention may improve function and quality of life. While the overall incidence of neuromuscular conditions is essentially static, progress in medical therapy has significantly altered the course for patients with

Chapter 64

Pediatric Musculoskeletal Infections, Inflammatory Disorders, and Nonaccidental Trauma

Amy L. McIntosh, MD

Pediatrics

ABSTRACT

Recently, musculoskeletal infections in children and adolescents have increased in incidence and severity. Bacterial behavior likely contributes to this rising disease burden. The variability of clinical presentations makes the diagnosis of musculoskeletal infections a challenge. Adhering to strict diagnostic and treatment algorithms while utilizing new classifications and scoring systems to determine the severity of illness can predict patient outcomes and improve patient care and resource utilization. The most common inflammatory conditions that affect pediatric patients are poststreptococcal reactive arthritis, juvenile idiopathic arthritis, and Lyme disease–associated arthritis. Treatments are specific to each disease, so accurate diagnosis is important. Fractures related to nonaccidental trauma are common, especially in children younger than 12 months. It is the duty of the orthopaedic surgeon to recognize and report suspected nonaccidental trauma to social services and local child protective service representatives.

Keywords: inflammatory arthritis; musculoskeletal infection; nonaccidental trauma

Introduction

Musculoskeletal infections in children generally occur during the first decade of life, and one-half of all cases present in children younger than 5 years. The majority of cases are caused by *Staphylococcus* species, followed by *Streptococcus* species. Early recognition and treatment by a coordinated multidisciplinary team that utilizes severity of illness (SOI) scores and disease classification systems can optimize resource utilization and improve patient outcomes.

Nonaccidental fractures resulting from the physical abuse of a child is also common and is a major public health concern. Traumatic injuries account for 18% of child abuse presentations, and 1,680 children die annually from abuse.[1] The physical abuse of children, especially those younger than year, frequently manifests as a fracture, which is second only to bruising as the most common sign of physical abuse.[2] Up to 20% of burns are nonaccidental in the pediatric population.[3]

Pediatric Musculoskeletal Infections

In recent decades, musculoskeletal infection (MSKI) have increased in incidence and severity.[4] However, substantial differences exist in the regional manifestations of MSKI. There is a higher incidence of MSKI in regions that have temperate climates (southern United States) compared with northern regions of the United States.[5] There is also seasonal variation with MSKI. Summer is the most common season for MSKI occurrence.[6]

Diagnosis

Traditionally, musculoskeletal infections were classified on the type of tissue infection: superficial abscess, septic joint, osteomyelitis, and deep abscess/pyomyositis. These conditions can occur in isolation, but MSKIs often occur in combination. A failure to recognize a complex MSKI that involves more than one tissue type and/or anatomic location can lead to treatment delays, prolonged hospitalizations, and increased risk for complications.[5] For these reasons, a novel stratification system has been proposed for MSKI based on the degree of system involvement, regardless of the type of tissue infection or causative bacteria.[7] This three-tiered classification system is based on the severity of the infection and the degree of dissemination. Pediatric MSKI patients should be classified into three groups: (1) inflammation, (2) local infection, or (3) disseminated infection (**Table 1**). The MSKI is classified as inflammation if all of the following were

---

Dr. McIntosh or an immediate family member is a member of a speakers' bureau or has made paid presentations on behalf of Globus Medical.

Table 1

Infection Severity Classification

	Definition	Example
Inflammation	All of the following must be true: • Negative blood culture • Negative local culture • The criteria for local or disseminated infection are not met	Transient synovitis
Local infection	One of the following must be true: • Osteomyelitis or pyomyositis in one anatomic site • Local culture positive AND/OR fluid/tissue consistent with infection • One positive blood culture • The criteria for disseminated infection are not met	Isolated distal femoral osteomyelitis with no subperiosteal abscess Isolated septic hip
Disseminated infection	Two or more anatomic sites, at least one of the following must be true: • Imaging diagnostic for osteomyelitis or pyomyositis • Local culture positive AND/OR fluid/tissue consistent with infection • Two or more positive blood cultures • Thromboembolic disease	Septic hip with surrounding muscle pyomyositis Distal fibular osteomyelitis with subperiosteal abscess

true: negative local culture, negative blood culture, and criteria for local or disseminated infection are not met. The MSKI is classified as a local infection, if imaging was characteristic of infection in one anatomic site or a single positive blood culture. Disseminated infection is defined as the presence of multiple positive blood cultures, positive tissue culture from different anatomic sites, imaging characteristic of infection in multiple anatomic sites, and/or thromboembolic disease.[7] The patients with disseminated infections are statistically more likely to undergo surgical débridement, have longer hospital stays, be admitted to the intensive care unit (ICU), and require a longer duration of antibiotic treatment. They also demonstrate higher C-reactive protein (CRP) levels, erythrocyte sedimentation rates (ESRs), white blood cell (WBC) counts, and temperature peaks.[7] Deep vein thrombosis (DVT) and pulmonary embolism (PE) are more likely to develop in patients with disseminated infections.[8] It is recommended that children who present with disseminated infection and are admitted to the ICU should undergo ultrasonograpic screening to assess for DVT.[8]

Pediatric patients with MSKI present with fever and focal tenderness, warmth, or swelling near the ends of long bones and decreasing ability to bear weight or use the extremity. Range of motion of the adjacent joint may be limited because of local inflammation or due to contiguous septic arthritis. All patients should undergo a through physical examination as well as appropriate laboratory tests and imaging studies. The routine laboratory tests to be performed are blood culture, complete blood count (CBC) with differential, ESR, and CRP. Plain radiographs of the involved bone are often negative initially, but they may demonstrate deep soft-tissue swelling when inspected carefully for this finding. Bone destruction is not observed on radiographs until an infection is present for at least 7 to 14 days. MRI is a key component to the workup of patients in whom an MSKI is suspected. MRI is an accurate and reliable modality to determine the anatomic and spatial extent of infection, provides a more complete understanding of the primary and contiguous tissues involved in the infection, and helps determine all foci of infection that require débridement and/or drainage. Disadvantages associated with MRI include its cost, the need for sedation in most children, and the logistics of obtaining the study in a timely fashion in busy pediatric medical centers. Ultrasonography is readily available and inexpensive. However, it is limited in its capability to identify deep infections of the muscle and bone (pyomyositis and osteomyelitis). In a recent study of pediatric patients evaluated in an emergency department to rule out septic hip arthritis, pelvis pyomyositis was twice as common as an isolated septic hip arthritis.[9] Another study reported that contiguous osteomyelitis was observed 68% of the time in patients who have septic hip arthritis.[10] The MRI can also be used to direct the approach for a joint aspiration. If the MRI demonstrates pelvic pyomyositis that affects the adductor musculature, then the joint aspiration should be approached anteriorly instead of from a medial approach to avoid contamination of the hip joint aspiration from the contiguous pyomyositis.[5]

For these and other reasons, MRI is the preferred imaging modality for the diagnosis of MSKI. At the institution of the author of this chapter, a noncontrast fast spin-echo sequence protocol is obtained from nonsedated pediatric patients with suspected MSKI in less than 30 minutes. This MRI protocol includes a coronal T1-weighted short tau inversion recovery MRI and an axial T2-weighted MRI. Both sequences provide the orthopaedic surgeon enough detail to make an accurate diagnosis as well as identify any foci of MSKI that are amendable to surgical or interventional radiologic débridement and/or drainage.[5]

Antibiotic Treatment

The timing of appropriate empiric antibiotic administration should balance the priorities of identifying the causative bacteria and avoiding unnecessary delay in antibiotic administration in children who may be demonstrating signs of sepsis. Antibiotics should not be administered until a blood culture is obtained.[11] If a specimen can be obtained from the specific site of infection in a timely manner, then antibiotics should be withheld until after that culture is obtained. Whenever clinical concern exists about the potential for evolving sepsis, which is discernible by the presence of fever, the ill appearance of the child, and hemodynamic changes, antibiotics should be administered regardless of the timing of anticipated advanced imaging or surgery. Empiric antibiotics should be selected on the basis of the most prevalent bacteria responsible for MSKI within the local community.[12] Currently, most children are treated effectively with a much shorter course of intravenous antibiotics, followed by 3 to 4 weeks of targeted oral therapy. Identifying oral antibiotics with good bioavailability to which the bacteria are susceptible offers flexibility in treatment options for the administration route. Sequential parenteral-to-oral antibiotic therapy is considered safe and effective and should be used in the absence of contraindications such as malabsorption, noncompliance, or antibiotic resistance of the causative organism that requires intravenous antibiotic therapy.

The duration of antibiotic treatment ideally should facilitate clinical and laboratory resolution of the MSKI. When the inflammatory indices have normalized within the antibiotic treatment timeframe, the antibiotic may be discontinued. If the inflammatory indices remain elevated, however, antibiotic treatment should be continued, with clinical and laboratory reassessment every 1 to 2 weeks until normalization occurs. If no trend toward improvement is seen, consideration should be given to further evaluation for a residual focus of infection such as an abscess or a sequestrum, which may be preventing resolution of the infection. The trough levels of antibiotics with the potential for systemic toxicity should be monitored in the laboratory periodically. Children taking antibiotics that are potentially nephrotoxic or hepatotoxic also should have periodic measurement of serum creatinine, alanine transaminase (ALT), and aspartate transaminase (AST) levels. The dosing of antibiotics should take into consideration the balance between achieving appropriate bactericidal activity within bone and avoiding systemic toxicity. Certain antibiotics such as clindamycin have excellent oral bioavailability and do not require routine serum concentration monitoring.

SOI Assessment and Surgical Treatment

An objective measurement of SOI in patients presenting with MSKI can help surgeons predict the likelihood of a disseminated infection and guide early antibiotic selection.[5] The SOI score from 0 (mild) to 10 (severe) has been used to guide resource utilization and intervention (**Table 2**). It has also allowed for the stratification of bacterial genomic variation in regard to virulence and severity of clinical disease burden.[12] Children with mild illness are unlikely to require surgery, whereas children with severe illness have a higher likelihood of requiring one or more surgical procedures to help resolve the infection. In the current era of methicillin-resistant *Staphylococcus aureus* (MRSA), a higher incidence of deep abscess formation appears to exist, which may be causing a higher rate of surgical intervention for children with MSKI.

Limited guidance in the existing literature exists regarding the specific surgical procedure(s) to perform to treat MSKI. Procedures include drainage of subperiosteal abscesses, drilling of the bone, or incision of the bone cortex with irrigation and débridement of the infected cancellous bone. If the child does not demonstrate appropriate clinical or laboratory improvement within 72 to 96 hours after surgical débridement, repeat irrigation and débridement should be considered. Additional imaging is of limited use unless another focus of infection that had not previously been addressed is suspected.

Recently, the SOI score has also been able to predict the likelihood of a long-term adverse outcome in patients with MSKI. A patient with a severe (7-10) SOI score at initial presentation was significantly more likely

Table 2

Modified Severity of Illness Score

Parameter	Point Value[a]
Initial CRP level (mg/dL)	
<10	0
10-15	1
>15	2
CRP level (mg/dL) 48 hr after presentation	
<5	0
5-10	1
>10	2
CRP level (mg/dL) 96 hr after presentation	
<5	0
5-10	1
>10	2
Band count (cells/µL)	
<1.5	0
≥1.5	1
Febrile days on antibiotics	
<2	0
≥2	1
ICU admission	
No	0
Yes	1
Disseminated musculoskeletal infection	
No	0
Yes	1

CRP = C-reactive protein; ICU = intensive care unit

[a]Range: 0-10 points.

to have osteonecrosis, chondrolysis, or bony deformity at 2-year follow-up compared with those patients with mild (0-2) or moderate (3-6) SOI scores.[13] By regression analysis, SOI score, plus age younger than 3 years, and MRSA predicted a severe outcome. The odds ratio of a long-term adverse outcome increased 1.34 per point increase in the SOI score. Therefore, children with the risk factors (young age, high SOI score, and MRSA) should be followed clinically and with plain radiographs, at least every 6 months, until it becomes clear whether or not severe sequelae of their MSKI will develop.[13]

Clinical Practice Guidelines

Children with bone and joint infections have benefitted from the development and implementation of guidelines to reduce variations in care. The new guidelines endorsed by the American Academy of Pediatrics (AAP), Pediatric Orthopaedic Society of North America (POSNA), Pediatric Infectious Disease Society (PIDS), and the Infectious Disease Society of America (IDSA) for the diagnosis and treatment of pediatric MSKI will be published in *Clinical Infectious Diseases*.

Pediatric Inflammatory Conditions Affecting the Musculoskeletal System

Poststreptococcal Reactive Arthritis Evaluation

Poststreptococcal reactive arthritis (PSRA) is considered in a school-age child who presents with pauciarticular or polyarticular arthritis that has been confirmed to not be septic arthritis and that does not meet the criteria for acute rheumatic fever.[14,15] The age distribution appears to peak between 8 and 14 years in children. Typically, a symptom-free period occurs after an episode of group A streptococcal pharyngitis, but some children with PSRA have no known prior history of streptococcal illness. The diagnosis of an antecedent group A streptococcal infection may be approached through throat culture or rapid antigen detection tests. The occurrence of symptoms remote to the primary infection typically requires serologic testing with acute and convalescent antibody titers. The most commonly used antibody titers are antistreptolysin O and antideoxyribonuclease-B.[14] The titers may remain elevated persistently for months or years after the streptococcal infection. Some challenges may occur in defining the normal cutoff values and avoiding overdiagnosis.[15] The serologic tests remain helpful in establishing a diagnostic and therapeutic direction for children with this condition.

Treatment

Because of concern for the possible evolution of carditis in the aftermath of PSRA, the American Heart Association recommends appropriate baseline cardiac screening and antibiotic prophylaxis for 1 year in cases of suspected PSRA.[16] Treatment is initiated for a period appropriate to cover an acute streptococcal illness (10 days with a semisynthetic penicillin or beta-lactam antibiotic). This regimen often is followed by monthly penicillin depot injections performed by the primary care physician, who also performs the baseline heart evaluation with an electrocardiogram and an echocardiogram. The inflammatory component of the condition typically is managed by a pediatric rheumatologist, who often initiates high-dose naproxen sodium treatment of a 10 mg/kg dose twice daily for several weeks and monitoring for improvement in the clinical symptoms and elevated inflammatory markers. The antibodies to *Streptococcus* (antistreptolysin O and antideoxyribonuclease-B) have an autoimmune behavior and appear to be cross-reactive with components of the joint synovium, which leads to the reactive arthritis. Overall, the long-term prognosis of PSRA is good, because it follows a self-limited course in most children.

Lyme Arthritis

Lyme arthritis in children is usually monoarticular and most commonly involves the knee joint. Lyme borreliosis is a tick-transmitted spirochetal infection caused by *Borrelia burgdorferi* in North America. Lyme disease is endemic in the Northeastern and the Upper Midwest regions of the United States. In 2016, a total of 26,203 confirmed cases of Lyme disease were reported in the United States (incidence = 8.1 cases per 100,000).[17] Early infection in children often manifests by a skin rash (erythema migrans), neurologic features (facial palsy, meningitis), and occasionally arthralgias and myalgias. Lyme arthritis does not need to be treated with urgent joint washout. Instead, it is treated on an outpatient basis with 4 weeks of oral antibiotics. Children presenting with a painful, swollen joint should be tested for the disease. Testing for Lyme disease involves the analysis of peripheral blood for antibodies through enzyme immunoassay and then a confirmatory Western blot analysis. There has been a recent proposal to eliminate the Western blot. Instead, the second-tier assay would also be an enzyme-linked immunosorbent assay (ELISA), but a different one from the first-tier assay.[18] This approach still has greater than 95% specificity and would make the performance of the tests easier, results would be available sooner, and it would eliminate the interpretation time of the Western blot.[18] In Lyme-endemic areas, the presentation of a child with an acutely swollen knee is more likely to be Lyme arthritis than traditional bacterial septic arthritis. Lyme arthritis in children has an excellent prognosis. In 2018, the AAP endorsed a short-term (21 day) use of doxycycline for Lyme disease in children younger than 8 years based on the low risk of dental staining.[19] Amoxicillin and cefuroxime are as effective as doxycycline in the treatment of Lyme arthritis.

Child Abuse and the Orthopaedic Surgeon

Nonaccidental fractures caused by physical abuse primarily occur in very young children (younger than 12 months). In children younger than 12 months, 25% of their fractures were caused by physical abuse compared with 7% of fractures in 12- to 23-month-old children and 3% of fractures in those 24 to 35 months old.[20] As children become ambulatory, a much smaller percentage of fractures are caused by physical abuse than by accidents such as falls.

Evaluation

No particular location or fracture morphology can identify abuse in isolation. The larger clinical picture is critical in distinguishing between an abusive and an accidental mechanism of injury. For example, an isolated, spiral femur fracture in an ambulatory toddler who presents acutely and with a clear story of a trip trip-and-fall episode while running demonstrates a very different clinical picture than one or more long bone fractures in an infant with no clear explanatory mechanism. **Table 3** lists the clinical and radiographic red flags that should prompt the orthopaedic surgeon to consider child abuse.

Table 3

Radiographic Findings in Infant and Toddlers With Nonaccidental Trauma Due to Physical Abuse

High specificity
Metaphyseal fractures
Rib fractures (posteromedial)
Spinous process fractures
Sternal fractures
Moderate specificity
Multiple fractures, especially bilateral
Fractures in different stages of healing
Epiphyseal separations
Complex skull fractures
Common, but low specificity
Subperiosteal new bone formation
Clavicular fracture
Lone bone shaft fracture
Linear skull fracture

Pediatrics

Table 4

Medical Conditions That Can Present With Multiple Fractures

Osteogenesis imperfecta
Osteopenia of prematurity
Scurvy
Copper deficiency
Menkes disease
Disuse osteopenia (nonambulatory or minimally ambulatory children)
Chronic disease (kidney or liver failure)

When a suspect or unexplained fracture is present in a child younger than 2 years, a skeletal survey should be ordered routinely to assess for other occult fractures. The prevalence of occult fractures ranged from 24.6% in infants aged 0 to 5 months to 3.6% in those aged 18 to 24 months.[21] The awareness and recognition of fractures potentially caused by physical abuse is critical for orthopaedic surgeons who care for children. Orthopaedic surgeons caring for children should utilize the help of multidisciplinary child abuse care teams. A careful examination and thorough history with detailed documentation by the orthopaedic surgeon are vital in assisting the differential diagnosis of fractures suspicious for physical abuse. Several medical conditions and bone diseases in infants and children may predispose to fracture. Osteogenesis imperfecta, in particular, can manifest as multiple fractures in young children. Relatively little literature compares the presentations in these two groups directly, but a genetic test for osteogenesis imperfecta can be performed if necessary. **Table 4** lists the diseases and conditions in the differential diagnosis for fractures presenting in very young children. Most of these can be distinguished easily from physical abuse with a thorough history and physical examination. The majority of the fractures associated with nonaccidental trauma can be treated with splints or casts.

Summary

The variability of clinical presentations makes the diagnosis of musculoskeletal infections a challenge. Adhering to strict diagnostic and treatment algorithms while utilizing novel SOI classifications and scoring systems can predict patient outcomes and improve patient care and resource utilization. The most common inflammatory conditions that affect pediatric patients are PSRA, juvenile idiopathic arthritis, and Lyme disease–associated arthritis. Treatments are specific to each disease, so accurate diagnosis is important. Fractures related to nonaccidental trauma are common, especially in children younger than 12 months. It is the duty of the orthopaedic surgeon to recognize and report suspected nonaccidental trauma to social services and local child protective service representatives.

Key Study Points

- Pediatric patients with musculoskeletal infection (MSKI) should be classified into three groups: (1) inflammation, (2) local infection, or (3) disseminated infection (**Table 1**).
- MRI is a key component to the workup of patients in whom an MSKI is suspected.
- When a suspicious or unexplained fracture is present in a child younger than 2 years, a skeletal survey should be ordered routinely to assess for other occult fractures.
- Lyme arthritis in children is usually monoarticular and most commonly involves the knee joint.
- Lyme arthritis does not need to be treated with urgent joint washout. Instead, it is treated on an outpatient basis with 4 weeks of oral antibiotics.

Annotated References

1. Nunez Lopez O, Hughes BD, Adhikari D, Williams K, Radhakrishnan RS, Bowen-Jallow KA: Sociodemographic determinants of non-accidental traumatic injuries in children. *Am J Surg* 2018;215(6):1037-1041.

   The authors studied the effects of sociodemographic factors associated with increased risk of mortality, increased occurrence, and higher use of resources in nonaccidental trauma cases.

2. Randel T, Loder JRF: Orthopaedic injuries in children with non-accidental trauma: Demographics and Incidence from the 2000 kids' inpatient database. *J Pediatr Orthop* 2007;27(4):421-426.

3. Nigro LC, Feldman MJ, Foster RL, Pozez AL: A model to improve dectection of nonaccidental pediatric burns. *AMA J Ethics* 2018;20(1):552-559.

   The authors developed a multidisciplinary method to identify suspected nonaccidental burns in pediatric patients in order to more consistently and reliably identify instances of abuse.

4. Sarkissian EJ, Gans I, Gunderson MA, Myers SH, Spiegel DA, Flynn JM: Community-acquired methicillin-resistant and methicillin sensitive *Staphylococcus aureus* musculoskeltal infections in children. *J Pediatr Orthop* 2016;36(3):323-327.

5. Rosenfeld SB, Copley LA, Mignemi M, An T, Benvenuti M, Schoenecker J: Key concepts of musculoskeltal infection. *Instr Course Lect* 2017;66:569-584.

   Management of musculoskeletal infections is dependent on accurate identification of organisms and thorough recognition of sites of infection and related tissues. MRI helps localize infection and identify areas of surgical débridement.

6. Lindsay EA, Tareen NT, Jo CH, Copley LA: Seasonal variation and weather changes related to the occurrence and severity of acute hematogenous osteomyelitis in children. *J Pediatric Infect Dis Soc* 2018;7(2):e16-e23.

   The authors determined that acute hematogenous osteomyelitis in children most commonly occurred in the summer.

7. Mignemi ME, Benvenuti MA, An TJ, et al: A novel classification system based on dissemination of musculoskeletal infection is predictive of hospital outcomes. *J Pediatr Orthop* 2018;38(5):279-286.

   The classification system for pediatric MSKI developed by the authors is advantageous because it can be applied to different types of MSKI and complements the previous practice of differentiating MSKI based on primary diagnosis. Level of evidence: II.

8. Ligon JA, Journeycake JM, Josephs SC, Tareen NG, Lindsay EA, Copley LAB: Differentiation of deep venous thrombosis among children with or without osteomyelitis. *J Pediatr Orthop* 2018;38(10):e597-e603.

   Children with DVT and osteomyelitis have higher SOI, rate of MRSA, occurrence of intensive care, and absence of comorbidities and postthrombotic syndrome than children with DVT only. Level of evidence: II.

9. Mignemi ME, Menge T, Cole HA, et al: Epidemiology, diagnosis, and treatment of pericapsular pyomyositis of the hip in children. *J Pediatr Orthop* 2014;34(3):316-325.

10. Monsalve J, Kan JH, Schallert EK, Bisset GS, Zhang W, Rosenfeld SB: Septic arthritis in children: Frequency of coexisting unsuspected osteomyelitis and implications on imaging workup and management. *Am J Roentgenol* 2015;204(6):1289-1295.

11. Section J, Gibbons SD, Barton T, Greenberg DE, Jo CH, Copley L: Microbiologic culture methods for pediatric musculoskeletal infection: A guideline for optimal use. *J Bone Joint Surg Am* 2015;97(6):441-449.

12. Collins A, Wakeland EK, Raj P, et al: The impact of *Staphylococcus aureus* genomic variation on clinical phenotype of children with acute hematogenous osteomyelitis. *Heliyon* 2018;4(6):e00674.

    The study authors introduced a novel reference strain along with detailed annotation of Staphylococcus aureus virulence genes in the hopes of devising future transcriptome investigations into osteomyelitis in children.

13. Vorhies JS, Lindsay EA, Tareen NG, Kellum RJ, Jo CH, Copley LA: Severity adjusted risk of long-term adverse sequelae among children with osteomyelitis. *Pediatr Infect Dis J* 2019;38(1):26-31.

    The authors determined that the long-term risk of severe adverse outcomes in children with osteomyelitis were predicted by initial SOI.

14. Uziel Y, Perl L, Barash J, Hashkes PJ: Post-streptococcal reactive arthritis in children: A distinct entity from acute rheumatic fever. *Pediatr Rheumatol Online J* 2011;9(1):32.

15. Moorthy LN, Gaur S, Peterson MG, Landa YF, Tandon M, Lehman TJ: Post-streptococcal reactive arthritis in children: A retrospective study. *Clin Pediatr* 2009;48(2):174-182.

16. Gerber MA, Baltimore RS, Eaton CB, et al: Prevention of rheumatic fever and diagnosis and treatment of acute streptococcal pharyngitis: A scientific statement from the American council on cardiovascular disease in the young. *Circulation* 2009;119:1541-1551.

17. Shapiro E: Lyme disease in 2018: What is new (and what is not). *JAMA* 2018;320(7):635-636.

    The authors discuss current concepts in the management of Lyme disease.

18. Moore A, Nelson C, Molins C, Mead PM: Current guidelines, common clinical pitfalls, and future directions for laboratory diagnosis of Lyme disease, United States. *Emerg Infect Dis* 2016;22(7):1169-1177.

19. Committee on Infectious Disease, American Academy of Pediatrics: *Report on the Committee on Infectious Diseases*, in *Red Book: 2018-2021*, Itasca, IL, American Academcy of Pediatrics, 2018, p 905.

20. Flaherty EG, Perez-Rossello JM, Levin MA, Hennrikus WL: Evaluating children with fractures for child physical abuse. *Pediatrics* 2014;133(2):477-489.

21. Wood JN, Henry MK, Berger RP, et al: Use and utility of skeletal surveys to evaluate occult fractures in young injured children. *Acad Pediatr* 2019;19(4):428-437.

    The authors recommend increasing the use of skeletal surveys in infants aged 0 to 5 months because of the high incidence of occult fractures in this age group.

Section 12

Oncology and Pathology

EDITOR

Matthew R. DiCaprio, MD FAOA

Chapter 65

Evaluation and Treatment of Musculoskeletal Tumors

Wakenda K. Tyler, MD, MPH, FAOA

ABSTRACT

Understanding the basics of appropriate evaluation and management of patients with neoplasms of the musculoskeletal system is an essential component in the education of orthopaedic surgeons. Good diagnostic acumen and appropriate early management can result in life- and limb-sparing surgical care. A decrease in unnecessary testing and undue worry is also accomplished if accurate diagnosis can be achieved early. We will discuss the following topics that are critical to adequate diagnosis and management of patients presenting with a suspected musculoskeletal tumor.

- Clinical presentation of patients with bone and soft-tissue tumors
- Imaging modalities used to assess musculoskeletal tumors
- Biopsy techniques and molecular diagnostics
- Staging of malignant bone and soft-tissue tumors
- Initial surgical management of patients with bone and soft-tissue tumors
- Adjuvant therapies and their role in management of patients
- The role of functional testing in musculoskeletal tumor patients

Keywords: biopsy; bone tumors; clinical presentation and imaging; oncology; sarcoma; soft-tissue tumors

Clinical Presentation

Patients with musculoskeletal tumors can present as an incidental asymptomatic finding to severely painful lesions with deformity and/or fractures. It is not infrequent for more aggressive tumors to present with significant pain and for more indolent tumors to be asymptomatic. Although, these are the general rules, many patients will fall outside of this norm. It is, therefore, imperative that the clinician assessing the patient incorporate all of the data available to determine a diagnosis. The presentation will vary depending on bone versus soft-tissue origin and often depending on age of the patient, as many very young children will not verbally express pain or discomfort.

Soft-Tissue Tumors

The vast majority of soft-tissue tumors will present without pain. Pain is not a determinant of a malignant versus benign process. In fact, more frequently, benign soft-tissue masses will present with pain. Examples of tumors that can present with pain are schwannomas and neurofibromas, which will often present with nerve-related pain, which will be sharp and shooting. Patients with nerve tumors will frequently have a Tinel's sign on examination, which will manifest as electric shooting pain at the site of the tumor when it is tapped. Vascular malformations and angiolipomas are also tumors that frequently present with pain. Patients will have pain directly over the mass. It is hypothesized that the vessels within these tumors have nerve endings within them that can be triggered from trauma or thrombosis of the vessels within the tumor.[1] Most malignant soft-tissue tumors will not cause pain unless they are directly invading a nerve, bone, or large vessel. Although possible, this is a rare event for most soft-tissue sarcomas.

Most soft-tissue sarcomas will present as growing masses. Rapid growth is often an ominous sign, but there are some sarcomas that will present with slower than expected growth, such as synovial sarcoma. Most benign soft-tissue tumors will often be slow growing or stable in growth. Some lipomas and fibromatosis can grow more rapid and still be benign. Vascular malformations may exhibit a waxing and waning pattern of growth with patients reporting rapid enlargement, followed by fairly rapid decrease in size. The lesion will rarely go away completely however.

Dr. Tyler or an immediate family member serves as an unpaid consultant to Musculoskeletal Transplant Foundation and Taithera; has stock or stock options held in Taithera, Inc.; and serves as a board member, owner, officer, or committee member of the American Academy of Orthopedic Surgeons, the J. Robert Gladden Society, and the Musculoskeletal Tumor Society.

Bone Tumors

Both benign and malignant bone tumors can present with pain. Unfortunately, the skeleton is a structure with a plethora of nerve endings throughout it components. Pain is a frequent finding in many active tumors, particularly when risk of fracture is present. When bone pain is present, patients often report pain at the site of the lesion and may describe this pain as achy and throbbing in nature (tooth ache–like). The patient may report feeling that the pain is deep seated. It is common for patients with bone pain to report night pain that will wake them from sleep. In situations where risk of fracture is imminent, patients will often report functional pain, such as pain with taking a step or getting up from a chair. Although many benign and malignant bone tumors will have pain associated with them, it is not uncommon for patients with inactive benign tumors to present with an incidental finding on imaging that was obtained for another reason, such as an acute transient injury or workup for some other process, such as arthritis or rotator cuff pathology.

Young children can be a challenge for assessing the presence of bone pain. Most young children will not report pain, but parents and caregivers may notice a limp or a sudden lack of use of a limb. In any child that presents in such a manner, a full workup, including thorough physical examination and imaging of any areas of concern is warranted. In one analysis of children diagnosed with malignancy, the number one presenting symptom was pain.[2] This points to the importance of care in assessing what pain is in the young child.

Occasionally, in the instance of bone tumors, the first presenting sign may be deformity of the limb involved. Osteofibrous dysplasia is a good example of such a presentation, in which case the parents may notice anterior bowing deformity of the shin (**Figure 1**). Other conditions such as isolated large osteochondromas or multiple hereditary exostosis will also often present with what is perceived as painless lumps or limb deformity.

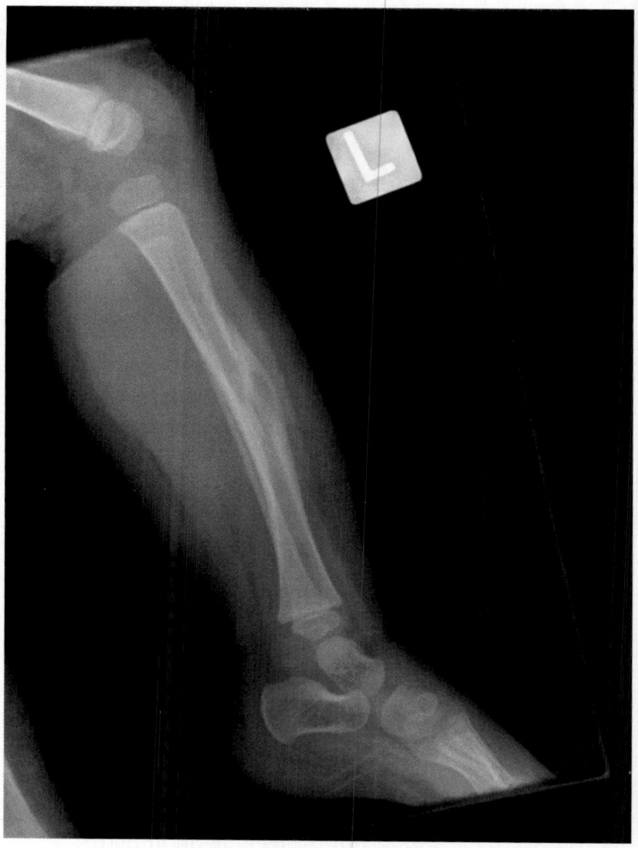

Figure 1 Radiograph showing osteofibrous dysplasia of the tibia in a 2-year-old boy. Note the mild anterior tibial bowing, which will likely get slightly worse with growth.

Imaging of Musculoskeletal Lesions

Radiographic features often play a key role in helping to diagnose many bone and soft-tissue tumors. Many tumors will have distinct radiographic features that are characteristic of a specific tumor. Such findings can often allow the clinician to limit further invasive and noninvasive testing. We will discuss the bone tumors and soft-tissue masses separately as radiographic classifications and diagnoses are very distinct for these two general groups.

Bone Tumors

Plain Radiographs

Plain radiographs are often the starting and ending point for many bone tumors. When imaging bone tumors, the plain orthogonal radiographs should always include the whole bone in question (full-length radiographs), as this may help identify an isolated condition versus a multifocal process. The radiographic presentation is frequently all that is needed for a diagnosis in many specific bone lesions. In a recent Dutch study looking at a universal country-wide registry, delays in diagnosis were often found to occur at the primary care or generalist level. The authors of the study point to the need to educate the generalist on the importance of early plain radiographs in the management of patient with musculoskeletal pain, as most bone sarcomas will be readily detected on plain radiograph.[3] The first question one should ask when assessing a plain radiographic lesion is whether the tumor has a matrix or not. This is often clearly seen on the plain radiographs. The two matrices one would see

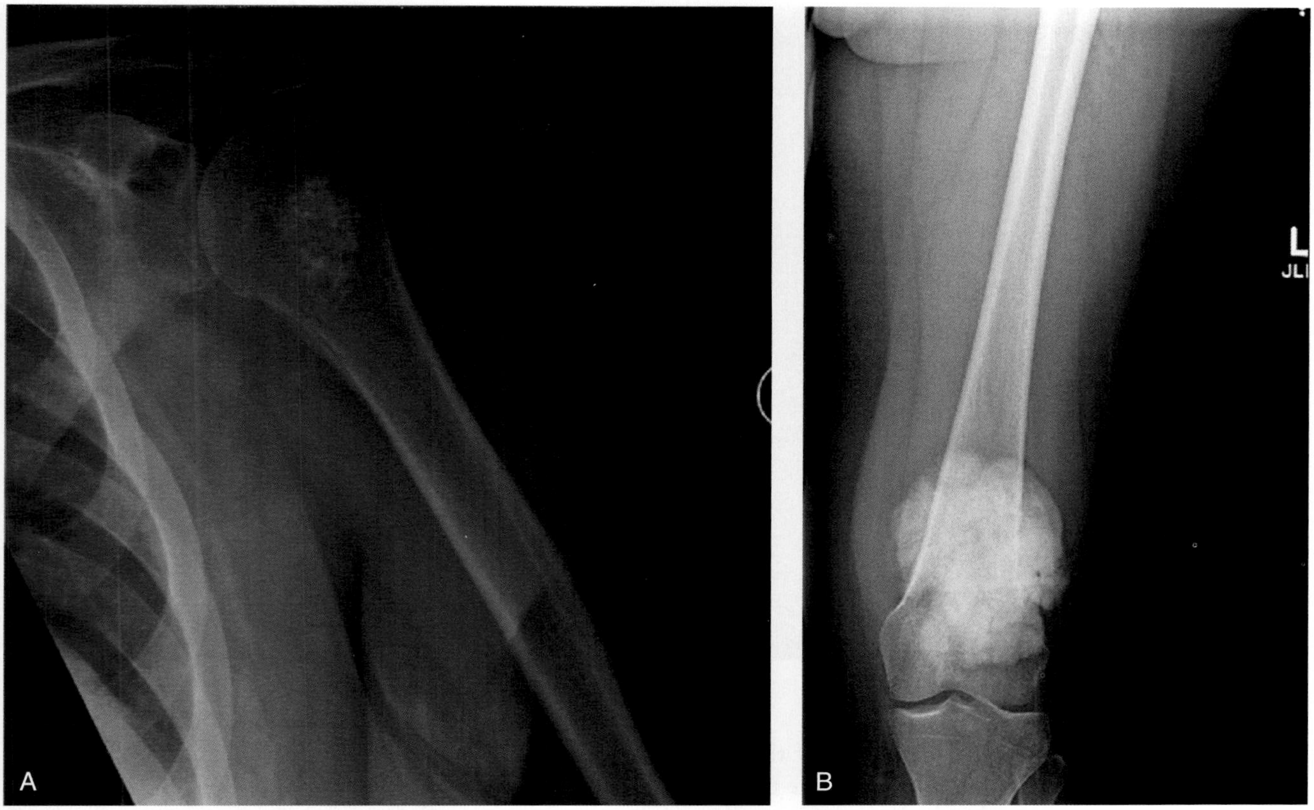

Figure 2 **A**, AP humerus with cartilaginous matrix tumor (enchondroma). Note the rings and stippled appearance of the cartilage matrix. **B**, Bone matrix tumor (osteosarcoma) of the distal femur. Note that the appearance is that of dense bone with extraosseous extension.

will be cartilage or bone (**Figure 2**). There can also be a fibrous tissue matrix, but this can be harder to discern from other lytic processes on plain radiograph. The matrix can then either be defined as aggressive appearing as in the case of chondrosarcoma or nonaggressive, such as an enchondroma. If no matrix is present, then the lesion is often described as radiolucent or lytic. It is important to keep in mind that in the case of a lytic lesion, greater than 30% of the calcium matrix needs to be lost before it will be seen on a typical plain radiograph. The Enneking's classification system for benign bone tumors is often a good starting point for classifying bone tumors[4] (**Table 1**). Enneking described three types of bone lesions, which he defined as latent, active, or aggressive based on plain radiographic features[5] (**Figure 3**). Latent tumors have clear and distinct borders, often with a sclerotic rim around the lesion. An example of a latent tumor is a nonossifying fibroma picked up as an incidental finding. Active lesions do not have a distinct border and will not have a sclerotic rim. They indicate a tumor that is growing, but not aggressively, such as unicameral bone cyst. Aggressive tumors will show expansion of the bone and destruction of one or more cortices with indistinct borders. Examples of aggressive tumors are frequently giant cell tumor of bone or aneurysmal bone cysts. Both active and aggressive imaging features can also be present in malignant bone tumors that are lytic, such as telangiectatic osteosarcoma.

Computer Tomography

CT utilizes multiple plain radiographs taken in different plains to generate a three-dimensional image of a particular body part being assessed. The benefits are that

Table 1

Enneking Staging for Benign Bone Tumors

Description	Radiographic Features
Latent	Clear and distinct sclerotic border
Active	Indistinct border, but contained within the cortex of bone
Aggressive	Indistinct border, no longer contained within the confines of the bony cortex

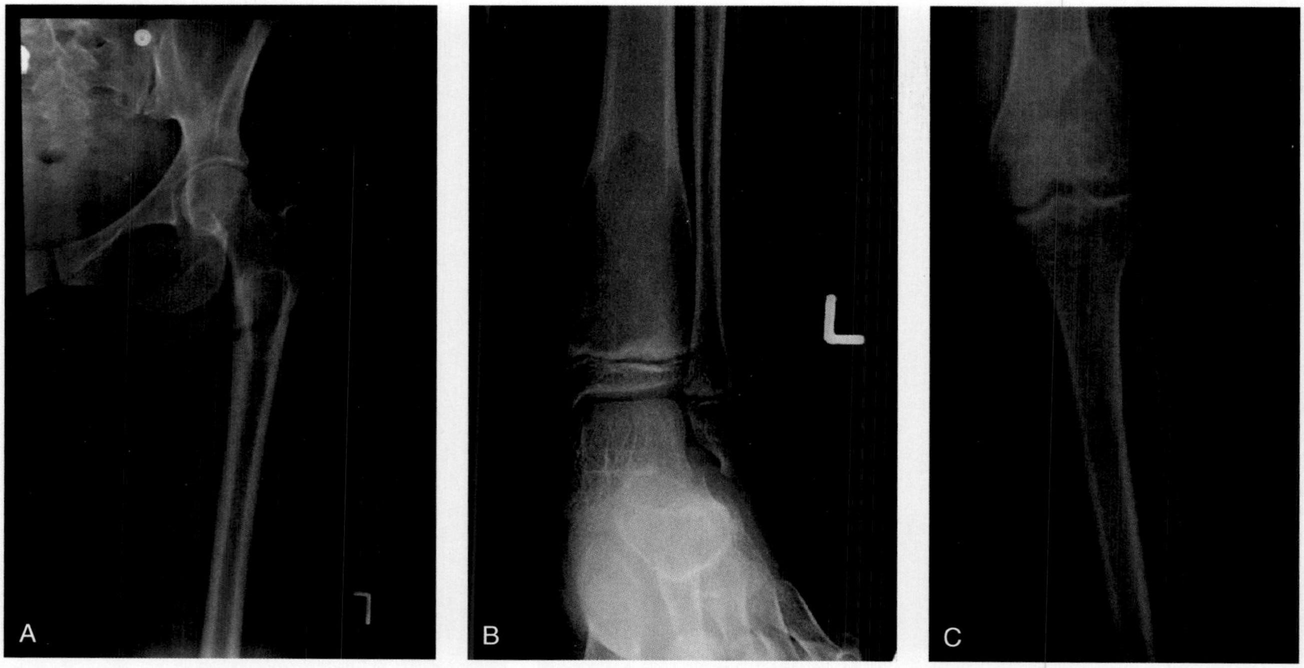

Figure 3 **A**, Inactive bone lesion. **B**, Active bone lesion. **C**, Aggressive bone lesion.

one can see the three-dimensional nature of the bone, and in that, assess the true relationship of the tumor to other surrounding bone and soft tissue. CT scans can allow for assessment of the structural integrity of the bone and the matrix of the tumor. CT scans are also less expensive than MRI and therefore may be favored in circumstances where cost containment is important. It does not provide the soft-tissue detail that can be assessed by MRI however. The other downside to CT scan is that, because one is effectively using numerous x-rays to generate an image, the radiation exposure is significantly higher than the typical two to four views one may obtain for a typical long bone. CT scans can carry up to 200-times more radiation exposure than a single plain radiograph. For this reason, it is important to use CT scans with some prudence, particularly in younger children where the exposure to multiple CT scans has been shown to have a theoretical risk of future cancer development.[6]

CT scans can be useful for certain tumors, particularly in situations where the three-dimensional nature of the cortical bone may need to be assessed. Osteoid osteomas, which are cortically based tumors, that frequently show a clear nidus on CT scan, are an example of a tumor for which CT scan can be extremely useful as a diagnostic tool. In other regions of the body where the complex nature of the bone is not well seen on plain radiographs, such as the sacrum and pelvis, a CT scan can be very helpful.

Magnetic Resonance Imaging

MRI can be a useful modality beyond plain radiographs, if plain radiographs do not definitively allow for determination of the lesion in question or if further information regarding soft-tissue involvement or marrow edema is warranted. It is often less informative about the structural integrity of the bone. When considering an MRI to assess a bone lesion, one should plan to order the MRI with intravenous gadolinium contrast, unless there is a contraindication. MRIs allow for detailed assessment of tumor-associated edema, which can be useful in distinguishing subtle pathologic fractures, as well as tumors showing aggressive behavior.

There is no better study than MRI when one is concerned about soft-tissue extension of a tumor and therefore should be considered when clear cortical disruption is seen on plain radiograph. The addition of gadolinium allows one to see more clearly the borders of a tumor and also allows for the distinction of a cystic versus a solid lesion. Gadolinium goes to sites of high vascularity and will also allow for determining the vascular nature of the tumor in question in some cases. This can be particularly important in the assessment of malignant tumors. An MRI of the whole bone in question is absolutely necessary for any malignant primary bone tumor. This is done to rule out metastases. MRI is unnecessary in the initial workup of an adult patient with presumed metastatic disease. Plain radiographs are usually adequate for assessing risk of fracture, and since wide resection is rarely performed for metastatic disease, knowing the exact margins of the tumor is unnecessary. In instances of an adult patient presenting with an unknown lesion in the bone, a specific algorithm that can be found in the metastatic bone disease chapter should be followed.

Bone Scans and Other Nuclear Imaging

Nuclear imaging is a modality that can often be helpful in the assessment of bone tumors, but are often more expensive tests and expose the patient to higher levels of radiation, so should be reserved for when a true need for further diagnostic assessment is determined. There are several different forms of nuclear imaging that can be used to assess bone tumors. The most common is a nuclear bone scan. This test utilizes a technetium-99 radiolabeled diphosphonate, which upon injection into the circulatory system will go to sites of rapid bone turnover. If a three-phase bone scan is performed, there will be three phases of image analysis, an initial perfusion phase, which allows for assessment of blood flow to the skeleton, followed by a blood pool phase, which can be helpful in distinguishing some inflammatory conditions. Finally there is a late phase, which assesses the osteoblastic activity within the skeleton.

A tagged white blood cell (WBC) scan is another nuclear imaging modality that allows for the assessment of WBC activity at a skeletal site. This can be helpful for determining the presence of an infection in bone. It should be noted that some inflammatory conditions, including some tumors, may also show increased uptake on a tagged WBC scan. Another nuclear test that we frequently see ordered by our medical oncology colleagues is positron emission tomography (PET) scan, which is a nuclear test that utilizes radiotracer labeled glucose (18F-fluorodeoxyglucose, FDG) to identify metabolically active areas of the entire body. This test is not just limited to the skeleton, but can detect high metabolic activity anywhere in the body. Tumors, as well as healing injuries and infections, will show increased FDG uptake, so this test can be very nonspecific and is usually reserved for patients with a known diagnosis of malignancy when one is in search of metastatic disease. Recent cost analysis comparing PET scan to other modalities, such as chest radiograph or chest CT scan to survey for recurrent or metastatic disease in primary bone sarcomas, found that PET was never found to be cost-effective.[7] Therefore, ordering of a PET should be coordinated with the medical or pediatric oncology teams and not as a first-line test for assessing for bone or soft-tissue malignancy.

Soft-Tissue Tumors

Plain Radiographs

Plain radiographs are often less helpful for diagnostic purposes in soft-tissue masses. There are a few instances where plain radiographs can be diagnostic or at least narrow the diagnostic possibilities. Lipomas, particularly large ones, are examples of tumors that are often seen on plain radiograph (**Figure 4**). This is because fat has a lower density than muscle. On plain radiograph, one can see the contrast of the lower density fat adjacent to or within the higher density muscle and skin. Soft-tissue calcifications on plain radiographs can also be helpful in narrowing the diagnosis. Certain benign conditions, such as synovial chondromatosis, heterotopic bone, and the phleboliths (vascular calcifications) within vascular malformations, will all exhibit soft-tissue calcification. Several malignant conditions will also show calcifications within the soft tissue, such as synovial sarcoma and extra-skeletal osteosarcoma. Both of these latter conditions will often have other concerning features on MRI or CT.

CT Scans

CT scans for soft-tissue masses can be used to delineate a calcified body, such as the case of heterotopic bone (HO). In the case of HO, the calcifications will start at the periphery of the mass and progress centrally as the mass matures. This is in contrast to malignant conditions with calcification, which will often show a more haphazard and nonzonal pattern of calcification. When MRI is contraindicated, then a CT scan with contrast can allow for an assessment of the nature of the mass and its relationship to surrounding structures. A CT

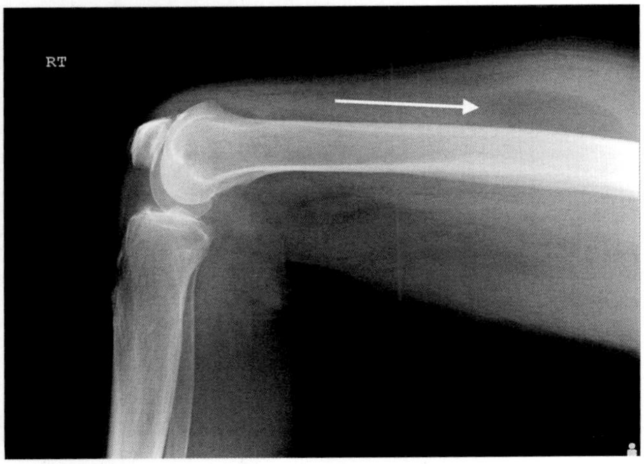

Figure 4 Plain radiograph of an intramuscular lipoma. White arrow points to an area of decreased density (the lipoma) within the muscle. The muscle having higher density than the lipoma allows one to see the lipoma on plain radiograph.

scan will often not give as much detail, such as subtle fat plane between the tumor and a nerve or vessel, but still can be very useful when MRI is not an option.

Magnetic Resonance Imaging

MRI with and without gadolinium contrast is the benchmark test for assessing soft-tissue masses. It allows for the clear distinction of fat versus denser fibrous tissue and allows for the determination of the water content of a mass. If done well, clear anatomic borders to a tumor can be determined, including assessing for the presence of peritumoral reactive edema. The addition of contrast allows for the detection of cystic versus solid masses and to determine degree of vascularity of a mass. All of this can help with the diagnostic process.

Unfortunately, even with a very well performed MRI, many masses will be considered indeterminate in nature and therefore will require a biopsy for final diagnosis. Some masses can be definitively diagnosed by MRI. A lipoma is one such example. A lipoma will have the same fat signal on all sequences, and in particular, will fully suppress on the fat suppression sequences. Cystic lesions, such as Baker's cysts, synovial cysts, and ganglion cysts, can almost always be determined with a contrast MRI as they will only exhibit contrast uptake at the very periphery of the lesion (**Figure 5**). Unfortunately, in many other instances, it may be difficult to distinguish benign versus malignant based on MRI alone. There are some features on MRI that may lead to concern for a more serious or malignant process. Invasion into surrounding structures, such as bone, tendon, vessel, or nerve, is often a worrisome sign. Similarly, heterogeneous enhancement with gadolinium is concerning for sarcoma. Peritumoral edema or less well defined borders to the tumor on MRI are both concerning findings. A large size greater than 5 cm and deep to the superficial fascia are also features that should raise suspicions for a sarcoma. These features taken together can indicate a very ominous process, but ultimately do not clinch the diagnosis. For any indeterminate mass, a biopsy will be required. No attempt should be made to resect an indeterminate mass without a biopsy first. An unplanned resection of a sarcoma will frequently increase the morbidity of the treatment required and increase the need for plastic surgery reconstruction following re-resection, and the risk of amputation.[8]

Biopsy, Grading, Molecular Diagnostics, and Staging of Tumors

Biopsy

As mentioned in the previous section, once a thorough investigation through history, physical examination, and imaging has been completed and the diagnosis is

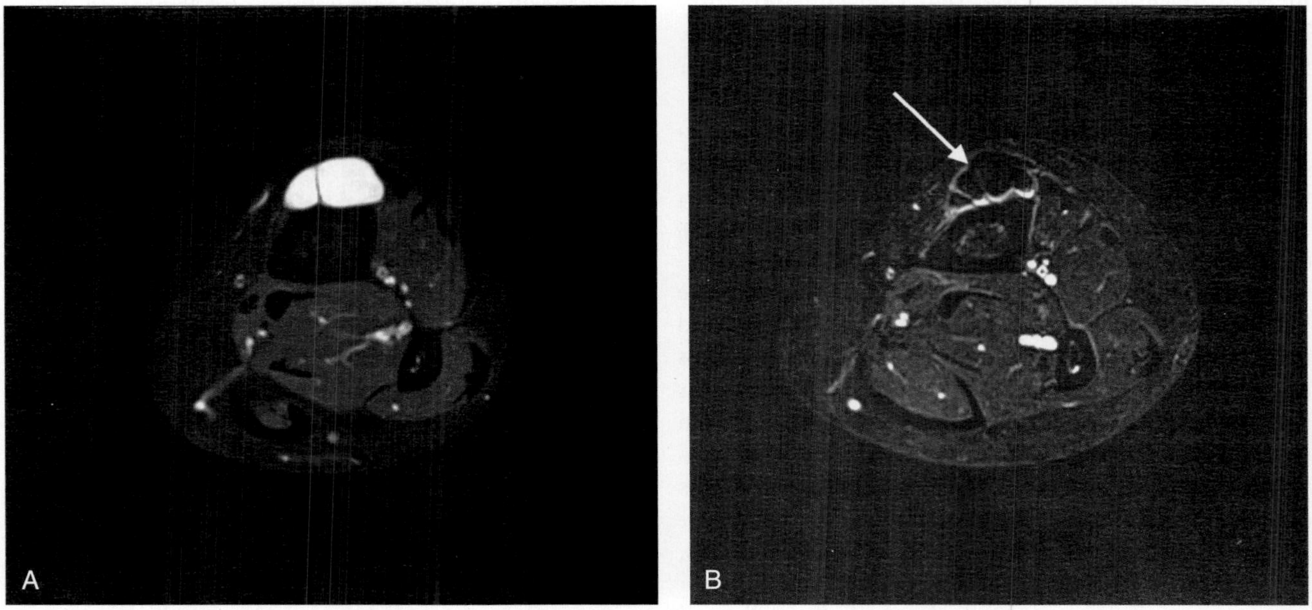

Figure 5 T2, fat saturated MRI without (**A**) and with (**B**) contrast. The white arrow in figure B points to the lesion in question, which can barely be seen in the contrast images because there is only minimal peripheral enhancement, confirming the cystic nature of the lesion. In A, the lesion can clearly be seen as a fluid containing lesion, but without contrast, one cannot confirm if it is solid with a lot of fluid or pure fluid.

still unclear, biopsy is usually necessary. The technique of biopsy for the musculoskeletal system is extremely important. Wrongly placed or performed biopsies can result in catastrophic outcomes for patients, including the need for amputation. Therefore, it is generally recommended that, whenever possible, the biopsy be performed at a tertiary care center with a skilled musculoskeletal oncologist and interventional radiologist. However, it is not uncommon for insurance companies to not cover the cost of a patient being seen at a tertiary care center without a specific diagnosis or a patient may have to travel a very long distance to obtain access to such centers, which may be infeasible for them. For this reason, every orthopaedic surgeon should have a basic understanding of biopsy technique.

There are several general principles to a musculoskeletal biopsy. First, avoid major nerves and vessels, as one does not want accidental contamination of these structures. Second, take the most direct route to the tumor in question, as long as there are no important structures in one's way. Thirdly, do not go between two muscle. This will contaminate both muscles and it is always best to only have to sacrifice one muscle at final resection. Fourthly, do not undermine skin or do extensive dissection outside of one's direct path to the tumor. This will only further contaminate the surrounding tissues. Remember, anything that is touched by the surgeon or the surgeon's instruments during the biopsy has to be resected at time of final resection. Fifthly, keep the biopsy tract and skin incision as small as possible to achieve acquisition of adequate tissue. Again, the biopsy tract must be resected with a 2 cm margin of normal tissue at time of final resection. If a drain must be used, it should never tunnel through the skin. Instead, it should be directly next to and in line with one's incision. All skin incisions should follow the same incision one would use for final resection. Many surgeons advocate drawing out your planned resection on the limb and then drawing out your biopsy along that resection incision if possible. Avoid horizontal incisions, except on the axial skeleton, as these generally do not follow an extensile approach in most cases. Finally, meticulous hemostasis should be achieved. This should be done with bovie, bipolar and sutures ties if necessary and any bone holes created that might bleed should be plugged with bone wax, bone cement, or gelfoam. Any hematoma that is present following biopsy is considered a site of contamination.

Tumor Grading

The grading of tumors is a histologic diagnosis. Benign tumors are not graded, but a pathologist may report histologic features, such as increased vascularity or increased mitotic activity to indicate a more aggressive tumor. These more aggressive features may be associated with a higher local recurrence rate or likelihood for "benign" hematogenous spread to the lungs. There are a few benign tumors that actually have a reported incidence of "benign" metastasis. This means the tumor can spread to the lungs, usually via hematogenous route, but once in the lung, the tumors nodules generally do not continue to grow or take over the lung parenchyma. This metastatic event is not thought to be a fatal event, as in the case of most malignant tumors. The two most common tumors in orthopaedics that will exhibit these pulmonary metastases are chondroblastoma and giant cell tumor of bone.[9,10]

All malignant tumors have a grade assigned to them, which is based on histologic features that have been shown to be associated with increased likelihood of metastatic disease or decreased disease specific survival. The grading system for mesenchymal tumors of the musculoskeletal system is normally G1 (low grade), G2 (intermediate grade), and G3 (high grade). The higher the grade, the greater the likelihood for metastatic disease and the lower the overall 5-year survival. Features that are generally associated with a higher grade are high mitotic activity, increased cellularity, nuclear atypia, greater cellular pleomorphism and heterogeneity, increased vascularity or vascular invasion, and decreased cellular features matching the original tumor tissue type (de-differentiation).

Molecular Diagnostics

Molecular diagnostics has changed the way we diagnose, and in many cases, even treat tumors. The genetic information often gleaned from molecular testing has allowed for much more precise diagnoses. The type of testing done can vary from immunohistochemistry, one of the more common and least costly forms of molecular testing, to more advanced chromosomal testing, such as fluorescent in situ hybridization (FISH). Immunohistochemistry can be used to detect a molecule produced by the tumor in its pathologic state. An antibody that is conjugated to a signaling substance, such as an enzyme, like horseradish peroxidase, or a beacon molecule, like a fluorescein, is used to identify the presence of a specific antigen. An example of such a test would be S-100 staining in nerve tumors. We now use a plethora of different molecular diagnostic tools to assist in the diagnosis of musculoskeletal tumors. **Table 2** provides examples of some of the more common examples, but is by no means an exhaustive list.

Oncology and Pathology

Table 2

Common Molecular Diagnostic Tests Used in the Musculoskeletal System

Tumor	Genetic Abnormality	Testing Used	Other Common Tests
Ewing sarcoma	Translocation 11:22 (FLi1:EWS) 21:22 (10% of cases)	FISH, RT-PCR	IHC for CD99
Synovial sarcoma	Translocation X:18 (SSX:SYT)	FISH, RT-PCR	IHC for epithelial membrane antigen and cytokeratin
Extraskeletal myxoid chondrosarcoma	Translocation 9:22 (CHN:EWS)	FISH, RT-PCR	
Rhabdomyosarcoma		IHC for desmin and myoglobulin	
Low-grade liposarcoma	MDM2 amplification	Quantitative PCR	
Dermatofibrosarcoma pertubans		IHC for CD34	
Langerhan's cell histiocytosis		IHC for CD1a and S100	
Elastofibroma		IHC for elastin	
Lymphoma		IHC for CD20	

The technique of FISH utilizes specific DNA probes that bind to regions of the cellular DNA.[11] These probes can be used to detect chromosomal rearrangements seen in translocations. If two probes are normally on separate chromosomes, if the FISH detects their presence side-by-side , then there has been a chromosomal rearrangement that has brought these two areas of the DNA together. This is an extremely sensitive test for looking for specific chromosomal translocations. Reverse transcriptase polymerase chain reaction (RT-PCR) is another useful diagnostic tool. This method allows for the detection of specific fusion proteins that are often formed as a result of a translocation.[11] The RNA is reverse transcribed into cDNA, which is then amplified to allow for visualization of this particular gene, which would normally not be detected in nonneoplastic tissue. Finally, one can do direct DNA sequencing or quantitative PCR to look for the presence of specific abnormal genes with a known mutation.

Staging of Tumors

Both bone and soft-tissue sarcomas have their own staging system, which is part of the American Joint Committee on Cancer staging system. Historically, both the bone and soft-tissue staging systems were developed by Dr. William Enneking and were referred to as the Enneking Staging for bone and soft-tissue sarcomas, respectively.[12] Enneking's staging system is based on grade of tumor, site of tumor (intra-compartmental versus extra-compartmental), and the presence of distant metastatic disease. Grading has been discussed above. The designation of intra-compartmental or extra-compartmental in the case of bone relates to whether the tumor has extended outside of the bone cortex. In the case of soft tissue, it refers to whether the tumor remains within the muscle compartment. A muscle compartment is defined as a muscle group that usually has its own fascial covering. An example would be the quadriceps muscle compartment. The final designation that Enneking believed was of clinical significance was whether the tumor was localized to one site or had regional or distant metastatic disease. This is still one of the most important factors for the determination of survival in patients with sarcomas.

The American Joint Committee on Cancer (AJCC) initially used the Enneking staging systems for bone and soft-tissue sarcomas, but as time went on, modifications were made to accommodate new knowledge pertaining to risk factors for survival. The AJCC staging system has become the standard staging used by both surgical and medical oncologists and is also widely used for research and clinical trial purposes. The most up-to-date versions of the AJCC staging systems for both bone and soft-tissue sarcomas now use size rather than compartment to designate the location of the tumor,[13] as that has been found to be more accurate and a more reproducible measure. Another more recent modification was the designation of intra-bone skip metastasis in bone sarcomas, which is associated with a poor prognosis, but not quite as poor as distant metastatic disease. The

Table 3

AJCC Staging for Bone Sarcomas[9]

Stage	Size (T)	Grade (G)	Node (N)	Metastatic (M)
Ia	<8c (T1)	Low grade (G1)	No nodal (N0)	No mets (M0)
Ib	>8 cm (T2) or skip met (T3)	Low grade (G1)	No node (N0)	No mets (M0)
IIa	<8 cm (T1)	Moderately differentiated high grade (G2) or high grade (G3)	N0	M0
IIb	>8 cm (T2)	G 2 or G3	N0	M0
III	Skip mets (T3)	G2 or G3	N0	M0
IV	Any T	Any G	Any N	Metastatic disease[a]

[a]AJCC breaks this down into stage IVa and IVb, with IVa being metastatic to lung and IVb representing metastatic to bone or other distant sites.

Data from AJCC Cancer Staging Manual, Eighth Edition (2017) published by Springer Science and Business Media LLC, www.springer.com.

most recent version of the AJCC (as of January 2018) also no longer uses intermediate grade designation and now uses moderately differentiated high grade (G2) and poorly differentiated high grade (G3)[13] for bone sarcomas only. For soft-tissue sarcomas, grade is separated out into low (G1), intermediate (G2), or high (G3) and also as a recent change the size designation is further characterized into less than 5 cm (T1), 5 to 10 cm (T2), 10 to 15 cm (T3), or greater than 15 cm (T4). This was done because of newer data pointing to the fact that a 5.5 cm tumor does not have the same prognosis as a 15.5 cm tumor. **Tables 3** and **4** provide the current simplified AJCC staging systems for bone and soft-tissue sarcomas, respectively.

Adjuvant Treatments

Adjuvant therapies often play a critical role in the management of patients with bone and soft-tissue sarcomas. As we will discuss below, they can dramatically affect local recurrence rates and overall survival for certain sarcomas. This means that the care of these patients must be closely coordinated with our radiation and medical oncology colleagues. These treatments are not without side effects and as surgeons, we need to be mindful of this in relation to our own treatments and counseling of patients. Unfortunately, not all sarcomas respond to adjuvant therapy, in which case surgery becomes the only curative option. Chondrosarcoma is

Table 4

AJCC Staging System for Soft-Tissue Sarcomas

Stage	Size (T)	Grade (G)	Node (N)	Metastatic (M)
Ia	<5 cm (T1)	Low (G1)	N0	M0
Ib	>5 cm (T1, 2, and 3)	Low (G1)	N0	M0
II	<5 cm (T1)	Intermediate or high (G2, G3)	N0	M0
IIIa	>5, but <10 cm (T2)	G2 or G3	N0	M0
IIIb	>10 cm (T3 and 4)	G2 or G3	N0	M0
IV	Any size	Any grade	Node positive or node negative with distant mets (N1, M0)	Distant mets or nodal mets (N0, M1)

Data from AJCC Cancer Staging Manual, Eighth Edition (2017) published by Springer Science and Business Media LLC, www.springer.com.

Table 5

Adjuvant Therapies in Treatment of Sarcomas

Sarcoma	Chemotherapy Sensitive	Radiation Therapy Sensitive
Osteosarcoma	Yes	No
Ewing sarcoma	Yes	Yes
Synovial sarcoma	Yes	Yes
Chondrosarcoma	No	No
High-grade soft-tissue sarcomas	Controversial	Yes

a clear example of a sarcoma that has no available systemic or regional adjuvant options, aside from what we do at the time of surgical resection. **Table 5** provides an overview of common sarcomas and the adjuvants that have been found effective in their treatment.

Chemotherapy

The story of chemotherapy is best told by looking at osteosarcoma. In the 1960s, the vast majority of patients received amputations for osteosarcoma and those patients went on to succumb to their diseases in about 80% of cases. In the early 1970s, physicians started exploring chemotherapeutic options, after seeing good results in leukemia and lymphoma patients. High-dose methotrexate (HDMTX) was one of the first agents used for this purpose. It then became evident that the use of multiagent therapy resulted in even better outcomes for patients. The three agents that stood out were HDMTX, Doxorubicin, and Cisplatin. With this three drug combination, 5-year survival rates jumped from a dismal 18% to around 65%. By the mid-1980s, this drug regimen had been established as the standard of care for high-grade osteosarcoma. This drug combination is still the backbone of all therapies for osteosarcoma today and unfortunately, we have not been able to move the survival rates further along with the addition of other agents or treatments thus far. Some institutions also add ifosfamide for high-risk or metastatic patients, but its benefit is controversial. Most patients receive neoadjuvant chemotherapy, which means two rounds of chemotherapy before surgery, followed by standard adjuvant chemotherapy of four rounds after surgery. This usually totals around 9 months of chemotherapy. The main purpose of the neoadjuvant chemotherapy is to allow for pathologist to provide an assessment of initial response to chemotherapy. Good responders (>90% necrosis) have a better prognosis than poor responders (<90% necrosis) and such data help guide further treatment and counseling to patients.

This same story can also be told for another bone sarcoma, Ewing sarcoma. Osteosarcoma and Ewing sarcoma make up the vast majority of the chemotherapy-sensitive cancers that we as orthopaedic surgeons primarily treat. It should be noted that all of these cytotoxic agents result in dysfunction of the immune system and therefore increase the risk of wound complications and infections. Other side effects that are important to note are doxorubicin which increases the risk of cardiomyopathy throughout the life of the patient. The next major advancement that will happen in the treatment of these and other bone sarcomas will be moving away from these cytotoxic agents, that simply blast the rapidly reproducing cells with poisons, and toward more targeted therapies with hopefully adverse effect profiles that can be tolerated better by patients.

One thing from a surgical standpoint that became evident in the era of chemotherapy discovery for osteosarcoma was that it was not the local disease that was resulting in the death of these often young children, but the microscopic systemic disease that was present at the time of initial evaluation. As a result, surgeons began using more limb-sparing techniques moving away from amputations as the surgical option. Today, less than 10% of patients receive an amputation for osteosarcoma.[14] The rate was above 80% 40 years ago.

Radiation Therapy

Like chemotherapy, the use of radiation therapy has greatly improved patient outcomes for certain sarcomas, primarily in the form of local control. There are now different forms of radiation therapy, but the general concept is that the tumor cells are exposed to particles or waves that lead to DNA damage and resultant cellular apoptosis. In an ideal world, those waves and particles would only be targeted to the cancer cells themselves and avoid normal tissues, but unfortunately, in most cases, the surrounding tissues are also exposed to the radiation. The smaller the field of radiation, the less exposure there is to the surrounding normal tissue. The standard dose of radiation for soft-tissue sarcomas is 50 to 66 Gray, which is double the dose given for most metastatic disease. The effects on the tissue are exponential and not linear, however, so the tissue damage as a result of this dose is significant.

In orthopaedic surgery, soft-tissue sarcomas are the most common cancer for which radiation is used. It was discovered through a series of trials that radiation therapy greatly reduced the risk of local recurrence in surgically resected soft-tissue sarcomas.[15] This was especially true for large and high-grade sarcomas and for sarcomas where surgical margins were negative. This latter finding points to the fact that even though surgeons felt they were doing an adequate job at resecting the soft-tissue sarcoma, in many instances, there were cells already outside of the surgical field. Radiation allows for the killing of those cells outside of the surgical field. It should be noted that although there is a reduction in local recurrence rate with the use of radiation therapy in soft-tissue sarcomas, there is not a direct association with overall survival. However, local recurrence is associated with poorer overall survival.

There is no difference in local recurrence rate with preoperative versus postoperative radiation. The use of preoperative versus postoperative radiation tends to be institution specific. Preoperative radiation therapy carries a significantly higher wound complication rate, so some surgeons prefer to give postoperative radiation. However, with postoperative radiation, the dose of radiation and field must be higher and bigger, respectively, to address the surgical edema. For this reason, many radiation oncologist advocate for preoperative radiation, especially with vital structures (bone, nerve, skin, etc).

As noted, radiation kills the cancer cells within the field of exposure; it also, unfortunately has deleterious effects on other tissues near or in the field of exposure. We have already mentioned wound complications due to skin and subcutaneous tissue damage. It is also not infrequent to see nerve damage, permanent lymphedema (lymphatic damage), and osteonecrosis and bone fragility. The nerve and bone damage can be very late complications, happening years later. Many surgeons will prophylactically stabilize a long bone that has been in the direct field of radiation for a soft-tissue sarcoma, for this reason. There is also a very low, but real, rate of postradiation sarcoma in areas that have received radiation. The incidence is thought to be less than 1% of patients who receive radiation for various reasons.[16]

Functional Outcome Measures

Functional outcomes have become an important part of any orthopaedic field. Analyzing and understanding function can afford surgeons a better understanding of the impact of a particular type of surgery on patients. Validated outcome measures can also allow for comparisons across surgeons, institutions, and countries, which will ultimately lead to better care for patients. There are several outcome measures used in orthopaedic oncology that warrant discussion. The musculoskeletal tumor society (MSTS) score is a scoring system that was created by members of the MSTS in 1985 and modified in 1993.[17] It takes the sum total of six measures (pain, function, emotional, supports, walking, and gait) in which patients are given a score from 0 to 5, with 0 representing worst possible outcome and 5 representing normal or societal baseline. A maximum score of 30 is possible. The major critique of the MSTS score is that in its original design, it was meant to be filled out by the surgeon, so it is not really a patient-reported outcome measure.[17] It also has a ceiling effect for looking at true outcome and some argue it is just not comprehensive enough to pick up subtle difference in function, pain, etc. It is still used by many researchers and surgeons today to obtain a global understanding of how a patient is doing after a sarcoma resection.

The Toronto Extremity Salvage Score (TESS) is a patient-reported outcome measure designed to determine functional outcomes in patients following limb salvage surgery for sarcoma treatment. The TESS has 29 questions for lower extremity and 28 questions for upper extremity. Activities of daily living are rated on a 5 point scale based on patient-reported experiences of not difficult at all to do to impossible to perform. This is thought to be a more comprehensive outcome measure, but may take longer for patients to fill out completely. The SF-36 (short-form 36) is a nondisease-specific patient-reported outcome measure with 36 questions. It has been validated and used extensively across many different disciplines of medicine. For this reason, it allows for comparison of patient-reported outcomes across diseases, not just oncologic or orthopaedic. It is commonly used by insurance companies and for research purposes.

The Patient-Reported Outcomes Measure Information System (PROMIS) is a validated nondisease-specific comprehensive outcome measure. It has multiple components to it that allow for physical as well as emotional satisfaction scores. Although relatively new compared with the other outcome measures discussed here, it is starting to have significant use in the United States. The main critique is that it can be a time-consuming test and for this reason, incomplete evaluations can be a problem. However, it can be easily loaded onto a computer or tablet and administered. In doing this, the program can skip questions that are irrelevant to a patient's particular circumstance. The PROMIS outcome measure has recently been used to look at patient progress following surgical management of metastatic bone disease with good success.[18] It will likely be a tool that continues to play an important role in follow-up of orthopaedic oncology patients. Several studies are underway currently looking at how well PROMIS compares to other older functional scoring systems, such as the MSTS and TESS. We will likely see the results of those studies in the near future. Much like the other outcome measures, it is simply a tool that physicians and researchers can use to gain a better understanding of the impact of diseases and our treatments on patient well-being. No test will be perfect, as subtle patient differences, experiences, and weighting of those experiences will be difficult to fully understand using a simple questionnaire. However, these tools can help guide therapies as we strive to improve patient care and surgical outcomes.

Summary

In this section, we discussed the clinical presentation and radiologic evaluation of patients presenting with musculoskeletal tumors. One can diagnose the vast majority of patients without invasive testing with the appropriate use of radiographs and judicious use of advanced imaging modalities. However, when clinical presentation and imaging fail to provide an answer, biopsy often with molecular testing is an extremely useful tool. The biopsy of tumors must be taken quite seriously, as performing a poor biopsy can lead to devastating consequences for patients.

Once a diagnosis is determined, an understanding of treatment is significant. We reviewed various treatments for malignant cancers, including chemotherapy and radiation therapy. Knowing when to use such approaches is necessary for good patient care. We have also discussed the future role of functional testing in orthopaedic oncology. In our current era focused on evidenced-based medicine, quality measures, and functional outcomes, these outcome measures will become increasingly more important in daily practice of orthopaedic oncology.

Key Study Points

- Distinguishing soft-tissue and bone tumors is a key starting point to the treatment of a patient with a musculoskeletal tumor.
- Pain, or lack thereof, is not indicative of malignancy in soft-tissue tumors.
- It is important to understand when various imaging techniques would be most helpful.
- Plain radiographs are an excellent starting point for most bone tumors.
- MRI is often helpful for soft-tissue tumors, bone masses with a soft-tissue component, and any malignant tumor.
- Understanding the key principles for performing a safe and effective musculoskeletal biopsy is paramount to care of patients with musculoskeletal tumors.
- Functional testing in orthopaedic oncology is gaining importance in the care and follow-up of patients.

Annotated References

1. Gokani VJ, Kangesu L, Harper J, Sebire NJ: Venous malformation associated nerve profiles and pain: An immunohistochemical study. *J Plast Reconstr Aesthet Surg* 2011;64(4):439-444.

2. Tatencloux S, Mosseri V, Papillard-Marechal S, et al: Care pathways before diagnosis in children and adolescents with malignancies. *Bull Cancer* 2017;104(2):128-138.

   A French hospital–based retrospective analysis of children presenting with malignancies anywhere in the body. The analysis retrospectively reviewed pediatric patients newly diagnosed with cancer at one major medical center over a 1-year period. One-hundred and six patients were identified and fit criteria for inclusion in the analysis. Greater than one-third of patients presented with pain as the primary complaint. Level of evidence: III.

3. Goedhart LM, Gerbers JG, Ploegmakers JJ, Jutte PC: Delay in diagnosis and its effect on clinical outcome in high-grade sarcoma of bone: A referral oncological centre study. *Orthop Surg* 2016;8(2):122-128.

   A single-institution retrospective review of patients diagnosed with high-grade bone sarcoma. Significant delays in diagnosis slightly greater than 160 days were identified for the diagnosis of osteosarcoma and Ewing's sarcoma, and greater than 600 days for chondrosarcoma. The authors found that most delays resulted before the patient was referred to a major medical center at the level of a general practitioner. Level of evidence: III.

4. Enneking WF: A system of staging musculoskeletal neoplasms. *Clin Orthop Relat Res* 1986;(204):9-24.

5. Jawad MU, Scully SP: In brief: Classifications in brief: Enneking classification: Benign and malignant tumors of the musculoskeletal system. *Clin Orthop Relat Res* 2010;468(7):2000-2002.

6. Brenner D, Elliston C, Hall E, Berdon W. Estimated risks of radiation-induced fatal cancer from pediatric CT. *AJR Am J Roentgenol* 2001;176(2):289-296.

7. Royce TJ, Punglia RS, Chen AB, et al: Cost-effectiveness of surveillance for distant recurrence in extremity soft tissue sarcoma. *Ann Surg Oncol* 2017;24(11):3264-3270.

   This study used a mathematical model, which simulates a cohort followed over time as the hypothetical cohort transitions through different phases of health states based on transition probabilities. The authors found that chest CT was most cost-effective and most effective at detecting disease, while standard CXR was still cost-effective, but less effective at detecting metastatic disease. PET was neither cost-effective nor better than chest CT at detecting metastatic disease. Level of evidence: II.

8. Traub F, Griffin AM, Wunder JS, Ferguson PC: Influence of unplanned excisions on the outcomes of patients with stage III extremity soft-tissue sarcoma. *Cancer* 2018;124(19):3868-3875.

   This was a single-institution retrospective review of patients referred for definitive management of a soft-tissue sarcoma after unplanned resection. Patient data were included from

1989 to 2010 with 94 patients meeting study criteria. The authors found a higher incidence of amputation and need for plastics coverage in patients with an unplanned resection. Eighty-three percent of re-resected specimens had residual tumor. The authors did not find a difference in overall survival or local recurrence after re-resection in this study population. Level of evidence: III.

9. Tamura M, Oda M, Matsumoto I, Sawada-Kitamura S, Watanabe G: Chondroblastoma with pulmonary metastasis in a patient presenting with spontaneous bilateral pneumothorax: Report of a case. *Surg Today* 2011;41(10):1439-1441.

10. Muheremu A, Niu X: Pulmonary metastasis of giant cell tumor of bones. *World J Surg Oncol* 2014;12:261.

11. Puls F, Niblett AJ, Mangham DC: Molecular pathology of bone tumours: Diagnostic implications. *Histopathology* 2014;64(4):461-476.

12. Enneking WF, Spanier SS, Goodman MA: A system for the surgical staging of musculoskeletal sarcoma. *Clin Orthop Relat Res* 1980;(153):106-120.

13. Amin MB, American Joint Committee on Cancer, American Cancer Society: in Amin MB, Edge SB, Gress DM, Meyer LR, ed: *AJCC Cancer Staging Manual*, ed 8. Chicago IL, American Joint Committee on Cancer, Springer, 2017.

    Most recent edition of the AJCC cancer staging manual. This simply outlines in full detail the new staging systems presented for all cancers. One can find the full updated sarcoma cancer staging system within this manual with some description of changes made to updated staging systems. Level of evidence: NA.

14. Tiwari A. Current concepts in surgical treatment of osteosarcoma. *J Clin Orthop Trauma* 2012;3(1):4-9.

15. Collin C, Godbold J, Hajdu S, Brennan M. Localized extremity soft tissue sarcoma: An analysis of factors affecting survival. *J Clin Oncol* 1987;5(4):601-612.

16. Mark RJ, Poen J, Tran LM, Fu YS, Selch MT, Parker RG: Postirradiation sarcomas. A single-institution study and review of the literature. *Cancer* 1994;73(10):2653-2662.

17. Uehara K, Ogura K, Akiyama T, et al: Reliability and validity of the musculoskeletal tumor society scoring system for the upper extremity in Japanese patients. *Clin Orthop Relat Res* 2017;475(9):2253-2259.

    This study used test-retest analysis to assess the reliability and internal consistency of the MSTS scoring system on patient treated with upper extremity tumors. The authors found that the MSTS was acceptable in comparison to TESS and SF-36 for functional outcomes, but fell short on global general health compared to TESS and SF-36. The MSTS scoring system was not originally designed to be a global health measure as the authors noted, which would explain this difference identified. Level of evidence: II.

18. Blank AT, Lerman DM, Shaw S, et al: PROMIS((R)) scores in operative metastatic bone disease patients: A multicenter, prospective study. *J Surg Oncol* 2018;118(3):532-535.

    A total of 13 patients with 9 data points for each patient collected over 6 months was reported by the authors. This a small prospective analysis of PROMIS scores among patients treated for metastatic pathologic and impending pathologic fractures. Scores showed appropriate improvement over time. The scores need comparison with MSTS, TESS, and SF-36, which was not accomplished in this study. Level of evidence: IV.

Chapter 66

Benign Bone Tumors

Sean V. McGarry, MD

ABSTRACT

Benign bone tumors are commonly encountered by practicing orthopaedic surgeons. Knowledge of the characteristic findings of the most common of these lesions is essential to appropriately observe or refer to an orthopaedic oncologist for further workup. This chapter will present the most common benign bone tumors grouped by the matrix being produced by the lesion. This will include (1) cartilage-producing tumors—osteochondroma, chondromas (including periosteal chondroma and enchondroma), chondroblastoma, and chondromyxoid fibroma; (2) bone-producing tumors—osteoid osteoma and osteoblastoma; (3) fibrous tumors—nonossifying fibroma and desmoplastic fibroma; (4) cystic tumors—unicameral bone cyst and aneurysmal bone cyst. Also included in this chapter will be a discussion of Langerhans cell histiocytosis, giant cell tumor of bone, and fibrous dysplasia, three lesions that do not fall into a distinct category. Discussion of treatment of benign bone tumors will focus on curettage and surgical adjuvants as well as radiofrequency ablation. Standard treatment of these lesions has not changed much in recent history, but recent trends in alternative treatments will be explored.

Keywords: benign bone tumors; bone lesion; curettage; radiofrequency ablation

Dr. McGarry or an immediate family member serves as a paid consultant to or is an employee of Musculoskeletal Transplant Foundation; has received research or institutional support from Musculoskeletal Transplant Foundation; and serves as a board member, owner, officer, or committee member of the National Comprehensive Cancer Center Bone Committee and the Soft Tissue Committee.

Introduction

The incidence of bone tumors is difficult to know. Many lesions are diagnosed incidentally on imaging for trauma or other aches and pains; probably many more lesions go undiagnosed. Additionally, many are only observed and a tissue diagnosis is never made. Regardless, most benign bone tumors have characteristic features that suggest their specific diagnosis. Familiarity with these characteristics will allow the practicing orthopaedic surgeon to follow with imaging to confirm radiographic stability or refer to an orthopaedic oncologist for diagnosis and treatment. Many of the characteristic findings are present on plain radiographs. All benign bone lesions should be imaged with at least orthogonal radiographs. Well-demarcated margins suggest a benign diagnosis, and observation of the matrix produced by the lesion will give a clue to the specific diagnosis. Other clues as to the diagnosis are that certain tumors occur in typical anatomic locations. Additionally, the location of the tumor within the bone itself is often helpful in making diagnoses. Most asymptomatic lesions can be treated conservatively. Symptomatic lesions are treated based on the natural history of the lesion. An osteochondroma causing mechanical popping of the hamstring tendons is not likely to improve and should be excised. A nondisplaced fracture through a phalangeal enchondroma with associated trauma can heal on its own with no further treatment.

Osteochondroma

Osteochondromas (or exostoses) are one of the most common of the benign bone tumors. In the Mayo clinic series they represented about one-third of all benign bone tumors.[1] Osteochondromas can present as either a solitary lesion or one of multiple lesions in a hereditary form of the disease MHE (multiple hereditary exostoses). The disorder is caused by a defect in either the EXT1 or EXT2 tumor suppressor genes and is inherited in an autosomal dominant pattern. Patients with MHE develop multiple exostoses throughout the skeleton.

They have a lifetime risk of malignant degeneration of an exostosis into a sarcoma of less than 2%.[2] They may also have short stature and gross deformity of the extremities in more severe cases. Patients with EXT1 mutations have been shown to have a higher risk of malignant degeneration than patients with mutations in the EXT2 gene.[3]

Patients present most commonly with a firm, nonmobile bump at or near a joint, most frequently the knee. It may be tender, but often is painless. They will occasionally describe mechanical symptoms that are caused by a muscle, tendon, or ligament moving over the lesion during activities.

On physical examination the mass is nonmobile and clearly attached to the underlying bone. Osteochondromas about the medial knee will often produce a visible and/or palpable clunk with motion of the knee. Occasionally, an overlying bursa will be palpable as a firm mass, raising concern for malignant degeneration. Imaging studies will generally demonstrate a fluid signal consistent with a fluid-filled bursa.

Plain radiographs demonstrate either a sessile (broad based) or pedunculated (stalk-like) growth off the metaphysis of a bone. Pedunculated exostoses point away from the epiphysis. CT scan or radiographs demonstrate the medullary bone flows into the base of the lesion without intervening cortex. CT scan or MRI will also demonstrate a cartilaginous cap over the top of the osteochondroma with a variable thickness, but normally a few millimeters. In growing children it is not uncommon to see a cartilage cap of 1 to 2 cm in thickness. In patients at skeletal maturity, a cartilage cap of greater than 2 cm raises concern for malignant degeneration to a chondrosarcoma (see **Figure 1**).

Most osteochondromas present as a bump. If the lesion is asymptomatic, it is not necessary to remove it. If the lesion is symptomatic, because of pain, mechanical symptoms, or appearance, the mass can be removed. Recurrence is uncommon in solitary pedunculated lesions. Recurrences more often occur in patients with sessile lesions or in patients with MHE.

Chondroma

Chondromas consist of both the more common enchondromas, which are intraosseous, and periosteal chondromas, which occur on the surface of the bone. These will be dealt with together, with differences noted as appropriate. Enchondromas are a relatively common benign bone, existing as 15.6% of the cases in the Mayo Clinic series.[1] Although their true incidence is probably higher, as many likely go undiagnosed because they are asymptomatic. Like osteochondromas they can occur as solitary lesions or in multiple skeletal locations (enchondromatosis or Ollier's disease). Enchondromatosis and multiple soft-tissue angiomas together are known as Maffucci's syndrome. Maffucci's syndrome and Ollier's disease both have an increased risk (reported rates vary greatly) of developing sarcomas or nonsarcomatous cancers over the course of their lifetime.[4]

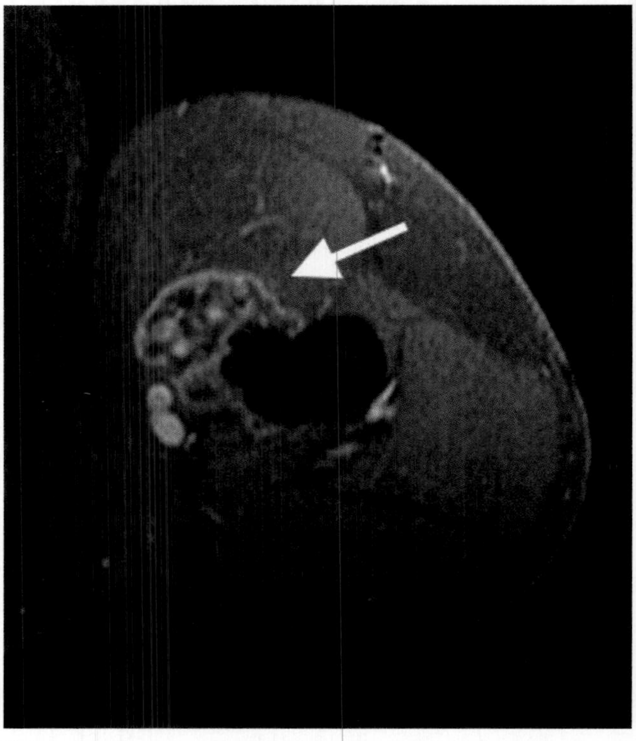

Figure 1 Axial cut MRI demonstrates thickened cartilage cap on a sessile osteochondroma (arrow), raising suspicion for a chondrosarcoma.

Most enchondromas present as incidental findings in the long bones. In general, they are thought to be painless. Frequently radiographs or MRI for adjacent pathology (eg, rotator cuff tear or osteoarthritis of the knee) will demonstrate a lesion unrelated to the symptoms for which the imaging was performed. Pathologic fracture is a much more common presentation in the small bones of the hands and feet. These are treated operatively more often, which probably explains the higher incidence of lesions in the hands and feet of the Mayo series.

On physical examination there are generally no outward signs of a bone lesion. There may be unrelated pain and examination findings from the underlying problem such as a frozen shoulder, rotator cuff pathology, or knee arthritis. Radiographs and CT scans of enchondromas typically show stippled or "popcorn" calcifications. Periosteal chondromas will show scalloping of the periosteal surface. MRI will usually show decreased homogenous signal on T1-weighted imaging and increased homogenous signal on T2-weighted imaging. Postcontrast images will show diffuse uptake throughout the lesion. Imaging should be surveyed for aggressive features suggesting a diagnosis of chondrosarcoma. Findings suspicious for malignancy include endosteal scalloping >50% of the cortical thickness, areas of radiolucency within the lesion, and cortical breakthrough or soft-tissue mass. Active lesions will show increased uptake on bone scan that has no correlation to a malignant diagnosis. A recent review looked at chondroid lesions in F-18 FDG PET and found that while SUVmax correlates with histologic grade in chondroid tumors, it was difficult to differentiate between benign and low-grade malignant lesions.[5]

Incidentally found lesions in the long bones are generally treated conservatively. Serial radiographs are obtained to confirm radiographic stability. Medical management with anti-inflammatories, and therapy or surgery is sought for the true pain generator. In patients seeking care for pathologic fracture in bones of the hands and feet, treatment may consist of conservative management to allow the fracture to heal or curettage, bone grafting, open reduction and internal fixation as needed for displaced or large lesions likely to refracture.

Chondroblastoma

Chondroblastomas are uncommon benign bone tumors, but often have a classic presentation. They represent about 5% of all benign bone tumors in the classic Mayo clinic series.[1] Patients present most commonly with localized pain. Often patients describe their pain as peri-articular, secondary to the lesions' frequent occurrence in the epiphysis. Other patients will complain of a stiff joint. Patients will sometimes have a long protracted history of symptoms.

Physical findings such as a lump or mass are often absent. More common is a vague tenderness or pain with motion of the involved joint, most frequently the knee or shoulder.

On plain radiographs almost all patients will show a radiolucent lesion either partially or completely within the epiphysis or apophysis. This is one of the hallmark findings that make chondroblastoma a diagnostic consideration for almost any apophyseal/epiphyseal lesion. Common locations include active long bone physes: proximal tibia, distal femur, proximal humerus, and proximal femur. Other locations include the talus, calcaneus, and patella. On CT scan the lesion is radiolucent, ovoid in shape, and well demarcated, and occasionally shows some punctate calcification. MRI shows increased central signal on T2-weighted imaging consistent with a chondroid matrix, a thin sclerotic rim, as well as surrounding edema.

Treatment consists of curettage with surgical adjuvants and bone grafting. The peri-articular location of these tumors can sometimes make an extended curettage challenging without violating the articular surface. Many of these patients go on to develop osteoarthritis and some even require arthroplasty at an early age as a result of these lesions. Because of its blood supply the proximal femur and talus are considered high-risk locations.[6] For this reason there has been an increase in the use of radiofrequency ablation (RFA) to treat chondroblastoma. A recent article presents results of RFA for chondroblastoma with success rates similar to those of RFA for treatment of osteoid osteoma.[7] Chondroblastoma is one of the rare benign bone tumors that can metastasize to the lungs. Typically it remains as a benign tumor in the lungs and can be resected for curative intent.

Chondromyxoid Fibroma

Chondromyxoid fibroma is a very rare benign bone tumor. Patients will typically present with pain in the area of concern, often describing long-standing symptoms. Sometimes patients will have a bump or tenderness in the area.

Physical examination findings are nonspecific, other than anatomic location. The most common location for chondromyxoid fibroma is the metaphysis of the proximal tibia. The next most common location is the distal femur. On radiographs the lesions are eccentrically located in the metaphysis, radiolucent, clearly demarcated from adjacent bone, and sometimes expansile of cortical bone. The radiographic appearance is often described as looking like "soap bubbles." The lobular organization of the tissue is also recognized on MRI.

Standard treatment is curettage, with surgical adjuvants as necessary. Small lesions can be excised en bloc without significant morbidity for better local control. Surgical defects can be bone-grafted.

Osteoid Osteoma

Osteoid osteoma and osteoblastoma share similar histologic features. They differ in anatomic distribution and size. Osteoid osteomas are less than 2 centimeters in size and osteoblastomas are larger. Osteoid osteoma represents about 13% of all benign bone tumors according to the Mayo Clinic series.[1]

Oncology and Pathology

Osteoid osteoma occurs two to three times more frequently in males than in females. It can present in nearly any bone of the body, but occurs most frequently in the femur and tibia. When it is located in the spine, it occurs typically in the posterior elements. Patients with osteoid osteoma classically present with localized pain, worse at night or at rest and significantly relieved by aspirin or NSAIDs. In the spine osteoid osteoma may produce a curvature of the spine.

Examination may not show more than tenderness or swelling in the area of concern. Late presenting osteoid osteoma may produce leg-length inequality (affected leg longer) and scoliosis.

Radiographs may show only periosteal thickening or nothing at all. When a radiograph shows a typical nidus, it can be diagnostic. When not obvious on radiographs, the nidus will be readily apparent on a CT scan (see **Figure 2**). Axial cuts clearly demonstrate a central radiolucency with thickened reactive rim around it. MRI findings are more subtle, but will also demonstrate the edema surrounding the lesion.

First line of treatment is aspirin or NSAIDs. Osteoid osteoma is a self-limited lesion that eventually burns out. Historically, surgery to completely remove the nidus was performed for lesions that failed conservative management. Surgery was challenging secondary to the small size of the lesion or associated with morbidity from fracture, from overzealous removal of bone. The introduction of radiofrequency ablation (either with CT-guidance or navigation) has equaled or bettered success rates of open surgery with less morbidity.[8,9] More recently, several groups have found similar results with a completely noninvasive technique known as magnetic resonance imaging–guided high-intensity focused ultrasound (MR-HIFU).[10-12]

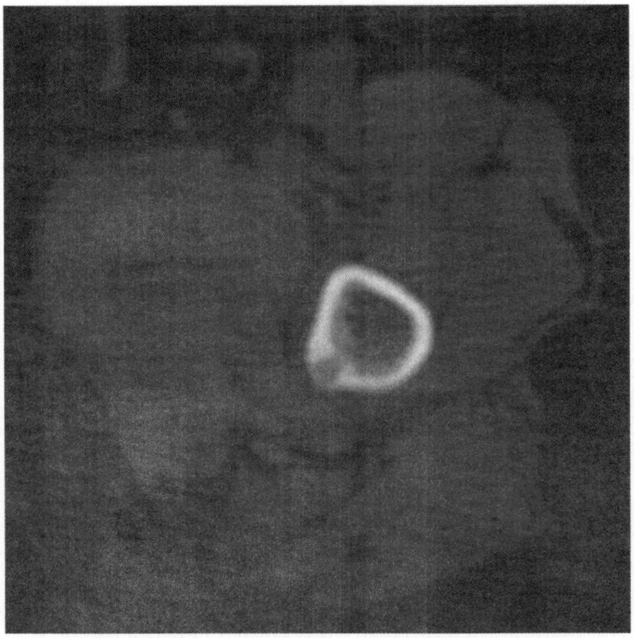

Figure 2 Axial cut CT shows osteoid osteoma. Note the radiolucent nidus with reactive sclerosis surrounding it.

Osteoblastoma

As noted in the prior section, osteoblastoma and osteoid osteoma share similar histologic features. Osteoblastomas are larger than 2 cm in size and osteoid osteomas are smaller. Osteoblastoma occurs less frequently than osteoid osteoma, accounting for 3.5% of all benign bone lesions. Osteoblastomas have been reported in almost all bones, but nearly half of them occur in the spine, most commonly in the posterior elements.[1]

Osteoblastoma shows a marked predilection for male patients. Nearly all patients with osteoblastomas present to their treating physician with pain. Occasionally patients with osteoblastoma of the spine will present with neurologic symptoms. Unlike osteoid osteoma, patients with osteoblastoma do not show a remarkable response to anti-inflammatory medications.

Physical examination findings may be limited to tenderness in the area of the lesion. Patients with spine lesions may have scoliosis or neurologic symptoms consistent with the level of involvement of the spine.

Radiographs show a radiolucent ovoid lesion with a thin reactive rim. Lesions of the long bones are typically located in the metaphysis. Lesions of the spine are most common in the posterior elements. Osteoblastomas can produce secondary aneurysmal bone cyst, with cystic features dominating the radiographic presentation.

Standard treatment consists of curettage of the lesion, with possible addition of intraoperative adjuvants such as high-speed burr and argon coagulopathy. Like chondroblastoma and giant cell tumor (GCT) of bone, osteoblastoma can metastasize to the lung. It is still considered benign, shows indolent growth, and can be resected with curative intent. A recent retrospective study showed success in a small number of patients with osteoblastomas treated with RFA.[13]

Nonossifying Fibroma

Nonossifying fibroma (also described as metaphyseal fibrous defect or fibrous cortical defect) is not a true neoplasm but rather a deficiency in ossification of the developing skeleton. The incidence of nonossifying fibromas (NOF) is unknown as they are most often found incidentally. It is estimated that up to one-third of all children have one or more of these lesions.[14] The most common location is around the knee, followed by the ankle. They are uncommon outside of the lower extremity. Most often patients with NOF are asymptomatic and the lesion is incidentally found on radiographs. Occasionally a patient will present with a pathologic fracture through a larger lesion (**Figure 3**).

Radiographic findings demonstrate an eccentric radiolucent and metaphyseal lesion that begins at the edge of the physis and grows away from it. Its multiloculated, bubbly appearance is somewhat similar to a chondromyxoid fibroma. Treatment is conservative observation in asymptomatic patients. Large lesions or pathologic fractures can be curetted, bone-grafted, and stabilized as necessary.

Desmoplastic Fibroma

Desmoplastic fibroma is the bony variant of soft-tissue fibromatosis or desmoid tumor. Desmoplastic fibroma is exceedingly rare. Presenting symptoms are pain and swelling in the area of concern. Occasionally in long-standing cases the patient will present with pathologic fracture. Physical findings are nonspecific. Radiographs demonstrate uneven, destructive, radiolucent lesions with expansion of the involved bone, sometimes described as a "honeycomb" pattern (see **Figure 4**). Desmoplastic fibroma is locally aggressive and has a high recurrence rate if not completely excised. Recommended treatment is marginal resection when possible without significant morbidity. If marginal resection would cause significant morbidity,

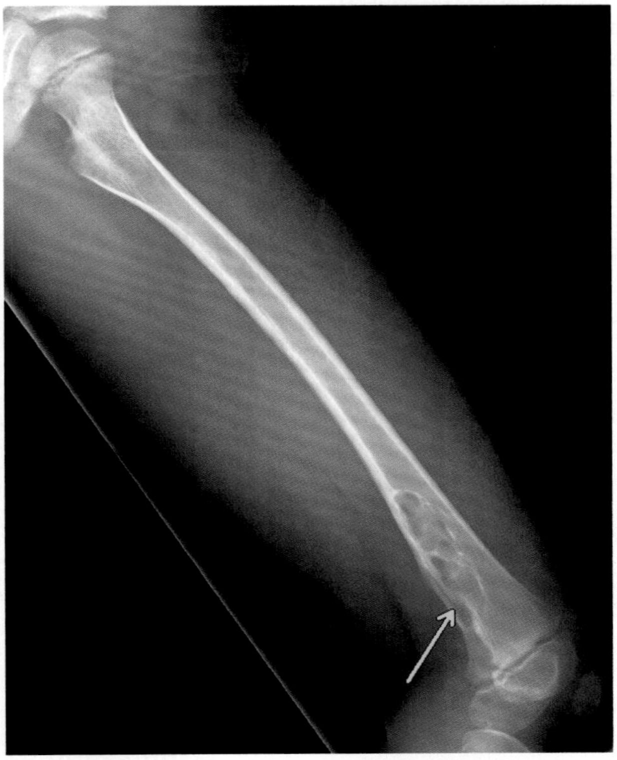

Figure 3 Lateral radiograph demonstrates a large femoral nonossifying fibroma. Arrow shows nondisplaced fracture through postero-lateral cortex.

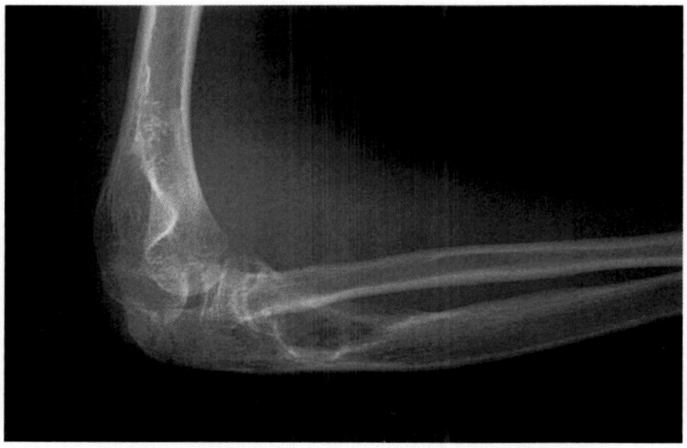

Figure 4 Lateral radiograph shows destructive, radiolucent, "honeycomb pattern" characteristic of desmoplastic fibroma.

an attempt is made at aggressive curettage. With multiple recurrences an amputation is occasionally needed for local control.

Unicameral Bone Cyst

A unicameral (or simple) bone cyst (UBC) is a fluid-filled cystic cavity arising on the metaphyseal side of the epiphyseal plate. It is not a true neoplasm. It is not known what causes UBCs. The true incidence of UBC is unknown, as many go undiagnosed.

Presentation

Patients may present with pain in the area likely secondary to microfracture. The more common presentation is after a pathologic fracture, often secondary to minor mechanism. Patient may or may not give a history of antecedent pain. Most common locations include (in order): proximal humerus, proximal femur, and proximal tibia.

On examination in a patient with pathologic fracture findings are similar to any other fracture—swelling, pain, and guarding of the extremity. Radiographs demonstrate a radiolucent lesion in the metaphysis of the involved bone with (or without) a fracture. If it is the initial presentation, there will not be any septations in the cyst (differentiating it from an aneurysmal bone cyst). Sometimes there is a fragment of cortical bone at the bottom of the cyst—"fallen leaf sign."

Unicameral bone cysts are graded as either active or latent. Active cysts occur in younger children (<10 years of age) and anatomically are adjacent to the physis. Latent cysts occur in older children (>10 years of age) and have grown some distance away from the physis. Latent cysts will often heal after a pathologic fracture. Active cysts are more likely to persist after pathologic fracture. In the setting of multiple pathologic fractures, an attempt at aspiration with injection of corticosteroid or demineralized bone matrix will sometimes stimulate a healing response. Cysts that have failed to heal after multiple attempts at injection may require a formal curettage and bone grafting. Incidentally found, asymptomatic cysts need no intervention, as their natural history is to heal with skeletal maturity.

Aneurysmal Bone Cyst

Whether aneurysmal bone cyst (ABC) is a true neoplasm or a reactive process is debatable. Historically it has been considered to be a reactive process. The fact that rearrangement of the USP6 gene occurs in 70% of all primary ABCs lends evidence to the former (that it is a neoplasm). Aneurysmal bone cyst can arise as a primary lesion in bone or as a reactive lesion in association with other neoplasms (chondroblastoma, osteoblastoma, or GCT of bone). This makes a discussion about the incidence of ABC problematic.

The lesion can be found anywhere in the skeleton but has a predilection for the posterior elements of the spine and metaphysis of the long bones (in particular around the knee). Patients will typically present with pain and swelling of the area of involvement. Patients present less commonly with pathologic fracture.

On physical examination the patient has a tender, swollen extremity. Occasionally an enlargement of the bone is palpable. Patients with tumors in their spine may or may not have neurological signs relating to their pathology.

Radiographs demonstrate an eccentric expansile radiolucent mass in the metaphysis. The cortical margin is often significantly thinned to absent. The central portion contains multiple septae. On MRI the cysts have classic "fluid-fluid levels" (see **Figure 5**). This is caused by the separation of blood into its fluid and cellular components.

Standard treatment is curettage with surgical adjuvants and bone grafting. Larger lesions may require temporary stabilization with plates and screws until the bone remodels. Recurrences are not uncommon but are treated the same.

Langerhans Cell Histiocytosis

Langerhans cell histiocytosis (LCH) is the term used to describe a spectrum of disease caused by a proliferation of macrophages. The different forms of the

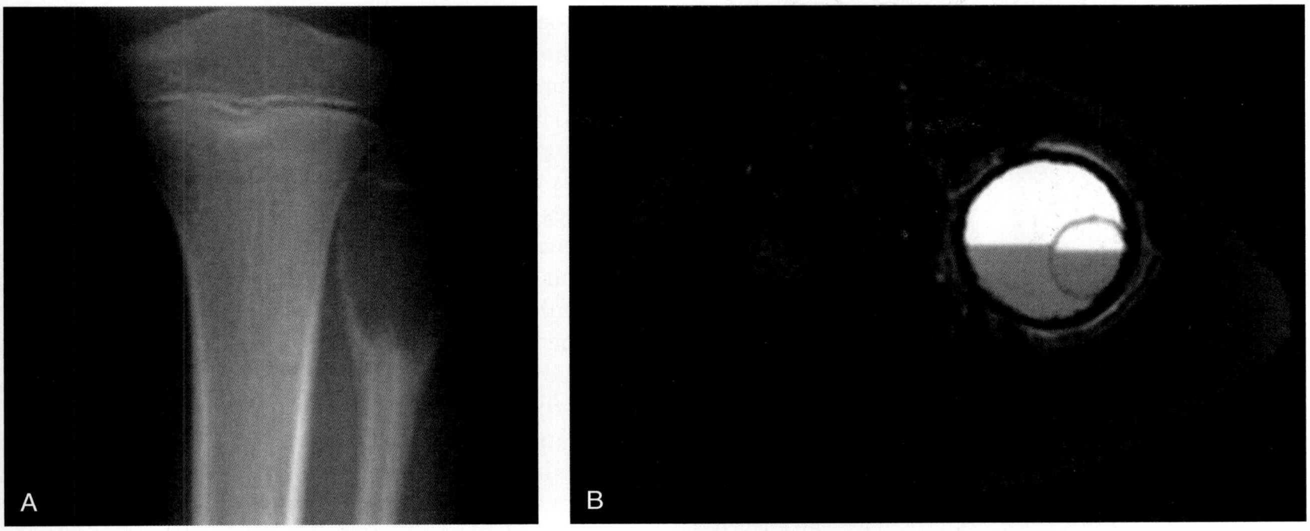

Figure 5 **A**, AP radiograph shows expansile lesion in the metaphysis of the proximal fibula, consistent with an aneurysmal bone cyst. **B**, Axial cut MRI shows the "fluid-fluid levels" characteristic of an aneurysmal bone cyst.

disease range from an isolated bone lesion to disseminated disease known as Schüller-Christian disease to rapidly fatal version of the disease known as Letterer-Siwe disease. The last two entities are more similar to leukemia or lymphoma. The focus of this discussion will be on the bone lesion described as Langerhans cell histiocytosis.

The lesions can occur anywhere in the skeleton, but have a propensity for the skull and anterior elements of the spine. When presenting in the long bones, they occur in the metaphysis and diaphysis. Patients generally present with pain or limp if it is a lower extremity lesion.

Physical findings are nonspecific in skeletal lesions. Children with disseminated disease may present with a variable presentation and appear quite sick. Spine lesions may present with focal neurologic findings based on level of lesion.

Radiographic findings can vary. Patients with disease in their spine often have a classic "vertebra plana" or flattened vertebral body. In flat bones LCH usually appears as a poorly marginated radiolucent lesion. In the long bones LCH tends to have a more distinct reactive rim. Because of its variable radiographic presentation Langerhans cell histiocytosis has been described as the "great imitator."

Treatment for LCH also varies depending on the level of involvement. Mono-ostotic lesions will often spontaneously regress after incomplete excision. Extended curettage and bone grafting is generally curative for bony lesions. Disseminated disease requires chemotherapy.

Giant Cell Tumor of Bone

Giant cell tumor (GCT) of bone is a unique tumor in many respects. It is one of the few benign bone tumors that have the capacity to metastasize. It also has the potential for malignant degeneration. It presents as one of the more common types of benign bone tumor but occurs most frequently in a population that is slightly older than most of the other benign bone tumors. In the Mayo series GCT represents just over 20% of all benign bone tumors.[1]

The exact cell of origin of GCT is not known. Historically the giant cells were thought to arise from the fusion of the mononuclear cells, but now it is thought that the mononuclear cells are what drives the dysregulation of the RANK pathway, disrupting the balance between the formation and resorption of bone.

GCT is very rare in skeletally immature patients. Almost all lesions occur in the epiphysis or epiphysis and metaphysis. Nearly half of all lesions in the Mayo series occurred about the knee, in either the distal femur or proximal tibia. The next most common sites of involvement were the distal radius and the sacrum. Pain is by far the most common presentation. Pathologic fracture is uncommon in GCT.

On physical examination patients have pain and swelling in the area. Frequently the examination overlaps with meniscal pathology or degenerative arthritis. Often the tumor has a soft-tissue component that can be appreciated on examination. Sometimes an effusion of the adjacent joint is present.

On plain radiographs the lesion appears as an eccentric, expansile, radiolucent mass involving the epiphysis

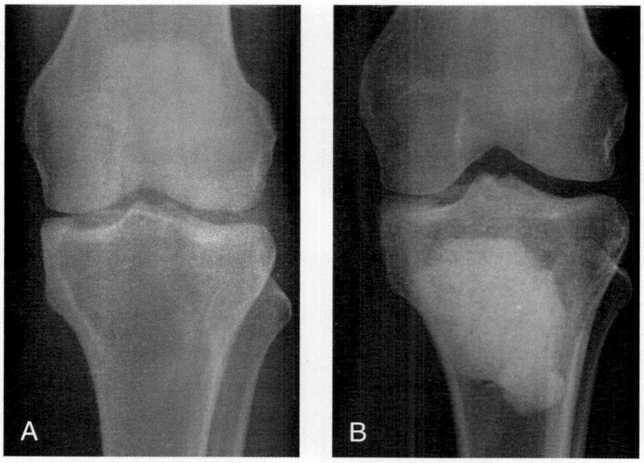

Figure 6 **A**, Pre-op radiograph of a large destructive giant cell tumor in the proximal tibia. **B**, Post-op radiograph of the same patient after treatment with extended curettage with argon beam coagulopathy. The defect was reconstructed with a combination of allograft bone in the subchondral region and bone cement in the metaphysis.

and metaphysis and frequently extending all the way to the subchondral bone (see **Figure 6**, **A** and **B**). Sometimes destruction of the cortex and a soft-tissue component will suggest a malignant diagnosis. CT imaging shows a similar picture of purely lytic eccentric lesion involving epiphysis, and metaphysis and expanding the cortex. MRI may better demonstrate the soft-tissue component, as well as adjacent bony edema.

Standard treatment consists of extended curettage with surgical adjuvants and bone grafting, cementation, or both. Often the large size of these lesions necessitates stabilization with plate and screws. The screws in the cement act as rebar to help stabilize the defect to adjacent normal bone. Intra-articular involvement requires osteo-articular or prosthetic reconstruction.

Denosumab is a monoclonal antibody that inhibits the RANKL ligand inhibitor that interferes with activation of osteoclasts. In 2013 the FDA approved denosumab for the treatment of GCT. Initial results of its use were encouraging for beneficial tumor response.[15-18] More recent studies have brought to light concerns of higher recurrence rates when therapy is stopped. Additionally, there is potentially an association of denosumab therapy and malignant transformation or novel development of sarcoma.[19,20]

Fibrous Dysplasia

Fibrous dysplasia is also not a true neoplasm. It is a deficiency in the development of bone. The trabecular bone in affected areas fails to organize along stress lines and does not mineralize normally. This leads to weakened bone prone to deformity and pathologic fracture. It occurs in either a mono-ostotic or polyostotic form. Often in the polyostotic variant overlying skin has brown pigmentation or "café au lait" spots. Polyostotic fibrous dysplasia in association with endocrine abnormalities is known as McCune-Albright syndrome. The incidence of fibrous dysplasia is unknown as many patients with this disease (especially the mono-ostotic version) are asymptomatic.

The lesions of fibrous dysplasia occur in all bones of the body, but commonly in the skull, jaw bones, ribs, and proximal femur. In mono-ostotic fibrous dysplasia, patients usually present with unrelated trauma or sports injuries. The lesion is an incidental finding on radiographs taken for other reasons. In polyostotic disease the patients present with stress fractures and pain in affected bones.

Physical examination findings include the café au lait spots. Patients with severe disease may demonstrate bowing of long bones. Involvement of the jaw bones causes visible deformity. Radiographic findings in fibrous dysplasia can vary significantly. Affected areas of the bone are often expansile with a thin cortical rim and a central homogenous gray "ground glass" appearance. In the proximal femur, constant fracture and remodeling will produce a bowing deformity classically described as a "shepherd's crook deformity."

Treatment of the incidental finding is unnecessary. Mono-ostotic lesions will often slowly remodel and mature after skeletal maturity. Progressive deformities can be corrected with osteotomies and intramedullary fixation. Deformities that have led to secondary arthritis will require joint replacement. Diphosphonates can be used to treat patients with painful lesions without fracture.[21]

Surgical Treatments of Benign Bone Lesions

Curettage and Surgical Adjuvants

In lesions that need surgery, curettage with or without surgical adjuvants has historically been the standard treatment for benign bone tumors and tumor-like conditions, with the exception of osteochondromas. Curettage is an intralesional excision. That is, tumor cells can be left behind, allowing for the lesion to recur. Surgical adjuvants are added to decrease that risk of recurrence.

The first step in curetting a benign bone tumor is gaining exposure. The key is a large bone window. The bone window must be at least as large as the base of the lesion. Any attempt at curettage with a smaller window will inevitably leave behind tumor on the endosteal surface of the bone around the corner from the existing window. By extending the window to the full size of the lesion the entire endosteal surface can be visualized and appropriately curetted. Once an adequate bone window/exposure is achieved, a large curet is used to debulk the lesion. Next the edge of the curet can be used to forcibly scrape across the entire surface of the cavity. Following the methodical curettage a high-speed burr is used in combination with irrigation and suction to extend the margin of the curettage. This is repeated after a thorough and aggressive irrigation, followed by another thorough and aggressive irrigation. It is at this point that a surgical adjuvant is added to the procedure.

The most common options for surgical adjuvants include phenol, liquid nitrogen, polymethyl methacrylate, and argon beam coagulation. Early reports on recurrence rate in simple curetting approached 45%.[22] When high-speed burring was added, the procedure was described as extended curettage and recurrence rates dropped.[23] Historically adjuvants such as phenol and liquid nitrogen were used to help lessen the recurrence rate. Various papers have shown improvements in recurrence rates; however, the use of these adjuvants was not without complications. Phenol is quite toxic to normal tissues, and it is difficult to keep it from coming into contact with adjacent tissue in the process of applying and then aspirating and then irrigating out the lesion cavity. Liquid nitrogen caused damage to adjacent normal bone and had unacceptably high rates of fracture. Neither option allowed for the surgeon to control the extension of the margin. A newer adjuvant termed "freezing nitrogen ethanol" is a semisolid material that may mitigate some of the shortcomings of these liquid adjuvants.[24] About 20 to 25 years ago argon beam coagulation began to be used to extend the margin of the curetted cavity. This allows the surgeon to control the thickness of the extension of the curettage and had fewer complications. Recurrence rates were comparable to other adjuvants.[25] Polymethyl methacrylate (PMMA) is also known to be an effective adjuvant. Polymerization of the cement effectively extends the margin and provides good radiographic contrast to adjacent cancellous bone for surveillance of recurrence.

Radiofrequency Ablation

The use of radiofrequency ablation in the treatment of osteoid osteoma was first reported in the early 1990s.[26] The procedure involves the use of CT imaging to localize placement of the tip of a radiofrequency probe in the center of an osteoid osteoma. Once the probe is appropriately placed a generator heats the tip of the probe to 90°C for 6 minutes. The lesion is thermally ablated and pain associated with the lesion stops almost immediately. This procedure is generally successful in 90% of patients. Osteoid osteoma is uniquely suited to this procedure because of its small size (usually <1 cm in diameter). With the success seen in osteoid osteoma RFA has been attempted in other benign bone tumors with mixed success. Its application is necessarily limited to smaller lesions.

Summary

In summary, benign bone tumors are commonly encountered by practicing orthopaedic surgeons. Although not common, they are often a common incidental finding when an orthopaedic surgeon is reviewing frequent imaging, particularly in a practice treating pediatrics, adolescents, and young adults. They often have a very familiar pattern that makes diagnosing and treating them relatively straightforward, often only radiographic observation. Bone tumors that are concerning or not recognizable to the practicing orthopaedic surgeon should be referred to an orthopaedic oncologist.

Key Study Points

- Many benign bone tumors can be treated conservatively (without surgery).
- The use of radiofrequency ablation has significantly altered the treatment of osteoid osteoma.
- Some benign bone tumors (specifically chondroblastoma and giant cell tumor) can metastasize, most commonly to the lungs.
- Denosumab is being used for the treatment of giant cell tumor of bone, particularly in tumors with a joint at risk. Length of therapy and its role in place of or in combination with surgery has yet to be fully elucidated.

Annotated References

1. Unni KK, Inwards CY, Research, MFME: *Dahlin's Bone Tumors: General Aspects and Data on 10,165 Cases*. Wolters Kluwer Health/Lippincott Williams & Wilkins; 2010.
2. Czajka CM, DiCaprio MR: What is the proportion of patients with multiple hereditary exostoses who undergo malignant degeneration? *Clin Orthop Relat Res* 2015;473: 2355-2361.

Oncology and Pathology

3. Porter DE, Lonie L, Fraser M, et al: Severity of disease and risk of malignant change in hereditary multiple exostoses. A genotype-phenotype study. *J Bone Joint Surg Br* 2004;86:1041-1046.

4. Verdegaal SHM, Bovée JVMG, Pansuriya TC, et al: Incidence, predictive factors, and prognosis of chondrosarcoma in patients with Ollier disease and Maffucci syndrome: An international multicenter study of 161 patients. *Oncologist* 2011;16:1771-1779.

5. Subhawong TK, Winn A, Shemesh SS, Pretell-Mazzini J: F-18 FDG PET differentiation of benign from malignant chondroid neoplasms: A systematic review of the literature. *Skeletal Radiol* 2017;46:1233-1239.

   The authors present a meta-analysis of the literature correlating SUVmax on F-18 FDG PET-CT with histologic grade in benign, low-grade malignant, and intermediate/high-grade chondroid lesions. Level of evidence: III.

6. Farfalli GL, Slullitel AI, Muscolo DL, Ayerza MA, Aponte-Tinao LA: What happens to the articular surface after curettage for epiphyseal chondroblastoma. A report on functional results, arthritis and arthroplasty. *Clin Orthop Relat Res* 2017;475:760-766.

   These authors review chondroblastoma treated with curettage and bone grafting and report on complications and functional outcomes. Level of evidence: III.

7. Xie C, Jeys L, James SLJ: Radiofrequency ablation of chondroblastoma: Long-term clinical and imaging outcomes. *Eur Radiol* 2015;25:1127-1134.

8. Rosenthal DI, Hornicek FJ, Wolfe MW, Jennings LC, Gebhardt MC, Mankin HJ: Percutaneous radiofrequency coagulation of osteoid osteoma compared with operative treatment. *J Bone Joint Surg* 1998;80:815-821.

9. Outani H, Hamada K, Takenaka S, et al: Radiofrequency ablation of osteoid osteoma using a three-dimensional navigation system. *J Orthop Sci* 2016;21:678-682.

   This group describes a retrospective review of the outcomes and complications of the treatment of osteoid osteoma using radiofrequency ablation guided by three-dimensional navigation. Level of evidence: IV.

10. Masciocchi C, Zugaro L, Arrigoni F, et al: Radiofrequency ablation versus magnetic resonance guided focused ultrasound surgery for minimally invasive treatment of osteoid osteoma: A propensity score matching study. *Eur Radiol* 2016;26:2472-2481.

    These authors present a retrospective comparison of successful outcome and complications in a matched cohort of patients treated for osteoid osteoma with radiofrequency ablation (RFA) versus magnetic resonance–guided focused ultrasound surgery (MRgFUS). Level of evidence: IV.

11. Napoli A, Bazzocchi A, Scipione R, et al: Noninvasive therapy for osteoid osteoma: A prospective developmental study with MR imaging-guided high-intensity focused ultrasound. *Radiology* 2017;285:186-196.

    This was a prospective review of a cohort of patients treated for osteoid osteoma by radiographic diagnosis with magnetic resonance imaging–guided high-intensity focused ultrasound. They reported on safety, clinical effectiveness, and radiographic tumor response. Level of evidence: IV.

12. Sharma KV, Yarmolenko PS, Celik H, et al: Comparison of noninvasive high-intensity focused ultrasound with radiofrequency ablation of osteoid osteoma. *J Pediatr* 2017;190:222-228.e1.

    The authors present a prospectively enrolled cohort with symptomatic radiographically diagnosed osteoid osteoma treated with magnetic resonance imaging–guided high-intensity focused ultrasound and compare it with a historical control of patients treated for osteoid osteoma by radiographic diagnosis with radiofrequency ablation. They compare safety and clinical response. Level of evidence: IV.

13. Wang B, Han SB, Jiang L, et al: Percutaneous radiofrequency ablation for spinal osteoid osteoma and osteoblastoma. *Eur Spine J* 2017;26:1884-1892.

    These authors present a retrospective review of patients with biopsy-proven, spinal osteoid osteoma or osteoblastoma treated with radiofrequency ablation. They compare pre-op and post-op pain via visual analog scale (VAS). Level of evidence: III.

14. Błaż M, Palczewski P, Swiątkowski J, Gołębiowski M: Cortical fibrous defects and non-ossifying fibromas in children and young adults: The analysis of radiological features in 28 cases and a review of literature. *Pol J Radiol* 2011;76:32-39.

15. Gaston CL, Grimer RJ, Parry M, et al: Current status and unanswered questions on the use of Denosumab in giant cell tumor of bone. *Clin Sarcoma Res* 2016;6:15.

    This paper is a review of the mechanism of action and historical use of Denosumab in the giant cell tumor of bone. The authors suggest their thoughts on appropriate use and future applications of the drug. Level of evidence: V.

16. Thomas D, Henshaw R, Skubitz K, et al: Denosumab in patients with giant-cell tumour of bone: An open-label, phase 2 study. *Lancet Oncol* 2010;11:275-280.

17. Chawla S, Henshaw R, Seeger L, et al: Safety and efficacy of denosumab for adults and skeletally mature adolescents with giant cell tumour of bone: Interim analysis of an open-label, parallel-group, phase 2 study. *Lancet Oncol* 2013;14:901-908.

18. Ueda T, Morioka H, Nishida Y, et al: Objective tumor response to denosumab in patients with giant cell tumor of bone: A multicenter phase II trial. *Ann Oncol* 2015;26:2149-2154.

19. Aponte-Tinao LA, Piuzzi NS, Roitman P, Farfalli GL: A high-grade sarcoma arising in a patient with recurrent benign giant cell tumor of the proximal tibia while receiving treatment with denosumab. *Clin Orthop Relat Res* 2015;473:3050-3055.

20. Broehm CJ, Garbrecht EL, Wood J, Bocklage T: Two cases of sarcoma arising in giant cell tumor of bone treated with denosumab. *Case Rep Med* 2015;2015:767198.

21. Simm PJ, Biggin A, Zacharin MR, et al: Consensus guidelines on the use of bisphosphonate therapy in children and adolescents. *J Paediatr Child Health* 2018;54:223-233.

    This paper presents guidelines on behalf of the Australian Paediatric Endocrine Group for the use of diphosphonates in children and adolescents for skeletal fragility. The guidelines are a consensus by this group after reviewing the existing literature using the GRADE system to give an objective level of evidence to those recommendations. Level of evidence: IV.

22. Dahlin DC, Cupps RE, Johnson EW: Giant-cell tumor: A study of 195 cases. *Cancer* 1970;25:1061-1070.
23. Blackley HR, Wunder JS, Davis AM, White LM, Kandel R, Bell RS: Treatment of giant-cell tumors of long bones with curettage and bone-grafting. *J Bone Joint Surg* 1999;81:811-820.
24. Wu PK, Chen CF, Wang JY, et al: Freezing nitrogen ethanol composite may be a viable approach for cryotherapy of human giant cell tumor of bone. *Clin Orthop Relat Res* 2017;475:1650-1663.

    The authors describe a unique surgical adjuvant—freezing nitrogen ethanol composite. After ex vivo and animal model validation, they describe outcomes in a small cohort of patients treated for giant cell tumor with curettage and this novel adjuvant. Level of evidence: IV.
25. Lewis VO, Wei A, Mendoza T, Primus F, Peabody T, Simon MA: Argon beam coagulation as an adjuvant for local control of giant cell tumor. *Clin Orthop Relat Res* 2007;454:192-197.
26. Rosenthal DI, Alexander A, Rosenberg AE, Springfield D: Ablation of osteoid osteomas with a percutaneously placed electrode: A new procedure. *Radiology* 1992;183:29-33.

Chapter 67

Malignant Primary Bone Tumors

Andre R.V. Spiguel, MD • Chung Ming Chan, MD, MBBS

ABSTRACT

Malignant primary tumors of bone are an exceedingly rare and varied group of diseases. These tumors can vary from low grade to high grade, and management is tailored to each specific tumor type. High-grade lesions are typically treated with neoadjuvant therapies, chemotherapy ± radiation therapy, and subsequent surgery, whereas low-grade lesions are usually managed with surgery alone. The three most common primary bone malignancies include osteosarcoma, Ewing sarcoma, and chondrosarcoma. Both osteosarcoma and chondrosarcomas have low-grade and high-grade variants, whereas Ewing sarcoma is high grade. Other rare low-grade malignancies of bone include chordoma and adamantinoma, classically treated with surgery alone. Radiation therapy has shown some promise as an adjuvant in the treatment of chordomas. Hematologic malignancies can also occur in bone. Lymphoma is a malignancy derived from lymphocytes. Multiple myeloma is a plasma cell malignancy characterized by clonal plasma cells. Chemotherapy and sometimes radiation therapy is the standard treatment for these cancers; surgical intervention is reserved for pathologic fractures or prophylactic fixation of impending fractures. Surgical management of primary bone tumors usually involves wide resection and reconstruction with limb-salvage the majority of the time. Commonly these tumors affect growing children which leads to unique challenges in surgical management.

Keywords: bone malignancy; chondrosarcoma; Ewing sarcoma; limb-salvage; osteosarcoma; surgical management

Neither of the following authors nor any immediate family member has received anything of value from or has stock or stock options held in a commercial company or institution related directly or indirectly to the subject of this chapter: Dr. Spiguel and Dr. Chan.

Osteosarcoma

Introduction

Primary malignant bone cancer is exceedingly rare and typically accounts for less than 0.2% of all malignancies in the United States. It is estimated that there will be 3,450 bone and joint cancers diagnosed in 2018 with an estimated 1,590 deaths in the United States.[1] Osteosarcoma is the most common primary bone tumor and is defined by malignant spindle cells of mesenchymal origin that produce osteoid.[2] It can occur anywhere in both the axial and appendicular skeleton and is seen most commonly in the metaphysis of long bones. A multidisciplinary approach is used in the treatment of osteosarcoma, which includes both surgery and chemotherapy. Before the 1970s, surgery was the only treatment modality and survival was 20%, with most patients succumbing to metastatic pulmonary disease. Today, survival rates are greater than 65% at 5 years, thanks to the discovery of multiagent chemotherapy, which is now the standard of care for high-grade lesions.[3]

Epidemiology

Osteosarcoma is the third most common cancer in adolescence with an annual incidence of 5.6 cases per million children younger than 15 years. It has a bimodal age distribution with the majority of the cases occurring in the second decade of life. A second peak occurs in the elderly, between the seventh and eighth decades, and it is rarely found before the age of 5.[4] Classically it is found near the metaphyseal growth plates of long bones and over 50% occurs around the knee, most commonly in the distal femur, followed by the proximal tibia and then the proximal humerus. The incidence has always been considered slightly higher in males than in females and more recent data show higher rates in Asian/Pacific Islanders and Hispanics.[5]

Pathogenesis

Osteosarcoma has a broad spectrum of histology and behavior with the common characteristic of neoplastic mesenchymal cells producing osteoid. They can be either primary or secondary and represent different entities based

Table 1

Osteosarcoma Types and Subtypes

Osteosarcoma	Types

Central—high grade	• Conventional
	  • Osteoblastic
	  • Chondroblastic
	  • Fibroblastic
	• Telangiectatic
	• Small cell
	• Epithelioid
	• Osteoblastoma-like
	• Chondroblastoma-like
	• Fibrohistiocytic
	• Giant cell rich

Central—low grade	• Fibrous dysplasia-like • Desmoplastic fibroma–like
Juxtacortical/surface based—high grade	• Dedifferentiated parosteal • High-grade surface
Juxtacortical/surface based—intermediate grade	• Periosteal
Juxtacortical/surface based—low grade	• Parosteal

on clinical, radiographic, or histological features. They can present as intramedullary or surface-based lesions and can include high-grade and low-grade variants (**Table 1**).

Conventional osteosarcoma (**Figure 1**) is the most common variant and represents 80% of all osteosarcomas. It is a primary neoplasm, high grade, and intramedullary, and depending on the predominant extracellular matrix present it is further classified as osteoblastic, chondroblastic, or fibroblastic. There are no significant differences regarding prognosis and clinical outcomes between the three subtypes. Other more rare high-grade subtypes include telangiectatic, small cell, and high-grade surface osteosarcoma. Small cell osteosarcoma is the only one with a slightly worse prognosis and theoretically this may be due to its relation to the Ewing sarcoma family of tumors.

Other primary osteosarcomas include low-grade central osteosarcoma and the juxtacortical or surface-based lesions such as parosteal and periosteal osteosarcoma. Periosteal osteosarcoma is typically intermediate grade and chondroblastic, it arises between the cortex and the cambium layer of the periosteum, and the cartilaginous component has varied degrees of cytologic atypia. Prognosis is excellent for low-grade tumors with survival approaching 90%.[6,7]

Osteosarcomas that result from an exposure or a prior condition are referred to as secondary osteosarcomas. These rare forms of osteosarcoma typically occur in older patients and are usually due to Paget's disease or exposures to ionizing radiation. Some other benign bone lesions such as fibrous dysplasia, chronic osteomyelitis, and bone infarcts may also rarely undergo malignant degeneration/transformation into secondary osteosarcomas.

The true etiology of osteosarcoma is largely unknown. Osteosarcoma cells have high genetic instability and significantly variable and complex karyotypes. Even though the majority of osteosarcomas are the result of sporadic mutations, there are several rare

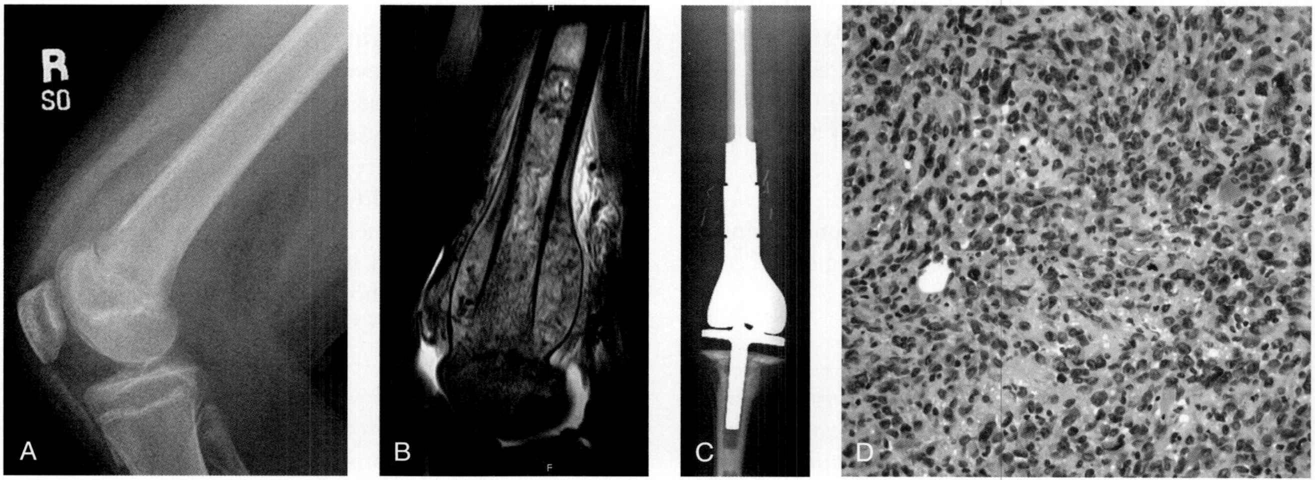

Figure 1 Distal femoral osteosarcoma. **A**, Soft-tissue swelling and subtle periosteal reaction. **B**, MRI depicting extent of tumor. **C**, Endoprosthetic reconstruction of defect from resection. **D**, Histology of conventional high-grade osteoblastic osteosarcoma.

genetic syndromes where an increased rate of osteosarcomas is found. Two such syndromes are retinoblastoma, which has a germline mutation of a tumor suppressor gene (RB1), and Li-Fraumeni, which has a mutation in the p53 gene responsible for cellular response to DNA damage. Rothmund-Thompson syndrome, Werner syndrome, and Bloom syndrome are a group of rare diseases associated with RECQ-helicase mutations, which are also at increased risk for osteosarcoma. RECQ-helicase is responsible for maintaining genomic stability by winding and unwinding DNA, and the instability caused by mutations is what likely drives tumorigenesis.[8,9]

Clinical Features

Most patients with osteosarcoma present with pain and swelling in the involved region, usually ongoing for the past few months. They commonly attribute it to trauma or physical exertion and over 50% of the time, it occurs around the knee as previously mentioned. On physical examination large palpable masses can be felt; patients can have swelling, erythema, induration, as well as limited ROM secondary to pain and mass size. Five to ten percent of patients present with a pathologic fracture and 20% of patients, although likely asymptomatic, have detectable pulmonary metastasis at presentation. There are no laboratory values to assist in diagnosis; however, alkaline phosphatase and lactate dehydrogenase can have some prognostic implications and are sometimes used to assess tumor response to chemotherapy.[10,11]

Imaging

Imaging is essential in the diagnosis, treatment, and surveillance of osteosarcoma. Plain radiographs of the affected area usually suggest the diagnosis. Common language used to describe the radiographs of a high-grade osteosarcoma includes mixed radiolucent and radiodense features with a permeative appearance and wide, poorly defined zones of transition. Periosteal new bone formation can be seen with lifting of the cortex and the appearance of Codman's triangle. Extension of tumor into the soft tissue has a "sunburst" pattern of ossification which is classic for osteosarcoma. Low-grade osteosarcomas have more narrow zones of transition and are more sclerotic or ossified on radiographs.

Axial imaging in the form of CT and MRI is also important in the management of this disease. Upon presentation, staging must be done using a CT scan of the chest to evaluate for pulmonary metastasis. An MRI of the entire bone is important to evaluate the soft-tissue mass, proximity to neurovascular structures, marrow involvement, and any skip metastasis that may be present. MRI is also helpful for surgical planning and is the imaging modality of choice to identify the osseous extent of tumor to achieve a margin negative resection, critical for local control.[12]

Whole body technetium bone scan is the benchmark for detecting the presence of extrapulmonary osseous metastasis at the time of diagnosis. The role of positron emission tomography (PET) scans for staging and to evaluate tumor response to chemotherapy is still evolving but looks promising and is now recommended by the Children's Oncology Group whenever possible.[13]

Current Treatments and Prognosis

The treatment of high-grade osteosarcoma today involves both surgery and chemotherapy. Historically, before the 1970s, when surgery was the only treatment, 2-year survival was 15% to 20% indicating that most patients had micro-metastasis at presentation. Patients underwent radical resections, frequently amputations, only to present 6 months to 1 year later with pulmonary disease. Important randomized control trials were established in the 1980s which defined the role of chemotherapy in the treatment of osteosarcoma. With the introduction of systemic chemotherapy and radical tumor resection, survival increased dramatically to 70% at 5 years in patients who presented without detectable metastasis. Patients with metastatic disease at presentation are treated with the same aggressive therapy, but survival at 5 years drops to less than 20%.[14] Low-grade and surface-based osteosarcomas are treated with surgery alone given their overall good prognosis and limited benefit of chemotherapy.

Osteosarcoma is a relatively radioresistant tumor and radiation therapy (RT) is not commonly used. It does have a role in the treatment of patients with inoperable tumors, positive margins after resection, and for palliation to treat pain due to bony metastasis. Given the comprehensive nature of the management of this disease, it is important that a multidisciplinary sarcoma program be involved in treatment, which includes medical and radiation oncology, musculoskeletal orthopaedic oncologists, surgical oncologists, musculoskeletal pathologists, and radiologists.

Emerging Therapies

Advances in the treatment of osteosarcoma have been stagnant over the past three to four decades, and although many clinical trials have been performed, no significant benefit in survival has been achieved. On the horizon is the use of immunotherapies to harness the patient's own immune system in the treatment of osteosarcoma.

Potentially using antibodies to target cancer cell surface proteins, tumor vaccines can be designed to induce an antitumor response through the exposure of tumor antigens. In addition, oncolytic attenuated viruses genetically engineered to only replicate in malignant cells are possible. Lastly, adoptive cell therapy, where cytolytic cells are introduced to counteract various ways tumor cells evade the host's immune system and cause an antitumor response are all potential targets.[15]

Tyrosine kinase inhibitors are also currently being evaluated in osteosarcoma, and promising results have been seen in vitro.[16] Recently, using a canine model, an attenuated *Listeria* vaccine was given to deliver and induce innate HER2/neu immunity, a tyrosine kinase receptor that is frequently overexpressed in aggressive phenotypes of carcinomas and pediatric canine osteosarcomas. This led to a significant reduction in metastatic disease and an overall increase in survival.[17] Current translation to clinical use is ongoing and remains a hopeful adjunct in the treatment of osteosarcoma.

Ewing Sarcoma

Introduction

Ewing sarcoma (ES) was originally described by James Ewing in 1918 as diffuse endothelioma and currently is classified together with primitive neuroectodermal tumors (PNETs) under the ES family of tumors. The majority of cases involve the bone; however, primary soft-tissue and visceral involvement is well documented but less common.

ES is the second most common primary bone malignancy in patients below 20 and the incidence rate is about three per million per year. There is a slightly higher incidence in males, and nine times higher incidence in African-Americans as compared with Caucasians. The site of disease is most commonly the lower extremities, followed by the pelvis, and then the chest wall.

Clinical Features

Patients with ES typically present with pain and swelling related to growth of the tumor, and these may be accompanied by systemic symptoms such as fever, malaise, anorexia, and weight loss. Back pain or neurologic symptoms may be the presenting symptoms for patients with involvement of the vertebral column. A large soft-tissue mass is often present at the time of presentation. ES can mimic an infectious process in both the systemic symptoms and the laboratory parameters on presentation. ES commonly affects the diaphysis or metadiaphysis of long bones, and plain radiographs typically show a permeative lytic process. Abundant periosteal reaction such as an "onion-skin" or "sunburst" pattern is often seen; however, this is not specific to ES. The anatomic extent of disease is best characterized on MRI, and extracortical extension into the surrounding soft tissues is common (**Figure 2**).

Histology and Genetics

ES appears microscopically as monotonous sheets of small round blue cells. Although no immunohistochemical stain is entirely specific for ES, CD99 is positive in

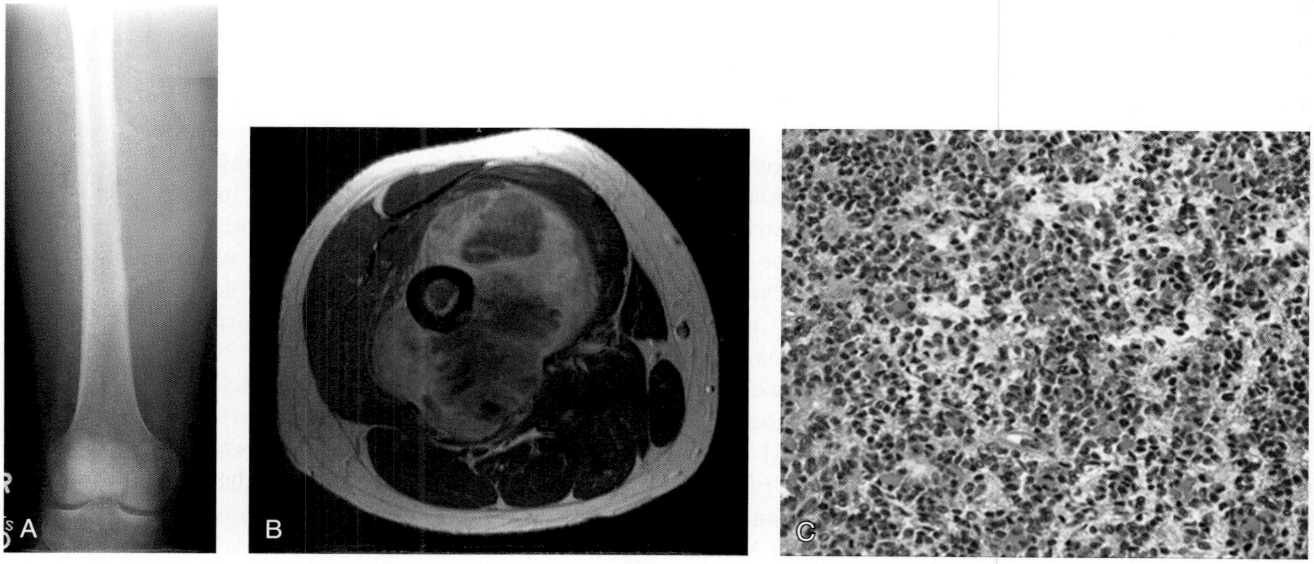

Figure 2 Ewing sarcoma. **A**, Periosteal reaction associated with large tumor. **B**, MRI depicting large extraosseous extent of tumor. **C,** Histology of Ewing sarcoma.

up to 99% of ES and its subtypes and is a very sensitive stain. The genetic hallmark of ES is a balanced translocation t(11;22)(q24;q12), which leads to the fusion of the EWS and FLI1 genes, and an EWSR1-FLI1 fusion transcript. The second most common translocation associated with ES is t(21;22)(q22;q12) resulting in the EWR1-ERG transcript.

Imaging

Staging studies to evaluate the extent of local disease and for the presence of systemic involvement should be performed on diagnosis. Recommended studies include radiographs and an MRI scan of the bone involved by the tumor, a chest CT scan, and a whole body technetium-99 bone scan. Apart from routine blood tests, lactate dehydrogenase should be considered, as elevated levels have been associated with increased risk of recurrence and an unfavorable outcome. Bone marrow biopsy has long been used as staging study to evaluate for microscopic marrow involvement, but the use of FDG-PET/CT in place of routine bone marrow biopsy has been proposed by current research.[18] The utility of FDG-PET/CT in ES has also been established for initial staging[19] and to detect recurrences.[20] It has been found to predict progression-free survival and correlates with the percentage of tumor necrosis on histologic assessment.

Treatment and Prognosis

The advent of multiagent chemotherapy was the most significant advance in the treatment of primary bone malignancies such as ES and osteosarcoma. Before the introduction of chemotherapy, 5-year survival rates ranged from 5% to 25%. First-line therapy currently comprises vincristine, adriamycin, and cyclophosphamide, alternating with ifosfamide and etoposide. Second-line multiagent regimens include temozolomide/irinotecan, topotecan/cyclophosphamide, and gemcitabine/docetaxel. Novel agents are being investigated for use in refractory cases, and these include insulinlike growth factor 1 receptor (IGF1R) inhibitors, and agents targeting the EWS-FLI1 fusion protein.[21,22]

ES is distinct from other primary bone malignancies in being sensitive to RT. RT is often employed in locations, such as the pelvis and spine, where surgical resection poses technical challenges and is accompanied with considerable surgical morbidity. The role of definitive RT compared with surgical resection is an area of some debate. Some studies have shown equivalent event-free survival and overall survival rates comparing definitive RT and resection for local control,[23] whereas other recent studies have found significantly better local control rates with surgery in patients with pelvic ES[24] and extremity ES.[25] The nature of the condition is such that these studies are largely retrospective studies or subset analyses of data from studies designed to investigate chemotherapeutic regimens. This makes these studies subject to selection bias for patients undergoing the different modes of treatment, that is, surgery, surgery and RT, definitive RT. Similarly, adjuvant RT following resection of ES is an area of current research, with some studies demonstrating benefit and others no benefit.[26]

Where wide resection is technically feasible, and where a reasonable functional result following reconstruction can be expected, surgical resection should be recommended. Adjuvant RT should be considered where there are positive surgical margins. Definitive RT in place of surgical resection is an option where resection is technically unfeasible, or excessively morbid. The risk of developing second malignancies in patients treated for ES is comparable with patients with other childhood cancers ranging from 3% to 6.5%. However, there is evidence that the risk of second malignancy is higher in patients who receive RT for local control.[27]

Five-year overall survival for patients treated with modern chemotherapy regimens range between 55% and 70% with negative prognostic factors including large tumor size and metastatic disease.[28,29] Notably, metastases to the bone are associated with a poorer prognosis than to the lung. Treatment for metastatic disease includes myeloablative chemotherapy, stem cell rescue, and total lung irradiation.

Chondrosarcoma

Introduction

Chondrosarcoma is a heterogeneous group of tumors, with diverse morphologic features and clinical behavior, which have neoplastic cells that produce hyaline cartilage. It is the second most common bone tumor after osteosarcoma with the majority of these being conventional chondrosarcomas. Other more rare subtypes of chondrosarcomas include mesenchymal chondrosarcoma, clear cell chondrosarcoma, and dedifferentiated chondrosarcoma. In 2013, the WHO made some important changes to the classification of malignant cartilage tumors. The term atypical cartilaginous tumor was introduced to replace grade 1 chondrosarcoma to better reflect its clinical behavior.[30] Cartilage tumors have a varied clinical presentation and are sometimes difficult to characterize between benign and malignant. The majority of these tumors are low grade, grow slowly, and rarely metastasize. It is especially important to have a multidisciplinary assessment combining pathology, radiology, and clinical features before a diagnosis is rendered.

Epidemiology

Chondrosarcomas represent 10% to 20% of all primary bone tumors. Conventional chondrosarcomas make up 80% to 85% of these tumors and include both primary and secondary chondrosarcomas. Secondary chondrosarcomas only account for 10% to 15% of conventional chondrosarcomas and are believed to arise from benign cartilage lesions such as enchondromas or osteochondromas. The remaining 15% to 20% of chondrosarcomas include the rare subtypes previously mentioned.

Chondrosarcomas are most commonly diagnosed in adults, in the fourth to sixth decades of life, and are extremely rare in children and adolescents. They can arise anywhere but are more commonly seen in the axial and proximal appendicular skeleton. Most commonly in the pelvis, followed by the proximal femur, proximal humerus, and the proximal tibia. There is a slight male predominance.[31]

Well-known rare syndromes associated with an increased risk of malignant degeneration and secondary chondrosarcomas include Maffucci's and Ollier's syndrome. These patients have enchondromatosis and carry a 25% to 30% lifetime risk of malignant degeneration.[32] Patients with multiple hereditary exostosis also have an increased risk of malignant degeneration with a lifetime risk of 1% to 6%.[33]

Clinical Features

Chondrosarcomas can present in a variety of ways. Sometimes patients present with persistent pain for a period of time and sometimes they are found incidentally. Given the frequently low-grade nature of this lesion, patients can present with very large tumors, especially in the axial skeleton and pelvis. High-grade lesions or dedifferentiated tumors can present with rapidly worsening pain, a growing soft-tissue mass, and even pathologic fractures due to cortical involvement and weakening of the bone. Patients with previously mentioned syndromes that are associated with secondary chondrosarcomas need to be followed up closely to assess for malignant transformation given their risk is far greater than the general population.

Imaging

Initial imaging involves orthogonal radiographs, which can be quite heterogeneous and shows a predominantly radiolucent lesion, usually metadiaphyseal, with mineralization within it with an "arc" and/or "ring" pattern of calcification. Evidence of endosteal changes or cortical disruption with an associated soft-tissue mass is highly suggestive of a chondrosarcoma. Serial radiographs are commonly used to decipher between benign enchondromas and low-grade chondrosarcomas, which can have similar radiographic appearances at diagnosis. Little change should be seen over time with enchondromas, whereas disease progression and cortical changes will be seen with chondrosarcomas.

Axial imaging can be very helpful in diagnosing and surgical planning for chondrosarcomas. CT scans are very helpful at assessing cortical integrity and endosteal changes. It allows us to see the interface between the lesion and the normal host bone to assess for changes concerning for a chondrosarcoma. MRI is also helpful in assessing the soft-tissue component of the lesion and neurovascular involvement. Cartilage is very water rich and the lesions are usually T2 hyperintense and have low signal on T1-weighted images (**Figure 3**). MRI is also useful in assessing the thickness of the cartilage cap on an osteochondroma with concern for malignant transformation. Once the diagnosis is made, both a bone scan and CT chest are necessary for staging the patient, which is standard of care for any primary bone sarcoma.

Histologic Characteristics

Conventional chondrosarcomas are histologically similar and fall into grades 1 to 3, which is an important clinical predictor of behavior. Grade 1 or atypical cartilaginous tumors make up the majority of tumors (60% to 70%), grade 2 lesions represent 20% to 30% of lesions, and grade 3 lesions are considered to be rare (less than 5%). Pathologists assess cellularity, pleomorphism, mitotic figures, presence of myxoid matrix, necrosis, and bony destruction in their evaluation of grade[34] (**Table 2**). While there are published criteria for pathologic grading of chondrosarcomas, there is poor interobserver reliability among experts at tertiary medical centers where many of these tumors are evaluated and diagnosed.[35]

Genetics

Like most sarcomas, there are no clear genetic events or molecular pathways known to result in chondrosarcomas. The most significant genetic finding in chondrosarcomas, are the mutations in the isocitrate dehydrogenase I (IDH1) and isocitrate dehydrogenase 2 (IDH2) genes. These genes code for metabolic enzymes IDH1 and IDH2 that are known to play a role in tumorigenesis. These mutations are found in the majority of primary and secondary central chondrosarcomas (70% to 80%), most periosteal chondrosarcomas, and 50%

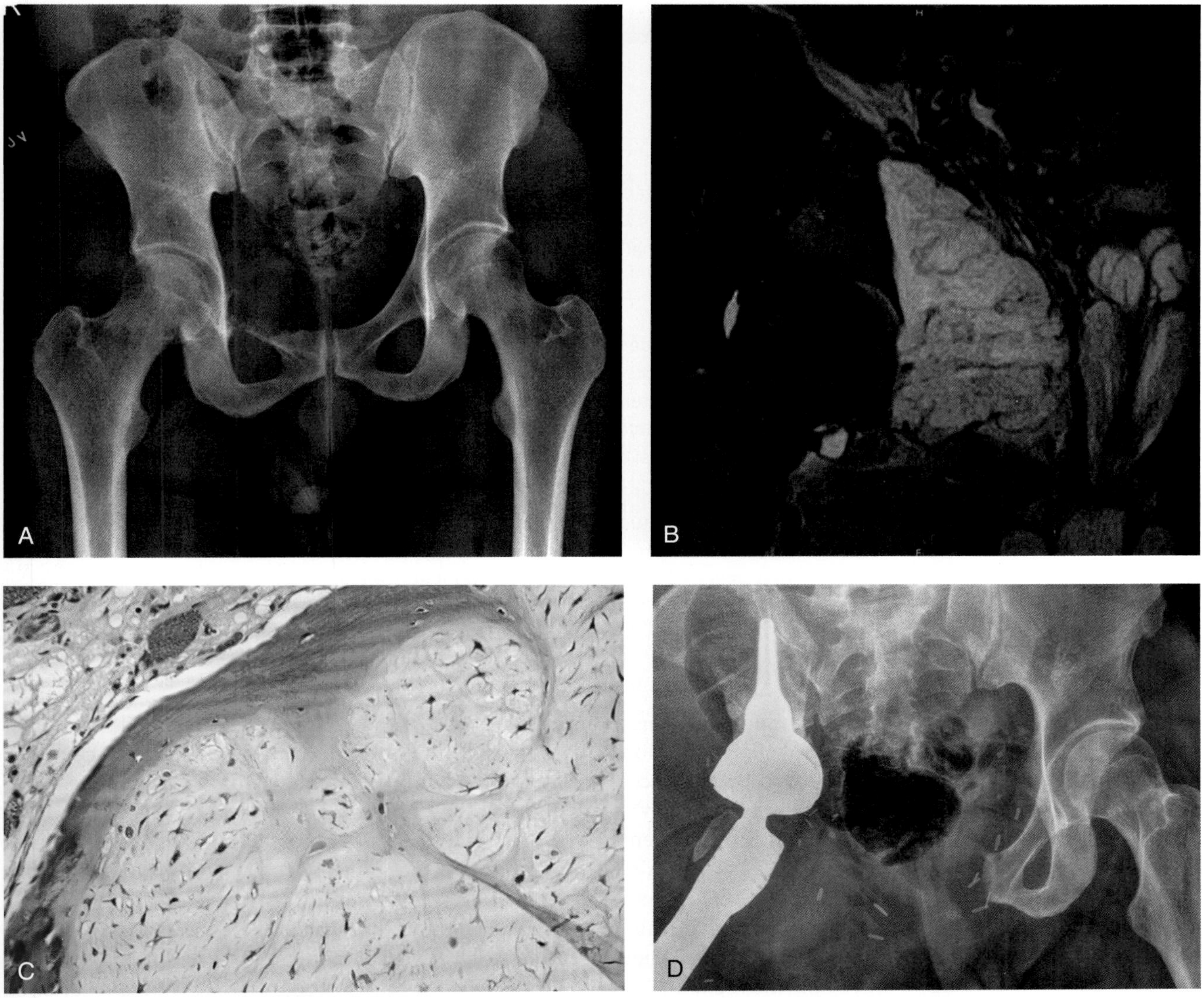

Figure 3 Chondrosarcoma. **A**, Destruction of superior pubic ramus by tumor seen on radiographs. **B**, MRI depicting extent of tumor and extension into hip joint, T2 water rich, hyperintense lesion with a notable hip effusion. **C**, Histology of high-grade chondrosarcoma. **D**, Endoprosthetic reconstruction of defect from resection.

of dedifferentiated chondrosarcomas. These findings can be helpful to pathologists in regard to diagnosis, which can sometimes be difficult, and have potential for future targeted therapies.[36]

Treatment and Prognosis

Surgery and wide resection continue to be the treatment of choice for conventional chondrosarcoma. Because of the low-grade nature of the majority of these tumors and their paucity of cells, mitotic figures, and limited vascularity, these tumors are relatively chemotherapy and RT resistant. With adequate surgical intervention and wide margins, prognosis is good with overall 5-year survival rates reported from 70% to 80% for low-grade lesions, and 40% to 50% for high-grade lesions.[37]

The controversy in the management of chondrosarcomas stems from surgical treatment of low-grade appendicular lesions with low rates of metastasis. Wide resection of these tumors can oftentimes be quite morbid and result in significant functional deficits. Some have advocated that these lesions should be treated with intralesional curettage and adjuvant treatments in the form of phenol, cryotherapy, or argon ablation with low local recurrence rates. Lesions amenable to this must be low grade, smaller, and confined to bone without soft-tissue extension.

Table 2

Grading of Conventional Chondrosarcoma

Grade	Histologic Features	10-yr Survival
I (Atypical cartilaginous tumor)	• Hyaline cartilage with paucity of cells with densely staining hyperchromatic plump nuclei, uniform in size • Small number of larger cells with pleomorphic nuclei • Predominantly chondroid matrix with minimal myxoid changes • Calcification seen • Infrequent binucleate cells	80%-90%
II	• Disorganized cells with moderately sized nuclei • More cellular areas with more myxoid stroma • Increased cellularity along tumor periphery • Greater degree of nuclear atypia, hyperchromasia, and nuclear size • Low mitotic rate (<2 mitoses/10 high power field [HPF])	65%-80%
III	• Greater than 2 mitoses/10 HPF in active areas • Increased cellularity along tumor periphery • Even larger nuclei in comparison to grade II lesions • Spindle shaped cells in high cellular areas without appreciable matrix (chondroid or myxoid) • Necrosis	30%-40%

A recent retrospective review of chondrosarcomas managed at a single institution over a 40-year period found that a positive margin did affect local recurrence-free survival; however, it did not affect overall survival because of low rates of metastasis.[38] Another recent meta-analysis looking at wide resection versus intralesional curettage for low-grade chondrosarcomas found that there is no scientific evidence to support intralesional curettage for low-grade chondrosarcomas. They recommend in their conclusion that the benchmark of wide resection with negative margins for malignant tumors continue to be applied.[39] When deciding the best option for each patient, one must balance the risk of surgical morbidity with the risk for local recurrence. Low-grade axial lesions of the spine and pelvis traditionally are more aggressive in behavior, and most would agree treatment with a wide resection when possible is necessary.

Rare Subtypes

Mesenchymal chondrosarcoma is a highly malignant tumor and represents approximately 4% of chondrosarcomas. Patients are typically much younger, second and third decade, and one-third of tumors are extraskeletal. Approximately 20% will have metastatic disease at presentation, and local and distant recurrences as well as metastatic disease can be seen up to 20 years after diagnosis. Survival at 5 and 10 years are 50% and 25% respectively. Tumor histology is biphasic with well-differentiated cartilage matrix and undifferentiated small round blue cells. Unlike other chondrosarcomas there seems to be a role for chemotherapy before surgical intervention when appropriate.

Dedifferentiated chondrosarcoma is another highly malignant lesion that represents anywhere from 2% to 10% of chondrosarcomas. It is also biphasic histologically with a high-grade, noncartilaginous sarcoma arising from a low-grade cartilage tumor with a sharp demarcation between the two components. Commonly diagnosed in patients older than 50 years, prognosis is dismal with 5-year survival ranging from 10% to 20%. Treatment is typically wide resection when possible, and the use of chemotherapy shows little to no benefit. Most patients develop widespread disease within 1 year of diagnosis.

Clear cell chondrosarcoma is very rare low-grade tumor, which represents less than 2% of chondrosarcomas. It is commonly diagnosed in young adults and found in the epiphysis of long bones, most commonly the proximal femur. Histologically, clear cells are seen with larger nuclei and an abundance of clear cytoplasm, in a background of varying amounts of mature cartilage. Prognosis is very good despite the propensity for late metastasis. Wide surgical resection is the treatment of choice.[40,41]

Other Primary Malignant Bone Tumors: Adamantinoma and Chordoma

Adamantinoma

Adamantinoma is a rare, low-grade malignancy representing <1% of primary malignant bone tumors that occurs in 90% of cases in the tibial diaphysis (**Figure 4**). Patients typically present in their second or third decade of life with pain, swelling, and deformity of the shin. The typical radiographic appearance is that of a "soap bubble" with juxtaposed areas of radiolucency and sclerosis. This is similar to the appearance of osteofibrous dysplasia (OFD), but its aggressive behavior is evidenced by the larger areas of radiolucency and associated soft-tissue mass. Histologically, nests of epithelial cells are seen in a background of osteofibrous tissue, while cytogenetic abnormalities such as trisomy of chromosomes 7, 8, and 12 are features. Resection with clear margins is key to local control,[42] and survival at 10 years of 80% to 90% with wide resection alone has been reported. Late local and distal recurrences have also been reported. The relationship of OFD, OFD-like adamantinoma, or differentiated adamantinoma is an area of current research.[43] These three conditions share similarities in presentation, radiologic, and pathologic findings. Studies have suggested that OFD-like adamantinoma may result from spontaneously regressing adamantinoma, or that it represents a precursor lesion in malignant transformation to adamantinoma.[44] The importance of clinical, pathologic, and radiologic correlation cannot be overstated as intralesional or marginal resection of adamantinoma is associated with local recurrence.

Chordoma

Chordoma is a rare primary bone malignancy that arises from the embryonic notochordal remnants. It is a low-grade slow-growing tumor that is characteristically midline in location and invades locally. The vast majority of chordoma arises in the axial skeleton; however, there have been reports of it occurring in the appendicular skeleton.

It is nearly equally distributed in the skull base, sacrococcygeal region, and mobile spine.[45] The estimated incidence is 0.08 per 100,000; with a peak incidence between 50 and 60 years of age, and males are affected slightly more commonly than females.

Chordoma is characterized by a slow and insidious course. Patients present with pain at the site of the primary tumor, and as the tumor progresses symptoms arising from local invasion and mass effect develop. The symptoms are very nonspecific, and this often results in a significant lag time for initial symptom onset to diagnosis. Owing to the frequent delays in diagnosis, it is not uncommon for patients with sacrococcygeal chordoma to present with large tumors and pelvic viscera displacement. Neural invasion causing bladder and bowel incontinence is a late symptom. The published metastatic rates range from 5% to 40%, and they can involve bone, lung, lymph nodes, and skin.[46,47]

Chordoma appears radiographically as a midline lytic bony lesion. On MRI, it displays high signal

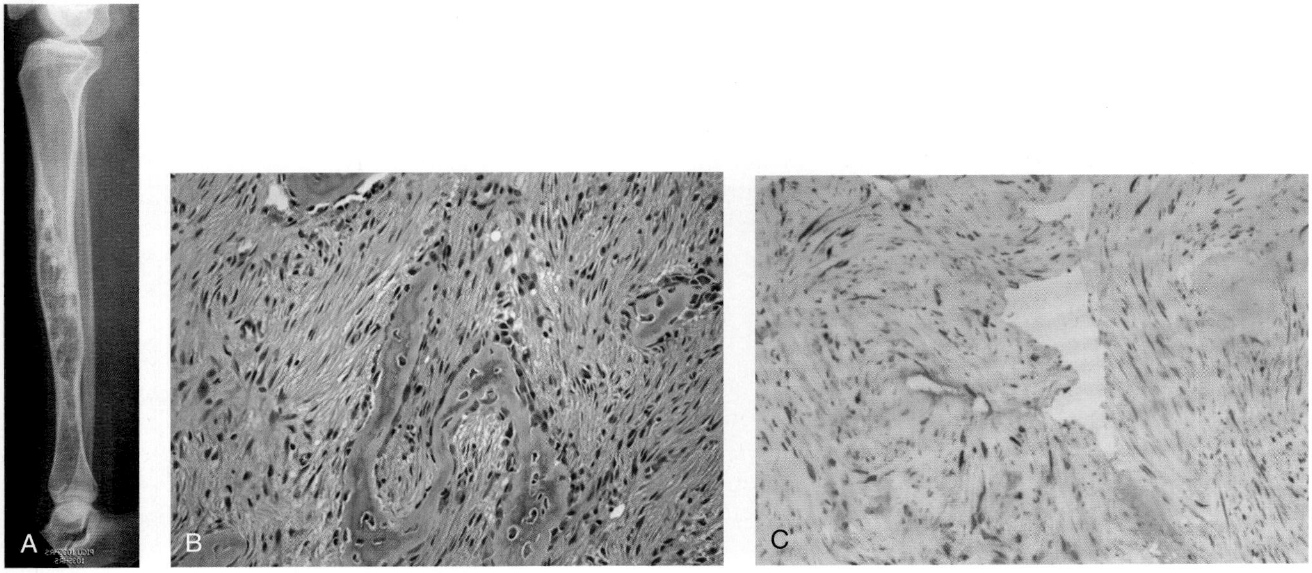

Figure 4 Adamantinoma. **A**, Radiographic appearance of tibia involved by adamantinoma. **B**, Histology depicting epithelial cells within osteofibrous tissue. **C**, Specimen staining positive for keratin.

intensity of T2-weighted images and contrast enhancement, while hypermetabolic activity is present on FDG-18 PET-CT.[48] Chordoma appears grossly as bluish gray myxoid tumor, and microscopically lobules of univacuolated physaliferous cells are separated by fibrous septae within a myxoid matrix (**Figure 5**). Regarding immunohistochemistry, chordoma is positive for S100, vimentin, EMA, and low-molecular-weight cytokeratin. Brachyury is a highly specific marker, which is overexpressed in chordoma and aids in distinguishing chordoma from other morphologically similar tumors.

Benign notochordal cell tumors are the benign counterpart to chordoma, which share morphological similarities, a similar immunophenotype, and cannot be distinguished by any single radiological criterion.[49] Clinical, radiological, and pathological findings need to be taken into consideration together for the diagnosis of chordoma.

Wide en-bloc resection of sacral lesions has been central to the philosophy of management of caudal lesions and contemporary studies of surgical management having clarified prognostic factors and functional results. The association between inadequate margins and local recurrence has been consistently reported and underscores the importance of adequate margins when undertaking resection. The extent of the lesion determines the surgical approach. A posterior approach is often reserved for lesions inferior to the SI joint, whereas lesions extending cranially require a combined anterior-posterior approach to obtain adequate margins. Sacral nerve involvement and the need to sacrifice these nerves can affect bladder and bowel function significantly. Sacrifice of either S2 nerve root is associated with at least the loss of voluntary control, with preservation of both S2 roots and a unilateral S3 root being associated with normal function.[50] Resection involving the SI joint not only requires a more extensive approach but also necessitates reconstruction to maintain stability of the pelvic ring.

The role of RT in the management of chordoma is an evolving area. Chordoma is a radioresistant tumor, and the proximity to the cord and nerve roots complicates the delivery of the high doses necessary to achieve local control. Proton beam therapy with highly conformed fields and better dose deposition permits higher doses to be delivered precisely and is increasingly employed

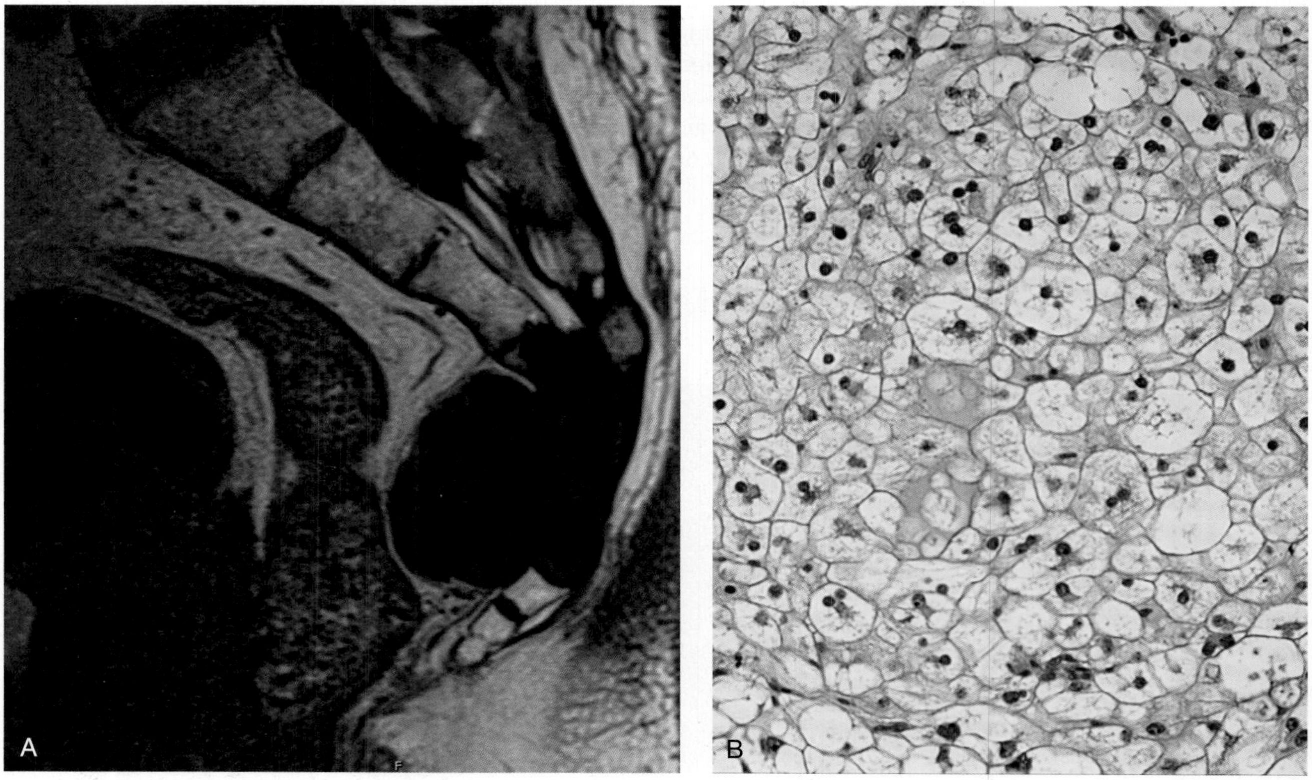

Figure 5 Chordoma. **A**, MRI depicting extent of tumor involving the sacrum. **B**, Histology of chordoma depicting prominent physaliphorous cells.

in the neoadjuvant and adjuvant setting. Charged particle therapy (eg, carbon ion therapy) is another option for RT in some of these challenging anatomic locations; however, there are limited centers in the world that offer this emerging therapy. In certain locations, such as the skull base, conventional photon beam therapy has not been very successful and stereotactic RT or charged particle therapy is preferred.

Although RT protocols vary, 91% 5-year local control rates in primary disease, and 57% local control rate for recurrent cases have been reported with a protocol including a preoperative dose of about 20 Gy, followed by surgical resection, and then a postoperative dose of about 50 Gy.[51] Definitive RT is performed less often, but may be necessary in inoperable disease. Outside of the caudal spine, wide resection is much more technically challenging, and in certain locations, such as the clivus, not feasible. In these situations, RT plays a central role. In the setting of disease in the sacrum and mobile spine, a local progression-free 5-year survival rate of 79.8% has been reported[52] with radiation alone.

Lymphoma

Lymphoma is a malignancy derived from lymphocytes, that is, B cells, T cells, and natural killer cells, and is broadly classified into Hodgkin lymphoma and non-Hodgkin lymphoma.

Hodgkin lymphoma accounts for around 10% of all new cases of lymphoma and is characterized by Reed-Sternberg cells on histology. Most patients are diagnosed in their 20s and 30s, but it can affect patients of all ages. Patients present with painless lymphadenopathy, and frequently with systemic symptoms known as B symptoms such as fever, chills, night sweats, and weight loss. Bone involvement is a feature of metastatic Hodgkin lymphoma, as it does not present with primary bone involvement. Treatment comprises chemotherapy and consolidative RT. Chemotherapy regimens are generally based on doxorubicin, bleomycin, vinblastine, and dacarbazine (ABVD).[53] RT has evolved from total lymphoid irradiation, to involved field RT, and most recently to involved site RT and involved node RT with the goal of reducing field size to minimize late toxicity from RT. Owing to the high rate of remission with 5-year survival rates of about 90% for adults with Hodgkin lymphoma, management of bony lesions should be as durable as possible to minimize the impact of late complications.

Non-Hodgkin lymphoma is a heterogeneous group of lymphoid malignancies that vary in their treatment and prognosis. Although risk factors include primary immunodeficiency, HIV infection, and organ transplantation, most newly diagnosed patients have no known causal factors. Arising from lymphocytes at various stages of development, non-Hodgkin lymphoma varies from the indolent to the aggressive. The most common subtypes of non-Hodgkin lymphoma are diffuse large B-cell lymphoma, chronic lymphocytic leukemia/small-lymphocytic lymphoma, and follicular lymphoma.[54] Patients may present similarly as patients with Hodgkin lymphoma with nonspecific systemic symptoms. It is estimated that 25% to 30% of patients with non-Hodgkin lymphoma have bone marrow involvement on presentation.[55] Complaints of bony, joint, or back pain in patients with non-Hodgkin lymphoma warrant workup as this may represent bony involvement, or a pathological fracture. Lymphoma may also occur primarily in the bone, and in cases of primary bone lymphoma, the diagnosis is that of diffuse large B-cell lymphoma in 90% of cases.

On radiographs, bony involvement by lymphoma appears as a permeative osteolytic lesion with ill-defined borders. MRI defines the extent of the lesion better than radiographs and may reveal a significant extraosseous soft-tissue component to the lesion with varying amounts of periosteal reaction.

Diagnosis of lymphoma requires biopsy of an involved lymph node, or in cases of primary bone lymphoma the primary bony lesion. The diagnosis and subtyping of lymphoma requires ancillary testing including immunohistochemistry, flow cytometry, and other techniques for cytogenetic analysis. These ancillary studies cannot be processed on formalin-fixed specimens, and thus it is important to have biopsy specimens appropriately handled by placing in normal saline and not in formalin. Adequate quantity of biopsy specimens should also be obtained when lymphoma is suspected to ensure sufficient material for all the required pathological studies to subtype the lymphoma.

Surgical management for bony lesions in the setting of lymphoma is mainly for pathologic fractures and impending pathologic fractures. Where surgery is required for diagnosis or in the setting of a fracture, the indication for surgery is often clear. However, as lymphoma frequently responds rapidly and profoundly to chemotherapy, the decision on whether to intervene surgically by way of prophylactic fixation of involved bone needs to take into consideration that surgery may delay the initiation of chemotherapy, and that the response to chemotherapy may diminish the need for surgical intervention. Antiresorptive therapy, that is, diphosphonates or anti-RANKL inhibitors, should be used to mitigate the risk of skeletal-related events (SRE).[56]

Myeloma

Multiple myeloma (MM) is a plasma cell malignancy characterized by clonal plasma cells. It is most often associated with secretion of a monoclonal immunoglobulin or M protein. However, in 15% to 20% of patients, only monoclonal free light chains are secreted and in less than 3% of patients, it is nonsecretory.[57] It lies on the spectrum of monoclonal gammopathies that include monoclonal gammopathy of undetermined significance (MGUS), smoldering multiple myeloma (SMM), and MM. Patients with MGUS and SMM are generally asymptomatic, and the diagnosis of MM requires at least 10% of clonal bone marrow plasma cells, or a biopsy-proven bony or extramedullary plasmacytoma, and the presence of end-organ damage of other myeloma-defining events (MDE). Signs of end-organ damage are known as CRAB features and include hypercalcemia, renal insufficiency, anemia, and bone disease. Apart from the CRAB features, the other MDEs are clonal bone marrow plasma cells ≥60%, serum free light chain (FLC) ratio ≥100 provided involved FLC level is 100 mg/L or higher, or more than one focal bone lesion on MRI.

The treatment for MM has changed significantly in the past decade with the advent of agents that have proved to be active against MM.[58] The standard chemotherapy regimen includes a proteasome inhibitor and an immunomodulatory drug, with the initial treatment of choice being bortezomib, lenalidomide and dexamethasone (known commonly by the acronym VRd representing the proprietary names Velcade, Revlimid, and dexamethasone). Where patients are deemed eligible for autologous stem cell transplant, they typically undergo transplant after four to six cycles of chemotherapy. For patients ineligible for transplant, a year of treatment with VRd is followed by maintenance therapy until disease progression using either bortezomib or lenalidomide.

RT can be valuable in the symptomatic management of symptomatic lesions including vertebral compression fractures, impending pathologic fractures, cord compression, and in combination with close observation in patients with an isolated plasmacytoma without evidence of systemic disease.

Surgical management for MM involves the same principles of management of osteolytic metastatic bone disease comprising the prophylactic fixation of impending pathologic fractures, and internal fixation or endoprosthetic reconstruction of pathologic fractures. Similar to the management of metastatic bone disease, antiresorptive therapy should be used when feasible.

Surgical Principles for Malignant Bone Tumors

The role of surgical management of malignant primary bone tumors varies according to extent of involvement of disease. In patients with localized disease without evidence of systemic involvement, complete removal of all involved tissue with a margin of normal tissue is the goal. In patients with metastatic involvement or multifocal disease, deciding on the specific goals of surgery is more nuanced as surgery potentially has less of an impact on overall survival.

Limb-Salvage Versus Amputation

The era of limb-salvage surgery in orthopaedic oncology was ushered in by the advent of multiagent chemotherapy regimens, which improved survival, and by studies documenting no compromise in survival with the limb-sparing tumor resections as compared with amputation. Short- and long-term studies have shown equivalent survival and quality-of-life outcomes with both approaches, but better functional outcomes have been found with limb-salvage.[59] The decision making surrounding whether to pursue limb-salvage versus an amputation is highly complex. Broadly, the following are factors to be taken into account: (1) whether the patient presents with localized or systemic disease, (2) the desire to optimize the patient's function, (3) the potential impact of the postoperative course on the patient's planned adjuvant treatment and/or remaining life, (4) the response of the patient's disease to neoadjuvant treatment when it is performed, (5) in skeletally immature patients the potential for future growth, and (6) the preferences of the patient.

In patients with localized disease, the priority in management is complete removal of the tumor, and the secondary consideration is function. This is due to the association of positive surgical margins with poorer overall survival. In patients with systemic disease, the goal of surgery may be optimizing the patient's short-term function with a resection and reconstruction that does not entail a complex rehabilitative course or in some cases palliation of symptoms.

The extent of involvement of the bony malignancy on the surrounding soft tissues and vital neurovascular structures may preclude removal of all tumor-bearing tissue without sacrificing vessels, nerves, or large amount of muscles and soft tissue. The expected functional outcome from the best reconstruction of all the structures requiring should be compared with that from an amputation (with a prosthetic where feasible and appropriate) to decide on whether to recommend limb-sparing surgery or amputation.

Certain reconstructive techniques are accompanied by higher risks of perioperative surgical complications, and this should be taken into consideration in patients whose treatment involves adjuvant chemotherapy that would be delayed by wound complications or other complications requiring revision surgery. The importance of chemotherapy on the overall survival outcome cannot be overstated in primary bone malignancies such as osteosarcoma and Ewing sarcoma.

In patients (such as those with osteosarcoma or Ewing sarcoma) who undergo neoadjuvant chemotherapy before surgery, do not have metastatic disease, and show localized disease progression on completion of neoadjuvant chemotherapy, amputation should be considered strongly over limb-sparing surgery. In this patient group where the tumor may have encroached further on surrounding soft tissues, amputation is often the best way to ensure complete removal of the tumor while minimizing the risk of positive surgical margins, and minimizing the risk of delaying resumption of adjuvant chemotherapy.

Consideration of the patient's preferences in choosing between amputation and limb-sparing surgery is significant where limb-sparing surgery although feasible from a technical perspective may be highly complex and has a high degree of unpredictability or where the best functional outcome is modest. Cultural norms and religious beliefs may cause patients to opt for limb-sparing surgery over amputation in such situations. Socioeconomic conditions, the cost of surgical reconstruction, and the availability and cost of prosthetic services and maintenance may also cause patients in certain situations and countries to opt for a certain mode of treatment.

Wide Resection and Margin Assessment

The foundational principles regarding surgical management of bone sarcomas were outlined by Enneking et al[60] with their surgical staging system. Margins are defined as intralesional, marginal, wide, and radical. An intralesional excision involves going through the tumor. A marginal excision involves excision of the tumor through the reactive zone of tissue surrounding the tumor. A wide excision involves excision of the tumor and a cuff of normal tissue surrounding it. A radical excision involves excision of the whole compartment within which the tumor is contained.

The actual size of the margin of normal tissue required to constitute a wide margin is a matter of debate. The association of local recurrence with inadequate surgical margins is well reported,[61] and studies have supported the practice of preserving vital neurovascular structures that may abut a tumor if not directly involved by the tumor when managed in the setting of adjuvant chemotherapy or RT.[62] The quality of the tissue constituting the surgical margins and not just the measured thickness of the margin of tissue around the tumor should be the consideration.

Following surgical resection of the bony tumor, the specimen should be examined for areas where the margins might be close or contaminated. Intraoperative pathologic consultation may be appropriate. Frozen section analysis of areas of concern, including bony resection margins, can be used to guide the need for additional resection of tissue to extend the area of resection. Once it is determined that the resection is adequate, the surgery switches focus from resection to reconstruction.

Surgical Management in the Skeletally Immature Patient

Treatment of primary bone tumors in skeletally immature patients presents a unique set of challenges and opportunities. Although there is no algorithm for this and each individual situation is unique, certain principles must be considered. Most primary tumors in children occur during the second decade of life, a time of accelerated growth. Given that limb-salvage is the treatment of choice after a resection, reconstructive options should strive to achieve a favorable, functional, and durable outcome. The decision on limb-salvage and the type of reconstruction is patient specific, regarding desired level of function and cosmesis, and location specific, with special attention to the extent of resection and remaining bone and soft tissue. Other important issues that must be considered include presence or absence of distant disease, response to neoadjuvant therapies, and potential for future limb-length discrepancies.

Several methods are available to calculate limb-length discrepancies, but the simplest is based on the normal growth rate of each specific physis per year (3 mm proximal femur, 9 mm distal femur, 6 mm proximal tibia, and 5 mm distal tibia). It is important to determine the anticipated discrepancy at skeletal maturity so that necessary steps can be taken to minimize this and provide some direction on the best option for the patient. Generally, a limb-length discrepancy of <2 cm is well tolerated and can be treated with a shoe lift if necessary. An anticipated discrepancy between 2 and 3 cm can be managed with an epiphysiodesis of the contralateral extremity. It is important to obtain serial imaging to determine optimal timing of such an intervention. In the very young patients, where the discrepancy will be >5 cm, options include an expandable endoprosthesis or secondary limb lengthening. Serious consideration for an amputation or rotationplasty should also be given to this patient population.

There are advantages and disadvantages to each reconstructive option available to the patient. Physeal sparing resection and reconstructions, including intercalary allografts, have the advantage of preserving the patient's native joints and physis allowing for continued growth. Disadvantages are infection risks due to length of technically demanding surgery and placement of allograft. In addition, junctional healing between the host and allograft can take up to 1 year. This requires patients to maintain weight-bearing restrictions, and nonunion rates can be as high as 50%, especially in patients undergoing chemotherapy. Endoprosthetic reconstruction has the advantage of immediate weight bearing, cosmetic appearance, and good function. Disadvantages include implant loosening, infection, and need for revision surgery in the future. Patient activity levels must also be modified for the rest of their lives to maximize durability of the implant and minimize complication risks. In the growing patient with an anticipated >5 cm discrepancy, an expandable endoprosthesis can be considered as previously mentioned. Unfortunately, revision surgery and complication rates are unacceptably high in this patient population, even with favorable emotional and physical results.[63] Lastly, amputation and rotationplasty is always an option in the growing child. Both options provide patients with potentially a single surgery and the ability to participate in high-impact activities. Amputations in children with significant remaining growth can lead to bony overgrowth, skin complications, and issues with prosthetic wear. Children who undergo a rotationplasty, the "nonamputation" amputation, are more likely to participate in preoperative hobbies and less likely to have activity restrictions (**Figure 6**). They also have no phantom limb pain, a significant advantage over amputations; however, social acceptance continues to be a significant issue.[64]

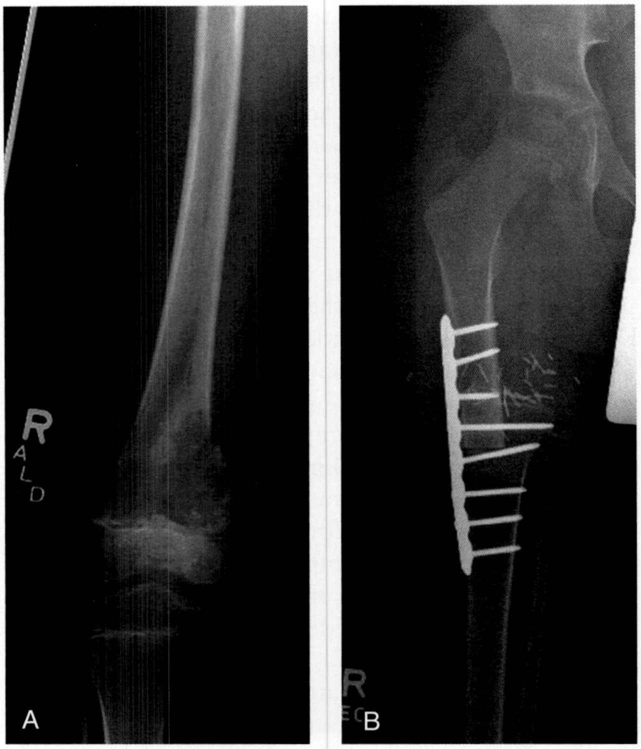

Figure 6 **A**, AP radiograph of a distal femoral osteosarcoma in an 8 year-old boy. **B**, AP radiograph status post distal femoral resection and rotationplasty.

Summary

Primary malignancies of bone comprise 0.2% of all cancers in the United States. A multidisciplinary approach is essential in the appropriate management of this disease. All of these tumors have a unique treatment algorithm which often includes surgery and sometimes chemotherapy and/or radiation therapy. Surgical management of these tumors is both patient and site specific and the majority of the time involves limb-salvage. These tumors often occur in the growing child, which possesses significant challenges when limb-salvage is performed. If the child survives, the durability of the reconstruction becomes important and they can develop significant limb-length discrepancies requiring further surgeries.

Key Study Points

- Osteosarcoma, chondrosarcoma, and Ewing sarcoma are the most common primary malignancies of bone, in that order.
- Lymphoma and myeloma are hematologic malignancies that can affect bone and need orthopaedic evaluation and intervention; prophylactic fixation of impending fractures and sometimes fracture fixation is required.
- Management for primary bone tumors usually involves tumor resection and limb-salvage. Most primary bone tumors occur in the second decade of life in skeletally immature individuals which presents the orthopaedic oncologist with a unique set of challenges when considering reconstructive options.

Annotated References

1. https://seer.cancer.gov/statfacts/html/bones.html.
2. Fletcher CDM, Bridge JA, Hogendoorn P, Mertens F: *WHO Classification of Tumours of Soft Tissue and Bone*, ed 4. IARC WHO Classification of Tumours. WHO, 2013.
3. Ottaviani G, Jaffe N: The epidemiology of osteosarcoma. *Cancer Treat Res* 2009;152:3-13.
4. Misaghi A, Goldin A, Awad M, Kulidjian AA: Osteosarcoma: A comprehensive review. *SICOT J* 2018;4:12.

   Recent review article summarizing osteosarcoma subtypes, diagnosis, clinical and histologic features, management, and future directions. Level of evidence: V (Review article).
5. Ottaviani G, Jaffe N: The epidemiology of osteosarcoma. *Cancer Treat Res* 2009;152:3–13.
6. Klein MJ, Siegal GP: Osteosarcoma: Anatomic and histologic variants. *Am J Clin Pathol* 2006;125(4):555-581.
7. Rose PS, Dickey ID, Wenger DE, Unni KK, Sim FH: Periosteal osteosarcoma: Long-term outcome and risk of late recurrence. *Clin Orthop Relat Res* 2006;453:314-317.
8. Hameed M, Mandelker D: Tumor syndromes predisposing to osteosarcoma. *Adv Anat Pathol* 2018;25(4):217-222.

   Recent review article summarizing rare hereditary cancer syndromes with an increased predisposition to osteosarcoma. Level of evidence: V (Review article).
9. Hanada K, Hickson ID: Molecular genetics of RecQ helicase disorders. *Cell Mol Life Sci* 2007;64(17):2306-2322.
10. Scully SP, Ghert MA, Zurakowski D, Thompson RC, Gebhardt MC: Pathologic fracture in osteosarcoma: Prognostic importance and treatment implications. *J Bone Joint Surg Am* 2002;84-A(1):49-57.
11. Marina N, Gebhardt M, Teot L, Gorlick R: Biology and therapeutic advances for pediatric osteosarcoma. *Oncologist* 2004;9(4):422-441.
12. Thompson MJ, Shapton JC, Punt SE, Johnson CN, Conrad EU III: MRI identification of the osseous extent of pediatric bone sarcomas. *Clin Orthop Relat Res* 2018;476(3):559-564.

    Retrospective study of 55 patients with either Ewing's sarcoma or osteosarcoma of the femur or tibia and comparison between MR-determined tumor extent and actual tumor extent. They concluded that one should account for a 1 cm difference when planning the resection using an MRI after neoadjuvant chemotherapy. Level of evidence: III (Retrospective comparative study).
13. Meyer JS, Nadel HR, Marina N, et al: Imaging guidelines for children with Ewing sarcoma and osteosarcoma: A report from the Children's Oncology Group Bone Tumor Committee. *Pediatr Blood Cancer* 2008;51(2):163-170.
14. Federman N, Bernthal N, Eilber FC, Tap WD: The multidisciplinary management of osteosarcoma. *Curr Treat Options Oncol* 2009;10(1-2):82-93.
15. Wedekind MF, Wagner LM, Cripe TP: Immunotherapy for osteosarcoma: Where do we go from here? *Pediatr Blood Cancer* 2018;65(9):e27227.

    Review outlining the mechanisms and status of immunotherapies currently in clinical trials and future therapies in osteosarcoma. Level of evidence: V (Review article).
16. Messerschmitt PJ, Rettew AN, Brookover RE, Garcia RM, Getty PJ, Greenfield EM: Specific tyrosine kinase inhibitors regulate human osteosarcoma cells in vitro. *Clin Orthop Relat Res* 2008;466(9):2168-2175.
17. Mason NJ, Gnanandarajah JS, Engiles JB, et al: Immunotherapy with a HER2-targeting *Listeria* induces HER2-specific immunity and demonstrates potential therapeutic effects in a phase I trial in canine osteosarcoma. *Clin Cancer Res* 2016;22(17):4380-4390.

    Phase I dose escalation trial on 18 canines with osteosarcoma that underwent amputation or limb-salvage and adjuvant chemotherapy as well as a recombinant *Listeria* vaccine expressing a chimeric HER2/neu fusion protein to induce immunity and prevent metastatic disease. Only low-grade transient toxicities were seen with variable dosing of the vaccine, and there was an increase in survival and a reduction in metastatic disease in these canines. The authors conclude that in patients with minimal residual disease, HER2/neu-specific immunity may reduce the incidence of metastatic disease and prolong survival in this large cancer animal model. Level of evidence: N/A.
18. Kasalak Ö, Glaudemans AWJM, Overbosch J, Jutte PC, Kwee TC: Can FDG-PET/CT replace blind bone marrow biopsy of the posterior iliac crest in Ewing sarcoma? *Skeletal Radiol* 2018;47:363-367.

    Retrospective study of 20 patients with Ewing's sarcoma who underwent both FDG-PET/CT and bone marrow biopsy (a total of 38 biopsies) which found agreement in 36 of 38 biopsies (94.7%, 95% confidence interval [CI]: 82.7%-98.5%) with FDG-PET/CT. Level of evidence: III (Retrospective study).
19. Newman EN, Jones RL, Hawkins DS: An evaluation of [F-18]-fluorodeoxy-D-glucose positron emission tomography, bone scan, and bone marrow aspiration/biopsy as staging investigations in Ewing sarcoma. *Pediatr Blood Cancer* 2013;60:1113-1117.
20. Sharma P, Khangembam BC, Suman KC, et al: Diagnostic accuracy of 18F-FDG PET/CT for detecting recurrence in patients with primary skeletal Ewing sarcoma. *Eur J Nucl Med Mol Imaging* 2013;40:1036-1043.
21. Pappo AS, Patel SR, Crowley J, et al: R1507, a monoclonal antibody to the insulin-like growth factor 1 receptor, in patients with recurrent or refractory Ewing sarcoma family of tumors: results of a phase II Sarcoma Alliance for Research through Collaboration study. *J Clin Oncol* 2011;29:4541–4547.
22. Tang SW, Bilke S, Cao L, et al: SLFN11 is a transcriptional target of EWS-FLI1 and a determinant of drug response in Ewing sarcoma. *Clin Cancer Res.* 2015;21:4184–4193.
23. Dunst J, Jürgens H, Sauer R, et al: Radiation therapy in Ewing's sarcoma: An update of the CESS 86 trial. *Int J Radiat Oncol Biol Phys* 1995;32:919-930.
24. Thorpe SW, Weiss KR, Goodman MA, Heyl AE, McGough RL: Should aggressive surgical local control be attempted in all patients with metastatic or pelvic Ewing's sarcoma? *Sarcoma* 2012;2012:953602.

Oncology and Pathology

25. Bacci G, Ferrari S, Longhi A, et al: Role of surgery in local treatment of Ewing's sarcoma of the extremities in patients undergoing adjuvant and neoadjuvant chemotherapy. *Oncol Rep* 2004;11:111-120.

26. Puri A, Gulia A, Crasto S, Vora T, Khanna N, Laskar S: Does radiotherapy after surgery affect outcomes in Ewing's sarcoma of the pelvis? *Indian J Orthop* 2018;52(1):73-76.

Retrospective study of 44 patients who underwent resection of pelvic Ewing's sarcoma, with postoperative RT (PORT) offered on a case-by-case basis. Five-year overall survival for patients with PORT was 74%, and without PORT was 78% ($P = 0.629$). Level of evidence: III (Retrospective study).

27. Kuttesch JF Jr, Wexler LH, Marcus RB, et al: Second malignancies after Ewing's sarcoma: radiation dose-dependency of secondary sarcomas. *J Clin Oncol* 1996;14:2818–2825.

28. Howlader N, Noone AM, Krapcho M, et al, eds: SEER Cancer Statistics Review 1975-2011. Bethesda, MD, National Cancer Institute. https://seer.cancer.gov/csr/1975_2016/.

29. Cotterill SJ, Ahrens S, Paulussen M, et al: Prognostic factors in Ewing's tumor of bone: Analysis of 975 patients from the European Intergroup Cooperative Ewing's Sarcoma Study Group. *J Clin Oncol* 2000;18:3108-3114.

30. Doyle LA: Sarcoma classification: An update based on the 2013 World Health Organization classification of tumors of soft tissue and bone. *Cancer* 2014;120(12):1763-1774.

31. Björnsson J, McLeod RA, Unni KK, Ilstrup DM, Pritchard DJ: Primary chondrosarcoma of long bones and limb girdles. *Cancer* 1998;83(10):2105-2119.

32. Schwartz HS, Zimmerman NB, Simon MA, Wroble RR, Millar EA, Bonfiglio M: The malignant potential of enchondromatosis. *J Bone Joint Surg Am* 1987;69(2):269-274.

33. Schmale GA, Conrad EU III, Raskind WH: The natural history of hereditary multiple exostoses. *J Bone Joint Surg Am* 1994;76(7):986-992.

34. Rozeman LB, Cleton-Jansen AM, Hogendoorn PC: Pathology of primary malignant bone and cartilage tumours. *Int Orthop* 2006;30(6):437-444.

35. Skeletal Lesions Interobserver Correlation among Expert Diagnosticians (SLICED) Study Group: Reliability of histopathologic and radiologic grading of cartilaginous neoplasms in long bones. *J Bone Joint Surg Am* 2007;89(10): 2113-2123.

36. Doyle LA: Sarcoma classification: an update based on the 2013 World Health Organization classification of tumors of soft tissue and bone. *Cancer* 2014;120(12):1763–1774.

37. Giuffrida AY, Burgueno JE, Koniaris LG, Gutierrez JC, Duncan R, Scully SP: Chondrosarcoma in the United States (1973 to 2003): An analysis of 2890 cases from the SEER database. *J Bone Joint Surg Am* 2009;91(5): 1063-1072.

38. Fromm J, Klein A, Baur-Melnyk A, et al: Survival and prognostic factors in conventional central chondrosarcoma. *BMC Cancer* 2018;18(1):849.

Retrospective review of 87 patients with central chondrosarcoma treated with resection. All patients were followed up and assessed for local recurrence, distant metastasis, and overall survival. They conclude that surgery remains the mainstay of therapy. Tumor grade, metastatic disease, age, and location significantly affect overall survival. Margin status affected local recurrence-free survival but not overall survival. Lastly, pelvic chondrosarcomas should be treated more aggressively and have a higher risk of local recurrence. Level of evidence: III (Retrospective study).

39. Zoccali C, Baldi J, Attala D, et al: Intralesional vs. extralesional procedures for low-grade central chondrosarcoma: A systematic review of the literature. *Arch Orthop Trauma Surg* 2018;138(7):929-937.

This is a meta-analysis and systematic review of the literature analyzing the results of curettage and resection for low-grade chondrosarcomas. The authors found 13 studies that fit their criteria, all of which were descriptive, retrospective, nonrandomized studies. The authors conclude that there is a lack of scientific evidence to support curettage for low-grade chondrosarcomas and that resection must be considered the general rule for these lesions. Level of evidence: III (Metanalysis of retrospective non-randomized studies).

40. Giuffrida AY, Burgueno JE, Koniaris LG, Gutierrez JC, Duncan R, Scully SP: Chondrosarcoma in the United States (1973 to 2003): An analysis of 2890 cases from the SEER database. *J Bone Joint Surg Am* 2009;91(5):1063–1072.

41. Leddy LR, Holmes RE: Chondrosarcoma of bone. *Cancer Treat Res* 2014;162:117-130.

42. Puchner SE, Varga R, Hobusch GM, et al: Long-term outcome following treatment of adamantinoma and osteofibrous dysplasia of long bones. *Orthop Traumatol Surg Res* 2016;102:925-932.

Study of 15 patients with adamantinoma or OFD with follow-up on OFD patients from 2 to 47 years and adamantinoma patients from 10 to 47 years. Local recurrence rates for both when surgically treated were 40% and distant disease occurred in 20% of adamantinoma patients. Level of evidence: IV (Case series).

43. Scholfield DW, Sadozai Z, Ghali C, et al: Does osteofibrous dysplasia progress to adamantinoma and how should they be treated? *Bone Joint J* 2017;99-B(3):409-416.

Retrospective study of 73 patients with OFD, OFD-like adamantinoma, or adamantinoma with a mean follow-up of 10.3 years. No evidence of progression from OFD to adamantinoma observed with conservative management often successful for patients with OFD and OFD-like adamantinoma. Level of evidence: III (Retrospective study).

44. Ramanoudjame M, Guinebretière JM, Mascard E, Seringe R, Dimeglio A, Wicart P: Is there a link between osteofibrous dysplasia and adamantinoma? *Orthop Traumatol Surg Res* 2011;97:877–880.

45. McMaster ML, Goldstein AM, Bromley CM, Ishibe N, Parry DM: Chordoma: Incidence and survival patterns in the United States, 1973-1995. *Cancer Causes Control* 2001;12:1-11.

46. Chambers PW, Schwinn CP: Chordoma. A clinicopathologic study of metastasis. *Am J Clin Pathol* 1979;72:765–776.

47. McPherson CM, Suki D, McCutcheon IE, Gokaslan ZL, Rhines LD, Mendel E: Metastatic disease from spinal chordoma: a 10-year experience. *J Neurosurg Spine* 2006;5:277–280.

48. Park SA, Kim HS: F-18 FDG PET/CT evaluation of sacrococcygeal chordoma. *Clin Nucl Med* 2008;33:906-908.

49. Kreshak J, Larousserie F, Picci P, et al: Difficulty distinguishing benign notochordal cell tumor from chordoma further suggests a link between them. *Cancer Imaging* 2014;14:4.

50. Samson IR, Springfield DS, Suit HD, Mankin HJ: Operative treatment of sacrococcygeal chordoma. A review of twenty-one cases. *J Bone Joint Surg Am* 1993;75:1476-1484.

51. Park L, Delaney TF, Liebsch NJ, et al: Sacral chordomas: Impact of high-dose proton/photon-beam radiation therapy combined with or without surgery for primary versus recurrent tumor. *Int J Radiat Oncol Biol Phys* 2006;65:1514-1521.

52. Chen YL, Liebsch N, Kobayashi W, et al: Definitive high-dose photon/proton radiotherapy for unresected mobile spine and sacral chordomas. *Spine* 2013;38(15):E930-E936.

53. Diefenbach CS, Connors JM, Friedberg JW, et al: Hodgkin lymphoma: Current status and clinical trial recommendations. *J Natl Cancer Inst* 2017;109(4). doi: 10.1093/jnci/djw249.

Review articles summarizing National Clinical Trials Network lymphoid malignancies clinical trials planning meeting consensus on current standard of care for Hodgkin lymphoma, unmet needs, and landscape of ongoing trials. Level of evidence: V (Review article).

54. Al-Hamadani M, Habermann TM, Cerhan JR, Macon WR, Maurer MJ, Go RS: Non-Hodgkin lymphoma subtype distribution, geodemographic patterns, and survival in the US: A longitudinal analysis of the National Cancer Data Base from 1998 to 2011. *Am J Hematol* 2015;90:790-795.

55. Conlan MG, Bast M, Armitage JO, Weisenburger DD: Bone marrow involvement by non-Hodgkin's lymphoma: the clinical significance of morphologic discordance between the lymph node and bone marrow. Nebraska Lymphoma Study Group. *J Clin Oncol* 1990;8:1163–1172.

56. Ottanelli S: Prevention and treatment of bone fragility in cancer patient. *Clin Cases Miner Bone Metab* 2015;12:116–129.

57. Kyle RA, Gertz MA, Witzig TE, et al: Review of 1027 patients with newly diagnosed multiple myeloma. *Mayo Clin Proc* 2003;78:21-33.

58. Rajkumar SV: Multiple myeloma: 2016 update on diagnosis, risk-stratification, and management. *Am J Hematol* 2016;91:719-734.

Review article summarizing state of the art regarding diagnosis and management of multiple myeloma. Level of evidence: V (Review article).

59. Rougraff BT, Simon MA, Kneisl JS, Greenberg DB, Mankin HJ: Limb salvage compared with amputation for osteosarcoma of the distal end of the femur. A long-term oncological, functional, and quality-of-life study. *J Bone Joint Surg Am* 1994;76:649-656.

60. Enneking WF, Spanier SS, Goodman MA: A system for the surgical staging of musculoskeletal sarcoma. *Clin Orthop Relat Res* 1980;153:106-120.

61. Nathan SS, Gorlick R, Bukata S, et al: Treatment algorithm for locally recurrent osteosarcoma based on local disease-free interval and the presence of lung metastasis. *Cancer* 2006;107:1607-1616.

62. Bertrand TE Cruz A, Binitie O, Cheong D, Letson GD: Do surgical margins affect local recurrence and survival in extremity, nonmetastatic, high-grade osteosarcoma? *Clin Orthop Relat Res* 2016;474:677-683.

Retrospective study of 31 patients analyzing margin status. Negative margins >1 mm compared with positive margins was a negative predictor of local recurrence, and positive margins had higher mortality than those with negative margins (HR, 6.26; 95% CI, 1.50-26.14; $P = 0.0119$). Level of evidence: III (Retrospective study).

63. Henderson ER, Pepper AM, Marulanda G, Binitie OT, Cheong D, Letson GD: Outcome of lower-limb preservation with an expandable endoprosthesis after bone tumor resection in children. *J Bone Joint Surg Am* 2012;94(6):537-547.

64. Levin AS, Arkader A, Morris CD: Reconstruction following tumor resections in skeletally immature patients. *J Am Acad Orthop Surg* 2017;25(3):204-213.

Review article discussing the current experience and results of limb-sparing surgery following bone sarcoma resections in growing children. Level of evidence: V (Review article).

Oncology and Pathology

Chapter 68

Soft-Tissue Tumors: Evaluation and Diagnosis

Bryan S. Moon, MD

ABSTRACT

Soft-tissue tumors are very common. Most of these tumors will be benign and can be managed appropriately by the primary orthopaedic surgeon. However, sarcomas will also be encountered, and it is important that they be identified before an unplanned resection. Fortunately, a thorough evaluation which includes quality imaging will result in appropriate management. MRI is the imaging modality of choice for the majority of soft-tissue tumors. When imaging is not definitive for a benign process, then needle biopsy or referral is indicated.

Keywords: benign; biopsy; chemotherapy; malignant; MRI; radiation therapy; resection; sarcoma; soft tissue; staging

Introduction

Soft-tissue tumors are very common. Although the exact incidence of benign tumors is unknown, and impossible to determine, it is estimated that benign soft-tissue tumors are at least 100 times more common than sarcomas. Although this is reassuring for orthopaedic surgeons and their patients, this commonality can lead to expectations of benignity which may result in unplanned resections of sarcomas. Unplanned resections, although still treatable, can cause a significant increase in morbidity for the patient. For this reason, adequate evaluation is essential.

History and physical are highly variable for soft-tissue masses. Size, consistency, depth, and absence or presence of growth are all important features to consider. Masses that are small, soft, superficial, and dormant are most likely benign and may be observed. Firm, deep, and enlarging masses require a higher level of suspicion. For masses that do not demonstrate a classic presentation, such as Dupuytren contracture or a dorsal wrist ganglion that transilluminates, imaging is indicated.

Quality imaging is critical in the evaluation of soft-tissue masses and criteria for the appropriateness of imaging exist.[1] Radiographs can be beneficial in certain cases such as identifying phleboliths in a hemangioma, a peripheral rim of calcification in myositis ossificans, or cortical involvement, but radiographs alone are rarely diagnostic. For small subcutaneous tumors, ultrasonography can be very useful. Ultrasonography can be an excellent modality for identifying superficial cystic and lipomatous masses, but its accuracy is dependent upon user experience and it may lack specificity.[2] MRI is the modality of choice for deep-seated masses and in certain situations, such as lipomas and vascular malformations, MRI can be diagnostic. Unfortunately, except for lipomas, most benign soft-tissue masses and sarcomas will demonstrate some degree of low signal on T1 images, high signal on T2 images, and contrast enhancement. So, although MRI is useful in raising suspicion for sarcoma or developing a differential diagnosis, it is not always diagnostic, and a systematic approach is encouraged.[3] One common error is trusting the diagnosis of a cyst on noncontrast MRI because a myxoid neoplasm (solid) can mimic a true cyst (fluid). In both cases MRI can demonstrate homogenous low signal on T1 images and high signal on T2 images (**Figure 1**). The important message is that contrast is needed for differentiation to avoid an unplanned sarcoma resection. A cyst will demonstrate only peripheral or septal enhancement, whereas myxoid lesions will have more diffuse enhancement.

For any mass that has not been definitively determined as benign following a thorough evaluation, biopsy before resection is warranted. Depending on the location, small (<3 cm) subcutaneous masses may be considered for excisional biopsy. For all other indeterminate masses, needle biopsy is warranted. Needle biopsy is preferred over an open biopsy because there is less potential for tumor contamination with a needle biopsy and diagnostic accuracy is excellent. Although needle biopsy is not technically demanding, the overall process that ranges from proper biopsy placement to accurate pathologic assessment is complex. A

Dr. Moon or an immediate family member serves as a board member, owner, officer, or committee member of the American Academy of Orthopaedic Surgeons and the Western Orthopaedic Association.

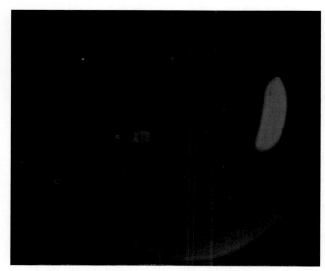

Figure 1 T2 fat-saturated image from noncontrast MRI. This is a myxoid liposarcoma that was interpreted and treated as a "cyst." (Courtesy of Behrang Amini, MD, PhD.)

reasonable guideline for the nononcologic orthopaedic surgeon is that any deep mass that is 4 cm or greater in size should be considered malignant and referral to an orthopaedic oncologist for assessment and biopsy is appropriate.[4]

Lipoma

Lipoma is the most common soft-tissue tumor that will be encountered by an orthopaedic surgeon and is one of the few soft-tissue masses that can be definitively identified on imaging. On MRI, the mass simply needs to be compared to the subcutaneous fat. A lipoma will demonstrate the same imaging features as subcutaneous fat on all MRI sequences (**Figure 2**). Lipomas can be solitary or multiple and can occur in an unlimited number of subcutaneous, intramuscular, intermuscular, and even intraosseous locations. Dormant, small (<5 cm), asymptomatic lipomas can be safely observed. Larger (>5 cm), deep, enlarging, or symptomatic lipomas can be marginally excised and rarely recur.

Atypical Lipoma

When treating the larger variety of lipoma, it is important to be aware of a variant known as atypical lipoma/well-differentiated liposarcoma (ALT/WDL). This variant can be classified as a low-grade malignancy with higher recurrence rates than typical lipomas but, when located in the extremity, rarely dedifferentiate or metastasize. For this reason, marginal resection is appropriate with the knowledge that the recurrence rate is higher than garden variety lipomas. On imaging, atypical lipomas tend to be larger, more septated, and less homogenous on MRI when compared with standard lipomas[5] (**Figure 3**). Following resection, atypical lipomas can be identified solely by histologic features, but when equivocal, the authors of a 2016 study have identified FISH for MDM2 as the ancillary study of choice.[6]

Lipoma Variants

Several variants of lipoma exist: angiolipoma, fibrolipoma, spindle cell lipoma, hibernoma. Not only do these variants differ histologically from a lipoma, they also display unique chromosomal aberrations. The imaging features can also be variable when compared with a classic lipoma. For example, a hibernoma, which is composed of brown fat, demonstrates high signal on T1 and T2 images. It is not uncommon for lipoma variants to require biopsy before definitive diagnosis. Despite the unique differences when compared with lipoma, the treatment for lipoma variants is the same and marginal resection is typically curable.

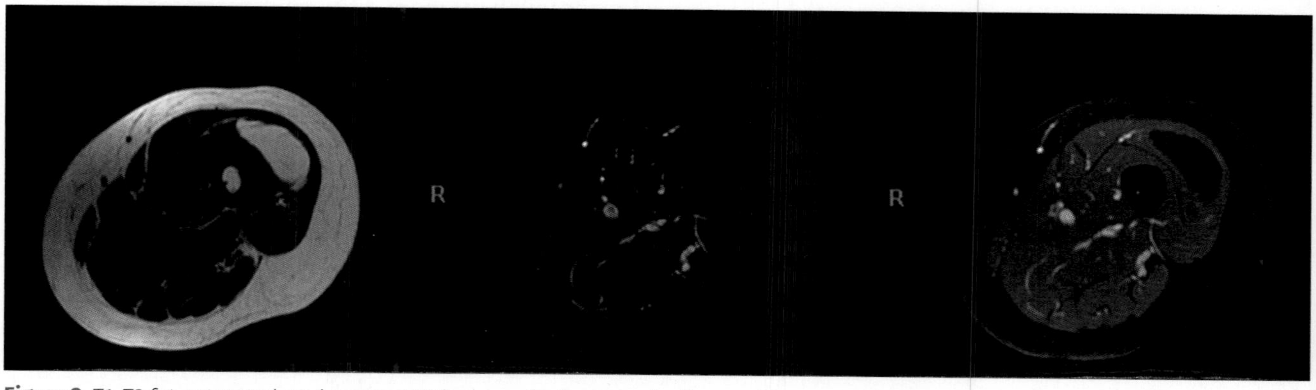

Figure 2 T1, T2 fat-saturated, and contrast T1 images of intramuscular lipoma. The magnetic resonance signal is same as subcutaneous fat on all sequences.

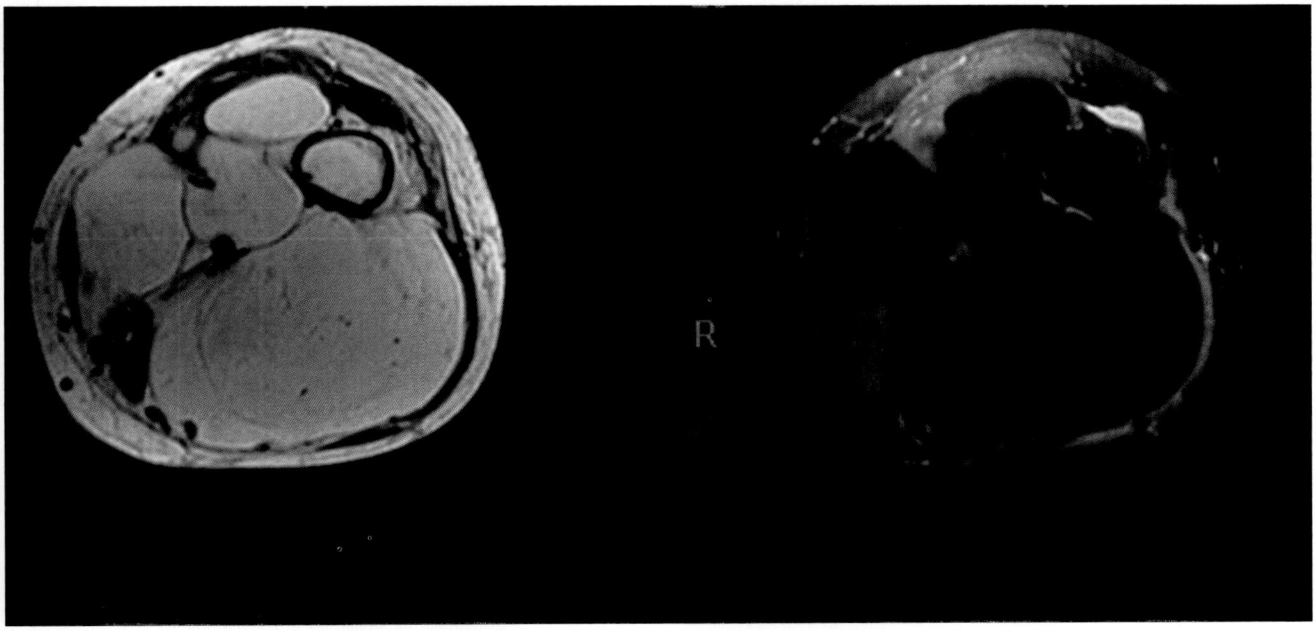

Figure 3 T1 and T2 fat-saturated images of large, septated atypical lipoma encasing the femoral artery.

Ganglion

Ganglion cysts arise from the joint capsule or tendon sheath and are the most common mass of the hand. They are typically firm, nonmobile, superficial mucin-filled masses with a classic predilection for the dorsum of the hand and foot although they can appear in any juxta-articular or peritendinous location. Physical examination can be diagnostic for most cases via transillumination or complete decompression at the time of aspiration. Ganglions are anechoic to hypoechoic on ultrasonography. MRI demonstrates low signal on T1 images and high signal on T2 images with peripheral or septal enhancement. For asymptomatic cysts, observation is appropriate whereas aspiration/injection or excision may be considered for symptomatic cysts.

Meniscal Cyst

Meniscal cysts are the result of joint fluid accumulation outside of the knee capsule and may present as a painful, firm mass along the joint line of the knee. This collection of fluid is due to a capsular defect that acts similar to a one-way valve. The meniscal cyst is formed secondarily and is merely a symptom of the true underlying problem. In most cases, a meniscal tear will be identified as the primary source of pathology. MRI is the imaging modality of choice because it can identify the cyst, meniscal tear, and communication of the cyst with the tear. Management of the symptomatic meniscal cyst typically involves management of the meniscal tear and aspiration or decompression of the cyst.

Popliteal/Baker Cyst

Popliteal cysts, also known as Baker cysts, are synovial lined cysts that form in the popliteal region of the knee. Patients may present with a pain or fullness in the posterior knee and will typically have symptoms of intra-articular pathology such as degenerative joint disease or meniscal tear. Like meniscal cysts, popliteal cysts develop secondarily via extravasation of joint fluid. These cysts typically can be easily identified on MRI because the classic cyst will demonstrate low T1 and high T2 signal with communication of joint fluid with the semimembranosus-gastrocnemius bursa. Popliteal cysts can become quite large and are not always homogenous on MRI because of debris, loose bodies, or hemorrhage that can accumulate in the cyst. The lining of the cyst will show enhancement on contrast MRI and can be quite thickened and septated because of inflammation. In such cases with atypical MRI features, clear communication with the joint should be verified before the assumption of a popliteal cyst. The primary treatment of the popliteal cysts requires management of the underlying intra-articular pathology. Following appropriate management, popliteal cysts may resolve without excision. For larger cysts that are causing symptoms in the popliteal fossa, excision through a posterior or posteromedial approach may be performed.

Popliteal cysts in children are considered separately because typically they are not associated with intra-articular pathology and may not always communicate with the joint. The fluid may involve the semimembranosus-gastrocnemius or subgastrocnemius bursa and usually resolve spontaneously without treatment.

Fibroma of Tendon Sheath

There is uncertainty regarding the classification of fibroma as a reactive or neoplastic process. However, this makes little difference as far as clinical management is concerned. Fibromas present as firm nodules, typically of the hands and feet, that overly tendinous structures. They are typically slow growing and may be painful. MRI will demonstrate a low signal mass on T1 and T2 images that is intimate with the tendon sheath. Nonpainful lesions that are not demonstrating growth can be observed. Enlarging or painful lesions can be marginally excised, but the local recurrence rate is not negligible. Therefore, management should be dictated by symptoms rather than the mere presence of the fibroma.

Plantar/Palmar Fibromatosis

Fibromatosis exists along the intermediate behavior spectrum of benign fibrous lesions and demonstrate infiltrative growth patterns. The palmar (Dupuytren) variant is more common than plantar (Ledderhose), but some patients may be affected by both variants. Palmar fibromatosis is more common in the elderly, whereas plantar fibromatosis can be seen in children.

Palmar fibromatosis tends to affect the ulnar aspect of the hand. There is typically slow progression that eventually results in contracture of the little and ring finger. Although not necessarily painful, the contracture can ultimately lead to significant dysfunction. Given the classic presentation, imaging is not typically required to make the diagnosis. Historically, the treatment of choice has been surgical resection. However, according to a 2018 meta-analysis, collagenase injection is equally efficacious.[7]

Plantar fibromatosis typically presents in the arch of the foot, arising from the plantar fascia. They typically arise as a small, isolated nodule but can progress to large, diffuse masses. The appearance is not as classic as the palmar variety and imaging can be beneficial to rule out a more threatening process. MRI will demonstrate a low-signal lesion arising from the plantar fascia. This process can often be self-limited and may be appropriately treated with shoe modification. Given the significant recurrence rate following surgical resection, wide margins is the goal. However, given the infiltrative nature, this is not always possible without associated morbidity. For this reason, more conservative treatment measures are encouraged.

Desmoid

Desmoid fibromatosis is the most locally aggressive of the "benign" fibrous tissue proliferations. It typically presents in the third decade and is more commonly found in women. Desmoid is a true neoplastic process with mutations identified in the CTNNB1 or the APC gene, and patients with familial adenomatous polyposis have a higher incidence than the general population. Desmoids present as deep-seated, firm, infiltrative mass that can be exquisitely painful. MRI demonstrates a mass with ill-defined margins and low signal on T1 and T2 images (**Figure 4**). Contrast enhancement is variable. Biopsy is required for definitive diagnosis. With no accurate means to predict clinical behavior, treatment for desmoids is highly variable and depends on location, symptoms, and signs of progression. Observation with or without NSAID therapy

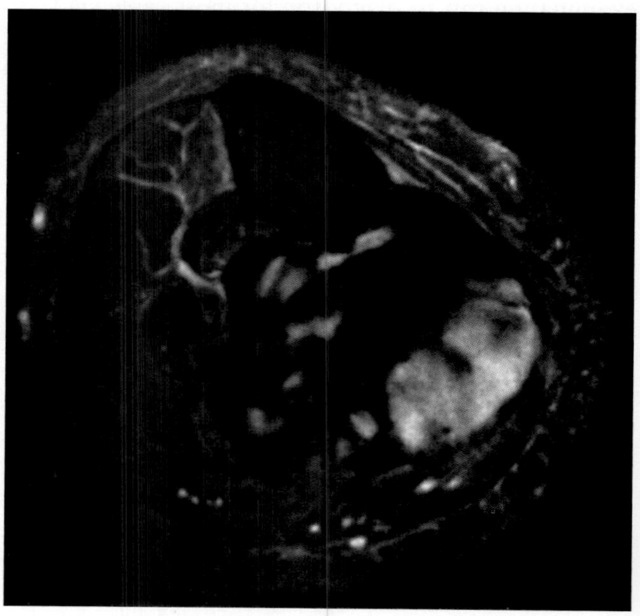

Figure 4 Axial T2 image of a desmoid tumor in the posterior compartment of the calf.

is appropriate for minimally symptomatic, indolent lesions. For lesions that are more clinically aggressive the options include surgical resection, radiation therapy, hormonal therapy, or chemotherapy. Surgery is typically reserved for masses that are accessible with negative margins and without significant morbidity. However, a desmoid's infiltrative nature should not be underestimated because negative margins can be difficult to achieve and recurrence rates are substantial.[8] For this reason, surgical resection should be considered cautiously. Radiation therapy and/or chemotherapy may be a more suitable option and an algorithmic approach should be considered.[9]

Pigmented Villonodular Synovitis

Pigmented villonodular synovitis (PVNS) is a true neoplastic process that affects the synovial lining of the joint. It is the result of a translocation that causes CSF1 overexpression. It can occur in any joint but is most commonly seen in the knee. The process can be highly variable ranging from an isolated, nodular form to a diffuse villonodular pattern. The patient typically presents with joint pain and recurrent effusion. Aspiration will typically result in hemorrhagic synovial fluid. Imaging and presentation alone can typically make the diagnosis, especially in cases with diffuse joint involvement. Radiographs may demonstrate articular erosions and, in later stages, loss of joint space. MRI demonstrates synovial proliferation that is low to intermediate signal on T1 and T2 images with variable contrast enhancement. The presence of bone erosion is also not uncommon. Blooming artifact can be seen on gradient echo images because of hemosiderin deposition. For most cases, surgical management is the treatment of choice. The isolated nodular form responds well to arthroscopic or open resection with a low recurrence rate. The villonodular form can be much more challenging for the patient and surgeon alike. In this case, extensive synovectomy is the treatment of choice. Whether this is performed arthroscopically or open depends on the extensiveness of the proliferation and the skill level of the arthroscopic surgeon and his or her ability to adequately access the entire joint. However, in a 2017 study, the authors found that recurrence rates for arthroscopic management of diffuse disease tend to be higher.[10] If advanced degenerative changes are present, then joint arthroplasty is indicated. Because of the recurrence rate and morbidity associated with radical synovectomy, the search for an effective adjuvant with supportive data and acceptable risk benefit ratio persists. Currently, tyrosine kinase inhibitors and monoclonal antibodies that target the CSF1 receptor continue to be explored. In a 2018 phase 2 trial, the authors report 90% disease control with the use of nilotinib.[11]

Synovial Chondromatosis

Synovial chondromatosis is a rare, metaplastic process of the synovial lining of the joint. In most of cases, its clinical course is benign; however, there have been reports of malignant degeneration. It most commonly affects the knee but can occur in various joints. Patients typically present with pain, swelling, and mechanical symptoms of the involved joint. Imaging alone can be diagnostic. Radiographs may demonstrate multiple lobular calcifications within the joint along with degenerative changes of the joint or, if no calcification has occurred, only a joint effusion may be noted. MRI will identify a joint effusion and lobular masses that demonstrate signal characteristics of cartilage, and calcifications are seen as signal voids. CT can also be useful if the nodules demonstrate calcification and can identify subtle joint erosions. Treatment involves surgical removal of the loose bodies and synovectomy through either an open or arthroscopic approach. If there are already advanced degenerative changes at the time of surgery, then joint arthroplasty is indicated.

Neurofibroma

Neurofibromas are benign tumors that originate from nonmyelinating Schwann cells. Most will present in solitary form with no genetic predisposition. Other forms include diffuse or plexiform which typically present in neurofibromatosis. Solitary neurofibromas may occur in any location ranging from the skin to peripheral nerves to bone. There are no distinctive clinical features for solitary neurofibromas, but neurofibromatosis has classic features that include café au lait spots on the skin, axillary/inguinal freckling, and Lisch nodules on the iris of the eye. Neurofibromas are hypointense on T1 images and hyperintense on T2 images. The target sign is highly suggestive of neurofibroma and can be seen as a hyperintense rim with a central area of low signal. MRI can also demonstrate the specific involvement of the affected nerve and is useful in planning treatment. The primary treatment for symptomatic neurofibromas is surgical resection. However, unlike schwannomas, neurofibromas are inseparable from the fibers of the involved nerve. This is of little consequence for neurofibromas that involve the skin or small nerve branches where resection will not result in any significant morbidity. However, for neurofibromas involving major peripheral nerves, conservative management is prudent because even meticulous, fiber-sparing resection can result in significant nerve dysfunction. According to a 2016 study, malignant degeneration has been reported for isolated neurofibromas but is more common when associated with NF1.[12]

Schwannoma

Schwannomas, as their name implies, are benign tumors that arise from Schwann cells. They most commonly present as isolated masses but can also rarely present as a form of schwannomatosis which has clinical overlap with NF2. Schwannomas can present in virtually any nerve fiber but are common in the head/neck and flexor surface of the extremities. They may range from painless to very painful and may exhibit a positive Tinel sign. Schwannomas are typically low signal on T1 and hyperintense on T2 and enhance diffusely with contrast. Other signs can also be very useful including the split-fat sign (thin, peripheral rim of fat) and the target sign (high signal rim with low signal center). Larger schwannomas may also show cystic degeneration or hemorrhage. For symptomatic schwannomas, surgical resection is the treatment of choice. Because schwannomas are encapsulated and are typically positioned eccentrically on the nerve, they can be marginally excised without associated nerve dysfunction. Marginal resection is typically curative and malignant degeneration is rare. A variant of schwannoma called cellular schwannoma also exists. This variant does demonstrate a higher rate of local recurrence especially with incomplete excision, but the overall prognosis is similar to schwannoma.

Intramuscular Hemangioma

Intramuscular hemangioma, also known as venous malformation, is a benign proliferation of excess blood vessels. The cause is unknown, but a history of trauma is not uncommon. When present in the extremity, this condition most commonly occurs in the thigh. The typical history is a mass that increases in size and pain level with activity but may be asymptomatic at rest. The mass is typically soft, compressible, and ill-defined on examination. Bluish discoloration may be noted when the location is superficial. Radiographs may demonstrate multiple phleboliths. On MRI, hemangiomas are low signal on T1 images with areas of high signal that indicate the presence of fat within the lesion. T2 images usually demonstrates high signal. The appearance is usually multilobulated and tubular structure can be seen. The "dot" sign, a central area of low intensity on T2 images, can be specific for hemangioma. Flow voids can also be seen in lesions with higher flow. Initial treatment should be conservative and may include observation, NSAIDs, and compressive garments. For more symptomatic lesions, surgery should be considered cautiously. Intramuscular hemangiomas tend to have an infiltrative growth pattern, so surgical resection should include tissue well beyond the palpable margins of the lesion. Given the significant morbidity and recurrence rates that may accompany surgical resection, other options such as sclerotherapy or embolization should be considered.[13]

Sarcoma

Sarcomas are malignant neoplasms that arise from mesenchymal cells which, embryologically, originate from the mesoderm. They have been classified by the World Health Organization into 12 different groups based on tissue type[14] (**Table 1**). They represent a heterogeneous group of tumors histologically and behaviorally that require aggressive management to result in cure.

Table 1

World Health Organization 2013 Soft-Tissue Tumor Categories

Adipocytic
Fibroblastic/myofibroblastic
So-called fibrohistiocytic
Smooth muscle
Pericytic
Skeletal muscle
Vascular
Chondro-osseous
Gastrointestinal stroma
Nerve sheath
Tumors of uncertain differentiation
Undifferentiated/unclassified sarcoma

Data from Jo VY, Fletcher CDM: WHO classification of soft tissue tumours: An update based on the 2013 (4th) edition. *Pathology* 2014;46(2):95-104.

Soft-tissue sarcomas are staged via the American Joint Committee on Cancer (AJCC) or Enneking staging systems. The AJCC staging system is more comprehensive in that it is based on tumor size and grade, lymph node involvement, and presence or absence of distant metastases (TNM), whereas the Enneking system is based primarily on grade, location within the anatomic compartment, and metastases.[15] Although staging is an important step with regard to standardized communication and development of treatment algorithms, the heterogeneous nature of sarcoma behavior limits the prognostic value of staging systems when compared with other cancers. The AJCC Cancer Staging Manual, Eighth Edition tries to address some of the issues of heterogeneity by creating different staging schemes depending on the anatomic location of the sarcoma, including additional size classifications, and grouping lymph node metastases with distant metastasis. In a 2017 study that discusses the AJCC changes, the authors indicate that it is yet to be seen whether or not these changes have improved the usefulness of the staging system.[16]

The typical presentation of a soft-tissue sarcoma is a painless mass in the fifth or sixth decade of life. Its innocuous presentation belies its aggressive nature and it is not uncommon for the sarcoma to go unrecognized until it becomes quite large. Although the most common location is the thigh, soft-tissue sarcomas can arise in any location. Adequate staging studies should be performed in the initial stages of presentation to guide treatment and assist in prognosis. Appropriate staging includes imaging of the primary site with a contrasted MRI as well as imaging of the lungs via radiographs or CT scan because the lungs are the most common site of metastatic disease. Lymph node imaging is not typically required but may be considered for certain sarcoma subtypes—clear cell, rhabdomyosarcoma, epithelioid, and angiosarcoma. Positron emission tomography CT scans are currently not indicated as a routine diagnostic tool. MRI, although not diagnostic, is the imaging modality of choice and is required for surgical planning because it accurately identifies the location of critical neurovascular structures. The treatment for sarcoma is usually multimodal by combining surgery with radiation therapy and/or chemotherapy.

Surgery

Negative margin surgical resection is the benchmark for sarcoma management. To achieve this goal an extracapsular, wide resection with a margin of normal tissue is required. These types of resections frequently result in large soft-tissue defects that require complex wound management including the use of muscle flaps. Although negative margin resections are the benchmark, a standard thickness of margin has not been established. Given a sarcoma's tendency to grow intimately adjacent to neurovascular structures, margins may be as small as a millimeter. In a 2017 study, the authors found that the quality of margin rather than the margin width was more predictive of prognosis.[17] For this reason, preservation rather than resection and reconstruction of vascular and neural structures can typically be achieved. Surgical resection alone may be considered for low-grade sarcomas, but because of higher rates of local recurrence for high-grade sarcomas, surgical resection is typically coupled with radiation therapy.

Radiation

The rationale for radiation therapy is the treatment of microscopic satellite disease that may extend beyond the surgical margin. Radiation therapy may be given preoperatively or postoperatively. Although both are equally effective in enhancing local control, each carries its own set of risks and benefits. Although preoperative radiation therapy is performed with a smaller dose and treatment field, the rate of wound complications is significantly higher than postoperative radiation. Postoperative radiation therapy has fewer wound complications, but it has a higher rate of soft-tissue fibrosis. The radiation doses range from approximately 50 to 65 Gy and are given in multiple small fractions over several weeks. In either scenario a break of several weeks between radiation and surgery is instituted to decrease the rates of adverse wound reactions.

Chemotherapy

Chemotherapy remains controversial for patients who present without metastatic disease. Survival rates for soft-tissue sarcoma continue to hover around 60% to 70%, and an effective chemotherapy is needed. When all soft-tissue sarcomas are evaluated as a group, most studies demonstrate survival benefits from chemotherapy to occur in a minority of patients. On the one hand, some subtypes such as Ewing sarcoma, rhabdomyosarcoma, and synovial sarcoma may demonstrate more chemosensitivity. On the other hand, chemotherapy may also be beneficial as far as local treatment is concerned. Myxoid liposarcoma, for example, is known as

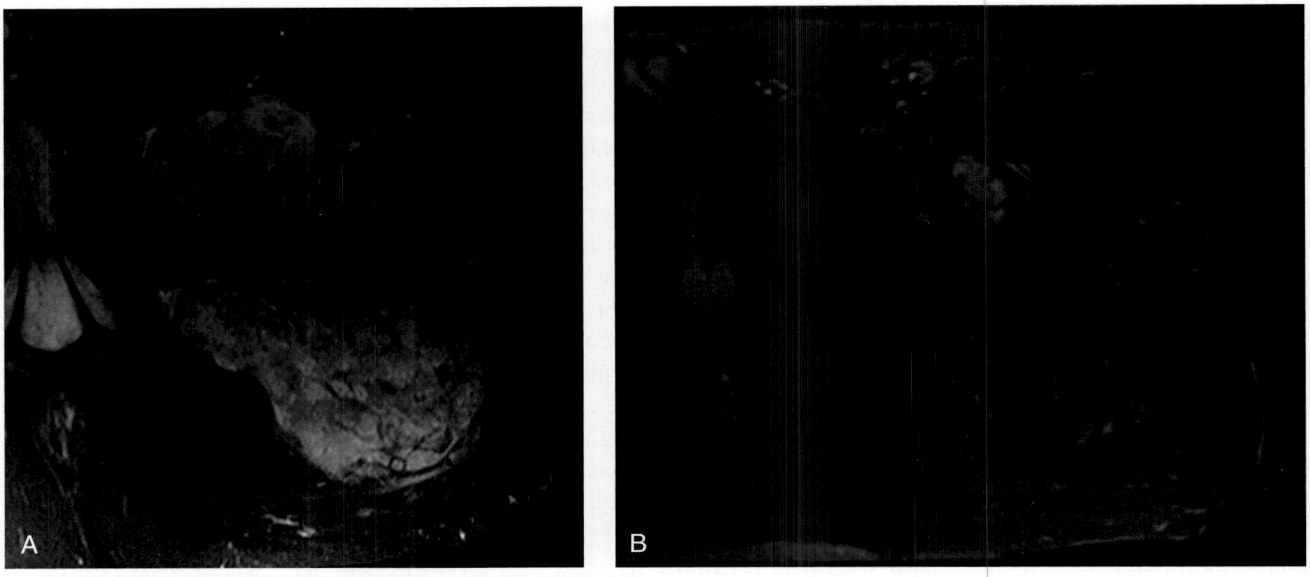

Figure 5 T2 images of myxoid liposarcoma before (**A**) and after (**B**) chemotherapy demonstrating dramatic local response.

one sarcoma subtype that can be exquisitely sensitive to preoperative chemotherapy with significant reduction in size of the tumor (**Figure 5**). This can be beneficial to the patient and surgeon by potentially leading to a less morbid resection. For these reasons, the risks and benefits of chemotherapy should be weighed for each patient's individual situation and judicious use may be employed. In a 2016 review, the authors identify that, when used, the first line of chemotherapy for soft-tissue sarcoma is a combination of doxorubicin and ifosfamide.[18] Targeted therapies and immunotherapy are alternatives to standard chemotherapy and continue to be explored. In a 2017 review of immunotherapy for sarcoma, the authors express high expectations with immunotherapy upon its maturation and better understanding of its mechanism of action.[19]

Summary

Soft-tissue tumors are extremely common and will be encountered by orthopaedic surgeons regardless of specialty. Although benign tumors are much more common than sarcomas, one should not assume that a mass is benign. In the majority of cases, a thorough history, physical, and appropriate imaging can lead to either a diagnosis or at least an appropriate level of suspicion for a malignancy. Masses smaller than 3 cm can be treated via excisional biopsy. Any other mass that cannot be definitively diagnosed on imaging should undergo needle biopsy before resection or direct referral to an orthopaedic oncologist.

Key Study Points

- Lipomas can be reliably diagnosed on MRI. A lipoma will have identical signal characteristics to subcutaneous fat on all sequences.
- Myxoid neoplasms can be mistaken for "cysts" on noncontrasted MRI.
- Diffuse PVNS continues to have high rates of local recurrence and open synovectomy continues to be standard treatment.
- Soft-tissue sarcomas most commonly present as a painless mass.
- High grade soft-tissue sarcomas are treated with a combination of surgery and radiation to improve rates of local control. Chemotherapy remains controversial for nonmetastatic soft-tissue sarcomas.
- The search continues to identify an effective, reliable adjuvant for desmoid tumors, diffuse PVNS, and soft-tissue sarcoma.

Annotated References

1. Kransdorf MJ, Murphey MD, Wessell DE, et al: *ACR Appropriateness Criteria®: Soft-Tissue Masses*. 2017, American College of Radiology. Available at: https://acsearch.acr.org/docs/69434/Narrative/. Accessed August 2018.

   The authors identify the most common clinical scenarios for soft-tissue tumors and recommend the most appropriate imaging for their assessment.

2. Bui-Mansfield LT, Chen DC, O'Brien SD: Accuracy of ultrasound of musculoskeletal soft-tissue tumors. *AJR Am J Roentgenol* 2015;204:W218.

3. Chung WJ, Chung HW, Shin MJ, et al: MRI to differentiate benign from malignant soft-tissue tumours of the extremities: A simplified systematic imaging approach using depth, size and heterogeneity of signal intensity. *Br J Radiol* 2012;85:831-836.

4. Grimer RJ: Size matters for sarcoma! *Ann R Coll Surg Engl* 2006;88:519-524.

5. Brisson M, Kashima T, Delaney D, et al: MRI characteristics of lipoma and atypical lipomatous tumor/well-differentiated liposarcoma: Retrospective comparison with histology and MDM2 gene amplification. *Skeletal Radiol* 2013;42:635-647.

6. Clay MR, Martinez AP, Weiss SW, Edgar MA: MDM2 and CDK4 immunohistochemistry: Should it Be used in problematic differentiated lipomatous tumors? A new perspective. *Am J Surg Pathol* 2016;40:1647-1652.

   The authors identify the most common clinical scenarios for soft-tissue tumors and recommend the most appropriate imaging for their assessment. The authors compared immunohistochemistry for MDM2 and CDK4 in a cohort of differentiated lipomatous tumor with ambiguous histologic/clinical features in which FISH was used to establish a final diagnosis. They concluded that FISH was more reliable and cost-effective. Level of evidence: IV.

7. Sanjuan-Cervero R, Carrera-Hueso FJ, Vazquez-Ferreiro P, Ramon-Barrios MA: Efficacy and adverse effects of collagenase use in the treatment of Dupuytren's disease: A meta-analysis. *Bone Joint Lett J* 2018;100-B:73-80.

   The authors identify the most common clinical scenarios for soft-tissue tumors and recommend the most appropriate imaging for their assessment. A meta-analysis was used to assess the safety and efficacy of collagenase compared with fasciectomy and percutaneous needle fasciotomy.

8. He XD, Zhang YB, Wang L, et al: Prognostic factors for the recurrence of sporadic desmoid-type fibromatosis after macroscopically complete resection: Analysis of 114 patients at a single institution. *Eur J Surg Oncol* 2015;41:1013-1019.

9. Bonvalot S, Desai A, Coppola S, et al: The treatment of desmoid tumors: A stepwise clinical approach. *Ann Oncol* 2012;23:158-166.

10. Patel KH, Gikas PD, Pollock RC, et al: Pigmented villonodular synovitis of the knee: A retrospective analysis of 214 cases at a UK tertiary referral centre. *Knee* 2017;24:808-815.

    The authors identify the most common clinical scenarios for soft-tissue tumors and recommend the most appropriate imaging for their assessment. Authors evaluate 214 cases of localized and diffuse PVNS. They concluded that recurrence rates are higher for diffuse PVNS when treated arthroscopically and recommend open synovectomy for diffuse PVNS. Level of evidence: III.

11. Gelderblom H, Copet C, Chevreau C, et al: Nilotinib in locally advanced pigmented villonodular synovitis: A multicenter, open-label, single-arm, phase 2 trial. *Lancet* 2018;19:639-648.

    The authors identify the most common clinical scenarios for soft-tissue tumors and recommend the most appropriate imaging for their assessment. The authors report the results of a phase 2 trial that evaluates the efficacy of nilotinib for the treatment of nonresectable PVNS. They report that 90% of patients achieved disease control after 12 weeks of treatment and recommend further study with randomized trials. Level of evidence: II.

12. James AW, Shurell E, Singh A, Dry SM, Eilber FC: Malignant peripheral nerve sheath tumor. *Surg Oncol N Am* 2016;25:789-802.

    The authors identify the most common clinical scenarios for soft-tissue tumors and recommend the most appropriate imaging for their assessment. The authors present a detailed review of malignant peripheral nerve sheath tumors including histologic criteria, molecular pathogenesis, and surgical management. Level of evidence: V.

13. Crawford EA, Slotcavage RL, King JJ, Lackman RD, Ogilvie CM: Ethanol sclerotherapy reduces pain in symptomatic musculoskeletal hemangiomas. *Clin Orthop Relat Res* 2009;467:2955-2961.

14. Doyle LA: Sarcoma classification: An update based on the 2013 World Health organization classification of tumors of soft tissue and bone: *Cancer* 2014;120:1763-1774.

15. Enneking WF, Spanier SS, Goodman MA: A system for the surgical staging of musculoskeletal sarcoma. *CORR* 1980;153:106-120.

16. Cates JM: The AJCC 8th edition staging system for soft tissue sarcoma of the extremities or trunk: A cohort study of the SEER database. *J Natl Compr Canc Netw* 2017;16:144-152.

    The authors identify the most common clinical scenarios for soft-tissue tumors and recommend the most appropriate imaging for their assessment. The author reviews the changes in the AJCC eighth edition staging system for soft-tissue sarcoma to determine if the performance of the system has been improved when compared with previous versions.

17. Harati K, Goertz O, Pieper A, et al: Soft tissue sarcomas of the extremities: Surgical margins can Be close as long as the resected tumor has No ink on it. *Oncologist* 2017;22:1400-1410.

    The authors identify the most common clinical scenarios for soft-tissue tumors and recommend the most appropriate imaging for their assessment. The purpose of this study was to determine the prognostic impact of surgical margins and clear margin widths in patients with soft-tissue sarcomas. They found that only the quality of surgical margin, but not the negative margin width had an influence on prognosis. Level of evidence: IV.

18. Ratan R, Patel SR: Chemotherapy for soft tissue sarcoma. *Cancer* 2016;122:2952-2960.

    The authors identify the most common clinical scenarios for soft-tissue tumors and recommend the most appropriate imaging for their assessment. The authors review current chemotherapy options for the treatment of soft-tissue sarcoma. They identify doxorubicin and ifosfamide as the most effective drugs for the majority of soft-tissue sarcomas and note that optimal dosing and administration influence outcomes.

19. Ghosn M, Rassy EE, Kourie HR: Immunotherapies in sarcoma: Updates and future perspectives. *World J Clin Oncol* 2017;10:145-150.

The authors identify the most common clinical scenarios for soft-tissue tumors and recommend the most appropriate imaging for their assessment. The authors present a targeted review of the published data and ongoing clinical trials in immunotherapies of sarcoma. Adoptive cell therapies, cancer vaccines, and immune checkpoint inhibitors are the primary treatment options discussed.

Chapter 69

Metastatic Bone Disease

Dieter M. Lindskog, MD • Izuchukwu Ibe, MD • Francis Y. Lee, MD, PhD

ABSTRACT

The bone is an organ that serves as a reservoir for metastatic cells that are able to invade and establish a microenvironment conducive for their proliferation. Tumor invasion of bone leads to many changes at the molecular level that translate to negative clinical outcomes for patients with bone metastasis. From an orthopaedic surgical point of view, metastatic cancers to bone cause pain, fractures, and neurologic deficit. Multifaceted approaches including surgical and nonsurgical options are vital in the management of metastatic bone disease with respect to prevention of pathological fractures or surgical stabilization of established fractures.

Keywords: bone loss; metastasis; metastatic disease

Introduction

Bones are a common site for cancer metastasis resulting in worsened morbidity and mortality for patients as well as a burden on the health care system. The axial and appendicular skeletons are affected with symptoms from bone metastases and are often the first indication of malignancy in patients.[1,2] Cancers arising in the breast, prostate, lung, kidney, and thyroid, and multiple myeloma show a particularly strong predilection for bone, inducing bone loss, and weakening the structure of bone. The effect on bone leads to negative events such as pathological fractures, spinal cord compression, pain, myelosuppression, and hypercalcemia.[3]

Pathophysiology of Disease

The theory of metastasis has evolved over the years; initial theories were the mechanistic theory and the seed and soil. The mechanistic theory involves the embolization to distal vasculature, with cancer cells traveling via lymphatics and blood vessels supported by Dr Rudolph Virchow and Dr James Ewing.[4] The seed and soil theory by Dr Stephen Paget suggested that certain tumor cells were able to spread and survive in specific conducive environments.[5] The combination of these theories led to the understanding of metastasis to include certain cells with a metastatic phenotype that escapes into the vasculature, travel to distant organs, and escape and create an environment that is conducive for their growth. This microenvironment or "niche" allows for continued immune evasion and tumor proliferation by manipulating various factors.

The metastatic cells are able to activate pathways and affect protein expression by imitating the already existent mechanisms of bone turnover, a term known as osteomimicry.

For example, invasive breast tumor tissue over expresses cadherin-11, a cell adhesion molecule normally found in the bone. This leads to an increased affinity for bone and increases the interactions of the metastatic cells with cells within bone.[6] Many other factors typically found in bone can be found in cancers that metastasize to bone including osteopontin (OPN), bone sialoprotein (BSP), alkaline phosphatase (ALP), osteoprotegerin (OPG), runt-related transcription factor-2 (Runx2), and receptor activator of nuclear factor kappa-B ligand (RANKL).[7] These osteomimetic mechanisms and mutations continue to be elucidated, but they play a role in affecting osteoblast and osteoclast interactions.

The osteoclast plays a central role in bone resorption; they are multinucleated cells formed from the fusion of multiple mononuclear myeloid precursors.[8]

Dr. Lindskog or an immediate family member serves as a board member, owner, officer, or committee member of the Musculoskeletal Tumor Society. Dr. Lee or an immediate family member has stock or stock options held in L&J BIO; has received research or institutional support from Musculoskeletal Transplant Foundation, National Institutes of Health (NIAMS & NICHD), and OREF. Neither Dr. Ibe nor any immediate family member has received anything of value from or has stock or stock options held in a commercial company or institution related directly or indirectly to the subject of this chapter.

Osteoclast precursors express RANK which is activated by the binding of the RANK ligand secreted by osteoblasts.

This activation leads to a resorption of bone beginning with the adherence of integrins with vitronectin and fibronectin leading to cytoskeletal rearrangement producing a sealing zone and creating a resorptive ruffled membrane.[9] Along the ruffled membrane protons are pumped into the lacunae between the osteoclast and the bone, proteases are secreted which degrade the collagen of the bone matrix.[9] Osteoclast regulation is accomplished through osteoblast secretion of osteoprotegerin (OPG). OPG binds to RANKL preventing the binding of RANKL to RANK and the subsequent development of osteoclasts.[10] Parathyroid hormone (PTH) stimulates RANKL upregulation and downregulates OPG. Calcitonin is another downregulator of osteoclast activity; it is secreted by the thyroid and inhibits osteoclasts by a mechanism that disrupts the cytoskeleton of osteoclasts inducing loss of polarity.[11]

Osteoblasts are the primary mediators of bone deposition and their differentiation is stimulated by Runx2. Runx2 is activated by bone morphogenic proteins (BMPs) and the transcription factor distal-less homeobox 5 (Dlx5).[12] Once activated, it upregulates osteocalcin (OCN), osteopontin (OPN), and bone sialoprotein (BSP).[9] Runx2 is downregulated by calcitriol, the biologically active form of vitamin D.[13] Osteoblasts are inhibited by sclerostin, a protein encoded by the SOST gene, secreted by osteocytes.[14] A mutation in the SOST gene leads to dysplastic disease such as sclerosteosis.[14]

Cancer cells are able to hijack this mechanism to affect bone structure molecularly. For example, approximately 90% of breast cancer bone metastases secrete parathyroid hormone-related peptide (PTHrP), causing the upregulation of RANKL and downregulation of OPG stimulating bone remodeling which in turn releases tumor growth factor beta (TGF-β). TGF-β induces the secretion of more PTHrP, leading to a continuous cycle of dysfunction and resultant bone loss.[15] Prostate cancer cells often lead to osteoblastic lesions; they frequently express both PTHrP and RANKL. Similar to osteolytic lesions, there is a cycle that involves osteoblast and osteoclasts.[7] PTH prevents osteoblast apoptosis and increases their activity, resulting in an increased rate of bone remodeling, but can increase bone deposition depending on the balance between osteoblast and osteoclast activity. Lung, kidney, and thyroid cancers most frequently produce osteolytic lesions, whereas metastases from prostate cancers tend to produce osteoblastic lesions.[16] This disjointed remodeling leads to a decrease in trabecular connectivity, bone volume, and alters bone architecture. These structural changes impact bone strength and integrity making bones affected by metastatic tumors at greater risk of fracture.

Nonsurgical Management of Patients

The management of skeletal metastases involves a multidisciplinary approach often combining various degrees of pharmacological interventions, radiation therapy, and surgery. The goals of these management options are to limit these effects and potentially prevent negative skeletal events.

Diphosphonates have long been the standard for treatment of bone loss. They function by inducing apoptosis or deactivating osteoclasts. Diphosphonates include non-nitrogen-containing agents such as clodronate which induce apoptosis by means of toxic metabolites and nitrogen-containing agents such as alendronate and risedronate which inhibit farnesyl pyrophosphate synthase in the osteoclast causing breakdown of its cytoskeleton.

Since their development, each generation of diphosphonates has increased in strength from the first-generation diphosphonates (ie, etidronate, tiludronate, and clodronate). They have been replaced by more potent drugs such as zoledronic acid.[17] Zoledronic acid is one of the most widely prescribed medications in the United States; current recommendations involve administering 4 mg of zoledronic acid intravenously every 3 to 4 weeks for maintenance of bone health in those with bone metastasis.[18] Diphosphonates have been associated with improved outcomes in patients with metastasis, decreasing their risk for skeletal-related events (SREs) such as fracture[19] and increasing bone density.[20]. Despite their potential benefit, diphosphonate administration has its drawbacks. They are renally excreted and should be limited in renally deficient patients;[21] they can cause hypocalcemia and can lead to atypical fractures of the femur[22,23] and osteonecrosis of the jaw, and, when taken orally, have been associated with esophagitis.[24] The optimal dosing for diphosphonates such as zoledronic acid is uncertain, but a recent randomized controlled trial showed no difference in skeletally related events when zoledronic acid was dosed every 4 weeks (standard) compared with a 12-week interval.[25] There was a trend toward less adverse events with the administration of zoledronic acid such as osteonecrosis of the jaw and elevated creatinine levels when zoledronic acid was administered at 12 week intervals.[25]

Denosumab is a monoclonal antibody against RANKL. It competitively binds with RANKL preventing the binding of RANK and therefore limiting osteoclastogenesis. Denosumab plays a similar role to OPG in down regulating bone resorption and shifting the bone remodeling balance toward bone deposition. Denosumab is an effective alternative to diphosphonates. Denosumab has been shown to reduce the risk of SREs in patients with bone metastasis. For SRE prophylaxis, 120 mg denosumab provided subcutaneously administered every four weeks[18] is recommended. Denosumab use, like diphosphonates, has been associated with hypocalcaemia and a similar rate of jaw osteonecrosis.[26] An advantage of denosumab is the fact it is not renally excreted and dosing does not need to be adjusted with worsening renal function in patients.

Other medications include teriparatide and romosozumab which unlike the mechanism of diphosphonates function by stimulating osteoblasts. Teriparatide is a portion of parathyroid hormone and leads to an overall increase in the rate of bone turnover.[27] Continuous teriparatide administration results in net bone loss, but intermittent dosing of PTH produces an inverse and anabolic effect through an increase in the expression of osteoblast transcription factors and downregulation of osteoblast inhibitors like sclerostin.[28] Romosozumab is an antisclerostin antibody that can promote osteoblastic bone formation, through its blockade of sclerostin. Future drugs targeting growth factors, chemokines, and integrins are being investigated for efficacy in treating and preventing skeletal related events in various cancers.[9]

Radiation Therapy

Radiation oncology and the improvements in the techniques of delivery have played a role in the improved outcomes for patients with cancer. Radiation therapy (RT) is an important tool in the treatment of metastatic bone disease. It is used to treat bone loss and is also effective in treating bone pain.[29] Radiation therapy can decrease the incidence of pathologic fractures in patients with osteolytic lesions.[30,31]

Radiation is not without its negative effects. It causes collateral damage to the tissue being radiated in a dose-dependent fashion. It limits bone quality and osteoprogenitors. Patients who receive radiation therapy are at risk for wound healing complications if they undergo any surgical intervention. Patients can also have fatigue, nausea, and vomiting, and myelosuppression can occur. Radiation therapy is versatile; it can be used in combination with the pharmacologic options such as diphosphonates and denosumab; and it can also be complimentary to surgical procedures provided before or after surgical intervention.

Prediction of Impending Fractures

The prediction of potential fractures is obtained through a combination of a clinical history, physical examination, and imaging studies. Findings such as pain and limitations in patient's activities of daily living (ADLs) as well as patient's baseline level are important. The primary cancer diagnosis if known and if not, allowing for appropriate staging workup to be performed including prostate-specific antigen, serum/urine protein electrophoresis (SPEP/UPEP), complete blood count (CBC), basic metabolic profile (BMP), and CT of the chest, abdomen, and pelvis. If patient is without known bone metastasis, a biopsy of the lesion should be performed to confirm metastasis to bone. Plain orthogonal radiographs remain the most reliable source of information in the analysis of metastasis to bone. It is estimated that a 25% to 75% loss of bone material occurs before lesions become visible on radiograph, indicating a significant loss of bone strength by the time of radiograph visibility; lysis of 50% of the diaphyseal cortex results in a 60% to 90% decrease in bone strength.[32]

In predicting the likelihood for patients presenting with a lesion to fracture, the Mirels criteria is widely used. The Mirels[33] criteria involve a combination of patient factors scored 1 to 3 such as pain level with radiographic factors, lesion type, lesion size, and location on the body. A score of 7 out of 12 was more likely to not fracture while a score of 10 out of 12 were more likely to fracture (**Figure 1**). Recently, CT scans can be used to predict the risk of fracture by evaluating the structural rigidity of bone. The use of CT based structural rigidity analysis tool has been shown to have a higher sensitivity, specificity, positive predictive value and negative predictive value when compared with Mirels criteria.[34] A reduction of 35% in axial, bending, or torsional rigidity was considered to be a risk for fracture.[34]

A patient who is at high risk either via the Mirels score or the structural analysis is often indicated for surgical intervention and prophylactic fixation. It is important to note that both lytic and blastic lesions can result in fracture (**Figures 2** and **3**).

Surgical Management of Metastatic Bone Disease

The goals of surgical management are the restoration and preservation of a patient's weight-bearing capacity, with as minimal collateral damage as possible. The resumption of function and the creation of a

Oncology and Pathology

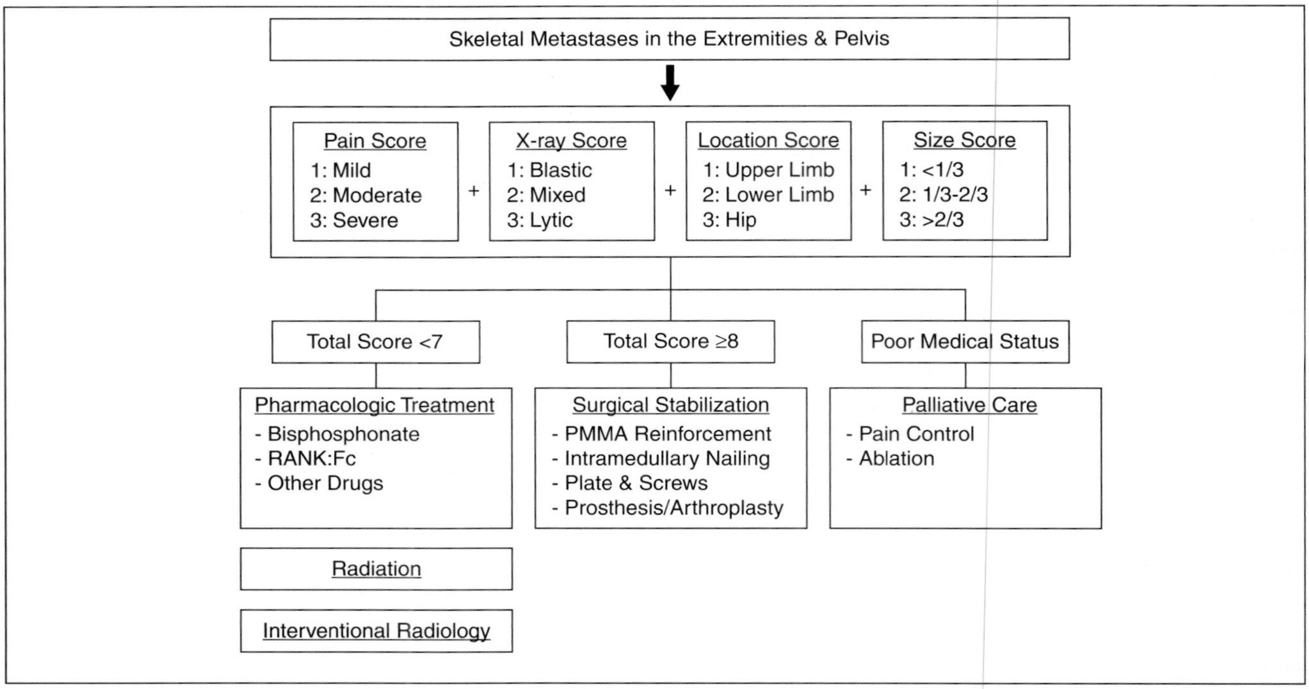

Figure 1 Schematic of Mirels criteria as well as an algorithm with management options.

stable construct that will outlive the patient is the ideal. Fracture management is dependent on many factors including the individual's goals of care and expectations, the location and the size of the metastatic foci. Preservation of as much host bone and the control of further metastatic disease are secondary goals. Preoperatively, use of embolization in patients with known hypervascular lesions, such as renal and thyroid metastases, can be helpful in decreasing blood loss. Information regarding previous radiation should also be considered when planning the surgery. Relative contraindications to surgery for metastatic disease to bone include moribund status, active wound infection within the surgical area, and expected patient survival shorter than the recovery window that would preclude the patient from benefitting from surgical management of the metastasis.[35]

The options for intervention are most commonly plate fixation, intramedullary nail (IMN) placement, and endoprosthetic reconstruction. IMNs are able to protect a large segment of bone while preserving periosteal blood supply and are often less technically demanding. Osteosynthesis or plate fixation can be used in

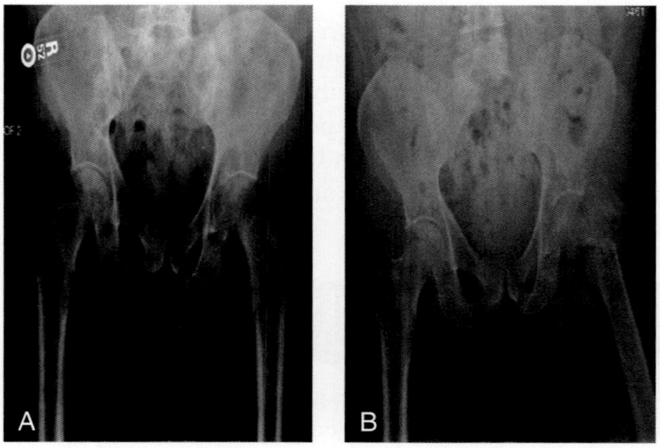

Figure 2 AP radiograph of pelvis in a patient with a blastic lesion of the left femur resulting in fracture. **A**, Pre fracture radiograph. **B**, Post fracture radiograph.

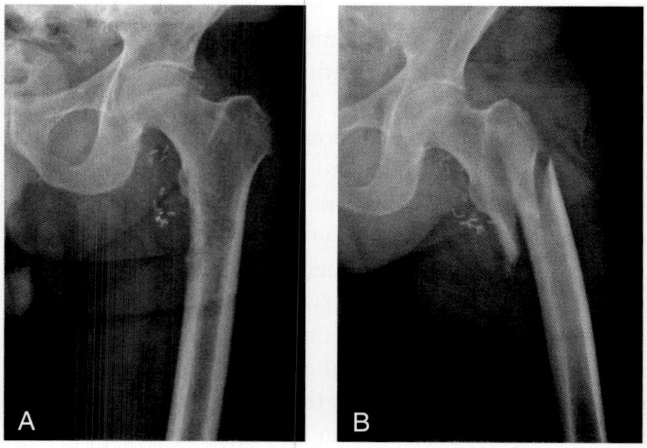

Figure 3 AP radiograph of the left femur in a patient with a lytic lesion of the proximal femur resulting in a fracture. **A**, Pre fracture radiograph. **B**, Post fracture radiograph.

different regions of the bone and provides proper visualization for curettage and the use of adjuvant such as cement but at a risk of the disruption of the periosteal blood supply. Endoprosthesis can be used periarticularly and in an intercalary fashion; they often require longer surgical times and larger dissections.

Lower Extremity

The femur is a common site of bone metastasis and the most frequent site of pathologic fracture due to the frequency of metastatic involvement and high physiologic stresses at this site.[36] Fractures are most likely to occur at the femoral neck, pertrochanteric region, diaphysis, and distal femur, respectively (**Table 1**).

Lesions of the femoral head and neck are mostly treated using hemiarthroplasty or total hip arthroplasty. The use of arthroplasty as the preferred option comes from the higher failure rate associated with internal fixation of the femoral head and neck region.[32] Prosthetic reconstruction allows for the removal of all gross metastatic disease. Total hip arthroplasty is favored if there is concomitant acetabular involvement. The management of lesions in the intertrochanteric region allows for the use of IMNs, internal fixation or resection of diseased bone, and endoprosthetic reconstruction can be used. The femoral diaphysis also allows for options that include an intercalary prosthesis, IMN, or plate fixation. Patients with long expected survivals and solitary metastasis or large destructive lesions of the diaphysis can be treated with a segmental prosthesis.[37] IMNs are recommended in the presence of multiple diaphyseal lesions and for impending fracture through small or solitary lesions.[37,38] Use of a retrograde femoral nail should be considered in patients with prior hip arthroplasty. Metastatic lesions to the distal femur and tibia are less common, but can be treated with plate fixation or an endoprosthesis depending on size. Endoprosthetic reconstruction around the knee can be challenging if the lesion compromises the extensor mechanism. Complications of surgical intervention with the specific interventions include deep wound infections, dislocations for arthroplasty, failure of fixation and nonunion with plate fixation, and failure of fixation with IMN.

Upper Extremity and Pelvis

Upper extremity metastases occur in approximately 7% of bone metastatic lesions behind 11% rate for the lower extremities.[39] Humeral metastases are the

Table 1

Lesion, Locations and Options for Lower Extremity Surgical Reconstruction

Location	Lesion	Reconstruction
Femoral head/neck	Small/solitary	Hemiarthroplasty ± cementation
	Large/diffuse	Hemiarthroplasty ± cementation
		Total hip arthroplasty ± cementation
Intertrochanteric/subtrochanteric	Small/solitary	IMN
		Plate ± cementation
	Large/diffuse	Proximal femur replacement ± cementation
		IMN ± cementation
Diaphysis	Small/solitary	IMN
		Plate ± cementation
		Intercalary prosthesis ± cementation
	Large/diffuse	IMN
		Intercalary prosthesis ± cementation
Distal femur/proximal tibia	Small/solitary	Plate ± cementation
		Distal femur replacement
	Large/diffuse	Distal femur replacement

IMN = intramedullary nail

Oncology and Pathology

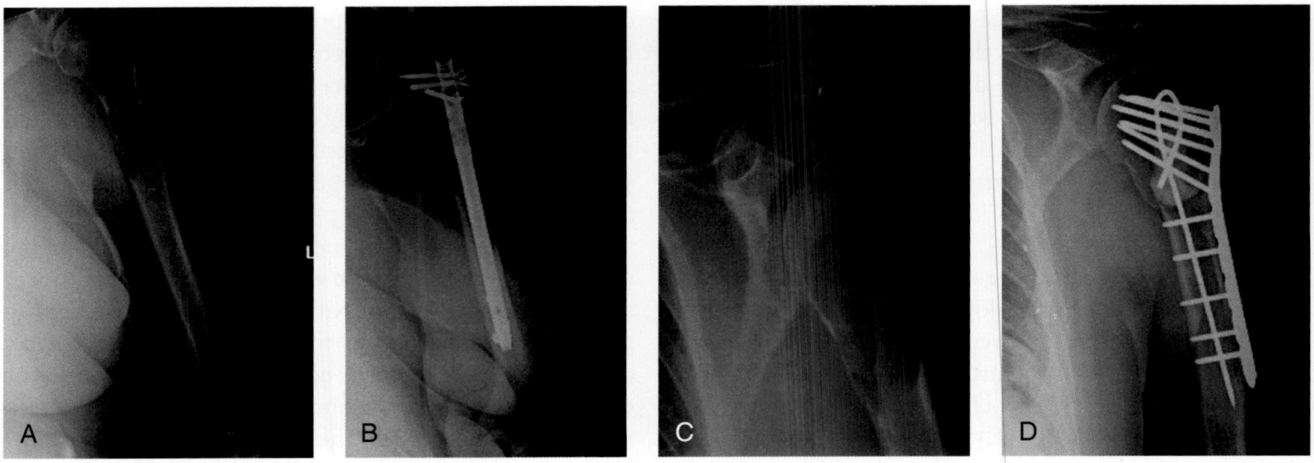

Figure 4 AP radiographs of proximal humerus lesions treated with augmentation and internal fixation (**C** and **D**) and with intramedullary nail (**A** and **B**).

most common location for upper extremity metastatic lesion. Similar to the lower extremity metastases, treatments are based on the location of the lesion as well as patients' symptomatology, prognosis, and extent of disease. Metastatic lesions to the humerus can be treated with internal fixation, intramedullary nailing, or resection and reconstruction (**Figure 4**). These provide pain control and an early return to activity for the patient. Metastasis to the hand or acral metastases are rare, but often associated with a poor prognosis. The common culprits are lung and renal primaries.[40] These patients often have limited life expectancy and are treated symptomatically.

The pelvis is the most common site of metastatic lesions outside of the axial skeleton.[39] These lesions can be very painful and can also pose a reconstructive dilemma for the surgeon. Many of these lesions are treated nonsurgically with radiation and/or antiresorptives. Surgical management is reserved for patients with symptoms resistant to nonsurgical treatment. Surgery involves minimally invasive techniques to reinforce the pelvis or larger more invasive procedures. Acetabular lesions can be addressed with a total hip arthroplasty. Surgical intervention in the setting of pelvic or acetabular lesions are associated with a complication profile that includes infections, instability, thromboembolic disease, loss of fixation, massive blood loss, and local progression.[39]

Summary

The advancements in medicine have allowed for increased survival and prolonged lifespan for patients with cancer. This has led to an increase in the number of patients with the long-term sequelae of cancer diagnoses such as bone metastasis. Tumor metastasis to bone is associated with poor outcomes for patients and can lead to poor bone quality and resultant fractures as well as poor quality of life. Combining pharmacologic, nonsurgical, and appropriate surgical plan for the patient to create a focused, patient-specific approach can improve patient outcomes related to bone metastasis.

Key Study Points

- Molecular mechanism of bone metastasis (PTH, RANK/RANKL, OPG)
- Mirels criteria
- Complications associated with antiresorptives
- Surgical goals include creating a durable, stable reconstruction that can allow immediate weight bearing, decrease pain, and improve patient function.

Annotated References

1. Coleman RE: Skeletal complications of malignancy. *Cancer* 1997;80:1588-1594.
2. Roodman GD: Mechanisms of bone metastasis. *N Engl J Med* 2004;350:1655-1664.
3. Cleveland C, Von Moos R, Walker MS, et al: Burden of symptoms associated with development of metastatic bone disease in patients with breast cancer. *Support Care Cancer* 2016;24:3557-3565.

   Retrospective study evaluating the patterns of patient reported outcomes in patients who developed bone metastasis. Level of evidence: IV.

4. Schultz M: Rudolf Virchow. *Emerg Infect Dis* 2008;14: 1480-1481.
5. Ribatti D, Mangialardi G, Vacca A: Stephen Paget and the 'seed and soil' theory of metastatic dissemination. *Clin Exp Med* 2006;6:145-149.
6. Tamura D, Hiraga T, Myoui A, Yoshikawa H, Yoneda T: Cadherin-11-mediated interactions with bone marrow stromal/osteoblastic cells support selective colonization of breast cancer cells in bone. *Int J Oncol* 2008;33:17-24.
7. Rucci N, Teti A: Osteomimicry: How tumor cells try to deceive the bone. *Front Biosci* 2010;2:907-915.
8. Burger EH, Van der Meer JW, Van de Gevel JS, Gribnau JC, Thesingh GW, van Furth R: In vitro formation of osteoclasts from long-term cultures of bone marrow mononuclear phagocytes. *J Exp Med* 1982;156:1604-1614.
9. Brook N, Brook E, Dharmarajan A, Dass CR, Chan A: Breast cancer bone metastases: Pathogenesis and therapeutic targets. *Int J Biochem Cell Biol* 2018;96:63-78.

   Reviews the mechanism of bone remodelling and the cellular responses that occur as a result of bone metastasis. Level of evidence: V.
10. Boyce BF: Advances in the regulation of osteoclasts and osteoclast functions. *J Dent Res* 2013;92:860-867.
11. Yamamoto Y, Noguchi T, Takahashi N: Effects of calcitonin on osteoclast. *Clin Calcium* 2005;15:147-151.
12. Samee N, Geoffroy V, Marty C, et al: Dlx5, a positive regulator of osteoblastogenesis, is essential for osteoblast-osteoclast coupling. *Am J Pathol* 2008;173:773-780.
13. Ducy P, Zhang R, Geoffroy V, Ridall AL, Karsenty G: Osf2/Cbfa1: A transcriptional activator of osteoblast differentiation. *Cell* 1997;89:747-754.
14. Balemans W, Ebeling M, Patel N, et al: Increased bone density in sclerosteosis is due to the deficiency of a novel secreted protein (SOST). *Hum Mol Genet* 2001;10:537-543.
15. Yin JJ, Selander K, Chirgwin JM, et al: TGF-β signaling blockade inhibits PTHrP secretion by breast cancer cells and bone metastases development. *J Clin Invest* 1999;103: 197-206.
16. Guise TA, Mohammad KS, Clines G, et al: Basic mechanisms responsible for osteolytic and osteoblastic bone metastases. *Clin Cancer Res* 2006;12:6213s-6216s.
17. Drake MT, Clarke BL, Khosla S: Bisphosphonates: Mechanism of action and role in clinical practice. *Mayo Clin Proc* 2008; 83(9):1032-1045.
18. Henry D, Vadhan-Raj S, Hirsh V, et al: Delaying skeletal-related events in a randomized phase 3 study of denosumab versus zoledronic acid in patients with advanced cancer: An analysis of data from patients with solid tumors. *Support Care Cancer* 2014;22(3):679-687.
19. Fuleihan GE-H, Salamoun M, Mourad YA, et al: Pamidronate in the prevention of chemotherapy-induced bone loss in premenopausal women with breast cancer: A randomized controlled trial. *J Clin Endocrinol Metab* 2005;90(6): 3209-3214.
20. Michigami T, Ihara-Watanabe M, Yamazaki M, Ozono K: Receptor activator of nuclear factor κB ligand (RANKL) is a key molecule of osteoclast formation for bone metastasis in a newly developed model of human neuroblastoma. *Cancer Res* 2001;61(4):1637-1644.
21. Miller PD, Jamal SA, Evenepoel P, Eastell R, Boonen S: Renal safety in patients treated with bisphosphonates for osteoporosis: A review. *J Bone Miner Res* 2013;28(10): 2049-2059.
22. Schilcher J, Michaëlsson K, Aspenberg P: Bisphosphonate use and atypical fractures of the femoral shaft. *N Engl J Med* 2011;364(18):1728-1737.
23. Shane E, Burr D, Abrahamsen B, et al: Atypical subtrochanteric and diaphyseal femoral fractures: Second report of a task force of the American Society for Bone and Mineral Research. *J Bone Miner Res* 2014;29(1):1-23.
24. Hoff AO, Toth BB, Altundag K, et al: Frequency and risk factors associated with osteonecrosis of the jaw in cancer patients treated with intravenous bisphosphonates. *J Bone Miner Res* 2008;23(6):826-836.
25. Himelstein AL, Foster JL, Khatcheressian JL, et al: Effect of longer-interval vs standard dosing of zoledronic acid on skeletal events in patients with bone metastases: A randomized clinical trial. *J Am Med Assoc* 2017;317(1):48-58.

   In patients with bone metastases secondary to breast cancer, prostate cancer, or multiple myeloma, the use of zoledronic acid every 12 weeks compared with the standard dosing interval of every 4 weeks did not result in an increased risk of skeletal events over 2 years. Level of evidence: I.
26. Stopeck AT, Lipton A, Body JJ, et al: Denosumab compared with zoledronic acid for the treatment of bone metastases in patients with advanced breast cancer: A randomized, double-blind study. *J Clin Oncol* 2010;28:5132-5139.
27. Chen YC, Sosnoski DM, Mastro AM: Breast cancer metastasis to the bone: Mechanisms of bone loss. *Breast Cancer Res* 2010;12:215.
28. Greenfield EM: Anabolic effects of intermittent PTH on osteoblasts. *Curr Mol Pharmacol* 2012;5:127-134.
29. Lutz S: The role of radiation therapy in controlling painful bone metastases. *Curr Pain Headache Rep* 2012;16(4): 300-306.
30. Bostel T, Förster R, Schlampp I, et al: Spinal bone metastases in colorectal cancer: A retrospective analysis of stability, prognostic factors and survival after palliative radiotherapy. *Radiat Oncol* 2017;12:115.

   The treatment of osteolytic metastasis to the spine with radiation, chemotherapy, and diphosphonates improves patients quality of life. Level of evidence: IV.
31. Schlampp I, Rieken S, Habermehl D, et al: Stability of spinal bone metastases in breast cancer after radiotherapy: A retrospective analysis of 157 cases. *Strahlenther Onkol* 2014;190(9):792-797.
32. Agarwal MG, Nayak P: Management of skeletal metastases: An orthopaedic surgeon's guide. *Indian J Orthop* 2015;49:83-100.

33. Mirels H: Metastatic disease in long bones. A proposed scoring system for diagnosing impending pathologic fractures. *Clin Orthop Relat Res* 1989;249:256-264.

34. Damron T, Nazarian A, Entezari V, et al: CT-based structural rigidity analysis is more accurate than Mirels scoring for fracture prediction in metastatic femoral lesions. *Clin Orthop Relat Res* 2016;474(3):643-651.

The use of CT-based structural rigidity analysis was found to be more sensitive and specific in predicting impending pathologic fractures in patients with skeletal metastasis. Level of evidence: II.

35. Ward WG, Spang J, Howe D: Metastatic disease of the femur. Surgical management. *Orthop Clin North Am* 2000;31:633-645.

36. Quinn RH, Randall RL, Benevenia J, Berven SH, Raskin KA: Contemporary management of metastatic bone disease: Tips and tools of the trade for general practitioners. *Instr Course Lect* 2014;63:431-441.

37. Willeumier JJ, van der Linden YM, van de Sande MAJ, Dijkstra PDS: Treatment of pathological fractures of the long bones. *EFORT Open Rev* 2016;1:136-145.

This article reviews bone metastasis of long bones, their evaluation, management, and treatment options. Options include radiotherapy and surgical intervention when necessary. Level of evidence: V.

38. Wedin R, Bauer HC: Surgical treatment of skeletal metastatic lesions of the proximal femur: Endoprosthesis or reconstruction nail? *J Bone Joint Surg Br* 2005;87(12):1653-1657.

39. Krishnan C, Han I, Kim HS: Outcome after surgery for metastases to the pelvic bone: A single institutional experience. *Clin Orthop Surg* 2017;9(1):116-125.

Complication rates for patients with pelvic metastasis occurred at a rate of 16%, and survival was influenced by primary cancer type, presence of visceral metastasis, and preoperative albumin levels. Level of evidence: IV.

40. Morris G, Evans S, Stevenson J, et al: Bone metastases of the hand. *Ann R Coll Surg Engl* 2017;99(7):563-567.

This study identified the rate of metastatic foci in the hand. Median time to death following acrometastasis was 18 months. Skin, lung, and kidney were the most common culprits. Level of evidence: IV.

INDEX

Note: Page numbers followed by "*f*" indicate figures and "*t*" indicate tables.

A

B

G

H

I

J

K

L

M

N

O

P

Q

R

S

T

U

V

W

X

Z